Editors

WILLIAM S. HAUBRICH, M.D.

Clinical Professor of Medicine, University of California,
San Diego; Senior Consultant, Division of Gastroenterology,
The Scripps Clinic and Research Foundation, LaJolla

MARTIN H. KALSER, M.D., Ph.D.

Professor of Medicine and Chief, Division of Gastroenterology,
University of Miami, Florida

JAMES L. A. ROTH, M.D., Ph.D.

Professor of Clinical Medicine, School of Medicine,
University of Pennsylvania; Director, Institute of Gastroenterology,
Presbyterian-University of Pennsylvania Medical Center

FENTON SCHAFFNER, M.D.

George Baehr Professor of Medicine and Professor of Pathology;
Chief, Division of Liver Disease, Mount Sinai School of Medicine
of City University of New York

Editorial Consultant

FRANCISCO VILARDELL, M.D., D.Sc.

Director, Escuela de Patologia Digestiva, Universidad Autonoma
de Barcelona, Spain

Editorial Associate

DANIEL PELOT, M.D.

Associate Professor of Medicine, University of California, Irvine

Volume 4

Bockus

GASTROENTEROLOGY

Fourth Edition

Editor-in-Chief

J. EDWARD BERK, M.D., D.Sc.

Distinguished Professor of Medicine
University of California, Irvine

W. B. SAUNDERS COMPANY 1985

Philadelphia London Toronto Mexico City Rio de Janeiro Sydney Tokyo

W. B. Saunders Company: West Washington Square
Philadelphia, PA 19105

1 St. Anne's Road
Eastbourne, East Sussex BN21 3UN, England

1 Goldthorne Avenue
Toronto, Ontario M8Z 5T9, Canada

Apartado 26370—Cedro 512
Mexico 4, D.F., Mexico

Rua Coronel Cabrita, 8
Sao Cristovao Caixa Postal 21176
Rio de Janeiro, Brazil

9 Waltham Street
Artarmon, N.S.W. 2064, Australia

Ichibancho, Central Bldg., 22-1 Ichibancho
Chiyoda-Ku, Tokyo 102, Japan

Library of Congress Cataloging in Publication Data

Bockus, Henry L. (Henry Le Roy), 1894–1982

Bockus GASTROENTEROLOGY.

1. Digestive organs—Diseases. 2. Gastrointestinal system—Diseases. I. Berk, J. Edward (Jack Edward) II. Title. [DNLM: 1. Gastrointestinal diseases. WI 100 B665g]

RC801.B663 1985 616.3 83–20120

ISBN 0–7216–1777–8

Listed here is the latest translated edition of this book together with the language of the translation and the publisher.

Italian (*2nd Edition*)—Editrice Universo, Rome, Italy

Spanish (*2nd Edition*)—Salvat Editores, Barcelona, Spain

Spanish (*3rd Edition*)—Salvat Editores S.A., Barcelona, Spain

Volume 1 ISBN 0-7216-1778-6
Volume 2 ISBN 0-7216-1779-4
Volume 3 ISBN 0-7216-1780-8
Volume 4 ISBN 0-7216-1781-6
Volume 5 ISBN 0-7216-1782-4
Volume 6 ISBN 0-7216-1783-2
Volume 7 ISBN 0-7216-1784-0
Bockus Gastroenterology 7 Volume set ISBN 0-7216-1777-8

Last digit is the print number: 9 8 7 6 5 4 3 2 1

Contributors

VOLUME 4

S. PHILIP BRALOW, M.D.
Clinical Professor of Medicine, School of Medicine, University of Pennsylvania, Philadelphia, Pa.

BRYAN N. BROOKE, M.D., M.Chir.
Emeritus Professor of Surgery, University of London at St. George's Hospital Medical School; Hon. Consultant, St. George's and St. James' Hospitals, London, England.

YORAM BUJANOVER, M.D.
Lecturer in Pediatrics, Sackler Faculty of Medicine, Tel-Aviv University; Pediatric Gastroenterologist, Tel-Aviv Medical Center, Tel-Aviv, Israel.

TE-WEN CHANG, M.D.
Associate Professor of Medicine, Tufts University School of Medicine, Boston, Mass.

WARREN E. ENKER, M.D.
Associate Professor of Surgery, Cornell University Medical College; Chief, Rectum and Colon Service, Department of Surgery, Memorial Sloan-Kettering Cancer Center, New York, N.Y.

RICHARD G. FARMER, M.D.
Chairman, Division of Medicine, Cleveland Clinic Foundation, Cleveland, Ohio.

VICTOR W. FAZIO, M.B., B.S.
Chairman, Department of Colorectal Surgery, Cleveland Clinic Foundation, Cleveland, Ohio.

TUVIA GILAT, M.D.
Profesor of Medicine, Sackler Faculty of Medicine, Tel-Aviv University; Chief, Department of Gastroenterology, Tel-Aviv Medical Center, Tel-Aviv, Israel.

STANLEY M. GOLDBERG, M.D.
Clinical Professor of Surgery and Director, Division of Colon and Rectal Surgery, University of Minnesota Medical School, Minneapolis, Minn.

FRANZ GOLDSTEIN, M.D.
Professor of Medicine, Jefferson Medical College of Thomas Jefferson University; Chief, Division of Gastroenterology, Lankenau Hospital, Philadelphia, Pa.

ADRIAN J. GREENSTEIN, M.B.B.Ch.
Professor of Surgery, Mount Sinai School of Medicine of the City University of New York, New York, N.Y.

STANLEY R. HAMILTON, M.D.
Associate Professor of Pathology, Johns Hopkins University School of Medicine, Baltimore, Md.

WILLIAM S. HAUBRICH, M.D.
Clinical Professor of Medicine, University of California, San Diego, School of Medicine; Senior Consultant, Division of Gastroenterology, Scripps Clinic and Research Foundation, La Jolla, Calif.

HENRY D. JANOWITZ, M.D.
Clinical Professor of Medicine, Mount Sinai School of Medicine of the City University of New York, New York, N.Y.

KATHERINE F. JETER, Ed.D., E.T.
Clinical Assistant Professor of Urology, Medical University of South Carolina, Charleston; Adjunct Professor of Psychology, University of South Carolina, Union, S.C.

JOSEPH B. KIRSNER, M.D., Ph.D.
The Lewis Block Distinguished Service Professor of Medicine, University of Chicago Pritzker School of Medicine, Chicago, Ill.

BURTON I. KORELITZ, M.D.
Clinical Professor of Medicine, New York Medical College; Chief, Section of Gastroenterology, Department of Medicine, Lenox Hill Hospital, New York, N.Y.

KLAUS J. LEWIN, M.D.
Professor and Vice Chairman of the Department of Pathology, University of California, Los Angeles, School of Medicine, Los Angeles, Calif.

CHARLES J. LIGHTDALE, M.D.
Associate Professor of Clinical Medicine, Cornell University Medical College; Director, Diagnostic Gastrointestinal Unit, Memorial Sloan-Kettering Cancer Center, New York, N.Y.

ARTHUR E. LINDNER, M.D.
Associate Professor of Medicine and Associate Dean, New York University School of Medicine, New York, N.Y.

DANIEL MAKLANSKY, M.D.
Associate Clinical Professor of Radiology, Mount Sinai School of Medicine of the City University of New York, New York, N.Y.

GERALD MARKS, M.D.
Professor of Surgery and Director, Department of Colorectal Surgery, Jefferson Medical College of Thomas Jefferson University; Head, Section of Colon and Rectal Surgery, Pennsylvania Hospital, Philadelphia, Pa.

RICHARD H. MARSHAK, M.D.
Late Clinical Professor of Radiology, Mount Sinai School of Medicine of the City University of New York, New York, N.Y.

GORDON McHARDY, M.D.
Emeritus Professor of Medicine, Louisiana State University Medical Center; Senior Visiting Physician, Louisiana State Charity Hospital, New Orleans, La.

ALBERT I. MENDELOFF, M.D., M.P.H.
Professor of Medicine, Johns Hopkins University School of Medicine; Senior Associate in Epidemiology, Johns Hopkins University School of Hygiene, Baltimore, Md.

SAMUEL MEYERS, M.D.
Associate Clinical Professor of Medicine, Mount Sinai School of Medicine of the City University of New York, New York, N.Y.

BASIL C. MORSON, D.M., F.R.C.(Path.)
Hon. Senior Lecturer in Pathology, Royal Postgraduate Medical School, University of London; Consultant Pathologist, St. Mark's Hospital, London, England.

SANTHAT NIVATVONGS, M.D.
Associate Professor of Surgery, Division of Colon and Rectal Surgery, University of Minnesota Medical School, Minneapolis, Minn.

ROBERT J. PRIEST, M.D.
Clinical Associate Professor of Internal Medicine, School of Medicine, University of Michigan; Division of Gastroenterology, Henry Ford Hospital, Detroit, Mich.

JOHN G. RAFFENSPERGER, M.D.
Professor of Surgery, Northwestern University Medical School; Surgeon-in-Chief, Children's Memorial Hospital, Chicago, Ill.

PHILIP J. SABRI, M.D.
Instructor in Radiology, School of Medicine, University of Pennsylvania, Philadelphia, Pa.

ARTHUR D. SCHWABE, M.D.
Professor of Medicine and Chief, Division of Gastroenterology, University of California, Los Angeles, School of Medicine, Los Angeles, Calif.

WILLIAM J. SNAPE, Jr., M.D.
Professor of Medicine, University of California, Los Angeles, School of Medicine; Chief of Gastroenterology, Harbor-UCLA Medical Center, Torrance, Calif.

GEORGE N. STEIN, M.D.
Professor of Radiology, School of Medicine, University of Pennsylvania, Philadelphia, Pa.

ALEXANDER J. WALT, M.B., Ch.B.
Professor and Chairman of the Department of Surgery, Wayne State University School of Medicine; Chief of Surgery, Harper-Grace Hospitals, Detroit, Mich.

SIDNEY J. WINAWER, M.D.
Professor of Clinical Medicine, Cornell University Medical College; Chief, Gastroenterology Service, Department of Medicine, Memorial Sloan-Kettering Cancer Center, New York, N.Y.

Contents

Bockus

GASTROENTEROLOGY

VOLUME 4

Intestine, Part Two

Chronic Inflammatory Bowel Disease; Colon

Chapter 124

Chronic Inflammatory Bowel Disease: Overview of Etiology and Pathogenesis

Joseph B. Kirsner

The inflammatory bowel diseases include a wide range of etiologically identified and idiopathic disorders as well as miscellaneous entities (Table 124–1). The "non-specific" inflammatory bowel diseases include ulcerative colitis and proctitis and Crohn's disease of the gastrointestinal tract.[1–5] Their designation as non-specific reflects the continuing mystery as to their origin. Ulcerative colitis and Crohn's disease share many clinical and laboratory features, but their status as interrelated or independent conditions remains unclear. The prevalence of ulcerative colitis generally has stabilized, whereas that of Crohn's disease, with 4 recent exceptions (Aberdeen, Cardiff, Stockholm, and Baltimore) has increased worldwide.

Multiple mechanisms rather than a single cause are involved in most human illnesses: clinical circumstances, genetic endowment, host defenses, adaptability to stress, immunologic resources, environmental pathogens, and individual behavioral patterns. Each of these requires consideration in assessing the etiology and pathogenesis of inflammatory bowel disease (IBD). It should be helpful, therefore, to summarize the principal clinical features of IBD before reviewing the various factors thought to play some etiologic or pathogenetic role.

Diagnostic Considerations

Problem of Differentiation Between Ulcerative Colitis and Crohn's Disease of the Colon. The small intestine and the colon of man respond to varied disease mechanisms (Table 124–1) with both distinctive and nonspecific features. Ulcerative colitis and Crohn's disease of the colon, in their fullest clinical and morphologic expressions, can be differentiated on the basis of composite clinical, endoscopic, radiologic, and pathologic findings in approximately 80% of patients.[6]

Table 124–1. CLASSIFICATION OF INFLAMMATORY BOWEL DISEASE

Idiopathic
- Ulcerative colitis
- Ulcerative proctitis
- Crohn's disease
- Ileojejunitis
- "Indeterminate" colitis

Bacterial
- Shigella
- Salmonella
- Gonococcal
- Syphilitic
- Tuberculosis
- Pathogenic *Escherichia coli*
- Staphylococcal enterocolitis
- *Yersinia enterocolitica*
- *Campylobacter* ssp. *jejuni*
- Pseudomembranous enterocolitis
- Other *(Aeromonas hydrophila)*

Parasitic
- Amebiasis
- Schistosomiasis
- Balantidiasis
- Cryptosporidiosis

Viral
- Lymphogranuloma venereum
- Cytomegalovirus
- Behçet's syndrome
- Herpesvirus proctitis
- Norwalk virus, other viruses, "viroids" (?)

Fungal
- Histoplasmosis
- Blastomycosis

Irradiation-induced
- Irradiation colitis

Drug, Chemical, Food-related
- Antibiotics
- Cytotoxic drugs (5-fluorouracil, oral contraceptives)
- Heavy metals (mercury)
- Milk protein allergy
- Soybean colitis (children)
- Cathartic colitis
- Chemicals
- Soaps, detergents
- Hydrogen peroxide
- Herbs, vinegar
- Brown sugar
- Gingko fruit

Miscellaneous
- Ischemic colitis
- Solitary ulcer, rectum
- Eosinophilic enterocolitis
- Collagenous colitis
- Uremic colitis
- Diverticulitis
- Allergic proctitis
- Metabolic (Fabry's disease, scleroderma)
- Hemolytic-uremic syndrome
- Obstructive colitis
- Myotonia dystrophica
- IgG myeloma
- Seat belt intestinal injury
- Acute "self-limited (evanescent) colitis"
- Leukemia-associated colitis

Differentiation may be difficult in 15% to 20% of patients because of the: (1) limited morphologic responsiveness of the bowel; (2) incomplete expression of IBD; (3) occurrence of an "indeterminate" colitis with features of both Crohn's disease and ulcerative colitis; and (4) mimicry of ulcerative colitis and Crohn's disease by other conditions.[7] None of the many abnormal laboratory findings, including protein alterations, endotoxemia, metabolic alkalosis, abnormal enzymes, and fecal fluid composition, is unequivocally distinctive for ulcerative colitis or Crohn's disease. Neither disorder has pathognomonic findings that are present in every instance of the one and absent in every instance of the other. Claims for the presence of "diagnostically specific" antigens and antibodies for either ulcerative colitis or Crohn's disease require confirmation.[8] The diagnostic enumeration of epithelial and connective tissue cells in biopsy tissue[9] has not been endorsed generally. It is now appreciated that involvement of the rectum, once considered exclusive to ulcerative colitis, occurs as well in Crohn's disease of the colon.[10] A sigmoidoscopically normal or minimally inflamed rectum, once regarded as inconsistent with ulcerative colitis, may indeed be associated with this disease.[11] Ulcerative colitis and Crohn's disease theoretically may occur simultaneously in the same patient, but this circumstance cannot be documented at present.

The precise differential diagnosis initially may be impossible, as in the case of a English female patient who was first seen in 1947 when she was 23 years old. At that time, rectal bleeding, diarrhea, and the proctoscopic findings prompted a diagnosis of ulcerative colitis. In 1965, roentgenograms revealed universal ulcerative colitis. In 1966, a narrowing in the transverse colon led to a subtotal colectomy and ileorectal anastomosis. Thorough examination of the resected colon by experienced pathologists confirmed a diagnosis of ulcerative colitis with "backwash ileitis." Re-operation was necessitated in 1973 by repeated flare-ups and partial bowel obstruction caused by 3 strictures proximal to the surgical anastomosis. Histologic examination of the strictures now revealed the characteristic findings of Crohn's disease, thereby capping what had been a diagnostic dilemma for 26 years.[12]

Indeterminate Colitis. The occurrence of "mixed" or "indeterminate colitis" with features of both ulcerative colitis and Crohn's disease, albeit uncommon, suggests a pathogenetic interrelationship. Indeterminate colitis is characterized histologically by: (1) extensive mucosal and submucosal ulceration separated by normal colonic mucosa; (2) an intact goblet cell population; (3) full-thickness inflammation; (4) increased vascularity in the base of ulcerations; (5) deep, slit-like fissures; and (6) absence of crypt abscesses, granulomas, and transmural lymphoid aggregates.[13]

Clinical Mimicry of IBD. Numerous inflammatory and other conditions of the colon and rectum with similar symptoms may mimic ulcerative colitis clinically and morphologically. These include Yersinia, Campylobacter,[14] and herpes simplex infections[15] of the rectum and colon, Behçet's syndrome,[16] amebiasis, toxigenic *E. coli* colitis, antibiotic-associated colitis, *Chlamydia trachomatis* (both non–lymphogranuloma venereum and lymphogranuloma strains[18]), syphilis,[19] gonorrhea, radiation injury, trauma, soybean colitis in infants, proctitis associated with IgG neoplasm, and vascular ischemia.[20] An allergic proctitis is characterized by increased numbers of IgE cells in the lamina propria[21] and apparently responds to disodium cromoglycate. Collagenous colitis is characterized by subepithelial collagenous deposits in the sigmoid colon, resembling the jejunal involvement in "collagenous sprue."[22] Fecal diversion colitis has the appearance of a mild ulcerative colitis in patients with diverting colostomies for diverticulitis or neoplasms of the colon.[23] A transient form of colitis that especially involves the right colon and is seen in patients less than 50 years of age probably represents vascular ischemia of the bowel.

The clinical mimicry of Crohn's disease is equally impressive, including acute appendicitis, infections with Yersinia, Campylobacter, and *Chlamydia trachomatis, Histoplasma capsulatum,*[24] as well as lymphoma,[25] endometriosis, ischemic enteritis, eosinophilic enteritis,[26] contraceptive enterocolitis,[27] sclerosing mesenteritis, and, rarely, actinomycosis, aspergillosis, and blastomycosis. Crohn's disease may be underdiagnosed,[28,29] as in patients mislabeled as having an irritable bowel, anorexia nervosa, or sigmoid diverticulitis. It also may be overdiagnosed,[30] as in patients with postappendiceal adhesions, endometrial implants, carcinoid of the ileum, and ovarian carcinoma.

Non-specific *ileojejunitis,* characterized by abdominal pain, fever, malabsorption, and undernutrition, is probably a heterogeneous collection of disorders of the jejunum and ileum. In some patients, it appears to be a clinical variant of celiac disease associated with villous atrophy of the small bowel and responding to a gluten-free diet. In other instances, diffuse ileojejunitis appears to be a variant of Crohn's disease, responding to sulfasalazine and steroids. In yet other rare circumstances, ulcerative ileojejunitis is a recurrent progressive independent illness with episodes of acute abdominal pain and fever and a poor prognosis.

The etiologic implications of these observations are unclear, but they are consistent with the concept of a limited morphologic response potential of the small and large intestine to varied disease processes.

Clinical Onset of IBD. The identifiable circumstances of the onset of IBD do not provide significant etiologic clues.[31] Patients generally are healthy individuals. Ulcerative colitis occurs at all times of the year, although individual patients note seasonal variations for any season. The onset of ulcerative colitis may be gradual or sudden. It may follow an emotional crisis, an acute viral illness (e.g., infectious mononucleosis), or the use of drugs (e.g., penicillin orally) or occur in the absence of any identifiable event.

The onset of Crohn's disease may be subtle, as in the slowing of growth in a child years before overt gastrointestinal symptoms, or acute, as in the clinical presentation of an apparent acute appendicitis. The early manifestations may be mistaken for the irritable bowel syndrome (Chapter 134) or anorexia nervosa or present as an unexplained fever with minimal or no gastrointestinal symptoms. The occasional onset of ulcerative colitis or Crohn's disease in one member of a family or a group, all of whom were exposed simultaneously to an acute enteric infection, indicates individual vulnerability to IBD.

Local Complications. The local complications of ulcerative colitis include hemorrhage, toxic dilatation, pericolitis, perforation, peritonitis, rectovaginal fistula, polyps, carcinoma of the colon and rectum, giant pseudopolyposis, filiform polyposis, colonic obstruction, and occasionally fibrous strictures of the rectum.[32] In regional enteritis (Crohn's disease), massive bleeding is less common. Toxic dilatation of the colon is infrequent in Crohn's disease of the colon but it does occur, and "toxic" dilatation of the ileum has also been described. Carcinoma of the colon likewise appears to be less common. Carcinoma of the small intestine statistically is more frequent in patients with regional enteritis than in the general population. Problems typical of regional enteritis include fistulas in at least 20% of patients (enteric, enteroenteric, duodenobiliary, enterocolonic, enterovesical, and enterocutaneous), abscess formation in 12% to 15% of patients at operation (abdominal, iliopsoas, hepatic), diminished bile acid pool, nephrolithiasis, obstructive hydronephrosis of the right ureter and kidney, and anorectal disease.

There are no obvious etiologic clues in this spectrum of complications, although they reflect a uniquely intense inflammatory process. The increased prevalence of colon and rectal cancer in ulcerative colitis directs attention to the colonic epithelium and its altered biologic state, including possible abnormalities in rectal-colonic epithelial mucin. The fistula formation in regional enteritis suggests the local action of a cytolytic microbial-enzymatic complex. The tendency for postoperative recurrences in regional enteritis to involve the small bowel immediately proximal to the surgical anastomosis and the widespread gastrointestinal distribution of Crohn's disease suggest the possibility of an etiologic agent in the bowel content.

Systemic Complications. The large number and variety of the systemic complications of IBD are unique,[32,33] reflecting significant but as yet unidentified associated pathogenetic mechanisms. They include arthritis, pyoderma gangrenosum,[34] autoimmune hemolytic anemia,[35] hypercoagulability of the blood,[36] iritis, myopericarditis,[37] obstructive pulmonary airway disease,[38] sclerosing cholangitis[39] (Chapter 164), phlebothrombosis, Takayasu's arteritis,[40] nephrolithiasis, aseptic necrosis of bone, and diverse nutritional and metabolic problems,[41] including pellagra and growth retardation in children. There are no demographic features identifying IBD patients at increased risk of complications other than early onset, positive family history, and severity of illness. Interestingly, autoimmune hemolytic anemia and sclerosing cholangitis tend to be more frequent in ulcerative colitis, while amyloidosis, cholelithiasis, nephrolithiasis, epidermolysis bullosa acquisita, and bronchiectasis are more common in Crohn's disease.

Since (1) the complications almost always are secondary to the bowel disease, (2) similar problems complicate jejunoileal bypass operations for morbid obesity, which is also associated with anaerobic bacterial overgrowth,[42] and (3) the complications subside with healing or resection of diseased bowel, the abnormal bacterial flora of the IBD bowel must play some role.[43] The presence of complications in some IBD patients and their continued absence in others reflect individual differences in host vulnerability and resistance to disease.

IBD in Children and Aged Persons. The course of IBD in the very young or very old individual provides no additional clues as to etiology. Crohn's disease of the small and/or large intestine occurs more frequently than ulcerative colitis in children and adolescents. The course of IBD in children is the same as in older patients. However, a surprisingly large number of pediatric patients with ulcerative colitis, after an initially favorable response to medical treatment, will relapse, progress, and later require surgery. Similarly, among older patients (greater than 60 years of age), the course of IBD is the same as in the younger age groups. Ischemic colitis mimics IBD and their differentiation can be difficult.

Demographic Considerations

The demographic aspects of imflammatory bowel disease offer interesting areas of speculation as to etiology and pathogenesis.[4,45–56] See Chapter 125 for a detailed discussion of these aspects.

Dietary Considerations

The evidence implicating certain foods (e.g., milk, corn flakes, chemically processed hydrogenated fats such as margarine, deficiency of dietary fiber) is faulted by genetic, immunologic, environmental, and other uncontrolled variables. The alleged causal relationship between excessive intake of refined sugar and Crohn's disease[57] lacks decisive evidence. IBD is rare in Morocco, Saudi Arabia, and other Moslem countries where the population consumes large amounts of sugar. Approximately 3000 chemical food additives are utilized in the food processing industry in the United States as preservatives, emulsifiers, stabilizers, thickeners, buffers, and flavor or color enhancers. Food additives are of interest chiefly because of the colitis induced in animals (mice, rats, rabbits, ferrets, monkeys, guinea pigs) whose drinking water contained extremely large amounts of carrageenan degraded by mild acid hydrolysis.[58] Ulcers developed in the cecums of these animals after 20 to 45 days and later involved the rest of the colon and rectum. The absence of colitis in germ-free animals and in carrageenan-fed animals given metronidazole implicates bacteria,[59] possibly Enterobacteriaceae or *Bacteroides vulgatus,* in the disease process. The response of animals with experimental carrageenan colitis to hydrocortisone and other therapeutic agents probably has no significance other than reflecting the non-specificity of the anti-inflammatory steroids. Since carrageenan decreases circulating complement levels, suppresses humoral immune responses, and exerts a cytolytic effect upon macrophages, immunologic mechanisms are also involved. Male and female infant baboons did not develop gastrointestinal lesions when reared from birth to 112 days on infant formulas containing concentrations of carrageenan 5-fold higher than the amounts in commercially available formulas for human infants.[60] The experimental conditions of the carrageenan model are so far removed from the circumstances of human IBD as to limit the clinical applicability of the experimental findings. There is no evidence at present to implicate food additives in the pathogenesis of IBD.[61]

Psychogenic Considerations

The central nervous system and the enteric nervous system[62] independently and jointly exercise important regulatory influences upon the motor, secretory, absorptive, and neuroendocrine functions of the gastrointestinal tract. The endocrine, paracrine, and neurocrine cells and opioid peptides in both the neuraxis and the gastrointestinal tract provide important neuroendocrine pathways for the expression of emotionally stimulated responses of the bowel.[63] The recognition of enteric neurotransmitters (e.g., acetylcholine, norepinephrine, 5-hydroxytryptamine) and neuropeptides (e.g., vasoactive intestinal polypeptide [VIP], substance P, somatostatin, enkephalins, bombesin, neurotensin)[64] further documents the close interrelationships between the nervous system and the digestive tract. Among individual patients, therefore, psychosocial stress may be as harmful to the body as extremes of temperature, pathogenic microorganisms, and physical trauma.[65] Indeed, significant changes in the levels of epinephrine, norepinephrine, cortisol, thyroxine, insulin, growth hormone, and testosterone occur under such circumstances.[66] Stress also may contribute to illness by altering host immune responses.[67] Such considerations provide a plausible basis for the participation of psychogenic stress in inflammatory bowel disease,[68] but the fundamental question of an initiating role remains unresolved.

Evaluation of emotional disturbances in the pathogenesis of inflammatory bowel disease is handicapped by the limitations of current psychiatric concepts and by insufficient "controlled" data. The chronologic associations between significant emotional events and the onset, recurrences, and intensification of IBD are not questioned, but such temporal relationships *per se* are indecisive. Antecedent emotional stresses apparently are no more common in patients with ulcerative colitis than in the general population and probably are less frequent than in patients with the irritable bowel syndrome.[69] Personality traits in patients with ulcerative colitis are approximately the same as in normal individuals. The incidence of suicide, divorce, psychosis, hospitalization for mental disorders, and the use of "psychotropic" drugs among ileostomy patients is no different than in the general population.[70] *The emotional disturbances in IBD patients probably reflect the impact of recurrent, unpredictable, at times life-threatening illness, rather than a specific antecedent psychiatric disturbance.*

Similarly, emotional difficulties are common in Crohn's disease, and are perhaps even more frequent than in ulcerative colitis. As with ulcerative colitis, they also represent consequences rather than causes. An alleged failure of "adaptive processes in particular individuals under specific circumstances" is a promising conceptual approach that requires sharper definition. Reversibility of the emotional difficulties after successful medical and surgical treatment of ulcerative colitis is consistent with the "secondary" nature of the psychogenic problems in IBD. The generally excellent health and successful careers of colectomy-ileostomy patients reflect an achieving and competent population group—certainly not the alleged ineffectual individuals cited psychoanalytically in earlier years.

The increased norepinephrene content of the rectal mucosa in ulcerative colitis[71] correlates with the increased perivascular adrenergic nerve plexus.[72] The reduced endorphin and enkephalin-like reactivity in the gut wall of patients with Crohn's disease presumably is secondary to the bowel damage. The thickened, intensely immunostained, VIP-containing nerves, dispersed in densely packed meshes and plexuses within the myenteric and submucosal plexuses and the muscle layer of the bowel in Crohn's disease, probably are also secondary developments.[73,74] Until psychiatrically directed clinical studies are carefully structured and controlled and are supported by appropriate pharmacologic, endocrine, and biochemical measurements, decisive correlations of IBD with psychogenic disturbances will be difficult. *As perceived presently, emotional stress or nervous tension, in all likelihood, does not directly cause ulcerative colitis or Crohn's disease. Undoubtedly, however, they can "non-specifically" precipitate or intensify IBD.*

Pathogenetic Implications of Therapeutic Approaches

Analysis of therapeutic responses in IBD does not provide substantial etiologic clues. Almost all aspects of therapy are arbitrary.[75] The relatively few "controlled" clinical trials thus far have failed to provide new insights. No single drug is curative, and a "non-specific" comprehensive therapeutic approach is most useful. Nutritional restoration improves body defenses generally and facilitates pharmacologic responses to medication, but the benefits are not specific to IBD.[76] While emotional support of the IBD patient is helpful in reducing the "burden of disability," the helpful effects are not exclusive to IBD.

Sulfasalazine appears to benefit patients with ulcerative colitis and, to a lesser degree, those with Crohn's disease by mechanisms that are apparently not confined to its antibacterial properties.[77–79] However, these mechanisms (e.g., inhibition of prostaglandin E_2 synthesis or inhibition of prostaglandin breakdown) and assessment of the action of its components (5-aminosalicylic acid vs. the entire sulfasalazine molecule) remain unsettled. Indeed, in several instances, sulfasalazine appears to have induced exacerbations of ulcerative colitis.[80] The generally erratic response of IBD to antibacterial agents, except in the presence of suppurative complications, does not conform to responses in known bacterial infections. The anti-anaerobic, and anti-protozoan properties of metronidazole do not provide lasting control of IBD.

The response of IBD to ACTH and to adrenocorticosteroids, while occasionally dramatic, is neither specific nor unique to IBD. All of the heterogeneous effects of steroids upon lymphoid cells and upon the immune response are also observed in other diseases. There is no evidence of an antecedent steroid deficiency in IBD; rather, prolonged steroid intake induces an adrenocortical insufficiency. Among the "effective" steroids (prednisone, prednisolone, methylprednisolone, hydrocortisone) and the ineffective steroids (cortisone, triamcinolone, dexamethasone), no unique therapeutic mechanism, or mechanisms, has emerged as being present or absent.

The continuing immunologic interest in IBD notwithstanding, there is no conclusive evidence of an underlying or abnormal immune reaction in IBD, at least one that is uniquely responsive to steroids. The apparent response of Crohn's disease to "immunosuppressant" medication (6MP-azathioprine), especially when given for periods as long as 6 months,[81] does not suggest a specific therapeutic mechanism. Moreover, the beneficial effect diminishes or disappears when the medication is discontinued. The alleged immunodeficiency in IBD, especially in Crohn's disease, may reflect secondary factors, including nutritional depletion, the presence of non-specific circulating inhibitors, and the dampening effect of drugs used in therapy (e.g., sulfasalazine). The ineffectiveness of transfer factor ("immune support") and the immunostimulants levamisole and bacille Calmette Guérin (BCG) in IBD does not support the concept of an immunodeficiency of significant degree. Attempted therapy with such diverse measures as plasmapheresis (removal of circulating immune complexes), disodium cromoglycate, superoxide dismutase, D-penicillamine, tranexamic acid (an anti-fibrinolytic agent), large doses of vitamin A, dapsone, limitation of carbohydrate intake, intestinal lavage, and the addition of fiber to the diet reflects the search for "effective" treatment rather than a supportable pathogenetic concept.

Analysis of the surgical treatment of IBD likewise does not yield significant etiologic clues.[82,83] Total colectomy and ileostomy is a curative operation for severe ulcerative colitis in virtually all patients, but it is an ablative procedure, removing the diseased bowel irrespective of etiology. The interesting pathogenetic aspect of the operation is the persistently normal status of the small bowel, i.e., its non-involvement in the ulcerative colitis process. *In Crohn's colitis, despite total colectomy and ileostomy, recurrences in the remaining small bowel range from 20% to 35%*. Even more significant is the exceedingly high recurrence rate of Crohn's disease of the small bowel after intestinal resection and re-anastomosis, with time approximating 80% to 90% or more. The morphologic, biochemical, and enzymatic evidences of disease in grossly uninvolved small bowel tissue indicate the diffuseness of Crohn's disease. This feature is perhaps consistent with alimentary tract exposure to a "transmissible agent" or a "cytotoxin."

Tissue Reactions

The diffuse inflammation and multiple superficial ulcerations, crypt abscesses, diminished goblet cells, disordered crypts, and augmented cellular infiltration of the lamina propria that characterize ulcerative colitis[84] are not pathognomonic. The apparent onset of ulcerative colitis on the mucosal surface of the colon suggests contact with cytotoxic substances within the bowel lumen. Potential sources of cytotoxins include the altered bacterial and viral flora of the gut, the damaged colonic epithelium, and the intense cellular infiltrate, including an increase in mast cells and Paneth cells, and the substances they release. The increased quantities of prostaglandin E_2 and its metabolites (see later) together with the kinins (bradykinin, kallidin, kininogen) are involved in various inflammatory reactions, including ulcerative colitis. The earlier observation of a proteolytic enzyme in fecal filtrates of patients with active ulcerative colitis, distinguishable from tryptic enzymes and capable of digesting epidermal cells, has never been confirmed. The colitis associated with *Clostridium difficile* toxin complicating the use of antibiotics, and found occasionally in active ulcerative colitis and in active Crohn's disease, is a secondary development. The possible involvement of other bacterial toxins has not been investigated.

The pronounced vascular congestion of the mucosa and submucosa and the virtually infarcted appearance of the colon in fulminating ulcerative colitis correlate with the intensity of the inflammation and are attributable to chemical and other mediators of the tissue reaction. The possible role of alterations in the microcirculation of the bowel producing a mucosal ischemia[85] has not been investigated adequately.

Histochemical studies of biopsied rectal and resected colonic tissues demonstrate depletion of various enzymes (e.g., alkaline phosphatase, lactic dehydrogenase, triphosphopyridine nucleotide phosphate–linked enzyme). This depletion, however, is a consequence of tissue injury[86] and not specific to IBD. The limited rectal biopsy studies of unaffected members of IBD families that have been made to date have not revealed enzymatic defects representing antecedent tissue vulnerability. The apparent deficiency of secretory IgA in normal-appearing sigmoid proximal to the visible demarcation of ulcerative proctitis suggests an antecedent local immune tissue defect.[87] This observation, however, also remains unconfirmed.

The continuously increased cell turnover in the large bowel mucosa in ulcerative colitis during remission, as well as during activity, is noteworthy in relation to the increased prevalence of carcinoma. The diminished incorporation of ^{14}C-labeled amino acids into colonic mucosal proteins in ulcerative colitis[88] suggests a defective mucosal regenerative capacity. The deficiency of fraction IV of colonic epithelial mucus in ulcerative colitis is of interest in this regard. The speed of maturation of goblet cells is decreased in ulcerative colitis but returns to normal with remission. Protective "trophic" substances promoting the regeneration of epithelium have been postulated for all areas of the digestive tract, but no information is available in relation to IBD specifically. The normal colon obviously possesses remarkable defenses against bacterial invasion and other sources of tissue injury, but the nature of this protection is unknown.

Prostaglandins and metabolites of arachidonic acid (lipoxygenases and cyclo-oxygenases) probably are involved in the inflammation and diarrhea of IBD but are not primary factors in the pathogenesis of the disease.[89–93] The increased synthesis of prostaglandin E_2 and of 6-ketoprostaglandin F_1 and thromboxane B_2 (the stable metabolites of prostacyclin I_2 and thromboxane A_2, respectively) during active colitis but not in biopsy specimens from patients in remission probably derives from stimulated local inflammatory cells. Prostaglandins stimulate small intestine adenylate cyclase activity, inhibit active sodium transport, and induce active ion secretion. Sulfasalazine and its constituents (5-aminosalicylic acid [5-ASA] and sulfapyridine) inhibit prostaglandin E_2 synthesis by cultured rectal mucosa, but only 5-ASA prevents the accumulation of thromboxane B_2 and 6-ketoprostaglandin F. The alleged cytotoxic effects of prostaglandins in ulcerative colitis are in contrast to the cytoprotective effects of the prostaglandins in preventing *C. difficile* toxin colitis in antibiotic-treated hamsters, the non-responsiveness of ulcerative colitis to flurbiprofen (a potent inhibitor of prostaglandin synthesis),[94] and the presence of prostaglandin E_2 in normal jejunal fluid.[95] Indeed, an alternative hypothesis suggests that sulfasalazine and its constituents inhibit the breakdown of prostaglandins, facilitating a cytoprotective action. The significance of the enhanced prostanoid synthesis by cultured peripheral blood monocytes from patients with active Crohn's disease, but not with ulcerative colitis, is not clear at present. The specificity of the increased mucosal prostanoid production in ulcerative colitis also is not established. The demonstration of bradykinin receptors in the mucosa and muscle layer of the small intestine indicates multiple additional mediators of intestinal function, including lipoxygenase and cyclo-oxygenase metabolites of arachidonic acid.

The remarkable localization of ulcerative colitis to the colon has been documented by an experiment of nature.[96] Severe ulcerative colitis in a 21-year-old Frenchman necessitated a total colectomy, but the patient died. A sigmoid colon duplication was found to be completely free of any pathologic changes, old or recent, despite the fact that (1) the lumen of the intestinal duplication communicated fully with that of the diseased colon, (2) the vascular supply was in common with that of the abnormal colon, and (3) the wall of the duplication included all the layers of the normal colon. In a contrary observation, ulcerative colitis apparently developed simultaneously in the rectum and in a discontinuous segment of colon utilized previously for colpopoiesis.

Implications of Tissue Reactions in Crohn's Disease. The pathologic features of Crohn's disease have been thoroughly documented[97–101] and are detailed in Chapter 127. Importantly, the same abnormalities are observed in the margins of surgically resected normal-appearing bowel.

The submucosal dilatation of lymphatics, endolymphangitis, and enlarged mesenteric lymph nodes of Crohn's disease imply that the lymphatics play some role in pathogenesis, perhaps as the site of entry of cytotoxic material (bacterial, viral, chemical) from the bowel lumen. Granuloma, although an important feature of Crohn's disease, is present in only 60% of patients[102] and, once present, may disappear. Its biologic significance in Crohn's disease is not clear. Granulomas also develop in response to foreign bodies (lipids, talc, sutures, beryllium) and certain infections (sarcoid, tuberculosis, histoplasmosis). Peripheral blood monocytes (presumably precursors of tissue macrophages) are normal, and macrophage turnover in ulcerative colitis and in Crohn's disease also is normal.[103]

Scanning and transmission electron microscopy demonstrates numerous intact and degranulated mast cells in proximity to eosinophils harboring increased numbers of arylsulfatase-containing granules but depleted of major basic protein-containing cores, findings consistent with an immune reaction. The augmented secretion of mucus by the bowel in Crohn's disease correlates with increased glucosamine synthetase activity.[104] Similarities in the histologic appearance of Crohn's disease and sarcoidosis, including the presence of epithelioid granulomas, suggest an etiologic relationship. However, except for a similarly decreased cell-mediated immunity (e.g., diminished responsiveness of circulating lymphocytes to mitogens), no pathogenetic relationship between the 2 disorders has been demonstrated. Levels of angiotensin-converting enzyme (ACE), reduced in sarcoidosis, are normal in Crohn's disease.[105] The association of ulcerative colitis and sarcoidosis in 5 patients is of interest in this regard.[106]

Regional enteritis–like morphologic features have been described in young women who develop mesenteric venous thrombosis after taking oral contraceptives and in individuals sustaining seat belt injuries to the abdomen. These are unusual circumstances, however, and are not representative of Crohn's disease. A genetically determined deficiency of erythrocyte and intestinal glucose-6-phosphate dehydrogenase as an indication of tissue vulnerability in Crohn's disease, especially among Ashkenazi Jews, has never been confirmed.

Unusual Sites of Crohn's Disease–like Lesions. The tendency of Crohn's disease to occur immediately proximal to sphincters (ileocecal, rectal), to recur immediately proximal to a surgically established bowel anastomosis, and to subside when the involved segment of bowel is diverted from the fecal stream is consistent with the action of a cytotoxic agent in the bowel content, but this etiologic clue remains unexplored.

The diffuse focal involvement of the gastrointestinal tract in Crohn's disease has now been documented by electron microscopy, tissue enzyme analysis,[107] immunofluorescent studies, abnormal jejunal surface pH, and changes in sodium flux and mucosal potential.[108] Crohn's disease of the appendix usually is in continuity with ileocecal disease. Rarely, the appendix is involved synchronously with Crohn's disease elsewhere in the gastrointestinal tract, as in the rectum. Involvement of the mouth may be an early indicator of intestinal disease.[109] Crohn's disease may also present in other unusual locations, including the skin,[110] vulva, femur,[111] synovial tissue,[112] gastrocnemius muscle,[113] epiglottis and vocal cords,[114] upper airway passages,[115] and lungs.[116] The implications of these observations are unclear, but suggest a systemic tissue response, at least in occasional patients.

In summary, attempts to clarify the pathogenesis of ulcerative colitis and Crohn's disease on the basis of the discernible tissue reactions, although intriguing, are hampered by (1) questions as to the specificity and constancy of the changes detected by light, scanning, and electron microscopy and by histochemical and immunofluorescent staining, (2) limitations in the methods of study, (3) the possible influence of antibacterial drugs, adrenocortical steroids, and other therapeutic agents, (4) the nutritional state of the patient, and (5) individual differences in morphologic response.

Natural Animal Occurrences and Experimental Reproduction

Spontaneous ulcerative colitis in animals comparable to that in man is unknown. Experimentally, inflammatory and ulcerative changes have been induced in the colon of dogs, monkeys, rabbits, guinea pigs, and other animals by various techniques[117,118]: (1) nutritional deficiencies (vitamin A, folic acid, pantothenic acid); (2) cytolytic enzymes (collagenase, lysozyme); (3) broad-spectrum antibiotics; (4) application of shigella and staphylococcal toxins to colonic explants; (5) injection of cholinergic drugs (methacholine, neostigmine, acetylcholine); (6) rectal instillation of 10% acetic acid (in rats); (7) exposure to staphylococcal toxin; (8) epinephrine, histamine, and histamine releasers; (9) various immunologic techniques,[119] including the Arthus, Shwartzman, and Auer-Kirsner reactions; (10) local application of dinitrochlorobenzene (DNCB) to the colonic mucosa in guinea pigs skin sensitized to DNCB[120]; (11) induction of runt disease in mice, rats, and guinea pigs; and (12) implantation of homologous fetal colon beneath the renal capsule of inbred rats. The lesions are acute, superficial, and transient. In rabbits with chronic serum sickness induced by daily injections of bovine serum albumin, deposits of bovine serum albumin, rabbit IgG, and complement 3 (C3), mainly in the vessel walls close to the intestinal glands and the surface epithelium[121] of the gastrointestinal tract, are consistent with localization of damaging immune complexes. Inflammation of both the small intestine and colon may be induced in highly inbred strains of rats injected with purified rat intestinal glycoproteins.[122]

A variety of inflammatory disorders in animals, involving especially the distal small bowel and the colon, undoubtedly are caused by infectious agents; none duplicates human IBD.[123,124] There is no evidence that animal species act as a reservoir for any putative infectious agents for IBD.[125] A terminal ileitis in swine, occurring especially in Scandinavian countries,[126] and a regional enterocolitis in cocker spaniel dogs[127] probably are caused by unidentified infectious agents. The granulomatous colitis of boxer dogs resembles Whipple's disease.[128] A granulomatous enteritis and enterocolitis in horses has been attributed to *Mycotuberculosis avium* and to *Strongyloides stercoralis.*[124] Johne's disease, a chronic enteritis in cattle, sheep, and goats caused by *Mycobacterium paratuberculosis,* is a chronic hyperplastic enterocolitis.[129] The lesions are characterized by pronounced infiltration with epithelioid cells and lymphocytes without caseation or ulceration. Infection of chickens with *E. coli* may lead to the development of granulomatous lesions in the intestines and the liver.

Crohn's disease also has not been duplicated experimentally. Lesions in the ileocecal region follow: (1) the intralymphatic injection of sclerosing solutions with and without bacteria[130]; (2) blunt trauma to the abdominal wall; (3) injection of ceramic spheres into small blood vessels supplying the small intestine and the colon of dogs; and (4) various immunologic procedures. Obstruction of the mesenteric lymphatics of the terminal ileum in pigs by the intralymphatic injection of formalin solution is followed after 3 weeks by growth retardation,[131] inflammation and mucosal ulcerations, and ileal fistulas. Although transmural inflammation with round cell aggregates, lymphoid accumulations, and occasional giant cells are noted, the process does not duplicate Crohn's disease. An ulcerative enterocolitis can be induced in dogs given cinchophen IV or indomethacin orally,[132] with a skip-like distribution of mucosal lesions corresponding to the distribution of lymphoid follicles. It is theorized that cells in Peyer's patches normally produce prostaglandins that protect the host from potentially dangerous responses to intestinal antigens. Presumably, prostaglandin synthetase inhibitors (e.g., indomethacin or cinchophen) abolish this protective effect, with release of lymphotoxins from sensitized lymphocytes reacting with antigen; this response leads to transmural penetration of lymphocytes and tissue injury.

Non-specific inflammation of the bowel has been induced in rabbits injected with filtrates of IBD intestinal tissue but has no relationship to the human disease. The direct injection of sterile non-viable bacterial (group A streptococci) cell wall fragments into the ileal wall and ileal mesentery of Sprague-Dawley rats produces a chronic granulomatous intestinal inflammation attributable to the peptidoglycan-polysaccharide (PG-PS) complex common to all bacterial cell walls.[133] The concept postulates that IBD develops in the setting of a damaged intestinal mucosa, allowing the transmigration of bacterial cell wall fragments and a resultant transmural granulomatous response that is maintained by the further entry of cell wall antigens. While constituents of the cell wall of intestinal bacteria are found in the bowel wall (e.g., diaminopimelic acid),[134] there is no evidence linking such findings to the pathogenesis of ulcerative colitis or Crohn's disease or to an altered immunologic responsiveness of the bowel.

In summary, despite varied and ingenious concepts and techniques, a completely acceptable and dependable animal model of either ulcerative colitis or Crohn's disease has not been developed. The suitability of the cotton-top marmoset for this purpose is under investigation.

Bacterial Infection

Neither ulcerative colitis nor Crohn's disease is contagious[135] or epidemic and their frequency correlates inversely with the prevalence of the infectious dysenteries.[136] An outbreak in one family has been reported that included ulcerative proctitis in the 30-year-old mother and Crohn's-type colitis in 2 sons (ages 11 and 14) and in a daughter (age 9).[137] All illnesses developed within a 5-year period and were attributed, without confirmatory information, to a questionable water supply in the German town where the family had resided. Person-to-person transmission is virtually impossible to document. IBD occurs, albeit rarely, in the initially healthy mate of an IBD patient, consistent with a slowly transmissible illness. Medical personnel in frequent or prolonged contact with IBD patients do not have an increased prevalence of either ulcerative colitis or Crohn's disease. Anti-bacterial drugs are helpful in therapy but are not curative. Despite these limitations, microbial infection remains an attractive concept in IBD because of: (1) the inflammatory process; (2) the enterocolitis caused by known bacteriologic and parasitic agents, such as bacillary dysentery, amebic dysentery, and lymphopathia venereum; (3) the microbially induced intestinal diseases in animals resembling human IBD; and (4) the recognition of new bacterial causes of intestinal inflammation (Yersinia,[138] Campylobacter,[139] *Aeromonas hydrophila,* and non-O group 1 *Vibrio cholerae.*[140]

Bacteriologic interest in ulcerative colitis originally involved Streptococcus, *Entamoeba histolytica,* hemolytic *E. coli,* Proteus, Mycoplasma, and *Sphaerophorus necrophorus.*[141] Attention currently is directed to intestinal anaerobes, variant cell wall–deficient bacteria, and mycobacteria. Studies of the bowel microflora in ulcerative colitis are highly variable and indecisive.[142] The numbers of bacteria are increased during active disease. However, no pathogenic organism exclusive to ulcerative colitis has been identified and bacterial distributions in the feces are non-specific. The findings range from increases in group D streptococci to *E. coli* with enhanced invasive properties.[143–145]

Microbial possibilities in Crohn's disease have included tuberculosis, lymphopathia venereum, and various anaerobes. Currently, the focus is on mycobacteria, including a newly described mycobacterium, Chlamydia, Campylobacter, and anaerobes. The gut microflora in Crohn's disease is characterized by bacterial overgrowth, especially anaerobes, including *Peptostreptococcus magnus* and *Eubacterium* strains C_{18}, Me_{46}, and Me_{47}.[146–148] These organisms, which are capable of activating the alternate complement pathway, are agglutinated more often and in higher titers by Crohn's disease serum than by serum from patients with ulcerative colitis, other intestinal disorders, and healthy persons,[149,150] but their role in Crohn's disease is unclear. Increases in *E. coli, Bacillus fragilis,* and lactobacilli in the gut do not correlate with histologic evidence of Crohn's disease.

Claims for *Mycobacterium kansasii,*[151] cell wall–deficient Pseudomonas-like bacteria[152] (including *Pseudomonas maltophilia),* and *Chlamydia trachomatis* in the pathogenesis of IBD[153] are unconfirmed. The presence of corynebacteria or propronibacteria in cultures of IBD lymph nodes and L forms of *E. coli, Streptococcus fecalis, Pseudomonas aeruginosa, Proteus mirabilis,* and *Enterobacter cloacae* in tissue biopsies and lymph nodes from patients with ulcerative colitis or Crohn's disease[154] primarily reflect the favorable environment of the small and large bowel in IBD for growth of many kinds of bacteria without a pathogenetic relationship to IBD. Except for one unconfirmed report, electron microscopic studies of resected Crohn's disease tissue have not demonstrated the presence of unusual bacteria.[155]

Agglutinating antibodies against *E. coli* O antigens are more frequent and in higher titers in patients with ulcerative colitis[156,157] and Crohn's disease[158] than in matched controls, but no specific O-serotype has been identified. Also, no correlation exists between the *E. coli* agglutinins and the site, extent, and severity of IBD.

Pseudomembranous colitis caused by *Clostridium difficile* and its toxins may complicate the administration of antibiotics and less often sulfonamides, including sulfasalazine.[159] A second more potent toxin (toxin A) produced by *C. difficile* has a similar molecular weight but different antigenic specificities and biologic activities.[160] While *C. difficile* toxin occasionally is found in the stools of patients with ulcerative colitis or Crohn's disease, there is no evidence to implicate this organism in the pathogenesis of either disorder.[160–162] The possible role of other bacterial enterotoxins in IBD has yet to be investigated.[163]

The variable and inconclusive bacteriologic observations in IBD reflect the technical difficulties involved in microbiologic studies of the gut. These difficulties include insufficient knowledge of: (1) the indigenous aerobic and anaerobic flora of the bowel; (2) the mechanisms of bacterial adherence and non-adherence to intestinal epithelium; and (3) host systemic and local (gut) defenses against microbial injury. The conflicting claims for various microbes recall earlier futile efforts to link ulcerative colitis with Shigella and *Sphaerophorus necrophorus* and to relate Crohn's disease to sarcoidosis or lymphopathia venereum. While present data remain inconclusive, a microbial mechanism in the etiology of IBD remains an attractive possibility—if not by means of a single agent or an altered gut reaction to a microbial constituent, then perhaps as a combination of bacterial and viral agents and microbial products altering normal bacterial relationships within the bowel of susceptible individuals.

Viral Etiology

Interest in a possible viral cause for IBD is supported by the clinical similarity of ulcerative colitis to a viral colitis (lymphopathia venereum), the occasional onset of ulcerative colitis or Crohn's disease soon after a viral illness (measles,[164] infectious mononucleosis), the prevalence of Norwalk virus and rotavirus enteritis in the general population,[165,166] and the experimentally induced infections of the small and large intestine with human viruses.[167,168] In contrast is the negative evidence of contagion,[169] the lack of a relationship between acute viral enteritis and IBD flare-ups, the absence of serologic evidence of excessive exposure to the currently identifiable viruses in ulcerative colitis and Crohn's disease and to rotavirus and Norwalk virus in Crohn's disease,[170] and the absence of adenovirus DNA in histologically normal and abnormal bowel from IBD patients.[171] The increased titers of cytomegalovirus in malnourished individuals with ulcerative colitis[172] are secondary consequences of the associated immune deficiency in such patients.

Earlier studies unsuccessfully sought to induce IBD-like lesions in the rectum and colon of rabbits, dogs, and monkeys by the injection of crude extracts of colitis and enteritis tissues and stool filtrates from IBD patients.[173] Based upon positive experiments with human sarcoid tissue, the injection of homogenates of Crohn's disease tissues and mesenteric lymph nodes produced epithelioid and Langhans' type giant cell granulomas in the footpads of normal and immunodeficient CBA mice; the lesions required as long as 500 days for complete evolution.[174,175] Similar changes were described in A_2G strain mice, in the ileum of NZW white rabbits injected intramurally, and most frequently among inbred C57BL/10 mice,[176] occasionally in bowel distant from the injection sites. Changes have also been produced in the bowel, liver, or spleen of normal A_2G mice and immunodeficient CBA mice injected with fresh or frozen filtrates of Crohn's disease homogenates from the ileum, colon, and lymph nodes. Utilizing the granulomatous lesions or the drainage lymph nodes, serial passage was accomplished in 4 successive generations of mice. These observations were "reproduced" partly or wholly by other investigators.[177,178] Subsequently, "RNA viral agents" were described in tissue cultures and by electron microscopy.[179] Cytopathic effects were demonstrated with 200-nm tissue filtrates for lung fibroblasts and for a 30-nm particle in rabbit ileal fibroblast cultures.

Other investigators subsequently were unable to: (1) induce granulomatous lesions with extracts of Crohn's disease tissue; (2) confirm a cell culture cytopathic effect related to IBD tissue homogenates in tissue culture cells not contaminated by *Mycoplasma hyorhinis;* and (3) identify virus particles in Crohn's disease tissues and biopsy specimens by electron microscopy, immunofluorescence search for specific antigens, interferon assay, and co-cultivation and reverse transcriptase assay for reovirus infections.[180–182] Multicenter reappraisal of the animal model and the "virus isolation" studies utilizing standardized methodology and the laboratory exchange of tissue homogenates also failed to confirm the original observations. Furthermore, granulomas were also induced in mouse footpads with tissues from control subjects.

The variable results raise numerous questions regarding the experiments, including the presence of foreign material in the injected homogenates, the status of the donors of the diseased tissues, and the most suitable animal species to serve as recipients. The "transmissible agent" now has been characterized as a cytotoxic protein of low molecular weight and not a virus. The "cytotoxins" are demonstrable in low titers in ulcerative colitis (heat stable), in Crohn's disease (heat labile), and also in carcinoma of the colon and in other bowel disorders. The "cytotoxins" in each disease apparently have different molecular weights and sensitivities to boiling. They are non-sedimentable at 148,000 g for 2 hours and resist inactivation by ultraviolet light. The source of this material is not yet known and its role, if any, in IBD is unclear.

Beeken[183] has pointed out that the possibility of innocent opportunistic viruses or bacteria occurring in diseased bowel with deficient mucosal barriers is real. Until it is clearly demonstrated that these organisms can induce disease and Koch's postulates are fulfilled, their significance cannot be judged. At the present time, there appears to be no conclusive evidence of a causative virus in the etiology of IBD. While accepting the validity of these considerations, the possible involvement of viral agents (e.g., a "slow virus" or "viroid")[184] cannot be excluded.

Approximately 8% of 10-week-old nu/nu mice develop lymphomas 10 to 28 weeks after the intraperitoneal injection of ultrafiltrates of mesenteric lymph node homogenates from patients with Crohn's disease. Similar lesions do not develop with preparations from patients with ulcerative colitis or sarcoid.[185] The induced lymphomas may be passed into a second generation of mice, presumably by means of an unidentified oncogenic agent. Indirect immunofluorescence staining of lymphoma cells occurs only with serum from Crohn's disease patients, not with serum from ulcerative colitis patients or other disease controls. The apparent antigen specificity of the lymphoma spleen antigen only for Crohn's disease and the question of a transmissible factor in Crohn's disease lymph nodes are intriguing, but the work requires confirmation in meticulously double-blind studies. Furthermore, no lymphomas developed in additional mice injected subsequently with lymph node homogenates from the 2 recent patients with Crohn's disease.

Genetic Aspects (See also Chapter 240)

Familial IBD. Ulcerative colitis and Crohn's disease are not conventional genetically transmitted disorders. Inheritable protein, enzymatic, metabolic, or antecedent chromosomal abnormalities have not been demonstrated as yet. ABO blood groups and secretor status are distributed normally.[186,187] Claims for glucose-6-phosphate dehydrogenase[188] and a rare isoenzyme of alkaline phosphatase[189] as markers of individual vulnerability to IBD are unconfirmed. No genetic "markers" of either ulcerative colitis or Crohn's disease have been revealed as yet (e.g., abnormal reaction to microbial or tissue antigens, cytotoxicity of peripheral blood mononuclear cells). The increased frequency of elevated antibody titers against enterobacterial common antigen among apparently unaffected female relatives of patients with ulcerative colitis or Crohn's disease is an unexplained observation.[190] Abnormalities in cultured lymphocytes from Crohn's disease patients are attributable to the accumulation of highly reactive superoxide radicals produced by macrophage elements of the tissue reaction rather than to a genetic mechanism.

Multiple occurrences of IBD in the same family are identified in from 20% to 40% of IBD cases. [191–193] As many as 3 generations and 5 or more family members may be involved. First-degree relatives (parents, siblings) are more vulnerable than second-degree relatives (aunts, uncles, nieces, nephews). IBD with high concordance ratios also occurs among monozygotic[194] and dizygotic twins. Ulcerative colitis is more likely to occur in families of probands with ulcerative colitis, and Crohn's disease is more likely among families of probands with Crohn's disease. However, the 2 disorders are intermingled in at least 25% of IBD families. A controlled Danish study of 152 patients with ulcerative colitis identified 8 families with additional affected members (5.3%) as compared with 1 family in the control group (0.73%).[195] In a Chicago study of 646 patients,[191] the familial occurrence rate of IBD was 17.5%. In 150 of the patients selected at random and then matched with 150 healthy people, the familial occurrence rate was 11% as compared with 4%. Genetically influenced susceptibility to IBD is further supported by the association of IBD with ankylosing spondylitis, an association found 10 to 20 times more often in men with IBD than in the general population.[196] Also, among patients with ankylosing spondylitis, the prevalence of IBD in many series was higher than could be anticipated by chance.[197]

A recessive gene influence is suggested by (1) the association of IBD with rare genetic syndromes, (2) the occurrence of Crohn's colitis in families with the Hermansky-Pudlak syndrome[198] (an autosomal recessive genetic disorder marked by tyrosine-positive albinism, a defect in the second phase of platelet aggregation, widespread accumulation of a ceroid-like pigment in tissue, and occasional pulmonary fibrosis), (3) the increased frequency of Crohn's disease and ulcerative colitis in patients with Turner's syndrome,[120] and (4) the occurrence of ulcerative colitis in a 13-year-old girl with $alpha_1$-antitrypsin deficiency and a structurally abnormal X chromosome.[200] However, Mendelian ratios are not observed, a generation is often skipped, and consanguinity is lacking.

One concept for the genetics of IBD recognizes ulcerative colitis and Crohn's disease as prototypes of a single disease process that encompasses a spectrum of intermediate tissue reactions with 2 polygenic systems determining liability and possessing a number of genes in common.[201] The possession of only a few of these genes presumably predisposes to ulcerative colitis, whereas a more complete genotype predisposes to Crohn's disease. This theory could explain not only familial IBD but also the increased frequency of IBD among families of probands with Crohn's disease. The genetic contribution presumably is to establish susceptibility, with the actual disease precipitated by external agents, including bacteria and viruses and their products, environmental pollutants, dietary antigens, and "stress."

The occurrence of IBD in family members living apart for long periods and the nonepidemic nature of IBD diminish the potential role of environmental influences. Nevertheless, non-genetic mechanisms also require consideration, e.g., a common family exposure to a "slow virus."

This possibility is indicated by a 22-year-old woman with a history of Crohn's disease for 6 years. The presence of Crohn's disease in the patient's grandmother, who lived in the same household, suggested a genetic relationship except for the critical fact that the patient was an adopted child and not a natural offspring of the family.

The appearance of IBD under circumstances of prolonged close contact or simultaneous exposure to possible sources of infection is infrequent, although 8 instances of IBD developing in the initially healthy spouse of an IBD mate now have been documented. In the family reported by Asquith,[202] Crohn's disease in the husband began approximately 2 years after marriage; the subsequent development of sacroiliitis in his wife was associated chronologically with the onset of ulcerative colitis that responded to sulfasalazine. Craxi et al.[203] describe the almost simultaneous development of chronic ulcerative colitis in a husband and wife living in Palermo, Sicily. Whorwell et al.[204] reported the development of Crohn's disease in both husband and wife after more than 30 years of marriage. Zetzel[205] recorded the presence of ulcerative colitis in the husband, Crohn's disease in the wife, and ulcerative colitis in 1 of 2 children. Also of note is the development in an American physician of ulcerative colitis after 10 years in gastroenterologic practice and the appearance of Crohn's disease in his wife 7 years later.[206]

IBD involvement of entire families is rare indeed. In a German family, the father, age 49, his 22-year-old son, and his two daughters, ages 25 and 21, each had Crohn's disease. In a Chicago family, the mother had ulcerative colitis that eventually required a total colectomy; this was followed by ulcerative colitis in her 7-year-old son 7 years later, who also required colectomy, and by regional enteritis in her husband 9 years later.[207] In a Mississippi family of 5 children, at least 4 had Crohn's disease. All 4 had the same maternal haplotype (A30/B17) and 3 had the same paternal haplotype (A2/B44).[208] In a French family, Crohn's disease was diagnosed in 32-year-old monozygous twin brothers who had been living apart for years preceding onset of the disease. In an American (California) family, monozygous twin brothers developed Crohn's disease within 8 months of each other.[194] In identical American male twins, age 22, ulcerative colitis in each was complicated by multifocal anaplastic carcinoma of the colon.[209]

The contact-transmission question has been examined utilizing lymphocytoxic activity (LCA) as a marker of exposure to an environmental agent, possibly a virus. LCA is determined by the presence of IgM antibodies with marked heterogeneity, reacting with both B and T lymphocytes. LCA was found in only 4% of control families in contrast to 50% among IBD family members (with both ulcerative colitis and Crohn's disease). The increased prevalence of IgM antibodies for synthetic polyribonucleotides, both synthetic single- and double-stranded RNA, in IBD patients (60%) and their spouses (40%) in comparison with controls (7%) suggests the presence of a viral agent. LCA antibodies are associated with viral and bacterial infections, but also have been detected in diseases of unknown etiology other than IBD, including systemic lupus erythematosus and multiple sclerosis.

Histocompatibility Haplotypes. The human leukocyte antigen system, HLA, is a highly polymorphic series of tissue antigens under the control of 4 genetic loci, each capable of determining a series of alternative genes at each gene locus, known as alleles (Chapter 243). The groups of alleles on a single chromosome are designated as haplotypes. The system has major immunoregulatory capacities.[213] With respect to IBD, however, except for the association between HLA-B27 and IBD with ankylosing spondylitis or iritis, studies from different parts of the world reflect varying ethnic-related haplotype distributions and are too inconsistent for decisive evaluation.

Ulcerative Colitis. The HLA-B5 phenotype was more common in 44 Japanese patients with ulcerative colitis, especially women and patients with total ulcerative colitis, than in 271 controls.[214] A Japanese survey noted a significant decrease in DW35 among patients with ulcerative colitis,[215] whereas no significant HLA phenotype was observed in 53 Italian patients with ulcerative colitis when compared with 2 control populations (269 Italians whose origins were in the Abruzzi and Emilia regions and 347 European whites).[216]

HLA-A2, Bw35, and Bw40 were more common among 30 Ashkenazi Jews from Haifa, Israel, with ulcerative colitis.[217,218] HLA-AW24 was common among those with early onset of severe disease. HLA phenotypes in patients with Crohn's disease, however, were unchanged from control groups.

Among 109 Dutch IBD patients (58 with ulcerative colitis, 51 with Crohn's disease), an increased frequency of A11 was noted in those with ulcerative colitis and B18 in those with Crohn's disease.[219] In 39 of the 109 patients who had both IBD and ankylosing spondylitis, 50% were B27-positive; Bw16 was increased in the B27-negative subgroup. HLA-DR2 was more common in 40 Japanese patients with ulcerative colitis (70%) than in 51 ethnically matched controls (31%). HLA-B5–DR also was more frequent (55% vs. 22%).[220]

Crohn's Disease. A sampling of HLA phenotypes in Crohn's disease also indicates wide variations. Among 70 members of 5 American kindreds, each having 2 or more patients with Crohn's disease, concordant segregation of HLA haplotypes and disease was not observed.[221] The study of HLA-A locus phenotypes in 64 additional patients with Crohn's disease also did not reveal any significant disease association.

In American kindreds containing 5 sibling pairs with regional enteritis, and in 22 patients with non-familial Crohn's disease, no unique HLA haplotype was identified when compared with 402 healthy blood donors.[222] The high frequency of HLA identity in affected siblings and the low frequency of identity in unaffected siblings suggest a linkage between the histocompatibility locus and the development of regional enteritis.

A study reported from Leiden, Holland, described the findings in 149 unrelated Dutch patients with Crohn's disease who were typed for HLA-A, B, C, and Dr antigens. Of these 149 patients, 65 were additionally typed for DR locus–controlled B cell alloantigens and compared with 148 healthy individuals.[223] No significant association with a particular antigen was identified. A segregation analysis of parental HLA haplotypes in 9 families with at least 2 children suffering from Crohn's disease did not reveal a significant deviation from the expected Mendelian segregation. HLA-DRW2 was less common in IBD patients than in the general population, but the significance of this observation is not yet known.

In a study of French patients, HLA-B27 was identified in only 5 of 15 patients with ankylosing spondylitis and Crohn's disease and in only a few of 11 individuals with asymptomatic ankylosing spondylitis and Crohn's disease. These findings suggest that sacroilitis and ankylosing spondylitis in Crohn's disease are controlled by a genetic factor different from the HLA-B27 marker. Among 50 IBD patients (12 with ulcerative colitis and 38 with Crohn's disease) with ankylosing spondylitis, HLA-B27 was found in 20 of the Crohn's disease patients and in 8 of the ulcerative colitis patients, also suggesting a combination of 2 types of ankylosing spondylitis in IBD.[224] An increased frequency of HLA-Bw16 was noted in the B27-negative patients. Observations on spondylitis, arthritis, and histocompatibility antigens thus vary.[225,226]

HLA-A, B, C, and Dr antigens were studied in 27 Viennese patients with Crohn's disease and 30 patients with ulcerative colitis.[227] The frequency of HLA-B12 was increased significantly in the Crohn's disease group as compared with healthy controls and with patients with ulcerative colitis. HLA-B12 and/or Cw5 and/or DR7 concomitantly were observed in 11 Crohn's disease patients but not in those with ulcerative colitis.

Possible linkage between certain HLA haplotypes (e.g., A10, B18) and the genetic transmission of a defect in the functional activity of the C2 component of complement is demonstrated in a 32-year-old female patient with regional enteritis and sacroiliitis who was homozygous for the A10, B18 haplotype and AW32, B18. She also had a C2 hemolytic complement deficiency but the levels of the remaining C1 to C9 components were normal.[228] The parents, both siblings, and an only child each had half-normal levels of C2 and carried either the A10, B18 or the AW32, B18 haplotype.

The family studied at the University of Chicago (known as the R family) also is of interest. The mother and her 13-year-old son both had a total proctocolectomy for ulcerative colitis. The father later developed regional enteritis involving the distal ileum. The mother had a haplotype of A10, B10 while the father and the son had a haplotype of A10, B18; each had normal serum levels of C1 and C2.

In summary, epidemiologic surveys support a role for genetic factors in the pathogenesis of IBD, probably in association with an external agent, or agents, such as bacteria and bacterial constituents and immunologic and other defense mechanisms. However, present evidence is incomplete. Definitive studies of HLA haplotypes, including the more precise characterization of possible subsets of ulcerative colitis or Crohn's disease, and improved immunogenetic techniques are necessary to clarify the possible immunoregulatory role of the major histocompatibility complex in IBD and to identify immunogenetic markers.

Host Cellular Defenses

Individual variations in susceptibility to IBD and its severity, complications, and familial incidence suggest individual differences in local (gut) and systemic host defenses, a little studied aspect of IBD. The apparently defective neutrophil and monocyte chemotaxis observed in occasional patients with ulcerative colitis or Crohn's disease, allegedly corrected by levamisole[229] and other immunostimulants, probably is attributable to non-immunologic factors: non-specific circulating cell-directed inhibitors in serum, severe zinc deficiency, or medication (e.g., sulfasalazine, 5-aminosalicylic acid, steroids)[230] rather than to a pathogenetically relevant immunodeficiency. Neutrophil migration may be diminished in Crohn's disease, not as a result of a cellular defect, but apparently as a consequence of a deficient local inflammatory response.[231]

In general, neutrophil and monocyte chemotaxis is normal in patients with Crohn's disease. Neutrophil chemotaxis is normal and monocyte chemotaxis may be increased in patients with ulcerative colitis.[232] The proposition that an antecedent of Crohn's disease is the inability of phagocytic leukocytes to adequately degrade antigens penetrating the intestinal mucosa from the bowel lumen[233] has not been proved. The possible modifying effects of polymorphonuclear leukocytes and other soluble products upon immune responses in IBD have yet to be studied. Increased phagocytosis and lysis of *E. coli* by polymorphonuclear leukocytes in the absence of opsonizing antibody, as seen in a 28-year-old man with Crohn's disease associated with progressive loss of alveolar bone, is an unusual phenomenon.[234] The association of hyperplastic ulcerative gingivitis and ulcerative colitis in one monozygotic twin is of related interest. Phagocytosis and intracellular killing of bacteria by peripheral monocytes are normal in ulcerative colitis and Crohn's disease.

The metabolism of ulcerative colitis colonic epithelial cells (colonocytes) allegedly differs from normal in that butyrate oxidation to CO_2 and ketone bodies is impaired and glucose and glutamine oxidation are increased, presumably as a compensatory response. The failure of fatty acid (N-butyrate) oxidation in ulcerative colitis is postulated as evidence of an energy-deficient state related to a tissue deficiency of coenzyme A (CoA) and pantothenic acid. The validity of this hypothesis has not been established.

Patients with active ulcerative colitis have an increased proportion of circulating monocytes phagocytic *in vitro* for sheep red blood cells coated by IgM antibody and complement, a phenomenon indicative of "activation."[218, 235] The isolation of an activated monocyte-macrophage population from colonic mucosa also has been reported. Whether this activated population gains access to the peripheral blood in IBD is not yet known. Patients with active IBD manifest significantly higher production and release of acid hydrolases from peripheral blood monocytes incubated *in vitro* either with or without stimulation by zymosan and unaffected by corticosteroids. These data reflect the multiple mechanisms, including immunologic stimuli releasing lysosomal enzymes from monocytes, in the chronic inflammation of IBD.

Immune Mechanisms

(See also Chapter 243)

The possible involvement of immune mechanisms in IBD was proposed by Kirsner and Palmer[141] in 1954 on the basis of suggestive clinical observations: (1) the association of IBD with immunologically mediated conditions such as iritis, thrombocytopenic purpura, systemic lupus erythematosus, and Hashimoto's thyroiditis; (2) the increased frequency of IBD among children and adolescents with potentially heightened immunologic responsiveness; (3) the immune-related concomitants of IBD (e.g., erythema nodosum, pyoderma gangrenosum, cutaneous vasculitis,[236] autoimmune hemolytic anemia); (4) the favorable therapeutic responses to adrenal corticosteroids; and (5) the rich immunologic resources and immunologic responsiveness of the gastrointestinal tract.[237, 238]

The digestive tract is well equipped for its important role in immunologic homeostasis of the body.[239–243] The gastrointestinal immune apparatus includes the gut-associated lymphoid tissue immune system (Peyer's patches, subepithelial lymphoid follicles, propriolymphocytes, theliolymphocytes, mast cells and Paneth's cells, and the gut secretory IgA), functioning in coordination with the systemic immune resources of the body. Abundant sources of dietary, microbial, and other antigens are present in the digestive tract and are capable of eliciting local immunologic responses. Immunoglobulin A is normally present within the mucosal epithelial cells[244, 245] as part of the local defense system. Secretory IgA participates in the gastrointestinal defenses by protecting the gut epithelium from the entry of intestinal antigens, immune complexes, and other substances, in the opsonization and agglutination of bacteria, antiviral effects, and perhaps by the masking of antigenic sites. Antibodies in the gastrointestinal tract are produced largely by the local lymphoid (plasma) cells, but some originate in the blood stream.

Autoimmune reactions may develop in patients with IBD under various circumstances: (1) an acquired abnormal or excessive humoral or cellular response without biologic alteration of the intestinal tissue; (2) a genetically influenced defect in immunologic regulation with an abnormal response to antigenic stimuli; (3) the access of intestinal or colonic tissue antigens to the peripheral circulation, thereby exposing sites of antibody formation to stimulation by antigens to which immunologic tolerance may never have been established; or (4) the alteration of the antigenic status of the small intestine and the colon. Although plausible, none of these mechanisms has been established in the pathogenesis of IBD. However, immunologic studies have revealed: (1) the importance of gastrointestinal lymphoid tissue in the immunologic homeostasis of the body; (2) the significant role of the digestive tract in the production of immunoglobulins; (3) the immunologic capacities of secretory IgA; and (4) the involvement of coliform bacteria in the immunologic response of the colon.[246, 247]

Experimentally, all known immunologic reactions have been induced in the gastrointestinal tract: (1) passive local sensitization in the mucosa of the ileum, cecum, colon, and rectum of monkeys;[248] and (2) immediate hypersensitivity, Arthus (immune complex), Shwartzman, Auer-Kirsner,[249, 250] and DNCB-mediated inflammatory responses in the colon.[251] Runt intestinal disease, a cell-mediated immunologic reaction evoked by the injection of adult parental strain or allogeneic spleen cells into newborn inbred mice, is associated with structural abnormalities in the small intestine and the colon.[252]

The potential role of increased cellular immunity to colonic and enterobacterial antigens, whether as a primary or a contributory event, is suggested by the colitis that develops in guinea pigs, swine, and rabbits sensitized to DNCB intrarectally. Animals receiving repeated instillations of DNCB converted delayed hypersensitivity skin reactions to rabbit colon extract from negative to positive. In effect, a non-specifically induced cellular immune reaction in the colon not only caused an experimental colitis but also generated T lymphocytes sensitized to colonic antigens.

An acute immune complex type of ulcerative colitis can be induced utilizing the Auer-Kirsner model of sensitization of guinea pigs to crystalline egg albumin and localization of the circulating egg albumin immune complexes into the colon by the rectal instillation of 1% formalin solution.[249] An extension of this principle involves the production of a mild chronic colitis in rabbits previously immunized with the enterobacterial common antigen of Kunin; the colonic mucosa of the rabbits had been irritated by the rectal instillation of dilute formalin, and they then received IV soluble immune complexes (BSA–anti-BSA [bovine serum albumin]) prepared in antigenic excess.[253] Sensitization to the antibacterial antigen alone did not lead to either acute or chronic colonic inflammation. In rabbits with chronic serum sickness induced by multiple daily injections of bovine serum albumin, immune complex glomerulonephritis developed in all rabbits with a pronounced antibody response. In approximately 50% of these rabbits, granular deposits of bovine serum albumin, rabbit IgG, and C3 also were found in the gastrointestinal tract, mainly in the vessel walls, close to the intestinal glands and the surface epithelium, and were associated with evidence of injury to these areas.

Although the precise role of the immune system in the pathogenesis of IBD remains unclear, a persuasive theory proposes an abnormal immune response precipitated by bacterial and/or viral agents.[254] The triggering antigens probably interact with a genetically susceptible host who already has clones of T or B cells capable of damaging the intestine but normally held in control. In the genetically susceptible host, however, the initiating event "unregulates" the clones of T or B cells or both and mounts a destructive immune reaction against the intestine.

Immediate Hypersensitivity (Allergic Reactions). The presence of eosinophils and increased histamine content of the rectal mucosa in ulcerative colitis and the degranulated mast cells in Crohn's disease are compatible with an immediate hypersensitivity reaction. Earlier emphasis upon gut allergic reactions to food allergens, especially cow's milk proteins (such as alpha-lactalbumin, beta-lactoglobulin, ovalbumin, and casein), has not been confirmed.[246] The prevalence and titers of circulating antibodies to such proteins are unchanged in IBD from healthy and disease controls. Circulating dietary-specific IgE immunocytes are normal.[256] If a monoclonal antibody to IgE is used, IgE immunocytes in the small and large intestine, though numerically variable, are probably normal in IBD.[257] Disodium cromoglycate, a therapeutic agent inhibiting the release of histamine from mast cells, is ineffective in ulcerative colitis.[258]

Humoral Immune Deficiency. *A significant humoral immune abnormality has not been demonstrated in IBD.* Antibody responses to standard bacterial immunizations, to upper respiratory tract viral agents, and to enteropathogens are normal. Minor alterations in C1q, C3, and C4 elements of complement and in C3PA (factor B) in patients with active IBD return to normal with clinical remission, responding like acute phase proteins.[259,260] Alterations of complement inhibitors and immunoconglutinins reflect secondary alterations in complement as a response to activity of IBD and subside with remissions.

Genetically mediated defective regulation of immunoglobulin production could be an important predisposing factor in the pathogenesis of IBD. However, current techniques thus far have failed to demonstrate quantitative or qualitative changes in immunoglobulins.[261,262] Serum levels of the major immunoglobulins are normal or slightly elevated non-specifically and are not correlated consistently with the severity of the disease. Serum secretory IgA occasionally is increased in patients with ulcerative colitis and other gastrointestinal disorders, presumably because of the reabsorption of intraluminal IgA through damaged intestinal epithelium or by way of the transfer of secretory IgA from the lamina propria of the bowel wall.[263] However, secretory IgA also is demonstrable in the serum of healthy individuals and in patients with disorders not involving secretory surfaces. The elevated serum IgM levels in some colitis patients after bowel resection[264] is not specific for IBD and probably reflects a response to bacterial or tissue antigens at the time of surgery. Although occurring in patients with immunoglobulin deficiencies, ulcerative colitis and Crohn's disease ordinarily are not associated with an immune deficiency.

Colon Antibodies. Ulcerative colitis serum contains antibodies reacting *in vitro* with antigens in the cytoplasm of mucus-secreting colonic epithelial cells. These antibodies react not only with autologous colon, but also with allogeneic fetal colonic tissues and colonic cells from other animal species, including germ-free rats.[265] The occurrence rate of anti-colon antibodies ranges from 15% in patients with ulcerative colitis and 0 in patients with Crohn's disease[266] (indirect immunofluorescence) to 90% in children with ulcerative colitis (passive hemagglutination with phenol water extract of human fetal colon as antigen) and somewhat lower in adult patients.[267, 268] High concentrations of anti-colon antibodies also have been found in colonic lymph nodes adjacent to diseased colon. Hemagglutinating anti-colon antibodies also are demonstrable in Crohn's disease, regardless of anatomic location, with frequency rates and titers comparable to those for ulcerative colitis. The hemagglutinating anti-colon antibodies are predominantly IgM, but those reacting with germ-free rat colon are of the IgA, IgG, or IgM class.[269, 270] The mucosa of patients with ulcerative colitis has demonstrated antibodies reacting with anaerobic but not aerobic bacteria from their own feces; reactants to anaerobic bacteria from other colitis patients also were demonstrable. The mucosa from occasional patients without colitis, although not containing antibodies against their own fecal bacteria, apparently may contain antibodies reacting with fecal anaerobes from colitis patients.

The presence and the titers of colon antibodies do not correlate with the age or sex of the patient, a family history of IBD, or the site, extent, duration, or activity of the IBD. Nor are the antibodies cytotoxic *in vitro* for colonic epithelial cells.[271] Furthermore, colon antibodies have been observed in the serum 2 to 10 years after total proctocolectomy. They also are detectable, albeit in low frequencies and in low titers, in healthy individuals and in patients with non-gastrointestinal disease, including systemic lupus erythematosus, urinary tract infections, cirrhosis of the liver, cancer of the colon, salmonella infections, pernicious anemia, and the irritable bowel syndrome.[268] Anti-colon antibodies have not been demonstrated in IBD colonic tissues, including colonic epithelial cells, but their lower occurrence rate in the bacillary and amebic dysenteries[272, 273] suggests that they may not merely represent an epiphenomenon.

An antigen immunologically related to the human colon antigen can be extracted in large amounts from the colon, cecum, and feces of germ-free rats. The antigenic determinants are carbohydrate in nature and probably include gastrointestinal mucopolysaccharides.[274] The colon antigen is gastrointestinal-specific but not colon-specific, and it differs from carcinoembryonic antigen (CEA), another glycoprotein. The shared antigenic determinants between germ-free rat colon or feces and a lipopolysaccharide extract of *E. coli* 014 imply that the colon antibodies originate from stimulation of the gut-associated lymphoid tissue by cross-reacting enterobacterial antigens. Patients with ulcerative colitis have elevated serum titers of hemagglutinating antibodies against *E coli* 014 lipopolysaccharide, but not against extracts from other coliform bacteria. Apart from somatic O-antigen, this extract contains the common antigen of Kunin (CA),[275] present in nearly all species of Enterobacteriaceae and not present in other gram-negative or gram-positive organisms. Because the lipopolysaccharide extract of *E. coli* 014 contains more of this antigen than extracts from other enterobacterial strains,[276] this material is used extensively in immunologic studies in IBD.

The presence of serum agglutinins against somatic O-antigens of greater numbers of *E. coli* strains and in increased titers among patients with IBD and the augmented humoral response to a dietary protein, bovine serum albumin (BSA), implicate intestinal mucosal damage in their production. The increased anti-colon antibody titers among first-degree healthy female relatives of patients with ulcerative colitis (44% of 157 relatives; 20 of 32 mothers and 32 of 61 sisters and daughters of colitis patients)[277, 278] also suggests a genetic influence in their synthesis. While colon antibodies are secondary developments in IBD, they may participate in its pathogenesis as constituents of immune complexes or, in cooperation with mononuclear cells, in a cell-mediated cytotoxic reaction.

The participation of coliform bacteria in the development of colon antibodies and the complexities of this association are reflected in such observations as (1) the presence of elevated antibody titers to *E. coli* 014 heterogenetic antigen in at least 30% of ulcerative colitis patients; (2) the production of anti-colon antibodies in rabbits injected with *E. coli*; (3) the inhibition of anti–rat colon antibodies by extracts of *E. coli* 014 or by colon antigen (obtained from germ-free rat colon and from rabbit and human colon); and (4) the production of similar anti-colon antibodies in germ-free rats mono-infected for 35 days or longer with *Clostridium difficile* or with the G62 Clostridium strain.

A wide variety of proteins, tissue antibodies, and other reactants also are demonstrable in the serum of IBD patients.[265] These include ceruloplasmin, haptoglobin, orosomucoid, pre-albumin, transferrin, $alpha_2$-macroglobulin, $alpha_1$-antitrypsin, $alpha_1$-antichymotrypsin, bovine albumin, antinuclear factors, antierythrocyte antibodies, antibodies to gastric and small intestinal mucous cells, antibodies to gastric parietal cells, antibodies to thyroglobulin, precipitins to pancreatic homogenates, antibodies to bile ductular cells, antibodies to phenol water extracts of liver or kidneys, antibodies to bacteria, viruses (CMV), and reticulin. Circulating oncofetal antigens (e.g., carcinoembryonic antigen) also are increased in IBD. Since they are found as well in non-IBD patients and in healthy controls, they presumably represent non-specific "secondary" responses to tissue injury and increased bowel permeability.

Antigen-Antibody Complexes.[279–286] Williams[279] has aptly pointed out that " . . . whether or not production of immune complexes serves some protective or modulating function . . . remains to be determined." Circulating antigen-antibody complexes have been reported in some patients with active ulcerative colitis or Crohn's disease, but evidence has also been advanced that denies the presence of such complexes in the circulation regardless of the clinical circumstances.[284] Moreover, *their demonstration does not correlate with the type, location, severity, or extraintestinal manifestations of IBD*. Beyond this, their antigenic composition is unknown. A recent observation suggests the presence in Crohn's disease patients of IgG and perhaps IgA complexed with antigen.[283] The absence of immune complexes in patients with Crohn's disease after successful bowel resection is consistent with a secondary phenomenon.

The involvement of both antigen-antibody complexes and host hypersensitivity to enterobacterial antigens in IBD is suggested by the chronic colitis following the IV injection of soluble immune complexes in rabbits previously sensitized to the common antigen and whose colonic mucosa had been irritated by the rectal instillation of dilute formalin.[285] Sensitization to the enterobacterial antigen alone did not lead to either acute or chronic colonic inflammation.

The immunohistochemical demonstration of IgG and complement (C1, C2) on the basement membrane of colonic epithelium and of lymphocytes and plasma cells clustered around activated macrophages in ulcerative colitis colon is consistent with the presence of immune complexes.[286] The formation of these complexes may represent a secondary response to bacterial penetration of the breached intestinal mucosa. Their occurrence in bacillary and amebic dysentery and in many other diseases is in accord with this view. Current tests for immune complexes are technologically imperfect, and their status in IBD thus remains uncertain. The immune complexes develop secondarily to IBD, although they may contribute to the severity and chronicity of the tissue reaction.

Circulating T and B Lymphocytes. Measurements of circulating T and B lymphocytes in patients with ulcerative colitis and Crohn's disease are highly variable, reflecting differences in methodology, disease activity, medication, and other clinical circumstances.[287–293] T-cell proportions usually are normal in ulcerative colitis; the decreased T-cell numbers noted occasionally are attributable to diminished total peripheral lymphocyte counts. T-cell numbers and proportions frequently are decreased in Crohn's disease, probably because of the gastrointestinal loss of cells and the sequestration of lymphocytes in the diseased bowel (T cells are increased considerably in Crohn's disease bowel compared with the bowel of ulcerative colitis patients or control subjects). However, T-cell numbers in Crohn's disease usually return to normal when the tissue reaction subsides, consistent with a secondary event. Reduced circulating T-cell numbers are not exclusive to Crohn's disease and are observed also in patients with chronic active liver disease or active sarcoidosis.

Total circulating immunoglobulin-bearing B lymphocytes are normal or increased in quiescent ulcerative colitis and Crohn's disease.[290, 291] B cell subpopulations, on the other hand, vary considerably, with reports of both increases and decreases in IgM-, IgA-, and IgG-bearing cells; decreased numbers of complement receptor–bearing lymphocytes in ulcerative colitis and Crohn's ileocolitis (but not in small bowel Crohn's disease); and diminished B cells associated with increased null cells in chronic active Crohn's disease, unrelated to the site of involvement. T- and B-cell numbers are unrelated to the activity of the disease, its anatomic location, duration of illness, or treatment with sulfasalazine or prednisone. Utilizing a cytofluorometric detection system to identify lymphocytes with homogeneous quantities of surface immunoglobulin, increased numbers of such monoclonal lymphocytes have been noted in the peripheral blood of some patients with IBD (both ulcerative colitis and Crohn's disease),[292] suggesting but not proving an abnormality in immunoregulation.

Defective regulation of immunoglobulin production, mediated genetically, and altered host responses to microbial, dietary, and other antigens could be important predisposing factors in the pathogenesis of IBD. Recent studies indicate significant alterations of *in vitro* synthesis and secretion of immunoglobulins IgA, IgG, and IgM, especially IgA, in patients with ulcerative colitis or Crohn's disease.[263] In comparison with normal peripheral blood mononuclear cells, intestinal mononuclear cells display moderately increased spontaneous secretion of IgG and IgM and markedly increased spontaneous secretion of IgA. By way of contrast, intestinal mononuclear cells from patients with active untreated ulcerative colitis or Crohn's disease exhibit decreased spontaneous antibody secretion, while peripheral blood mononuclear cells manifest a greatly increased synthesis and secretion of IgA. One possible explanation is that IgA precursor cells are in a highly activated state in normal intestinal lamina propria and, because of the intestinal inflammation, migrate from the intestine into the peripheral blood. An alternative explanation infers a primary mucosal immunodeficiency in the intestine of patients with IBD, allowing agents to penetrate the intestinal mucosa and subsequently initiate both a local inflammation and a heightened systemic immune response.

Cell-Mediated Immune Reactions. Cell-mediated immune responses in IBD have been studied by 3 principal techniques: (1) skin tests; (2) the response of circulating lymphocytes to mitogens; and (3) the effects of various antigens upon the *in vitro* migration of leukocytes. Of these, the skin tests are the least reliable.[294–296] The intradermal injection of mumps antigen and of extracts of *Candida albicans* and *Trichophyton gypsum* evoked the same number of positive responses in patients with ulcerative colitis and Crohn's disease as in normal controls. Positive "allergic" skin reactions to autologous leukocytes and their extracts have been reported in active and quiescent ulcerative colitis, but the significance of this observation is dubious. Skin test responses to bacterial and fungal antigens are normal in ulcerative colitis and are normal or temporarily diminished in Crohn's disease.[255] Skin reactivity to DNCB may be diminished in Crohn's disease, but normal results also are reported. The earlier variably positive Kveim reactions in Crohn's disease resulted from differences in the test splenic suspensions; those suspensions yielding false-positive results in diseases other than sarcoidosis have been withdrawn.[296]

Circulating and lymph node lymphocytes

from patients with ulcerative colitis respond normally *in vitro* to various mitogens, including fetal colonic antigens. The decreased responsiveness noted infrequently in ulcerative colitis patients disappears after total proctocolectomy and ileostomy. Diminished lymphocyte responsiveness is more common in patients with Crohn's disease,[297] but normal responses also are observed.[298] While such observations have been interpreted in Crohn's disease as indications of an immune deficiency, undernutrition, including trace metal (zinc) deficiency,[299–301] and circulating inhibitors of lymphocyte responsiveness often are implicated. Lymphocytes from regional lymph nodes in both ulcerative colitis and Crohn's disease respond normally to various mitogens.[302]

Leukocyte Migration.[303–311] Extracts of human fetal large and small bowel and extracts of autologous rectal mucosa inhibit the migration of peripheral leukocytes from patients with ulcerative colitis, but only rarely inhibit leukocytes from patients with Crohn's disease or from control subjects. Positive migration inhibition also may be demonstrated with the colon-related glycoprotein from *E. coli* 0114, but not with extracts of liver, kidney, or adrenal gland. The migration inhibition tests directly correlate with the clinical activity of the colitis and are negative in colitis patients who have undergone total proctocolectomy.

In contrast, antigens contained in small bowel contents and Crohn's colon homogenate, or its mitochondrial fraction, inhibit the migration of leukocytes in Crohn's disease but not leukocytes in ulcerative colitis. A lipopolysaccharide extract of *E. coli* 0119:B14 inhibits leukocyte migration in both healthy subjects and patients with IBD, but to a greater degree in IBD. Common antigen also elicits greater release of macrophage and leukocyte migration inhibitory factors (MMIF:LMIF) from active ulcerative colitis lymphocytes and macrophage-depleted colonic mononuclear cells than from Crohn's disease lymphocytes or lymphocytes from healthy controls.[308]

Macrophage migration inhibitory factor (MIF) is released by lymphocytes from patients with ulcerative colitis when these cells are incubated *in vitro* with the enterobacterial common antigen; in contrast, MIF is not released from control lymphocytes. Colitis lymphocytes and, to a lesser extent, lymphocytes from normal controls release MIF when exposed to a lipopolysaccharide extract of *E. coli* 019.B14, suggesting the presence of cell-mediated immunity to the extract. A lipopolysaccharide extract of *E. coli* 014, especially rich in the common antigen of Kunin, readily differentiated patients with active ulcerative colitis from a healthy control group. LMIF release *in vitro* by macrophage-depleted colonic mononuclear cells from patients with severe ulcerative colitis also increased when the cells were stimulated by common antigen. Noteworthy as well is the inhibition of leukocyte mobility by medications commonly prescribed in the treatment of ulcerative colitis[310] and by microorganisms.[311] The nature and clinical significance of leukocyte inhibition factor, apparently more abundant in patients with quiescent than with active Crohn's disease, await further study.

Despite the complexities of cell-mediated immunity, the technologic difficulties, and the variable results, present data suggest an increased cellular immunity to colonic and enterobacterial antigens, whether as a primary or a secondary event, in patients with IBD compared with healthy controls and control patients with other diseases. The potential importance of such cell-mediated immune reactions in inducing IBD-like bowel damage is illustrated by the DNCB colitis animal model. However, the significance of such a relationship in the pathogenesis of IBD remains unsettled.

Lymphocyte Cytotoxicity. Circulating lymphocytes of patients with ulcerative colitis and Crohn's disease are cytotoxic *in vitro* for autologous and allogeneic colonic epithelial cells.[312–318]

1. The cytotoxic effect is demonstrable only in patients with IBD, regardless of anatomic distribution and extent. It is specific for colonic epithelial cells and does not occur with gastric or intestinal epithelial cells, kidney or liver cells, and experimental cell lines.

2. The effect is rapid (2 hours), does not require complement, and occurs also with cell-free extracts of lymphocytes.

3. The cytotoxic effect persists during clinical remission of IBD, disappears within 10 days after the resection of diseased bowel, and returns with reappearance of the IBD.

4. The cytotoxic effect can be induced in normal lymphocytes by prior incubation with colitis serum, by incubation with a high molecular weight factor present in the sera of some IBD patients (possibly a cytophilic IgM antibody or small circulating immune com-

plex), and also by a lipopolysaccharide extract of *E. coli* 019.B14.

5. The cytotoxic effect can be abolished or diminished by prior incubation of colitis lymphocytes with isologous ulcerative colitis serum, coliform extract, or anti-IgM.

6. The lymphocytes involved are Fc-receptor K cells, stimulated by cross-reacting enterobacterial antigen. In IBD, these cells are presumably "armed" for cytotoxicity either by cytophilic IgM antibody or by immune complexes, since each can induce specific cell-mediated cytotoxicity *in vitro* in other systems.

The pathogenetic significance of lymphocyte cytotoxicity *per se* in IBD remains unclear. The degree of lymphocyte cytotoxicity appears to be similar in all IBD patients and is not correlated with the extent or severity of the disease. The phenomenon is demonstrable in patients with Crohn's disease limited to the small intestine, even though their lymphocytes are cytotoxic only for colonic epithelial cells and have no effect upon ileal cells. Nevertheless, *the observations suggest a link between antibodies (or antigen-antibody complexes) and cellular immune responses to cross-reacting enterobacterial antigens.* Killer (K) cells are responsible for antibody-dependent cell-mediated cytotoxicity (ADCC) and are one of the body's immune defense mechanisms. Natural killer cell activity has been reported as deficient in patients with IBD, possibly as a consequence of decreased lymphocyte production of interferon. It has also been noted to be normal, again reflecting the variability of immunologic observations in IBD.

Suppressor Cell Activity.[319–332] Acquired or genetically mediated imbalances in immunoregulatory T cell subsets could be important in the pathogenesis of IBD through enhanced expression of damaging immune responses.[68] Current observations on regulator suppressor cell activity in IBD are too few and too variable for decisive evaluation.

There apparently is no antecedent deficiency of circulating suppressor T cells regulating antibody synthesis in IBD. Patients with Crohn's disease may have reduced numbers of T cells, but T_M, T_G, and B cells appear to be normal. Concanavalin A–stimulated suppressor T cell activity is decreased in the peripheral blood of some patients with active ulcerative colitis or Crohn's disease,[321] but returns to normal with quiescence of IBD, consistent with a secondary event. Circulating covert suppressor T cells are demonstrable in some patients with Crohn's disease; these can be activated *in vitro* to inhibit the synthesis of IgM.[322] The absence of an inhibitor of suppressor cell activity in IBD sera also has been noted but not yet confirmed.[323] The diminished natural killing *in vitro* by circulating mononuclear cells from patients with Crohn's disease (for LIK [lymphoblastoid] cells or for K562 cell line cells) may be related to suppressor cell activity,[324, 325] but the significance of this observation also is unclear. Monoclonal antibody studies of circulatory lymphocytes in Crohn's disease in comparison with other acute and chronic illnesses yielded no evidence for underlying abnormalities of circulating lymphocyte subpopulations. Reduced suppressor cell activity in intestinal lymphocytes from patients with Crohn's disease has been reported, suggesting a diminished immunoregulation at the mucosal level.[327]

Despite suggestions of increased suppressor cell activity and alterations in helper/suppressor ratios, significant abnormalities in circulating lymphocyte subpopulations and in helper/suppressor T cell ratios have at present not been demonstrated consistently in IBD.[326–328]

Gut Immunologic Events.[333–349] Because immunologic studies of the blood do not necessarily reflect events in the bowel wall, various immunologic activities of the gut are under investigation.

Studies of the gut-associated lymphoid tissue thus far are highly variable. T cell predominance in the deeper layers of the bowel wall is noted in Crohn's disease, but not in ulcerative colitis. The increased numbers of B cells (mostly IgG cells) in the lamina propria of Crohn's disease ileum and colon have been both denied and affirmed.[257] Both T and B cells have been identified in the augmented intraepithelial lymphocyte populations.[341] Lamina propria lymphocytes obtained by mechanical isolation from patients with small bowel Crohn's disease were larger than lymphocytes from control patients with other diseases and manifested higher basal DNA synthesis. Sequential chemical and enzymatic procedures have identified proportionally more B lymphocytes (IgA and IgG cells), with equal or decreased numbers of T lymphocytes. Null cells in colonic lamina propria lymphocytes have been both affirmed and denied.[338]

The cytotoxicity of gut lymphocytes for autologous or allogeneic colonic epithelial cells, important in relation to a possible antibody-dependent, cell-mediated cytotoxic mechanism, has not been studied in IBD as yet. However, the ability of gut mucosal mononuclear cells to mediate either antibody-dependent, cell-mediated cytotoxicity or natural killer cell acitvity for other targets, including chick erythrocytes and Chang hepatoma cells, has been tested, with both positive and negative results.[334, 335, 343–346] Other inconsistencies include increased or absent K cell activity in the blood and the intestinal mucosa in Crohn's disease. Since cytotoxic lymphocytes are also demonstrable in patients with ulcerative colitis, in patients with colon-rectal carcinoma, in the gut mucosal cells of guinea pigs,[337] and in normal human intestinal mucosa, their disease specificity is unclear. These preliminary observations on gut lymphocytes again are handicapped by numerous technical artefacts and are impossible to evaluate at present.

Protection against the attachment and entry of microorganisms and their toxins is provided by an intact bowel wall and by the secreted antibodies on the luminal surfaces of intestinal epithelial cells. A primary mucosal immunodeficiency in the intestinal wall of IBD patients is suggested by the observation of decreased spontaneous synthesis of IgM, IgG, and IgA associated with a moderately increased spontaneous synthesis and secretion of these immunoglobulins, especially IgA. Such an intestinal immunodeficiency could allow the penetration of antigens, facilitating both a local inflammation and an accentuated systemic immune response. Other studies, however, demonstrate significant increases in IgA-IgM-, and especially IgG-containing cells 3 to 5 weeks before clinical relapse was apparent. This would suggest a role for mucosal antibody production in the pathogenesis of ulcerative colitis. Although specific antigens have not been identified, IgG antibodies against fecal anaerobic bacteria are demonstrable in the colonic mucosa of ulcerative colitis patients; these antibodies are produced locally by mucosal immunocytes.[88]

Quantitation of the different classes of immunoglobulin-producing lamina propria immunocytes in IBD depends, in part at least, upon the histopathologic changes. There is no defect in the *in vivo* local production and epithelial transport of IgA and IgM in IBD. The more definitive studies demonstrate increased immunocytes producing IgA, IgG, or IgM in the intestinal mucosa of patients with ulcerative colitis and Crohn's disease. IgG cells predominate in the deeper layers of the Crohn's disease bowel, suggesting local stimulation of gut-associated B cells.[348, 349] In both diseases, the deeper layers of the bowel wall are densely infiltrated by IgA and IgM, 2- to 5-fold more than normal, and are infiltrated by IgG at least 30-fold greater than normal. In Crohn's disease, about 80% of the immunoglobulin-containing cells are in the muscularis propria and the submucosa.

Increased numbers of immunocytes containing IgE have been identified in rectal biopsies of patients with allergic proctitis. This form of "colitis" may respond to disodium cromoglycate. Even though numerous IgE immunocytes may be observed in ulcerative colitis and Crohn's disease, they are not characteristic of either of these diseases.

The interepithelial intestinal lymphoid tissue includes lymphocytes and occasional neutrophils and eosinophils. Preliminary observations suggest that they are more numerous in patients with IBD than in normal persons and that they may be abnormal in IBD (increased size, leptochromatic nuclei, frequent lysosomes). Whereas intestinal lymphocytes from normal persons respond readily to concanavalin A and poorly or not at all to phytohemagglutinin (PHA), intraepithelial lymphocytes from patients with Crohn's disease respond poorly to concavavalin A and normally to PHA. Lamina propria and intraepithelial lymphocytes in patients with IBD contain higher proportions of cells bearing IgA and fewer numbers of cells bearing IgM or IgD. Macrophages also are found intraepithelially in the IBD colon and in disease controls.

The local "activation" of intestinal macrophages releasing tissue-damaging enzymes and lysosomal acid hydrolases on exposure to bacterial antigens could contribute to the tissue damage of IBD. However, the role of intestinal macrophages in IBD has not been determined as yet. The many variable observations of T and B lymphocytes, null cells, killer cells, and activated T cells in the bowel wall reflect the limitations of current methodology. Further information is needed on the importance of Peyer's patches, the priming process for a secretory IgA response, the role of M cells in facilitating the entry of antigens, the mechanism of "homing" of lymphocytes to mucosal surfaces, and the role of cytotoxic lymphocytes and monocytes, killer cells, and natural killer cells in the pathogenesis of IBD.

Immunodeficiency in IBD. Primary immunodeficiency syndromes are a heterogeneous group of diseases characterized by impairment of the B cell system (humoral immunity), the T cell system (cell-mediated immunity), or both. Ulcerative colitis infrequently has been associated with primary immunodeficiency states (e.g., Swiss type of agammaglobulinemia, primary hypogammaglobulinemia accompanied by diminished or absent free secretory component of salivary IgA, thymic alymphoplasia, Hashimoto's disease, selective IgA deficiency).[350] However, *there is no conclusive evidence for a primary immune deficiency in ulcerative colitis.* Interestingly, immunoglobulin-synthesizing cells are present in the intestinal mucosa of immunoglobulin-deficient individuals. The impaired primary and secondary responses to bacteriophage ø 174 in ulcerative colitis appear to be related to hyposplenism.[351]

Immunoglobulin deficiencies also are associated with Crohn's disease,[95, 96, 352, 353] possibly as a consequence of increased suppressor cell activity. In some patients with Crohn's disease, hypogammaglobulinemia may be attributable to the action of covert suppressor T cells. The concept of an underlying immunodeficiency state in Crohn's disease rests upon such observations as: (1) reduced skin responsiveness to various antigens (PPD-S, mumps, Candida, or Trichophyton antigens, and Mantoux test to 2,4-DNCB and to streptokinase); (2) response to a "cocktail" of antigens, including streptokinase-streptodornase (Varidase), Trichophyton, Candida, mumps, and PPD; (3) diminished responsiveness of circulating lymphocytes to PHA, concanavalin A, and pokeweed mitogen; (4) the reduced proportion and absolute numbers of T cells in the blood of some patients with Crohn's disease, regardless of steroid therapy; (5) the lack of stimulation to DNA synthesis by isolated autologous rectal epithelial cells in a few Crohn's disease patients with rectal involvement; and (6) the lack of inhibition of leukocyte migration with intestinal antigens. Parallel experiments in patients with ulcerative colitis, in contrast, yield positive results, and in those colitis patients with lowered lymphocyte responsiveness to mitogens, a positive response is restored by colectomy. On the other hand, a study of 38 patients with Crohn's disease indicated qualitatively normal immunity, as estimated by skin tests and lymphocyte responses to PHA and pokeweed mitogen, in addition to absolute lymphocyte counts, measurement of the serum immunoglobulins, and antibody response to bacteriophage ø174.[354]

The conflicting observations, the varying techniques employed, and the limitations of available methods again reflect the incomplete understanding of cellular energy in Crohn's disease. Question also might be raised as to how representative of the integrity of the total body lymphocytes are observations of a relatively few lymphocytes obtained from peripheral venous blood by methods as yet not allowing completely pure separations of B and T lymphocytes. Other important factors include cell-inhibiting substances in the serum and the concurrent use of sulfasalazine, adrenocortical steroids, azathioprine, or 6-MP. In addition, a variety of gut-associated gram-negative bacteria, bacterial enzymes, bacterial endotoxins, and mycoplasmal, protozoan, and metazoan parasites are all known *per se* to suppress immune responsiveness in man.

Lymphocyte responses are highly variable and are influenced by a wide variety of nonimmunologic circumstances, including undernutrition, smoking, advancing age, and operations such as cholecystectomy. Clarification of this aspect of immunity requires further investigation of cellular activity, including monocyte/macrophage and helper/suppressor cell relationships.[355]

Conclusions

Present evidence suggests that ulcerative colitis and Crohn's disease are interrelated prototype conditions (perhaps as "cousins" rather than as "siblings"), probably occurring among genetically mediated vulnerable individuals in response to environmental agents and encompassing a multiplicity of intermediate tissue reactions grouped heterogeneously as IBD.

The available evidence does not establish a fundamental disorder of immunologic homeostasis as the primary cause of either ulcerative colitis or Crohn's disease. Antecedent abnormalities in humoral and cell-mediated immunity have not been demon-

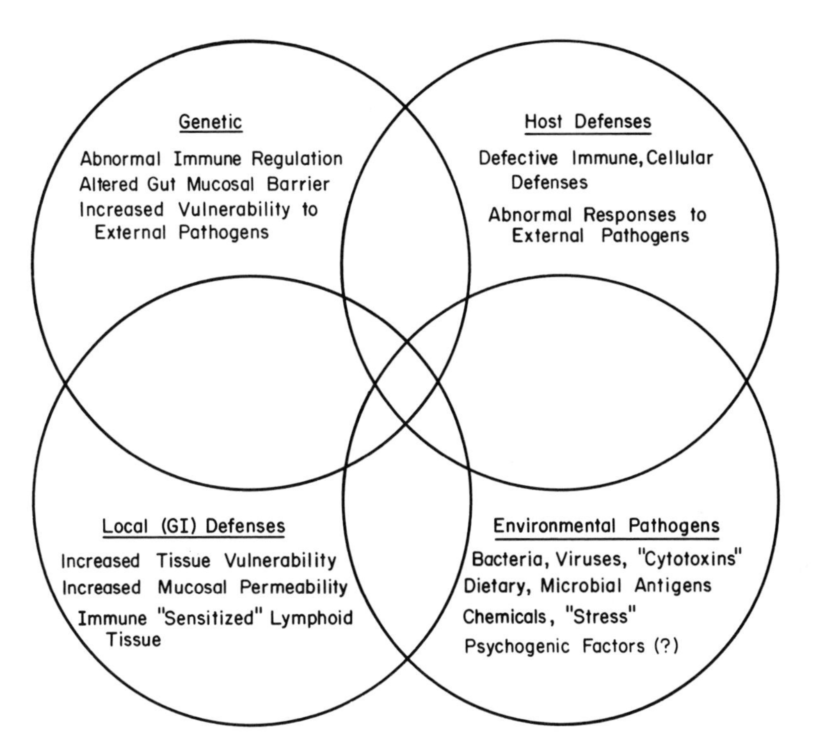

Figure 124–1. Schematic overview of interactions of genetic, host defense, local (GI) defenses, and environmental factors in the etiology of inflammatory bowel disease.

strated. Indeed, most, if not all, of the immunologic observations identified thus far in IBD patients could be epiphenomena, although contributing to the IBD tissue reaction secondarily. Nevertheless, the remarkable expansion of knowledge of immune processes holds much promise for the future clarification of immune mechanisms in IBD.

An attractive hypothesis involves external agents, such as bacteria or viruses, and genetically mediated altered host immune responses in the pathogenesis of IBD, incorporating the following considerations (Fig. 124–1):

1. Ulcerative colitis and Crohn's disease are prototypes of a single disease process, encompassing a spectrum of intermediate tissue reactions, with the differing tissue manifestations depending in part upon the site of immunologic interaction and individual host responses.

2. An external agent or agents, possibly microbial or viral agents or their metabolites, host immune responses, and genetic immunoregulatory influences are involved. Cross-reactivity between the "external" antigens and the host account for many of the "autoimmune" features of IBD.

3. If the external agent is a microbe normally residing within the bowel of the affected individual, sensitization of the host to its antigens may occur early in life during the period of "colonization" of the gut. Enterobacterial and other antigens normally gain access to the lymphoid tissues in the bowel wall and to the regional lymph nodes probably early in infancy, before the regulation of such absorption by the bowel mucosa achieves maturity. This, in effect, constitutes an "immunologic priming" of the gut-associated lymphoid tissue. Presumably, all individuals become sensitized to the antigens of indigenous gut bacteria. However, genetic factors impose a potentially harmful hypersensitivity state only on those at risk of developing IBD later in life, perhaps by means of genetically determined abnormalities of antigen absorption by gut mucosa and of host responses. Histocompatibility antigens might serve as cell surface receptors for microbial agents and facilitate their attachment to, and penetration of, epithelial surfaces. A similar sequence of events can be postulated for other antigens (e.g., dietary, as in infant feeding formulas or possibly in breast milk).

4. Once such hypersensitivity is established, any "insult" increasing intestinal mucosal permeability to microbial and other antigens could result in an interaction between these antigens and the "immunologically primed" gut-associated lymphoid tissues. All this could lead to immune-induced inflammation in the bowel wall. The nature and quantity of antigen or antigens, the host immune responses (systemic and gut), the site of challenge, and the genetic influences presumably determine the type of inflammatory response: ulcerative colitis, Crohn's disease, or "indeterminate colitis." Japanese investigators already have identified HLA-linked control of immune responses to microbial antigens. The inciting event might include an acute bacterial or viral illness, drugs, vascular ischemia, or anxiety-stimulated stress. Host immune responses also are likely to be involved by analogy with hepatitis B virus infections. In these, the virus is present in hepatocytes of healthy carriers who demonstrate no evidence of liver disease and no immunologic responses either to the virus or to viral autoantigens. The viral organism alone apparently is not enough, and host immune responses seem to determine both the occurrence and the nature of the liver disease. Limitations in methodology probably account for the failure thus far to demonstrate fundamental alterations in host immunoglobulins and in antibody responses among IBD patients.

The prospects for clarification of the etiology and pathogenesis of IBD seem brighter today than ever before, in part because of the heightened investigative as well as clinical interest in this problem and in part because of the remarkable expansion in the understanding of immune mechanisms and of human illness generally.

References

1. Kirsner JB, Shorter RG. Recent developments in "nonspecific" inflammatory bowel disease. N Engl J Med 1982; 306:775–85.
2. Kirsner JB, Shorter RG. Inflammatory Bowel Disease. 2nd Ed. Philadelphia: Lea & Febiger, 1980.
3. Schachter H, Kirsner JB. Crohn's Disease of the Gastrointestinal Tract. New York: J Wiley & Sons, 1980.
4. Kirsner JB. Inflammatory bowel disease—considerations of etiology and pathogenesis. Am J Gastroenterol 1978; 69:253–71.
5. Sachar DB, Ausland MO, Walfish JS. Aetiological theories of inflammatory bowel disease. Clin Gastroenterol 1980; 9:231–57.
6. Schachter H, Goldstein MJ, Rappaport H, Fennessy JJ, Kirsner JB. Ulcerative and granulomatous colitis—validity of differential diagnositic criteria; A study of 100 patients treated by total colectomy. Ann Intern Med 1970; 72:841–51.

7. Kirsner JB. Problems in the differentiation of ulcerative colitis and Crohn's disease of the colon: The need for repeated diagnostic evaluation. Gastroenterology 1975; 68:187–91.
8. Nagai T, Das KM. Detection of colonic antigen(s) in tissues from ulcerative colitis using purified colitis colon tissue–bound IgG (CCA-IgG). Gastroenterology 1981; 81:463–70.
9. Sommers SC, Korelitz BI. Mucosal cell counts in ulcerative and granulomatous colitis. Am J Clin Pathol 1975; 63:359–65.
10. Ritchie JK, Lennard-Jones JE. Crohn's disease of the distal large bowel. Scand J Gastroenterol 1976; 11:433–6.
11. Burnham WR, Ansell ID, Langman MJS. Normal sigmoidoscopic findings in severe ulcerative colitis: An important and common occurrence. Gut 1980; 21:A460.
12. Marks, CG, Riddell RH, Lennard-Jones J. Clinical pathological conference: A problem of inflammatory bowel disease. Proc R Soc Med 1975; 68:32–3.
13. Price AB. Overlap in the spectrum of non-specific inflammatory bowel disease—colitis indeterminate. J Clin Pathol 1978; 31:567–77.
14. Blaser MJ, Reller LB. Campylobacter enteritis. N Engl J Med 1981; 305:1444–52.
15. Siegal FP, Lopez C, Hammer GS, Brown AE, Kornfeld SJ, Gold J, Hassett J, Hirschman SZ, Cunningham-Rundles C, Adelsberg BR, Parham DM, Siegal M, Cunningham-Rundles S, Armstrong D. Severe acquired immunodeficiency in male homosexuals, manifested by chronic perianal ulcerative herpes simplex lesions. N Engl J Med 1981; 305:1439–44.
16. Dilsen N, Konice M, Ovul C, eds. Behçet's disease—International Symposium, Istanbul (September, 1977). Amsterdam: Excerpta Medica, 1979.
17. Bartlett JG, Gorbach SL. Pseudomembranous enterocolitis (antibiotic-related colitis). Adv Intern Med 1977; 22:455–76.
18. Quinn TC, Goodell SE, Mkrtichian E, Schuffler MD, Wang SP, Stamm WE, Holmes KK. Chlamydia trachomatis proctitis. N Engl J Med 1981; 305:195–9.
19. Akdamar K, Martin RJ, Ichinose H. Syphilitic proctitis. Am J Dig Dis 1977; 22:701–4.
20. Duffy TJ. Reversible ischaemic colitis in young adults. Br J Surg 1981; 68:34–7.
21. Rosekrans PCM, Meijer CJLM, Van Der Wal AM, Lindeman J. Allergic proctitis: A clinical and immunopathological entity. Gut 1980; 21:1217–23.
22. Bogomoletz WV, Adnet JJ, Birembaut P, Feyoy P, Dupont P. Collagenous colitis: An unrecognized entity. Gut 1980; 21:164–8.
23. Glotzer DJ, Glick ME, Goldman H. Proctitis and colitis following diversion of the fecal stream. Gastroenterology 1981; 80:438–41.
24. Miller DP, Everett ED. Gastrointestinal histoplasmosis. J Clin Gastroenterol 1979; 1:233–6.
25. Hyams JS, Goldman H, Katz AJ. Differentiating small bowel Crohn's disease from lymphoma: Role of a rectal biopsy. Gastroenterology 1980; 79:340–3.
26. Tedesco FJ, Huckaby B, Hauckley-Allen M, Ewing GC. Eosinophilic ileocolitis. Dig Dis Sci 1981; 26:943–8.
27. Bernardino ME, Lawson TL. Discrete colonic ulcers associated with oral contraceptives. Am J Dig Dis 1976; 21:503–6.
28. Chang SF, Burrell MI, Belleza NA, Spiro HM. Borderlands in the diagnosis of regional enteritis. Gastrointest Radiol 1978; 3:67–72.
29. Admans H, Whorwell PJ, Wright R. Diagnosis of Crohn's disease. Dig Dis Sci 1980; 25:911–5.
30. Nugent W, Fromm D, Silen W. Pseudo Crohn's disease. Am J Surg 1979; 137:566–71.
31. Kirsner JB. Clinical observations on inflammatory bowel disease. Med Clin North Am 1969; 53:1195–217.
32. Kirsner JB. Local and systemic complications of inflammatory bowel disease. JAMA 1980; 242:1177–83.
33. Greenstein AJ, Janowitz HD, Sachar DB. The extra-intestinal complications of Crohn's disease and ulcerative colitis: A study of 700 patients. Medicine (Baltimore) 1976; 55:401–12.
34. Holt PJA, Davies MG, Saunders KC, Nuki G. Pyoderma gangrenosum: Clinical and laboratory findings in 15 patients with special reference to polyarthritis. Medicine (Baltimore) 1980; 59:114–33.
35. Shashaty G. Hemolytic anemia and ulcerative colitis. Dig Dis Sci 1980; 25:154–5.
36. Juhlin L, Krause U, Shelley WB. Endotoxin-induced microclots in ulcerative colitis and Crohn's disease. Scand J Gastroenterol 1980; 15:311–4.
37. Becker SA, Wishnitzer R, Botwin S, Eliraz A, Bass DD. Myopericarditis associated with inflammatory bowel disease. J Clin Gastroenterol 1981; 3:267–70.
38. Butland RJA, Cole P, Citron KM, Turner-Warwick M. Chronic bronchial suppuration and inflammatory bowel disease. Q J Med 1981; 197:63–75.
39. Sivak MF Jr, Farmer RG, Lalli AF. Sclerosing cholangitis: Its increasing frequency of recognition and association with inflammatory bowel disease. J Clin Gastroenterol 1981; 3:261–6.
40. Owyang C, Miller LJ, Tihie J, Fleming CR. Takayasu's arteritis in Crohn's disease. Gastroenterology 1979; 76:825–8.
41. Sitrin M, Rosenberg IH, Chawla K, Meredith S, Sellin J, Rabb JM, Coe F, Kirsner JB, Kraft SC. Nutritional and metabolic complications in a patient with Crohn's disease and ileal resection. Gastroenterology 1980; 78:1069–79.
42. Drenick EJ, Ament E, Finegold SM, Passaro E Jr. By-pass enteropathy: An inflammatory process in the excluded segment with systemic complications. Am J Clin Nutr 1977; 30:76–89.
43. Thayer WR Jr, Kirsner JB. Enteric and extra-enteric complications of intestinal by-pass and inflammatory bowel disease: Are there some clues? (Editorial). Gastroenterology 1980; 78:1097–9.
44. Rogers BHG, Clark LM, Kirsner JB. The epidemiologic and demographic characteristics of inflammatory bowel disease: An analysis of a computerized file of 1400 patients. J Chronic Dis 1971; 24:743–73.
45. Garland CF, Lilienfeld AM, Mendeloff AI, Markowitz JA, Terrell KB, Garland FC. Incidence rates of ulcerative colitis and Crohn's disease in fifteen areas of the United States. Gastroenterology 1981; 81:1115–24.
46. Langman MJS. Chronic Nonspecific Inflammatory Bowel Disease in the Epidemiology of Chronic Digestive Disease. Chicago: Year Book Medical Publishers, 1979: 80–102.
47. Segal I, Tim LO, Hamilton DG, Walker ARP. The rarity of ulcerative colitis in South African blacks. Am J Gastroenterol 1980; 74:332–6.
48. Sinclair TS, Brunt PW, Mowat NAG. Natural history of proctocolitis in the northeast of Scotland: A community study. Gut 1980; 21:A924.
49. Sedlack RE, Whisnant J, Elveback LR, Kurland LT. Incidence of Crohn's disease in Olmsted County, Minnesota (1935–1975). Am J Epidemiol 1980; 112:759–63.
50. Brahme F, Lindstrom C, Wenckert A. Crohn's disease in a defined population: An epidemiological study of incidence, prevalence, mortality and secular trends in the city of Malmo, Sweden. Gastroenterology 1975; 69:342–51.
51. Gilat T, Rozen P. Epidemiology of Crohn's disease and ulcerative colitis: Etiologic implications. Israel J Med Sci 1979; 15:305–8.
52. Rozen P. Crohn's disease in the Jewish population of Tel-Aviv-Yafo: Epidemiologic and clinical aspects. Gastroenterology 1979; 76:25–30.
53. Kyle J, Stark G. Fall in the incidence of Crohn's disease. Gut 1980; 21:340–3.
54. Cited by Hellers G. Crohn's disease in Stockholm County (a study of epidemiology, results of surgical treatment and long-term prognosis). 1955–1974. (Thesis). Stockholm: 1979.
55. Das SK, Montgomery SD. Chronic inflammatory bowel disease in Asian immigrants. Practitioner 1978; 221:747–9.
56. Watanabe H, Hiwatashi N, Yamagata S. Clinical observations on ulcerative colitis. Tokohu J Exp Med 1977; 123:197–213.
57. Martini GA, Braudes JW. Increased consumption of refined carbohydrates in patients with Crohn's disease. Klin Wochenschr 1976; 54:367–71.
58. Watt J, Marcus R. Experimental ulcerative disease of the colon. Meth Exp Pathol 1975; 7:56–71.
59. Onderdonk AB, Hermos JA, Dzink JL, Bartlett JG. Protec-

tive effect of metronidazole in experimental ulcerative colitis. Gastroenterology 1978; 74:521–6.
60. McGill HC Jr, McMahan A, Wigodsky HS, Sprinz H. Carrageenan in formula and infant baboon development. Gastroenterology 1977; 73:512–7.
61. Carstensen J. Food additives and their possible role in Crohn's disease. Z Gastroenterol 1979; 17(Suppl):145–53.
62. Gershon MD, Erde SM. The nervous system of the gut. Gastroenterology 1981; 80:1571–94.
63. Ambinder RF, Schuster MM. Endorphins: New gut peptides with a familiar face. Gastroenterology 1979; 77:1132–40.
64. Grossman MJ, Brazier MAB, Lechago J. Cellular Basis of Chemical Messengers in the Digestive System. New York: Academic Press, 1981.
65. Lipowski ZJ. Psychosomatic medicine in the seventies: An overview. Am J Psychiatr 1977; 134:233–44.
66. Riley V. Psychoneuroendocrine influences on immunocompetence and neoplasia. Science 1981; 212:1100–9.
67. Keller SE, Weiss JM, Schleifer SJ, Miller NE, Stein M. Suppression of immunity by stress: Effect of a graded series of stressors on lymphocyte stimulation in the rat. Science 1981; 213:1397–1400.
68. Almy TP. Psychosocial aspects of chronic ulcerative colitis and Crohn's disease. *In*: Kirsner JB, Shorter RG, eds. Inflammatory Bowel Disease. 2nd Ed. Philadelphia: Lea and Febiger, 1980: 44–54.
69. Mendeloff AI, Monk M, Siegel CI, Lilienfeld A. Illness experience and life stresses in patients with irritable colon and with ulcerative colitis. N Engl J Med 1970; 282:14–7.
70. Liedtke R, Tschirch L, Zepf S. Studies in ulcerative colitis patients by MMPI Saarbrucken. Med Klin 1976; 71:807–13.
71. Kwaan HC, Cocco A, Mendeloff AI, Astrup T. Fibrinolytic activity in the normal and inflamed rectal mucosa. Scand J Gastroenterol 1969; 4:441–5.
72. Kyosola K, Penttila O, Salaspuro M. Rectal mucosal adrenergic innervation and enterochromaffin cells in ulcerative colitis and irritable colon. Scand J Gastroenterol 1977; 12:363–7.
73. Davis DR, Dockerty MB, Mayo CW. The myenteric plexus in regional enteritis: A study of ganglion cells in the ileum in 24 cases. Surg Gynecol Obstet 1955; 101:208–16.
74. Bishop AE, Polak JM, Bryant MG, Bloom SR, Hamilton S. Abnormalities of vasoactive intestinal polypeptide–containing nerves in Crohn's disease. Gastroenterology 1980; 79:853–60.
75. Kirsner JB, Goodman MJ. The medical treatment of inflammatory bowel disease. *In*: Kirsner JB, Shorter RG, eds. Inflammatory Bowel Disease. 2nd Ed. Philadelphia: Lea and Febiger, 1980: 413–46.
76. Kirschner BS, Klich JR, Kalman SS, DeFavaro MV, Rosenberg IH. Reversal of growth retardation in Crohn's disease with therapy emphasizing oral nutritional restitution. Gastroenterology 1981; 80:10–5.
77. Lennard-Jones JE, ed. Symposium on azulfidine (salazopyrin)—11th International Congress of Gastroenterology, Hamburg, West Germany—June 11, 1980. Z Gastroenterol 1981; 19(Suppl):3–48.
78. Van Hees PAM, Bakker JH, Van Tongeren JHM. Effect of sulphapyridine 5-amino salicylic acid and placebo in patients with idiopathic proctitis: A study to determine the active therapeutic moiety of sulphasalazine. Gut 1980; 21:632–5.
79. Klotz U, Maier K, Fischer C, Heinkel L. Therapeutic efficacy of sulphasalazine and its metabolites in patients with ulcerative colitis and Crohn's disease. N Engl J Med 1980; 303:1499–502.
80. Schwartz AG, Targan SR, Saxon A, Winstein WM. Sulfasalazine-induced exacerbation of ulcerative colitis. N Engl J Med 1982; 306:409–12.
81. Present DH, Korelitz BI, Wisch N, Glass JL, Sachar DM, Pasternack BS. Treatment of Crohn's disease with 6-mercaptopurine. N Engl J Med 1980; 302:981–7.
82. Kirsner JB. Current medical-surgical opinions on important therapeutic issues in inflammatory bowel disease. Am J Surg 1980; 140:391–5.
83. Block GE. Surgical management of Crohn's colitis. N Engl J Med 1980; 302:1068–70.
84. Morson BC. Pathology of ulcerative colitis. *In*: Kirsner JB, Shorter RG, eds. Inflammatory Bowel Disease. 2nd Ed. Philadelphia: Lea and Febiger, 1980:281–95.
85. Fairburn RA. On the aetiology of ulcerative colitis: A vascular hypothesis. Lancet 1973; 1:697–9.
86. Monis B, Mendeloff AI. Studies in ulcerative colitis: TPH-linked dehydrogenases and nonspecific esterase in rectal biopsy specimens. Gastroenterology 1965; 48:173–84.
87. Das KM, Erber WF, Rubinstein A. Immunohistochemical changes in morphologically involved and uninvolved colonic mucosa of patients with idiopathic proctitis. J Clin Invest 1977; 59:379–85.
88. Lipkin M, Bell B, Sherlock P, Bertino JR. Cell proliferation kinetics in the gastrointestinal tract of man. I. Cell renewal in colon and rectum. J Clin Invest 1963; 42:767–76.
89. Smith PR, Dawson DJ, Swan CHJ. Prostaglandin synthetase activity in acute ulcerative colitis: Effects of treatment with sulphasalazine, codeine phosphate and prednisolone. Gut 1979; 20:802–5.
90. Ligumsky M, Karmeli F, Sharon P, Zor U, Cohen F, Rachmilewitz D. Enhanced thromboxane A_2 and prostacyclin production by cultured rectal mucosa in ulcerative colitis and its inhibition by steroids and sulfasalazine. Gastroenterology 1981; 81:444–9.
91. Hawkey CJ, Truelove SC. Effect of prednisolone on prostaglandin synthesis by rectal mucosa in ulcerative colitis: Investigation by laminar flow bioassay and radioimmunoassay. Gut 1981; 22:190–3.
92. Rachmilewitz D, Ligumsky M, Haimovitz A, Treves AJ. Prostanoid synthesis by cultured peripheral blood mononuclear cells in inflammatory disease of the bowel. Gastroenterology 1982; 82:673–9.
93. Johansson C, Kollberg B, Nordemar R, Samuelson K, Berkstrom S. Protective effect of prostaglandin E_2 in the gastrointestinal tract during indomethacin treatment of rheumatic disease. Gastroenterology 1980; 78:479–83.
94. Rampton DS, Sladen GE. Prostaglandin synthesis inhibitors in ulcerative colitis: Flurbiprofen compared with conventional treatment. Prostaglandins 1981; 21:417–25.
95. Bukave K, Rask-Madsen J. Prostaglandin E_2 in jejunal fluids and its potential diagnostic value for selecting patients with indomethacin-sensitive diarrhea. Eur J Clin Invest 1981; 11:191–7.
96. Nouel O, Galian A, Hugent C, Vilde JL, Rambaud JC. Colite ulceronecrosante idiopathique extendue d'evolution mortelle associee a une duplication sigmoidiene. Gastroenterol Clin Biol 1978; 2:507–11.
97. Whitehead R. Pathology of Crohn's disease. *In*: Kirsner JB, Shorter RG, eds. Inflammatory Bowel Disease. 2nd Ed. Philadelphia: Lea and Febiger, 1980: 296–310.
98. Dourmashkin RR, Davies H, Wells C, Shah D, Price A, O'Morain C, Levi J, Hall THA. *In*: Pena AS, Weterman IT, Booth CC, Strober W, eds. Recent Advances in Crohn's Disease: Early Epithelial Lesions in Crohn's Disease Revealed by Electron Microscopy. The Hague: Martinus-Nijhoff, 1981: 117–23.
99. Dvorak AM. Ultrastructural evidence for release of major basic protein-containing crystalline cores of eosinophil granules in vivo: Cytotoxic potential in Crohn's disease. J Immunol 1980; 125:460–2.
100. Dvorak AM, Dickersin GR. Crohn's disease: Transmission electron microscopic studies. I. Barrier function. Possible changes related to alterations of cell coat, mucous coat, epithelial cells and Paneth cells. Hum Pathol 1980; 11(Suppl):561–71.
101. Dvorak AM, Monahan RA, Osage JE, Dickersin GR. Crohn's disease: Transmission electron microscopic studies. II. Immunologic inflammatory responses. Alterations of mast cells, basophils, eosinophils and the microvasculature. Hum Pathol 1980; 11:606–17.
102. Surawicz CM, Meisel JL, Ylvisaker T, Saunders DR, Rubin CE. Rectal biopsy in the diagnosis of Crohn's disease: Value of multiple biopsies and serial sectioning. Gastroenterology 1981; 80:66–71.
103. Meuret G, Bitzi A, Hammer B. Macrophage turnover in Crohn's disease and ulcerative colitis. Gastroenterology 1978; 74:501–3.
104. Goodman MJ, Kent PW, Truelove SC. Glucosamine syn-

thetase activity of the colonic mucosa in ulcerative colitis and Crohn's disease. Gut 1977; 18:219–28.
105. Nunez-Gornes JF, Tewksbury DA. Serum angiotensin-converting enzyme in Crohn's disease. Am J Gastroenterol 1981; 75:384–5.
106. Theodoropoulos D, Archimandritis A, Davaris P, Plataris J, Melissinos K. Ulcerative colitis and sarcoidosis: A curious association—Report of a case. Dis Colon Rectum 1981; 24:308–10.
107. Dunne WT, Cooke WT, Allan RN. Enzymatic and morphometric evidence for Crohn's disease as a diffuse lesion of the gastrointestinal tract. Gut 1977; 18:290–4.
108. Allan R, Steinberg DM, Dixon K, Cooke WT. Changes in the bidirectional sodium flux across the intestinal mucosa in Crohn's disease. Gut 1975; 16:201–4.
109. Beitman RG, Frost SS, Roth JLA. Oral manifestations of gastrointestinal disease. Dig Dis Sci 1981; 26:741–7.
110. McCallum DI, Gray WM. Metastatic Crohn's disease. Br J Dermatol 1976; 95:551–4.
111. Nugent FW, Glaser D, Fernandez-Herlihy L. Crohn's colitis associated with granulomatous bone disease. N Engl J Med 1976; 294:262–3.
112. Frayha R, Stevens MD, Bayless TM. Destructive monarthritis and granulomatous synovitis as the presenting manifestations of Crohn's disease. Johns Hopkins Med J 1975; 137:151–5.
113. Menard DB, Haddad H, Blain JG, Beaudry R, DeVroede G, Masse S. Granulomatous myositis and myopathy associated with Crohn's colitis. N Engl J Med 1976; 295:818–9.
114. Kelly JH, Montgomery WW, Goodman ML, Mulvaney TJ. Upper airway obstruction associated with regional enteritis. Ann Otol 1979; 88:95–9.
115. Wilder WM. Crohn's disease of the epiglottis, aryepiglottic folds, anus and rectum. J Clin Gastroenterol 1980; 2:87–91.
116. Shah SM, Texter EC Jr, White HJ. Inflammatory bowel disease associated with granulomatous lung disease. Gastrointest Endosc 1976; 23:98–9.
117. Cave DR, Kirsner JB. Animal models of inflammatory bowel disease. Z Gastroenterol 1979; 17(Suppl):125–35.
118. MacPherson BR, Pfeiffer CJ. Experimental colitis. Digestion 1976; 14:424–52.
119. Kirsner JB. Experimental colitis with particular reference to hypersensitivity in the colon. Gastroenterology 1961; 40:307–12.
120. Rabin BS, Rogers SJ. A cell-mediated immune model of inflammatory bowel disease in the rabbit. Gastroenterology 1978; 75:29–33.
121. Accini L, Brentjens JR, Albini B, Ossi E, O'Connell DW, Pawlowski IB, Andres GA. Deposition of circulating antigen-antibody complexes in the gastrointestinal tract of rabbits with chronic serum sickness. Am J Dig Dis 1978; 23:1098–106.
122. Roche JK, Cook SR, Day ED. Cellular cytotoxicity and gastrointestinal inflammation in inbred rats: Induction with gut organ–specific antigens. Immunology 1981; 44:489–97.
123. Catcott EJ. Feline Medicine and Surgery; A Text and Reference Work; The Work of 31 Authors. Santa Barbara, Cal: American Veterinary Publications, Inc., 1964.
124. Camprich RE. Equine granulomatous enteritis. Vet Pathol 1974; 11:535–47.
125. Mayberry JF, Rhodes J, Heatley RV. Infections which cause ileocolic disease in animals: Are they relevant to Crohn's disease? Gastroenterology 1980; 78:1080–4.
126. Emsbo P. Terminal or regional ileitis in swine. Nord Vet Med 1951; 3:1–28.
127. Strande A, Sommers SC, Petrak M. Regional enterocolitis in cocker spaniel dogs. Arch Pathol 1954; 57:357–62.
128. Van Kruiningen HG. Granulomatous colitis of boxer dogs: Comparative aspects. Gastroenterology 1967; 53:114–22.
129. Johne AH, Frothingham I. Chronic mycobacterial enteritis in ruminants. Proc R Soc Med 1895; 65:998–1001.
130. Reichert FL, Mathes ME. Experimental lymphoedema of the intestinal tract and its relation to regional cicatrizing enteritis. Ann Surg 1936; 104:601–14.
131. Kalima TV, Saloniemi H, Rahko T. Experimental regional enteritis in pigs. Scand J Gastroenterol 1976; 11:353–62.
132. Steward TH, Hetenyi C, Rowsell H, Onzaga M. Ulcerative enterocolitis in dogs induced by drugs. Pathology 1980; 131:363–78.
133. Sartor RB, Schwab JH, Powell DW, Cromartie WJ. Granulomatous enterocolitis induced by bacterial cell wall fragments (Abstract). Gastroenterology 1981; 80:1271.
134. Bregman E, Kirsner JB. Amino acids of colon and rectum: Possible involvement of diaminopimelic acid of intestinal bacteria in antigenicity of ulcerative colitis colon. Proc Soc Exp Biol Med 1965; 118:727–31.
135. Miller DS, Keighley A, Smith PG, Hughes AO, Langman MJS. A case control method for seeking evidence of contagion in Crohn's disease. Gastroenterology 1976; 71:385–7.
136. Walker ARP, Segal I. Epidemiology of non-infective intestinal diseases in various ethnic groups in South Africa. Israel J Med Sci 1979; 15:309–13.
137. Gelfand MD, Krone CL. Inflammatory bowel disease in a family. Ann Intern Med 1970; 72:903–7.
138. Vantrappen G, Agg HO, Ponette E, Geboes K, Bertrand PH. Yersinia enteritis and enterocolitis: Gastroenterological aspects. Gastroenterology 1977; 72:220–7.
139. Drake AA, Gilchrist MJR, Washington JA, Huizenga KA, Van Scoy RE. Diarrhea due to campylobacter fetus subspecies jejuni (A clinical review of 63 cases). Mayo Clin Proc 1981; 56:414–23.
140. Morris JJG, Wilson R, Davis BR, Wachsmuth IK, Riddle CF, Wathen HG, Pollard RA, Blake PA. Non O Group 1 vibrio cholerae gastroenteritis in the United States: Clinical, epidemiologic and laboratory characteristics of sporadic cases. Ann Intern Med 1981; 94-656–8.
141. Kirsner JB, Palmer WL. Ulcerative colitis (considerations of its etiology and treatment). JAMA 1954; 155:341–6.
142. Gorbach SL. Intestinal microflora in inflammatory bowel disease: Implications for etiology and therapy. *In*: Kirsner JB, Shorter RG, eds. Inflammatory Bowel Disease. 2nd Ed. Philadelphia: Lea and Febiger, 1980: 55–70.
143. Vander Wiel-Korstanje J, Winkler KC. The faecal flora in ulcerative colitis. J Med Microbiol 1975; 8:491–501.
144. Keighly MRB, Arabi Y, Dimock F, Burdon DN, Allan RN, Alexander-Williams JA. Influence of inflammatory bowel disease on intestinal microflora. Gut 1978; 19:1099–104.
145. Dickinson RJ, Varian SA, Axon ATR, Cooke EM. Increased incidence of fecal coliforms with in vitro adhesive and invasive properties in patients with ulcerative colitis. Gut 1980; 21:787–92.
146. Vince A, Dyer NH, O'Grady FW, Dawson AM. Bacteriological studies in Crohn's disease. J Med Microbiol 1972; 5:219–29.
147. Wensinck F. The fecal flora of patients with Crohn's disease. Van Leeuwenhoek Arch 1975; 41:214–5, cited by Van de Merwe JP. A possible role of eubacterium and peptostreptococcus species in the aetiology of Crohn's disease. *In*: Pena AS, Weterman IT, Booth CC, Strober W, eds. Recent Advances in Crohn's Disease. The Hague: Martinus-Nijhoff, 1981: 201–6.
148. Bourgault AM, Rosenblatt JE, Fitzgerald RH. Peptococcus magnus: A significant human pathogen. Ann Intern Med 1980; 93:244–8.
149. Van de Merwe JP. Agglutination of eubacterium and peptostreptococcus species as a diagnostic test for Crohn's disease. Hepato Gastroenterol 1981; 28:155–6.
150. Van de Merwe JP. A possible role of eubacterium and peptostreptococcus species in the aetiology of Crohn's disease. *In*: Pena AS, Weterman IT, Booth CC, Strober W, eds. Recent Advances in Crohn's Disease. The Hague: Martinus-Nijhoff, 1981:201–6.
151. Burnham WR, Lennard-Jones JE, Stanford JL, Bird RG. Mycobacteria as a possible cause of inflammatory bowel disease. Lancet 1978; 2:693–6.
152. Parent K, Mitchell PD. Bacterial variants: Etiologic agent in Crohn's disease. Gastroenterology 1976; 71:365–8.
153. Elliott PR, Forsey T, Darongar S, Trehorne JD, Lennard-Jones JE. Chlamydiae and inflammatory bowel disease. Gut 1981; 22:25–7.
154. Peach S, Lock MR, Katz D, Todd IP, Tabaqchali S. Mucosal-

associated bacterial flora in the intestine of patients with Crohn's disease and in a control group. Gut 1978; 19:1034–42.
155. Whorwell PJ, Davidson IW, Beeken WL, Wright R. Search by immunofluorescence for antigens of rotavirus, *Pseudomonas maltophilia* and *Mycobacterium kansasii* in Crohn's disease. Lancet 1978; 2:697–8.
156. Heddle RJ, Shearman DJC. Serum antibodies to *Escherichia coli* in subjects with ulcerative colitis. Clin Exp Immunol 1979; 38:22–30.
157. Tabaqchali S, O'Donoghue DP, Bettelheim KA. *Escherichia coli* antibodies in patients with inflammatory bowel disease. Gut 1978; 19:108–13.
158. Matthews N, Mayberry JF, Rhodes J, Neale L, Munro J, Wensinck F, Lawson GHK, Rowland AC, Berkhoff GA, Barthold SW. Agglutinins to bacteria in Crohn's disease. Gut 1980; 21:376–80.
159. Moskovitz M, Bartlett JG. Recurrent pseudomembranous colitis unassociated with prior antibiotic therapy. Arch Intern Med 1981; 141:663–4.
160. Viscidi R, Willey S, Bartlett JG. Isolation rates and toxigenic potential of *Clostridium difficile* isolates from various patient populations. Gastroenterolog 1981; 80:693–6.
161. Trnka YM, La Mont JT. Association of *Clostridium difficile* toxin with symptomatic relapse of chronic inflammatory bowel disease. Gastroenterology 1981; 80:693–6.
162. Meyers S, Mayer L, Bottone E, Desmond E, Janowitz HD. Occurrence of *Clostridium difficile* toxin during the course of inflammatory bowel disease. Gastroenterology 1981; 80:697–700.
163. Thorne GM, Gorbach SL. New bacterial enterotoxins and human diarrheal diseases. *In*: Janowitz HD, Seebar DB, eds. Frontiers of Knowledge in the Diarrheal Diseases. Upper Montclair, New Jersey: Projects in Health, Inc., 1979: 165–76.
164. Monif JRG, Hood CI. Ileocolitis associated with measles (rubeola). Am J Dis Child 1970; 120:245–7.
165. Gomez-Barretto J, Palmer EL, Nahmias AJ, Hatch MH. Acute enteritis associated with reovirus-like agents. JAMA 1976; 235:1857–60.
166. Shepherd RW, Butler DG, Cutz E, Gall DG, Hamilton JR. The mucosal lesion in viral enteritis. Gastroenterology 1979; 76:770–7.
167. Davidson GP, Gall DG, Petric M, Butler DG, Hamilton JR. Human rotavirus enteritis induced in conventional piglets: Intestinal structure and transport. J Clin Invest 1977; 60:1402–9.
168. Mohanty SB, Dutta SK. Feline viruses. *In*: Mohanty JB, Dutta SK, eds. Veterinary Virology. Philadelphia: Lea and Febiger, 1981: 225–34.
169. Miller DS, Keighley A, Smith PG, Hughes AD, Langman MJS. Crohn's disease in Nottingham: A search for time-space clustering. Gut 1975; 16:454–7.
170. Greenberg HB, Gebhard RL, McClain CJ, Soltis RD, Kapikian AZ. Antibodies to viral gastroenteritis viruses in Crohn's disease. Gastroenterology 1979; 76:349–50.
171. Roche JK, Wold WSM, Sanders PR, Mackey JK, Green M. Chronic inflammatory bowel disease: Absence of adenovirus DNA as established by molecular hybridization. Gastroenterology 1981; 81:853–8.
172. Cooper HS, Raffenberger EC, Jones L, Mackey JK, Green M. Cytomegalovirus inclusions in patients with ulcerative colitis and toxic dilatation requiring colon resection. Gastroenterology 1977; 72:1253–6.
173. Victor R, Kirsner JB, Palmer WL. Failure to induce ulcerative colitis experimentally with filtrates of feces and rectal mucosa. Gastroenterology 1950; 14:398–400.
174. Mitchell DN, Rees RJW. Agents transmissible from Crohn's disease tissue. Lancet 1970; 2:168–71.
175. Cave DR, Mitchell DN, Brooke BN. Crohn's disease and ulcerative colitis: A review of the evidence for transmissibility. *In*: Jerzy-Glass GB, ed. Progress in Gastroenterology. New York: Grune and Stratton, 1977: 839–55.
176. Cohen Z, Cook G, Festenstein H. The transmission of human Crohn's disease in inbred strains of mice. Ann R Coll Phys Surg Can 1978; 2:51.
177. Donnelly BJ, Delaney PV, Healy TM. Evidence for a transmissible factor in Crohn's disease. Gut 1977; 18:360–3.
178. Aronson MD, Phillips CA, Beeken WL, Forsyth BR. Isolation and characterization of a viral agent from intestinal tissue of patients with Crohn's disease and other intestinal disorders. Prog Med Virol 1975; 21:165–76.
179. Gitnick GL, Rosen VJ, Arthur MH, Hertweck SA. Evidence for the isolation of a new virus from ulcerative colitis patients: Comparison with virus derived from Crohn's disease. Dig Dis Sci 1979; 24:609–19.
180. Heatley RV, Bolton PM, Owen E, Williams WJ, Hughes LE. A search for a transmissible agent in Crohn's disease. Gut 1975; 16:528–32.
181. Ahlberg J, Bergstrand O, Gillstrom P, Holmstrom P, Kroneri T, Reiland S. Negative findings in search for a transmissible agent in Crohn's disease. Acta Chir Scand 1978; 482:45–57.
182. Phillpotts RJ, Hermon-Taylor J, Teich NM, Brooke BN. A search for persistent virus infections in Crohn's disease. Gut 1980; 21:202–7.
183. Beeken WL. Infectious agents in inflammatory bowel disease. *In*: Berk JE, ed. Developments in Digestive Diseases, Vol. 2. Philadelphia: Lea and Febiger, 1979: 57–71.
184. Prusiner SB. Novel proteinaceous infectious particles cause scrapie. Science 1982; 216:136–44.
185. Das KM, Valenzuela I, Morecki R. Crohn's disease lymph node homogenates produce murine lymphoma in athymic mice. Proc Natl Acad Sci USA 1980; 77:588–92.
186. Kirsner JB. Inflammatory bowel disease: Clinical, etiological and genetic aspects. *In*: Rotter JI, Samloff IM, Rimoin DL, eds. Genetics and Heterogeneity of Common Gastrointestinal Disorders. New York: Academic Press, 1980: 261–80.
187. McConnell RB. The Genetics of Gastrointestinal Disorders. London: Oxford University Press, 1966: 128–42 (cited in Genetics of Gastrointestinal Disorders). Clin Gastroenterol 1973; 2:489–724.
188. Katsaros D, Truelove SC. Regional enteritis and glucose-6-phosphate dehydrogenase deficiency. N Engl J Med 1969; 281:295–6.
189. Streifler C, Schnitzer N, Harell A. A rare isoenzyme of alkaline phosphatase in 4 patients with ulcerative colitis. Clin Chem Acta 1972; 38:244–6.
190. Polcak J, Skolova M. Immunologic manifestations of healthy consanguineous relatives of patients suffering from ulcerative colitis. Am J Proctol 1968; 19:197–203.
191. Singer HC, Anderson JGD, Frischer H, Kirsner JB. Familial aspects of inflammatory bowel disease. Gastroenterology 1971; 61:423–30.
192. Kirsner JB. Genetic aspects of inflammatory bowel disease. Clin Gastroenterol 1973; 2:557–75.
193. Farmer RG, Michener WM, Mortimer EA. Studies of family history among patients with inflammatory bowel disease. Clin Gastroenterol 1980; 9:271–8.
194. Klein GL, Ament ME, Sparkes RS. Monozygotic twins with Crohn's disease: A case report. Gastroenterology 1980; 79:931–3.
195. Binder V, Weeks E, Olson JH, Anthonisen P, Riis P. A genetic study of ulcerative colitis. Scand J Gastroenterol 1966; 1:49–56.
196. McConnell RG. Inflammatory bowel disease and ankylosing spondylitis. Birth Defects, Original Article Series 1972; 8:42–5.
197. Costello PB, Alea JA, Kennedy AC, McCheskey RJ, Green FA. Prevalence of occult inflammatory bowel disease in ankylosing spondylitis. Ann Rheum Dis 1980; 39:453–6.
198. Schinella RA, Creco MA, Gobert BL, Denmark LW, Cox RP. Hermansky-Pudlak syndrome with granulomatous colitis. Ann Intern Med 1980; 92:20–3.
199. Price WH. A high incidence of chronic inflammatory bowel disease in patients with Turner's syndrome. J Med Genet 1979; 16:263–6.
200. Pedersen JK. Deficiency of alpha-1-antitrypsin, fatty liver and ulcerative colitis: A hitherto unknown symptom-complex with account of familial predisposition. Ugeskr Laeger 1974; 136:2741–4.
201. McConnell RB. Inflammatory bowel disease: Newer views

of genetic influence. *In*: Berk JE, ed. Developments in Digestive Disease, Vol 3. Philadelphia: Lea and Febiger, 1980: 129–38.
202. Asquith P. Birmingham, England: Personal communication, 1976, 1977.
203. Craxi A, Oliva L, Distenfano G. Ulcerative colitis in a married couple. Ital J Gastroenterol 1979; 11:184–6.
204. Whorwell PJ, Eade OE, Hossenbocus A, Bamforth J. Crohn's disease in a husband and wife. Lancet 1978; 2:186–7.
205. Zetzel L. Crohn's disease in a husband and wife. Lancet 1978; 2:583.
206. Goodman MJ. Bury, England: Personal communication, 1981.
207. Rosenberg JL, Kraft SC, Kirsner JB. Inflammatory bowel disease in all three members of one family. Gastroenterology 1976; 70:759–60.
208. Achord JL, Gunn CH Jr, Jackson JF. Multiple occurrences of regional enteritis in a family. Dig Dis Sci 1982; 27:330–2.
209. Bisordi W, Lightdale CJ. Identical twins discordant for ulcerative colitis with colon cancer. Am J Dig Dis 1976; 21:71–3.
210. Strickland RG, Friedler EM, Henderson CA, Wilson ID, Williams RC Jr. Serum lymphocytotoxins in inflammatory bowel disease: Studies of frequency and specificity for lymphocyte subpopulations. Clin Exp Immunol 1975; 21:384–93.
211. DeHoratious RJ, Miller WC, Gaeke RF, Strickland RG, Volpicelli NA, Kirsner JB, Williams RC Jr. Antibodies to synthetic polyribonucleotides in spouses of patients with inflammatory bowel disease. Lancet 1978; 1:1116–9.
212. Kuiper I, Weterman IJ, Biemond I, Van Rood JI, Pena AS. Lymphocytotoxic antibodies in patients with Crohn's disease and family members. *In*: Pena AS, Weterman IJ, Booth CC, Strober W, eds. Recent Advances in Crohn's Disease. The Hague: Martinus-Nijhoff, 1981: 341–7.
213. McDevitt HO. Current concepts in immunology. Regulation of the immune response by the major histocompatibility system. N Engl J Med 1980; 303:1514–7.
214. Tsuchiya M, Yoshida T, Asakura H, Hibi T, Ono A, Mizuno Y, Tsuji K. HLA antigens and ulcerative colitis in Japan. Digestion 1977; 15:286–94.
215. Hiwatashi N, Kikuchi T, Masamune O, Watanabe H, Goto Y. HLA antigens in inflammatory bowel disease. Tokohu J Exp Med 1980; 131:381–5.
216. Corazza GR, Tabacchi P, Colaneri F, Ionatay R, Borbori F, Gasparrini G. HLA antigens and ulcerative colitis: Is there any link? Ital J Gastroenterol 1978; 10:139–41.
217. Nahir M, Gidconi D, Eidelman S, Barzilai A. HLA antigens in ulcerative colitis. Lancet 1976; 2:573.
218. Delpre G, Kadish U, Gazit E, Joshua H, Zamir R. HLA antigens in ulcerative colitis and Crohn's disease in Israel. Gastroenterology 1980; 78:1452–7.
219. Pena AS. Immunogenetic aspects of inflammatory bowel disease. *In*: Rotter JI, Samloff IM, Rimoin DL, eds. The Genetics and Heterogeneity of Common Gastrointestinal Disorders. New York: Academic Press, 1980: 281–9.
220. Asakura H, Tsuchiya M, Aiso S, Watanabe M, Kobayashi K, Hibi T, Ando K, Takata H, Sekiguehi S. Association of the human lymphocyte DR_2 antigen with Japanese ulcerative colitis. Gastroenterology 1982; 82:413–8.
221. Schwartz SE, Siegelbaum SP, Fazio TL, Hubbell C, Henry JB. Regional enteritis: Evidence for genetic transmission by HLA typing. Ann Intern Med 1980; 93:424–7.
222. Eade OE, Moulton C, MacPherson BR, St. Andre-Ukena, Albertini RJ, Beeken WL. Discordant HLA haplotype segregation in familial Crohn's disease. Gastroenterology 1980; 79:271–5.
223. Pena AS, Biemond I, Kiuper J, Weterman IT, Van Leeuwen A, Schreuder I, van Rood JJ. HLA antigen distribution and HLA haplotype segregation in Crohn's disease. Tissue Ant 1980; 16:56–61.
224. Van den Berg-Loonen EM, Dekker-Saeys BJ, Meuwissen SGM, Nijenhuis LE, Engelfriet CP. Histocompatibility antigens and other genetic markers in ankylosing spondylitis and inflammatory bowel disease. J Immunogenet 1977; 4:167–75.
225. Acheson ED. An association between ulcerative colitis, regional enteritis and ankylosing spondylitis. Q J Med 1969; 29:489–99.
226. Mallas EG, Mackintosh P, Asquith P, Cooke WT. Histocompatibility antigens in inflammatory bowel disease: Their clinical significance and their association with arthropathy with special reference to HLA-B27. Gut 1976; 17:906–10.
227. Smolen JS, Gangl A, Polterauer P, Menzel EJ, Mayr WR. HLA antigens in inflammatory bowel disease. Gastroenterology 1982; 82:34–8.
228. Slade JD, Luskin AT, Gewurz H, Kraft SC, Kirsner JB, Zeitz HJ. Inherited deficiency of second component of complement and HLA haplotype $A_{10}B_{18}$ associated with inflammatory bowel disease. Ann Intern Med 1978; 88:796–8.
229. Segal AW, Lowei G. Neutrophil dysfunction in Crohn's disease. Lancet 1976; 2:219–21.
230. Rhodes JM, Bartholomew TC, Jewell DP. Inhibition of leucocyte motility by drugs used in ulcerative colitis. Gut 1981; 22:642–7.
231. Morain CO, Segal AA, Walker D, Levi AJ. Abnormalities of neutrophil function do not cause the migration defect in Crohn's disease. Gut 1981; 22:817–22.
232. Wandall JH, Binder V. Leucocyte function in Crohn's disease. Gut 1982; 23:173–80.
233. Ward M. The pathogenesis of Crohn's disease. Lancet 1977; 2:903–5.
234. Lamster I, Sonis S, Hannigan A, Kolodkin A. An association between Crohn's disease, peridontal disease and enhanced neutrophil function. J Peridontol 1978; 49:475–9.
235. Mee AS, Jewell DP. Monocytes in inflammatory bowel disease: Monocyte and serum lysosomal enzyme activity. Clin Sci 1980; 58:295–300.
236. Gillam JH III, Challa VR, Agudelo CA, Albertson DA, Huntley CC. Vasculitis involving muscle associated with Crohn's colitis. Gastroenterology 1981; 81:787–90.
237. Kirsner JB, Goldgraber MB. Hypersensitivity, autoimmunity and the digestive tract. Gastroenterology 1960; 38:536–62.
238. Kraft SC, Kirsner JB. Immunological apparatus of the gut and inflammatory bowel disease. Gastroenterology 1971; 60:922–51.
239. Kraft SC, Kirsner JB. Ulcerative colitis. *In*: Samter M, ed. Immunological Diseases, Vol II, 2nd Ed. Boston: Little, Brown, 1971: 1346–66.
240. Kraft SC, Kirsner JB. The immunology of ulcerative colitis and Crohn's disease: Clinical and humoral aspects. *In*: Kirsner JB, Shorter RG, eds. Inflammatory Bowel Disease, 2nd Ed. Philadelphia: Lea and Febiger, 1980: 86–120.
241. Goldgraber MG, Kirsner JB. The histopathology of the experimental hypersensitive state in the gastrointestinal tract. Arch Intern Med 1958; 102:134–48.
242. Kraft SC. Inflammatory bowel disease (ulcerative colitis and Crohn's disease). *In*: Asquith P, ed. Ulcerative Colitis and Crohn's Disease in Immunology of the Gastrointestinal Tract. London: Churchill Livingstone, 1979: 95–128.
243. Shorter RG, Tomasi TB Jr. Gut immune mechanisms. Adv Intern Med 1982; 27:247–80.
244. Gelzayd EA, Kraft SC, Fitch FW. Immunoglobulin A: Localization in rectal mucosal epithelial cells. Science 1967; 157:930–1.
245. Gelzayd EA, Kraft SC, Fitch FW, Kirsner JB. Distribution of immunoglobulins in human rectal mucosa. II. Ulcerative colitis and abnormal mucosal control subjects. Gastroenterology 1968; 54:341–7.
246. Goldgraber MB, Kirsner JB, Palmer WL. The histopathology of chronic ulcerative colitis and its pathogenetic implications. Gastroenterology 1960; 38:596–604.
247. Kirsner JB. The immunologic response of the colon. JAMA 1965; 191:809–14.
248. Goldgraber MB, Kirsner JB. The Arthus phenomenon in the colon of rabbits. Arch Pathol 1959; 67:556–71.
249. Kirsner JB, Elchlepp J. The production of an experimental colitis in rabbits. Trans Assoc Am Phys 1957; 70:102–19.
250. Kraft SC, Kirsner JB, Fitch FW. Histologic and immunohistochemical features of Auer colitis in rabbits. Am J Pathol 1963; 43:913–27.

251. Rabin BS, Rogers SJ. A cell-mediated immune model of inflammatory bowel disease in the rabbit. Gastroenterology 1978; 75:29–33.
252. Reilly RW, Kirsner JB. Runt intestinal disease. Lab Invest 1965; 14:102–7.
253. Hodgson HFJ, Potter BJ, Skinner J, Jewell DP. Immune complex–mediated colitis in rabbits. Gut 1978; 19:225–32.
254. Shorter RG, Huizenga KA, Spencer RJ. A working hypothesis for the etiology and pathogenesis of nonspecific inflammatory bowel disease. Am J Dig Dis 1972; 17:1024–32.
255. Bleumink E. Food allergy and the gastrointestinal tract. *In*: Asquith P, ed. Immunology of the Gastrointestinal Tract. London: Churchill Livingstone, 1979: 195–213.
256. Jones DB, Parker JH, Kerr GD, Wilson RSE. Dietary allergy and specific IgE in ulcerative colitis. J R Soc Med 1981; 74:292–3.
257. O'Donoghue DP, Kumar P. Rectal IgE cells in inflammatory bowel disease. Gut 1979; 20:149–53.
258. Binder V, Elsborg L, Greibe J, Hendriksen C, Hoj L, Jensen KB, Kristensen E, Madsen JR, Marner B, Riis P, Willumsen L. Disodium cromoglycate in the treatment of ulcerative colitis and Crohn's disease. Gut 1981; 22:55–60.
259. Ward M, Eastwood MA. Serum C_3 and C_4 complement components in ulcerative colitis and Crohn's disease. Digestion 1975; 13:100–3.
260. Lake AM, Stitzel AE, Urmson JR, Walker WA, Spitzer RE. Complement alterations in inflammatory bowel disease. Gastroenterology 1979; 76:1374–9.
261. Bergman L, Johansson SG, Krause U. The immunoglobulin concentrations in serum and bowel secretions in patients with Crohn's disease. Scand J Gastroenterol 1975; 8:401–6.
262. Hodgson HJF, Jewell DP. The humoral immune system in inflammatory bowel disease. II. Immunoglobulin levels. Am J Dig Dis 1978; 23:123–8.
263. MacDermott RP, Nash GS, Bertovich MJ, Seiden MV, Bragdon MJ, Beale MG. Alterations of IgM, IgG and IgA synthesis and secretion by peripheral blood and intestinal mononuclear cells from patients with ulcerative colitis and Crohn's disease. Gastroenterology 1981; 81:844–52.
264. Gelernt IM, Present DH, Janowitz HD. Alterations in serum immunoglobulins after resection for ulcerative and granulomatous disease of the intestine. Gut 1972; 13:21–3.
265. Kraft SC, Kirsner JB. The immunology of ulcerative colitis and Crohn's disease: Clinical and humoral aspects. *In*: Kirsner JB, Shorter RG, eds. Inflammatory Bowel Disease, 2nd Ed. Philadelphia: Lea and Febiger, 1980: 86–120.
266. Harrison WJ. Autoantibodies against intestinal and gastric mucous cells in ulcerative colitis. Lancet 1965; 1:1346–50.
267. Broberger G, Perlmann P. Autoantibodies in human ulcerative colitis. J Exp Med 1959; 110:657–74.
268. Carlsson HE, Lagercrantz R, Perlmann P. Immunological studies in ulcerative colitis. VIII. Antibodies to colon antigen in patients with ulcerative colitis, Crohn's disease and other diseases. Scand J Gastroenterol 1977; 12:707–14.
269. Permann P, Hammarstrom S, Lagercrantz R, Gustafsson BE. Antigens from colon of germfree rats and antibodies in human ulcerative colitis. Ann NY Acad Sci 1965; 124:377–94.
270. Zeromski J, Perlmann P, Lagercrantz R, Hammarstrom S, Gustafsson BE. Immunological studies in ulcerative colitis. VII. Anticolon antibodies of different immunoglobulin classes. Clin Exp Immunol 1970; 7:469–75.
271. Broberger G, Perlmann P. In vitro studies of ulcerative colitis. I. Reactions of patients' serum with human fetal colon cells in tissue cultures. J Exp Med 1963; 117:705–16.
272. Lagercrantz R, Hammarstrom S, Perlmann P, Gustafsson BE. Immunological studies in ulcerative colitis. III. Incidence of antibodies to colon antigen in ulcerative colitis and other gastrointestinal diseases. Clin Exp Immunol 1966; 1:263–76.
273. Lagercrantz R, Hammarstrom S, Perlmann P, Gustafsson BE. Immunological studies in ulcerative colitis. IV. Origin of autoantibodies. J Exp Med 1968; 128:1339–52.
274. Perlmann P, Hammarstrom S, Lagercrantz R, Campbell D. Autoantibodies to colon in rats and human ulcerative colitis: Cross-reactivity with *Escherichia coli* 0114 antigen. Proc Soc Exp Biol Med 1967; 125:975–80.
275. Kunin CM. Separation, characterization and biological significance of a common antigen in enterobacteriaceae. J Exp Med 1963; 118:565–86.
276. Hammarstrom S, Carlsson HE, Perlmann P, Svensson S. Immunochemistry of the common antigen of enterobacteriaceae (Kunin): Relation to lipopolysaccharide core structure. J Exp Med 1971; 134:565–76.
277. Lagercrantz R, Perlmann P, Hammarstrom S. Immunological studies of ulcerative colitis. V. Family studies. Gastroenterology 1971; 60:381–9.
278. Bartnik W, Kaluzewski S. Cellular and humoral responses to the Kunin antigen (CA) in ulcerative colitis and Crohn's disease. Arch Immunol Ther Exp 1979; 27:531–8.
279. Williams RC Jr. Immune complexes: A clinical perspective (Editorial). Am J Med 1981; 71:743–5.
280. Fiasse R, Lurhuma AZ, Cambiaso CL, Masson PL, Dive C. Circulating immune complexes and disease activity in Crohn's disease. Gut 1978; 19:611–7.
281. Hodgson HJF, Potter BJ, Jewell DP. Immune complexes in ulcerative colitis and Crohn's disease. Clin Exp Immunol 1977; 29:187–96.
282. Kemler BJ, Alpert E. Inflammatory bowel disease associated with circulating immune complexes. Gut 1980; 21:195–201.
283. Richens ER, Thorp CM, Bland PW, Hall ND. Circulating immune complexes in Crohn's disease: Their characterization and interrelationship with components and the complement system. Dig Dis Sci 1982; 27:129–38.
284. Soltis RD, Hasz D, Morris MJ, Wilson ID. Evidence against the presence of circulating immune complexes in chronic inflammatory bowel disease. Gastroenterology 1979; 76:1380–5.
285. Mee AS, McLaughlin JE, Hodgson HJF, Jewell DP. Chronic immune colitis in rabbits. Gut 1979; 20:1–5.
286. Gebbers JO, Otto HF. Immunohistochemical and electron microscopic observations on the local immune response in ulcerative colitis. Virchows Arch [Pathol Anat] 1977; 374:271–3.
287. Strickland RG, Husby G, Black WC, Williams RC Jr. Peripheral blood and intestinal lymphocyte subpopulations in Crohn's disease. Gut 1975; 16:847–53.
288. Auer IO, Wechsler W, Ziemer E, Malchow H, Sommer H. Immune status in Crohn's disease. I. Leukocyte and lymphocyte subpopulations in peripheral blood. Scand J Gastroenterol 1978; 13:561–71.
289. Auer IO, Gotz S, Ziemer E, Malchow H, Ehms H. Immune status in Crohn's disease. III. Peripheral blood B lymphocytes, enumerated by means of $F(ab)_2$-antibody fragments, null and T lymphocytes. Gut 1979; 20:261–8.
290. Eckhardt R, Kloos P, Dierich MP, Zum Buschenfelde KHM. K-lymphocytes (killer-cells) in Crohn's disease and acute virus B-hepatitis. Gut 1977; 18:1010–6.
291. Meijer CJLM, Bosman FT, Lindeman J. Evidence for predominant involvement of the B cell system in the inflammatory process in Crohn's disease. Scand J Gastroenterol 1979; 14:21–32.
292. Ginsburg CH, Ault KA, Falchuk ZM. Monoclonal B lymphocytes in the peripheral blood of patients with inflammatory bowel disease. Gastroenterology 1981; 81:1111–4.
293. Raeman F, DeCock W, DeBenkelaar T, DeCree J, Verhaegen H. Enumeration of T lymphocytes and T lymphocyte subsets in autoimmune disease using monoclonal antibodies. Clin Exp Immunol 1981; 45:475–9.
294. Thayer WR Jr, Fixa B, Komarkova O, Charland C, Field CE. Skin test reactivity in inflammatory bowel disease in the United States and Czechoslovakia. Am J Dig Dis 1978; 23:337–40.
295. Meuwissen SGM, Schellekens PTA, Huismans L, Tytgat GN. Impaired anamnestic cellular immune response in patients with Crohn's disease. Gut 1975; 16:854–60.
296. James DG. Kveim revisited, reassessed. N Engl J Med 1975; 292:859–60.
297. Meyers S, Sachar DB, Taub RN, Janowitz HD. Significance of anergy to dinitrochlorobenzene (DNCB) in inflammatory

bowel disease: Family and postoperative studies. Gut 1978; 19:249–52.
298. Bird AG, Britton S. No evidence for decreased lymphocyte reactivity in Crohn's disease. Gastroenterology 1974; 67:926–32.
299. Allen JI, Kay KE, McClain CJ. Severe zinc deficiency in humans: Association with a reversible T-lymphocyte dysfunction. Ann Intern Med 1981; 95:154–7.
300. Hsu CCS, Wu MB, Rivera-Arcilla J. Inhibition of lymphocyte reactivity in vitro by autologous polymorphonuclear cells (PMN). Cell Immunol 1979; 48:288–95.
301. Surrenti, Ramarli D, Casini A, Scarabelli S, Campi P, Fauci A, Nieri S. Studies of cell-mediated immunity in patients with Crohn's disease. Hepato Gastroenterol 1981; 28:157–9.
302. Skinner JM, Whitehead R. A morphological assessment of immunoreactivity in colonic Crohn's disease and ulcerative colitis by a study of lymph nodes. J Clin Pathol 1974; 27:202–6.
303. Bendixen G. Cellular hypersensitivity to components of intestinal mucosa in ulcerative colitis and Crohn's disease. Gut 1969; 10:631–6.
304. Fixa B, Komarkova O, Skaunic V, Nerad M, Kojecky Z, Benysek L. Inhibition of leucocyte migration by antigens from human colon and *E. coli* 014 in patients with ulcerative colitis. Scand J Gastroenterol 1975; 10:491–3.
305. Dykes PW. Delayed hypersensitivity in Crohn's disease. Proc R Soc Med 1970; 63:906–8.
306. Richens ER, Williams MJ, Gough KR, Ancill RJ. Mixed lymphocytic reaction as a measure of immunologic competence of lymphocytes from patients with Crohn's disease. Gut 1974; 15:24–38.
307. Bull DM, Ignaczak TF. Enterobacterial common antigen-induced lymphocyte reactivity in inflammatory bowel disease. Gastroenterology 1973; 64:43–50.
308. Eckhardt R, Heinisch M, Meyer zum Buschenfelde KH. Cellular immune reactions against common antigen, small intestine, and colon antigen in patients with Crohn's disease, ulcerative colitis and cirrhosis of the liver. Scand J Gastroenterol 1976; 11:49–54.
309. Bartnik W, ReMine SG, Shorter RG. Leucocyte migration inhibitory factor (LMIF) release by human colonic lymphocytes. Arch Immunol Ther Exp (Warsaw) 1981; 29:397–405.
310. Rhodes JM, Bartholomew TC, Jewell DP. Inhibition of leukocyte motility by drugs used in ulcerative colitis. Gut 1981; 22:642–7.
311. Schwab JH. Suppression of the immune response by microorganisms. Bacteriol Rev 1975; 39:121–43.
312. Perlmann P, Broberger G. In vitro studies of ulcerative colitis. II. Cytotoxic action of white blood cells from patients on human fetal colon cells. J Exp Med 1963; 117:717–33.
313. Watson DW, Quigley A, Bolt RJ. Effect of lymphocytes from patients with ulcerative colitis on human adult colon epithelial cells. Gastroenterology 1966; 51:985–93.
314. Shorter RG, Spencer RJ, Huizenga KA, Hallenbeck GA. Inhibition of in vitro cytotoxicity of lymphocytes from patients with ulcerative colitis and granulomatous colitis for allogeneic colonic epithelial cells using horse anti-human thymus serum. Gastroenterology 1968; 54:227–31.
315. Shorter RG, Cardoza M, Spencer RJ, Huizenga KA. Further studies of in vitro cytotoxicity of lymphocytes from patients with ulcerative and granulomatous colitis for allogeneic colonic epithelial cells, including the effects of colectomy. Gastroenterology 1969; 56:304–9.
316. Shorter RG, Huizenga KA, Spencer RJ, Aas J, Guy SK. Inflammatory bowel disease: Cytophilic antibody and cytotoxicity of lymphocytes for colonic cells in vitro. Am J Dig Dis 1971; 16:673–80.
317. Stobo JD, Tomasi TB, Huizenga KA, Spencer RJ, Shorter RG. In vitro studies of inflammatory bowel disease: Surface receptors of the mononuclear cell required to lyse allogeneic colonic epithelial cells, Gastroenterology 1976: 70:171–6.
318. Kemler BJ, Alpert E. Inflammatory bowel disease: Study of cell-mediated cytotoxicity for isolated human colonic epithelial cells. Gut 1980; 21:353–9.
319. Waldmann TA, Broder S. Suppressor cells in the regulation of the immune response. *In*: Schwartz R, ed. Progress in Clinical Immunology. New York: Grune and Stratton, 1977: 155–99.
320. Hodgson HJF, Wands JR, Isselbacher KJ. Decreased suppressor cell activity in inflammatory bowel disease. Clin Exp Immunol 1978; 32:451–8.
321. Ginsburg CH, Master JT, Falchuk ZM. Defective autologous mixed-lymphocyte reactions and suppressor T-cell generation in patients with inflammatory bowel disease (Abstract). Gastroenterology 1980; 78:1173.
322. Victorino RMM, Hodgson HJF. Alteration in T lymphocyte subpopulations in inflammatory bowel disease. Clin Exp Immunol 1980; 41:156–65.
323. Kemler BJ, Alpert E. Immune regulation in inflammatory bowel disease: Absence of a serum inhibitor of suppressor cell function. Clin Exp Immunol 1980; 42:280–4.
324. Auer IO, Ziemer E, Sommer H. Immune status in Crohn's disease. V. Decreased in vitro natural killer cell activity in peripheral blood. Clin Exp Immunol 1980; 42:41–9.
325. Ginsburg CH, Ault KA, Falchuk ZM. Defective natural killer cell activity in patients with inflammatory bowel disease: Evidence for a primary defect (Abstract). Gastroenterology 1981; 80:1156.
326. Holdstock G, Chastenay BF, Krawitt EL. Increased suppressor cell activity in inflammatory bowel disease. Gut 1981; 22:1025–30.
327. Hanauer SB, Kluskens LF, Yan SZ, Kraft SC. Monoclonal antibody studies of circulating lymphocytes in Crohn's disease (Abstract). Chicago: American Gastroenterological Association, May, 1982.
328. Goodacre RL, Bienenstock J. Reduced suppressor cell activity in intestinal lymphocytes from patients with Crohn's disease. Gastroenterology 1982; 82:653–8.
329. Shorter RG, ReMine SG, Bartnik W. T cells and concanavalin A–induced suppressor cell activity in vitro in colonic inflammatory bowel disease. *In*: Pena AS, Weterman IT, Booth CC, Strober W, eds. Recent Advances in Crohn's Disease. The Hague: Martinus-Nijhoff, 1981.
330. Pena AS, Cnossen J, Damsteeg WGM, Weterman IT, Meijer CJLM. T-cell subpopulations in Crohn's disease. *In*: Pena AS, Weterman IT, Booth CC, Strober W, eds. Recent Advances in Crohn's Disease. The Hague: Martinus-Nijhoff, 1981.
331. Victorino RMM, Hodgson HJF. Spontaneous suppressor cell function in inflammatory bowel disease. Dig Dis Sci 1981; 26:801–6.
332. Elson CO, Graeff AS, James SP, Strober W. Covert suppressor T cells in Crohn's disease. Gastroenterology 1981; 80:1513–21.
333. Clancy R. Isolation and kinetic characteristics of mucosal lymphocytes in Crohn's disease. Gastroenterology 1976; 70:177–80.
334. Bookman MA, Bull DM. Characteristics of isolated intestinal mucosal lymphoid cells in inflammatory bowel disease. Gastroenterology 1979; 77:503–10.
335. Bland PW, Richens ER, Britton DC, Lloyd JV. Isolation and purification of human large bowel mucosal lymphoid cells: Effect of separation technique on functional characteristics. Gut 1979; 20:1037–46.
336. Chiba M, Shorter RG, Thayer WR, Bartnik W, ReMine S. K-cell activity in lamina proprial lymphocytes from the human colon. Dig Dis Sci 1979; 24:817–22.
337. Arnaud-Battandier F, Bundy BM, O'Neill M, Bienenstock J, Nelson DL. Cytotoxic activities of gut mucosal lymphoid cells in guinea pigs. J Immunol 1978; 121:1059–65.
338. Fiocchi C, Battisto JR, Farmer RG. Gut mucosal lymphocytes in inflammatory bowel disease (isolation and preliminary functional characterization). Dig Dis Sci 1979; 24:705–17.
339. Goodacre R, Davidson R, Singal D, Bienenstock J. Morphologic and functional characteristics of human intestinal lymphoid cells isolated by a mechanical technique. Gastroenterology 1979; 76:330–8.
340. Bartnik W, ReMine SG, Chiba M, Thayer WR, Shorter RG.

Isolation and characterization of colonic intraepithelial and lamina proprial lymphocytes. Gastroenterology 1980; 78:976–85.
341. Selby WS, Janossy G, Jewell DP. Immunohistological characterization of intraepithelial lymphocytes of the human gastrointestinal tract. Gut 1981; 22:169–76.
342. Fiocchi C, Battisto JR, Farmer RG. Studies on isolated gut mucosal lymphocytes in inflammatory bowel disease. Dig Dis Sci 1981; 26:728–38.
343. MacDermott RP, Franklin GO, Jenkins KM, Kodner IJ, Nash GS, Weinrieb, IJ. Human intestinal mononuclear cells. I. Investigation of antibody-dependent, lectin-induced and spontaneous cell-mediated cytotoxic capabilities. Gastroenterology 1980; 78:47–56.
344. MacDermott RP, Bragdon MJ, Jenkins KM, Franklin GO, Shedlofsky S, Kodner IJ. Human intestinal mononuclear cells. II. Demonstration of a naturally occurring sub-class of T cells which respond in the allogeneic mixed leukocyte reaction but do not affect cell-mediated lympholysis. Gastroenterology 1981; 80:748–57.
345. MacDermott RP, Jenkins KM, Franklin GO, Weinrieb IJ, Nash GS, Kodner IJ. Antibody-dependent (ADCC), spontaneous (SCMC) and lectin induced (LICC) cellular cytotoxicity by human intestinal lymphocytes (Abstract). Gastroenterology 1979; 76:1190.
346. Chiba M, Bartnik W, ReMine SG, Thayer WR, Shorter RG. Human colonic intraepithelial and lamina proprial lymphocytes: Cytotoxicity in vitro and the potential effects of the isolation method on their functional properties. Gut 1981; 22:177–86.
347. Monteiro E, Fossey J, Shiner M, Drasar BJ, Allison AC. Anti-bacterial antibodies in rectal and colonic mucosa in ulcerative colitis. Lancet 1971; 1:249–51.
348. Brandtzaeg P, Baklien K. Immunohistochemical studies of the formation and epithelial transport of immunoglobulins in normal and diseased human intestinal mucosa. Scand J Gastroenterol 1976; 11(Suppl 36):1–45.
349. Baklien K, Brandtzaeg P. Comparative mapping of the local distribution of immunoglobulin-containing cells in ulcerative colitis and Crohn's disease of the colon. Clin Exp Immunol 1975; 22:197–209.
350. Engstrom JF, Arvanitakis C, Sagawa A, Abdou NI. Secretory immunoglobulin deficiency in a family with inflammatory bowel disease. Gastroenterology 1978; 74:747–51.
351. Ryan FP, Verrier-Jones J, Wright JK, Holdsworth CD. Impaired immunity in patients with inflammatory bowel disease and hyposplenism. The response to intravenous ø174. Gut 1981; 22:187–9.
352. Soltoft J, Petersen L, Kruse P. Immunoglobulin deficiency and regional enteritis. Scand J Gastroenterol 1972; 7:233–6.
353. Hodgson HJF, Jewell DP. Selective IgA deficiency and Crohn's disease: Report of two cases. Gut 1977; 18:644–6.
354. Thayer WR Jr, Charland C, Field CE. *Escherichia coli* 014 and colon hemagglutinating antibodies in inflammatory bowel disease. Gastroenterology 1976; 71:369–84.
355. Surrenti C, Ramarli D, Cassini A, Scarabelli S, Campi P, Fauci A, Nieri S. Studies of cell-mediated immunity in patients with Crohn's disease. Hepato Gastroenterol 1981; 28:157–9.

Chapter 125

Epidemiologic Aspects of Inflammatory Bowel Disease

Albert I. Mendeloff

In this chapter we propose to deal with those forms of inflammatory bowel disease for which no specific etiologic agent or agents can be identified. Although exact data are not available, experience with amebiasis, lymphopathia venereum, and shigellosis persuades that each one can on occasion result in various chronic inflammatory reactions which may persist long after the initial inciting pathogen has disappeared, or at least cannot be isolated. At some stages of this progression to chronicity it is possible to confuse the clinical, radiologic, proctoscopic, and perhaps biopsy appearance of the bowel so affected with the lesions one associates with Crohn's disease or with ulcerative colitis. In epidemiologic investigations, the varying percentages of the total inflammatory bowel diseases in the population that actually represent chronic features of these specific etiologic entities may serve to distort the true state of events. In fact, some of the earliest clinical data obtained on poorly defined population groups were those on patients having "chronic bacillary dysentery" and those with chronic "thromboulcerative colitis" in which a diplostreptococcus was supposedly isolated. Unfortunately, errors in diagnosis are difficult to correct during the course of epidemiologic studies. These must be completed within a finite time period. Furthermore, all such studies are subject to classification errors which may, if sufficiently unidirectional or of great magnitude, mislead the investigators.

This chapter discusses those more recent studies of the distribution in populations of: (1) Crohn's disease (CD); (2) ulcerative colitis (UC), as carefully defined by the investigators; and (3) those small numbers of patients in whom the total clinical picture resembles both of the diseases in one respect or another and must therefore be classified as indeterminate or mixed. The discussion will be limited to studies in which a reasonable attempt to define the population at risk has been carried out and rigorous diagnostic criteria have been applied to classification of the diseases in the patients. In some studies, not only have data for incidence and prevalence been acquired, but other characteristics of the population suffering from these disorders have been compared with control populations of various types. Although such investigations have been carried out for only 3 decades, a surprising degree of agreement on many details has been obtained.

Methodologic Problems

Subjects with chronic disease move from an undifferentiated pool of "normal" subjects into the category of patients carrying a definite "diagnosis." This fact provides the background for the statistical treatment of clinical data which can then be translated into epidemiologic terms. The term "clinical" refers to the bedside, and clinical data refer to manifestations of disease in people who are ill. "Epidemiologic" data refer to the total population, both well and sick; techniques are available for predicting or identifying certain features of the population which are more or less concentrated in the ill, as compared to healthy members of that population.

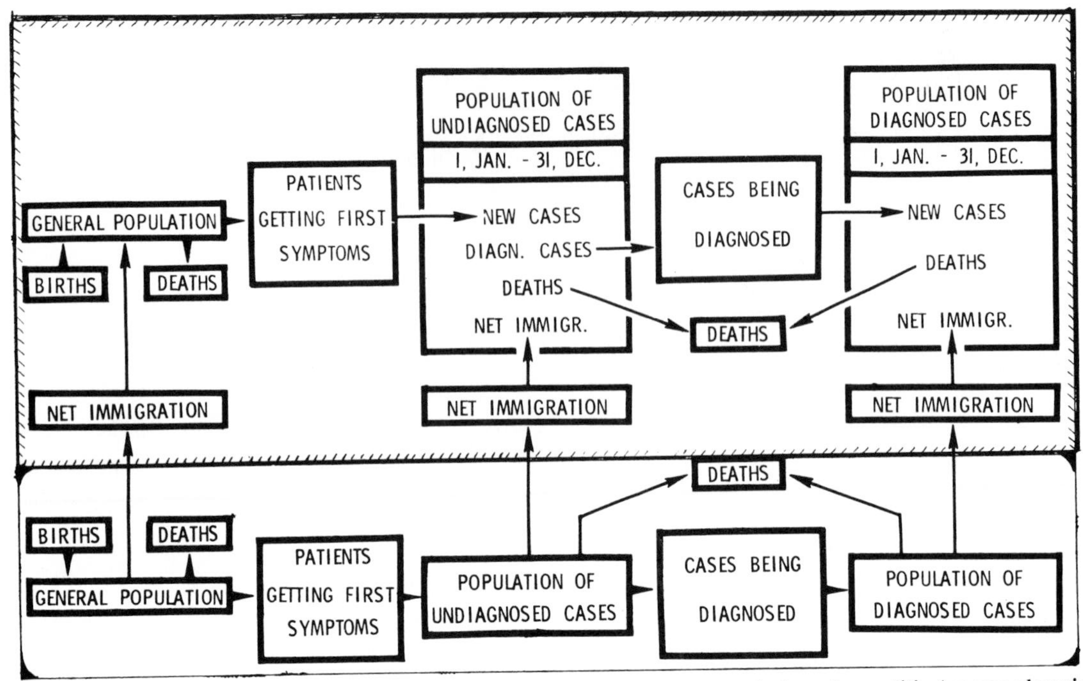

Figure 125–1. Scheme for identifying diagnosed and undiagnosed areas of ulcerative colitis (or any chronic disease) in a total population. The upper rectangle represents the population in one geographic area. The lower rectangle represents the remainder of the country of which the smaller population is a part (Adapted from Iversen et al.[16])

An excellent example of the use of such a hypothesis has been published by Iversen et al.[16] for ulcerative colitis in the entire country of Denmark and is reproduced with some modifications as Figure 125–1. In Table 125–1 the same authors tabulate the number of cases diagnosed definitely as ulcerative colitis per year against the number of years of symptoms preceding the point in time at which the diagnosis was made. Such data can be plotted in a diagram which, when compared with general population data, gives a dynamic concept of the rate of occurrence of this disease per 100,000 persons at risk per year, i.e., *the annual incidence rate.* In this same total population there is, furthermore, a number which represents all the patients afflicted with disease at any one point in time, i.e., the *prevalence* of the disorder per 100,000 persons at risk. Furthermore, there is a movement *into* the population under study of those persons who have already been diagnosed elsewhere, as well as a movement *out* of the study group of those persons physically emigrating or dying, whether from the disease in question or from other causes.

A properly conceived study of the magnitude of the problem created by any disease requires: (1) careful criteria for ascertainment of cases; (2) reasonably good data for the time of onset of the disorders; (3) demographic characterization of the specific population from which the patients are drawn;

Table 125–1. DECREMENT TABLE FOR UNDIAGNOSED CASES OF ULCERATIVE COLITIS IN COPENHAGEN COUNTY*

Years After First Symptoms	Remaining Patients	Diagnosis	Deaths	Diagnosis Rate
0	1000	387	13	0.39
1	600	109	9	0.18
2	482	75	7	0.16
3	400	47	6	0.12†
4	347	39	5	0.11
5	303	89	19	0.07
10	195	67	12	0.08
15	116	35	8	0.07†
20	73	22	5	0.07
25	46	19	3	0.10
30	24	21	3	—
Total	—	910	90	—

*From Iversen ED et al. Scand J Gastroenterol 1968; 3:593. Reproduced with permission.

†Three years after onset of first symptoms, 12% of the total group of patients are first diagnosed, and even 15 years after first onset of symptoms 7% of patients are first diagnosed.

Table 125–2. INCIDENCE OF ULCERATIVE PROCTOCOLITIS (UP) AND CROHN'S DISEASE (CD) PER 100,000 POPULATION

Area	Reference No.	Years	Average Incidence (Both Sexes)	
			UP	*CD*
Oxford, United Kingdom	9	1951–1960	6.5	0.8
Baltimore, United States	27	1960–1963	4.6	1.8
Copenhagen, Denmark	6	1961–1967	7.3	
	15	1960–1970		1.3
Norway	30	1964–1969		0.9
Rochester, Minnesota, United States	33	1935–1964	7.2	
Tel Aviv, Israel	12	1961–1970	3.7	
Malmö, Sweden	7	1958–1973		4.3
Uppsala and Västmanland, Sweden	4	1956–1961		1.8
		1962–1968		3.3
Aberdeen, United Kingdon	19	1960–1969		4.5
	20	1973–1975		2.6
15 areas, United States	11	1973	5.7	4.8

(4) some idea of the natural history of the disease, e.g. its severity, case-fatality rate, modification by treatment; and (5) educated guesses about the possible errors which might distort the results, including temporal trends in reporting, ascertainment, and treatment. Such a study would provide minimal but essential data which could contribute to ideas concerning possible etiologic factors; not to *prove* them to be true, but to provide evidence that they are or are not *likely* to be true.

In the diseases here discussed, the childhood population is usually rather poorly studied because of the reluctance of physicians to submit children to radiologic, endoscopic, and biopsy procedures. In the total population, patients with the mildest symptoms will probably not consult physicians and thus will be missed completely; hospitalized cases tend not to include patients who are minimally ill, especially in those countries which do not provide ready hospitalization at no out-of-pocket cost to the patient. In countries in which private practitioners of radiology see many patients in their offices, full tabulations of diagnosed cases are less likely to be attained, especially in urban areas, by those conducting the epidemiologic study. The fatality rates generally reflect what happens to those most severely ill patients seen in the larger treatment centers.

Incidence and Prevalence

In Tables 125–2 and 125–3 are summarized data thought by the author to be based on what I consider to be the best population information in published studies. Although there are many reports now in the literature from many parts of the world recording incidence and prevalence rates, insufficient confidence can be placed either in their reference population bases, or on the rigor with which the diagnoses were arrived at, to warrant including them with other more precisely defined studies.

Table 125–3. RANGE OF INCIDENCE AND PREVALENCE OF IBD WORLDWIDE IN 1980 PER 100,000 WHITES*

Disease	Incidence	Prevalence
Ulcerative proctitis	3–8	40–100
Ulcerative proctocolitis	2–7	40–100
Crohn's disease	1–7	10–100
Total	6–22	90–300

*Composite of 11 reports (data among non-white populations too scanty for inclusion).

Significance of Epidemiologic Data

It is the purpose of this chapter to ask certain key questions, and then to see whether epidemiologic data are available to answer them.

Geographic Areas. Are there geographic areas or climatic belts which are characterized by very high or very low frequencies of patients with these disorders? Although there are highly varying differences in the reported incidence of inflammatory bowel diseases throughout the world, there are no areas which careful search has found to be free of these disorders. High frequencies of specific infections and parasitic infestations have tended to obscure underlying non-specific inflammations, especially of the colon. When knowledgeable experts have looked for the latter, they have found them even in the presence of active parasitization. Chronic disorders of the colon (e.g., polyps, diverticulosis, and cancer) have been noted most often in Western populations, and it is in the Western part of the world that the most reliable health data have been acquired. There are no significant reasons to believe that geography or climatic variables, *per se*, play decisive roles in determining the incidence and prevalence of chronic inflammatory bowel diseases. However, dietary factors, by influencing both the frequency of stools and the bacterial population of the colon, may well contribute to the variable course of the diseases and the development of malignancy in the bowel harboring such chronic disorders.

Age-Sex Factors. Is there a definable population which is specially subject to one or the other of these inflammatory bowel disorders? In order to assemble the data needed to answer questions about a population, one would first of all look into the age-sex distribution of the patients. Among countries with population stock of predominantly English origin, there is a distinct female preponderance in UC and possibly also in CD. In countries with a heavy admixture of other racial and ethnic backgrounds, Crohn's disease appears about equally in men, and the female predominance in UC is less marked. Both disorders affect children, with those under age 6 years more often attacked by UC. Unselected series show the bulk of cases first being identified between ages 15 and 35 for both disorders, although new cases are identified at all ages.

For UC, a number of series, but by no means all, have shown a secondary peak of incidence for new cases beginning about age 50[11,21] (Fig. 125–2). Since this secondary peak is rather inconstant and numerically low, it has been thought by some workers that perhaps a different population is being attacked. This could be a population with vascular susceptibility, so that, accordingly, the disease in these older subjects may actually be a variant of ischemic colitis. The evidence to support this supposition is not convincing,

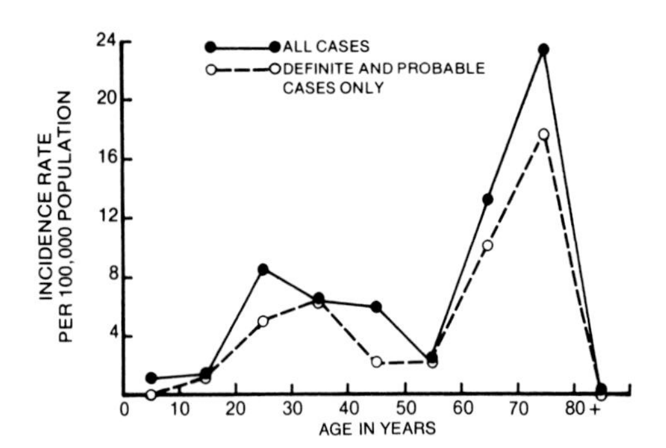

Figure 125–2. Annual age-specific incidence rates in ulcerative colitis per 100,000 population; white males, 15 PAS areas, 1973. (From Garland C et al. Gastroenterology 1981; 81:1115. Reproduced with permission.)

but the behavior of inflammatory bowel disease (IBD) among the elderly does merit careful study.[21] For both CD and UC, data from 1965 to 1980 show that bimodality in women is clear (Fig. 125–3). The sharp increase in the rates for women aged 15 to 40 may be related to worldwide use of oral contraceptives in that population. In the age group over 60, CD of the descending colon can certainly coexist with diverticulitis, or can simulate it. The occasional small localized lesion of CD of the descending colon may also look like an ischemic lesion and progress to stricture.

In summary, both these diseases occur at all ages, with maximal onset in the second through fourth decades in both sexes; later onset is not uncommon, but may result from predisposing factors of which the most rea-

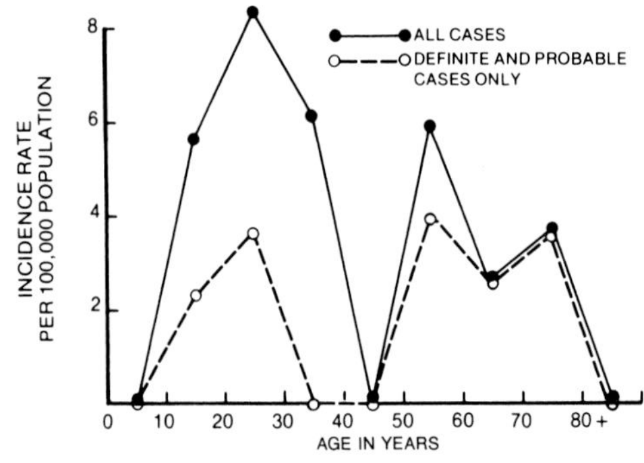

Figure 125–3. Annual age-specific incidence rates of Crohn's disase per 100,000 population; white female, 15 PAS areas, 1973. (From Garland C et al. Gastroenterology 1981; 81:1115. Reproduced with permission.)

sonable may be vascular disease. There are no epidemiologic data suggesting that a transmissible causative agent is responsible for either disease.

On the basis of age-sex data, except for the diseases in early childhood, there is no convincing evidence that a different population is affected by CD as compared with UC.[22, 23]

Race. Are certain racial and ethnic groups especially vulnerable? In those few studies in which it has been possible to characterize populations of meaningful size into such rubrics, the data strongly suggest that, from 1960 to 1970, United States blacks and American Indians were at low risk for both these diseases. In the Baltimore study,[28] the black population, which has good access to hospital facilities, was one-third as likely to be affected by UC and one-fifth as likely to have CD as was the white population. There is no inherent reason to expect this ratio to remain low, nor is there evidence that the diseases behave differently in blacks than whites. In fact, both diseases increased in United States blacks in the 1970s.[11] There are too few cases so far reported to determine if familial clusters also are more common among blacks than chance would warrant. Deaths in the United States by race and sex from 1959 to 1961 have been specially analyzed by Mendeloff and Dunn[24] and appear in Table 125–4.

Reports of inflammatory bowel disease among other non-white peoples in South America, Africa, and Asia cannot be given in statistically meaningful terms, but do indicate that the diseases are noted in these populations. In New Zealand, whose white citizens have prevalence figures for UC similar to those of their English forebears, that disease occurs perhaps one-twentieth as frequently among native full-blooded Maoris.[36]

Ethnic Groups. In England, in 1950, Paulley[31] compared the proportion of Jewish patients with UC in 2 London hospitals. He found a 2-fold increase of the disease in Jews as compared with the proportion of total Jewish patients discharged from the 2 hospitals. In the United States, Acheson[1] found that of 2320 male veterans discharged between 1953 and 1957 from Veterans Administration hospitals with a diagnosis of either UC or CD, there were 4 times as many Jews as occurred in a 12.5% sample of all patients discharged in October, 1956, from these same hospitals. This predominance of Jews in the IBD group occurred regardless of their United States region of birth and even foreign country of origin. A study of CD among United States soldiers by Rappaport et al.[32] also noted a 4-fold increase among Jews in the population at risk. Brahme et al.[7] found a 5-fold increase in Jews with CD in Malmö, Sweden.

Monk et al.,[28] using 1960 census tract data in Baltimore, interviewed patients with UC, CD, irritable colon, diverticulitis of the colon, and cancer of the colon admitted to Baltimore hospitals from 1960 to 1963. They compared the findings to a census tract general population and to control populations matched for sex, age, ethnic group, and socioeconomic status. The frequency of UC among Jews was found to be about 3½ times the rate among non-Jews. For CD, the rate was 6 times higher for Jewish men and 3 times higher for Jewish women than the corresponding rates for non-Jews. In fact, if one subtracted all the Jewish patients with CD, the rates for the remaining white Baltimore population were

Table 125–4. DEATHS AND CRUDE DEATH RATES FOR CHRONIC ENTERITIS AND ULCERATIVE COLITIS (COMBINED) ACCORDING TO RACE, BY SEX (UNITED STATES 1959–1961)*

(ISC Code 572)

Race	Deaths			Death Rate/100,000		
	Total	*Male*	*Female*	*Total*	*Male*	*Female*
White	8832	4083	4739	1.9	1.7	2.0
Non-white	586	269	317	1.0	0.9	1.0
Black	544	241	303	1.0	0.9	1.0
Indian	16	8	8	1.0	1.0	1.0
Chinese	7	6	1	1.0	1.5	0.3
Japanese	12	8	4	0.8	1.2	0.5
Other	7	6	1	0.6	0.9	0.2

*From Mendeloff AJ, Dunn JP. Digestive Diseases. A Vital and Health Statistics Monograph of the American Public Health Association. Cambridge, Mass: Harvard University Press, 1971. Reproduced with permission.

identical to those found by Evans and Acheson[9] in their excellent study of the area around Oxford, England. A repeat study in Baltimore in 1973 confirmed the increased susceptibility of Jews to both diseases.[23]

Such findings must be considered highly significant and should contain leads concerning etiology. Additionally, familial cases are also more frequently encountered among Jewish patients, and these appear to have an earlier onset than those cases not clustered in families.[34] The reported failures of other investigators in Continental Europe and in England to identify a preponderance of Jews in the population subject to these diseases,[13,19] whether valid or not, do not make the data for United States Jews less impressive. Such striking differences ought to stimulate further efforts to identify genetic and environmental factors in the vulnerable population in the United States.[12,23]

Urban-Rural Distribution. Studies of the United States Army dischargees by Acheson and Nefzger[3] in 1944 showed a predominantly urban origin for those developing UC. More recent reports from many countries are somewhat unclear by virtue of difficulties in keeping urban-rural dwelling status separate from occupational factors. That both diseases exist in rural populations and may be increasing can be documented in a number of reports.[11,14] In the Baltimore study, urban-rural migration was not a significant feature; studies from the Uppsala district of Sweden and from Olmstead County, Minnesota, show very nearly comparable data for incidence and prevalence, and both are close to the figures generally accepted for urban areas[4,33] (Table 125–5). Only in Scotland has Kyle[19] reported what appear to be data to favor urban over rural frequency in CD, and this finding has disappeared more recently.[20]

Socioeconomic Factors. An exhaustive treatment of these data was carried out in Baltimore.[29] Once again, these features were not greatly different among those with IBD than among the control populations. In Denmark a high socioeconomic group characterized those with UC.[5] Others have likewise reported less controlled data to indicate that upper social classes are more vulnerable. I remain skeptical on this point and believe that little important new information is likely to be derived from pursuing this factor.

Familial Groupings. There is no simple mendelian genetic mechanism at work in the transmission of IBD.[18] Aggregate studies of familial occurrence almost invariably include families in which both UC and CD occur, although it is not unusual to have a family in which only UC or only CD is noted in more than one member. When this does occur, it is more likely to be CD. Since ferreting out cases of either disease in relatives of index cases is a function of the interest of the physician and of the cooperation of the families in submitting to the expensive and rather unpleasant studies necessary to document the diseases, the literature on familial incidence of these disorders almost certainly represents an underestimation of its magnitude.

A study of a selected population attending the University of Chicago Clinics has been reported by Singer et al.[34] The bias introduced by the selective nature of referrals to this group was counteracted in part by a random number selection of 150 controls without IBD, who were matched to 150 patients with these diseases. Of patients with these diseases, 17.5% reported definitely positive family histories; 4% of the control population had IBD in their families, and the diseased patients to whom the controls were

Table 125–5. INFLAMMATORY BOWEL DISEASE IN RELATIVES OF PATIENTS WITH THESE DISORDERS*

Condition	Number Studied	Positive Family History of IBD		Relative's Condition		
		No.	*%*	*Crohn's*	*UC*	*IBD*
Crohn's disease	165	35	21.2	20	18	2
Ulcerative colitis	171	25	14.6	3	21	6
IBD	12	1	8.3	0	1	0
Total	348	61	17.5			

*From McConnell RB, Lewkonia RM. Gut 1976; 17:235. Reproduced with permission.

matched had a family history of disease of 11.3%. Of the total familial occurrences, 16% were in 2 or more affected relatives per family group. In this entire study population, onset of disease among affected families was significantly at lower ages (i.e., less than age 20 rather than between the ages of 20 and 40) than among those without family histories. Jewish patients predominated in the total group (44% of the total) and significantly ($p < 0.01$) among the patients with positive family histories.

At the Cleveland Clinic, Farmer et al.[10] have investigated the family histories of 838 patients with IBD onset before the age of 21. Of 316 patients with UC, 29% had family histories positive for IBD. Of 522 patients with CD, 35% had positive family histories. Of all first-degree family members, 15% had IBD. There was a mean of 2.4 siblings per family. If one takes the prevalence of IBD to be 100/100,000, there is a 0.1% chance that any family member will have IBD. This experience is a convincing demonstration of the heightened risk for IBD in the families of subjects whose IBD occurs in childhood. Unfortunately, data from control families which would make these comparisons more precise are not available.

If more family members of all patients are investigated, the frequency of familial cases is much less. A more characteristic frequency distribution can be seen in Table 125–5. Nevertheless, there seems little question that these 2 forms of IBD are intermingled in families peculiarly susceptible to the development of these disorders; it would be reasonable to assume that special studies of families would be of great importance.

Studies of distribution of ABO blood groups, secretor status, and HLA types in the IBD population have yielded either conflicting results or negative associations with either UC or CD.[10,18,21]

Further Epidemiologic Studies

It is probable that further understanding of the determinants which cause certain persons to manifest these disorders will not come from the rather gross and imprecise classifications I have attempted to define above. It will probably be necessary to make more intensive studies of families and to analyze the prevalence of other better understood disorders in these families, as well as more sophisticated studies of genetic and metabolic markers. More intensive psychologic studies also are called for, but can be carried out only in small numbers. The few family constellation studies by psychiatrists are totally uncontrolled.[17]

Interrelationships with Other Diseases. It is of significance that the same kinds of systemic and local "complications" characterize both UC and CD.[35] Aphthous stomatitis, erythema nodosum, uveitis, and pyoderma gangrenosum are observed in patients with either of these inflammatory bowel diseases, and complications such as liver enlargement and various hepatic inflammatory responses may be found in each. The common denominator here may be colonic involvement, with implication of colonic bacterial flora as the mediators. It is true that in the present stage of our knowledge the frequencies with which such phenomena are observed differ in the 2 diseases. This is unlikely to prove to be of fundamental importance, however, and may reflect physician interest and assiduity rather than anything else.

Of the tissue responses known to have an existence independent of their relationship to bowel inflammation, the most fascinating are the arthritides (Chapters 126, 127, 253). Only one well characterized disease in the general population seems to occur with increased frequency in patients with bowel disorders, i.e., ankylosing spondylitis.[26] The association between HLA-B27 and ankylosing spondylitis is about 80%. The spondylitis is thought to be transmitted as an autosomal dominant trait, with the presence of IBD making the development of this disorder much more likely. The reasons for this are not clear,[2,18,22] and the association between ankylosing spondylitis and IBD may or may not have epidemiologic inferences.

The problem of defining sacroiliitis as a form of ankylosing spondylitis is not an easy one; many of the observations made thus far have used the spine as it appears on barium enema radiographs as the basis for diagnosis.

The *irritable colon syndrome* was formerly thought by some physicians to be a predisposing factor, if not an early stage, in the genesis of IBD. This is actually a very rare situation provided rigorous criteria are maintained for diagnosis. Since both irritable colon syndrome and IBD tend to have their onset in adolescence and early adult life, the disorders are usually fairly distinct from each other by the time the patients consult physicians. There are no convincing studies that demonstrate a transition from one to the other when proper diagnostic methods are used. Studies derived from the Baltimore surveys by Mendeloff et al.[25] show that the irritable colon group differs in many important ways from patients with UC. Lactose intolerance, which has been reported in subjects with a wide variety of bowel disorders and is probably the norm rather than the exception for the world's non-white population, probably has no specific relationship to the pathologic processes identified in IBD, although it may contribute to the presenting symptoms.

There is probably good reason to pursue sophisticated attempts with genetic markers and linkage patterns to characterize the entire population at risk and to follow up such leads (Table 125–6). Although the state of the art does not permit identification as yet of those specific markers that are likely to be of greatest importance, it does not make good sense to abandon our efforts when the science of immunogenetics is making such rapid progress. A comparison of Jews in the United States suffering from IBD with their relatives in other countries would seem to be a study of considerable importance, for example, inasmuch as environmental factors may also be more precisely evaluated when genetic factors are held in control.[12]

The most intriguing and most difficult area to evaluate in terms of population dynamics is that of psychosocial influences. Few would deny that most chronic disorders, once established, fluctuate in intensity in accordance with overt or repressed reactions to interpersonal conflicts and to anxieties arising in the course of daily life. It may never be possible to arrive at etiologic hypotheses with studies directed at populations larger than single families. It is unlikely that the kinds of information obtained from subjects queried as to the established facts of their lives (their childhood, their schoolings, their "stresses," the loss of close friends or relatives) will be able to provide evidence for serious internal disharmony at a level which will permit serious hypotheses and attempts to test them.[17] Data of this type were acquired in Baltimore[29] and analyzed both in patients and in control populations, including those suffering from various serious disorders of the gastrointestinal tract other than IBD and from the irritable colon syndrome. Analyses of these data did not provide evidence that patients who went on to suffer the complications of IBD had "unhealthy" past histories, or that their lives contained significantly more "precipitating factors" than did the controls. In fact, the irritable bowel group showed a marked predominance in their "stress index" over all the other groups. For those students of IBD who believe that the "helplessness" of such patients can only be brought out in the setting of intensive psychologic probing, results of this sort might be anticipated. For those who would like to be able to apply mental health techniques at levels applicable to populations larger than the single patient, such results are disappointing.

Table 125–6. GENERAL CHARACTERISTICS OF POPULATION AT HIGH RISK FOR INFLAMMATORY BOWEL DISEASE

1. Roughly equal in men and women
2. Worldwide, but with marked variations: more common in Western and Eastern European stock
3. Slightly more urban than rural
4. More white than non-white
5. More Jewish than expected on the basis of proportion of population
6. Definite familial aggregations of both ulcerative colitis and Crohn's disease
7. Associated disorders (spondylitis)

Epilogue

What directions, then, is the epidemiologic approach to IBD to take if meaningful data bearing on etiology and control are to be gained? First, it would be helpful to be able to define a group of people at high risk of acquiring the disease. Thus far the best way for doing this is to identify those families in which multiple cases have already appeared. A very intensive study of the members of such families, preferably when young and existing as a family group, may entail genetic, psychologic, and certain metabolic analyses (including gut content measurements) of those still unaffected, with follow-up at various intervals and attempts to correlate initiation of the disease process with some change in environment—physical or psychologic.

For those whose illness appears sporadically, it would be desirable to confirm associations with other disorders, such as spondylitis, or with an enteric infection, drug reaction, or other identifiable illness.

For children who show full-blown evidence of UC, data on the prevalence of malignancies of the gut in their ancestors would be of value. Tests revealing inability to detoxify known carcinogens, or the presence of unusual immunologic reactions (including those to oncogenic viruses) are needed.

Children who first manifest UC before age 15 develop carcinoma of the colon before age 40 at rates far greater (10% to 33%) than those found in persons first diagnosed as having colitis at age 20 or above (perhaps 1% to 4%).[8] Since almost all carcinoma is first identified 10 years or more after the diagnosis of the underlying IBD is established, the sheer longevity of the inflammation is probably important in carcinomatous change, but other factors promoting neoplasia must also be at work. Crohn's disease also is beginning to show evidence of malignant associations we aquire more familiarity with its natural history, and it will be important to acquire from such patients as much information as can be of benefit to the proper management of their illness.

It is necessary to prevent confusion between the features of the naturally occurring disease and those which result from interactions of unknown constitutional factors with the potent anti-inflammatory and possibly immunologically destructive therapeutic agents we employ to treat them. Epidemiologic methods can serve as guides in such an endeavor. They help us to set up the criteria that permit us to determine the trends in incidence and prevalence which will throw further light on these vexing problems. Most Western gastroenterologists are convinced that both UC and CD have been increasingly prevalent in Western populations. There is now evidence, however, that plateaus have been reached and the diseases may actually be declining in frequency.[14,20] Although not apparent in earlier studies, an association with non-smoking of cigarettes has been recently reported for patients with ulcerative colitis.[37,38] In contrast to patients with Crohn's disease, who smoke cigarettes as frequently as does the general population, patients with ulcerative colitis have significantly higher rates for never having smoked, and some patients have reported remission of disease after beginning to smoke.[39] How these new findings can be reconciled with the failure in the past 25 years to identify any association, positive or negative, with cigarette smoking or how they bear on the emergence of the disease in children or in the elderly is unclear. However, if data can be replicated in other studies, some new hypothesis must be developed, *viz.* that cigarette smoking does play a role, in a genetically susceptible population, in determining which disease is likely to be manifested.

References

1. Acheson ED. The distribution of ulcerative colitis and regional enteritis in United States veterans with particular reference to the Jewish religion. Gut 1960; 1:291–3.
2. Acheson ED. An association between ulcerative colitis, regional enteritis, and ankylosing spondylitis. Q J Med 1960; 29:489–99.
3. Acheson ED, Nefzger MD. Ulcerative colitis in the United States Army in 1944. Gastroenterology 1963; 44:7–19.
4. Bergman L, Krause U. The incidence of Crohn's disease in central Sweden. Scand J Gastroenterol 1975; 10:725–9.
5. Bonnevie O. A socioeconomic study of patients with ulcerative colitis. Scand J Gastroenterol 1967; 2:129–36.
6. Bonnevie O, Riis P, Anthonisen P. An epidemiological study of ulcerative colitis in Copenhagen county. Scand J Gastroenterol 1968; 3:432–8.
7. Brahme F, Lindstrom C, Wenckert A. Crohn's disease in a defined population. Gastroenterology 1975; 69:342–51.
8. Devroede G, Taylor WF, Sauer WG, Jackman RJ, Stickler GB. Cancer risk and life expectancy of children with ulcerative colitis. N Engl J Med 1971; 285:17–21.
9. Evans JG, Acheson ED. An epidemiological study of ulcerative colitis and regional enteritis in the Oxford area. Gut 1965; 6:311–24.
10. Farmer RG, Michener WM, Mortimer EA. Studies of family history among patients with inflammatory bowel disease. Clin Gastroenterol 1980; 9:271–8.
11. Garland C, Lilienfeld A, Mendeloff AI, Markowitz JA, Terrell KB, Garland FC. Incidence rates of ulcerative colitis and Crohn's disease in fifteen areas of the United States. Gastroenterology 1981; 81:1115–24.
12. Gilat T, Ribak J, Benaroy Y, Zemishlany Z, Weissman I. Ulcerative colitis in the Jewish population of Tel Aviv-Jaffa. Gastroenterology 1974; 66:335–42.
13. Goligher JC, deDombal FT, Watts JM, Watkinson G. Ulcerative Colitis. Baltimore: Williams & Wilkins, 1968.
14. Hellers G. Crohn's disease in Stockholm County 1955–74. Scand J Gastroenterol (Supp 490), 1979.
15. Höj L, Brix-Jensen P, Bonnevie O, Riis P. An epidemiological study of regional enteritis in Copenhagen County and Gentofte municipality. Scand J Gastroenterol 1973; 8:381–4.
16. Iversen EO, Bonnevie O, Anthonisen P, Riis P. An epidemiological model of ulcerative colitis. Scand J Gastroenterol 1968; 3:593–610.
17. Jackson DD, Yalom I. Family research on the problem of ulcerative colitis. Arch Gen Psychiatry 1966; 15:410–8.
18. Kirsner JB. Genetic aspects of inflammatory bowel disease. Clin Gastroenterol 1973; 2:557–75.
19. Kyle J. An epidemiological study of Crohn's disease in northeast Scotland. Gastroenterology 1971; 61:826–33.
20. Kyle J, Stark G. Fall in the incidence of Crohn's disease. Gut 1981; 21:340–3.
21. Langman MJS. Epidemiology of Chronic Digestive Disease. Chicago: Year Book Medical Publishers, 1979, Chapter 4.
22. Lewkonia RM, McConnell RB. 1976 familial inflammatory bowel disease—heredity or environment? Gut 1976; 17:235–43.
23. Mendeloff AI. The epidemiology of inflammatory bowel disease. Clin Gastroenterol 1980; 9:259–70.

24. Mendeloff AI, Dunn JP. Digestive Diseases. A Vital and Health Statistics Monograph of the American Public Health Association. Cambridge, Mass, Harvard University Press, 1971: 53.
25. Mendeloff AI, Monk M, Siegel CI, Lilienfeld A. Illness experience and life stresses in patients with irritable colon and with ulcerative colitis. N Engl J Med 1970; 282:14–7.
26. Moll JMH, Haslock I, Macrae IF, Wright V. Associations between ankylosing spondylitis, psoriatic arthritis, Reiter's disease, the intestinal arthropathies and Behcet's syndrome. Medicine 1974; 53:343–64.
27. Monk M, Mendeloff AI, Siegel CI, Lilienfeld A. An epidemiological study of ulcerative colitis and regional enteritis among adults in Baltimore. I. Hospital incidence and prevalence. Gastroenterology 1967; 53:198–210.
28. Monk M, Mendeloff AI, Siegel CI, Lilienfeld A. An epidemiological study of ulcerative colitis and regional enteritis among adults in Baltimore. II. Social and demographic factors. Gastroenterology 1969; 56:847–57.
29. Monk M, Mendeloff AI, Siegel CI, Lilienfeld A. An epidemiological study of ulcerative colitis and regional enteritis among adults in Baltimore. III. Psychological and possible stress-precipitating-factors. J Chron Dis 1970; 22:565–78.
30. Myren J, Gjone E, Hertzberg JN, Rygvold O, Semb L, Fretheim B. Epidemiology of ulcerative colitis and regional enterocolitis (Crohn's disease) in Norway. Scand J Gastroenterol 1971; 6:511–4.
31. Paulley JW. Ulcerative colitis: Study of 173 cases. Gastroenterology 1950; 16:566–76.
32. Rappaport HF, Burgoyne H, Smetana HF. The pathology of regional enteritis. Milit Surg 1951; 109:463–501.
33. Sedlack RE, Nobrega FT, Kurland LT. Inflammatory colon disease in Rochester, Minnesota, 1935–1964. Gastroenterology 1972; 62:935–41.
34. Singer HC, Anderson JGD, Frischer H, Kirsner JB. Familial aspects of inflammatory bowel disease. Gastroenterology 1971; 61:423–30.
35. Truelove SC. Course and prognosis. *In*: Engel A, Larsson T, eds. Regional Enteritis (Crohn's Disease). Skandia International Symposia. Stockholm: Nordiska Bokhandeln Forlag, 1971: 116.
36. Wigley RD, MacLurin BP. A study of ulcerative colitis in New Zealand, showing a low incidence in Maoris. Br Med J 1962; 2:228–31.
37. Harris AD, Baird A, Rhodes J. Non-smoking: a feature of ulcerative colitis. Br Med J 1982; 281:706.
38. Vick H, Walker AM. Cigarette smoking and ulcerative colitis. N Engl J Med 1983; 308:261–83.
39. Vick H, Walker AM. Cigarette smoking and ulcerative colitis. N Engl J Med 1983; 308:1477–8.

Chapter 126

Ulcerative Colitis

Richard G. Farmer • Stanley R. Hamilton • Basil C. Morson • George N. Stein • Philip J. Sabri • Victor W. Fazio

History and Epidemiology

Richard G. Farmer

Inflammation of the colon and rectum with predominant ulceration can be found clinically under many different circumstances. Included among these are specific infections, association with systemic diseases, and an idiopathic condition for which no specific cause is as yet known. For over 100 years the last condition has been referred to as "ulcerative colitis" and has become one of the major chronic digestive diseases encountered in clinical practice in the Western world. Because the illness affects a predominantly young population and is associated with remissions and exacerbations, the numerous facets of the disease can create many different types of problems that are difficult for the physician to manage and the patient to endure.

Specific infectious agents (e.g., ameba, *Shigella, Campylobacter,* and the toxin-producing *Clostridium difficile*) can be associated with a type of ulcerative colitis. In recent years, a colonic inflammation has been found with the acquired immunodeficiency syndrome (AIDS) (Chapter 121). Systemic diseases such as uremia, sickle cell anemia, vasculitis, or the so-called collagen diseases (Chapter 244) may also have colonic ulcerations as one of their manifestations. A form of hemorrhagic enterocolitis has been associated with food allergy (Henoch-Schönlein purpura) (Chapter 239), as a toxic reaction to mercury and gold compounds, and in association with radiation injury (Chapter 142). In addition, although not entirely similar clinically, are the colorectal inflammatory changes associated with ischemic colitis (Chapter 116), diverticulitis (Chapter 135), and Crohn's disease (Chapter 127).

Many different terms have been used to define ulcerative colitis in the past; most frequently either "non-specific" or "idiopathic" was used to emphasize the fact that no specific cause of the illness is known. Older terms included colitis gravis, colitis ulcerosa, and thrombo-ulcerative colitis. Ulcerative colitis may be defined as an acute, subacute, or chronic inflammation of the colon and rectum (proctocolitis) of unknown etiology or pathogenesis with the following features: (1) a variable course, unpredictable prognosis, and many local and systemic complications; (2) rectal bleeding, diarrhea, cramping abdominal pain, fever, anorexia, and weight loss as the principal symptoms; and (3) proctosigmoidoscopic and roentgen features that are usually diagnostic. It is predominantly a diffuse mucosal disease with continuous involvement without skip areas and is characterized pathologically by crypt abscesses, ulcerations, increased capillary formation, and vascular congestion.

History

The term "simple ulcerative colitis" first appeared in the literature in 1875, but, according to Goligher et al.,[1] a non-contagious type of diarrhea associated with colonic inflammation was recognized as early as about A.D. 300:

One fascinating and detailed early description of ulcerative colitis–like disease is attributed to Aretaeus of Cappadocia (c. A.D. 300). He described a large number of different types of diarrhea including one which consisted of chronic non-contagious diarrhea of a foul type found chiefly in adults, more common in women than in men, occasionally seen in elderly persons and in older children, but never found in infants! It is arguable that some cases of Crohn's disease or idiopathic steatorrhea might have been included under this heading but Aretaeus' account is one which many present day clinicians would accept as descriptive of ulcerative colitis. Certainly he has reproduced the age specific instances of this latter disease with uncanny precision! Similar though less precise descriptions of a condition like ulcerative colitis were recorded by a number of other physicians in Roman times including one from Ephesus (c. A.D. 117), whose name "Soranus" seems curiously apt.[42]

In 1859 Sir Samuel Wilks reported the necropsy findings of what we know as toxic megacolon in a letter to the Medical Times and Gazette.[2] In his description of "the morbid appearance of the intestine of Miss Banks" he observed "an erosion of the mucosa throughout all regions of the rectum and colon and terminal ileum with massive sloughing and hemorrhage." The medical officers of the Union Army during the American Civil War in 1865 described the pathologic and clinical features of what is now called ulcerative colitis in cases of "chronic diarrhea."[1] They emphasized changes in the crypts in their differentiation of this group of cases from others that were most likely due to dysentery or paratyphoid fever.

Credit, however, is usually given to Wilks and Moxon for naming and defining ulcerative colitis. In the second edition of their book, *Lectures on Pathologic Anatomy,* published in 1875, they described simple ulcerative colitis in a section on "Inflammations of the Large Intestine."[2]

The term colitis is sometimes used as though synonymous with dysentery. Our usual language has indeed been too indefinite, made incorrect in speaking of all affections of the large intestine as dysenteric; for the true dysenteric process, although in many features like simple ulcerative colitis, yet it is a disease having certain definite characters.

There is quite as much reason to regard febrile epidemic dysentery as a disease distinct from simple ulcerative colitis as there is to regard febrile epidemic dyphtheria as a disease distinct from croup. . . .

Cases of idiopathic colitis are rare and stand, as we have said, in the same relation to true dysentery as croup does to dyphtheria, from the absence of those peculiar features which give dysentery the characters of a specific fever. For example, we have seen a case attended by discharge of mucus and blood where, after death, the whole internal surface of the colon presented a highly vascular, soft, red surface, covered with tenacious mucus and adherent lymph, and here and there showing a few points of ulcerations; the coats, also were much swollen by exudation into the mucous and submucous tissues. In other examples there has been extensive ulceration, commencing in the follicles, and spreading from them to destroy the tissue around, thus producing a ragged ulcerated surface.

Within a decade other reports appeared in the literature calling attention to the association of liver disease with "simple ulcerative colitis." The observations of White[3] in 1895 remain an excellent description of the disease as it is now recognized.

Epidemiology

The frequency of ulcerative colitis differs geographically. Mendeloff[4] found the incidence (new cases/year/100,000 population) to be between 4.6 and 7.3 in various locations in North America and Europe. Ulcerative colitis has also been encountered with relative frequency in Australia, South Africa, Japan, and South America.

Over the past 25 years the number of new cases of ulcerative colitis has appeared to reach a plateau, in striking contrast to rapid increase in the observed numbers of new cases of Crohn's disease during the same period of time[5, 6] (Chapter 127). The fact that Crohn's disease appears to affect a similar population has created confusion in the interpretation of epidemiologic data. In addition, patients with ulcerative colitis have frequently been found to have a milder distal form of the disease, i.e., proctitis or proctosigmoiditis. This has been especially true in recent years. Incidence figures for ulcerative pancolitis have varied from 2 to 7 new cases/100,000 population in contrast with 3 to 8 new cases for the milder distal form of the disease. There is poor correlation, however, between patients having ulcerative colitis and those who have other types of colitis, particularly infectious colitis such as amebic dysentery, bacillary dysentery, and other specific forms of colitis.

Mendeloff[4] has described 6 characteristics of patients with ulcerative colitis: (1) sex distribution is nearly equal; (2) patients are more commonly Western than Oriental and more often Northern European, Anglo-Saxon, or Eastern European; (3) the disease is more prevalent among those living in urban areas; (4) the disease is more common among whites than blacks; (5) it is more common among Jews living in Europe and North America than among non-Jews, but is not common among Israelis; and (6) the disease is more common in families than occurrence by chance alone.

It is difficult to obtain epidemiologic data in the United States because of the difficulty of defining a specific population and because of referral patterns of patients with ulcerative colitis.[7] In other countries, however, this has been possible, and data from Denmark have shown findings similar to those of Mendeloff.[4] Binder and her colleagues[8] studied a total of 909 patients seen in Copenhagen County from 1962 to 1978; the mean incidence was 8.1/100,000 population. It should also be noted that because of the chronic nature of the illness, prevalence figures are much higher than incidence figures.

References

1. Goligher JC, deDombal FT, Watts JMcK, et al. Ulcerative Colitis. London: Bailliere, Tindall & Cox, 1968.
2. Wilks S, Moxon W. Lectures on Pathological Anatomy. 2nd Ed. London: J & A Churchill, 1875.
3. White WH. Colitis. Lancet 1895; 1:537.
4. Mendeloff AI. The epidemiology of inflammatory bowel disease. Clin Gastroenterol 1980; 9:259–70.
5. Hellers G. Crohn's disease in Stockholm County 1955–1974. A study of epidemiology, results of surgical treatment and longterm prognosis. Acta Chir Scand 1979; 490(Suppl):1–84.
6. Mayberry J, Rhodes J, Hughes CE. Incidence of Crohn's disease in Cardiff between 1934 and 1977. Gut 1979; 20:602–8.
7. Kirsner JB, Shorter RG. Recent developments in "nonspecific" inflammatory bowel disease. N Engl J Med 1982; 306:775–85.
8. Binder V, Both H, Hansen PK. Incidence and prevalence of ulcerative colitis and Crohn's disease in the county of Copenhagen 1962–1978. Gastroenterology 1982; 83:563–8.

Pathology

Stanley R. Hamilton • Basil C. Morson

Gross Pathologic Appearances

The pathologic findings in ulcerative colitis depend upon the severity, the clinical phase, and the duration of the disease.[1] The dominant features of ulcerative colitis are its predominance of involvement in the left colon and its continuous distribution (Fig. 126–1).

Ulcerative colitis virtually always involves the rectum to produce proctitis, although steroid enemas may mask this distribution.[2] The more proximal regions of the colon are variably involved to produce proctosigmoiditis or proctocolitis, which may be left-sided, subtotal, or even total. The rectum generally shows the greatest evidence of chronicity of the process. The involvement of the proximal areas occurs in continuity with the rectum, although the intensity of the abnormalities may show some variation. The transition from grossly abnormal to grossly normal colon at the proximal end of the diseased area may be either gradual over several centimeters or abrupt.

In the early phases, ulcerative colitis shows only mucosal congestion and increased peristalsis *in vivo*. With active chronic disease, the mucosa becomes granular, velvety, and friable with superficial erosions such that the mucosa can be wiped off. As the disease continues, the involved areas lose their haustra and become flat (Fig. 126–1). Oozing of blood from the mucosa provides gross pathologic evidence of increased vascularity associated with active disease. When ulceration occurs in ulcerative colitis, the ulcers are usually in the midst of grossly abnormal mucosa. They are usually irregular, but linear longitudinally oriented ulcers that overlie the taenia coli occasionally occur. With inactive longstanding ulcerative colitis, the mucosa becomes thin, pale, and smooth, referred to as featureless and atrophic (Fig. 126–2).

The mucosa sometimes shows polyps, i.e., structures that protrude into the lumen from a mucosal surface. These develop in ulcerative colitis as a result of ulceration combined with mucosal regeneration. Inflammatory

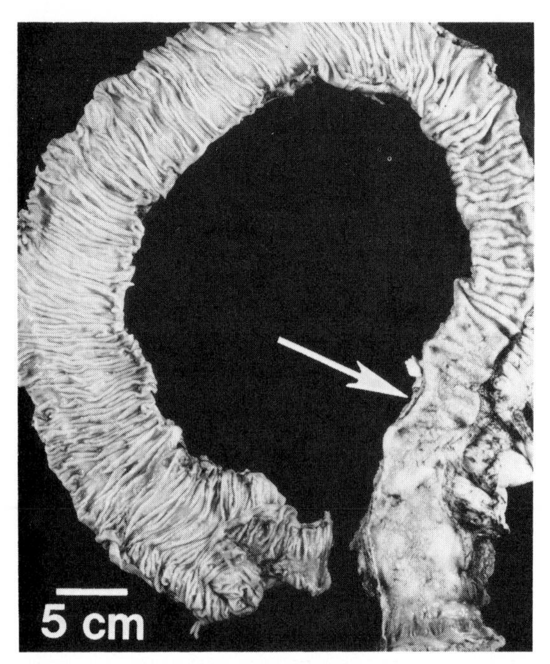

Figure 126–1. Ulcerative colitis in total proctocolectomy specimen demonstrating left-sided predominance and continuous distribution. The rectum and sigmoid colon show absence of folds and coarsely granular mucosa *(arrow)*. The descending colon has reduced numbers of abnormal, thickened folds with finely granular, congested mucosa that blends into the grossly normal mucosa of transverse and right colon.

polyps are often referred to as "pseudopolyps" because they are not adenomas; however, "inflammatory polyp" is the preferable term. Inflammatory polyps are more common in the colon than in the rectum in ulcerative colitis, suggesting that mechanical factors play a role in pathogenesis. Inflammatory polyps may be single or multiple, sessile or pedunculated. When large numbers are present, the term "inflammatory polyposis" is often applied (Fig. 126–3). Pedunculated inflammatory polyps sometimes form mucosal bridges across the colonic lumen. In rare instances, exuberant giant inflammatory polyps develop.[3]

The colonic wall in ulcerative colitis is usually grossly normal, as the condition is for the most part a disease of the mucosa. The colonic length and diameter may be reduced, however, owing to contracture of the muscularis mucosae and muscularis propria associated with abnormal muscle function. Strictures and fistulas are rare. The serosal surface usually shows only vascular congestion beneath areas of active inflammation.

The terminal ileum is normal in the vast majority of cases. In about 10% of cases,

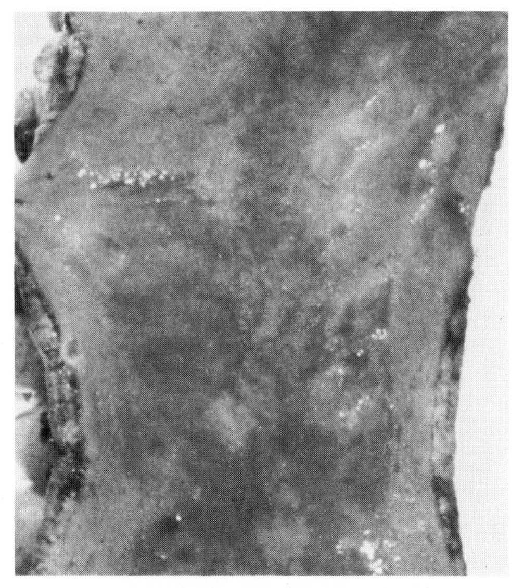

Figure 126–2. Atrophic, "featureless" mucosa in longstanding ulcerative colitis. Haustra are absent and the mucosal surface is smooth. See Figure 126–7*B* for histopathologic findings. (Shown 1/2 ×.)

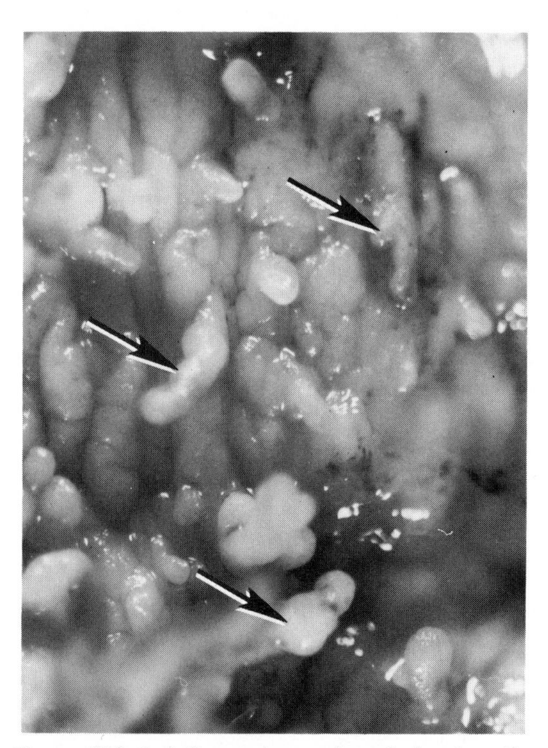

Figure 126–3. Inflammatory polyposis in ulcerative colitis. Numerous irregularly shaped fronds *(arrows)* extend into the lumen from the mucosal surface. (Shown actual size.)

dilatation of the terminal ileum for several centimeters proximal to the ileocecal valve is present. The mucosa is usually reddened and granular without plicae. This abnormality, termed "backwash ileitis," is usually associated with a rigidly dilated incompetent ileocecal valve, which allows backflow of colonic contents into the terminal ileum. Erosions, ulcers, and inflammatory polyps occasionally occur.

The appendix is involved in many cases, but the inflammation is confined to the mucosa and does not usually produce transmural appendicitis with peritonitis.[4]

The anus is usually normal in patients with ulcerative colitis. The abnormalities, when present, include acute fissures, abscesses, and excoriations, but ordinarily not deep fistulas.

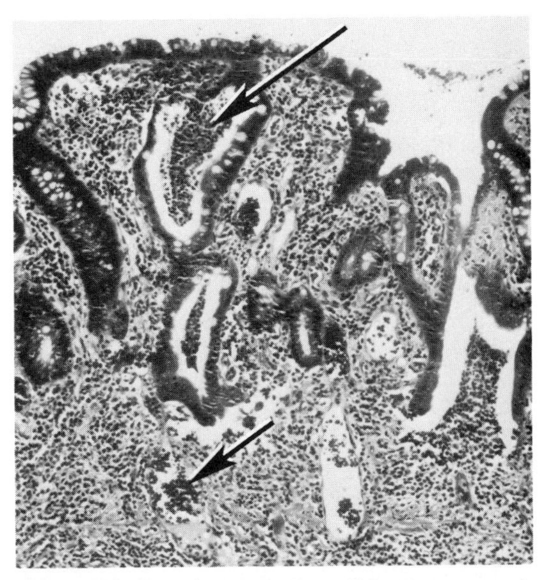

Figure 126–4. Active ulcerative colitis. Numerous dilated, congested capillaries *(short arrow)* and multiple crypt abscesses containing acute inflammatory exudate *(long arrow)* are present. The goblet cell population and mucin content are markedly reduced. The lamina propria is diffusely and uniformly infiltrated by acute and chronic inflammatory cells. Distortion of crypt architecture is apparent. (Hematoxylin and eosin, × 100.)

Histopathology

Ulcerative colitis is a dynamic disease characterized by remissions and exacerbations. The histopathologic findings show great variability related to disease activity, duration, and site examined. For purposes of clinical correlation, the spectrum of histopathologic features can be divided into findings of: (1) active disease; (2) low-grade active disease, which sometimes represents a spontaneous or therapeutically induced remission; and (3) inactive disease.

Active disease is defined by the presence of prominent acute inflammation (Fig. 126–4). Striking vascularity characterized by dilatation and congestion of blood vessels occurs in the mucosa and submucosa, accompanied by relatively little edema. The inflammatory infiltrate includes prominent neutrophils in crypt and surface epithelium as well as in the lamina propria. Crypt abscesses are conspicuous and are characterized by crypt epithelial necrosis with fibrinoinflammatory exudate filling the dilated lumen. Surface epithelial erosions with exudate may also be seen. Goblet cell numbers and mucin content are characteristically reduced or absent in active disease. Reactive epithelial changes with enlarged, hyperchromatic nuclei and prominent mitotic figures are a manifestation of increased epithelial proliferation in response to injury. Chronic inflammation involves the lamina propria in a diffuse manner with all areas relatively uniformly infiltrated. The chronic inflammatory infiltrate includes prominent plasma cells with an admixture of lymphocytes and eosinophils. Foreign body giant cells are occasionaly seen in areas of ulceration. Crypt destruction and loss with distortion of remaining crypts are prominent in chronic disease (Fig. 126–5). Mucosal erosions and ulcers, when present, occur in the midst of such mucosa. Dense fibrosis is not usually seen with ulcerative colitis, but villiform and polypoid regeneration of the mucosa sometimes produces irregularity of the mucosal surface. The muscularis mucosae may show chronic inflammation and hypertrophy. Because ulcerative colitis is a mucosal disease, the submucosa is often normal but sometimes shows chronic inflammation of the superficial portions, particularly with severe active disease (Fig. 126–5). Mucosal inflammation exceeds submucosal inflammation in such cases. The submucosa and muscularis propria are not inflamed in uncomplicated ulcerative colitis (see later discussion of Fulminant Colitis). Regional lymph nodes usually show non-specific reactive hyperplasia.

Low-grade active ulcerative colitis shows lessening of the findings associated with active inflammation (Fig. 126–6). Heavy infiltration

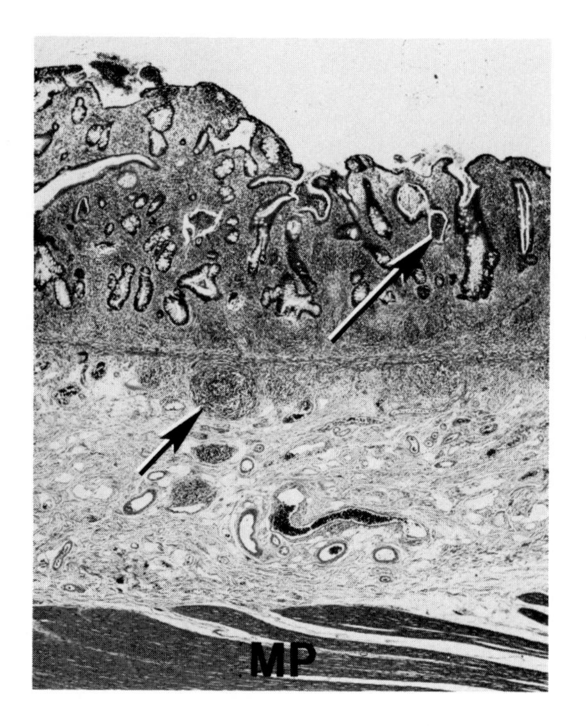

Figure 126–5. Active longstanding ulcerative colitis. The mucosa shows multiple crypt abscesses *(long arrow)*, marked crypt distortion, and regeneration that produce irregularity of the luminal surface; diffuse acute and chronic inflammation involving the lamina propria in a uniform fashion; and reduced epithelial mucin. The superficial submucosa shows aggregates of chronic inflammatory cells *(short arrow)* beneath the muscularis mucosae, but the deep submucosa and muscularis propria (MP) are uninvolved. (Hematoxylin and eosin, × 18.)

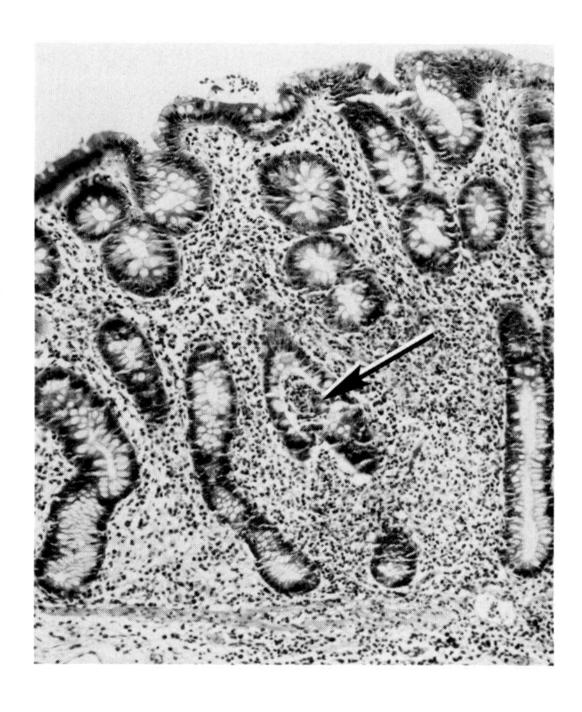

Figure 126–6. Low-grade active ulcerative colitis. A crypt abscess with acute inflammatory exudate *(arrow)* in the lumen is present, but the goblet cell population and mucin content are greater than in active disease. In addition, inflammation of the lamina propria is less intense and patchy in distribution. Distortion of crypt architecture is apparent. (Hematoxylin and eosin, × 100.)

of the mucosa by neutrophils, crypt abscesses, and vascularity are no longer prominent features. The population of goblet cells and their mucin content return toward normal. Reactive epithelial changes are often prominent in the bases of crypts where epithelial proliferation occurs. The chronic inflammatory cell infiltrate becomes patchy, with a reduction in the numbers of plasma cells and lymphocytes and with uneven distribution. Eosinophils, however, often remain prominent.[5] Crypt distortion usually persists.

Inactive ulcerative colitis is defined by lack of acute inflammation (Fig. 126–7). Chronic inflammation of the lamina propria, including prominent eosinophils, may persist for long periods of time after cessation of activity. Crypt architectural changes are even more persistent and may be found in the absence of chronic inflammation (Fig. 126–7*A*). Mucosal atrophy with decreased numbers of crypts and thinning of the distance between the muscularis mucosae and the surface epithelium is usually accompanied by crypt distortion with loss of parallel arrangement, uneven distribution, and branching of remaining crypts (Fig. 126–7*B*). Shortfall of crypts with increased distance between the bases of the crypts and the muscularis mucosae also occurs. Other findings in inactive ulcerative colitis include Paneth cell metaplasia[6] of crypt epithelium, increased epithelial mitoses, and thickening of the muscularis mucosae, particularly in the rectum. On the other hand, the muscularis mucosae is often absent in areas of previous ulceration where mucosal regeneration occurs on the submucosa.

The temporal sequence of active, then low-grade active, and finally inactive ulcerative colitis may be seen in one anatomic site (e.g., the rectum) with therapeutically induced or spontaneous remission of active disease. Some patients, however, continuously have low-grade active disease in which the features of active disease are muted. An anatomic sequence of active, then low-grade active, and finally inactive disease can usually be seen as one proceeds proximally to examine the colon of an individual patient. In particular, grossly normal mucosa proximal to evident ulcerative colitis often shows findings of inactive disease, characterized by crypt distortion, chronic inflammation of the lamina propria, and reactive epithelial changes including increased crypt mitoses. As a result, *endoscopic and radiographic examinations underestimate the extent of abnormal mucosa in ulcerative colitis.*

Inflammatory polyps show a spectrum of histopathologic findings. Some are composed only of inflamed granulation tissue devoid of epithelial elements. Most show redundant proliferation of glands in a stroma of fibrous connective tissue with inflammation. The glands are often misshapen and dilated. The surface of inflammatory polyps frequently shows areas of ulceration, and reactive epithelial changes may be striking. Inflammatory polyps appear to develop as a consequence of ulceration combined with regeneration; they do not represent merely remnants of non-ulcerated mucosa. Evidence

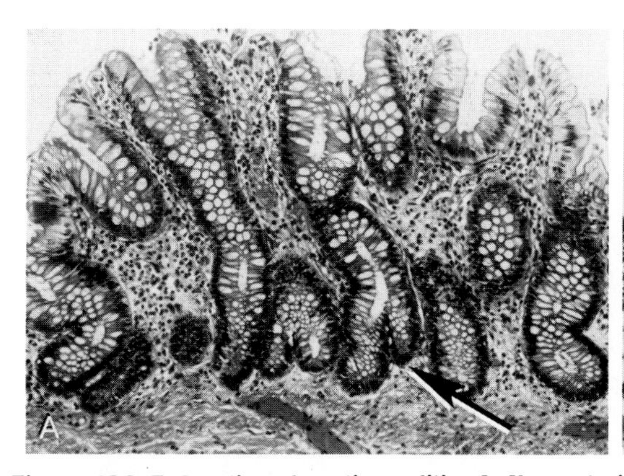

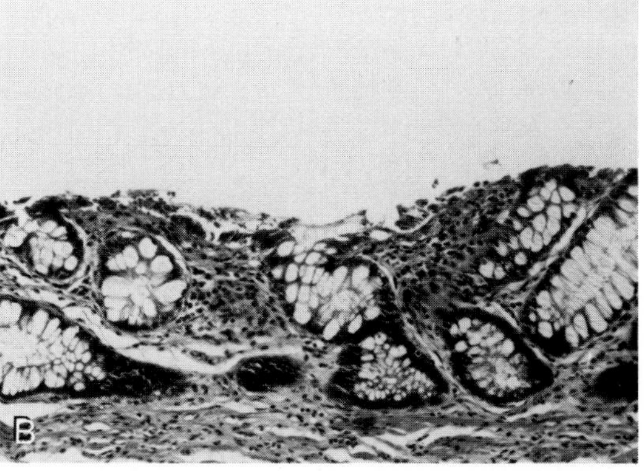

Figure 126–7. Inactive ulcerative colitis. *A,* No acute inflammation is present and the lamina propria shows only mild chronic inflammation in this example. Distortion of crypt architecture, including forked crypts *(arrow)*, is present. *B,* Mucosal atrophy is characterized by marked thinning of the mucosa with distorted crypt architecture. Specimen is from same patient as in Figure 126–2. (Hematoxylin and eosin, × 100.)

of regeneration is often seen in flat mucosa, but the formation of a polyp protruding into the bowel lumen depends upon exuberance of the regeneration and mechanical factors associated with movement of feces. Mechanical traction on the mucosa and submucosa contiguous to an area of regeneration that is pulled into the lumen by peristalsis leads to the formation of the stalk.

Benign strictures, when present, usually show hypertrophy of the muscularis mucosae[7] and sometimes the muscularis propria, rather than fibrosis. Strictures can also result from malignancy (see subsequent discussion of Carcinoma and Dysplasia).

Lymphoid hyperplasia is a prominent feature in some cases of ulcerative colitis. A striking increase in the rectum of the number of lymphoid nodules, many with prominent germinal centers, sometimes leads to displacement and distortion of the remaining crypts. This histopathologic pattern of ulcerative colitis is termed "follicular proctitis."

On histopathologic examination, "*backwash ileitis*" shows flat, atrophic ileal mucosa devoid of villi and with reduced numbers of crypts. Vascular dilatation with congestion and chronic inflammation is characteristic, but acute inflammation is usually absent, except when ulcers are present. Reactive epithelial changes are usually found, and the epithelium may acquire the characteristics of colonic epithelium, referred to as "colonic metaplasia" or "colonification."

Colonoscopic Biopsy. Biopsy of the terminal ileum, colon, and rectum through the colonoscope is now widely used in the assessment of patients with inflammatory bowel disease.[8–14] Biopsies are useful in primary diagnosis to demonstrate and document the presence of inflammatory bowel disease and to attempt to establish a diagnosis as to type. Differential diagnostic possibilities that can be evaluated in biopsy specimens include inflammatory bowel disease of known causes (e.g., infections and ischemia) as well as ulcerative colitis and Crohn's disease (Chapter 127). Colorectal biopsies are also useful for follow-up in patients with inflammatory bowel disease. Response of active disease to therapy can be evaluated, and development of dysplasia and malignancy complicating chronic inflammatory bowel disease can be detected (see later discussion of Carcinoma and Dysplasia).

Optimal interpretation of endoscopic biopsies requires communication and cooperation between endoscopists and pathologists. Endoscopists are responsible for the sampling procedures, which include the number and sites of the tissue specimens, and for documentation of the endoscopic findings, the biopsy sites, and the clinical history. Pathologists must decide upon the laboratory procedures to be used, including choice of fixative, specimen orientation procedure, and numbers of sections and stains (Chapter 47). Finally, the pathologist is responsible for assessing the clinical information and histopathologic findings to provide an accurate diagnosis and answers to the clinical questions to be answered by the examination of biopsy specimens.

Many of the pathologic findings of ulcerative colitis can be demonstrated in colonoscopic biopsy samples. The continuous nature of the disease is manifested by similarity in the histopathologic findings in specimens from the same region of the colon. The left-sided predominance of ulcerative colitis can be identified if multiple biopsies from various anatomic sites are submitted as separate specimens. In this way the proximal colon can be shown to be normal or less severely abnormal than the left colon and rectum. Ileal biopsy specimens usually lack active inflammation in ulcerative colitis. In addition to the anatomic distribution of findings, the histopathologic characteristics and distribution of inflammation in the lamina propria can also be assessed by biopsy. The findings in ulcerative colitis, however, are nonspecific; biopsy diagnosis rests upon the presence of consistent histopathologic features in a patient with an appropriate clinical history in whom other causes for the changes have not been identified.

Pathologic Features of Complications

Fulminant Colitis. In occasional patients, ulcerative colitis enters a fulminant phase. The transverse colon is most commonly affected, although there may have been no clinical evidence of previous ulcerative colitis there. The sigmoid colon is also a frequent site (Fig. 126–8). In advanced phases, the affected area is dilated (termed "toxic megacolon") and the wall is markedly thinned. The latter also is often extremely friable and may disintegrate with handling. Perforation with fibrinous or fibrinopurulent peritonitis is common. In the early phases, the colon

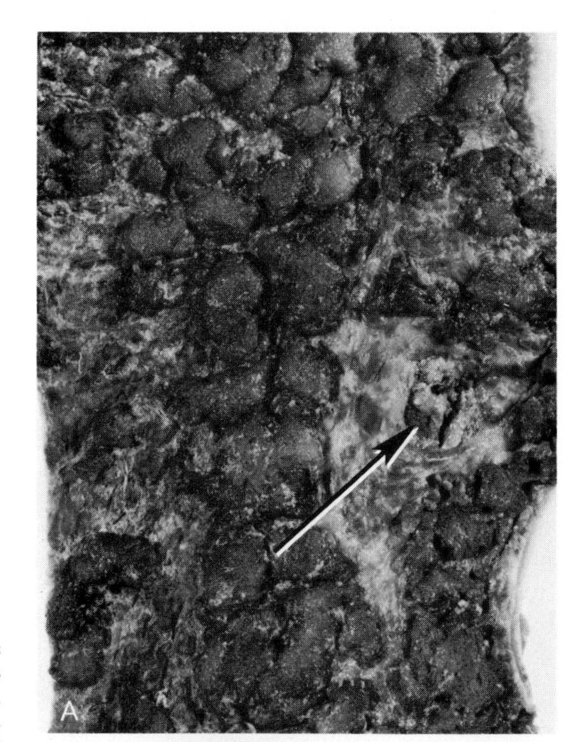

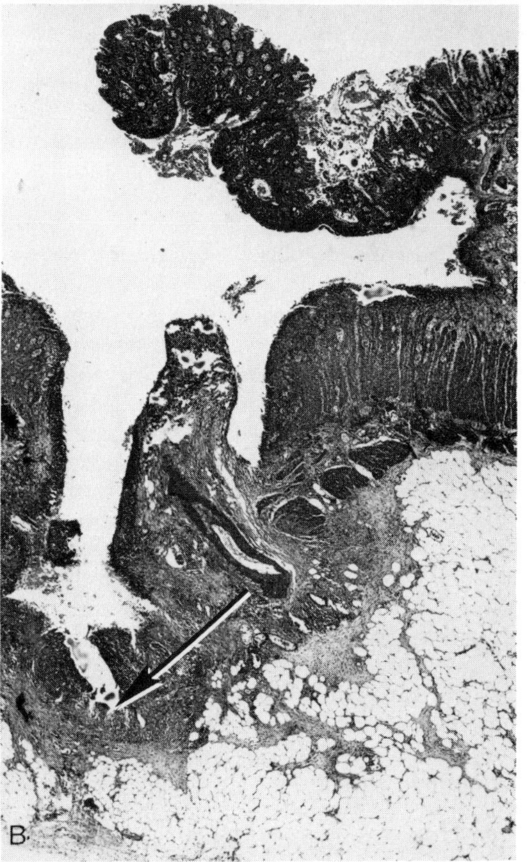

Figure 126–8. Fulminant ulcerative colitis. *A*, The sigmoid colon has irregular interconnecting ulcers surrounding islands of congested mucosa. Only mild dilatation of the colon is present, but perforation had occurred *(arrow)*. (Shown actual size.) *B*, Fissure-like ulcers undermine adjacent mucosa and extend through the muscularis propria into the pericolonic soft tissue *(arrow)*, representing incipient perforation. Striking vascular dilatation and congestion are present. The mucosa shows chronic but no acute inflammation; crypt architecture and goblet cell mucin are preserved. (Hematoxylin and eosin, × 18.)

may be of normal caliber but with intense serosal vascularity. The mucosal surface shows striking, extensive ulceration with congestion and hemorrhage (Fig. 126–8*A*). Sloughing of large areas of mucosa may occur, with islands of intact mucosa in their midst. The ulcers are often discrete and irregular.

On histopathologic examination, the ulcers appear acute with necrosis accompanied by marked vascular dilatation and congestion. However, there are relatively few inflammatory cells and little granulation tissue. The ulcers frequently extend through the submucosa into the muscularis propria and may appear fissured (Fig. 126–8*B*). The muscularis propria is often thin, with the fibers separated by edema and congested blood vessels. Muscle fiber necrosis is common and inflammation of blood vessels may be seen. Perforation results from transmural extension of ulcers into the peritoneal cavity. The islands of mucosa remaining in the midst of fulminant disease frequently show little active disease and maintenance of the goblet cell population. Submucosal edema is often prominent.

Fulminant ulcerative colitis may be mistaken for Crohn's disease because it frequently gives the appearance of proximal, discontinuous involvement on gross examination.[2, 14, 15] Furthermore, the transmural extension of the inflammation and the fissured appearance of the ulceration in fulminant ulcerative colitis may suggest Crohn's disease if the acute nature of the process is not recognized. However, evidence of proctitis is usually present, and recognition that the inflammatory bowel disease is in an acute phase allows circumspection in classification. Nonetheless, fulminant colitis is the most common factor leading to categorization of a resection specimen as colitis of indeterminate type (Chapter 127). Evaluation of previous or subsequent biopsy and resection specimens may be necessary to classify a patient with fulminant idiopathic colitis as having either ulcerative colitis or Crohn's disease.

Postoperative and Superimposed Inflammatory Bowel Diseases. Following total colectomy for ulcerative colitis, unrelated inflammatory bowel disease may develop in an ileostomy stoma or continent ileostomy pouch.[16, 17] These forms of inflammatory bowel disease may lead to confusion with Crohn's disease. In addition, colitis can occur in a rectal pouch from which the fecal stream has been removed after subtotal colectomy.[18] This form of inflammatory bowel disease has been termed "diversion colitis." Finally, infection with a number of pathogens (e.g., *Campylobacter, Clostridium difficile,* and cytomegalovirus) may be superimposed upon ulcerative colitis.[19–21]

Carcinoma. The pathologic and clinical features of large bowel carcinoma in many patients with idiopathic inflammatory bowel disease, particularly ulcerative colitis, are similar to those of usual large bowel carcinoma. Such similarity makes classification of these tumors as a complication of the inflammatory bowel disease uncertain, particularly in countries where large bowel carcinoma occurs frequently. On the other hand, the majority of colorectal carcinomas in patients with ulcerative colitis have pathologic features that distinguish them from usual large bowel cancer. First, the tumors arise in areas of colon involved by inflammatory bowel disease, which may either inactive or active, and may be multiple, in contrast to the usual rarity of synchronous colonic carcinomas. Unlike usual colorectal carcinoma, the tumors frequently are flat, infiltrating, and ill-defined on gross examination. Infiltration of the wall without formation of an exophytic luminal mass makes these carcinomas difficult to visualize, more like carcinoma of the stomach than usual large bowel carcinoma. Some of the tumors produce strictures, which appear benign on radiographic examination (Fig. 126–9*A*). In addition, the carcinomas are more commonly poorly differentiated and mucinous than the usual large bowel carcinomas (Fig. 126–9*B*). Finally, the carcinomas often appear to invade from areas of epithelial dysplasia, which may be flat, poorly circumscribed, and involve relatively large areas of mucosa (Fig. 126–10). These features of the precursor to the carcinomas complicating inflammatory bowel disease contrast with the discrete, well-demarcated, and typically polypoid areas of dysplasia, termed "adenomas," which are the precursor to the usual large bowel carcinoma.

Dysplasia. "Dysplasia" is the morphologic term applied to epithelial fetures that represent neoplastic alteration capable of giving rise to invasive carcinoma. The presence of dysplasia thus indicates that a patient's mucosa has acquired a neoplastic abnormality of the epithelium. The term "dysplasia" should

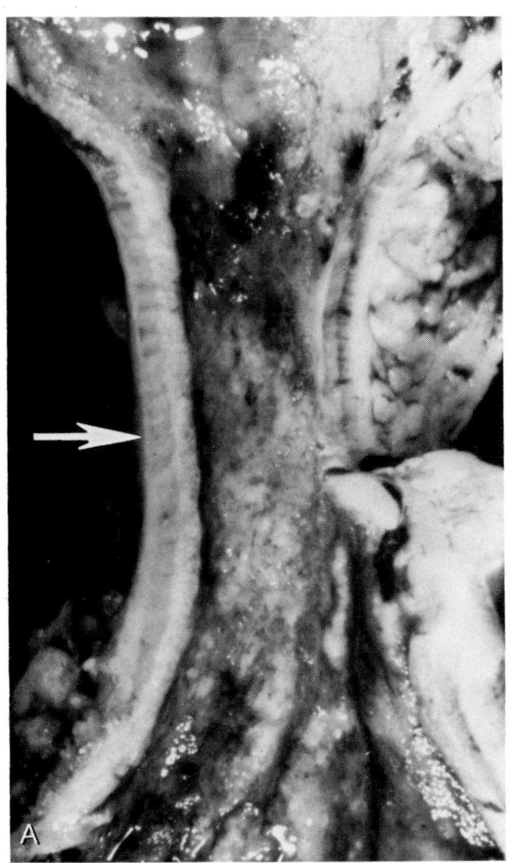

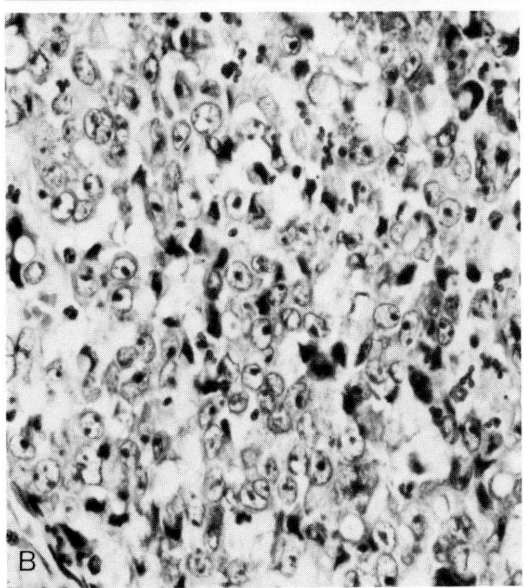

Figure 126–9. Carcinoma complicating ulcerative colitis. *A,* The carcinoma presented as a stricture in the sigmoid colon. The mucosal surface is granular without an intraluminal mass. The colonic wall is thickened *(arrow)* owing to hypertrophy of the muscularis propria associated with infiltration by carcinoma. *B,* On histopathologic examination, the tumor is a poorly differentiated adenocarcinoma. (Hematoxylin and eosin, × 390.)

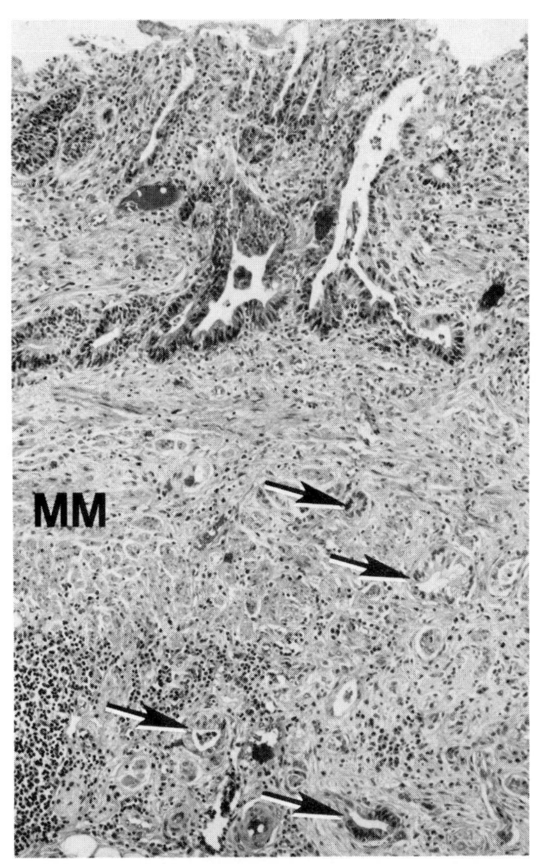

Figure 126–10. Carcinoma complicating ulcerative colitis. Adenocarcinoma *(arrows)* infiltrates insidiously through the thickened muscularis mucosae (MM) into the submucosa beneath a flat area of dysplasia. (Hematoxylin and eosin, × 100.)

not be used to describe reactive epithelial changes associated with active inflammation (which may be difficult to distinguish).

Accelerated colonic epithelial proliferation occurs in both active and inactive ulcerative colitis.[22] Of even greater interest, in long-standing disease inhibition of proliferation *in vitro* does not occur under conditions that are normally inhibitory.[23] The diagnosis of dysplasia, however, is based upon histopathologic criteria that include abnormal glandular or villiform architecture of the mucosa and abnormal epithelial characteristics. The epithelial criteria include increased size of nuclei with increased nuclear-to-cytoplasmic ratio, variation in nuclear size and shape, abnormal nuclear chromatin, increased size and number of nuclei, increased numbers of mitotic figures with abnormal forms, increased numbers of cells in the epithelium with pseudostratification and loss of nuclear polarity, and abnormal cytoplasmic differentiation. An example of abnormal differentiation is the occurrence of goblet cells with mucin vacuoles at the base, referred to as "upside-down" or "inverted" goblet cells. In addition, immunohistologic studies have demonstrated reduced immunoglobulin A and secretory component in dysplastic as compared with normal and reactive colonic epithelium.[24, 25]

For the most part, the histopathologic features of dysplastic epithelium complicating inflammatory bowel disease are similar to those in epithelium of adenomas. As a result, dysplasia complicating inflammatory bowel disease is often described as "adenomatous epithelium." Similarity of the features leads to problems in classifying polypoid adenomatous lesions in older patients with inflammatory bowel disease who are in the adenoma-bearing age range. The presence of dysplastic epithelium on the stalk suggests that the lesion represents polypoid dysplasia complicating inflammatory bowel disease, while the presence of normal epithelium on the stalk favors a usual adenoma.

On gross (and therefore endoscopic) examination, areas of dysplasia show a variety of appearances. Visible lesions are commonly nodular (Fig. 126–11), verrucous, or granular rather than pedunculated, but dysplasia in flat mucosa may not be detectable except by histopathologic examination. Dysplasia often has a patchy distribution. In patients with carcinoma complicating inflammatory bowel disease, dysplasia is commonly found in the rectum and surrounding or overlying the carcinoma; however, dysplasia may not be detected in these sites in some patients with carcinoma despite extensive histopathologic study. Nonetheless, development of dysplasia in inflammatory bowel disease appears to precede development of carcinoma by an interval of years.[26] As a result, detection of

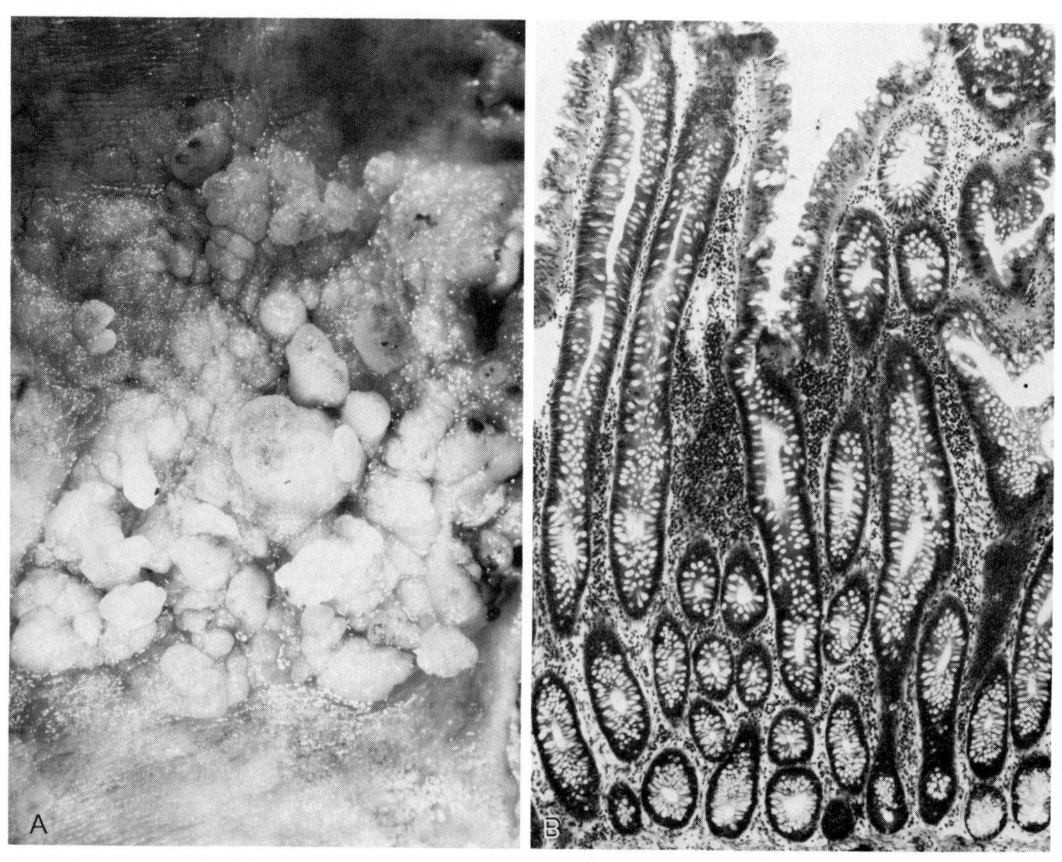

Figure 126–11. Dysplasia in ulcerative colitis. *A,* This nodular area of dysplasia was located in the transverse colon. (Shown 2 ×) *B,* On histopathologic examination, the area showed marked thickening of the mucosa by villiform low-grade dysplasia but no carcinoma. (Hematoxylin and eosin, × 60.)

dysplasia by endoscopic biopsy is an important strategy in the prevention or early detection of large bowel carcinoma in patients with longstanding inflammatory bowel disease (Chapter 128).

Interpretation of epithelial abnormalities in colorectal biopsy specimens as dysplasia sometimes poses a considerable problem. First, determining whether or not the abnormalities represent dysplasia is often complicated by the features of the underlying inflammatory bowel disease. With active inflammation, infiltration of epithelium and lamina propria by neutrophils results in cellular injury and reactive epithelial proliferation. The histopathologic features of these abnormalities may be difficult to differentiate from neoplastic epithelial proliferation. In addition, even with inactive disease, striking abnormalities of mucosal architecture with crypt distortion, inflammatory polyp formation, and villiform regeneration may simulate dysplasia (adenomas) of patients without inflammatory bowel disease. Although pathologists are generally facile in distinguishing neoplastic lesions, the variety of inflammatory and reparative findings in biopsies from patients with inflammatory bowel disease may pose a problem for those who do not deal with such biopsies on a regular basis. Furthermore, published criteria for dysplasia in inflammatory bowel disease vary. As a second aspect to the problem, once the pathologist decided that a lesion was dysplastic, no standardized terminology was available to express the findings.

To attempt to solve these problems, a group of pathologists from 10 institutions in the United States, England, and Sweden, where studies of dysplasia complicating inflammatory bowel disease were underway, formed the Inflammatory Bowel Disease Dysplasia Morphology Study Group.[27, 28] Based upon exchanges of histopathologic slide sets and discussions, the group developed a classification system and tentative management implications (Table 126–1).[29]

The classification system is composed of 3 main categories of findings: NEGATIVE, INDEFINITE, and POSITIVE (Fig. 126–12). NEGATIVE biopsies include normal tissue and the findings of inactive and active disease without any features raising the possibility of dysplasia. INDEFINITE biopsies include those with technical problems, such as artifacts of improper histopathologic procedures and insufficient tissue, as well as lesions for which a firm decision regarding the nature of the abnormalities cannot be made. Such lesions most commonly include atypical epithelium that could be considered dysplastic but is present in the setting of active disease (Fig. 126–12). The presence of abnormal epithelium of unknown significance also results in classification as INDEFINITE (e.g., epithelium with incomplete maturation characterized by prominent basal nuclei and absence of cytoplasmic mucin in cells along the entire crypt length, atypical epithelium associated with follicular proctitis, a polypoid lesion that would be classified as a hyperplastic polyp if the patient did not have

Table 126–1. INFLAMMATORY BOWEL DISEASE DYSPLASIA MORPHOLOGY STUDY GROUP CLASSIFICATION

Category and Subcategories	Management Recommendations*	
	No Endoscopic Lesion	*Endoscopic Lesion*
NEGATIVE for dysplasia		
Normal	Surveillance†	Surveillance†
Inactive disease	Surveillance†	Surveillance†
Active disease	Surveillance†	Surveillance†
INDEFINITE for dysplasia		
Probably negative	Surveillance†	Early rebiopsy‡
Unknown	Early rebiopsy‡	Early rebiopsy‡
Probably positive	Early rebiopsy‡	Early rebiopsy‡
POSITIVE for dysplasia		
Low-grade	Early rebiopsy‡ or consider colectomy§	Consider colectomy§
High-grade	Consider colectomy†	Consider colectomy§

*Management recommendations are subject to revision as data become available.

†Surveillance = continued regular yearly surveillance (Chapter 128).

‡Early rebiopsy = repeat colonoscopy with multiple biopsies in 3 to 6 months to reassess findings, preferably during quiescence of inflammatory bowel disease.

§Consider colectomy = consideration of colectomy *after confirmation* by multiple biopsies and/or by concurrence between 2 or more pathologists familiar with the classification system and criteria.

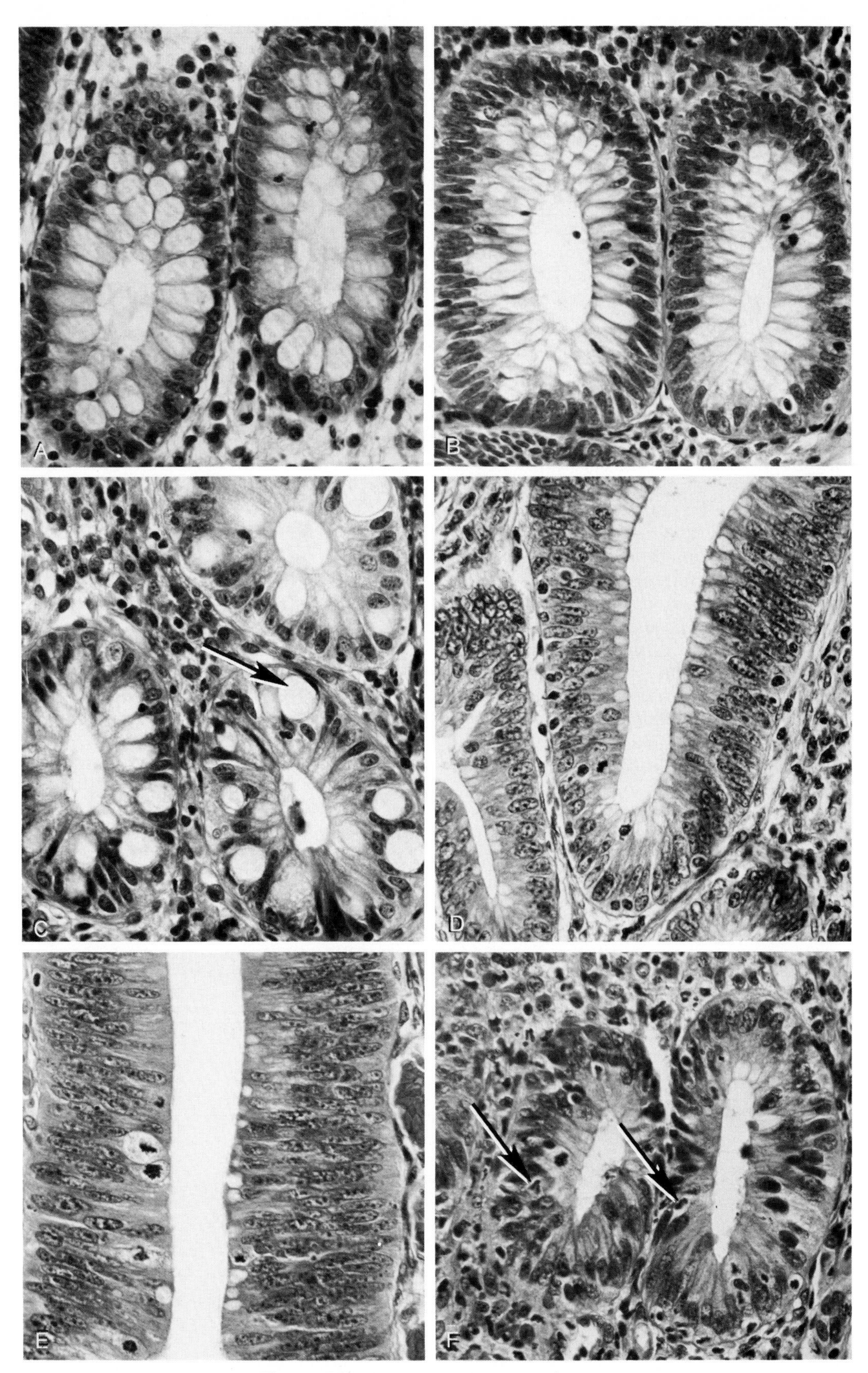

Figure 126–12. *See legend on opposite page*

inflammatory bowel disease). The INDEFINITE category is helpful in permitting pathologists to express uncertainty about a lesion that nonetheless causes them concern. The subgroups within the category are used to indicate the depth of their concern: INDEFINITE biopsies can be classified as probably negative, unknown, and probably positive.

POSITIVE biopsies are those that appear to have definite dysplasia representing unequivocal neoplastic changes. This category is subdivided into low-grade and high-grade, based upon the severity of the architectural and cytologic abnormalities. POSITIVE biopsies must be assessed carefully for the presence of invasive carcinoma accompanying the dysplasia.

Despite the development of histopathologic criteria for each category, disagreement over individual cases is expected because application of criteria is subjective in the final analysis. Experience with the system indicates that while NEGATIVE and high-grade POSITIVE biopsies generally show good intra- and inter-observer agreement, disagreements are more likely in the INDEFINITE and low-grade POSITIVE categories. As a result, review of the histopathologic findings in biopsies classified as INDEFINITE or POSITIVE by pathologists familiar with the classification system and criteria may be required before a decision is made regarding clinical management.

The suggested clinical responses to biopsy reports using the Inflammatory Bowel Disease Dysplasia Morphology Study Group Classification are summarized in Table 126–1 and are discussed later in this chapter. Modification of these tentative recommendations may occur as more data become available, but currently patients with NEGATIVE and INDEFINITE but probably negative biopsies taken randomly from flat mucosa are recommended for continued regular surveillance if no endoscopically or radiographically suspicious lesions are present. Patients with random biopsies from flat mucosa classified as INDEFINITE but unknown, INDEFINITE but probably positive, and low-grade POSITIVE are recommended for repeat examination with multiple additional biopsies from the suspicious areas. Biopsies taken during quiescence of the inflammatory bowel disease are preferred. Patients with random biopsies from flat mucosa classified as high-grade POSITIVE are recommended for colectomy after confirmation of the histopathologic findings by multiple biopsies and/or concurrence between 2 or more pathologists familiar with the classification system and criteria. When carcinoma is present in this situation, the tumors are often early (Dukes A).[30, 31] Patients with biopsies from suspicious endoscopic lesions classified as INDEFINITE are recommended for repeat examination with multiple additional biopsies, preferably during quiescence of the inflammatory bowel disease. If biopsies of suspicious lesions are POSITIVE, colectomy is advised after confirmation of the biopsy findings, because endoscopically evident lesions appear to result from dysplasia at a more advanced stage of development than dysplasia in flat mucosa. In addition, such lesions are associated with a higher proportion of invasive carcinoma,[32] and the carcinomas appear to be more advanced (Dukes B and C).[30, 31]

Differential Diagnosis

Distinction between ulcerative colitis and Crohn's disease of the colon poses a common

Figure 126–12. Illustrations of the Inflammatory Bowel Disease Dysplasia Morphology Study Group Classification. All photomicrographs show crypts and are at the same magnification. *A,* NEGATIVE for dysplasia. Crypt epithelium in inactive inflammatory bowel disease has small, rounded, regular nuclei located in the basal portion of the cells along the basement membane. *B,* POSITIVE for dysplasia. Low-grade dysplasia in this example shows hypercellular crypt epithelium with elongated nuclei, some of which are no longer located in the basal portion of the cells. The epithelial thickness is increased. Cytoplasmic mucin is abundant. *C,* POSITIVE for dysplasia. Low-grade dysplasia in this example shows enlarged rounded nuclei and prominent inverted goblet cells with mucin vacuoles in the basal rather than the apical portion of the cytoplasm. *D,* POSITIVE for dysplasia. High-grade dysplasia in this example shows hypercellular epithelium with enlarged nuclei having prominent chromatin clumps and parachromatin clearing. The epithelium is thickened and many nuclei are no longer located in the basal portion of the cells. Cytoplasmic mucin is reduced. *E,* POSITIVE for dysplasia. High-grade dysplasia in this example is histopathologically equivalent to carcinoma in-situ in an adenoma of a patient without inflammatory bowel disease. *F,* INDEFINITE for dysplasia. Epithelial findings resemble those in dysplasia (see panel *D* above for comparison), but numerous neutrophils *(arrows)* are present in the epithelium and lamina propria. The activity of the inflammatory bowel disease results in uncertainty regarding the classification of the epithelial findings as dysplasia. (All hematoxylin and eosin, × 355.)

problem in gastrointestinal pathology. The contrasting salient features are presented here and are considered as well in Chapter 127, which deals with Crohn's disease.

Ulcerative colitis begins in the rectum and spreads proximally in continuity for variable distances. Crohn's disease, on the other hand, is discontinuous. The rectum is often spared and, in contrast to ulcerative colitis, predominantly right-sided disease is more common than disease of the distal colon.

Disease of the terminal ileum is more common in Crohn's disease of the colon than in ulcerative colitis and the features are different. "Backward ileitis" in ulcerative colitis involves the terminal few inches of ileum, which is usually dilated with an incompetent ileocecal valve. The mucosal surface is usually granular and hemorrhagic. In contrast, the ileum involved by Crohn's disease is usually narrowed and shows ulceration, which is often serpiginous and fissuring with normal intervening mucosa.

Shortening of the colon, resulting from hypertrophy of the muscularis mucosae and muscularis propria, is prominent in ulcerative colitis, whereas fibrosis is the usual finding in Crohn's disease. Similarly, the strictures that occasionally occur in ulcerative colitis are due to muscle abnormality or malignancy, whereas fibrous strictures are common in Crohn's disease.

Fulminant colitis with toxic megacolon is an important complication of ulcerative colitis but is rare in Crohn's disease of the colon. Inflammatory polyposis is frequent in ulcerative colitis, but such polyps are seen only occasionally in Crohn's disease and then in fewer numbers and with a less uniform distribution. The anal lesions of ulcerative colitis are usually acute, whereas chronic anal involvement with fistulas and abscesses is frequent in Crohn's disease.

In histopathologic sections, ulcerative colitis shows inflammation confined to the mucosa for the most part, except in fulminant colitis. Crohn's disease is characterized by transmural inflammation accompanying fissuring ulcers or in the form of aggregates of lymphocytes. Non-caseating granulomas are the hallmark of Crohn's disease but are not seen in ulcerative colitis, although foreign body giant cell granulomas are occasionally found.

The quantitative as much as the qualitative differences in pathologic findings must be recognized in the differential diagnosis of inflammatory bowel disease. In some cases, classification is uncertain owing to conflicting combinations of features. Such cases are classified as *"colitis of indeterminate type."* Examination of previous as well as subsequent pathologic and radiographic evidence often results in categorization of such cases as either ulcerative colitis or Crohn's disease.

References

1. Morson BC, Dawson IMP. Gastrointestinal Pathology. 2nd Ed. Oxford: Blackwell Scientific, 1979: 523–74.
2. Price AB. Difficulties in the differential diagnosis of ulcerative colitis and Crohn's disease. *In*: Yardley JH, Morson BC, Abell MR, eds. The Gastrointestinal Tract. Baltimore: Williams and Wilkins, 1977; 1–14.
3. Kovalcik, PJ, Szydlowski TR. Localized giant pseudopolyposis of the colon in ulcerative colitis. Dis Colon Rectum 1980; 23:268–70.
4. Lumb, G, Protheroe, RHB. Ulcerative colitis: a pathologic study of 152 surgical specimens. Gastroenterology 1958; 34:381–407.
5. Willoughby CP, Piris J, Truelove SC: Tissue eosinophils in ulcerative colitis. Scand J Gastroenterol 1979; 14:395–9.
6. Watson AJ, Roy AD. Paneth cells in the large intestine in ulcerative colitis. J Pathol Bacteriol 1960; 80:309–16.
7. Goulston SJM, McGovern WJ. The nature of benign strictures in ulcerative colitis. N Engl J Med 1969; 281:290–5.
8. Yardley JH, Donowitz M. Colo-rectal biopsy in inflammatory bowel disease. *In*: Yardley JH, Morson BC, Abell MR, eds. The Gastrointestinal Tract. Baltimore: Williams and Wilkins, 1977: 50–94.
9. Whitehead R. Mucosal Biopsy of the Gastrointestinal Tract. 2nd Ed. Philadelphia: WB Saunders, 1979.
10. Mitros FA. The biopsy in evaluating patients with inflammatory bowel disease. Med Clin North Am 1980, 64:1037–57.
11. Rotterdam H, Sommers SC. Biopsy Diagnosis of the Digestive Tract. New York: Raven Press, 1981.
12. Haggitt RC. Handling of gastrointestinal biopsies in the surgical pathology laboratory. Lab Med 1982; 13:273–8.
13. Frei JV, Morson BC. Medical audit of rectal biopsy diagnosis of inflammatory bowel disease. Gut 1982; 35:341–4.
14. Hamilton SR. Diagnosis and comparison of ulcerative colitis and Crohn's disease involving the colon. *In*: Norris HT, ed. Contemporary Issues in Surgical Pathology. Vol. 2. New York: Churchill-Livingstone: 1983; 1–19.
15. Price AB, Morson BC. Inflammatory bowel disease. The surgical pathology of Crohn's disease and ulcerative colitis. Human Pathol 1975; 6:7–29.
16. Knill-Jones RP, Morson BC, Williams R. Prestomal ileitis: clinical and pathological findings in five cases. Q J Med 1970; 39:287–97.
17. Bonello JC, Thow GB, Manson RR. Mucosal enteritis: A complication of the continent ileostomy. Dis Colon Rectum 1981; 24:37–41.
18. Glotzer DJ, Glick ME, Goldman H. Proctitis and colitis following diversion of the fecal stream. Gastroenterology 1981; 80:433–7.
19. Barlett JG. *Clostridium difficile* and inflammatory bowel disease. Gastroenterology 1981; 80:863–5.
20. Day DW, Mandal BK, Morson BC. The rectal biopsy appearances in Salmonella colitis. Histopathology 1978; 2:117–31.
21. Keren DF, Milligan FD, Strandberg JD, Yardley JH. Intercurrent cytomegalovirus colitis in a patient with ulcerative colitis. Johns Hopkins Med J 1975; 136:178–82.
22. Serafini EP, Kirk AP, Chambers TJ. Rate and pattern of epithelial cell proliferation in ulcerative colitis. Gut 1981; 22:648–52.
23. Alpers DH, Philpott G, Grimme Nl, Morgolis DM. Control

of thymidine incorporation in mucosal explants from patients with chronic ulcerative colitis. Gastroenterology 1980; 78:470–8.
24. Rognum TO, Elgjo K, Fausa O, Brandtzaeg P. Immunohistochemical evaluation of carcinoembryonic antigen, secretory component, and epithelial IgA in ulcerative colitis with dysplasia. Gut 1982; 23:123–33.
25. Isaacson P. Synthesis of secretory component (SC) by dysplastic colonic mucosa with special reference to precancerous dysplasia in ulcerative colitis (UC). Gastroenterology 1981; 80:1182.
26. Kewenter J, Hulten L, Ahren C. The occurrence of severe epithelial dysplasia and its bearing on treatment of longstanding ulcerative colitis. Ann Surg 1982; 195:209–13.
27. Inflammatory Bowel Disease Dysplasia Morphology Study Group. International cooperative study of epithelial dysplasia in ulcerative colitis (UC). Gastroenterology 1981; 80:1181.
28. Goldman H. Dysplasia and carcinoma in inflammatory bowel disease. *In*: Rachmelewitz D, ed. Inflammatory Bowel Diseases. Developments in Gastroenterology Vol 3. The Hague: Martinus Nijhoff, 1982: 27–40.
29. Riddell RH, Goldman H, Ransohoff DF, et al. Dysplasia in inflammatory bowel disease: Standardized classification with provisional clinical applications. Human Pathol 1983; 14:931–68.
30. Butt JH, Morson BC. Dysplasia and cancer in inflammatory bowel disease. Gastroenterology 1981; 80:865–8.
31. Butt JH, Konishi F, Morson BC, Lennard-Jones JE, Ritchie JK. Macroscopic lesions in dysplasia and carcinoma complicating ulcerative colitis. Dig Dis Sci 1983; 15:18–26.
32. Blackstone MO, Riddell RH, Rogers BHG, Levin B. Dysplasia-associated lesions or mass (DALM) by colonoscopy in long-standing ulcerative colitis: An indication for colectomy. Gastroenterology 1981; 80:366–74.

Clinical Features

Richard G. Farmer

Symptoms

The initial and most common symptom of ulcerative colitis is *rectal bleeding*. A blood stain on the toilet tissue or the appearance of bloody mucus on the outside of the stools is the first symptom. Often both the patient and the physician initially consider the bleeding to be from hemorrhoids. This is especially true when the discharge of bloody mucus accompanies and follows a bout of constipation, which occasionally may persist throughout a mild attack. When constipation occurs as a presenting complaint, it is most often associated with disease limited to the rectum and rectosigmoid, where spasm probably prevents feces from entering the involved area. A tendency to constipation or normal bowel behavior initially may be a hallmark of patients with ulcerative proctosigmoiditis.[1] Diarrhea, on the other hand, occurs with or follows more extensive colonic involvement, and blood is mixed with feces. Usually the onset is relatively abrupt, with the entire symptom complex appearing within 1 or 2 months.

Diarrhea may vary considerably in severity from 3 to 4 bowel discharges/day to as often as one every 1 or 2 hours throughout the 24-hour period. The nocturnal occurrence of bowel discharges is an important distinguishing feature of diarrhea caused by organic disease. The stools in ulcerative colitis are usually small in volume and may be soft, formed, mushy, or loose brick-red slush with a mixture of blood. The diarrhea is frequently associated with considerable urgency, and often the patient will pass only a small amount of bloody mucus.

The principal mechanism for diarrhea in ulcerative colitis is exudation and secretion of mucus, which increase the fecal solute and result in increased fecal water. Only a relatively small increase above normal in stool water (100 to 200 ml/day) is required to produce diarrhea (Chapter 8). Reduced absorption of sodium and water has also been demonstrated in colonic loops affected by the disease.[2] In addition, the blood and mucus that exude into the lumen not uncommonly cause frequent bowel evacuations due to "pseudodiarrhea," i.e., rectal discharges consisting largely of blood and exudate.

In patients with mild involvement, the bloody mucoid discharge may be minimal or entirely absent in the early stages of the disease. Infrequently, the onset will be of the acute fulminating type, with the entire symptom complex developing within 2 or 3 days. The patient may have almost continuous liquid evacuations, frequently containing little fecal material and composed almost entirely of blood, pus, and mucus ("bloody flux"). Rectal incontinence may develop under these circumstances. Rectal tenesmus is one of the most annoying subjective complaints in those patients with frequent bowel movements.

Abdominal pain is a very common complaint, although it is minimal or absent in mild attacks or in patients who have an insidious onset. Usually the pain is colicky or crampy in character and most often is confined to the left lower abdominal quadrant or hypogastrium, but it may be generalized. Characteristically, the pain occurs in association with the desire to defecate and is relieved by bowel evacuation. As the colon becomes a scarred, inflexible, shortened tube, cramping abdominal pain diminishes as the urge to defecate is no longer associated with the gastrocolic reflex or transport motility of the colon. In this advanced stage of damage to the colonic wall, the patient may lose the warning signal for defecation, or the urge to defecate may occur unexpectedly, as with turning over in bed (gravitational filling of the rectum with liquid feces). Low back ache may be a distressing symptom in some patients, but it is not as commonly encountered as in Crohn's disease.

Other gastrointestinal symptoms such as anorexia, fullness, nausea, epigastric discomfort, and, at times, actual vomiting may be present. These are probably reflex and vary with the severity of colitis. In the mild insidious form of the disease, they may be entirely absent; in the very acute fulminating type, they can be so severe that it is difficult to maintain normal nutrition.

Loss of weight and *strength* depend entirely upon the severity of the disease and the associated systemic toxemia. In very mild cases with little or no diarrhea and no bleeding of consequence, the patient may feel entirely well, whereas in the acute fulminating form, loss of weight and progressive weakness are very prominent from the onset of the disease. Varying degrees of protein, water, electrolyte, and vitamin depletion are evident.

Fever may or may not be present, depending upon the severity of the attack and the extensiveness of colonic involvement. In severe cases with malabsorption and interference with nutrition, a septic temperature and rapid pulse are found. The majority of patients have a very moderate elevation of pulse or temperature during the acute phase of the disease. The tachycardia is usually out of proportion to the degree of temperature elevation and is attributed, in part, to dehydration. The latter frequently is more profound than clinical signs would suggest.

Personal and Family History

Much effort has been expended to find antecedent factors that might be of importance, if not the precipitating cause, for either the onset or a recurrence of ulcerative colitis. However, information gleaned from these studies remains contradictory and controversial. The relationships of breast feeding, dietary and nutritional factors, allergies, associated illnesses, and psychologic problems have all been assessed with inconclusive results.

Many clinicians have observed that emotional conflicts appear to provoke exacerbations of the disease,[3] and the work of Engel[4] is usually quoted. In the 1950s, Engel and co-workers observed that "the onset and relapses of the disease were found to occur in settings which represented to the patient, real, threatened, or fancied interruptions of key relationships." These interruptions included the death of or separation from a parent or other relative to whom the patient was attached, disruption of marital or other emotional ties, related anxiety or depression, and problems associated with friends at school. The mother/child relationship has been emphasized, with the mother representing a dominant figure. Whether or not these relationships represent cause or effect, however, has never been proved. In recent years, the tendency has been to downplay the etiologic importance of family and interpersonal relationships in either onset or exacerbations of the disease, if for no other reason than to decrease the guilt reaction by the patient. The ability to cope with the illness may be adversely affected if the patient has the impression that his or her actions or relationships have brought on the disease.

The specificity of emotional disturbances in patients with ulcerative colitis appears to be no different from patients with many chronic illness or those with the irritable bowel syndrome. Mendeloff and co-workers[5] showed that no differences could be demonstrated between patients with ulcerative colitis and those with Crohn's disease or irritable bowel syndrome and healthy controls in respect to personality types, evidence of psychiatric illness, or precipitating psychologic factors or stress before an attack.

Attempts have been made to characterize the personalities of patients with ulcerative colitis, but as Engel says of his own description,[4] "It would be misleading to say that the character traits here listed are specifically associated with ulcerative colitis. Most people with such character traits do not have ulcerative colitis."

A high proportion of patients are described as manifesting obsessive-compulsive character traits, including neatness, orderliness, punctuality, conscientiousness, indecision, obstinacy, and conformity. With these are often noted a guarding of affectivity, overintellectualization, rigid attitudes toward morality and standards of behavior, meticulousness of speech, avoidance of "dirty" language, defective sense of humor, obsessive worrying, and timidity. Some patients are petulant, querulous, demanding, and provocative, but well-directed aggressive action and clear-cut expressions of anger are uncommon. Many observers have been impressed by the extreme sensitivity of these patients and their almost uncanny perception of hostility or rejecting attitudes in others. They are easily hurt, are constantly alert to the attitudes and behavior of others toward them, and tend to brood and withdraw. Much activity is devoted to warding off or avoiding rebuffs, including placating attitudes, submission, politeness, attempts to please and conform, and seductive behavior. Others use denial, remaining proud, nonchalant, haughty, and aloof.[4]

Another factor that has been thought to be associated with either onset or exacerbation of the disease is an upper respiratory tract infection. While the infection may well act as a non-specific stress, there is little scientific documentation as to the validity of this relationship. However, the observation that upper respiratory tract or other infections seem to be associated with an exacerbation of ulcerative colitis is relatively frequent.

A flare of colitis may likewise follow the ingestion of certain foodstuffs or bowel irritants, and much study of the relationship of milk and lactase deficiency has occurred in recent years. However, once again, no specific relationship has been established, and it has not been possible to correlate lactase deficiency with colitis. Although it is well established that a milk-free diet or one low in milk products may be beneficial for some patients with ulcerative colitis, this may relate more to severity of illness than to a specific reaction to a substance in one of the foodstuffs.

The taking of strong laxatives or other irritating drugs (e.g., colchicine and certain antibiotics) may produce sufficient irritability of the colon to cause an exacerbation of symptoms when the disease has been clinically latent. Use of irritant enemas, such as soap suppositories, may also be associated with relapse. Similarly, barium enema or colonoscopic examination may also be associated with a relapse, although, once again, the exact mechanism is unclear.

Familial clustering of ulcerative colitis has been recognized for many years[6]; whether or not there are genetic implications, however, is poorly understood. In a study of 316 patients with childhood onset of ulcerative colitis,[7] 29% were found to have a positive family history for a similar illness involving a first-degree relative or an immediate family member. Disease affecting an immediate family member was present in 15% of those studied, but there was no pattern established that could be defined as "genetic." Distribution was both vertical (from one generation to another) and horizontal (within the same generation to the level of first-degree relative). The importance of clustering of the disease in families is that it created yet another problem for the patient as well as for other members of the family. In addition to concern over the symptoms and prognosis for the individual patient, as well as long-term concerns over the development of cancer or the need for surgery, the potential for development of ulcerative colitis in other relatives or children only adds to the psychologic burden carried by the patient and his or her family. Although both environmental and genetic factors may theoretically be of some significance, there are no data at present to indicate the need for or value of genetic counseling. Furthermore, racial, cultural, and ethnic factors do not convey specific implications. Thus, the status of family clustering of ulcerative colitis, while of obvious importance, remains to be further elaborated.

Ulcerative Colitis and Pregnancy

This aspect is reviewed in detail in Chapter 129. It will suffice here, therefore, to state by way of summary that: (1) fertility is only minimally, if at all, diminished in the patient (man or woman) with ulcerative colitis; (2) women with inactive disease have an excellent prognosis for a normal delivery; (3) there is a certain risk for a flare of the colitis in the first trimester or in the puerperium, but the patient can be safely treated with corticosteroids and sulfasalazine without adverse effects on the fetus; and (4) the prognosis for pregnant patients with ulcerative colitis appears to be better than for those with Crohn's disease.[8–13]

Physical Findings

Physical examination of a patient with ulcerative colitis may be completely normal between attacks and even in the presence of low-grade disease activity. However, in the hospitalized patient, the examiner may be impressed first by the apprehensive, tense appearance and the pallor, weakness, and evident weight loss. These are particularly noticeable in a young patient and create the impression (accurate in most cases) that the patient is chronically ill.

Abdominal examination may reveal no abnormality, but even in mild cases tenderness may be elicited by palpation over the left colon or may be generalized throughout the abdomen. Rebound tenderness may be elicited and may reflect serosal involvement of the colon, peritoneal irritation, or impending perforation. The descending or sigmoid colon may be palpated as a rigid tube that often cannot be differentiated from a spastic colon. There may be voluntary muscle guarding, particularly in patients with active disease involving the entire colon. The abdomen is usually flat but soft. Distention, particularly in the upper half of the abdomen overlying the transverse colon, will develop with the complication of toxic megacolon. Occasionally the liver is palpably enlarged because of fatty infiltration or other hepatic abnormality. Auscultation of the abdomen may reveal increased bowel sounds and, in some cases, audible borborygmi. With toxic megacolon, bowel sounds are quiet or absent.

Rectal examination is frequently painful, so that gentleness is important. The anal sphincter is often spastic, but it may also be relaxed and patulous in the acutely ill, toxic patient. The experienced examiner may be able to detect gritty or coarse granular changes in the rectal mucosa on digital palpation. Pseudopolyps may also be palpated, and a rectal stricture may be detected. In addition, it may be possible to feel a carcinoma. Rectal and perianal complications are far less frequent and less destructive than in Crohn's disease and ordinarily consist only of minor fissuring. The gloved finger may demonstrate the characteristic exudate consisting of mucus, pus, and blood.

Examination of the skin and joints is important to detect the most common extraintestinal manifestations: erythema nodosum, pyoderma gangrenosum, and arthritis. The skin may also be dry and show loss of turgor. Arthritic changes ("colitic arthritis"), somewhat similar to rheumatoid arthritis, may be noted in the large joints, particularly the knees, ankles, elbows, and wrists. Occasionally, ankylosing spondylitis is found in conjunction with ulcerative colitis.

Complete physical examination may reveal other findings, including ocular manifestations (in the form of iritis, iridocyclitis, or episcleritis), pallor of the skin, aphthous ulcers of the mouth, evidence of nutritional anemia, pretibial edema secondary to hypoalbuminemia, evidence of hypocalcemia and/or hypomagnesemia, fever and tachycardia, growth retardation in children, and thrombophlebitis. In addition, there may be noticeable apathy, lethargy, anxiety, and depression or psychosis.

Laboratory Studies

There is no single laboratory test or group of tests that will specifically confirm the diagnosis of ulcerative colitis. Much effort has gone into attempts to find such tests, and the search for a "marker," either for the diagnosis of ulcerative colitis or for assessment of its disease activity, has not been successful. The most common laboratory findings are anemia, leukocytosis, and elevation of the erythrocyte sedimentation rate. The degree and severity of anemia generally reflect the severity of blood loss; the hemoglobin and hematocrit usually are normal in cases of proctitis and progressively abnormal with increasing severity of the colitis. In addition to iron deficiency anemia secondary to blood loss, superimposed effects of chronic inflammation and hemolytic anemia may be present. Leukocytosis generally is not severe and is not a good prognostic feature to detect severity of illness. The erythrocyte sedimentation rate and other non-specific markers of inflammation generally are abnormal in cases of active disease but seldom provide a clue for disease that cannot be detected by other means.

Patients with severe ulcerative colitis may have electrolyte abnormalities with hypokalemia, metabolic acidosis or alkalosis, hypocalcemia, or hypomagnesemia. Serum protein electrophoresis may demonstrate hypoalbuminemia, and there may be non-specific elevations of globulins.

Despite considerable interest in liver disease associated with ulcerative colitis, hepatic enzyme abnormalities are not common. Asymptomatic elevation of serum alkaline phosphatase activity may be the first manifestation of sclerosing cholangitis (Chapter 164). Elevation of the serum aminotransferases, serum bilirubin, and other liver tests may follow. Blood cultures are rarely positive in patients with ulcerative colitis, except for those with bacteremia in association with toxic megacolon.

Examination of a stool specimen is important in patients with ulcerative colitis for a variety of reasons. The specimen is best obtained during proctosigmoidoscopy and when significant symptoms are present. The typical stool in ulcerative colitis patients is quite distinctive. During the active stage of the disease, the bowel evacuations often consist almost entirely of mucus, purulent exudate, and blood. With different degrees of activity, varying amounts of liquid, soft, or even formed feces may be present together with blood, pus, and mucus. In the acute phase, examination of the stool specimen microscopically reveals large numbers of leukocytes. This finding, of course, is not pathognomonic of ulcerative colitis and may be found in cases of bacterial diarrhea (Chapter 24). Stool culture for enteric pathogens should be done in all cases of ulcerative colitis, with specific attention to the possibility of *Shigella, Campylobacter, Salmonella,* and the toxin of *Clostridium difficile.* Examination of several stool specimens for parasites is necessary, particularly to exclude amebic dysentery. Rectal biopsy may also be helpful, but frequently demonstrates only non-specific inflammatory changes.

References

1. Farmer RG. Long-term prognosis for patients with ulcerative proctosigmoiditis (ulcerative colitis confined to the rectum and sigmoid colon). J Clin Gastroenterol 1979; 1:47–50.
2. Duthie HL, Watts JM, deDombal FT, et al. Serum electrolytes and colonic transfer of water and electrolytes in chronic ulcerative colitis. Gastroenterology 1964; 47:525.
3. Lepore MJ. The importance of emotional disturbances in chronic ulcerative colitis. JAMA 1965; 191:819.
4. Engel GI: Psychological factors in ulcerative colitis in man and gibbon. Gastroenterology 1969; 57:362.
5. Mendeloff AI, Monk M, Siegal CI, et al. Illness experience and life stresses in patients with irritable colon and with ulcerative colitis. N Engl J Med 1970; 282:14.
6. Kirsner JB. Genetic aspects of inflammatory bowel disease. Clin Gastroenterol 1973; 2:557.
7. Farmer RG, Michener WM, Mortimer EA. Studies of family history among patients with inflammatory bowel disease. Clin Gastroenterol 1980; 9:271–8.
8. Jarnerot G. Fertility, sterility and pregnancy in chronic inflammatory bowel disease. Scand J Gastroenterol 1982; 17:1.
9. Mogadam M, Korelitz BI, Ahmad SW. The course of inflammatory disease during pregnancy and postpartum. Am J Gastroenterol 1981; 75:265.
10. Mogadam M, Dobbins WO, Korelitz BI, et al. Pregnancy in inflammatory bowel disease: Effect of sulfasalazine and corticosteroids on fetal outcome. Gastroenterology 1981; 80:72.
11. Sorokin JJ, Levine SM. Pregnancy and inflammatory bowel disease: A review of the literature. Obstet Gynecol 1983; 62:247–52.
12. Webb MJ, Sedlack RE. Ulcerative colitis in pregnancy. Med Clin North Am 1974; 58:823.
13. Zetzel L. Fertility, Pregnancy, and Idiopathic Inflammatory Bowel Disease. *In:* Kirsner JB, Shorter RG, eds. Inflammatory Bowel Disease. 2nd Ed. Philadelphia, Lea and Febiger, 1980: 241–53.

Roentgen Features

George N. Stein • Philip J. Sabri

All patients in whom ulcerative colitis has been diagnosed endoscopically, or in whom it is strongly suspected clinically, should have a barium enema examination. However, if the diagnosis is firmly established and the colitis is fulminant, barium enema examination should be delayed until there is improvement in the severity of the disease in order to ensure a technically satisfactory study and to maximize patient comfort and safety. Repeat barium studies are useful to help exclude the possibility of carcinoma, particularly in patients who have had the disease for more than 5 years. They are also important in the evaluation of patients in whom significant progression of the disease is suspected or when clinical concern exists about the possibility of complications such as stricture.[1]

While barium enema examination is the primary radiologic method for diagnosing ulcerative colitis, the importance of plain films must not be overlooked. The barium meal, the small bowel enema, and the peroral pneumocolon study may also be useful, particularly in differentiating ulcerative colitis from Crohn's colitis.[2] Other types of diagnostic imaging have yet to play an important role, although ^{67}gallium citrate scintigraphy and ^{111}indium-tagged leukocytes show potential as non-invasive techniques to demonstrate the extent of activity of the disease, particularly in patients too ill for barium enema examination or colonoscopy.[3–5]

Survey Film

Roentgenologic evaluation of the patient suspected of having ulcerative colitis must include a preliminary film of the abdomen. This is especially important in severely ill patients, inasmuch as toxic dilatation or perforation should be excluded before a barium enema examination is performed. The survey film may also provide other useful information. For example, evaluation of colonic residue can be helpful. Although the amount and distribution of colonic fecal residue are quite variable, some residue is almost always present in normal persons, particularly in the cecum. Since residue does not accumulate adjacent to inflamed mucosa,[6] the complete absence of residue suggests total colitis and the distribution of residue can give clues to the areas of involvement.[7, 8]

The presence of air within the lumen allows assessment of the mucosal outline and haustral pattern. Unlike the normal mucosa, which has a smooth interface with retained intraluminal air, the mucosal edge may be fuzzy or finely irregular with widened haustral clefts or absent haustrations in diseased segments. Narrowed gas-filled segments of colon also suggest involvement,[9] as does an irregular contour with multiple deep projections indicative of ulceration. Nodular intraluminal protrusions due to pseudopolyps, as well as shortening or lack of redundancy of the colon, may be identified (Fig. 126–13). Scout films may also disclose changes indicative of ankylosing spondylitis or sacroilitis, which may be associated with ulcerative colitis.

Toxic Dilatation and Perforation. Plain films are particularly important in the diagnosis of toxic megacolon. This serious complication may occur at any time during the acute or chronic phase of ulcerative colitis. While toxic dilatation is most commonly seen in ulcerative colitis, it may also occur in Crohn's colitis, ischemic colitis, salmonellosis, amebiasis, and rarely in other infectious diseases and in pseudomembranous colitis.[10, 11]

The anteroposterior recumbent film of the abdomen is generally diagnostic and usually

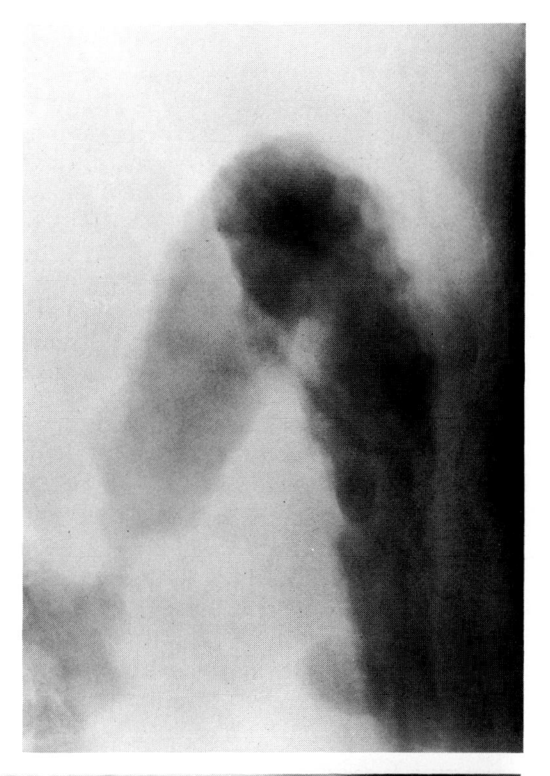

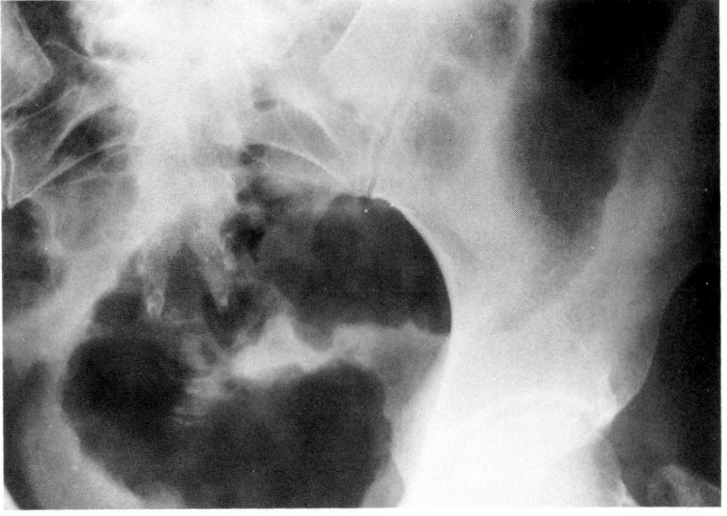

Figure 126–13. *A,* Survey film suggesting ulcerative colitis. The splenic flexure as seen in the erect film shows marginal irregularity, polypoid changes, and loss of haustral markings. *B,* Survey film in another patient demonstrating similar findings in rectosigmoid.

demonstrates the transverse colon to be the most prominently dilated segment. This probably is due in part to the fact that this segment possesses a mesentery and therefore is the most anterior portion of the colon in the supine position (Fig. 126–14). The descending colon and sigmoid colon are also often distended, but less so than the transverse colon; the rectum is rarely distended.[12] Dilatation beyond 5.5. cm is generally considered abnormal,[13] but strict criteria cannot be applied because the caliber of the distended segments can vary greatly. Moreover, some patients with longstanding ulcerative colitis may develop chronically dilated colons in the absence of any clinical signs or symptoms of toxic dilatation.[1] A continuous column of air throughout the entire colon indicates toxic dilatation regardless of the degree of distention.[14]

Typically, the lengths and locations of the visualized portions of colon are relatively normal despite the dilatation. There is no remarkable redundancy and the location of the splenic and hepatic flexures is usually normal. Decubitus or erect films, which should obtained to exclude free intraperitoneal air, demonstrate fluid levels that are typically few in number and unusually long.

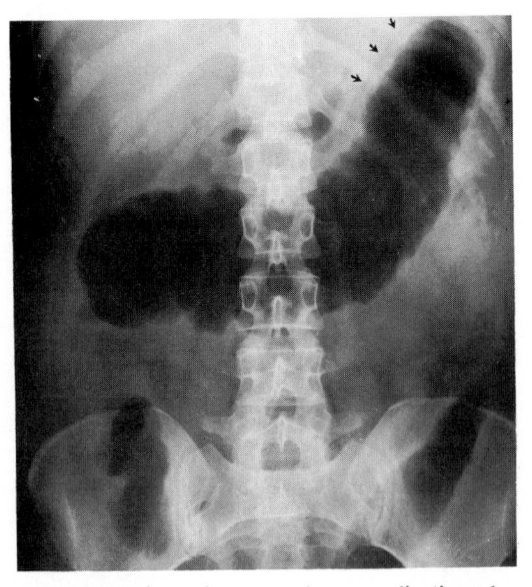

Figure 126–14. Toxic megacolon complicating ulcerative colitis. A radiolucent line *(arrows)* paralleling the bowel wall in this patient with toxic megacolon probably represents intramural dissection of air. The transverse colon is moderately distended with air and dilated.

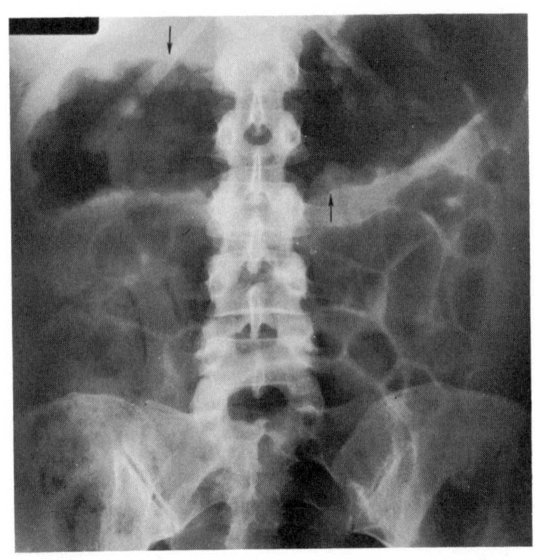

Figure 126–15. Pseudopolyps in toxic megacolon. Supine film demonstrating a dilated transverse colon that contains multiple nodular densities due to pseudopolyps. Arrows indicate particularly prominent pseudopolyps.

These films also aid in the differentiation of toxic megacolon from mechanical distal colonic obstruction. Haustra may be absent or thickened in the involved segments. Multiple broad-based nodular intraluminal protrusions due to pseudopolyps may be seen. These can appear as circular shadows when projected *en face* within the air column (Fig. 126–15). Air-filled crevices that may project from the bowel into adjacent soft tissues evidently represent ulcerations. A common finding is the presence of numerous air-filled loops of small bowel, sometimes with air-fluid levels; these possibly are due to aerophagia.[12] Occasionally, a radiolucent line paralleling the bowel lumen is demonstrated. This is evidence of intramuscular dissection of air and suggests that perforation may be imminent.[8]

Although perforation is rare in the absence of toxic dilatation, it is more likely to occur during the initial attack of colitis than in subsequent severe attacks. Perforation is most common in patients with total involvement of the colon with ulcerative colitis. The sigmoid is the most frequent site of perforation.[15] When free air is in the intraperitoneal cavity, it is easily demonstrated on erect or left lateral decubitus views. However, sealed localized perforations may be undetectable radiologically.[7]

Barium Enema Examination

Indications, Contraindications, and Complications. Barium enema study is indicated to establish the diagnosis of ulcerative colitis, to determine the extent or severity of the disease, and, as a follow-up examination, to determine any complications that may be present. Follow-up examinations are also useful to assess the success of therapy. The frequency of repeat examinations depends on whether or not there is clinical suspicion of an increase in the severity or extent of the disease or if there is a change in the symptoms suggestive of a particular complication. Of course, patients with severe disease of long duration require more frequent screening for carcinoma.

There are few, if any, indications for performing a barium enema study in the severely ill patient with bloody diarrhea, abdominal pain, and systemic findings. The study is generally thought to be contraindicated in toxic megacolon (and, of course, in perforation).[14, 16, 17] Because of the friability of the bowel wall in toxic megacolon and the frequency of spontaneous perforation, the risk of iatrogenic perforation would seem to be high. Although Wolf and Marshak[12] noted no apparent complications from barium enema examinations performed on patients with toxic megacolon, they concluded that this was due to the fact that it was not possible to introduce much barium into the colon without inducing evacuation. They, like other investigators, concluded that such a study not only provided little information but was undesirable.[12, 18]

Some observers consider a barium enema to be a predisposing factor in the development of toxic megacolon.[1, 19, 20] Others, however, contend that this has never been conclusively demonstrated.[2, 14, 21] While a barium enema is occasionally followed by an exacerbation of symptoms, many more patients have exacerbations without having barium enemas. In those few patients who do develop increased symptoms following barium study, other factors such as the method of bowel preparation may be of importance.

Perforation is a rare complication of barium enema examination in either diseased or normal colons and may be either extraperitoneal or intraperitoneal. In the latter case, severe peritonitis may result. Perforation is most often due to trauma secondary to an inflatable rectal balloon or to the enema tube itself. Rupture of the colon by hydrostatic pressure is even rarer.[22] Since the frequency of occurrence is increased when an inflated balloon tip is used, it is particularly important to avoid using balloon tips in the presence of rectal disease associated with ulcerative colitis.

Other complications of barium enemas include barium granulomas, barium emboli, and transient bacteremia.[22–25] All these complications are rare, and many investigators report large series of patients with diseased colons in whom barium enemas resulted in no apparent complications.[9, 26–28] It does seem prudent, nevertheless, to avoid performing barium enema studies in patients with fulminant disease because of the potential risks and the difficulty obtaining a satisfactory study.

Single versus Double Contrast. Rigler and Weiner[29] noted that Schüle performed the first opaque enema examination of the colon in 1904 with the use of bismuth subnitrate. Later, barium was substituted for bismuth. According to Margulis,[30] Fisher, in 1923, first popularized a form of the double contrast enema examination using barium and air.[30] A variety of modifications have developed over the years, including the single contrast enema, the Malmö secondary double contrast enema, and a variation of the Malmö technique called the "instant enema," in which the patients are given no bowel preparation.[31, 32] Over the last decade, Laufer and others[8, 26, 33, 34] have done much to popularize the primary double contrast enema examination in the United States.

The primary double contrast enema technique utilizes high-density barium together with immediate injection of air. In the secondary double contrast technique, the colon is filled with barium, the patient evacuates, and air is insufflated. Laufer[34] argues that the primary technique is superior because the secondary technique often results in poor coating by the thinner barium as well as variable evacuation. In addition, the delay during evacuation may result in deterioration of the quality of the mucosal coating. However, those who prefer the secondary double contrast technique argue that it affords a better view of the rugal pattern.

In recent years there has been much discussion concerning which method is best for evaluation of inflammatory bowel disease. Numerous comparisons have been made between the primary double contrast technique and the conventional single contrast examination, but there still is divergent opinion about the role of the double contrast examination in inflammatory bowel disease. Many of the single contrast advocates have had little experience with the primary double contrast technique. On the other hand, the double contrast group often has unfairly compared the accuracy of their examinations performed after meticulous bowel cleansing with the results obtained in older studies using single contrast techniques in which bowel preparation was often less than optimal.[9] A number of investigators have reported that the double contrast technique is considerably more sensitive in the detection of inflammatory bowel disease. It allows better differentiation between ulcerative and granulomatous colitis, particularly early in the course of the disease, because it can better demonstrate superficial changes in the mucosa, such as granularity and ulceration.[17, 26, 27, 33–35] We believe that the primary double contrast examination is superior for the diagnosis of early disease and allows differentiation between ulcerative colitis and Crohn's colitis with more confidence.

In 1971, Margulis et al.[36] found in a retrospective study that only 70% of patients with Crohn's colitis and 79% with ulcerative colitis were correctly diagnosed using a conventional single contrast barium enema study. In about 25% of cases, it was not possible to differentiate between the 2 entities by radiologic criteria.[10] Kirsner[37] reported similar diagnostic difficulty with the single contrast study. However, Brazeau-LaMontagne et al.[38] stated that with adequate bowel preparation and careful attention to diagnostic criteria a 90% diagnostic accuracy rate was possible with this technique in distinguishing ulcerative from Crohn's colitis. In contrast to this, others reported that in early and mild cases of ulcerative colitis, the conventional single contrast barium enema study may be normal in 15 to 80%.[33, 39, 40, 41]

Results have been better with the double contrast method. For example, Kelvin et al.[27] made a positive radiologic diagnosis in 83% of patients with ulcerative colitis and 98% of patients with Crohn's colitis. Laufer and Hamilton[26] evaluated 50 patients with idiopathic colitis and their radiologic diagnosis of Crohn's or ulcerative colitis was in agreement with the endoscopic or pathologic report in each case.

Comparisons have also been made between the correlation of the 2 methods with endoscopic findings, with reports of poor correlation between the single contrast technique and endoscopy. Single contrast studies have been found to underestimate the extent of the disease in many cases.[42–44] Somewhat contradictory results have been obtained for the double contrast method, but generally there has been better correlation with endoscopic findings. Laufer et al.,[26, 34] for example, reported using the primary both contrast technique in 80 patients with inflammatory bowel disease and showed a 95% correlation with endoscopic findings. Fraser and Findlay[42] graded the severity of inflammatory bowel disease as seen on both double and single contrast studies and compared the grading with the endoscopic appearances. They found the findings of the double contrast barium enema examination and endoscopy to be in agreement in 77% of cases; there was disagreement of only one grade (on a scale utilizing 4 grades) in another 23% of the patients. On the other hand, they judged the single contrast examination to be unreliable in assessing the severity of the disease.

Other investigators have found that even using the double contrast technique there was a tendency to underestimate the extent of involvement when compared with endoscopic and particularly with histologic evaluation.[35, 43, 44] Williams et al.[35] thought that while double contrast examination was less sensitive than endoscopy, it was more specific in differentiating ulcerative from granulomatous colitis. In addition, it seemed to add complementary information to that obtained endoscopically.

Barium enema examination is more sensitive for the detection of minor changes in haustrations and distensibility than colonoscopy and can also reveal lesions within the endoscopically blind areas, such as behind the flexures and sharp bends. Double contrast study offers greater specificity than proctosigmoidoscopy in differentiating ulcerative colitis from Crohn's disease, probably owing, in part, to its ability to display the entire colon.[35] Miller[45] noted that the double contrast examination and colonoscopy are complementary studies, with each technique having its distinct advantages and limitations.

As a consequence of these reports and observations, most radiologists have accepted the double contrast technique as being superior for the demonstration of subtle mucosal abnormalities and thus early mucosal disease. However, there still is reluctance on the part of some radiologists and gastroenterologists to use the examination in patients with inflammatory bowel disease for fear of a higher risk of inducing toxic megacolon or perforation. This fear has not been substantiated,[8] and it is believed by some that any patient fit enough to have a barium enema examination is fit enough to have double contrast study.[27, 35, 42] We agree that the danger is minimal and with gentle bowel preparation and careful handling of the patient during the procedure, a double contrast study can be performed safely and satisfactorily.

Preparation. Bowel preparation must be tailored to the individual patient. In patients with quiescent disease, a mild laxative such as mineral oil or bisacodyl is frequently recommended in combination with a clear liquid diet for 1 to 2 days days prior to the examination. A tapwater or saline enema on the morning of the examination is usually preferred, and Bartram and Laufer[8] think this is the most important part of the preparation. In patients with active disease in whom a barium enema examination is felt to be both necessary and safe, use of laxatives should be omitted.[1, 2, 8, 27, 34] These patients usually have diarrhea and hence clear liquids in combination with the enema suffice. Glucagon, 1 mg IV, is frequently given prior to the study to assure adequate colonic relaxation and minimal discomfort from spasm. Performance of proctosigmoidoscopy and barium enema examination on the same day should be avoided. If a rectal biopsy is performed, the barium enema study should be delayed at least 5 days.[1] Use of a rectal balloon should be avoided in patients with suspected inflammatory bowel disease.

Radiologic Appearances. It is convenient to divide the radiologic findings of ulcerative colitis into mucosal and secondary changes. Since ulcerative colitis is predominantly a mucosal disease, the initial radiologic changes are particularly well demonstrated by the double contrast technique.[8] Secondary changes that occur largely because of smooth muscle spasm or muscular hypertrophy are readily seen in both conventional and double contrast examinations.

With the use of double contrast examination, mucosal changes such as granularity, ulceration, and pseudopolyps may be recognized. The normal *en face* appearance is smooth and featureless (Fig. 126–16). The contour of the bowel is seen as a smooth white line. The earliest abnormality demonstrated by double contrast study is a finely granular mucosa due to edema and hyperemia (Fig. 126–17) that is diagnostic of active disease.[33] The contour remains smooth initially.[8, 33] This stage of the disease is probably not detectable on single contrast examinations. With progression, superficial erosions develop, resulting in a stippled appearance consequent to the adherence of flecks of barium to the erosions. On occasion, this may be simulated by barium caught between adherent fecal particles, making bowel preparation crucial.

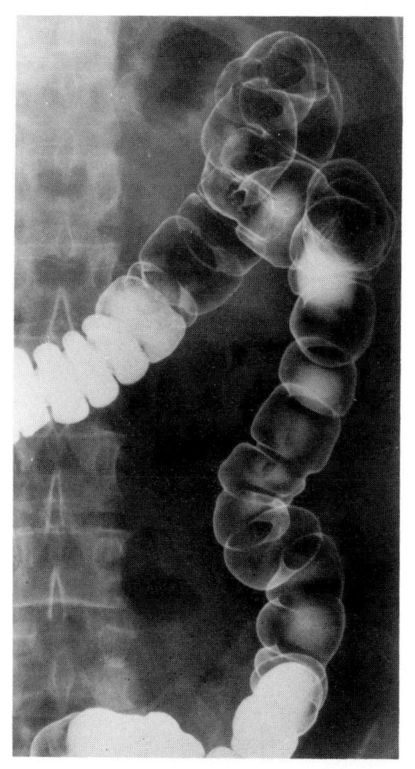

Figure 126–16. Double contrast film of splenic flexure and descending colon in normal person demonstrating the contour of bowel to be smooth and featureless. The bowel appears as a smooth white line.

Further progression is marked by ulceration. This initially is superficial and, when shallow, can be seen only *en face* (Fig. 126–18). When deeper, these ulcerations, unlike the granular mucosa just discussed, result in disruption of the mucosal outline and can be seen in profile (Fig. 126–19). When ulceration occurs on a background of diffuse

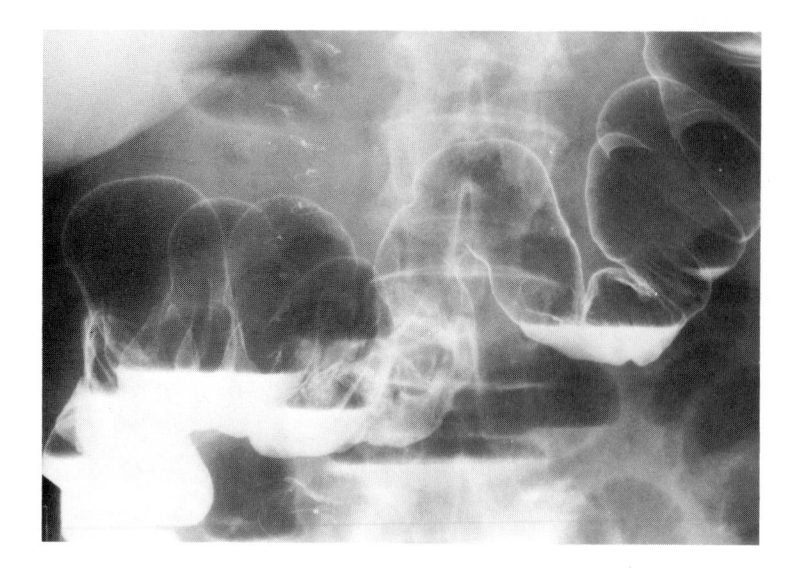

Figure 126–17. Double contrast film demonstrating finely granular mucosa in the transverse colon of patient with ulcerative colitis.

fine granularity, the appearance is considered characteristic of ulcerative colitis. The presence of ulceration implies severe disease. With chronicity, the granular appearance coarsens as the mucosa is replaced by granulation tissue. Ulcerations superimposed upon a coarsely granular background are viewed as indicative of chronic disease with an acute exacerbation.[8] Polypoid changes noted in all stages of ulcerative colitis are also well demonstrated by air contrast studies and are seen as round, oval, or irregular radiolucencies both *en face* and in profile.

The foregoing changes are most often seen in the rectosigmoid. Even in patients with universal disease, the inflammatory changes are usually most pronounced in the left colon. Rectal sparing is unusual, and the diagnosis of ulcerative colitis should be questioned when there is a normal-appearing rectum. Rectal mucosal changes can be documented in 95% to 97% of patients with ulcerative colitis by using double contrast examination.[31, 33, 35] The alterations are usually diffuse and feature granularity or a stippled appearance. Ulceration of the rectum is relatively rare, and this may account for the fact that Margulis[10] noted the absence of rectal involvement in 22% of patients studied by single contrast examination. Isolated involvement of the right colon or segmental involvement of the intervening bowel is considered by many not to occur,[9] but Williams et al.[35] reported 12 examples of segmental disease and one instance of disease isolated to the right colon. The affected segments were symmetrically involved. Our experience parallels that of Williams and his co-workers. We have seen histologically proven ulcerative colitis isolated to the right colon. In addition, we have noted one case with "skip areas," i.e., discontinuous disease (Fig. 126–20).

Evaluation of the colon with the single contrast technique requires observation of the marginal outline, including the haustral configuration, the caliber and length of the colon, and, in particular, the mucosal pattern as judged by the postevacuation film. Roentgen findings, of course, vary with the severity of the inflammation. Early roentgen findings may be extremely subtle on single contrast examination and thus may escape detection.[28] The radiologic changes result from edema, secretions, ulceration, and altered motility.[14]

Edema is one of the earliest changes and is manifested by alteration of the mucosal pattern, so that there is a coarsening of the normal delicate, sharply outlined, crinkled, or rosetted appearance of the mucosal folds on the postevacuation films. The folds may be smudged or indistinct. There is a tendency for the folds to assume a linear pattern. While linear folds may also be seen in the normal distal colon, the linear folds that occur in ulcerative colitis are wider and more indistinct[28] (Fig. 126–21). Abundant secretions, particularly in more fulminant disease, may cause the barium to assume a granular or flocculent appearance. Secretions and

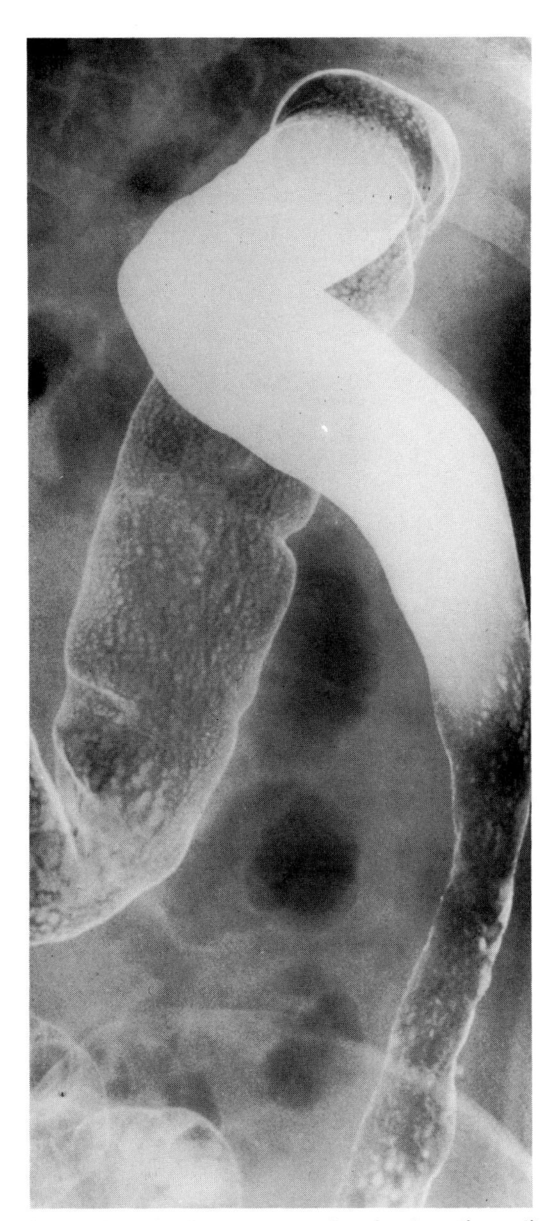

Figure 126–18. Ulcers seen *en face* in ulcerative colitis. Ulcerations appear as small dots of barium in this double contrast film of the splenic flexure.

edema can cause the margin of the barium-filled colon to appear fuzzy. Severe mucosal edema may produce "thumbprinting," similar to that seen in ischemic colitis or other inflammatory processes (Fig. 126–22). Tiny irregular spicules of barium may project from the outline of the colon, representing barium in small superficial ulcer craters. These spiculations may involve only the distal colon or may spread to involve the entire colon, depending on the severity of the attack. When present, the spiculations tend to involve the bowel wall circumferentially. Spiculations due to ulceration can usually be differentiated from spiculations due to barium penetration of the glands of Lieberkühn or the innominate grooves because ulcerations have a less uniform and more irregular and indistinct appearance (Fig. 126–23). Superficial ulcers may also be noted on postevacuation films as tiny projections from the thickened folds.

Alterations in the haustral configuration, such as widening of the haustral clefts or flattening or squaring of the normally smoothly rounded haustrations, may be observed. These may be due to muscle spasm or edema rather than to fibrosis, since they are often reversible. Irregular or absent haustrations are seen in more advanced disease (Fig. 126–24). Absence of haustrations in the descending and sigmoid colon, however, is a common normal finding, so undue significance should not be placed upon this finding unless it is accompanied by other signs of

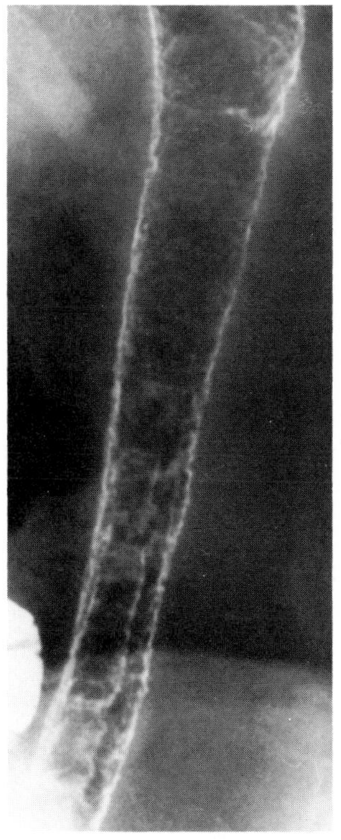

Figure 126–19. Double contrast film of the descending colon demonstrating disruption of the mucosal outline seen with deeper ulcers in ulcerative colitis.

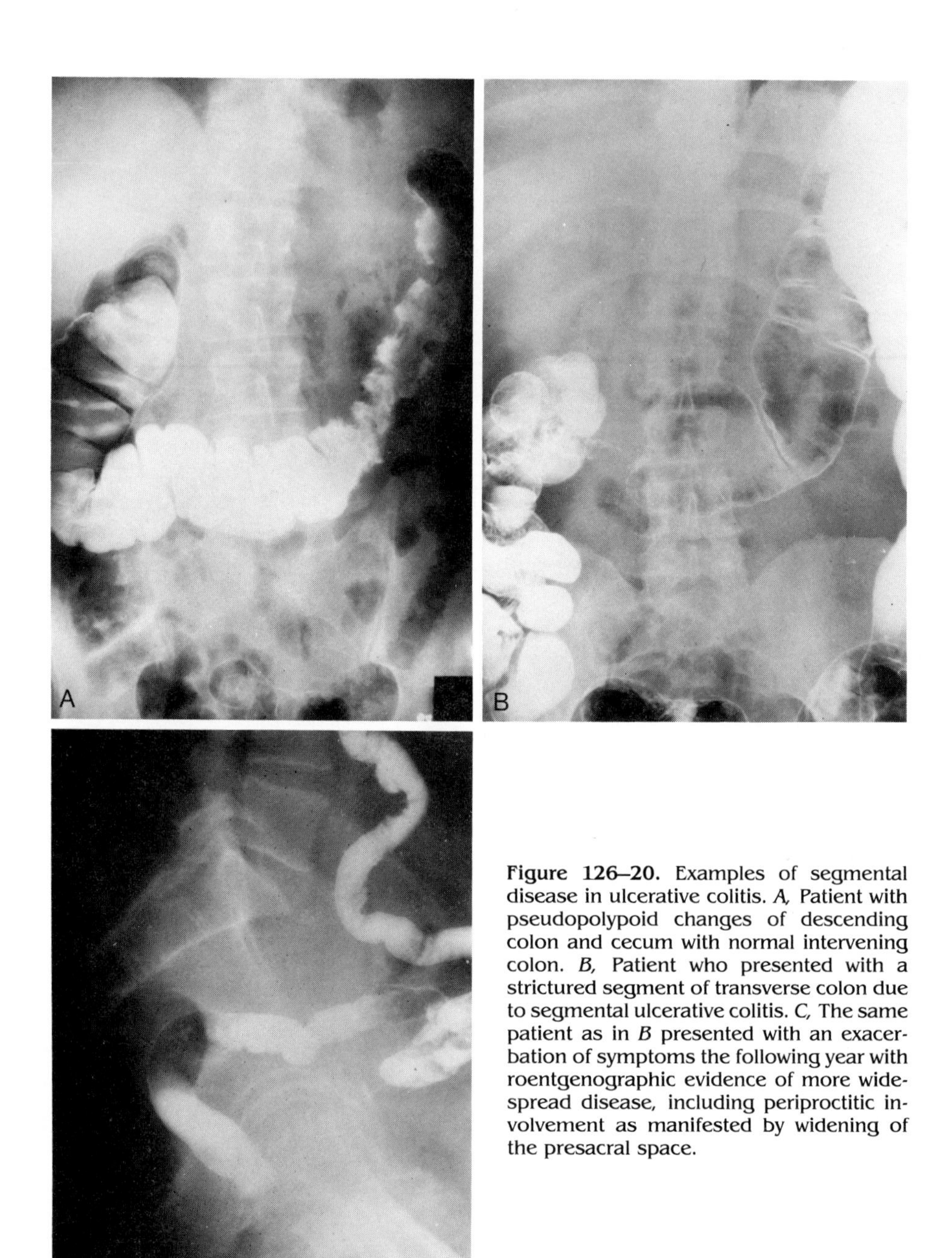

Figure 126–20. Examples of segmental disease in ulcerative colitis. *A*, Patient with pseudopolypoid changes of descending colon and cecum with normal intervening colon. *B*, Patient who presented with a strictured segment of transverse colon due to segmental ulcerative colitis. *C*, The same patient as in *B* presented with an exacerbation of symptoms the following year with roentgenographic evidence of more widespread disease, including periproctitic involvement as manifested by widening of the presacral space.

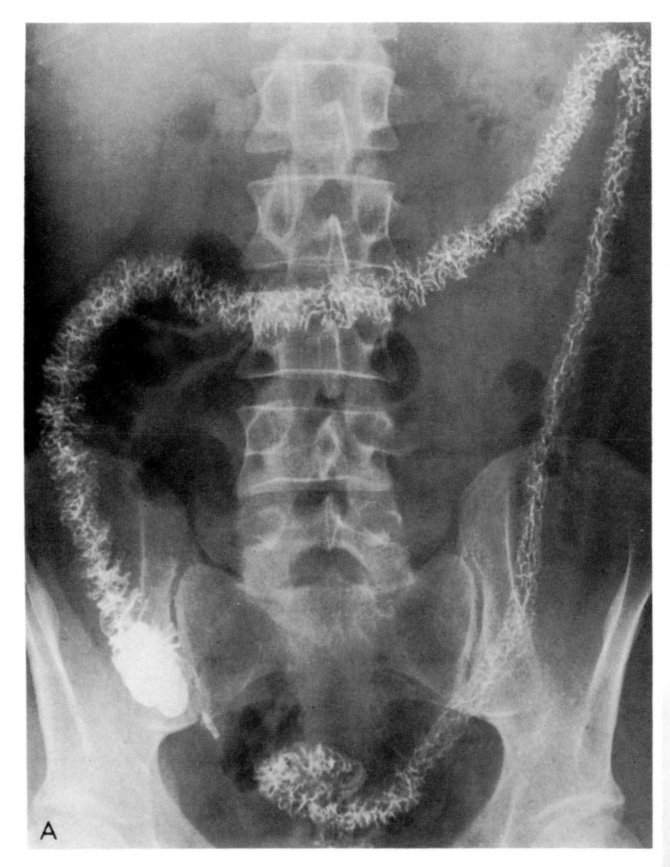

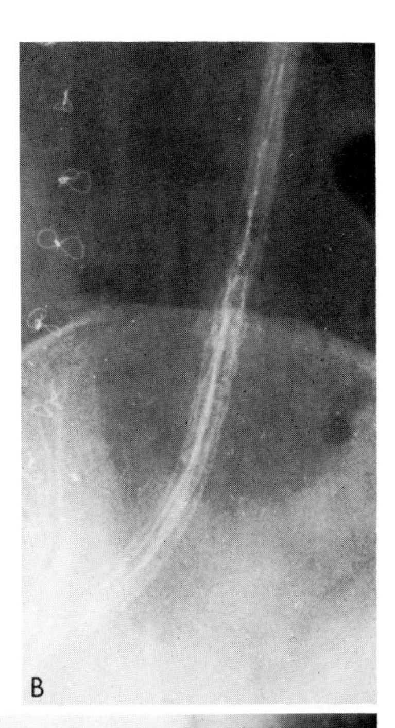

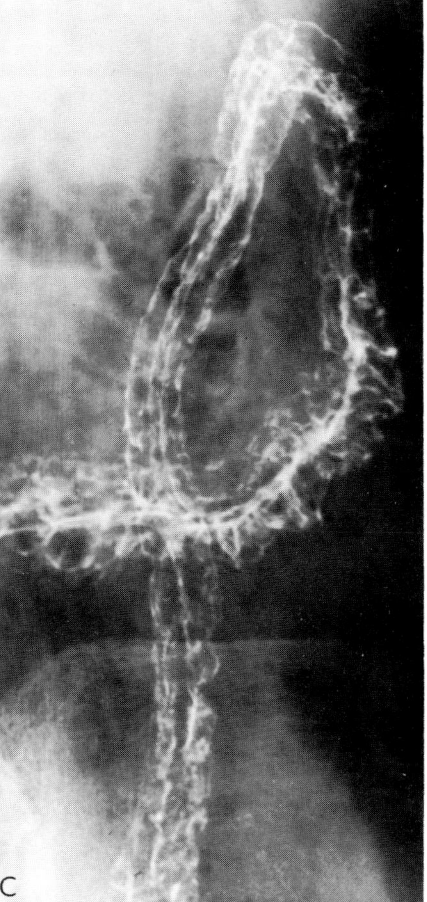

Figure 126–21. Mucosal evaluation in postevacuation films. *A,* Normal crinkled and sharply distinct mucosa. *B,* Postevacuation view of the linear mucosa seen in a significant number of normal persons. The folds are thin and well defined. *C,* Coarsened, crinkled, and linear mucosa in a patient with ulcerative colitis. The edematous folds are wider and less distinct than normal (compare with *B*).

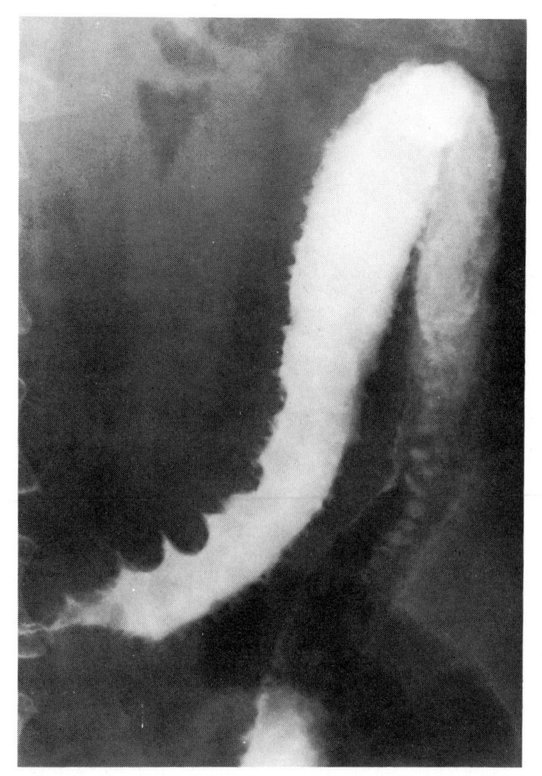

Figure 126–22. Thumbprinting in ulcerative colitis. Severe mucosal edema has resulted in thumbprinting of the distal transverse colon. Note the irregular marginal spiculations and loss of haustrations.

colitis. In more fulminant disease, altered motility is reflected by spasm and irritability, which result in narrowing and incomplete filling of the colon. With progression, ulcerations become more prominent and the spiculated marginal outline is replaced by an irregular serrated border. More deeply penetrating ulcers are seen as larger projections of barium that may be broader at their termination than at their base—so-called "collar-button" ulcers. Although variable in size and shape, they are usually symmetrically distributed throughout the involved portions of the bowel. They are not pathognomonic of ulcerative colitis and, in fact, are seen just as frequently in Crohn's colitis. They have also been reported in tuberculous, *Salmonella, Shigella,* and staphylococcal infections and in amebiasis (Fig. 126–25). Rarely, the "collar-button" ulcers may coalesce to form a longitudinal tract of barium that parallels the lumen (Figs 126–26 and 126–27). This is much more frequently seen in Crohn's colitis, however, or in diverticulitis.[9, 14, 39, 46] Rarely, pneumatosis coli may be seen in an area of severe ulceration.

In severe attcks with considerable ulceratin, polypoid formations may develop as a result of the combination of ulceration and mucosal regeneration (as described in the earlier section on Pathology). These inflammatory polyps ("pseudopolyps") are demonstrated as filling defects or radiolucencies within the barium column. They can be of variable size, shape, and pattern. Mucosal bridging may also be seen.[47] Occasionally, it is difficult to differentiate inflammatory polyps from the cobblestone appearance seen in Crohn's colitis. One distinguishing feature is that the so-called pseudopolyps tend to be more uniform in size and appearance[9] (Fig. 126–28).

Polypoid change may be seen as well in the absence of acute disease and ulceration, possibly as a result of re-epithelialization. Some authors use the terms "inflammatory" or "postinflammatory" polyp to refer to polypoid change occurring in low-grade and quiescent disease,[8] and "pseudopolyp" for the polypoid change seen in active disease with marked ulceration. Inflammatory polyps are usually nodular but may take the form of filiform polyposis seen as long filamentous radiolucent defects.[48] When localized, such inflammatory polyps can simulate a neoplasm, particularly a villous adenoma; rarely, they may cause obstruction. They may be difficult to differentiate from adenomatous polyps except that they tend to have a slightly irregular surface (best demonstrated on double contrast examination) and are rarely pedunculated.[8]

Widening of the retrorectal (presacral) soft tissue space, as seen in the lateral view, is a sign of periproctitic involvement. When measured on films showing normal rectal distention, the retrorectal space seldom exceeds 0.5 cm in normal subjects.[49] Measurements greater than 1 cm are taken as abnormal. As the retrorectal space widens in more severe involvement, the caliber of the rectum tends to narrow. This is most often seen late in the disease (Fig. 126–29). Thickening, blunting, or absence of the rectal valves of Houston may also be seen. However, neither widening of the presacral space nor loss of the valves of Houston is a reliable indicator of early ulcerative colitis.

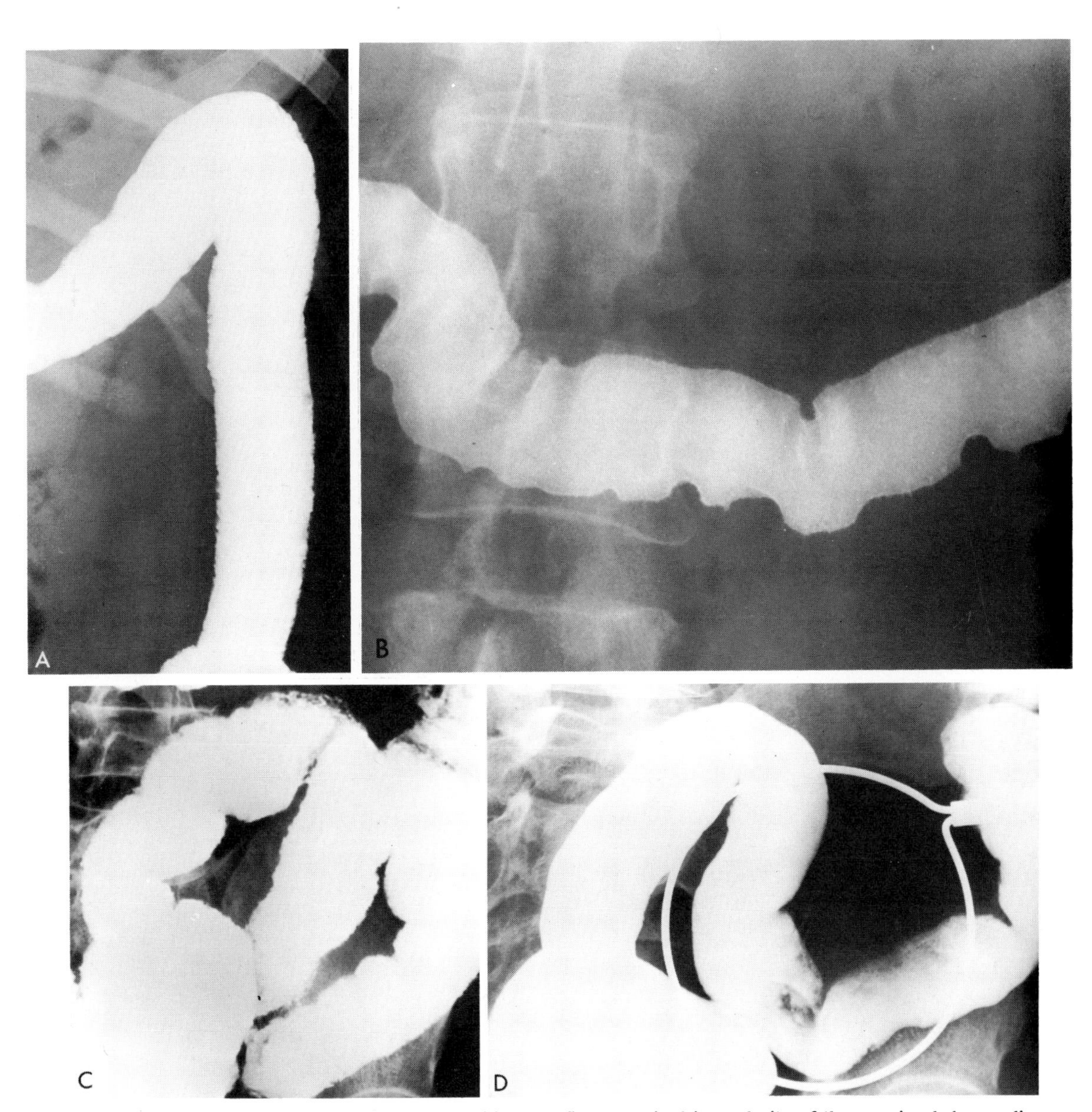

Figure 126–23. *A,* Spiculation in ulcerative colitis. The fine marginal irregularity of the proximal descending colon is due to tiny ulcers. *B,* Postevacuation film showing spiculation in a normal transverse colon due to unusually good penetration of the glands of Lieberkühn with barium. *C,* Non-opaque residue is adherent to the bowel wall, causing irregularity in outline and simulating ulcerative colitis. *D,* Same patient as in C, 8 days later, following cleansing enemas. The marginal outline is now smooth and regular.

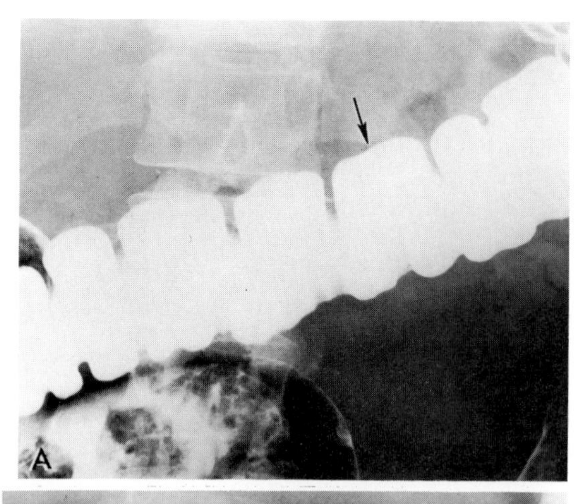

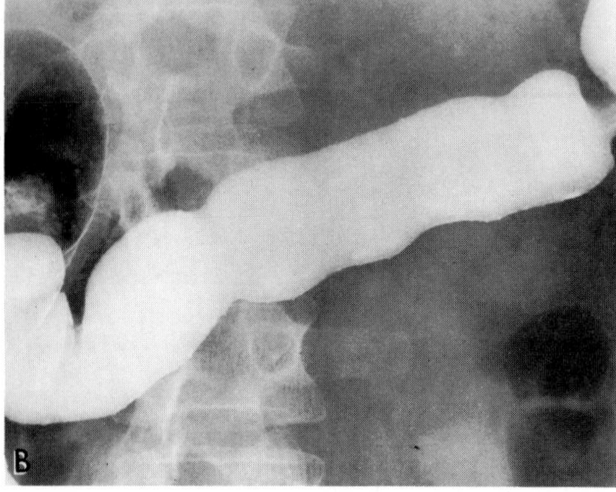

Figure 126–24. Haustral changes in ulcerative colitis. *A*, Squaring of the haustra in the transverse colon *(arrow)* is seen in a patient with clinical findings of ulcerative colitis. *B*, Same patient, 3 years later, showing progression of disease with loss of haustra in the same segment of colon.

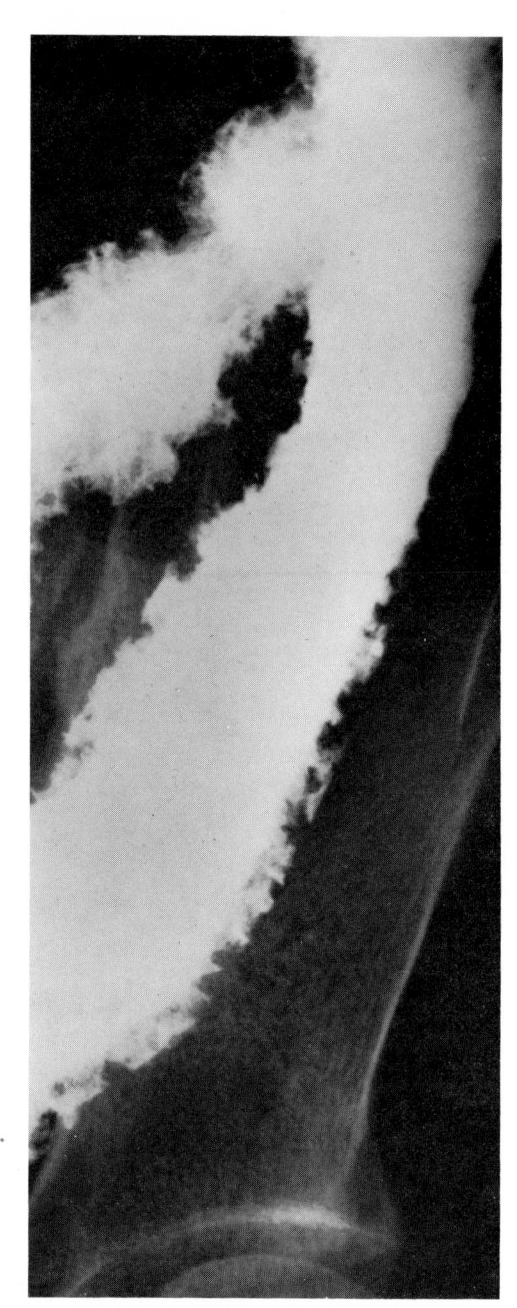

Figure 126–25. Deep ulcers in ulcerative colitis. The ulcers in the descending colon assume a "collar-button" configuration in this patient with moderately advanced disease.

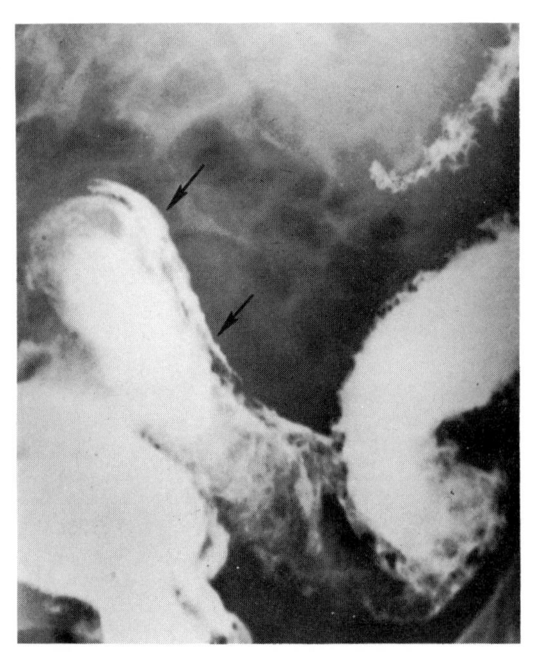

Figure 126–26. Deep ulcers in the sigmoid colon of patient with ulcerative colitis that have coalesced to form a linear collection of barium parallel to the bowel lumen *(arrows)*.

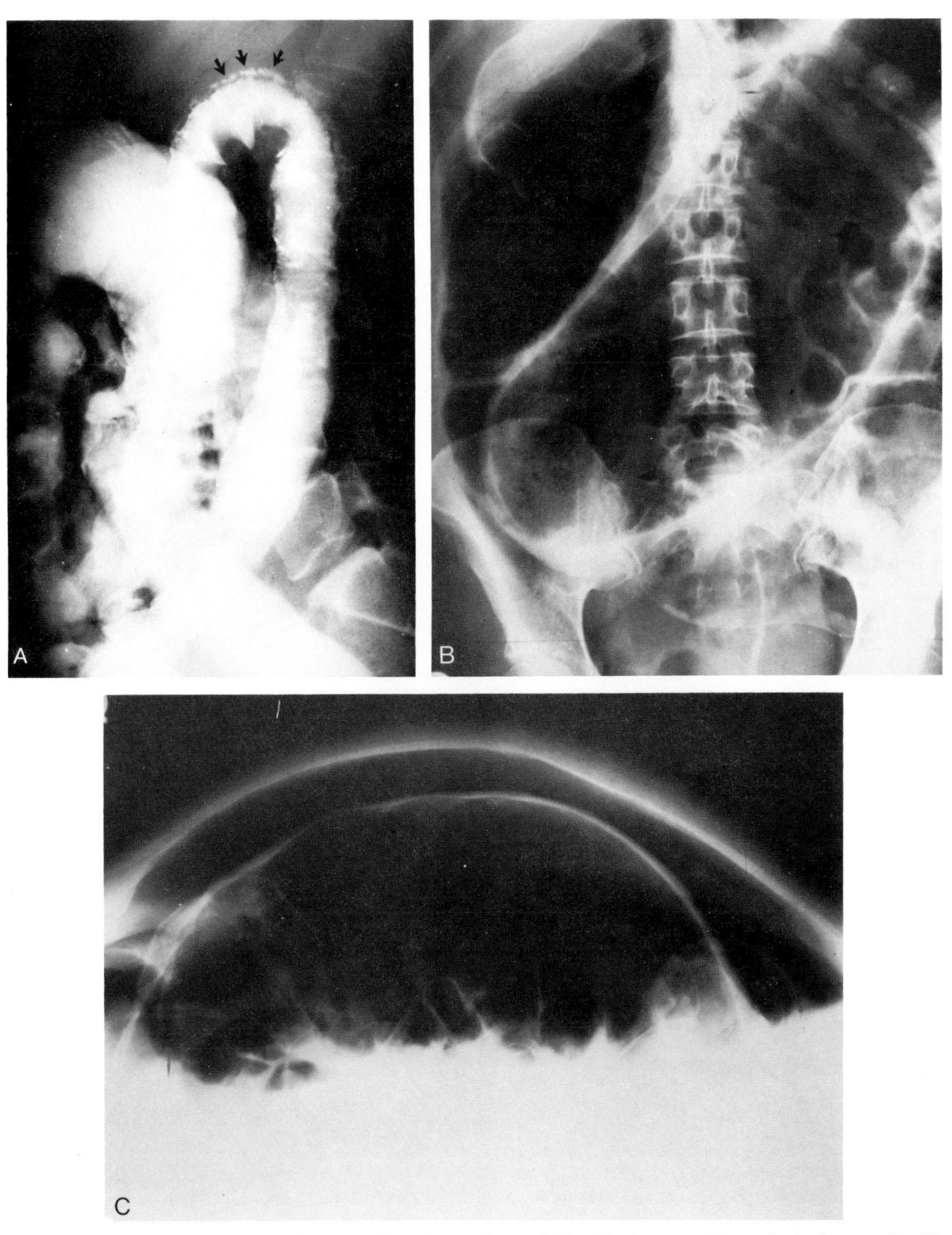

Figure 126–27. *A,* A linear collection of barium *(arrows)* paralleling the lumen of the splenic flexure of a 32-year-old patient with ulcerative colitis evidently due to coalescence of deep ulcers. *B* and *C,* Anteroposterior and crosstable lateral plain films of the same patient obtained 2 years later during an acute exacerbation of symptoms. These demonstrate toxic dilatation and perforation with pneumoperitoneum.

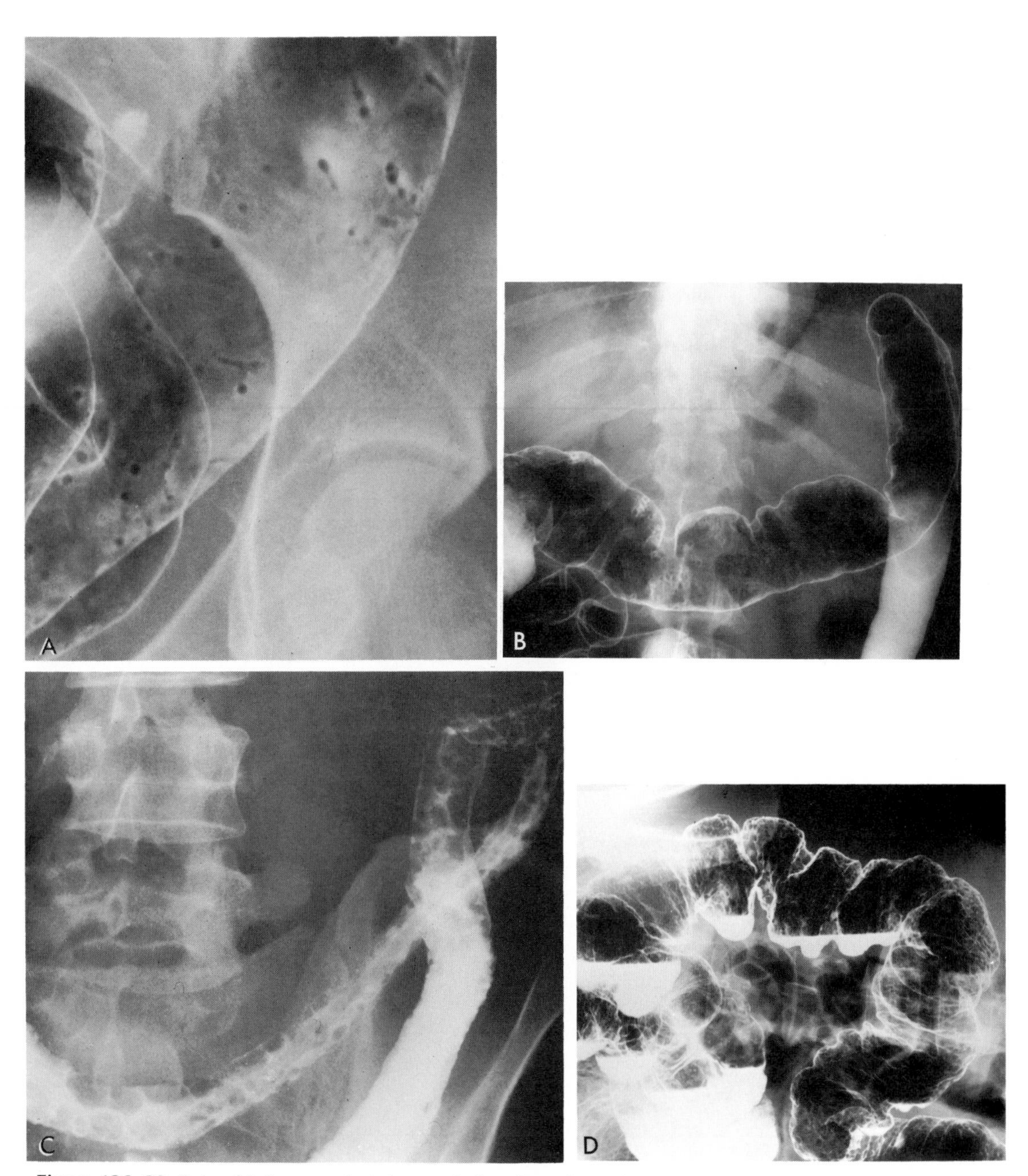

Figure 126–28. Polypoid changes. *A,* Anteroposterior view of the sigmoid colon as seen by air contrast study reveals many small rounded and linear radiolucencies that were demonstrated throughout the colon and represent mucosal bridges. *B,* Another patient with long filamentous radiolucent filling defects due to inflammatory polyps seen on double contrast film of the transverse colon. *C,* Posteroanterior view of the transverse colon of a patient with ulcerative colitis showing diffuse pseudopolypoid mucosa that simulates the "cobblestone" appearance of granulomatous colitis. *D,* Decubitus double contrast film of the ascending and transverse colon of a fourth patient with ulcerative colitis showing numerous barium-coated pseudopolyps involving the entire colon.

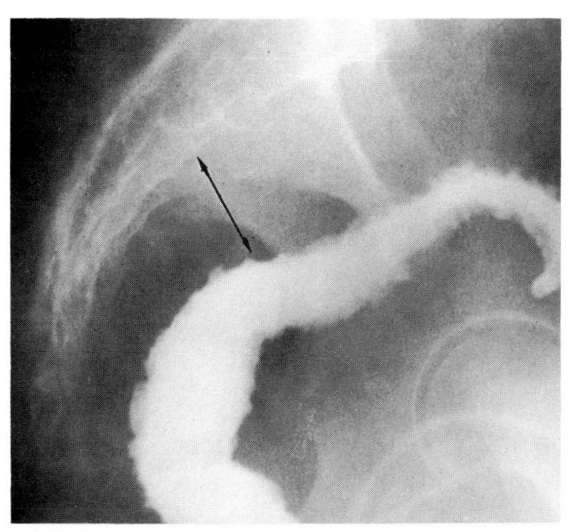

Figure 126–29. Increase in the presacral space in ulcerative colitis. Lateral film of the barium-filled rectosigmoid reveals the presacral space *(arrow)* to be widened to twice normal diameter. Extensive marginal ulcerations are evident.

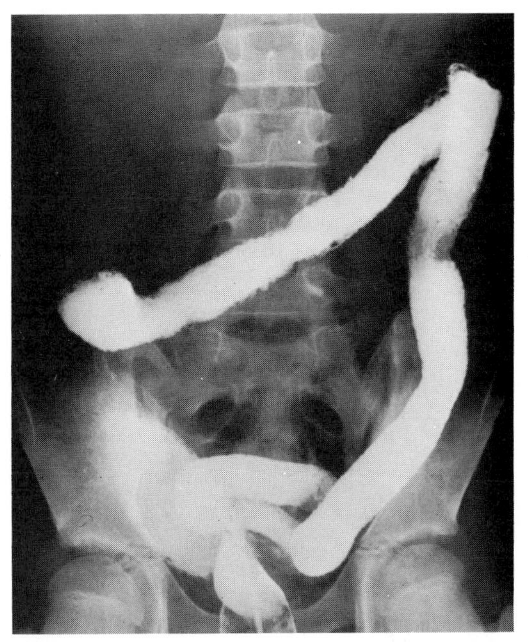

Figure 126–30. Chronic ulcerative colitis with shortening of the colon. The flexures are depressed and the entire colon was shortened as a result of repeated inflammatory attacks in this 12-year-old patient. There are marginal ulcerations throughout the colon, indicating an acute exacerbation.

As the disease becomes chronic, epithelial regeneration, inflammatory polyps, muscular hypertrophy, spasm, and possibly fibrosis progress and account for changes in the roentgenologic appearance. The colon develops a fixed configuration with absent haustrations; shortening occurs, resulting in downward placement and uncoiling of the flexures; and narrowing of the lumen frequently is present. This is the "lead-pipe" colon appearance of chronic ulcerative colitis (Fig. 126–30). Only rarely does a colon of this configuration return to a more normal caliber and length on subsequent examinations.[9]

In patients with longstanding pancolitis, abnormalities of the terminal ileum may be demonstrated, such as a gaping ileocecal valve, dilatation, stiffness, absent peristalsis, and a granular mucosa in a segment measuring 5 to 25 cm. This "backwash ileitis" (Fig. 126–31) is seen in approximately 10% of patients undergoing colectomy for ulcerative colitis.[8] The contraction, fissuring, and evidence of fistulization and an inflammatory mass that are frequently present in Crohn's disease are not seen.

Regardless of the method of examination and the stage of the disease, the hallmarks of ulcerative colitis are uniform and continuous involvement of the affected bowel. The rectum is almost always involved in continuity with the left colon when the colon is not totally involved. Granularity and ulceration tend to be continuous over the involved

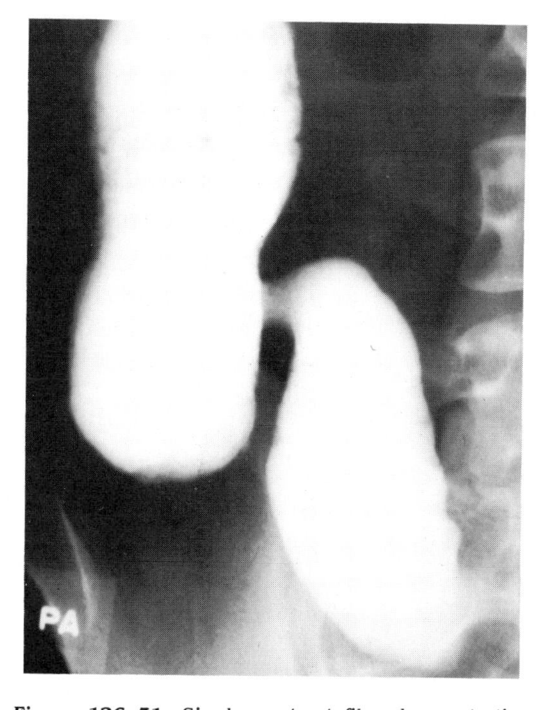

Figure 126–31. Single contrast film demonstrating backwash ileitis in ulcerative colitis. There is a gaping ileocecal valve with dilatation of the terminal ileum.

colon without normal segments of bowel intervening between 2 diseased segments of colon.

Strictures. Benign strictures, defined as localized, rigid narrowings that produce antegrade obstruction, are rare in ulcerative colitis; when seen, they are associated with longstanding disease. Marshak et al.[50] observed strictures in 1% of 1700 patients, whereas deDombal et al.[51] report a prevalence rate of 11.2%. The left colon and ileocecal valve are the most frequent sites. Stricturing of the ileocecal valve with resultant dilatation of the terminal ileum may simulate a carcinoma of the ascending colon. Strictures were previously thought to be secondary to local fibrosis. However, the occasional disappearance of a stricture on follow-up radiographic examination, as well as some evidence based on pathologic findings, together suggest that hypertrophy and contraction of the muscularis mucosae may be the cause in some cases. Areas of spasm can be differentiated from the strictures by the IV administration of 1 mg of glucagon prior to the examination.

The typical benign stricture has a concentric lumen with smoothly contoured, pliable, tapering margins (Fig. 126–32). Double contrast examinations show the mucosa within the stricture to be identical to that on either side of it. Benign strictures occasionally are eccentric, with irregularity of the mucosa and marginal outline making the roentgen differentiation between a benign and a malignant stricture impossible. It has been advocated, therefore, that strictures in ulcerative colitis be presumed to be malignant until proved otherwise.[52]

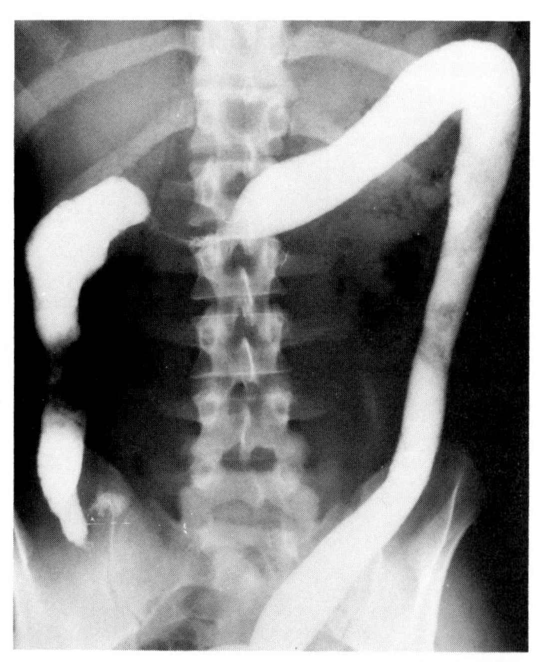

Figure 126–32. Single contrast film showing benign inflammatory stricture in ulcerative colitis. The gradual tapered narrowing at either end of this localized stricture of the proximal transverse colon suggests that this is most likely a benign complication rather than carcinoma.

Carcinoma. The distribution of carcinoma of the colon complicating ulcerative colitis differs from that in non-colitic colons in that fewer rectosigmoid lesions are seen in patients with inflammatory bowel disease. In addition, the tumors associated with ulcerative colitis are more evenly distributed throughout the bowel,[58] and there is a tendency for them to be multiple. The roentgenographic appearance is often atypical, probably because of the superimposed inflammatory process. Scirrhous carcinoma often produces a narrowing that is difficult, if not impossible, to differentiate radiographically from a benign stricture (Fig. 126–33). Occasionally, however, eccentricity of the lumen and irregularity of the mucosa, which differs from the mucosa adjacent to the stricture, are seen. Uneven narrowing or shouldering may also be present. These features would suggest malignancy.

Cancer developing in a colon involved by ulcerative colitis may sometimes form an annular constricting lesion typical of adenocarcinoma seen in non-colitic colons (Fig. 126–34). Still a third form that cancer in association with ulcerative colitis may assume is that of a polypoid tumor.

Differential Diagnosis

In the United States, Canada, and Western Europe the great majority of cases of inflammatory disease involving the colon are idiopathic. Ischemic disease of the colon and infectious diseases, such as blastomycosis, amebiasis, shigellosis, tuberculosis, and lymphogranuloma venereum among others, may also produce colonic changes that radiologically resemble inflammatory bowel disease of the idiopathic variety.[59] These diseases simulating idiopathic ulcerative colitis generally can be distinguished on clinical, bacteriologic, and histologic grounds.

Diffuse pseudopolyposis in ulcerative colitis occasionally resembles familial polyposis. However, patients with familial poly-

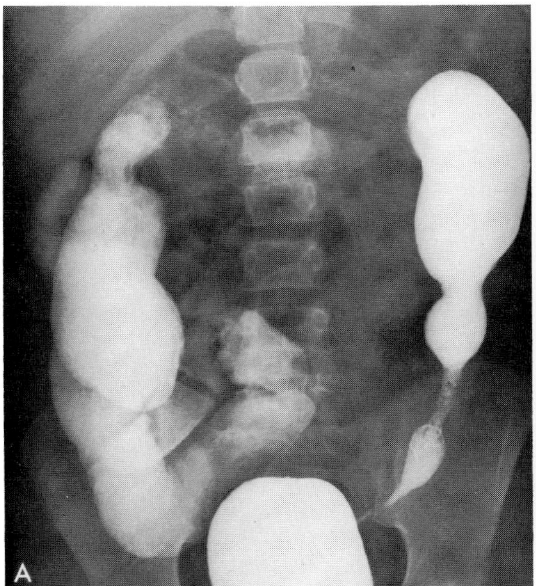

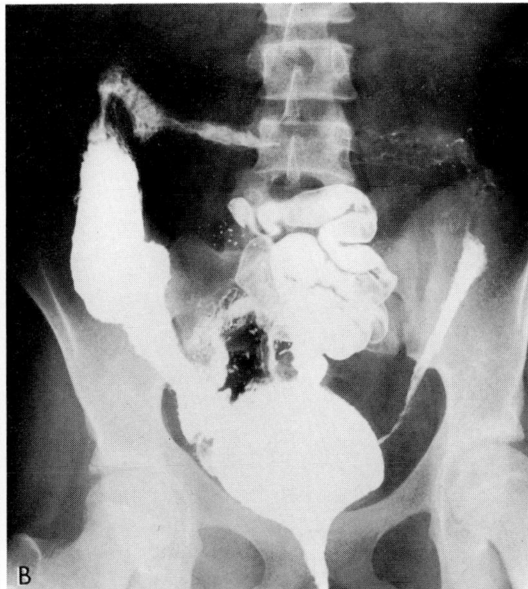

Figure 126–33. Carcinoma complicating ulcerative colitis. *A*, Barium enema study in this young patient with a prolonged history of ulcerative colitis shows a shortened, stiff colon with narrowing in the distal descending colon, evidently due to benign stricture. *B*, Re-examination 4 years later reveals progression of the narrowing and shortening of the colon and a change in the caliber of the ascending colon at the hepatic flexure, which proved to be due to carcinoma.

posis generally have no radiologic evidence of inflammation. Hence, ulcerations, contraction of the colon, and absence of haustrations are not seen.

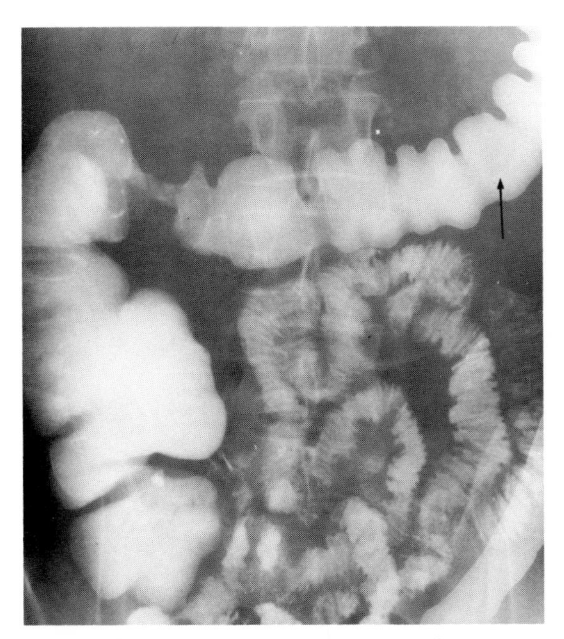

Figure 126–34. Typical annular constricting adenocarcinoma of proximal transverse colon in 29-year-old male with a 12-year history of ulcerative colitis. Note also the synchronous neoplasm in the distal transverse colon *(arrow)*, which proved to be an inflammatory pseudopolyp.

Chronic ingestion of irritant laxatives, particularly cascara and podophyllin, may result in the entity known as cathartic colon. The roentgen changes in such a colon are often similar to those seen in advanced ulcerative colitis. Backwash ileitis may also be simulated. The changes are usually most extensive in the right colon (Fig. 126–35). The paradox of roentgen findings suggestive of chronic ulcerative colitis in the presence of constipation should raise the suspicion of chronic laxative abuse.[60, 61]

The principal differential diagnosis that most often must be made is between the 2 idiopathic forms—ulcerative colitis and Crohn's disease of the colon. As mentioned previously, double contrast radiographic examination of the colon has greatly facilitated differential diagnosis of these 2 entities, particularly early in the disease. Sensitivities of 90% and better have been reported.[17, 26, 27, 33–35] Nevertheless, diagnostic difficulty is still encountered, especially late in the course of the disease, as numerous exacerbations, remissions, and various modes of therapy alter the roentgenographic appearance. Moreover, reports have appeared of coexistent Crohn's disease and ulcerative colitis in the same patient[62, 63] (Fig. 126–36).

The radiographic features of Crohn's disease are presented in detail in Chapter 127.

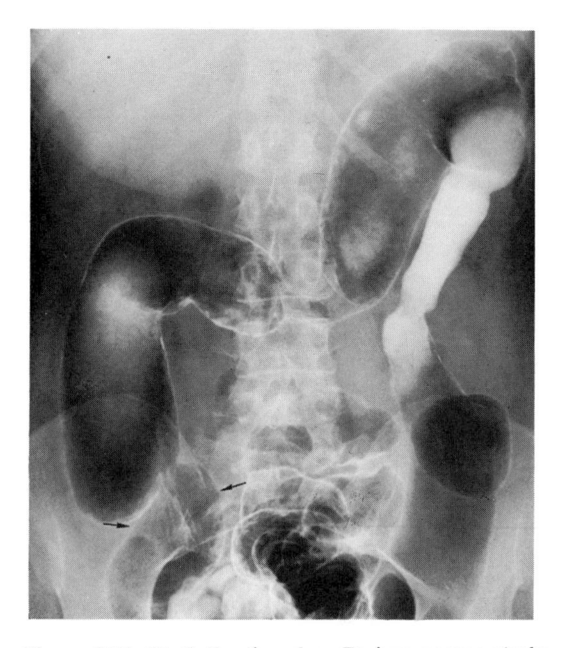

Figure 126–35. Cathartic colon. Barium enema study in a patient without clinical or proctosigmoidoscopic evidence of ulcerative colitis but with a history of chronic cathartic ingestion shows shortening and stiffening of the colon with loss of haustral markings. The ileocecal area is patulous and the terminal ileum is dilated *(arrow)*. The roentgenographic picture is indistinguishable from that of ulcerative colitis with backwash ileitis.

To be emphasized here is that in contrast to the diffuse continuous granular mucosal pattern of early ulcerative colitis, early Crohn's colitis is characterized by discrete aphthoid ulcers superimposed upon a normal mucosa and is typically discontinuous, with skip areas and asymmetric involvement. Also, there is a greater tendency to involve the terminal ileum and right colon. Therefore, a small bowel study is often valuable in the differential diagnosis. Rectal involvement is less frequent (approximately 50%). The aphthoid ulcer, which is seen as a fleck of barium surrounded by a radiolucent halo of edema, is the first detectable change in Crohn's colitis and probably cannot be seen on the single contrast examination. Although this ulcer is not seen in ulcerative colitis,[27] it is not pathognomonic of Crohn's disease, since it may be seen in amebiasis, Behçet's disease, and infection by *Yersinia entercolitica*.[59] Of note is the fact that there have been reports that the diffuse, continuous, granular mucosal pattern typical of ulcerative colitis may also be seen in rare cases of Crohn's colitis.[13, 64] Contrasting features that help distinguish between ulcerative colitis and Crohn's disease affecting the colon are summarized in Table 126–2.

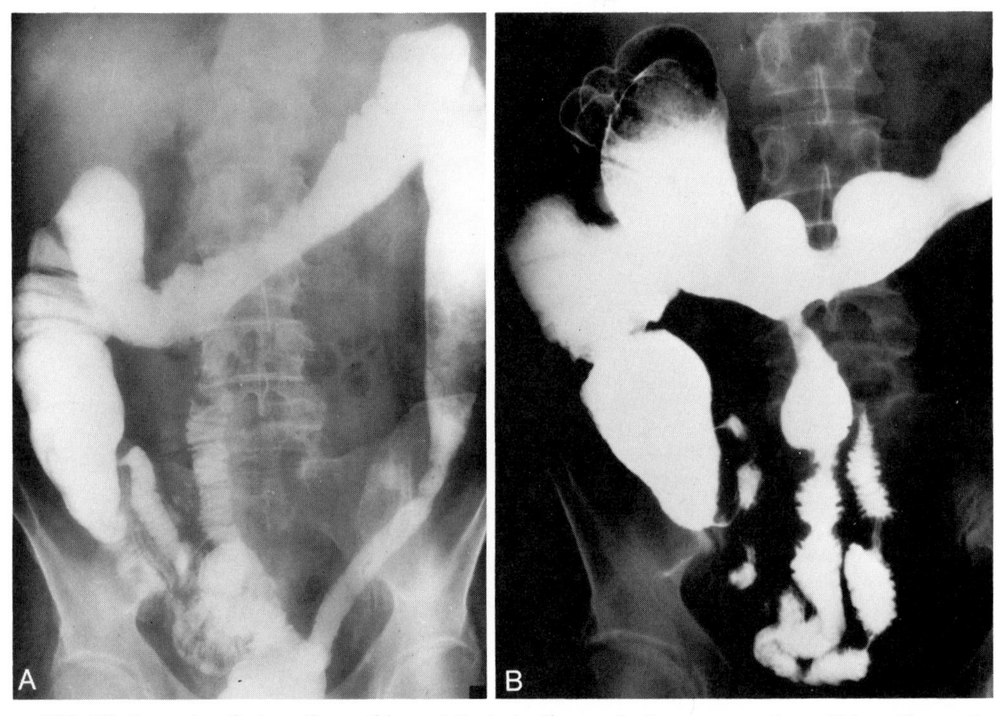

Figure 126–36. Example of ulcerative colitis and Crohn's disease in the same patient. This patient, who had had a previous ileotransverse colostomy without resection for Crohn's ileitis *(A)*, presented later with changes in the small bowel due to Crohn's disease and involvement of the colon with ulcerative colitis *(B)* proved by gross and microscopic findings on pathologic examination.

Table 126–2. SOME RADIOGRAPHIC FEATURES DIFFERENTIATING ULCERATIVE COLITIS FROM CROHN'S COLITIS

Ulcerative Colitis	Crohn's Colitis
1. Diffusely granular mucosa: Ulceration, if present, is superimposed upon granularity and is diffusely and symmetrically distributed	1. Aphthoid ulcers superimposed on normal mucosa: asymmetric distribution
2. Symmetric and continuous involvement: Extends proximally from rectum; total involvement in approximately 50%	2. Asymmetric and discontinuous involvement: Skip lesions; tendency to involve right colon and terminal ileum
3. Rectum almost always diffusely involved (95%)	3. Rectum frequently normal: 50% have patchy involvement; anal lesions and pericecal sinuses frequent
4. Fistulas and abscesses very rare	4. Fistulas and abscesses common
5. Small bowel involvement: Terminal ileum involved in 10% to 20%, but short segments are involved; superficial involvement without narrowing; gaping ileocecal value	5. Small bowel involvement: More frequent (50%) and extensive narrowing, ulceration, skip lesions, and mesenteric thickening frequent; thickened ileocecal valve often with cecoileal fistulization
6. Other features:	6. Other features:
a. Strictures—rare (2% to 11%), consider malignancy	a. Strictures—more common and generally more severe
b. Malignant potential—much higher than normal	b. Malignant potential—probably increased incidence
c. Pseudopolyps and hyperplastic polyps—more common and more extensive	c. Pseudopolyps and hyperplastic polyps—less common, less extensive
d. Cobblestoning—less frequent	d. Cobblestoning—more frequent
e. Deep ulcers—less frequent	e. Deep ulcers—more common; transverse and longitudinal fissuring seen
f. "Collar-button" ulcers—similar frequency	f. "Collar-button" ulcers—similar frequency
g. Thumbprinting—similar frequency	g. Thumbprinting—similar frequency
h. Toxic dilatation—rarely occurs but ulcerative colitis is the most common cause	h. Toxic dilatation—less common
i. Chronically contracted colon with abnormal or absent haustrations—more frequent	i. Chronically contracted colon with abnormally or absent haustration—less frequent
j. Thickened bowel wall—less prominent	j. Thickened bowel wall—more prominent

References

1. Goodman MJ, Sparberg M. Ulcerative Colitis. 1st Ed. New York: John Wiley, 1978.
2. Goldberg HI, Jeffrey RB. Recent advances in the radiologic evaluation of inflammatory bowel disease. Med Clin North Am 1980; 64:1059–79.
3. Jones B, Abbruzzese AA, Hill TC, Adelstein SJ. Gallium-67-citrate scintigraphy in ulcerative colitis. Gastrointest Radiol 1980; 5:267–72.
4. Sty JR, Boedecker RA, Thorp SM. Abdominal imaging in ulcerative colitis. Clin Nucl Med 1979; 4:427.
5. Segal AW, Munro JM, Ensell J, Sarner M. Indium-111 tagged leucocytes in the diagnosis of inflammatory bowel disease. Lancet 1981; 2:230–2.
6. Halls J, Young AC. Plain abdominal films in colonic disease. Proc Roy Soc Med 1964; 58:859–60.
7. Bartram CI. Plain abdominal x-ray in acute colitis. Proc Roy Soc Med 1976; 69:617–8.
8. Bartram CI, Laufer I. Inflammatory bowel disease. *In:* Laufer I, ed. Double Contrast Radiology with Endoscopic Correlation. 1st Ed. Philadelphia: WB Saunders, 1979: 601–88.
9. Janower ML. Ulcerative colitis. *In:* Dreyfuss JR, Janower ML, eds. Radiology of the Colon. 1st Ed. Baltimore: Williams and Wilkins, 1980: 199–242.
10. Margulis AR. Radiology of ulcerative colitis. Radiology 1972; 105:251–63.
11. Schofield PF, Mandal BK, Ironside AG. Toxic dilatation of the colon in salmonella colitis and inflammatory bowel disease. Br J Surg 1979; 66:5–8.
12. Wolf BS, Marshak RH. "Toxic" segmental dilatation of the colon during the course of fulminating ulcerative colitis: Roentgen findings. Am J Radiol 1959; 82:985–95.
13. Bartram CI. Radiology in the current assessment of ulcerative colitis. Gastrointest Radiol 1976/1977; 1:383–92.
14. Marshak RH, Linder AE, Maklansky D. Radiology of the Colon. Philadelphia: WB Saunders, 1980.
15. deDombal FT, Watts JMcK, Watkinson G, Goligher JC. Intraperitoneal perforation of the colon in ulcerative colitis. Proc Roy Soc Med 1965; 58:713–5.
16. Roth JLA. Ulcerative colitis. *In:* Bockus HL, ed. Gastroenterology. 3rd Ed. Philadelphia: WB Saunders, 1976: 645–749.
17. Thoeni RF, Margulis AR. Radiology in inflammatory disease of the colon: An area of increased interest for the modern clinician. Invest Radiol 1980; 15:281–92.
18. Marshak RH, Lindner AL. Radiologic diagnosis of chronic ulcerative colitis and Crohn's disease. *In:* Kirsner JB, Shorter RG, eds. Inflammatory Bowel Disease. 2nd Ed. Philadelphia: Lea and Febiger, 1980: 341–409.
19. Binder SC, Patterson JF, Glotzer DJ. Toxic megacolon in ulcerative colitis. Gastroenterology 1974; 66:909–15.
20. Roth JLA, Valdes-Dapena A, Stein GN, Bockus HL. Toxic megacolon in ulcerative colitis. Gastroenterology 1959; 37:239–55.
21. Goldberg HI. The barium enema and toxic megacolon: Cause-effect relationship? Gastroenterology 1975; 68:617–8.
22. Seaman WB, Wells J. Complications of the barium enema. Gastroenterology 1965; 48:728–37.
23. Nelson JA, Daniels AV, Dodds WJ. Rectal balloons: Complications, causes and recommendations. Invest Radiol 1979; 14:48–59.
24. LeFrock J, Ellis CA, Klainer AS, Weinstein L. Transient bacteremia associated with barium enema. Arch Intern Med 1979; 135:835–7.
25. Schimmel DH, Hanelin LG, Cohen S, Goldberg HI. Bacteremia and the barium enema. Am J Radiol 1977; 128:207–8.
26. Laufer I, Hamilton J. The radiological differentiation between ulcerative and granulomatous colitis by double contrast radiology. Am J Gastroenterol 1976; 66:259–69.
27. Kelvin FM, Oddson TA, Rice RP, Garbutt JT, Bradenham

BP. Double contrast barium enema in Crohn's disease and ulcerative colitis. AJR 1978; 131:207–13.
28. Stein GN, Roy RH, Finkelstein AK. Roentgen changes in ulcerative colitis. Semin Roentgenol 1968; 3:3–26.
29. Rigler LG, Weiner M. History of roentgenology of the gastrointestinal tract. *In:* Margulis AR, Burhenne HJ, eds. Alimentary Tract Roentgenology. 2nd Ed. St. Louis: CV Mosby, 1973: 3–17.
30. Margulis AR. Examination of the colon. *In:* Margulis AR, Burhenne HJ, eds. Alimentary Tract Radiology. 2nd Ed. St. Louis: CV Mosby, 1973: 923–62.
31. Simpkins KC, Stevenson GW. The modified Malmö double contrast enema in colitis: An assessment of its accuracy in reflecting sigmoidoscopic findings. Br J Radiol 1972; 45:486–92.
32. Young AC. The "instant" barium enema in proctocolitis. Proc Roy Soc Med 1963; 56:491–4.
33. Laufer I. The radiologic demonstration of early changes in ulcerative colitis by double contrast technique. J Assoc Can Radiol 1975; 116–21.
34. Laufer I, Mullens JE, Hamilton J. Correlation of endoscopy and double contrast radiography in the early stages of ulcerative and granulomatous colitis. Radiology 1976; 118:1–5.
35. Williams HJ, Stephens DH, Carlson HC. Double-contrast radiography: Colonic inflammatory disease. Am J Radiol 1981; 315–22.
36. Margulis AR, Goldberg HI, Lawson TL, Montgomery CK, Rambo ON, Noonan CD, Amberg JR. The overlapping spectrum of ulcerative and granulomatous colitis: A roentgenographic-pathologic study. Am J Radiol 1971; 113:325–34.
37. Kirsner JB. Problems in differentiation of ulcerative colitis and Crohn's disease of the colon: The need for repeated diagnostic evaluation. Gastroenterology 1975; 68:187–91.
38. Brazeau-Lamontagne L, Strom BG, Devroede G. Reliability of radiologic diagnosis in colitis. J Assoc Can Radiol 1980; 31:40–2.
39. Welin S, Welin G. The Double Contrast Examination of the Colon. Experience with the Welin Modification. Stuttgart, Thieme, 1976.
40. Fennessey JJ, Sparberg M, Kirsner JB. Early roentgenologic manifestations of mild ulcerative colitis and proctitis. Radiology 1966; 87:848–58.
41. Nugent FW, Veidenheimer MC, Zuberi S, Garabedian MM, Parikh NK. Clinical course of ulcerative proctosigmoiditis. Am J Dig 1970; 15:321.
42. Fraser GM, Findlay JM. The double contrast enema and Crohn's colitis. Clin Radiol 1976; 27:103–12.
43. Gabrielsson N, Grangvist S, Sundelin P, Thorgeirsson T. Extent of inflammatory lesions in ulcerative colitis assessed by radiology, colonoscopy, and endoscopic biopsies. Gastrointest Radiol 1979; 4:395–400.
44. Bartram CI, Walmsley K. A radiological and pathological correlation of the mucosal changes in ulcerative colitis. Clin Radiol 1978; 29:323–8.
45. Miller RE. Barium enema versus colonoscopy. Gastrointest Endosc 1982; 28:40–1.
46. Marshak RH, Lindner AE, Maklansky D. Paracolic fistulous tracts in diverticulitis and granulomatous colitis. JAMA 1980; 243:1943–6.
47. Hammerman AM, Shatz BM, Susman N. Radiographic characteristics of colonic "mucosal bridges": Sequelae of inflammatory bowel disease. Radiology 1978; 127:611–4.
48. Zegel HG, Laufer I. Filiform polyposis. Radiology 1978; 127:615–9.
49. Edling NPG, Eklof O. The retrorectal soft tissue space in ulcerative colitis. Radiology 1963; 80:949–53.
50. Marshak RH, Block C, Wolf BS. The roentgen findings in stricture of the colon associated with ulcerative and granulomatous colitis. AJR 1963; 90:709–16.
51. deDombal FT, Watts JMcK, Watkinson G, Golingher JC. Local complications of ulcerative colitis: Stricture, pseudopolyposis and carcinoma of colon and rectum. Br Med J 1966; 1:1442–7.
52. Fennessy JJ, Sparberg MB, Kirsner JB. Radiological findings in carcinoma of the colon complicating chronic ulcerative colitis. Gut 1968; 9:338–97.
53. MacDougall IPM. The cancer risk in ulcerative colitis. Lancet 1964; 2:655–8.
54. Greenstein AJ, Sachar DB, Smith H, Janowitz HD, Aufses AH. A comparison of cancer risk in Crohn's disease and ulcerative colitis. Cancer 1981; 48:2742–5.
55. Greenstein AJ, Sachar DB, Smith H, Pucillo A, Papatestas AE, Kreel I, Geller SA, Janowitz HD, Aufses AH Jr. Cancer in universal and left sided ulcerative colitis: Factors determining risk. Gastroenterology 1979; 77:290–4.
56. Sauer WG, Barger JA. Chronic ulcerative colitis and carcinoma. JAMA 1949; 141:982–5.
57. Hodgson JR, Sauer WG. The roentgenologic features of carcinoma in chronic ulcerative colitis. AJR 1961; 86:91–6.
58. Edling NPG, Lagercrantz R, Rosenquist H. Roentgenologic findings in ulcerative colitis with malignant degeneration. Acta Radiol 1959; 52:123–7.
59. Theoni RE, Margulis AR. The radiology of inflammatory disease of the colon. Postgrad Radiol 1981; 1:187–212.
60. Urso FP, Urso MJ, Lee CH. The cathartic colon: Pathological findings and radiological/pathological correlation. Radiology 1975; 116:557–9.
61. Heilbrun N, Bernstein C. Roentgen abnormalities of the large and small intestine associated with prolonged cathartic ingestion. Radiology 1955; 65:549–56.
62. Voitk AJ, Owen DR, Lough J. Coexistent regional enteritis and ulcerative colitis. Int Surg 1976; 61:535–7.
63. Eyer S, Spadaccini C, Walker P, Ansel H, Schwartz M, Sumner HW. Simultaneous ulcerative colitis and Crohn's disease. Am J Gastroenterol 1980; 73:345–9.
64. Joffe N. Diffuse mucosal granularity in double-contrast studies of Crohn's disease of the colon. Clin Radiol 1981; 32:85–90.

Endoscopy

Richard G. Farmer

Proctosigmoidoscopy

Proctosigmoidoscopic examination should ordinarily be carried out promptly. It is best performed without prior preparation with laxatives or enemas because these can cause mucosal irritation and perhaps increase the inflammation present. Proctosigmoidoscopic examination should be diagnostic in almost 100% of patients with ulcerative colitis.[1] The proximal extent of the disease may be beyond the reach of the instrument, or it may be sharply demarcated and readily viewed with normal-appearing mucosa above the upper limit of involvement (proctitis or proctosigmoiditis). The activity of the disease and the response to therapy may also be determined quite satisfactorily by serial proctosigmoidoscopic observation. At times, the patient may be so ill that the sigmoidoscope is inserted for only a few inches while the patient lies in the left lateral position, but the examination can be safely performed on virtually all patients with ulcerative colitis, no matter how ill.

Gross changes in the endoscopic appearance of the mucosa in ulcerative colitis are characteristically diffuse and continuous, not spotty or patchy. In observing activity of ulcerative colitis, attention is given to the type of exudate (mucoid, mucopurulent, sanguinopurulent, or grossly bloody); the degree of edema and hyperemia; the mucosal texture, which reflects the presence and size of ulcerations ("ground glass," fine, or coarse granularity); and the friability of the mucosa ("contact bleeding"). Edema is revealed in the swollen, succulent appearance of the mucosa, but most frequently in the thickened, rounded edges of the valves. The granular appearance of the mucosa is due to "highlights" from lymphoid hyperplasia in the submucosa, to intervening islands of the mucosa between pinpoint ulcerations, or to pock-like scarring of petechial ulcerations. Friability of the mucosa refers to the ease with which bleeding is provoked by gentle swabbing with a cotton-tipped applicator or by the sigmoidoscope. Bleeding may also occur spontaneously and may be seen on the initial inspection of the mucosa or observed coming down from above the advancing instrument. These endoscopic observations are somewhat subjective, and considerable variation in descriptive interpretation can be expected from different observers. Baron et al.[2] found the greatest agreement (82% of cases) among experienced colleagues in the assessment of friability, spontaneous bleeding, and the presence or absence of the vascular network. Less agreement (60% of cases) was reported for the descriptions of the shades of color, the surface of the mucosa, and the appearance of the valves of Houston.

Proctosigmoidoscopic Appearances (Table 126–3)

Acute Phase (Fig. 126–37). In the acute phase of ulcerative colitis, the "stages" described correspond to the severity of the disease. The patient may be observed initially at one of these stages, their relationship to time being extremely variable (days to weeks). As the disease process subsides and remission occurs, the reverse order of the "stages" may be observed. The changes in the acute phase are believed to be reparable, at least to a great extent, but not in patients with fulminating disease.

Stage 1 (minimal activity): The earliest change visualized is mottled discoloration due to a shower of petechiae under the mucosal surface. These hemorrhagic spots are all small and some are almost pinpoint in size. Edema may be noted in applying a cotton swab, which causes elevation of the membrane. The membrane may have a granular character ("ground glass").

Stage 2 (mild activity): The next change visualized is hyperemia and the mucosa may appear somewhat swollen. It has a moist, glistening character and there is an excess of mucoid secretion. The surface, after swabbing, looks granular (fine granularity) and shows frank bleeding points. Ulcerations

Table 126–3. PROCTOSIGMOIDOSCOPIC FEATURES OF ULCERATIVE COLITIS

Severity of Activity	Acute Phase				Chronic Phase	
	Minimal	*Mild*	*Moderate*	*Severe*	*Active*	*Quiescent*
Stage	1	2	3	4		
Exudate	Nil	Mucoid	Mucopurulent	Sanguino-purulent	Purulent	Nil
Edema	± Minimal	+ + (hyperemia)	+ + or + + + (red mucosa)	+ + + or + + + +	+ + (congestion)	Nil (pale)
Texture (surface)	Glistening or "ground glass"	Fine granularity; ± ulcerations, small, shallow	Coarse granularity; ulceration, extensive	Coarse pitting; denuded areas, hyperplastic islands	Polypoid hyperplasia or denudation; ± stenosis	Polypoid changes frequently persist; less stenosis
Friability (bleeding)	± Pinpoint hemorrhagic spots	+ or + + Bleeding points	+ + or + + + Oozing blood	+ + + + Free bleeding	+ + ± Diffuse ooze	0 No bleeding

may or may not be present. If present, they are usually small and shallow and likely to be located on the lower valve of Houston or just within the rectum; however, they may be diffusely distributed throughout the rectum.

Stage 3 (moderate activity): In the next phase, the mucosa is red and edematous, showing the characteristic pitted, granular appearance (coarse granularity). Usually there is a constant oozing of blood from the surface; swabbing is likely to result in such a free flow of blood that visualization of the mucous membrane is difficult. Ulceration is extensive and variable in size and depth, with little or no normal-appearing mucosa. Much of the surface may be covered with a thick mucopurulent exudate, which is frequently quite adherent. The valves of Houston become less prominent but very thick in appearance. At this stage, proctosigmoidoscopy may be difficult because of excessive spasm.

Stage 4 (severe or fulminating activity): In the very severe or fulminating cases, great difficulty is experienced in passing the sigmoidoscope, which must be inserted carefully. Little or no normal mucosa will be seen in the involved area of the rectum and sigmoid. There may be mucopurulent, sanguineous exudate. The mucosal surface is more or less constantly obscured by hemorrhage, and when visualized appears coarsely pitted, edematous, and ulcerated. Edema can be recognized despite bleeding and extreme congestion.

Chronic Phase (Fig. 126–38). The time necessary to produce the chronic stage is variable and depends on the tissue response to the disease process. In some patients the chronic changes may appear 2 or 3 months after onset.

Active digital examination of the anal canal may reveal stenosis. The rectal lumen may be narrowed and tubular, with complete loss of normal architecture. The rectal valves are blunted. The mucosal surface has a granular character, and although diffuse oozing of blood may be noted, edema and congestion are more characteristic. Purulent exudate is prominent. Hyperplastic polypoid areas are common, although denudation of the mucosa may be widespread.

Quiescent Phase. The appearance in the quiescent stage is very similar to that just described for the active stage with the exception that the evidence of congestion and edema is lacking. The mucosa appears dull and the normal vascular pattern is lost. Little or no evidence of exudate is noted. The surface is pale and able to withstand moderate trauma without bleeding. Although the rectum has usually increased somewhat in diameter, stenosis may persist. Evidence of polypoid change is frequently noted. This picture may persist for years without much change except during acute exacerbations.

Polypoid Hyperplasia (Fig. 126–39). Inflammatory polyps or so-called pseudopolyps (see earlier section on Pathology) are soft in comparison with true adenomas and show evidence of irregular growth on their surface; i.e., they are frequently only incompletely covered with membrane. These polypoid formations generally do not bleed easily. When the disease has been quiescent for a long period of time, they may become

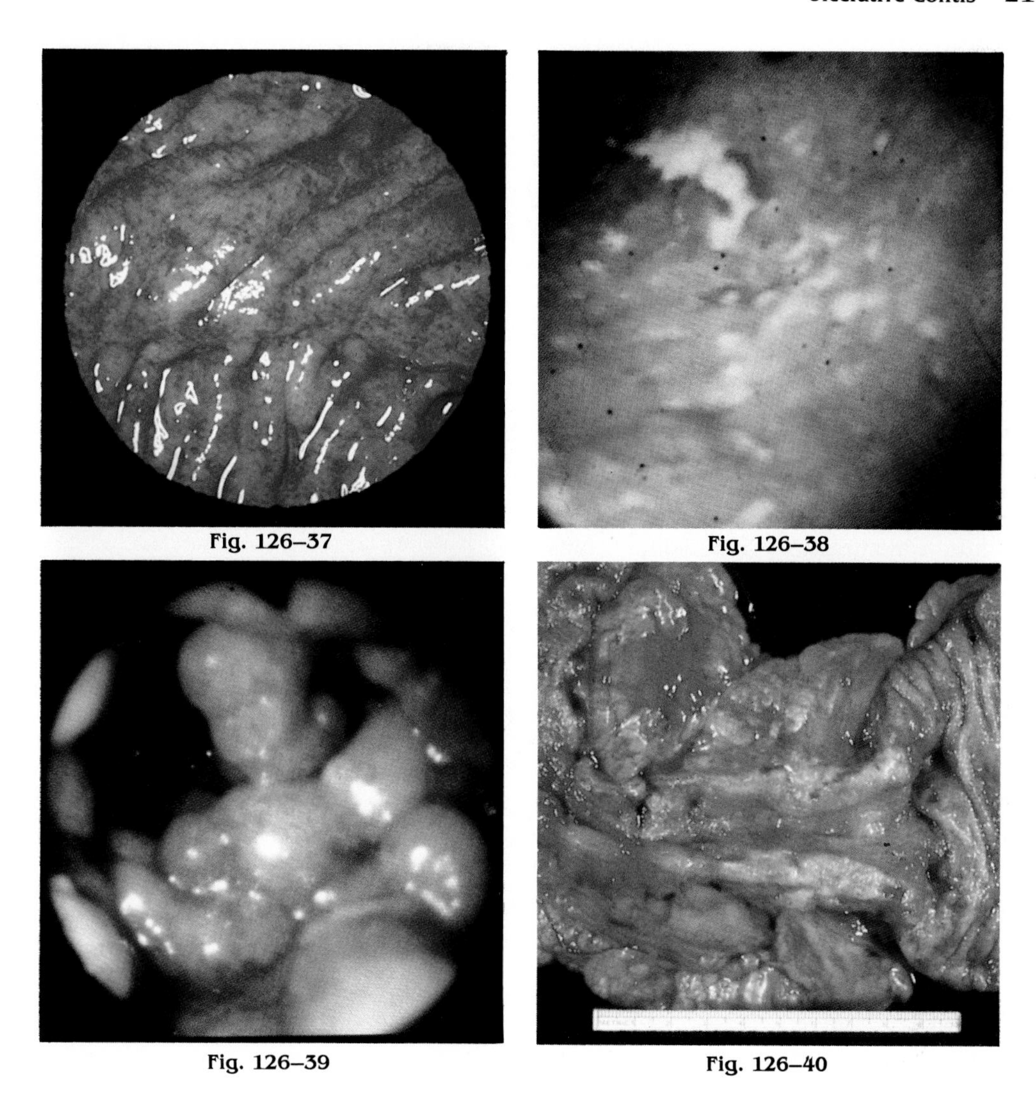

Fig. 126–37

Fig. 126–38

Fig. 126–39

Fig. 126–40

Figure 126–37. Active ulcerative colitis with fine diffuse mucosal ulcerations; active ulcerative colitis ulceration and friability, diffuse and uniform in distribution.

Figure 126–38. "Granular" mucosa in ulcerative colitis, with pus and some friability; chronic state.

Figure 126–39. Chronic ulcerative colitis with inflammatory polypoid formations (pseudopolyposis); surgical specimen showing extensive pseudopolyposis.

Figure 126–40. Surgical specimen showing cancer in ulcerative colitis.

smaller and even gradually disappear. Since they represent a combination of ulceration and an attempt at mucosal repair (see earlier section on Pathology), they may be found in recurrences in association with any of the previously described proctosigmoidoscopic appearances. They are frequently seen in greatest numbers in the region of the valves of Houston.

Colonoscopy

The ability to visualize and biopsy the entire mucosal surface of the colon by means of colonoscopy is of great benefit, particularly in long-term management and in cancer surveillance. Because the mucosal changes during acute inflammation are usually most noted in the rectosigmoid, proctosigmoidoscopy or fiberoptic sigmoidoscopy is beneficial in following the progress of the disease and the response to therapy. At times, however, it may be important to visualize the more proximal mucosa, particularly to determine the upper extent of the disease as well as its severity. One of the most frequent indications for colonoscopy in a patient with ulcerative colitis is to differentiate this disease from Crohn's disease of the colon. Perhaps the greatest value for colonoscopy, however, is in long-term surveillance and attempts at detection of dysplasia or other pre-cancerous changes (see earlier section on Pathology).

References

1. Crohn BB, Rosenberg H. Sigmoidoscopic picture of chronic ulcerative colitis (non-specific). Am J Med Sci 1925; 170:220.
2. Baron JH, Connell AM, Lennard-Jones JE. Variation between observers in describing mucosal appearances in proctitis. Br Med J 1964; 1:89.

Clinical Types and Differential Diagnosis

Richard G. Farmer

Clinical Types

The clinical picture of ulcerative colitis often develops in 1 of 2 ways: (1) an early acute or fulminating onset with great severity of symptoms, or (2) a rather indolent and often chronic course associated with frequent recurrences of symptoms, leading to chronic illness and malnutrition.

Various classifications have been used to evaluate patients with ulcerative colitis. Classifications according to severity of attack (mild, moderate, or severe), clinical course (acute fulminating, relapsing-remitting, or chronic continuous), or anatomic type based upon topographic localization (proctosigmoid, left colon, entire colon) are useful for orientation and prognostic significance. While there is considerable overlap (Fig. 126–41), the concept is helpful and difficulty is rarely encountered in fitting a given case into these classifications.

Severity. Since the clinical severity of an attack of ulcerative colitis has a profound influence on prognosis, each attack should be classified according to the grade of severity. Many clinicians utilize the criteria of Truelove and Witts[1]:

Severe: Diarrhea with 6 or more movements/day with macroscopic blood in the stools; either a mean evening temperature above 99.5°F or a temperature of 100°F or more on at least 2 days out of 4; tachycardia with a mean pulse rate of more than 90/minute; anemia with a hemoglobin concentration 75% of normal or less, allowance being made for recent blood transfusions; and an erythrocyte sedimentation rate greater than 30 mm/hour.

Mild: Diarrhea with 4 or fewer movements/

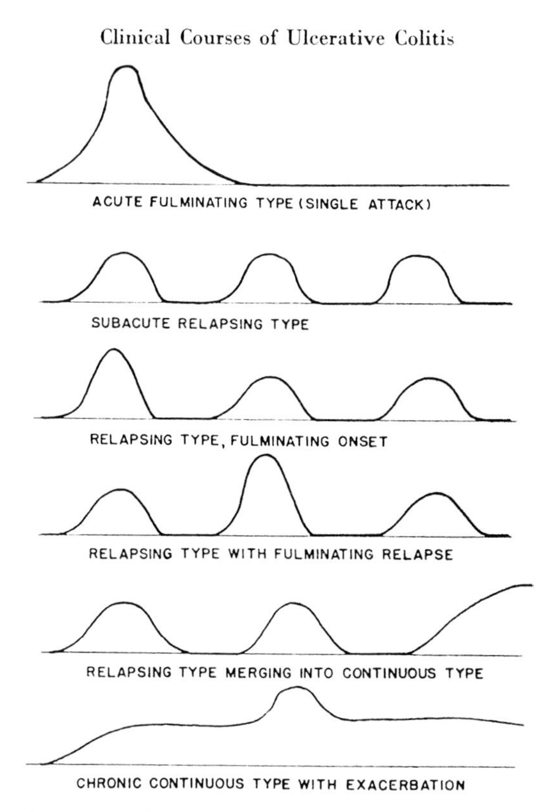

Figure 126–41. Principal clinical types of ulcerative colitis with clinical variants. (From Bockus HL et al. Gastroenterologia 1956; 86:560. Reproduced with permission.)

day and only small amounts of macroscopic blood in the stools; no fever; no tachycardia; anemia not severe; and an erythrocyte sedimentation rate less than 30 mm/hour. Jalan et al.[2] attempted to assess severity reported by a group of experienced clinicians more objectively by the use of a formula:

$$Y = 0.84\, X_2 + 0.12\, X_4 + 0.34\, X_6 - 0.59$$

where X_2 is temperature, X_4 the number of bowel movements, and X_6 the erythrocyte sedimentation rate. They pointed out that severity should be graded at the time of hospital admission rather than at the peak of severity, before which time decision regarding need for surgery should be made.

Table 126–4 shows the relative distribution of patients according to grade of severity of the first attack for which the patient was seen as recorded in 3 different groups. Table 126–5 graphically portrays the principal clinical types and their clinical courses.

A problem that bears on the classification according to anatomic location is the possibility that disease initially confined to the distal colon may extend proximally. This has generally been regarded to occur in about 10% of patients after 10 or more years of distal disease.[3] However, before the advent of fiberoptic sigmoidoscopy and colonoscopy, it was often difficult, if not impossible, to fix the upper limit of disease. We evaluated 100 consecutive patients who were considered clinically to have ulcerative colitis localized in the distal colon.[4] Overlap was found among patients with proctitis, proctosigmoiditis, and distal colon ulcerative colitis, but all had a more favorable prognosis than patients with total colon involvement.

Differential Diagnosis

The principal disorder from which ulcerative colitis needs to be distinguished is Crohn's disease of the colon.[5] In addition, a whole host of other conditions may simulate ulcerative colitis and must also enter into differential considerations (Table 126–6).

Crohn's Disease. Distinction between ulcerative colitis and Crohn's disease is reviewed extensively in Chapter 124, in the section on Pathology in this chapter, and in Chapter 127, which is concerned with Crohn's disease. As a supplement to these discussions, it may simply be noted here that because of the anatomic distribution of ulcerative colitis, proctosigmoidoscopic examination is abnormal in virtually all cases. In contrast, even when Crohn's disease affects the colon, it frequently does not involve the rectum. In addition, perianal fistulas are much more characteristic of Crohn's disease.[6, 7] Although diarrhea and weight loss occur with approximately equal frequency in

Table 126–4. SEVERITY OF FIRST REFERRED ATTACKS (Percentage)

	Edwards and Truelove[17]	***Watts et al.***[18] ***(203 patients)***	*Jalan et al.*[2] *(399 patients)*
Mild	64.7	37.4	50.0
Moderate	23.6	26.6	17.0
Severe	11.7	36.9	33.0

Table 126–5. CLASSIFICATION OF CLINICAL TYPES*

1. Relapsing-remitting type:	
a. Mild variety	Site of involvement: commonly rectum and rectosigmoid Clinical course often mild, afebrile Duration of attack often 4–12 weeks (self-limited)
b. Severe variety	Fever, toxemia, blood loss (1) With complete remission of symptoms and complete proctosigmoidoscopic resolution of lesion, or (2) With complete or almost complete remission of symptoms but continuation of activity by proctosigmoidoscopy Either mild or severe varieties (a or b) may merge into chronic continuous type or relapse may be acute fulminating type
2. Chronic continuous type:	Symptoms continuous for 6 months or longer Site of involvement: usually rectum and above; eventually entire colon All grades of severity: may be relatively mild without fever; often fluctuating Usually colon deteriorates progressively, with increasing fibrosis; irreversible changes eventually Colonic complications frequent; carcinoma more common after 5 years Surgery required in the majority
3. Acute fulminating type:	Relatively uncommon (5%) Left colon or entire colon involved Hyperpyrexia, nutritional deficit, and hemorrhage common Penetrating ulcers and colonic dilatation produce signs of impending perforation or obstruction

*From Bockus HL et al. Gastroenterologia 1956; 56:549. Reproduced with permission.

Table 126–6. CONDITIONS OTHER THAN CROHN'S DISEASE THAT MAY SIMULATE ULCERATIVE COLITIS

A. Specific infections
  1. Bacterial
    a. *Campylobacter* enterocolitis
    b. Salmonellosis
    c. Shigellosis
    d. *E. coli* enterocolitis
    e. Staphylococcal enterocolitis
    f. Antibiotic-associated colitis
  2. Fungal
    a. Histoplasmosis
  3. Viral
    a. Lymphogranuloma venereum
  4. Protozoan
    a. Amebic dysentery
    b. Schistosomiasis
    c. Infections associated with autoimmune deficiency syndrome (AIDS)
B. Other specific diseases
  1. Radiation proctitis
  2. Diverticulitis
  3. Ischemic colitis
C. Neoplasms and premalignant diseases
  1. Lymphoma; carcinoma
  2. Familial polyposis
D. Miscellaneous disorders
  1. Behçet's disease
  2. Polyarthritis
  3. Solitary ulcer of rectum
  4. Cathartic colon
  5. Irritable colon
  6. Hemorrhoids
  7. Diseases of malabsorption

both diseases, abdominal pain is much more a feature of Crohn's disease. Extraintestinal manifestations occur in about the same proportion in both diseases.[8]

In 1979 Farmer et al.[9] evaluated 366 consecutively resected specimens from patients who had undergone operation at the Cleveland Clinic for inflammatory bowel disease. Of these, 121 patients were diagnosed as having ulcerative colitis and 245 as having Crohn's disease. The contrasting pathologic features are shown in Table 126–7. Experience at this institution has continued to be that the characteristic clinical features of the disease are accompanied by characteristic pathologic features as well.

In many clinical circumstances, a mucosal biopsy is all that is possible, and it can be difficult to differentiate between ulcerative colitis and Crohn's disease in these cases.[10]

While there is a certain degree of overlap in the histologic features of the 2 diseases, it is probably possible to differentiate over 90% of cases histologically by means of an adequate tissue specimen.[11] To aid in this differentiation, attempts have been made to apply objective pathologic criteria.[12] However, differentiation between ulcerative colitis and Crohn's disease must be made not only from the histologic findings but also from a

Table 126–7. COMPARISON OF PATHOLOGIC FEATURES OF ULCERATIVE COLITIS AND CROHN'S DISEASE

	Ulcerative Colitis		Crohn's Disease	
Pathologic Features*	*Cases*	%	*Cases*	%
Transmural inflammation	34	28	240	98
Serositis	33	27	235	96
Granulomas	0	0	122	49
Lymphedema	4	3	215	88
Fissuring	0	0	186	76
Crypt abscess	115	95	137	56
Mucosal dysplasia	56	46	5	2

*Based on Cleveland Clinic series of 366 consecutive resected surgical specimens.[9]

combination of clinical features[7, 13, 14] (Table 126–8).

Infectious Agents (Chapter 118). *Campylobacter enterocolitis* both clinically and in macroscopic appearance may closely resemble ulcerative colitis and at times Crohn's disease.[15] *Campylobacter fetus* may cause a diffusely granular and friable rectal mucosa and a non-specific colitis similar to that of ulcerative colitis. However, it is generally self-limited and does not result in the chronic course typical of ulcerative colitis. Although experience with this form of colitis is limited, evidence of subsequent development of ulcerative colitis has not been shown.

Salmonella gastroenteritis is an acute self-limited disorder developing 8 to 48 hours after the ingestion of the organisms and subsiding in 2 to 5 days. Diarrhea, abdominal pain and tenderness, blood-tinged mucus, and fever are features that are common to both salmonellosis and ulcerative colitis. However, the proctosigmoidoscopic picture is completely different, the self-limited clinical course of salmonellosis is different, and there usually is little difficulty differentiating the 2 conditions.

Shigellosis (bacillary dysentery) is another acute, self-limited enteric infection with bloody stools, diarrhea, cramping abdominal pain, fever, nausea, and vomiting. At times, the degree of illness may be severe. The proctosigmoidoscopic appearance in the acute phase of a strawberry-red, hyperemic distal bowel with profuse bleeding and edematous, slightly nodular, friable mucosa is similar to that seen in ulcerative colitis. However, the infection is usually acute and may be associated with male homosexuality at times. Fecal leukocytes may be present in both shigellosis and ulcerative colitis, so that stool culture is important for differentiation of the 2 conditions.

Infection with *Escherichia coli* may also

Table 126–8. CLINICAL DIFFERENTIATION OF ULCERATIVE FROM CROHN'S COLITIS

Feature	Ulcerative Colitis	Crohn's Colitis
Rectal bleeding	Very common—90% Usually minor Massive—3%	Uncommon: may be only occult; rarely massive
Diarrhea	Early, frequent, small stools	Less distressing or absent
Abdominal pain	Predefecatory urgency	Colicky, postprandial
Fever	Uncommon if uncomplicated	30% to 50%
Palpable mass	Rare	Frequent, right lower quadrant
Proctosigmodoscopy	Diffuse pinpoint ulcerations continuous "diagnostic" changes	Normal or patches of lumpy edema or discrete aphthoid ulcerations
Rectal biopsy:		
Inflammation	Diffuse mucosal	Submucosal, more severe edema, fibrosis
Granulomas	Uncommon—7%	Common— 50%, deep
Clinical course	Relapses-remissions, 65% Chronic-continuous—20% to 30% Acute fulminating—5% to 8%	Usually slowly progressive; rarely fulminant
Longitudinal spread	Proctosigmoiditis—10% to 13% Left colon—20%	Rarely preoperative; 50% postoperative
Recurrence after resection	Rare	Frequent—50%

cause acute diarrhea, but seldom creates a problem in differentiation from ulcerative colitis. Enterotoxigenic *E. coli,* now known to be the most common cause of traveler's diarrhea (Chapter 118), is usually a self-limited, watery diarrhea without bleeding and without proctosigmoidoscopic findings similar to ulcerative colitis.

Amebic dysentery may simulate ulcerative colitis clinically, and at times differentiation by proctosigmoidoscopy may be somewhat difficult (Chapter 232). However, the discrete, punched-out ulcers in amebiasis, undermining of the ulcer margins with a rolled edge, and normal-appearing intervening mucosa make differentiation from Crohn's disease more of a problem than differentiation from ulcerative colitis. Search for *Entamoeba histolytica* trophozoites in a stool specimen in a patient with an "atypical" colitis is important.

Antibiotic-Associated Colitis (Chapter 141). This condition has received a great deal of attention with the recognition of the causative role of the toxin of *Clostridium difficile.* The proctosigmoidoscopic features, including the development of a pseudomembrane, may simulate Crohn's disease more than ulcerative colitis. Nonetheless, the possibility of coexistence of *C. difficile* infection and ulcerative colitis,[16] as well as the fact that patients with ulcerative colitis may receive antibiotic therapy for other reasons, makes this condition important in the differential diagnosis.

Autoimmune Deficiency Syndrome (AIDS) (Chapters 98 and 121). With the recognition of AIDS as a significant clinical entity among male homosexuals and other specific subgroups of the population, certain gastrointestinal infections have also been recognized to be associated with this syndrome. Among these are infections caused by *Shigella, Entamoeba histolytica,* and *Giardia lamblia.* In addition, infection with chlamydiae and cryptospordia may be associated with severe systemic disease and fatality in patients with AIDS. The clinical picture is dominated by the other manifestations of the syndrome (fever, weight loss, and lymphadenopathy), but watery diarrhea may also be an important feature. The endoscopic appearance of the rectal mucosa is that of diffuse edema without significant ulceration or friability. Thus, differential diagnosis would more likely be with Crohn's disease than with ulcerative colitis.

Radiation Proctitis (Chapter 142). The rectosigmoid is particularly the site of radiation injury because many patients with carcinoma of the cervix receive radiation therapy. Clinical features of radiation proctitis include diarrhea, mucoid discharge, tenesmus, and cramping abdominal pain developing 4 to 12 months following radiation exposure. The typical proctosigmoidoscopic picture is that of telangiectases that bleed easily. In addition, solitary shallow rectal ulcers can appear that simulate Crohn's disease more than ulcerative colitis. However, the mucosal changes may be relatively diffuse and resemble ulcerative colitis. To be emphasized is that the effects of radiation may center at a distance from the radiation itself, so that a careful history to disclose previous radiation exposure is important.

Diverticulitis (Chapter 135). This disorder seldom is of serious differential diagnostic concern. The age differential that usually is present in patients with these 2 conditions helps to separate them. However, diverticulitis can simulate ulcerative proctitis or proctosigmoiditis, and these can occur in an older population. Bleeding is relatively uncommon in diverticulitis, and on proctosigmoidoscopic examination the distal rectal mucosa is usually normal. When complicated by perforation and fistula formation, diverticulitis may simulate Crohn's disease more than ulcerative colitis.

Ischemic Colitis (Chapter 116). The acute onset of left lower quadrant pain, tenesmus, and diarrheal stools mixed with bloody mucus in an elderly patient with co-existing vascular disease is the typical clinical picture of ischemic bowel disease. Proctosigmoidoscopic examination may be normal, may show patchy friability, or may only give evidence of blood coming from the more proximal portion of the colon.

Behçet's Disease. This rare, chronic, relapsing, idiopathic symptom complex consists of oral ulceration, genital ulceration, and ocular inflammation. Its diagnosis requires at least 2 features of this clinical triad. In some cases, a type of colitis may occur that simulates Crohn's disease more than it does ulcerative colitis. However, some of the extraintestinal manifestations of ulcerative colitis, particularly arthritis, erythema nodosum, uveitis, and aphthous stomatitis, are also characteristic features of Behçet's disease.

References

1. Truelove SC, Witts IJ. Cortisone in ulcerative colitis. Report on therapeutic trial. Br Med J 1953; 2:375; 1955; 2:1041.
2. Jalan KN, Prescott RJ, Sircus W, et al. An experience of ulcerative colitis. II. Short-term outcome. Gastroenterology 1970; 59:589.
3. Farmer RG. Long-term prognosis for patients with ulcerative proctosigmoiditis (ulcerative colitis confined to the rectum and sigmoid colon). J Clin Gastroenterol 1979; 1:47–50.
4. Farmer RG, Whelan G, Sivak MV Jr. Colonoscopy in distal colon ulcerative colitis. Clin Gastroenterol 1980; 9:297–306.
5. Farmer RG. Differentiating ulcerative colitis and transmural colitis. Am Fam Phys 1972; 5:78–84.
6. Farmer RG, Hawk WA, Turnbull RB. Regional enteritis of the colon: A clinical and pathologic comparison with ulcerative colitis. Am J Dig Dis 1968; 13:501–14.
7. Kirsner JB. Problems in the differentiation of ulcerative colitis and Crohn's disease of the colon: The need for repeated diagnostic evaluation. Gastroenterology 1975; 68:187–91.
8. Greenstein AJ, Janowitz HD, Sachar DB. The extra-intestinal complications of Crohn's disease and ulcerative colitis: A study of 700 patients. Medicine 1976; 55:401–12.
9. Farmer RG, Hawk WA, Turnbull RB Jr. Clinical and pathological correlations in inflammatory bowel disease: A reaffirmation of histologic criteria for diagnosis. Clev Clin Q 1979; 46:36–7.
10. Chambers TJ, Morson BC. Large bowel biopsy in the differential diagnosis of inflammatory bowel disease. Invest Cell Pathol 1980; 3:159–73.
11. Price AB. Overlap in the spectrum of non-specific inflammatory bowel disease—"colitis indeterminate." J Clin Pathol 1978; 31:567–77.
12. Cook MG, Dickson MF. An analysis of the reliability of detection and diagnostic value of various pathological features in Crohn's disease and ulcerative colitis. Gut 1973; 14:255–62.
13. Farmer RG. Clinical features and natural history of inflammatory bowel disease. Med Clin North Am 1980. 64:1103–15.
14. Roth JLA. Diagnosis and differential diagnosis of chronic ulcerative colitis and Crohn's colitis. *In:* Kirsner JB, Shorter RG, eds. Inflammatory Bowel Disease. 2nd Ed. Philadelphia: Lea and Febiger, 1980.
15. Loss RW Jr, Mangla JC, Periera M. Campylobacter colitis presenting as inflammatory bowel disease with segmental colonic ulcerations. Gastroenterology 1980; 79:138–40.
16. Bartlett JG. Clostridium difficile and inflammatory bowel disease. Gastroenterology 1981; 80:863–5.
17. Edwards FC, Truelove SC. The course and prognosis of ulcerative colitis. Part II. Long-term prognosis. Gut 1963; 4:309.
18. Watts JMcK, deDombal FT, Watkinson G, et al. Early course of ulcerative colitis. Gut 1966; 7:16.

Complications

Richard G. Farmer

In the course of ulcerative colitis, numerous and varied complications may develop. Although the primary disease process is limited to the colon, the complications are not confined to the bowel but may occur systemically and constitute one of the most challenging and perplexing aspects of the disease. Complications may be divided into local (colonic), "specific" (general), or systemic (extraintestinal).

Local (Colonic) Complications

Under this heading are considered those complications that occur either within the colon or by direct extension from the colon.

Pseudopolyposis (Fig. 126–39; see page 2181). As discussed in the earlier section on Pathology, inflammatory polyps ("pseudopolyps") represent a combination of reactive hyperplasia and mucosal ulceration. Because of the non-epithelial nature of the histologic structure of the inflammatory polyp, it is not precancerous. Reported frequency rates of pseudopolyposis have varied considerably. Edwards and Truelove[1] encountered pseudopolyposis in 14.9% of their patients, deDombal et al.[2] in 20.5%, and Jalen et al.[3] in 19%. While it is thought that pseudopolyposis is more likely to be present in patients who have experienced a severe episode of ulcerative colitis, this is not always the case. Furthermore, the pseudopolyps tend to be found more in patients with extensive colitis

Table 126–9. INCIDENCE OF PSEUDOPOLYPOSIS WITH VARYING EXTENT OF COLITIS*

Extent	No. of Patients	No. with Pseudopolyps
Rectum alone	84	0
Rectum and left colon	134	13 (9.7%)
Rectum and left and right colon	210	41 (19.5%)

*From de Dombal FF et al. Br Med J 1966; 1:1442. Reproduced with permission.

Difference between the left-sided colonic involvement and total colonic is significant ($\times^2$ = 5.96; n = 1; P<0.02).

Table 126–10. INFLUENCE OF THE EXTENT OF COLITIS UPON THE INCIDENCE OF STRICTURE*

Extent	No. of Patients	No. with Stricture
Rectum	84	3 (3.6%)
Rectum and left colon	134	10 (7.5%)
Rectum and left and right colon	210	36 (17.1%)

*From de Dombal FF et al. Br Med J 1966; 1:1442. Reproduced with permission.

Excludes 37 patients with other or unknown extent of colitis. Difference between left-sided colonic involvement and total colonic involvement is significant ($\times^2$ = 6.61; n = 1; P <0.01).

and with disease over a reasonably long period of time (Table 126–9).

Pseudopolyps are most common in the rectosigmoid and left colon. While they may regress, the usual pattern is for them to persist following their development. Adenomatous polyps may co-exist with pseudopolyps and may be difficult to differentiate colonoscopically. This can present a dilemma as to which polyp to biopsy. Pseudopolyposis *per se* is not an indication for surgery.

Stricture. Benign stricture of the colon is occasionally encountered in patients with ulcerative colitis, although it is more common in those with Crohn's disease. Edwards and Truelove[1] and deDombal et al.[2] reported a prevalence of 6.3% and 11.2%, respectively, in their series. Strictures may be detected clinically by rectal examination, proctosigmoidoscopy, colonoscopy, or barium enema examination and are typically found in the distal colon. The narrowing of the lumen most often is localized to 2 or 3 cm. Concern always exists about carcinoma when a stricture is present. However, the ability to obtain biopsy specimens by means of endoscopy, the clinical experience that most strictures are benign, and the rarity of a carcinoma under such circumstances are somewhat reassuring. Nonetheless, because of the frequency of carcinoma as a complication of ulcerative colitis, the finding of a stricture requires full diagnostic attention. As with pseudopolyposis, stricture formation is more common with extensive disease and with relatively longstanding ulcerative colitis (Table 126–10).

Perianal Inflammation. Perianal inflammation, fistula formation, and abscess formation are more characteristic of Crohn's disease than of ulcerative colitis. Indeed, such complications are now appreciated to be rare in patients with ulcerative colitis. Minor fissuring may occur and hemorrhoids may also develop in ulcerative colitis patients. In addition, rectal prolapse occurs rarely.

Cancer (Fig. 126–40) (see also Chapter 128). Colonic carcinoma has been known to occur as a more frequent complication of ulcerative colitis than of Crohn's disease. It is also known to be associated with illness that is of long duration[4, 5] and that involves the total colon.[6–10] The exact frequency and the factors that predispose to the development of colonic carcinoma in ulcerative colitis, however, remain somewhat uncertain.[11, 12] These aspects and other details concerning this highly important complication are the subject of Chapter 128. No further discussion is needed here, therefore, other than to note that 2 important advances have improved our understanding of cancer development in ulcerative colitis and have aided in its earlier recognition: the evolution of the concept of dysplasia,[13] and the development of fiberoptic colonoscopy and its application to a surveillance program.[14]

The morphologic features, terminology, and significance of *dysplasia* were discussed earlier in the section on Pathology. As a corollary to that discussion, it is of interest that studies conducted at the Cleveland Clinic in which one of us (RGF) participated[15] emphasized the significance of atrophic and non-inflamed mucosa and the following 6 characteristics of epithelial dysplasia: atrophic mucosa, goblet cell depletion, pseudostratification of nuclei, enlargement of nuclei, increased mitotic activity, and minimal inflammation. It is also worthy of emphasis that the proposal regarding classification and terminology advanced in 1983 by a group of pathologists interested in dysplasia[16] provides a reasonable and orderly basis for interpreting and applying the findings in dysplasia to the vexing problem of cancer of the colon complicating ulcerative colitis. The provisional schema of patient management that was recommended (and was given in detail in the section on Pathology) deserves clinical application: (1) continuing regular follow-up for patients whose dysplasia classification is negative or indefinite (probably negative), (2) a short interval follow-up for those whose biopsy classification fits into the unknown or "probably positive" category as well as those with low-grade dysplasia, (3) consideration of colectomy if patients with low-grade dysplasia have a gross lesion, (4) serious consideration of colectomy for all patients with high-grade dysplasia after confirmation of this interpretation.

Surveillance schemas designed to identify disposition toward malignant transformation or actual malignancy in its earliest stages based on dysplastic changes are considered in Chapter 128 and referred to as well in Chapter 139. It is now generally accepted that total colon colonoscopy should be carried out at an appropriate (although not entirely defined) interval for patients determined to be at high risk for the development of colonic carcinoma, i.e., duration of ulcerative colitis of approximately 10 years or more and disease of the total colon.[17] Multiple sequential biopsies are taken for histologic presence and grading of dysplasia. The location of colonic carcinoma in patients with ulcerative colitis has been found to be more proximal than that occurring in the general population (Table 126–11), which only emphasizes the need and value of total colon endoscopic examinations in patients with ulcerative colitis. Surveillance is also wise in patients with inactive disease, usually associated with mucosal atrophy,[15] and in patients who have undergone ileorectal anastomosis and are at risk of developing carcinoma in the rectal stump.[18–20]

Table 126–11. PERCENTAGE ANATOMIC DISTRIBUTION OF COLONIC CARCINOMA*

	Ulcerative Colitis	General Population
No. of cases	379	6277
Colon		
Ascending	16.4%	10.9%
Transverse	25.9%	8.5%
Descending	10.3%	4.5%
Sigmoid and rectum	47.4%	76.1%

*After Langman MJS. Proc R Soc Med 1966; 59:132.

"Specific" (General) Complications

Massive Hemorrhage. Diffuse oozing of blood from the actively diseased bowel may be expected to occur in the majority of patients with ulcerative colitis, but massive hemorrhage is encountered infrequently, probably in no more than 2% or 3% of patients. Massive hemorrhage is defined as bleeding of such magnitude as to require at least 4 units of blood. Occasionally, emergency colectomy is necessary under such circumstances. While continued blood loss with anemia is common among patients with acute or severe ulcerative colitis, massive hemorrhage may occur, albeit rarely, without significant activity of disease.

Chronic Illness. From 1955 to 1974, 838 patients with inflammatory bowel disease diagnosed before the age of 21 years (505 with Crohn's disease and 333 with ulcerative colitis) received medical and surgical therapy at the Cleveland Clinic.[21] During this period, chronicity was the only complication seen in more than 10% of the patients with ulcerative colitis; in Crohn's disease, by contrast, in addition to chronicity, perianal disease, intestinal obstruction, and internal fistulas all occurred with a prevalence of greater than 10% (Table 126–12). These observations reaffirm the chronic and recurrent nature of inflammatory bowel disease with onset in childhood and adolescence. They also indicate considerable divergence in the clinical course and prognosis for patients with Crohn's disease and ulcerative colitis.

The nutritional status of a given patient may be difficult to assess objectively other than by the use of relatively general parameters: weight, serum albumin levels, hemoglobin concentration, and hematocrit. However, search for protein depletion and other nutritional deficits should always be made.

Toxic Megacolon. Toxic megacolon represents the most immediate life-threatening complication of inflammatory bowel disease.[22] While usually associated historically with ulcerative colitis, Crohn's colitis and ileocolitis are emerging as other important causes of toxic megacolon. Even though mortality and morbidity have tended to decrease over the last decade, is still true that "the results of treatment in relation to both mor-

Table 126–12. COMPLICATIONS IN INFLAMMATORY BOWEL DISEASE—CLEVELAND CLINIC

	Crohn's Disease	Ulcerative Colitis
Number of patients	505	333
Complications	361 (71.5%)	113 (33.8%) ($p<0.001$)
Perianal disease	137 (27.1%)	6 (1.8%) ($p<0.001$)
Intestinal obstruction	123 (24.4%)	11 (3.3%) ($p<0.001$)
Internal fistulas	83 (16.4%)	3 (0.9%) ($p<0.001$)
Growth retardation	40 (7.9%)	7 (2.1%) ($p<0.001$)
Megacolon	32 (6.3%)	10 (3.0%) ($p<0.05$)
Chronicity	75 (14.9%)	73 (21.9%) ($p<0.01$)
Surgery	311 (62.8%)	118 (35.6%) ($p<0.01$)

bidity and mortality remain far from satisfactory."[23] Colonic dilation superimposed on acute fulminant colitis may occur as a complication in a patient with a short or long-standing history of inflammatory bowel disease; it commonly occurs as the initial presentation of the illness. Furthermore, the dilation may fluctuate or disappear, leaving the patient still ill with toxic colitis. For this reason, megacolon may be regarded as a phase of toxic colitis.

The actual frequency of toxic megacolon is difficult to ascertain. Thus, Edwards and Truelove[1] reported a prevalence of 1.6% in 624 cases of chronic ulcerative colitis, McInerney and associates[24] reported a 9.5% prevalence in 370 hospitalized patients, and Roth et al.[25] reported toxic megacolon in 13% of 399 patients with ulcerative colitis.

Toxic megacolon is defined as a severe attack of colitis with total or segmental dilation of the colon. When the term "toxic" is used, one thinks of a desperately ill individual with fever, tachycardia, and shock. The literature, however, demonstrates a paucity of an exact definition of the "toxic" state. The febrile patient with tachycardia and hypotension may be desperately ill, independent of the leukocyte response. For that matter, the patient may be just as ill with or without colonic dilation. It is clear that morbidity and mortality can be devastating in either circumstance, as observed by Glotzer and Silen.[26] Nevertheless, in reporting series of cases it is important to define the criteria used for toxicity and megacolon. Jalen et al.[23] considered toxicity to be present when at least 3 of the following 4 conditions obtained: pyrexia greater than 101.5°F, tachycardia greater than 120 beats/minute, leukocytosis with a white blood cell count greater than 10,500/mm^3, and anemia with a hemoglobin concentration less than 60% of normal. In addition, one of the following 4 conditions had to be present: dehydration, mental changes, electrolyte disturbance, and hypotension. This degree of toxicity, coupled with clinical or radiologic evidence of colonic distention, completed the picture of toxic megacolon. At the Cleveland Clinic,[27] the patient is considered toxic if, in addition to a chart notation to that effect, there is evidence of at least 2 of the following: tachycardia with a pulse rate greater than 100 beats/minute, temperature greater than 101.5°F, leukocytosis with a white blood cell count greater than 10,000 cells/mm^3, and hypoalbuminemia with a concentration of serum albumin less than 3.0 g/dl. Furthermore, the presence of abdominal distention is documented in each patient. Other features commonly present, although not necessary for the diagnosis, include abdominal tenderness, hypotension, electrolyte imbalance, and anemia. Megacolon is defined as being present if the diameter of the colon measures 5 cm or more and the haustral pattern is disturbed or absent.

In the Cleveland Clinic series,[27] there were 50 female and 65 male patients with an age range from 7 years to 73 years and a mean age of 30 years. Tachycardia greater than 100 beats/minute occurred in 90% and was greater than 120 beats/minute in 60% of the patients. While almost all patients had elevated temperature at the time of diagnosis, only 37 patients (32%) had fever greater than 101.5°F. No patient had a normal serum albumin concentration; in 47% the value was 1.9 g/dl or less and in 90% it was less than 2.9 g/dl. A high mortality was noted with profound depression of serum albumin values. Of the 9 deaths that occurred, 8 were in patients with a serum albumin value of less than 1.9 g/dl.

The features observed in toxic megacolon represent a spectrum of illness[28] and depend upon the rapidity of onset of this complication, the duration of the illness, the presence of underlying malnutrition, and the fulminant nature of the attack. While the patient usually complains of abdominal pain, this is not always present, as delirium or administration of steroids or analgesics may modify this symptom. The patient usually has had symptoms and signs of acute colitis for at least a week before megacolon supervenes, including severe diarrhea, frequently of bloody nature. Indeed, a sinister feature is "improvement" in the patient's diarrhea to the point of absolute constipation. The corollary is also true that diarrhea occurring during medical treatment of toxic megacolon implies an improvement in the patient's condition. Colonic hemorrhage may accompany toxic megacolon; in addition, hypotension, prostration, signs of dehydration and electrolyte imbalance, anemia, and hypoalbuminemia are commonly present. Abdominal distention is present, and the contour of the dilated transverse colon is frequently seen or felt on inspecting and percussing the abdomen. Localized tenderness, especially in the left upper quadrant, implies local peritonitis and impending colonic perforation. Generalized tenderness, rebound tenderness, guarding, and complaints of shoulder-tip pain indicate free perforation. Bowel sounds are usually disminished. The clinician's appreciation of some of these findings may be modified by disturbances of the patient's sensorium. Toxic psychosis and delirium are themselves sinister signs and are a reflection of toxemia.

Gram-negative septicemia may be present, but unrecognized. Hypoprothrombinemia, hypokalemia, hyponatremia, and hypochloremia may also be present to a greater or lesser extent.

Systemic (Extraintestinal) Complications

Certain lesions of the joints, skin, liver, and eyes occur with relative frequency in association with ulcerative colitis. It remains unproved whether these are systemic manifestations of the host's response to an etiologic agent responsible for the colonic disease or complications secondary to the colonic lesion, or whether they all result from an autoimmune mechanism in which body proteins are made "foreign" by changes occurring in the diseased bowel.

In a study of the extraintestinal manifestations of Crohn's disease and ulcerative colitis from Mount Sinai Hospital (New York),[29] the most common manifestation was found to be arthritis with active synovitis (Chapter 253). Three categories were defined: (1) those related to the activity of the colitis, including joint, skin, mouth, and eye manifestations; (2) those related to the pathophysiology of the small intestine and thus largely associated with Crohn's disease (Chapter 127); and (3) those related to non-specific manifestations, including osteoporosis, hepatic complications, peptic ulcer, and amyloidosis. In this study, by far the largest number of extraintestinal manifestations for patients who had ulcerative colitis occurred in the "colitis-related" group, in which joint and skin manifestations predominated. The single most commonly affected joint was the knee, and non-articular synovitis was a frequent finding. This observation was confirmed by results of a Cleveland Clinic analysis of 336 children who had ulcerative colitis.[30] This study also indicated that arthritis was the most common extraintestinal manifestation.

The occurrence of extraintestinal manifestations cannot be used to differentiate clinically between patients who have ulcerative colitis and those who have Crohn's disease (Table 126–13); in the Mount Sinai Study,[29] patients with Crohn's colitis were found to have a distribution of "colitis-related" extraintestinal manifestations that was similar to that of patients with ulcerative colitis.

Arthritis. Bargen,[31] in 1929, called attention to peripheral arthritis as a sequel of chronic ulcerative colitis. Studies indicate that 15% to 22% of patients with ulcerative colitis have arthritic involvement in one form or another: peripheral arthritis, spondylitis, or coincidental rheumatoid arthritis.[31] A form of peripheral arthritis (*"colitic arthritis"*), which differs from rheumatoid arthritis, also occurs in patients with ulcerative colitis. Larger joints are usually affected, especially the knees, ankles, elbows, and wrists. There is a tendency for this form of arthritis to flare and subside with exacerbations and remissions of the colitis. The peripheral arthritis occurs after or simultaneously with the onset of colitis in approximately 90% of the patients. Furthermore, in most instances when the arthritis antedates the colitis, the arthritis tends to flare during subsequent exacerbations.

Men and women have been affected

Table 126–13. EXTRACOLONIC COMPLICATIONS IN INFLAMMATORY BOWEL DISEASE—CLEVELAND CLINIC[21]

	Crohn's Disease	Ulcerative Colitis
Number of Patients	505	33
Arthritis	37 (7.3%)	24 (7.2%) ($p>0.9$)
Pyoderma	7 (1.4%)	6 (1.8%) ($p>0.4$)
Iritis	1 (0.2%)	3 (0.9%) ($p>0.3$)
Liver disease	3 (0.6%)	5 (1.5%) ($p>0.3$)
Erythema nodosum	14 (2.8%)	11 (3.3%) ($p>0.8$)

equally by the peripheral arthritis, and the age of onset is usually between 25 and 45 years. Wright and Watkinson[32] found the prevalence of arthritis greater in patients with severe, extensive colonic disease having a chronic continuous or chronic relapsing course. However, Jalan et al.[33] were unable to make such correlations. A significant association between colitic arthropathy and pseudopolyposis, perianal disease, uveitis, erythema nodosum, aphthous ulcerations, and massive hemorrhage was observed by both of these groups of investigators.

In comparison with rheumatoid arthritis, McEwen[34] pointed out the following differences in the peripheral arthritis that accompanies ulcerative colitis: (1) the onset tends to be abrupt in 85% of the attacks, reaching a peak in 12 to 24 hours; (2) although the joints tend to be more severely affected, fewer joints (no more than 3 in 85% of attacks) are involved in a given attack of colitic arthritis; (3) when the spread is migratory, involvement in one joint usually subsides as the next joint is affected; (4) the ankles are more commonly affected in patients with ulcerative colitis, while the hands, wrists, and small joints of fingers and toes are involved far more often in those with rheumatoid arthritis, and in both groups the knees, elbows, shoulders, and hips are about equally affected; (5) symmetrical involvement of joints on both sides of the body is observed in 88% of patients; (6) serologic tests for rheumatoid factors are usually negative; and (7) there is a tendency to recover with no permanent articular damage and with minimal clinical or radiographic evidence in 25% of patients.[34] Symptoms of the peripheral arthritis are transient and may remit for long periods. Such long asymptomatic periods make it difficult to evaluate the effect of bowel surgery on the articular manifestations of chronic inflammatory bowel disease. However, most observers agree that recurrence of peripheral arthritis symptoms is rare after proctocolectomy.[33, 34] Although the presence of arthritis should not unduly influence a decision regarding surgery in the management of ulcerative colitis, when proctocolectomy is required because of severity or persistence of the colitis, it can be anticipated that the peripheral joint disease will disappear following surgery.

The *spondylitic* form of arthritis occurs with considerably greater frequency in patients with ulcerative colitis (4.2% to 5.5%) than in the general population.[33, 35] In a prospective radiologic analysis of 234 patients with ulcerative colitis, Wright and Watkinson[32] found sacroiliitis in 18%, in contrast to 4% in a matched control population. They also found a significant association of sacroiliitis and colitic arthritis in women but not in men. Although the predilection for men was less marked than in the control subjects, Wright and Watkinson[32] found a florid picture of fusion of sacroiliac joints and intervertebral bridging much more common in men with ulcerative colitis.

The onset of the spondylitic form of articular involvement is insidious and gradual. For this reason it is more difficult to recognize flares of the spondylitis associated with activity of the ulcerative colitis, but McEwen[34] observed a simultaneous association of colitic and spondylitic exacerbations in about 25% of his patients; the onset of spondylitis occurred after or simultaneously with the onset of ulcerative colitis in about 75% of patients. Thus, there is a slightly greater tendency for spondylitis than for colitic arthritis to antedate the onset of ulcerative colitis.[36]

There appears to be no significant relationship between the spondylitis and the severity, extent, or duration of the colitis. The joints are damaged progressively over many years, eventually resulting in sacroiliac obliteration and typical "bambooing" or ligamentous ossification of the spine in most patients.

The hips and shoulders similarly show progressive damage when they are affected, but involvement in the more peripheral joints usually subsides. The unrelenting course of the spondylitis is reflected in its failure to regress after proctocolectomy.[34, 36] Furthermore, the response of the spondylitis to corticosteroid therapy is limited, in contrast to the dramatic improvement in colitic arthritis following steroid therapy.

Clubbing of the fingers was encountered in 5% of the 399 patients reviewed by Jalan et al.[33] The clubbing is related to the extent of colonic involvement and to the duration and severity of the disease, the latter being evidenced by association of the clubbing with toxic megacolon, pseudopolyposis, carcinoma, and colitic arthritis and spondylitis.

Skin Lesions. The prominent skin lesions found in patients with ulcerative colitis are erythema nodosum[37] and pyoderma gangrenosum.[38] Other less striking or characteristic skin lesions also occur. A description of these lesions is found in Chapter 18.

Aphthous Ulcerations of the Mouth. These lesions are not unusual and may be found together with other extraintestinal manifestations in patients with ulcerative colitis (Chapter 17).

Liver Disease. Liver dysfunction and disease are relatively frequent in ulcerative colitis. Antemortem studies are generally in agreement that the primary hepatic alteration in patients with chronic ulcerative colitis and associated disease of the liver is cholestasis (Chapter 148). In keeping with this, most observers report an "obstructive" profile featuring elevation of serum alkaline phosphatase activity, disproportionate rise of direct-reacting bilirubin when jaundice is present, the common occurrence of hypercholesterolemia, and only slight to moderate elevations of aminotransferase activities or gamma globulin. Although Perrett et al.[39] observed some abnormality of liver function in 15% of 300 patients with ulcerative colitis, approximately one-third of these had no histologic abnormality on liver biopsy. Conversely, when biopsy specimens have been obtained from patients with normal liver tests, mild fatty change or pericholangitis has been observed in up to 40%.[40] Severe chronic liver disease is almost always associated with elevated serum alkaline phosphatase and alanine aminotransferase activities.[39]

Involvement of the liver in ulcerative colitis has been recognized since the report by Thomas in 1874[41] of a postmortem examination that revealed severe fatty hepatic degeneration. In more recent years, considerable attention has been focused on the spectrum of hepatic diseases in ulcerative colitis, and the types are becoming fairly well defined. The frequency of acute and chronic liver disease is greater in patients with ulcerative colitis than in the general population, and fatty change is the most common lesion found at necropsy. Thus, postmortem observations of Palmer et al.[42] revealed a much greater frequency of fatty liver (about 50%) in patients with ulcerative colitis than in a control series. However, a comparable proportion of matched controls who died of equally debilitating disease also had fatty liver. Fatty change appears to occur less commonly in the living patient (19% to 38%), as evidenced by patients selected for needle biopsy of the liver.[39, 43, 44] At the time of colectomy, fatty change occurs in about 45% of patients, being moderate to severe in only 14%. The extent of the fatty infiltration frequently correlates with the severity of colitis, but not all observers have found this to be the case. Perrett et al.,[39] for example, found fatty changes to be independent of the extent of colonic disease, the presence of other systemic complications, a past history of other systemic complications, a past history of jaundice or transfusion, and the type of past medical treatment.

Fatty infiltration may be diffuse or focal, tending to begin at the periphery of the lobule and spreading centrally. The fatty change has been ascribed to malnutrition, toxemia, and anemia anoxia; generally, it is a reversible lesion, disappearing as remission occurs and the patient's general health improves. Extensive fatty changes have been found in some patients, however, who are free of symptoms at the time of biopsy; in other patients who were seriously ill, no fatty change has been observed in the liver biopsy.[39]

Pericholangitis (triaditis) is the most characteristic and perhaps the most common hepatic lesion in the living patient with ulcerative colitis. This inflammatory change of the portal tracts is not limited to the bile ducts (pericholangitis), but also involves the connective tissues around the hepatic artery and portal vein (portal triaditis). The term pericholangitis, however, has become accepted by dint of usage. Hepatic parenchymal cells are commonly involved, so that histologically pericholangitis may merge with chronic active hepatitis, and both may sometimes appear to progress to postnecrotic cirrhosis. Mistilis[45] observed progression from acute to subacute and chronic pericholangitis, but biliary cirrhosis did not appear to be the end result. Mistilis et al.[46] observed cholangitis alone in 24 of 49 patients selected for biopsy and cholangitis associated with chronic active hepatitis in an additional 4 patients. Stauffer et al.[47] described portal triaditis with cholestasis in 14 and triaditis without bile stasis in 7 of their 30 patients in whom biopsy material was available. Dordal et al.[44] encountered pericholangitis in 20 of their 76 patients who had biopsies, while Perrett et al.[39] reported this histologic lesion in 15 of 50 patients selected for biopsy.

It is not possible to define the precise frequency of this hepatic lesion in ulcerative colitis, since many factors influenced the availability of biopsy material in the reports that have appeared. Biopsy was performed for the most part in asymptomatic patients if there were persistently abnormal liver tests or unexplained hepatomegaly; in other patients, symptomatic evidence of cholestasis or cholangitis was the indication for biopsy.

Ulcerative colitis usually precedes the onset of pericholangitis, and by the time the liver disease becomes established, the colitis is in a chronic inactive phase. There appears to be no correlation between the presence and severity of pericholangitis and the severity of ulcerative colitis. Although this hepatic lesion seems to be associated with more extensive colonic disease, it does occur as well with limited distal colitis.[39, 46] The frequency and clinical manifestations of pericholangitis do not appear to be related to the duration of the colitis or to previous medical treatment. Likewise, colectomy has not appeared to have a significant effect on the progression, or lack of progression, of the hepatic lesion.[47a]

Once the disease is established in the portal tracts, it tends to be recurrent and self-perpetuating. The cause of the self-perpetuation is not clear. Recurrent portal bacteremia or an autoimmune phenomenon has been suggested. Immunologic studies are inconclusive and do not establish ulcerative colitis or associated pericholangitis as an autoimmune disease; no relationship has been found between the hepatic lesions and any of the positive immunologic tests.[39, 44] There is general agreement that there is no evidence to indict post-transfusion hepatitis or drugs used in the treatment of ulcerative colitis as etiologic factors in the development of pericholangitis.[39, 44]

Although fatty liver and pericholangitis are much more common in patients with ulcerative colitis, overt chronic liver disease in the form of chronic active hepatitis,[39, 45] and the cirrhoses are far more serious, accounting for 10% of the deaths in one large series of patients with ulcerative colitis.[45] The frequency of cirrhosis in patients with ulcerative colitis has varied greatly in different series, but it is questionable whether this frequency is higher than in the general population because of the selectivity of the patients.[39] Perrett et al.[39] concluded that "the true incidence is probably in the 2% to 3% range." No consistent histopathologic pattern of the cirrhosis has been described, but the dominant form seems to be postnecrotic cirrhosis. Serial biopsies have not shown progression in the severity of established pericholangitis or cirrhosis,[44] but the transition from portal fibrosis to cirrhosis, or from pericholangitis to postnecrotic cirrhosis has been observed.[46, 48]

Sclerosing Cholangitis. Recognition of sclerosing cholangitis in association with ulcerative colitis[49] has increased with more frequent use of methods for imaging the bile ducts, particularly endoscopic retrograde cholangiopancreatography (ERCP).[50, 51] The subject of sclerosing cholangitis in all its aspects is fully addressed in Chapter 164. Comment here, therefore, will be confined to the disorder as it specifically relates to ulcerative colitis.

Weisner and LaRusso,[52] in a study of 50 patients with sclerosing cholangitis, noted that 50% also had inflammatory bowel disease (IBD), chiefly ulcerative colitis. Asymptomatic elevation of serum alkaline phosphatase activity in a patient with ulcerative colitis, usually of long duration, was the predominant presenting feature of sclerosing cholangitis in a study done at the Cleveland Clinic,[53] as well as in studies made by others.[52, 54] Blackstone and Nemchausky[54] described 20 cases of IBD (16 of ulcerative colitis, 3 of Crohn's disease, 1 indeterminate) in which liver function and ERCP were abnormal. They emphasized that abnormalities of the intrahepatic cholangiogram are relatively common in this group of patients, that intrahepatic ductular obstruction appears to be more common than extrahepatic, that ERCP is the best method for diagnosis, and that the lesion tends to be non-progressive with a clinical course not unlike that with pericholangitis.

The heightened awareness of the association of sclerosing cholangitis with IBD has generally led to an emphasis on early ERCP. This examination is distinctly more valuable than many others commonly employed in the past. Thus, for example, liver biopsy in a series of patients examined at the Cleveland Clinic[53] was of less value than ERCP in defining the type and extent of biliary tract involvement. No progression was apparent in the 4 patients who had serial biopsies. The changing microscopic picture in a few patients, including an occasional reversion to normal, is probably related to sampling. Unless another disease involving the liver is suspected, liver biopsy is largely restricted to a confirmatory role.

Our more recent experience[53] emphasizes that patients with longstanding ulcerative colitis represent the group most likely to develop sclerosing cholangitis. As there is no evidence that colectomy improves the status of the biliary tract, this procedure should not be performed in an attempt to improve the state of the liver or biliary tract. Despite earlier enthusiasm, there is little evidence that corticosteroid therapy alters the clinical course, and steroid therapy could prove harmful if biliary tract infection is present. The prognosis for sclerosing cholangitis, in our experience, appears to be relatively good,[55] although our follow-up period has not been long. The clinical status remains stable for long periods, and secondary biliary cirrhosis does not appear to be inevitable or may take many years to develop.

Ocular Lesions. The occurrence of ocular disease in association with ulcerative colitis is uncommon. Billison et al.[56] observed ocular complications in 3.6% of 465 patients during an ongoing study. The most common lesions were *episcleritis* and *iritis* (non-granulomatous anterior uveitis). Other eye diseases were also encountered (conjunctivitis, blepharitis, keratitis, choroiditis) but were considered to be unrelated to the colitis. The eye lesions commonly occur during a severe exacerbation of colonic symptoms, but in some cases uveitis has been noted during remission or appears to precede the onset of colitis.[57] This observation, as well as the frequency with which colitic arthritis (84%), erythema nodosum (38%), and aphthous ulcerations (17%) have been associated with the uveitis, has been interpreted as evidence in favor of these being systemic manifestations (immune phenomena) of the same disease process rather than resulting from colitis.

The frequency of uveitis does not appear to be related to the extent of the colitis, and there is disagreement about its relationship to the duration of the disease. Billison et al.[56] observed uveitis most frequently during the first year of colitis symptoms. The mean duration of ulcerative colitis at the time eye lesions developed was 4 years. However, Wright et al.[58] reported evidence of past or current iritis in nearly one-third of their patients with a history of ulcerative colitis of 10 or more years. It may be that such a high prevalence of eye lesions in this group with longstanding ulcerative colitis is attributable to the inclusion of cases of uveitis occurring 10 or more years previous to the study and before corticosteroids were widely used to control the ulcerative colitis. Uveitis occurs more commonly in women and tends to subside within 6 to 8 weeks regardless of therapy, but may recur (in more than 50% of patients) and may eventually lead to blindness in a few patients.[57] Although uveitis is unlikely to recur after colectomy, most observers agree that its occurrence *per se* does not constitute an indication for colonic surgery.[56, 57] The majority of patients with uveitis will come to surgery for other reasons, and its occurrence should support the other indications for colonic surgery.

Growth Retardation in Children. Childhood onset of ulcerative colitis presents 2 special problems: (1) chronic disease occurring during the normal growth period can affect the patient beyond the clinical expressions of the disease,[59] and (2) the longer potential duration of disease makes the problem of subsequent development of cancer of the colon even more significant.[60] Additional problems can occur as a result of a costly, debilitating, and perhaps disfiguring illness occurring at a time when a young person is attempting to attain psychologic and economic independence. In addition, with the current mobility of the population, those who have childhood onset of ulcerative colitis are likely to move, probably change physicians, and thus be lost to follow-up. In a study at the Cleveland Clinic of 316 patients who developed ulcerative colitis before the age of 21 years,[30] it was found that the disease was more one of adolescence than of childhood, with a mean age at onset of 15 years. There was no sex preponderance and the predominant clinical picture was that of chronic but incapacitating illness. Growth retardation was present in 7 patients (less than the third percentile in height and weight as compared with their peers) and was statistically less frequent than in a comparable group of patients with Crohn's disease. This study, which covered the period 1955 to 1975, showed a statistically significant decrease in the number of operations performed in the second decade as compared with the first (from 49% to 26%). Overall, 38% of patients required an operation. There were 18 deaths (5%), half of which were caused by colonic carcinoma. Patients were asked to assess their quality of life after a mean follow-up of more than 10 years; only 21% evaluated the quality as "good." The vast majority (72%) considered that they were functioning suboptimally as compared with their peers.

Thus, while ulcerative colitis with childhood onset has many features similar to those associated with onset at an older age, there are characteristics peculiar to the younger age group that must be recognized by the managing physician. In addition to the various medical aspects, a child with ulcerative colitis can have a highly negative psychologic and social impact on the family. The physician must be aware of these potential problems to be of optimal help to the patient and family in coping with the illness.

Renal Lesions. Pyelonephritis and nephrolithiasis occur with relative frequency in patients with ulcerative colitis, but not as commonly as in those with Crohn's disease. *Pyelonephritis* has been reported in 2% to 6% of patients with ulcerative colitis, *nephrolithiasis* in 1.9% to 6.4%.[61, 62] Maratka and Nedbal[62a] have emphasized the frequency (13%) with which renal calculi develop after ileostomy. Stone formation has been attributed to (1) loss of water and sodium through the ileostomy with resultant decrease in urinary output, and (2) increase in urinary crystalloid excretion, particularly calcium and uric acid. There has been emphasis on the role of uric acid in the development of kidney stones, with the possibility that urinary tract infection may increase the likelihood of stone development. In patients seen at the University of Chicago,[63] there was an increased frequency of uric acid stones, particularly following ileostomy. Hyperoxaluria, as reported in patients with Crohn's disease who develop calcium oxalate stones, is not as common among patients with ulcerative colitis.

Other Systemic (Extraintestinal) Manifestations. Pulmonary complications are relatively rare in patients with ulcerative colitis except under the following circumstances: (1) as a terminal event in patients with severe toxemia and inanition (pneumonitis), (2) in the seriously ill patient with an acute fulminating type of disease (embolism, pneumonitis), and (3) as complications following operations (atelectasis, embolism, pneumonitis). Myocardial changes are noted consistently in patients dying of ulcerative colitis. The muscle fibers show fatty changes and vacuole formation. The thickness of the myocardial walls is often decreased, and clinical evidence of disturbed myocardial function is manifested by persistent tachycardia in severely ill patients. Other rare complications have been reported, such as pulmonary vasculitis,[64] amyloidosis,[65] and sideropenic dysphagia[66] associated with a very low serum iron level due to chronic blood loss. Disturbances of menstrual function, particularly amenorrhea, are common during severe activity of the disease.

In addition to personality changes, seriously ill patients with ulcerative colitis may exhibit any of the cerebral manifestations of a severe toxemia. Somnolence, poor cerebration, tendency to disorientation, coma, and even delirium may be encountered. Acute toxic psychosis, however, is rare.

Associated Diseases

The co-existence of lupus erythematosus,[67] scleroderma,[68] chronic active hepatitis, and thymoma[69] with ulcerative colitis has supported speculation of an autoimmune phenomenon in these diseases. A genetic predisposition has been postulated for the association of eczema, hay fever (allergic rhinitis), and ankylosing spondylitis and polyarthritis (rheumatoid type) with ulcerative colitis.[69] No causal interrelationship has been suggested for the occurrence of peptic ulcer disease with ulcerative colitis, but their potential co-existence must be considered in making therapeutic decisions.

Cancer Surveillance

Colonic carcinoma has been known to be a complication much more frequently associated with ulcerative colitis than with Crohn's disease and has been found to be associated with a long duration of illness, as well as with total disease of the colon. However, the exact incidence and the factors that predispose to development of colonic carcinoma remain somewhat uncertain. In the past the carcinoma associated with ulcerative colitis has been found to have a poor prognosis. More recent evidence[70] indicates that this may have been due to delayed detection; the incidence is lower if the disease involves less than the entire colon.[71]

Two important advances in the understanding of cancer development in ulcerative colitis have been the evolution of the concept of *dysplasia*[13] and the development of the technique of fiberoptic colonoscopy to carry out a surveillance program. Dysplasia has been known to occur in ulcerative colitis for many years, but there has been confusion regarding the morphology, terminology, and significance of the dysplastic lesion.

A major step forward in the understanding and definition of the histologic significance of mucosal dysplasia occurred with the publication "Dysplasia in Inflammatory Bowel Disease: Standardized Classification with Provisional Clinical Applications" by a group of pathologists under the chairmanship of Riddell and Yardley.[16] This work was a cooperative effort that resulted from a series of workshops sponsored by the National Foundation for Ileitis and Colitis and culminated in publication in November 1983 of the manuscript. Prior to this, there had been much confusion about the terminology, definition, and clinical significance of dysplasia. The authors discussed the classification system and its clinical significance.

> The classification system that has been devised appears to be reproducible and easy to demonstrate and has the potential for clinical application. Dysplasia is defined as an unequivocal neoplastic ulceration of the colonic epithelium. It should be stressed that such dysplastic epithelium not only may be a marker or precursor of carcinoma but may itself be malignant and associated with direct invasion into the underlying tissue. This definition is analogous to the definition of dysplasia and adenomas of the colon in the absence of inflammatory bowel disease, in neoplastic lesions of the rest of the gastrointestinal tract, and in other epithelia. The classification consists of three major categories: Negative, indefinite, and positive for dysplasia. Dysplasia is identified on the basis of a combination of microscopic features including (1) architectural alteration exceeding that resulting from repair in chronic colitis, often resembling glandular arrangement of adenomas; (2) cytologic abnormalities, principally cellular and nuclear pleomorphism, nuclear hyperchromatism, loss of nuclear polarity, and marked stratification of nuclei.

It has been noted that the active and resolving phases of ulcerative colitis cause most of the problems in the interpretation of biopsy findings with regard to the presence or absence of dysplasia. Furthermore, "mucus depletion resulting from acute inflammation or bowel preparation must be excluded before a diagnosis of dysplasia is considered."[16] It is possible, using the criteria established, to separate out changes as a result of inflammation alone and those relating to the regenerative process. This work emphasizes the importance of including in the category "positive for dysplasia" only cases with unequivocally neoplastic mucosa. It has been observed that most tumors do not pass through a morphologically recognizable phase of in-situ carcinoma and that similar observations have been made in the adenoma-carcinoma sequence in non-colitis patients. In this classification, dysplasia is divided only into low and high grades, the former having histologic characteristics similar to those of tubular adenomas. The authors stated that "whether dysplasia affects predominantly the superficial part of the crypt or the crypt base, the grade is always determined by the features of the most dysplastic portion."[16] It has been observed that adenomatous polyps may at times be present in a patient with ulcerative colitis, but dysplasia in inflammatory pseudopolyps is rare. Over 500 readings by 10 pathologists measured inter-observer variability with careful assessments of results in this study.[16]

Although the data derived from this important study need to be applied clinically, the authors recommended a provisional schema of patient management related to the classification of dysplasia. This included continuing regular follow-up for patients whose biopsy classification is negative (normal mucosa), inactive "quiescent" colitis, active colitis, or indefinite (probably negative) category. A short interval follow-up should be instituted for those patients whose biopsy classification fits into the unknown or "probably positive" category as well as those patients with low-grade dysplasia. However, if patients with low-grade dysplasia have a gross lesion, colectomy should be considered. For all patients with high-grade dysplasia, colectomy should be seriously considered after the dysplasia is confirmed more than once. This classification is the one that we have been using at the Cleveland Clinic as an integral part of the surveillance program for patients with ulcerative colitis.

Dysplasia is also discussed and the histologic characteristics illustrated in the earlier section on Pathology.

References

1. Edwards FC, Truelove SC. The course and prognosis of ulcerative colitis. Part III. Complications. Gut 1964; 5:1–15.
2. deDombal FT, Watts JMcK, Watkinson G, et al. Local complications of ulcerative colitis. Stricture, pseudopolyposis and carcinoma of colon and rectum. Br Med J 1966; 1:1442.
3. Jalan KN, Walker RJ, Sircus W, et al. Pseudopolyposis in ulcerative colitis. Lancet 1969; 2:555.
4. Devroede GJ, Dockerty MB, Sauer WG, et al. Cancer of the colon in patients with ulcerative colitis since childhood. Can J Surg 1972; 15:369–74.
5. Devroede GJ, Taylor SF, Sauer WG, et al. Cancer risk and life expectancy of children with ulcerative colitis. N Engl J Med 1971; 285:17.
6. Aylett S. Cancer and ulcerative colitis. Br Med J 1957; 2:489.
7. Bargen JA, Gage RP. Ulcerative colitis leading to cancer. Gastroenterology 1960; 39:385.
8. Bargen JA, Sauer WG, Sloan WP, et al. The development of cancer in chronic ulcerative colitis. Gastroenterology 1954; 26:32.
9. Bargen JA. Chronic ulcerative colitis associated with malignant disease. Arch Surg 1928; 17:561
10. Counsell PB, Dukes CE. Association of chronic ulcerative colitis and carcinoma of rectum and colon. Br J Surg 1952; 39:485.
11. Gyde SN, Prior P, MacCartney JC, et al. Malignancy in Crohn's disease. Gut 1980; 21:1024.
12. Whelan G. Cancer risk in ulcerative colitis. Why are results in the literature so varied? Clin Gastroenterol 1980. 9:469–76.
13. Morowitz DA, Kirsner JB. Mortality in ulcerative colitis: 1930 to 1966. Gastroenterology 1969; 57:481.
14. Riddell RH, Morson BC. Value of sigmoidoscopy and biopsy in detection of carcinoma and premalignant change in ulcerative colitis. Gut 1979; 20:575.
15. Fuson JA, Farmer RG, Hawk WA, et al. Endoscopic surveillance for cancer in chronic ulcerative colitis. Am J Gastroenterol 1980; 73:120–6.
16. Riddell RH, Goldman H, Ransohoff DF, et al. Dysplasia in inflammatory bowel disease. Standardized classification with provisional clinical applications. Human Pathol 1983; 14:931–68.
17. Farmer RG, Hawk WA, Turnbull RB. Carcinoma associated with mucosal ulcerative colitis and with transmural colitis and enteritis (Crohn's disease). Cancer 1971; 28:289–92.
18. Baker WNW, Glass RE, Ritchie JK, Aylett SO. Cancer of the rectum following colectomy and ileorectal anastomosis for ulcerative colitis. Br J Surg 1978; 65:862–8.
19. Grundfest SF, Fazio VW, Weiss, RA, et al. The risk of cancer following colectomy and ileorectal anastomosis for extensive mucosal ulcerative colitis. Ann Surg 1981; 193:9–14.
20. Lavery IC, Chiulli RA, Jagelman DG, et al. Survival with carcinoma arising in mucosal ulcerative colitis. Ann Surg 1982; 195:508–12.
21. Michener WM, Greenstreet RL, Farmer RG. Comparison of the clinical features of Crohn's disease and ulcerative colitis with onset in childhood and adolescence. Cleve Clin Q 1983; 49:13–6.
22. Korelitz BI, Janowitz HD. Dilatation of colon: Serious complications of ulcerative colitis. Ann Intern Med 1960; 53:153.
23. Jalan KN, Sircus W, Card WI, et al. An experience of ulcerative colitis. Toxic dilation in fifty-five cases. Gastroenterology 1969; 57:68–82.
24. McInerney GT, Sauer WG, Baggenstoss AH, et al. Fulminating ulcerative colitis with marked colonic dilatation. A clinico-pathologic study. Gastroenterology 1962; 42:244–57.
25. Roth JLA, Valdes-Dapena A, Stein GN, et al. Toxic megacolon in ulcerative colitis. Gastroenterology 1959; 37:329.
26. Glotzer DJ, Silen W. Indications for surgical treatment in chronic ulcerative colitis and Crohn's disease of the colon. *In:* Kirsner JB, Shorter RG, eds. Inflammatory Bowel Disease. Philadelphia: Lea and Febiger, 1975: 322–37.
27. Fazio VW. Toxic megacolon in ulcerative colitis and Crohn's colitis. Clin Gastroenterol 1980; 9:271–8.
28. Caprilli R, Verina P, Colaneri O, Frieri G. Risk factors in toxic megacolon. Dig Dis Sci 1980; 25:817–22.
29. Greenstein AJ, Janowitz HD, Sachar DB. The extra-intestinal complications of Crohn's disease and ulcerative colitis: A study of 700 patients. Medicine 1976; 55:401–12.
30. Michener WM, Farmer RG, Mortimer EA. Long-term prognosis of ulcerative colitis with onset in childhood or adolescence. J Clin Gastroenterol 1979; 1:301–5.
31. Bargen JA. Complications and sequelae of chronic ulcerative colitis. Ann Intern Med 1929; 3:335.
32. Wright V, Watkinson G. Articular complications of ulcerative colitis. Am J Proctol 1966; 17:107.
33. Jalan KN, Prescott RJ, Walker RJ, et al. Arthropathy, ankylosing spondylitis, and clubbing of fingers in ulcerative colitis. Gut 1970; 11:748.
34. McEwen C. Arthritis accompanying ulcerative colitis. Clin Orthop 1968; 57:9.
35. Fernandez-Herlihy L. The articular manifestations of chronic ulcerative colitis. N Engl J Med 1959; 261:6.
36. Palumbo PJ, Ward IE, Sauer WG, et al. Musculoskeletal manifestations of inflammatory bowel disease. Mayo Clin Proc 1973; 48:411.
37. Kelley ML, Logan VW. Erythema nodosum in association with chronic ulcerative colitis. Gastroenterology 1956; 31:285.
38. Brunsting LA, Gockerman WH, O'Leary PA. Pyoderma (erythema) gangrenosum. Arch Dermatol Syp 1930; 22:655.
39. Perrett AD, Higgins G, Johnson HH, et al. The liver in ulcerative colitis. Am J Med 1971; 40:211.
40. Anthonisen P, Christoffersen P, Riis P, et al. Liver function and histology in patients with non-specific hemorrhagic proctocolitis (hemorrhagic proctitis and ulcerative colitis). Ugeskr Laeg 1966; 128:471.
41. Thomas CH. Ulceration of the colon with a much enlarged fatty liver. Trans Path Soc 1874; 4:87.
42. Palmer WL, Kirsner JB, Goldgraber MB, et al. Disease of the liver in chronic ulcerative colitis. Am J Med 1964; 36:856.
43. Kleckner MS, Stauffer MH, Bargen JA, et al. Hepatic lesions in living patient with chronic ulcerative colitis as demonstrated by needle biopsy. Gastroenterology 1952; 22:13.
44. Dordal E, Glagov S, Kirsner JB. Hepatic lesions in chronic inflammatory bowel disease. Gastroenterology 1967; 52:239.
45. Mistilis SP. Pericholangitis and ulcerative colitis. I. Pathology, etiology and pathogenesis. Ann Intern Med 1965; 63:1.
46. Mistilis SP, Skyring AP, Goulston SJM. Pericholangitis and ulcerative colitis. II. Clinical aspects. Ann Intern Med 1965; 63:17.
47. Stauffer MH, Sauer WG, Dearing WH, et al. The spectrum of cholestatic hepatic disease. JAMA 1965; 191:829.

47a. Eade MN, Cooke WT, Brooke BN. Liver disease in ulcerative colitis. I. Analysis of operative liver biopsy in 138 consecutive patients having colectomy II. The long-term effect of colectomy. Ann Intern Med 1970; 72:475.

48. Vinnik IE, Kern F. Liver disease in ulcerative colitis. Arch Intern Med 1963; 112:41.
49. Warren KW, Athanassiades S, Monge JI. Primary sclerosing cholangitis. A study of forty-two cases. Am J Surg 1966; 111:23.

50. Chapman RWG, Arborgh BAM, Rhodes JM, Summerfield JA, et al. Primary sclerosing cholangitis: A review of its clinical features, cholangiography and hepatic histology. Gut 1980; 21:870–77.
51. Thrope MEC, Scheuer PJ, Sherlock S, et al. Primary sclerosing cholangitis: The biliary tree and ulcerative colitis. Gut 1967; 8:435.
52. Wiesner RH, LaRusso NF. Clinicopathologic features of the syndrome of primary sclerosing cholangitis. Gastroenterology 1980; 79:200–6.
53. Sivak MV Jr, Farmer RG, Lalli AF. Sclerosing cholangitis. Increasing frequency of recognition and association with ulcerative colitis. J Clin Gastroenterol 1981; 3:261–6.
54. Blackstone MO, Nemchausky BA. Cholangiographic abnormalities in ulcerative colitis associated pericholangitis which resemble sclerosing cholangitis. Am J Dig Dis 1978; 23:579–85.
55. Wood RAB, Cuschieri A. Is sclerosing cholangitis complicating ulcerative colitis a reversible condition? Lancet 1980; 2:716–8.
56. Billison FA, deDombal FT, Watkinson G, et al. Ocular complications of ulcerative colitis. Gut 1967; 8:102.
57. Korelitz BI, Coles RS. Uveitis (iritis) associated with ulcerative and granulomatous colitis. Gastroenterology 1967; 52:78.
58. Wright R, Lumsden K, Luntz MH, et al. Abnormalities of the sacroiliac joints and uveitis in ulcerative colitis. Q J Med 1965; 34:229.
59. McCaffery TD, Nasr K, Lawrence AM, et al. Severe growth retardation in children with inflammatory bowel disease. Pediatrics 1970; 45:386.
60. Stickler GB. Cancer of the colon in patients with ulcerative colitis since childhood. Can J Surg 1972; 15:368–74.
61. Gelzayd EA, Breuer RI, Kirsner JB. Nephrolithiasis in inflammatory bowel disease. Am J Dig Dis 1968; 13:1027.
62. Deren JJ, Proush JG, Levitt MF, et al. Nephrolithiasis as a complication of ulcerative colitis and regional enteritis. Ann Intern Med 1962; 56:843.
62a. Maratka Z, Nedbal J. Urolithiasis as a complication of the surgical treatment of ulcerative colitis. Gut 1964; 5:214.
63. Kirsner JB. Clinical observations on inflammatory bowel disease. Med Clin North Am 1969; 53:1204.
64. Isenberg JI, Goldstein H, Korn AR, et al. Pulmonary vasculitis—An uncommon complication of ulcerative colitis. N Engl J Med 1968; 279:1376.
65. Forshaw JWB, Moorehouse EH. Amyloidosis secondary to chronic ulcerative colitis. Br Med J, 1964; 2:94.
66. Wright R. Sideropenic dysphagia in a patient with ulcerative colitis. Roentgen findings. AJR 1959; 82:985.
67. Alarcon-Segovia D, Herskovic T, Dearing W, et al. Lupus erythematous cell phenomenon in patients with chronic ulcerative colitis. Gut 1965; 6:39.
68. DeLuca VA, Spiro HM, Thayer WR. Ulcerative colitis and scleroderma. Gastroenterology 1965; 49:433.
69. Kirk BW, Freedman SO. Hypogammaglobulinemia, thymoma and ulcerative colitis. Can Med Assoc J 1967; 96:1272.
70. Yardley JH, Bayless TM, Diamond MP. Cancer in ulcerative colitis. Gastroenterology 1979; 76:221 (Editorial).
71. Greenstein AJ, Sachar DB, Smith R, et al. Cancer in universal and left-sided ulcerative colitis. Factors in determining risk. Gastroenterology 1979; 77:290–4.

Medical Management

Richard G. Farmer

In considering the treatment of a patient with ulcerative colitis, 4 general factors must be taken into account:

1. *Location of disease.* Ulcerative colitis affects only the colon and does not extend into the small intestine, except for the occasional instance of "backwash ileitis" discussed earlier. Within the colon, the disease may involve only certain segments or the entire colon (pancolitis). The extent (location) of the disease correlates with prognosis and is a significant factor in response to therapy.

2. *Activity of disease.* Patients whose disease has an acute onset and those with chronically active inflammatory symptoms present different clinical pictures, and the response to therapy is likewise affected. Therapeutic regimens must be tailored to deal with the varying severity (activity) of disease.

3. *Duration of disease.* Although it has become increasingly apparent that longstanding ulcerative colitis may be associated with the subsequent development of colonic carcinoma, the duration of disease may also play a role in the therapeutic response. Factors include the previous response to therapy, whether the patient has been on chronic continuous therapy, and whether the disease has been quiescent.

4. *Overall impact of the disease on the patient and his adaptation to the disease state.* A patient in a suboptimal state of nutrition, function, and general health may respond less predictably to therapy than a patient in better con-

dition. This is often the situation in which "psychologic" factors are allegedly present but which may in reality be factors of chronic illness.

Certain other features must also be taken into account in planning a therapeutic regimen for the patient with ulcerative colitis. The age of onset may be a factor, particularly if it occurs in childhood or prepubescence. Likewise, patients who are over 50 frequently have a milder course of illness or may have another systemic disease complicating the situation. The severity of the previous course of ulcerative colitis in a given patient needs to be considered in relation to potential response to therapy as well as the patient's attitude about therapy.

Any therapeutic regimen must assume that a correct diagnosis has been made, and the most common disorder from which ulcerative colitis must be distinguished is Crohn's disease, as noted earlier. Assuming a correct diagnosis has been established, the physician must then define the goals of therapy and relate these to the patient's quality of life. The physician and the patient must have a mutual understanding of what it means to have a "failure of response" to therapy. Unrealistic expectations may be an important limiting factor in therapeutic response and may lead to impaired rapport between the patient and the physician. Breakdown of communication can lead to lack of patient compliance with the therapeutic program. Thus, the cornerstones of therapy to be laid at the outset are rapport with the patient and patient education. Because the symptoms of rectal bleeding, diarrhea, and malnutrition may be so troublesome to the patient, "simple" solutions may be sought unsuccessfully, leading to further frustration. In such circumstances, various psychologic problems and difficulties with interpersonal relationships have tended to dominate the therapeutic response by the patient. Many of these can be prevented by patient education about both the disease and its symptoms and by the patient's adaptation to the state of illness, insofar as this may be possible to attain.

Therapeutic Modalities

Functional Activity. It is important for the patient to be as physically and mentally active as possible and to pursue normal daily activity patterns as regularly as possible. Chronic fatigue, disappointment in the state of health, depression, and anxiety may be dominant factors. These can be minimized if the patient is able to function as normally as possible. When there is a general "poor state of health," there is a tendency for both physician and family to encourage lack of work activity by the patient, but patients who are able to function in relationship to their peer group often have an improved adaptation to the disease. This can lead (potentially) to greater therapeutic benefit.

Hospitalization. Hospitalization is indicated for the following reasons:

1. Failure of apparently mild disease to improve significantly within 1 month on outpatient treatment. Hospitalization serves 2 purposes: it removes the patient from an aggravating environment and provides the physician with an opportunity to initiate a more effective and intensive therapeutic program.

2. Severe illness with anorexia, nausea, vomiting, fever, and uncontrolled diarrhea (acute fulminant disease). Prompt hospitalization for such patients is essential not only to provide the measures necessary for control of the disease, but also to prevent complications or recognize their occurrence promptly (e.g., toxic megacolon).

3. Development of local or systemic complications, including severe hemorrhage, persistent anemia necessitating transfusions, profound hypoalbuminemia, or suspicion of carcinoma. Consideration of the need for surgery not only for colonic complications (toxic megacolon, impending perforation), but also because of refractoriness to the prolonged administration of a comprehensive medical regimen, should be reason for hospitalization.

4. To remove a patient with emotional problems from an upsetting home environment or the burdens of decision-making.

Nutrition. The patient's general state of nutrition relates to his well-being and adaptation and, if good, perhaps facilitates therapeutic response. Many patients are 10% to 20% under their optimal weight, and others may have more specific nutritional deficiencies. Much emphasis was placed in the past on diet, with avoidance of roughage and institution of a bland, high-protein diet. While avoidance of fresh fruits and vegetables as well as poorly digested skins and other fiber is likely desirable during the acute state of illness, permitting the patient to have a normal (for him) nutritional intake can be psychologically beneficial, particularly for a young patient. There are more convincing data showing an association between a good general nutritional state and therapeutic response than equivalent data supporting multiple specific dietary restrictions. Thus, most patients are instructed to avoid certain foods that might cause diarrhea or abdominal cramping (e.g., coffee, alcohol, skins, nuts, seeds), but to try to maintain a diet that is both "normal" for them and generally nutritious. For the patient who is chronically malnourished (i.e., 20% below optimal body weight), consultation with a nutritionist can be helpful. Many patients, however, resist the emphasis on "food as medicine."

Some patients may be lactase-deficient and thus lactose-intolerant. The ability to tolerate milk should be specifically discussed, although this may be related more to dose and stage of illness than to lactose intolerance.

Anxiety or Depression. Rapport between the treating physician and the patient over a long period of time is important, but specific consultation with a psychiatrist or psychologist is seldom indicated. Emphasis on psychologic factors may not be beneficial to a patient who is already concerned about his physical health and his chronic symptoms. Likewise, the use of tranquilizers and antidepressants should be reserved for those patients with clinically significant evidence of anxiety or depression. This is particularly true for patients who are relatively young and helps them avoid the simplistic thinking that "drugs" can, in and of themselves, make them feel better.

Supportive Therapy. Supportive therapy consists of medications that either improve the patient's general state of health and nutrition or alleviate symptoms. To achieve the latter, patients may tend to overutilize prescribed medications, and agents with a habit-forming propensity can themselves become a problem. In addition to their habit-forming potential, narcotics can cause hypomotility and may precipitate toxic megacolon. Nonnarcotic analgesics can be used, although they may be associated with gastrointestinal upset. A small number of patients with ulcerative colitis who take aspirin products develop peptic ulceration.

Anticholinergics also have the ability to precipitate toxic megacolon and may or may not be helpful for alleviating abdominal cramping. In general, it is thought best to avoid this group of agents for patients with ulcerative colitis, except on a short-term basis for a patient with relatively quiescent or moderate disease.

The key "supportive" medications are *antidiarrheal agents,* especially diphenoxylate (Lomotil) or loperamide (Imodium). Although both drugs are "controlled" and require narcotic numbers on prescriptions, loperamide seems to have fewer side effects. Nevertheless, the habit-forming potential of antidiarrheal agents is one of the most important problems relating to drug use in ulcerative colitis. Because of the effectiveness of the agents and the desire to control the symptom of diarrhea, patients frequently use more medication than prescribed. In a sense, the relative effectiveness of these drugs tends to perpetuate their use. Therefore, there must be a frank discussion with the patient as to the number of tablets or capsules utilized to control diarrhea and the circumstances under which these medications are used.

Multiple vitamin and iron supplements are frequently prescribed for patients with ulcerative colitis, but there is relatively little scientific data to support their use other than for "general nutritional" reasons or for iron replacement if there is iron deficiency. Patients often report that they feel better taking vitamins, but the use of vitamins, minerals, and other supplements (except in the case of iron deficiency) remains relatively empiric, and there is little evidence to support "megavitamin" therapy.

Patients who are acutely or severely ill may require IV fluid replacement, blood transfusions, and, at times, *antibiotics.* However, the need for antibiotics in patients with ulcerative colitis is infrequent. Moreover, there is no evidence to support long-term use of antibiotics in the therapy of ulcerative colitis. The primary indication for antibiotics is the presence or suspected existence of intra-abdominal infection[1, 2] with evidence of peritonitis, as may occur in patients with toxic megacolon. As noted earlier, mortality due to toxic megacolon increases in the presence of sepsis and malnutrition. Therefore, the appropriate use of antibiotics under these circumstances can be life-saving. As noted by McHenry,[3] most intra-abdominal infections are caused by a mixture of aerobic and anaerobic bacteria, and there is evidence in both man and animals that the antibiotic treatment of intra-abdominal infections should incorporate drugs to cover both the aerobic and the anaerobic bacteria present[4] (Chapter 228). There is general agreement that an amino glycoside antibiotic, such as gentamicin, is an appropriate agent for the aerobic gram-negative bacilli, while drugs such as chloramphenicol, clindamycin, cefoxitin, metronidazole, and ticarcillin or carbenicillin are appropriate for anaerobic coverage. It has been shown that gentamicin administered conjointly with clindamycin is effective and relatively safe for the treatment of intra-abdominal infections; response rates of 68% to 93% have been reported.[2] Favorable response rates have also been noted with the combinations of gentamicin and metronidazole and with tobramycin and metronidazole. Harding and colleagues[5] reported results of a prospective randomized comparative study indicating that clindamycin, chloramphenicol, and ticarcillin, each in combination with gentamicin, are equally effective in the treatment of intra-abdominal sepsis.

Hyperalimentation. Hyperalimentation (total parenteral nutrition, TPN) (Chapter 235) has been shown to be quite valuable under 2 specific circumstances: (1) as a preoperative adjunctive form of treatment for the patient who is severely malnourished and protein-depleted and who requires colectomy, and (2) postoperatively for the patient who has undergone colectomy under similar circumstances.[6] In general, TPN should be continued for 2 to 3 weeks. It has been found to have relatively little place in the long-term management of ulcerative colitis. Our experience with TPN is that it is seldom beneficial as "primary" therapy but is often valuable in an adjunctive role.[7]

For patients who are seriously ill and/or malnourished, total bowel rest and adequate nutritional support are the cornerstones of nutritional therapy. There have been relatively few studies comparing the 2 modalities of TPN and elemental diets (Chapter 234) in ulcerative colitis. Votik et al.[8] reported a 72% remission rate with elemental diets in patients with inflammatory bowel disease, and Axelsson et al.[9] achieved a 40% remission rate in 15 of 34 patients with inflammatory bowel disease using an elemental diet. However, despite the isolated successes, the use of an elemental diet in the treatment of patients with ulcerative colitis remains of limited value. In order to achieve total bowel rest, IV TPN is generally considered to be preferable.

Fischer et al.[10] used TPN as primary therapy for patients with ulcerative colitis, and 25% of these patients were able to avoid surgery. The authors noted weight gain, improved hematocrit, and elevated serum albumin level, but all patients needed blood transfusions. Truelove and Jewell[11] reported on 49 patients with acute ulcerative colitis treated with a 5-day course of IV therapy consisting of saline, glucose, and blood. They found that 73% of their patients went into complete remission by the end of the 5-day period. Failure to improve was taken to be an indication for colectomy. Fazio et al.[12] reported their experience with emphasis on the adjunctive nature of TPN. Others[13–15] have reported that TPN improved the nutritional status, prevented clinical deterioration, and was beneficial for decreasing the significance of infections. Workers at the University of Chicago, reporting their experience with TPN, noted that a substantial number of their patients with ulcerative colitis achieved an initial clinical remission.[16] Seashore et al.[17] reported on the use of TPN in children; 50% of the children failed to respond and required total colectomy. They stated that although TPN may induce remission or clinical improvement in children with ulcerative colitis, the response is usually short-lived. Others,[18] however, noted growth after TPN in patients with growth retardation.

To summarize, TPN can improve the nutritional status as measured by improvement in sense of well being, weight gain, positive nitrogen balance, and decreased requirements for albumin and blood transfusions.[13] However, long-term remissions are uncommon and the response generally is unpredictable. TPN and total bowel rest do not appear to alter the course of the disease and do not appear to be effective as a primary form of treatment in ulcerative colitis. TPN serves rather as an adjunctive means of nutritional support to prepare the patient for colectomy.

Hydrocortisone Enemas and Other Forms of Topical Therapy. For patients with distal ulcerative colitis, particularly those with proctitis and proctosigmoiditis, hydrocortisone enemas (consisting of 100 mg of hydrocortisone in 60 ml of saline solution or water) have been shown to be quite successful both in alleviating the symptoms of distal ulcerative colitis (rectal bleeding, tenesmus, and diarrhea) and in effecting a decrease in the degree of inflammation observed in the rectal mucosa. Furthermore, if consecutive daily administration is continued for 3 weeks or less, there is insufficient absorption to cause adrenal suppression.[19] While there are no good studies comparing the efficacy of topical steroids with either placebo or oral steroids, there is enough clinical evidence to support the use of hydrocortisone enemas as the sole therapeutic modality for patients with proctitis or proctosigmoiditis. Hydrocortisone enemas may also be valuable in an adjunctive role for patients with pancolitis who have significant tenesmus and rectal bleeding.

Sulfasalazine or various sulfasalazine derivatives, notably 5-aminosalicylic acid, given in enema form have aroused interest. Studies[20, 21] have indicated the efficacy of 5-aminosalicylic acid for patients with proctitis or distal colon ulcerative colitis used in either enema[22] or suppository form. The medication in such forms can be administered over a longer period of time[23] without concern for adrenal suppression due to steroid absorption,[19] as is the case with hydrocortisone enemas. At present, therefore, there is considerable optimism about the use of these forms of topical therapy.

Management of Refractory Proctosigmoiditis. About 15% of patients with distal colon ulcerative colitis may have a relapsing course and appear to be refractory to most forms of therapy.[24] Patients with refractory proctosigmoiditis have rectal bleeding, but usually do not have diarrhea or other symptoms. The factors that make the situation "refractory" are usually (1) frequent recurrences of rectal bleeding and tenesmus, or (2) persistent rectal bleeding. If the patient has had symptoms or an established diagnosis for several years, the risk of extension is quite low; in most patients in our experience, extension, when it does occur, appears within 2 years after the original diagnosis. While it might seem to be a paradox, the physician may be in the position of reassuring the patient that rectal bleeding is not a serious symptom!

In cases that appear to be refractory, it is particularly important to: (1) be certain that other infectious processes are not present, looking especially for *Campylobacter* and other organisms, as well as for *Clostridium difficile toxin;* and (2) perform a colonoscopic examination to determine, if possible, the upper limit of the inflammatory process and to be certain that the disease has not extended higher than determined clinically or by proctosigmoidoscopic or barium enema examination.[24a] Furthermore, refractory cases are more likely to be seen in patients with proctosigmoiditis rather than simple proctitis.

Almost all "refractory" patients will already have received some form of topical steroid agent and perhaps sulfasalazine. However, the seeming failure to respond to these agents previously does not preclude their being used again, often in combination. Thus, the use of hydrocortisone enemas on a regular basis for approximately 3 weeks, the use of steroid suppositories, and the combination of these with oral sulfasalazine in the 2- to 3-g range constitute the most commonly employed therapeutic regimen for this situation. In addition, assuming that lack of extension has been established, reassurance of the patient can also be beneficial.

Specific Drug Therapy

Sulfasalazine. Sulfasalazine is probably the medication most frequently used to treat ulcerative colitis.[25] Many therapeutic trials[26, 27] and experimental evidence[28–30] have indicated the value of its use, but the exact mechanism of action remains incompletely understood.[31] Sulfasalazine is a conjugate of 5-aminosalicylic acid and sulfapyridine linked by an azo-bond. Most of the ingested dose is absorbed from the small intestine intact and about 10% of the drug is excreted into the urine. The remainder is returned to the bowel unchanged by way of the bile. On reaching the colon, sulfasalazine is cleaved by bacterial action into 5-aminosalicylic acid and sulfapyridine[32]; little of the parent drug remains in the stool. Azo-bond cleavage depends solely on colonic bacteria; the liberated sulfapyridine is largely absorbed and excreted in the urine, while the 5-aminosalicylate moiety remains in the colon and is excreted in the stool. It was originally thought that the drug was bound by connective tissue and that its anti-inflammatory effects were based on this mechanism. Another hypothesis was that sulfasalazine altered intestinal flora in a way that decreased inflammation. However, little, if any, bacterial effect of the drug has been shown, although there is some evidence that it may decrease the number of anaerobic bacteria present in the large intestinal lumen. A more recent postulate is that sulfasalazine inhibits the production of prostaglandins or affects the migration of inflammatory cells into the bowel wall.[33] It would appear from available evidence that 5-aminosalicylate is the active moiety of sulfasalazine,[34] that it acts topically in the lumen of the intestine, and that it inhibits the inflammatory process.

The usual oral dose of sulfasalazine is 1 g (2 tablets of 0.5 g each) twice daily, increasing to a total of 4 g (2 tablets of 0.5 g 4 times daily). Improvement and therapeutic response may take up 3 to 4 weeks after initiation of sulfasalazine therapy. A number of patients (perhaps as many as 25%) have some gastric upset and headache associated with ingestion of the drug. However, lowering the dose and gradually increasing it again will usually permit the drug to be tolerated. In the National Cooperative Crohn's Disease Study (carried out in the United States) in which sulfasalazine was used,[35] side effects were observed in 12% to 14% of the patients treated. Nausea, vomiting, and loss of appetite occurred in one-third of the patients in that study. Side effects involve dose-independent hypersensitivity reactions, which include the dyspeptic symptoms and headache already mentioned. Hematologic complications have occurred, including hemolysis and leukopenia. An important side effect is that of reduction in sperm count and motility with resultant temporary infertility.[36] This is reversible, however. There does not appear to be any special relationship between intolerance or allergy to sulfasalazine and a similar reaction to other sulfa agents or to other salicylates. There is a correlation between therapeutic response (as well as side effects) and plasma sulfapyridine levels. There also is a correlation between therapeutic response and 5-aminosalicylic acid content in the colon.

Therapy with sulfasalazine is usually long-term, most often 1, 2, or more years,[37] with a dose of 4 g daily initially, gradually tapering to 2 g daily. This form of therapy has been most effective in patients with mild to moderate disease. Long-term (even indefinite) use of sulfasalazine has been advocated as beneficial in patients with ulcerative colitis.[26] However, the exact duration of therapy is a source of controversy. Convincing data have accrued that at least 1 year of maintenance therapy is beneficial following remission of primary symptoms.[37] Despite conflicting data, it is probably best to continue sulfasalazine in a patient in remission for a longer period of time than only 1 year, but whether one should treat for 2 years, 5 years, some arbitrary point in time, or indefinitely remains unclear.

Sulfasalazine is frequently used in conjunction with prednisone because of the latter's more rapid onset of therapeutic benefit and the more sustained benefit from sulfasalazine without concern about long-term effects. Several new forms of oral delivery of 5-aminosalicylate are under investigation, the most promising of which appears to be sodium azodisalicylate. Preliminary studies have indicated the efficacy of maintenance of remission with both oral 5-aminosalicylic acid and azodisalicylate.[20] The value of these agents remains to be established.

Corticosteroids. These agents are the drugs of choice for the acute stage of ulcerative colitis, the severe form of the disease, or the fulminant form.[38] One of the initial hopes was that steroid therapy, in addition to its effectiveness on a short-term basis, might enable patients to avoid colectomy, but this has generally not been the case. However, even in patients who do require colectomy, such as those with toxic megacolon, steroid therapy has been shown to be beneficial and not harmful.[39] Prednisone has become the most frequently used steroid form, and dosage levels for moderate to severe disease are in the range of 40 to 60 mg daily, with a gradual tapering over a period of weeks to 20 mg or less, at times using alternate-day dosage.[40] Patients on 20 mg or less will typically have fewer steroid side effects and can gradually be weaned from the dose, often while maintaining a dosage of sulfasalazine of 2 to 4 g daily. Long-term use of prednisone,[41] unlike sulfasalazine, has not been shown to prevent relapse. Also, side effects make its use beneficial on a short-term basis rather than for long-term therapy.

Whether treating with steroids, sulfasalazine, or a combination of these agents, the physician must be able to assess the therapeutic response.[42] The activity of the disease plays a major role in assessing both the need for therapy and the therapeutic response. Objective data that help assay activity include (1) the weight of the patient, (2) the visual appearance of the rectal mucosa on endoscopic examination, (3) the blood hemoglobin level, and (4) the serum albumin level. Subjective symptoms are more difficult to correlate with therapeutic response. Extraintestinal manifestations can be useful guidelines clinically, but fewer than 10% of patients will actually have such manifestations.

For patients with more severe disease (malnutrition, fever, abdominal pain and tenderness, bloody diarrhea, anemia, and hypoalbuminemia), the use of IV hydrocortisone, 100 to 400 mg/day, may be necessary.[11] Concern has been expressed in the past that these dosage levels might "mask" a perforation of the colon and lead to peritoneal sepsis and death; therefore, careful monitoring of the patient on such high doses is quite important. Generally, however, mortality rates have been lower over the past decade than in previous years for patients with severe ulcerative colitis.[43]

For patients with fulminant colitis, with or without toxic megacolon, parenteral steroids should be utilized for 48 to 72 hours. If there is insufficient response, surgery should be seriously considered. A useful guideline for ill patients, but not those with fulminant colitis or toxic megacolon, is that therapy should be continued for approximately 3 weeks and surgical consultation should be considered if there is a lack of response.

Whether or not there is an advantage of adrenocorticotropic hormone (ACTH) over other parenteral steroids or oral agents is not well established or understood.[44] The phenomenon of a patient responding to one form of steroid when there was no or poor response to another form is well known. Evidence has been advanced by Meyers et al.[45] suggesting that ACTH administered IV is most effective when given to patients with severe ulcerative colitis who have not previously received oral steroids, and in such circumstances is probably the agent of choice.

Riis[46] has advocated the following therapeutic guidelines: (1) Fulminant cases or an acute exacerbation should be treated with systemic prednisone, 60 to 80 mg, and sulfasalazine, 3 to 5 g, daily. If no response occurs in 3 to 4 days, colectomy should be considered. (2) For chronic intermittent activity of disease, sulfasalazine, 2 to 3 g daily, is used with a low dose (less than 20 mg) of prednisone for several weeks to months. (3) For chronic continuous ulcerative colitis, sulfasalazine, 2 to 3 g daily, is given with systemic prednisone in a dose of 20 to 40 mg daily, with or without local steroid therapy, for a period of 3 months.

Immunosuppressive Agents. Although there is some evidence from English studies[47, 48] indicating the value of azathioprine in the treatment of ulcerative colitis, there has been much more interest and emphasis on immunosuppressive therapy in Crohn's disease. However, the many side effects of immunosuppressive agents have deterred widespread use. In addition to leukopenia, there is concern about the possible development of lymphoma. In a study of over 1300 British and Australian patients on immunosuppressive agents, including patients with Crohn's disease on azathioprine,[49] there was a 12-fold increase in lymphomas compared with the expected number in the general population. Because of concern over side effects of immunosuppressive agents, because of the relative effectiveness of the aforementioned therapeutic regimens, and because of the relative effectiveness of colectomy in the treatment of ulcerative colitis, there has been less interest in immunosuppressive agents for treatment of ulcerative colitis than for Crohn's disease.[50–52]

Other Therapeutic Agents. Unlike Crohn's disease, in which some antibiotic agents (notably *metronidazole*) have apparently been successful in treatment under certain circumstances, this has not been the case for patients with ulcerative colitis. Because eosinophils have been observed in the inflammatory infiltrate of ulcerative colitis and because mast cells increase in number during relapse, it has been speculated that there might be therapeutic benefit from a mast cell stabilizer, such as *disodium cromoglycate.* However, this has not proved to be the case.

Indications for Surgery

The primary operation for ulcerative colitis is colectomy, either total or subtotal. Segmental resections of the colon are invariably associated with failure. Any decision regarding surgery, therefore, is important because of the magnitude of the operation.[53] Indications for surgery in ulcerative colitis include a severe or acute fulminating course, development of toxic megacolon, severe hemorrhage, or chronicity.[54] The last is the most common indication for surgery in our experience in the last decade and includes persistence of malnutrition, diarrhea, rectal bleeding, extracolonic manifestations, anemia, and hypoalbuminemia. Patients who might be satisfactory candidates for ileorectal anastomosis are those with longstanding and quiescent disease and inactive inflammation in the rectal mucosa. Patients for whom the Kock pouch has been successful include those with a fairly good nutritional state and chronic disease and those for whom the decision for colectomy can be made on a relatively elective basis. The same holds true for the technically difficult ileoanal anastomosis.

Surgical management is discussed in detail in the following section.

References

1. Altemier WA, Culbertson WR, Fullen WD, et al. Intraabdominal abscess. Am J Surg 1973; 125:70.
2. Levison ME. Peritonitis and intra-abdominal abscess. *In:* Mandell GL, Douglas RG Jr, Bennett JE, eds. Principles and Practices of Infectious Diseases. New York: John Wiley and Sons, 1979: 609–43.
3. McHenry MC. Therapeutic aspects of aminoglycosides. *In:* Barnes WG, Hodges GP, eds. The Aminoglycoside Antibiotic—Colon: A Guide to Therapy. New York: CRC Press, 1984: 87–151.
4. Pitcher WD, Musher DM. Critical importance of early diagnosis and treatment of intra-abdominal infection. Arch Surg 1982; 117:328.
5. Harding GKM, Buckwold FJ, Ronald AR. Prospective, randomized, comparative study of clindamycin, chloramphenicol, and ticarcillin, each in combination with gentamicin in therapy for intraabdominal and female genital tract sepsis. Infect Dis 1980; 142:384.
6. Mullen JL, Hargrove WC, Dudrick SJ, et al. Ten years experience with intravenous hyperalimentation and inflammatory bowel disease. Ann Surg 1978; 187:523–9.
7. Diehl JT, Steiger E. Hoolei RD. The role of intravenous hyperalimentation in intestinal disease. Surg Clin North Am 1983; 63:11–26.
8. Votik AJ, Echave V, Feller JH, Brown RA, et al. Experience with elemental diet in the treatment of inflammatory bowel disease. Arch Surg 1973; 107:329–33.
9. Axelsson C, Jarnum S. Assessment of the therapeutic value of an elemental diet in chronic inflammatory bowel disease. Scand J Gastroenterol 1977; 12:89–95.
10. Fischer JE, Foster GS, Abel RM, et al. Hyperalimentation as primary therapy for inflammatory bowel disease. Am J Surg 1973; 125:165–75.
11. Truelove SC, Jewell DP. Intensive intravenous regimen for severe attacks of ulcerative colitis. Lancet 1974; 1:1067–70.
12. Fazio VW, Kodner IJ, Jagelman DG. Parenteral nutrition as primary or adjunctive treatment in inflammatory bowel disease. Dis Colon Rectum 1976; 19:574–78.
13. Elson CO, Layden JJ, Nemchausky BB, et al. An evaluation of total parenteral nutrition in the management of inflammatory bowel disease. Dig Dis Sci 1980; 25:42–8.
14. Riddell RH, Morson BC. Value of sigmoidoscopy and biopsy in detection of carcinoma and premalignant change in ulcerative colitis. Gut 1979; 20:575.
15. Reilly J, Ryan J, Strole W, et al. Hyperalimentation in inflammatory bowel disease. Am J Surg 1976; 131:192–200.
16. Driscoll RH, Rosenberg IH. Total parenteral nutrition in inflammatory bowel disease. Med Clin North Am 1978; 1:185–201.
17. Seashore JH, Hillemier AL, Gryboski JD. Total parenteral nutrition in the management of inflammatory bowel disease in children. A limited role. Am J Surg 1982; 143:504–7.
18. Layden T, Rosenberg J, Nemchausky B, et al. Reversal of growth arrest in adolescents with Crohn's disease after parenteral alimentation. Gastroenterology 1976; 70:1017–21.
19. Farmer RG, Schumacher OP. Treatment of ulcerative colitis with hydrocortisone enemas. Dis Colon Rectum 1970; 13:355.
20. Dew MJ, Hughes MB, Harries AD, et al. Maintenance of remission in ulcerative colitis with oral preparation of 5-aminosalicylic acid. Br Med J 1982; 285:1012.
21. Willoughby CP, Piris J, Truelove SC. The effect of tropical N-acetyl-5-aminosalicylic acid in ulcerative colitis. Scand J Gastroenterol 1980; 15:715–9.
22. Jansens J, Geboes K, Delanote C, et al. 5-Aminosalicylic acid (5-ASA) enemas are effective in patients with resistant ulcerative rectosigmoiditis. Gastroenterology 1983; 84:1198 (Abstract).
23. Campieri M, Lanfranchi GA, Bazzocchi G, et al. Treatment of ulcerative colitis with high-dose 5-aminosalicylic acid enemas. Lancet 1981; 2:270–1.
24. Farmer RG. Long-term prognosis for patients with ulcerative proctosigmoiditis (ulcerative colitis confined to the rectum and sigmoid colon). J Clin Gastroenterol 1979; 1:47–50.

24a. Farmer RG, Whelan G, Sivak MV Jr. Colonoscopy in distal colon ulcerative colitis. Clin Gastroenterology 1980; 9:297–306.

25. Klotz U, Maier K, Fischer C, et al. Therapeutic efficacy of sulfasalazine and its metabolites in patients with ulcerative colitis and Crohn's disease. N Engl J Med 1980; 303:1499–1502.
26. Dissamayake AS, Truelove SC. A controlled therapeutic trial of long-term maintenance treatment of ulcerative colitis with sulphasalazine (salazophron). Gut 1973; 14:923–6.
27. Moertel CG, Bargen JA. A critical analysis of the use of salicylazosulfapyridine in chronic ulcerative colitis. Ann Intern Med 1959; 51:879.
28. Azad-Kach AK, Piris J, Truelove SC. An experiment to determine the active therapeutic moiety of sulphasalazine. Lancet 1977; 2:892–5.
29. Das KM, Sternlieb I. Salicylazosulfapyridine in inflammatory bowel disease. Dig Dis 1975; 20:971–6.
30. Van Hees PAM, Bakker JH, Van Tongeren JHM. Effect of sulphapyridine 5-ASA and placebo in patients with idiopathic proctitis: A study to determine the active therapeutic moiety of sulphasalazine. Gut 1980; 11:632–5.
31. Goldman P, Peppercorn MA. Sulfasalazine. N Engl J Med 1975; 293:20–3.
32. Peppercorn MA, Goldman P. The role of intestinal bacteria in the metabolism of salicylazo-sulphapyridine. J Pharmacol Exp Ther 1972; 181:556–62.
33. Hodgson HJF. Assessment of drug therapy in inflammatory bowel disease. Br J Clin Pharmacol 1982; 14:159–70.
34. Sack DM, Peppercorn MH. Drug therapy of inflammatory bowel disease. Pharmacotherapy 1983; 3:158–76 (Review).
35. Singelton JW, Summers RW, Kern F Jr, et al. A trial of sulfasalazine as adjunctive therapy in Crohn's disease. Gastroenterology 1979; 77:870–82.
36. Toovey S, Hudson E, Hendry WF, et al. Sulphasalazine and male infertility: reversibility and possible mechanism. Gut 1981; 1:22:445–51.
37. Misiewicz JJ, Lennard-Jones JE, Connell AM, et al. Controlled trial of sulphasalazine in maintenance therapy for ulcerative colitis. Lancet 1965; 1:185.
38. Spencer JA, Kirsner JB. Mlynaryk P, et al. Immediate and prolonged therapeutic effects of corticotrophin and adrenal steroids in ulcerative colitis. Observations in 340 cases for periods up to 10 years. Gastroenterology 1962; 42:113.
39. Jalan KN, Prescott RJ, Smith AN, et al. Influence of corticosteroids on the results of surgical treatment for ulcerative colitis. N Engl J Med 1970; 283:588.
40. Powell-Tuck J, Brown RL, Chambers TJ, Lennard-Jones JE. A controlled trial of alternate day prednisolone as maintenance treatment for ulcerative colitis in remission. Digestion 1981; 22:263–70.
41. Lennard-Jones JE, Misiewicz JJ, Connell AM, et al. Prednisone as maintenance treatment for ulcerative colitis in remission. Lancet 1965; 1:188.
42. Riis P. A critical survey of controlled studies in the treatment of ulcerative colitis and Crohn's disease. Clin Gastroenterol 1980; 9:351–70.
43. Truelove SC, Willoughby CP, Lee EG, et al. Further expe-

rience in the treatment of severe attacks of ulcerative colitis. Lancet 1978; 2:1086–8.
44. Powell-Tuck J, Bucknell NA, Lennard-Jones JE. A controlled comparison of corticotropin and hydrocortisone in the treatment of severe proctocolitis. Scand J Gastroenterol 1977; 12:971–5.
45. Meyers S, Sachar DB, Goldberg JD, Janowitz HD. Corticotropin versus hydrocortisone in the intravenous treatment of ulcerative colitis: A prospective, randomized, double-blind clinical trial. Gastroenterology 1983; 85:351–7.
46. Riis P. Therapy of ulcerative colitis—a critical evaluation. Scand J Gastroenterol 1982; 88(Suppl):24–9.
47. Jewell DP, Truelove SC. Azathioprine in ulcerative colitis: final report on controlled therapeutic trial. Br Med J 1974; 4:627–30.
48. Kirk AP, Lennard-Jones JE. Controlled trial of azathioprine in chronic ulcerative colitis. Br Med J 1982; 284:1291–2.
49. Kinlen LJ, Sheil AGR, Peto J, et al. Collaborative United Kingdom–Australasian study of cancer in patients treated with immunosuppressive drugs. Br Med J 1979; 2:1461–6.
50. Korelitz BI. Editorial: The treatment of ulcerative colitis with "immunosuppressive" drugs. Am J Gastroenterol 1981; 76:297.
51. Lennard-Jones JE. Azathioprine and 6-mercaptopurine have a role in the treatment of Crohn's disease. Dig Dis Sci 1981; 26:364–8.
52. Present DH, Korelitz BI, Wisch N, et al. Treatment of Crohn's disease with 6-mercaptopurine: a long-term, randomized, double blind study. New Engl J Med 1980; 302:981–7.
53. Fazio VW, Turnbull RB Jr. Ulcerative colitis and Crohn's disease of the colon—a review of surgical options. Med Clin North Am 1980; 64:1135–59.
54. Goligher JC, deDombal FT, Grahm RG, et al. Early surgery in the management of severe ulcerative colitis. Br Med J 1967; 3:193.

Surgical Management

Victor W. Fazio

Evolution

Keetley[1] introduced the concept of appendicostomy for the treatment of ulcerative colitis in 1895. This opening was used to instill a warm solution of sodium bicarbonate into the colon. Little popular support developed for this procedure,[2, 3] and it is now of historical significance only. Brown,[4] in 1913, recommended ileostomy as a means of bypassing the diseased colon (although he used a cecostomy as well to provide colonic irrigation). Two major problems were encountered after this procedure. The first was the frequent development of a clinical syndrome termed "ileostomy dysfunction"[5] (discussed later in the section on Complications). The immediate problem could be managed somewhat by leaving an indwelling catheter in the ileostomy (below the fascial level), and gradual "maturation" of the stoma would occur by a process of epithelialization of the serosal surface from the ileal mucosa.[6] Prevention, however, was found to require a biologic cover for the exposed serosa.[7–10]

The second problem with ileostomy as a method for the surgical treatment of ulcerative colitis was that the defunctionalized colon could still develop activity at a later date. Moreover, colonic cancer could supervene and extraintestinal manifestations of the disease could persist. In addition, ileostomy closure invariably was associated with reactivation of the disease.[11] Despite these limitations, ileostomy alone remained the premier operation for ulcerative colitis in the 1930s and 1940s.

In 1948, Ferguson and Stevens[12] noted that many patients with fulminant disease required colectomy in addition to ileostomy. At this time there was popular support for a 3-stage procedure, i.e., ileostomy, subtotal colectomy, and abdominoperineal resection at 3-month intervals.[11] In 1949, Miller et al.[13]

combined colectomy with ileostomy, and in a few cases proctocolectomy, as a single-stage procedure for ulcerative colitis. Crile and Thomas,[14] in 1951, advocated primary colectomy and ileostomy rather than ileostomy for toxic megacolon complicating ulcerative colitis. In the same year, Ravitch and Handelsman[15] reported performing total proctocolectomy and ileostomy in a series of patients without a death.

Advances since that time have been directed toward improving the patient's quality of life with respect to avoiding a permanent ileostomy (ileorectal anastomosis) or providing a continence mechanism for the ileostomy (Kock pouch).[16] While ileosigmoid anastomosis was practiced as early as 1903,[17] and popularized for a time by Devine,[18] this operation has been replaced in favor of ileorectal anastomosis because the latter provides removal of the extrasigmoid segment, so commonly involved in a significant way with inflammatory changes.

Other significant contributions are of more contemporary interest. Included in these are the "blow-hole" procedure of colonic diversion and decompression,[20] the continent ileostomy (Kock),[21] and ileoanal pull-through operation,[22] and the ileoanal pull-through with pelvic ileal reservoir.[23]

Frequency of Surgical Treatment

The frequency with which surgery has been reported to be used in the treatment of ulcerative colitis ranges from 16.7% to 48%.[11, 24–28] Lennard-Jones,[29] in 1982, reported experience with 269 newly diagnosed cases of ulcerative colitis analyzed over a period of up to 11 years. The cumulative probability of operation in the entire group was 8±2% at 5 years and 15±4% at 10 years. One-third of the patients with extensive colitis required surgery within the first year, usually as an urgent procedure. For patients with proctitis, the probability of upward extension of the disease was 5±3% at 5 years; for patients with proctosigmoiditis, the likelihood of proximal extension of the disease was 18±5% at 5 years.

Preoperative Preparation

General Considerations. In previous decades, surgery for ulcerative colitis invariably meant that the patient would be left with a permanent ileostomy. Proctocolectomy with end ileostomy is still the most commonly performed procedure for ulcerative colitis.

In the early discussion with patients about to undergo an operation, the aim is to develop a climate of trust and provide accurate information about an ileostomy so as to maximize the psychologic acceptance of a stoma. The more acute or debilitating the illness before operation, the higher the rate of acceptance. When possible, illustrative material is given to the patient and, more importantly, an interview is arranged with an ileostomate of the same sex and approximate age who has made a good recovery (Chapter 130).

There are instances, however, when despite all these efforts, the patient is reluctant and even refuses to have surgery performed. In these situations, surgical alternatives, such as the continent ileostomy or the internal pelvic reservoir with ileoanal anastomosis, may be broached. Intelligent, informed patients will often have heard about these alternatives before consulting the surgeon. Additionally, many patients will ask about the sequelae of an operation—what the operation will achieve for them, limitations with respect to work or social activities, and the various complications that may occur. The extent to which information is given to the patient varies from one clinician to another. In my view, a patient is entitled to be told that a small risk exists for impotence, non-healing of the perineal wound, and certain ileostomy complications (see later discussion of Complications).

Systemic Preparation. Anemia is corrected by whole blood or packed red blood cell transfusions. Electrolyte imbalance is similarly corrected. Hypokalemia may be particularly severe in patients with acute attacks of colitis. Hypoalbuminemia may reflect either chronic disease with malnutrition or be secondary to an acute fulminant episode of colitis with resultant large losses of protein in the colonic exudate. Preoperative albumin transfusion may be given to such individuals to restore normal values, or the clinician may consider the use of total parenteral nutrition (TPN) (Chapter 235). TPN is indicated if significant malnutrition exists or if there is a reasonable possibility of carrying a patient through an acute attack and improving the condition at the time of surgery.[30] The value of TPN given as a single course in the hope of producing a sustained remission is debatable or at least uncertain. While short-term remissions of several months occur in perhaps three fourths of patients so treated (in combination with conventional medical therapy, including steroids), we were unable to demonstrate a significant long-term remission rate.[31]

Prothrombin defects are corrected by vitamin K administration. Because thromboembolic phenomena occur fairly often following elective proctocolectomy, my practice is to use "mini" heparin therapy (5000 units subcutaneously, twice daily) through the perioperative and postoperative periods.

Steroids are used during the pre- and postoperative periods if the patient had been treated with corticosteroids within 6 months of the operation. Goligher[28] has advocated steroid therapy if the patient had been taking corticosteroids within 2 years of the operative date.

Antibiotics are used both systemically and orally. On the day before surgery, erythromycin base and neomycin, 1 g each, are given at 1 PM, 2 PM, and 10 PM. Antibiotics effective against both aerobic and anaerobic gram-negative bacilli are given IV, as a single drug or in combinations, immediately before the operation and are continued for 24 hours afterward. If operative contamination occurs, treatment with antibiotics is continued for 5 days. A combination of an aminoglycoside, such as tobramycin, and an antianaerobic agent, such as clindamycin or metronidazole, is particularly effective. However, coverage with one of the third-generation cephalosporins as a single agent is becoming popular.

The activity of the colitis determines the vigor with which catharsis is employed. A small dose (100 ml) of magnesium citrate or 25 ml of 10% mannitol is usually well tolerated in elective cases. Use of an elemental or semi-elemental diet for 2 to 3 days before operation is also of value.

Stoma Marking. For patients who are to have a conventional end ileostomy or loop ileostomy proximal to an ileorectal or ileoanal anastomosis, preoperative stoma marking is mandatory. Perhaps this is the most important factor in determining successful long-term rehabilitation of the patient (Chapter 130). The site is chosen with the patient in the supine position and in the sitting position with hips flexed in an exaggerated fashion. This maneuver, in turn, exaggerates any folds or skin creases that may not be obvious in the supine position. The site is chosen in an area that is visible to the patient, on the summit of the right infraumbilical fat mound away from scars, creases, bony prominences, and planned incision lines and within the surface marking of the rectus abdominis muscle. Using standard-sized face plates corresponding to stoma plates of available appliances, an indelible mark is made over the chosen site.

Surgical Procedures

Ileostomy. This is rarely performed today without colectomy or proctocolectomy. When used, it would probably be in the following special situations: (1) when the nature of the colitis is in doubt (and potentially reversible); (2) in a patient who is malnourished and in whom systemic or enteral hyperalimentation is undesirable or impossible; such a patient may benefit from an ileostomy alone to "rest" the colon and permit better preparation for a staged definitive second operation;[32] (3) as a staging procedure in the treatment of toxic megacolon (see later discussion on Colonic Decompression); and (4) as a "double-barreled" ileostomy created to provide intestinal "rest" and an access point to irrigate the distal colon with anti-inflammatory agents, as advocated by Truelove et al.[33] There is controversy, however, about all of these uses.

Total Proctocolectomy and Ileostomy. This surgical procedure is the standard one at this time for patients with ulcerative colitis. The patient is freed of all colitic symptoms and the threat of recurrence, the risk of cancer is negated, health is restored, and the operation can be done in the elective situation with minimal morbidity and mortality. Hawley and Ritchie[34] stated in a report published in 1979 that there had been no deaths after surgery for colitis at St. Mark's Hospital in London since 1974, and there have been no operative deaths in my own series of 108 patients. Mortality, on the other hand, can be high for urgent operations, especially in institutions where such seriously ill patients are rarely seen.[35] In specialized institutions, the mortality from urgent colectomy has been reported to range from 7% to 15%.[36, 37] When the patient's condition permits, a one-stage procedure is preferred. For urgent or emergency situations or when the patient is significantly debilitated, abdominal or subtotal colectomy and ileostomy are done, with a second-stage proctectomy performed several months later. Certain experienced surgeons maintain that even in emergency situations, total proctocolectomy done in a one-stage procedure is safe in their hands and that any morbidity incurred is outweighed by that of leaving a rectum affected by disease.[28, 38]

In most cases, the extraintestinal manifestations of ulcerative colitis are alleviated by proctocolectomy, although no surgical procedure will reliably reverse certain hepatobiliary or spinal arthritic complications.

Certain technical points are important. A midline incision is chosen so that both lower quadrants are left undisturbed—one for construction of the ileostomy and the other for use in the unlikely event that ileostomy relocation becomes necessary. The midline incision also allows for extension upward or for left upper quadrant lateral extension if needed to allow safe delivery of a high splenic flexure. Generally, conservative resection of the colon is done with little disturbance to the retroperitoneum. The exception is when one operates on a patient known to have cancer of the colon or a patient with longstanding disease (e.g., more than 15 years) in whom an occult cancer may be present. Whenever possible, the omentum is preserved to quarantine the viscera from the incision. A conservative resection of the rectum is performed without wide lateral, anterior, and posterior dissection in order to minimize injury to the nervi erigentes and presacral sympathetic nerves with consequent sexual and bladder dysfunction. Primary closure of the perineal wound minimizes the risk of delayed perineal wound healing and sinus formation. The exception is in the case of inadvertent pelvic contamination with enteric content. The presacral space is drained of its obligatory exudate with sump suction drains. The ileostomy is constructed so that a segment of 5 to 6 cm of ileum is delivered, free of tension, beyond the skin level through an aperture that accommodates the tips of the operator's index and middle fingers. The length of bowel and this particular aperture size allows for both easy application of a pouch and freedom from obstruction. The cut end of the ileum is observed to assure that there is an excellent blood supply. The internal mesenteric defect around the ileostomy is obliterated to prevent internal volvulus, and the stoma is sewn to the skin ("matured") primarily after the main incision is closed.

Subtotal (Abdominal) Colectomy and Ileostomy. This procedure has been used for patients who are debilitated or malnourished or who have an urgent or emergency indication for surgery. Since the extra procedure of proctectomy adds more time and trauma to the operation, morbidity and mortality can be expected to be greater compared with abdominal colectomy alone. Fulminant disease, whether or not associated with toxic megacolon, is rarely associated with rectal perforation. Hence, the rectum need not be removed, as detoxification occurs with abdominal colectomy alone. A debatable issue is the need for proctectomy when major colonic hemorrhage compounds the clinical state of toxic colitis. Since bleeding of significant degree may be occurring from the rectal segment as well, it may be supposed that proctectomy must be done despite the poor condition of the patient. This is a matter of surgical judgment, taking into account the age and general condition of the patient and the proctoscopic appearance of the rectum. The rarity of continued significant bleeding from the rectal segment in such situations is impressive.

Goligher[28] has correctly pointed out that construction of a mucous fistula in the rectosigmoid after abdominal colectomy is not trouble-free. While it is rare for the retained segment to continue to produce systemic effects, drainage of pus, blood, and mucus can be so great that a second stomal pouch needs to be used. Furthermore, unless special care is taken, the sigmoid stump can recede into the peritoneal cavity and produce localized peritonitis. In patients with fulminant colitis, suturing the open end of the sigmoid colon to the skin cannot be relied on because of this very problem. Instead, the stump is exteriorized for several inches and wrapped in gauze so that recession is impossible. After a week or so, the excess bowel can be trimmed back to skin level and a delayed maturation of the mucous fistula made with safety. For patients with less acute presentations, in whom malnutrition is present or in whom a future ileorectal or ileoanal anastomosis is being considered, the rectal stump may be stapled across and implanted into the subcutaneous space of the lower part of the incision; this makes for easier management by the patient.

With the recent interest of many surgeons in the various forms of ileoanal anastomosis, several authorities, including Parks et al.,[23] have made a plea for leaving the rectal stump intact. Despite the severity of the disease in the rectum, the advocates of ileoanal anastomosis state that an anastomosis through the trimmed rectal stump (after mucosal proctectomy) can be done.

Colonic Decompression (Diversion) ("Blow-Hole" Procedure) (Fig. 126–42). Crile and Thomas[14] showed that colectomy was superior to ileostomy alone in the management of toxic megacolon and reduced the mortality rate from 68% to 14%. Mortality in patients with toxic megacolon is due to abnormal sepsis and bowel perforation. Turnbull et al.[20] and Fry and Atkinson[39] noted that perforation and sepsis can be encountered not only with spontaneous disruption of the colon, but also with iatrogenic perforation at the time of colectomy. This was especially likely in the region of the splenic flexure when the surgeon manipulated the inflamed, distended, edematous, and fragile colon. For this reason, Turnbull et al.[20] advocated a non-manipulative approach in patients with sealed perforations. Klein et al.[40] had success using colonic decompression (cecostomy) in 4 patients; Turnbull et al.[20] reasoned that adding colonic diversion (loop ileostomy) to colonic decompression (skin level—"blow-hole" colectomy) would be of additional value. This procedure was advocated as a preliminary or staging operation to allow detoxification prior to elective colectomy.

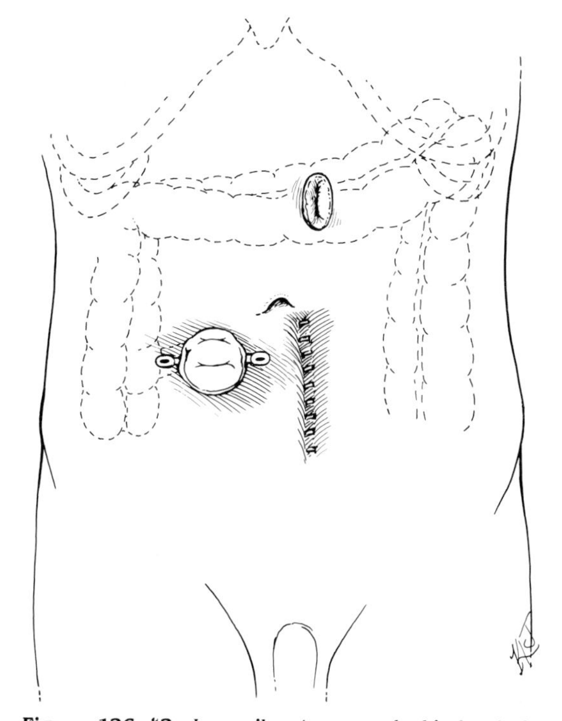

Figure 126–42. Loop ileostomy and skin-level decompression transverse colostomy. Completion colectomy or proctocolectomy is performed in 3 to 6 months.

Timing of Surgery for Toxic Megacolon. Following resuscitation of the patient by means of IV fluids, protein, blood (if needed), and steroids, immediate surgery is indicated in the following situations; (1) free colonic perforation; (2) signs of general peritonitis; (3) severe localized tenderness, usually in the left upper quadrant; (4) initial presentation with endotoxemic shock; (5) evidence of deterioration over the preceding 24 hours if referred from another institution; and (6) massive dilatation of the colon. In most cases, however, the patient may be observed for 24 to 72 hours to identify a pattern of response to treatment. During this period, attention is given to changes in signs of toxicity, fever, tachycardia, blood pressure, and leukocytosis and to changes in the diameter of the colon on the daily (sometimes twice daily) plain films of the abdomen. If there is clinical improvement, medical therapy is continued; however, illusory "improvement" is frequently noted. Toxicity parameters may fluctuate, as may the degree of colonic dilatation. Sometimes signs of toxicity persist and colonic dilatation disappears. Unless there is improvement in toxicity parameters within 72 hours, surgical treatment is indicated.

The indications for diversion decompression as opposed to colectomy are: (1) the presence of sealed or "contained" perforations of the colon; (2) obesity; (3) a "high" splenic flexure, in which iatrogenic injury to the spleen or colon is a significant risk; (4) inexperience of the surgeon in performing emergency colectomy; and (5) an extremely dilated colon. Contraindications include: (1) the presence of a free perforation (although occasionally this can be exteriorized); (2) associated major hemorrhage from the colon; and (3) individualized situations in which the surgeon deems that colectomy poses no unusual difficulties. In our experience, morbidity has been minimal with the "blow-hole" procedure. Three of 83 patients required colectomy during the same hospitalization following the "blow-hole" procedure because of colonic hemorrhage. Hospital mortality with the procedure was 3.6%, although an

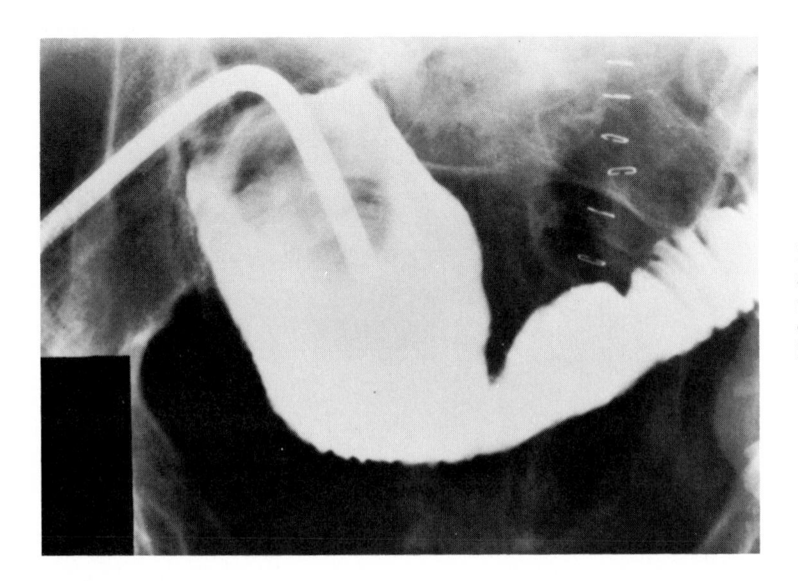

Figure 126–43. Barium study of a 3-loop continent ileostomy. The nipple valve is seen as a filling defect through which the catheter is passing.

additional 2 deaths after definitive colectomy gave an overall mortality rate of 6%.[41]

Continent Ileostomy (Kock Pouch) (Fig. 126–43). Kock[16] introduced the concept of an internal ileal reservoir in 1969 and later (1973) added a valve mechanism[21] (Fig. 126–44) to provide continence. This spared the patient the need to wear an external appliance to collect fecal discharge. Instead, the reservoir is intubated and its contents evacuated 2 to 4 times a day. The procedure may be done either at the time of definitive proctocolectomy or as a conversion procedure by revising an established conventional ileostomy. Sense of body image and sexuality are improved when the patient is freed of the need to wear an external pouch. Other advantages over conventional ileostomy include less noise from the stoma, less odor, lack of skin excoriation, a non-phallic appearance, improved social activities, and ability to wear close-fitting garments. Equipment costs, per annum, for the conventional and the continent ileostomy are $500 and $100, respectively.

The operation adds nothing to the patient's physical well-being, but is sought by those with an aversion to wearing an external pouch. With the use of this and other procedures as alternatives to conventional ileostomy, patients will frequently undergo an operation at a somewhat earlier time in the course of their colitis, rather than live with increasing degrees of disability on continued medical therapy. Surgeons are divided in their support for the operation, but as experience with it is amassed, enthusiasm for the procedure appears to increase.

Complications of the operation are mainly related to the construction of the valve mechanism. There is a tendency for the intussuscepted nipple valve to slide or extrude on its mesenteric aspect (Fig. 126–45). This, in turn,

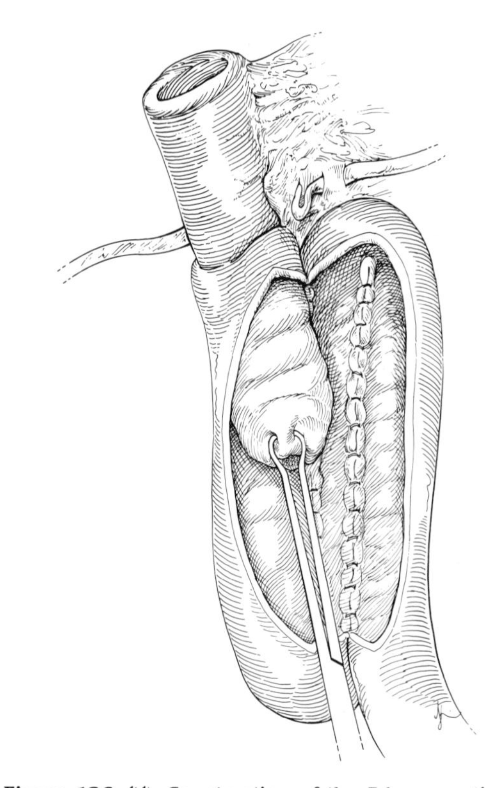

Figure 126–44. Construction of the 3-loop continent ileostomy. After anastomosing 3 loops of terminal ileum, the nipple valve is made by intussuscepting the exit conduit. Three rows of staples are applied to the valve to maintain its reduction. A fascial or mersilene sling applied at the mesentery assists in maintaining reduction.

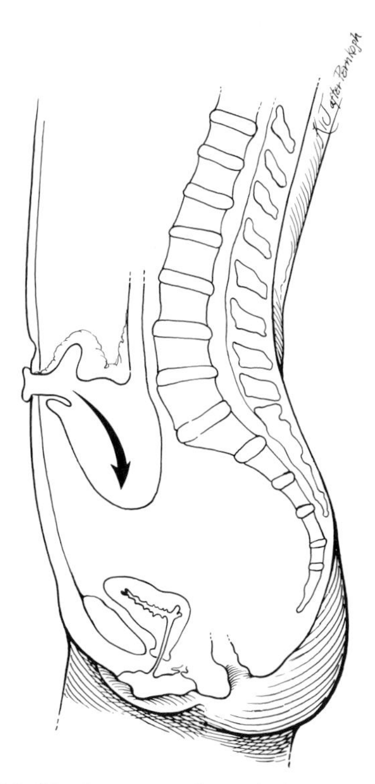

Figure 126–45. Desussception of the valve on its mesenteric aspect produces incontinence and sometimes difficulty in intubation.

produces difficulty in intubation and incontinence or obstruction. One review[42] reported an average occurrence rate of 16.5% for these complications. Fistulas from the pouch to the skin or through the nipple valve (bypassing the continence mechanism) are uncommon. Rarer still are ischemic necrosis of the valve, reservoir perforation by the catheter, and extrusion (prolapse) of the entire valve through the external skin aperture. Nonspecific ileitis, or "pouchitis," is seen in about 10% of patients. The etiology of this change is unclear, but it is thought to occur as the result of stasis and anaerobic bacterial overgrowth; constant drainage of the pouch and oral antibiotics produce resolution in 4 to 7 days. Mortality rates of 2% have been reported,[42] although several series, including my own, have been without operative deaths.

The indications for the continent ileostomy are not universally accepted. Patients with ulcerative colitis may reasonably be offered this procedure when no contraindications are present and when the patient is given an accurate, candid account of the operation and its possible sequelae. No patient should be "talked into" having such a sophisticated procedure.

A high rate of complications can be expected in obese patients, those taking large doses of steroids or immunosuppressive drugs, aged patients, and those with fulminant or acute colitis. The operation is contraindicated in patients with a psychotic tendency. It also should not be done in association with abdominal colectomy and rectal preservation because reservoir adherence to the rectal stump may make subsequent proctectomy very difficult.

Overall results have improved as experience with the operation has increased. Continence rates of 60%[43] to 90%[44] were reported in the 1970s. These reports related to total continence, including those patients who had minor or infrequent problems. Gelernt[45] reported rates of complete continence, minimal incontinence, and significant incontinence (appliance needed) of 94%, 5.5%, and 0.5%, respectively, in 200 patients. Our own experience has been similarly encouraging.

Absorption studies of continent ileostomy patients[46] have disclosed normal levels of hemoglobin, serum iron, serum folate, creatinine, electrolytes, and serum vitamin B_{12}. Fecal fat excretion on a standard daily 100-g fat diet exceeded the upper limit of normal (6 g/24 hours) in 8 of 10 patients; urinary D-xylose excretion was reduced in 5 of 10 patients.

Abdominal Colectomy and Ileorectal Anastomosis (Fig. 126–46). The controversies relating to this operation stem not so much from whether it should be used, but rather from the frequency with which it can be performed with reasonable assurance of a satisfactory outcome. Some have denied any significant role for ileorectal anastomosis in the treatment of ulcerative colitis,[47] while others perform the procedure in 50% to 80% of surgically treated cases.[19, 48, 49] The proportion of cases in which it may profitably be employed probably lies somewhere between these extremes.

In determining whether to recommend the procedure, consideration is given to the appearance of the rectum and perianal tissues and the reliability of the patient in returning for regular long-term follow-up. In 2% to 10% of patients with ulcerative colitis, the rectum is relatively spared from disease.[50] Topical steroid administration and exclusion of the rectum from the fecal stream may also significantly lessen the inflammatory process. The surgeon is guided not only by the mucosal appearance but also by the disten-

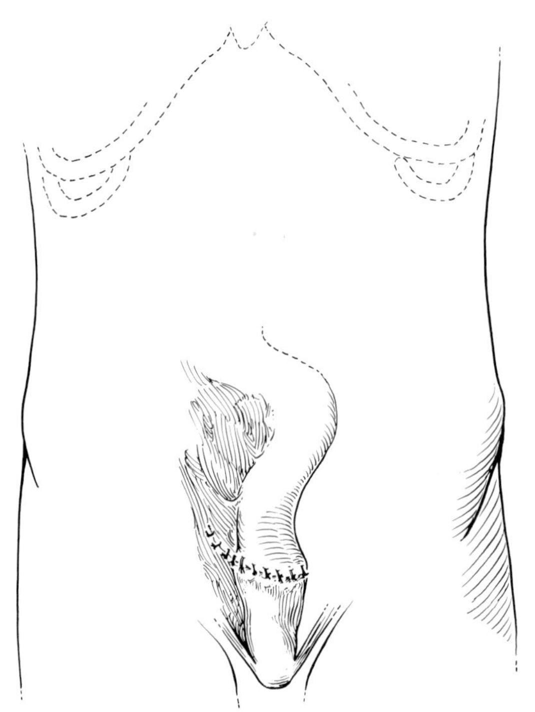

Figure 126–46. Ileorectal anastomosis. The rectosigmoid is divided at the sacral promontory, leaving approximately 15 cm of distal large bowel. The ileum has been previously transsected at the ileocecal valve.

sibility of the rectum (i.e., the possibility of future reservoir function as opposed to a rigid conduit). This is tested by air insufflation at proctoscopy. Additionally, anal or perianal disease and poor sphincter control should deter the surgeon from considering this option. Other contraindications include the presence of dysplasia or cancer in the proximal colon, inasmuch as the rectal segment is then at a much greater risk for the development of metachronous cancer.[51] As a rule, the younger the patient, the more acceptable the functional result.

It is apparent to surgeons experienced with this operation that the degree of inflammation observed in the rectum, both before and after ileorectal anastomosis, correlates poorly with the functional result. Aylett[19] popularized this procedure and was one of the first to point out that a good result can be obtained even with significant degrees of rectal inflammation. The surgeon may "stage" the operation by initial abdominal colectomy and ileostomy with preservation of the rectal stump before anastomosis is done. Disease in the retained stump may then be treated locally by the use of steroid suppositories. A decreased rate of anastomotic problems as compared with problems due to primary anastomosis and temporary ileostomy was observed in our patients. The one-stage procedure is reserved for patients whose disease is quiescent, whose nutritional state is satisfactory, and in whom the rectal mucosa is minimally inflamed.

As mentioned earlier, the frequency with which this operation is used in the surgical treatment of ulcerative colitis varies. Alexander-Williams and Buchmann[52] reported that 7% of 480 patients operated on for ulcerative colitis had a primary or secondary ileorectal anastomosis. Hawley[53] reported a 33% rate of ileorectal anastomosis in their ulcerative colitis patients. At the Cleveland Clinic, 24% of such patients have been considered suitable for ileorectal anastomosis.

Of major concern in those treated by this method are: (1) rectal function and disability due to diarrhea, urgency, and incontinence and (2) cancer risk in the retained rectum. Patient satisfaction with the operation is surprisingly greater than would be expected based on interviews with patients and learning of the frequency of bowel actions. Thus, Watts and Hughes,[48] in a review of 81 patients having ileorectal anastomosis for inflammatory bowel disease, found that satisfactory results were achieved in 61% and 51%, respectively, as assessed by the patient and the interviewer. A salutary result, but with some reservations, was achieved in 23% and 28% of patients, respectively. Binder and co-workers[54] reported that of 27 patients with ulcerative colitis so treated, 16 had an excellent result and 6 had a good result. At the Cleveland Clinic, 12 of 89 patients with ileorectal anastomosis for ulcerative colitis had subsequent proctectomy because of poor rectal function. In Alexander-Williams' group,[52] 8 of 34 patients underwent subsequent proctectomy.

The cancer risk in the rectal segment after ileorectal anastomosis is less than that when the colon is in place. Nevertheless, the risk mandates close surveillance of the rectal segment for the patient's lifetime, including annual or biannual endoscopy and biopsy for dysplasia. This, in turn, requires careful selection and total compliance by the patient. Aylett[55] found that 7 of 350 patients with ileorectal anastomosis developed rectal cancer. Baker et al.[56] found 22 cancers in 374 patients. Grundfest et al.[51] described the experience at the Cleveland Clinic, where 4 of 89 patients developed rectal cancer. Since 2 of these 4 patients had colon cancer and the other 2 had dysplasia at the time of colectomy and ileorectal anastomosis, we regard these as contraindications to rectal-sparing operations unless the operations are for palliation (e.g., the presence of liver metastasis).

Proctocolectomy with Ileoanal Anastomosis. In this operation, the entire colon and the upper two-thirds of the rectum are removed. The mucosa is stripped from the lower rectal segment and the ileum is pulled through this rectal shell and anastomosed to the dentate line of the anal canal. The operation, therefore, removes the epithelium at risk for developing both cancer and flares of inflammation, both of which may occur with ileorectal anastomosis. Furthermore, in contrast to operations that preserve the rectum, this procedure appreciably diminishes, if it does not entirely negate, the persistence of certain extraintestinal manifestations of colitis. Another obvious advantage over traditional proctocolectomy is that permanent ileostomy is obviated. Ravitch and Sabiston[22] described this operation in 1947, but it failed to gain support because of associated disabling incontinence. Interest was rekindled in later years in light of the favorable report by Martin et al.[57] of good function in 15 of 17 patients under the age of 21 years. They caution against the operation in the presence of severe rectal inflammation, advising preoperative parenteral nutrition, systemic and local steroids, and occasionally initial fecal diversion to render the rectal inflammation quiescent. While continence was ultimately obtained in Martin's patients, it could take several months to achieve and operative complications were considerable. Nevertheless, others were stimulated to consider this form of sphincter preservation. Telander and Perrault[58] reported the findings at the Mayo Clinic with this procedure in 25 patients; all patients had a covering temporary ileostomy. Results were excellent in 11 patients, good in 7, fair in 3, and poor in 3; one patient had not undergone closure of the loop ileostomy. Although some soiling and leakage occurred, especially during the night, these complications decreased with time. Peck[59] reported good to excellent continence in 87% of 56 patients; 36 of these had ulcerative colitis. Beart,[60] however, strongly favors the addition of a reservoir (see following section).

The complications of ileoanal anastomosis are still considerable at this phase in its development. Pelvic sepsis, hemorrhage, fistulas, and questionable sphincter function will likely deter most surgeons from choosing this procedure over conventional proctocolectomy until reproducible good results are obtained.

Proctocolectomy and Ileoanal Pull-Through with Ileal Reservoir (Fig. 126–47). Parks and Nicholls[61] felt that an ileal reservoir, if sutured to the anal canal, would provide an improved functional result compared with proctocolectomy with ileoanal anastomosis. They presented data on 21 patients in whom mucosal proctectomy was done transanally.[23] The mean frequency of evacuation for a 24-hour period was 3.8. Ten patients evacuated spontaneously, but 10 required pouch intubation per rectum. All patients had daytime continence, but 10 had discharge of mucus during sleep (one had discharge of stool as well).

A number of technical points have emerged as a result of this and other experience with the procedure. The exit conduit from the reservoir that is pulled through the rectal cuff and anastomosed to the anal canal must be minimal in length inasmuch as kinking of this conduit can produce difficulty in evacuation. Only a minimal rectal cuff is now used; this, in turn, reduces the extent of a tedious and bloody separation of rectal mucosa from the underlying muscle and lessens the risk of leaving islands of rectal epithelium behind. While the 3-loop pouch, arranged in an "S" fashion, has its protagonists, the simpler "U" loop has decided advantages. Difficulties with advancement of the ileum sufficient to reach the anal canal have been encountered on occasion. Careful release of the distal superior mesenteric artery, relying on the vascular arcades of its proximal branches, enables sufficient bowel length to be obtained.

A number of sophisticated procedures are emerging that may find a greater or lesser place in the surgical treatment of ulcerative colitis. It is likely that this quest for continence will take several years before a definitive position can be adopted, especially concerning the pull-through procedures. The performance of these techniques is best reserved for those who are not only experienced in

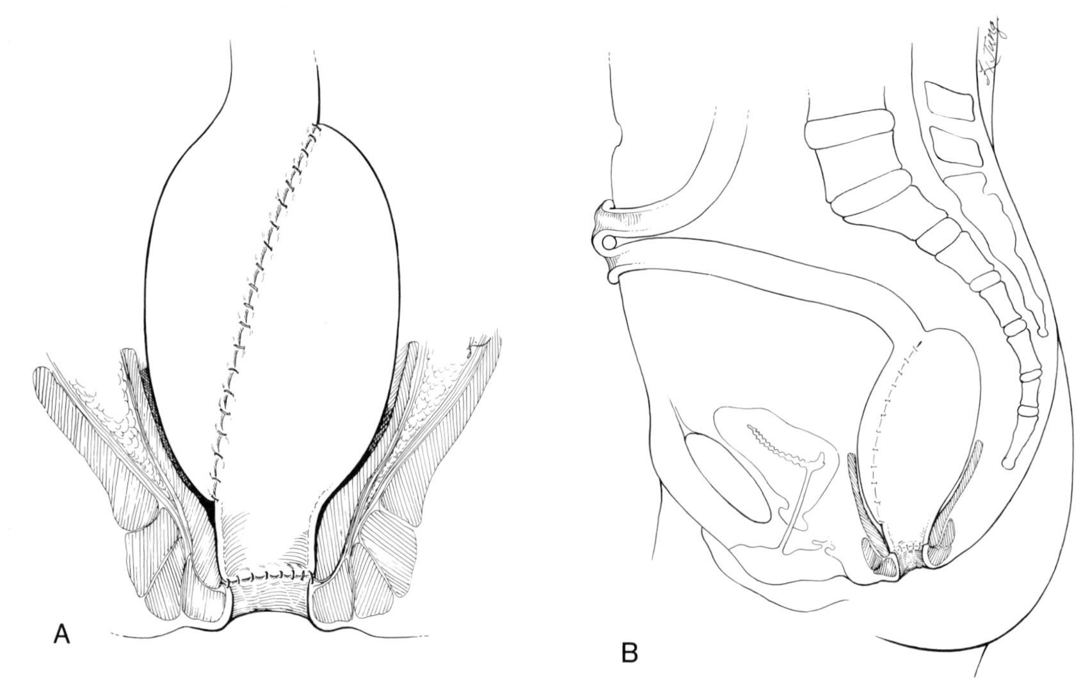

Figure 126–47. *A,* Ileoanal anastomosis with pelvic reservoir. After the muscoa is removed from the distal anorectal segment, an "S"-shaped ileal reservoir is constructed and is brought through the rectal muscular cuff. The end of the ileal exit conduit is sewn to the dentate line. *B,* The lateral view shows a proximal loop ileostomy performed to minimize the effects of distal anastomotic leakage. The ileostomy is closed after 3 months.

the surgical treatment of ulcerative colitis, but are also able to evaluate results in a critical manner.

Postoperative Care

The same general guidelines are followed as with any major intestinal operation. Intravenous fluids and electrolytes are given until intestinal function returns, with intake and output monitored on a flow sheet. Nasogastric suction is maintained until peristalsis is evident. Ileostomy function appears 2 to 4 days postoperatively; however, caution is required in assessing this return of function. A thin, bluish effluent, especially if mixed with whitish particulate matter (mucus), indicates ileus or high intestinal obstruction, and nasogastric suction should be maintained. This effluent of succus entericus can similarly occur early after ileorectal anastomosis. After the ileostomy begins normal function, there may be a period of 2 to 3 weeks when it is particularly active, with outputs of 1200 to 2000 ml/day (normal effluent volume is about 750 ml/day). During this time an antidiarrheal medication, such as diphenoxylate (Lomotil) or loperamide (Imodium), is useful.

Postoperative antibiotics are continued for 24 hours unless operative contamination has occurred. In this case, antibiotics are continued for 5 to 7 days. Heparin, 5000 units every 12 hours, is given by subcutaneous injection until the patient is discharged. There is a period early in the postoperative course after ileorectal anastomosis when diarrhea occurs. It is unwise to provide medication for this, however, until diarrhea has been present for 2 or 3 days for fear of a rebound effect that could induce ileus.

The urinary catheter is left indwelling for 7 days if rectal resection has been part of the operative procedure; premature removal may be associated with urinary retention. Cultures are taken at the time of removal of the catheter. Patients are continued on steroids on a reducing schedule, depending upon the dosages used before surgery. A typical program is hydrocortisone acetate, 100 mg IV every 12 hours for 2 days, tapered to 50 mg every 12 hours for 2 days, and then prednisone, 20 mg by mouth daily until discharge from the hospital. At that time a further tapering program is planned, dependent upon the individual case.

Continent ileostomy patients require special attention. A tube is left indwelling in the pouch, and its patency must be assured by checking every 2 hours for the first 48 hours after surgery by means of irrigation of small volumes of saline. The stabilizing sutures around the tube are cut on the third day, and a face plate is used to fix the tube into position. This provides greater comfort. Prior to discharge, the patient is shown how to intubate the pouch (in the event that the tube becomes dislodged inadvertently before the patient's scheduled follow-up appointment). A leg bag is fitted so that continuous drainage can be obtained in the ambulant patient. Upon return after 1 month, the patient is carefully instructed in a program of catheterization, e.g., every 3 hours for 3 weeks, then every 4 hours for 4 weeks, before *ad lib* catheterization is permitted.

Most patients will have a conventional end or loop ileostomy. From the practical standpoint, these function in much the same way. Postoperatively, a karaya washer is applied to the stoma and a clear plastic pouch, open-ended, is then applied (Chapter 130). Tincture of benzoin is not used owing to the frequency of skin irritation it induces; Skin-Prep is an excellent substitute. From the second or third day, a skin barrier is used (Stomahesive)* to which one of several appliances can be applied. The Hollister pouch is simple to use, although others, such as Surefit,* are also excellent. The patient begins learning about care of the stoma on the sixth or seventh postoperative day and is then permitted to go home about 3 to 4 days later after demonstrating expertise in stomal care. Appropriate literature, introduction to the local ostomy association, and, most importantly, the phone number of a stomatherapist is given to the patient before going home. Nothing is quite so distressing to a patient as having the appliance leak after discharge from the hospital and then attempting to solve the problem on his own. Instructions are kept simple. Permanent equipment is ordered and is ready for the patient at the time of the postoperative check-up (Chapter 130).

*Squibb Pharmaceuticals.

Complications

The mortality rate following elective surgery is about 2%. In special centers, rates ranging from 7% to 15% have been reported in urgent cases,[36, 37] with low rates or even no mortality being reported from certain centers in more recent years.[62, 63] In 108 patients of my own who underwent proctocolectomy for ulcerative colitis, there were no operative deaths. An additional 28 patients with toxic megacolon associated with both ulcerative colitis and Crohn's disease, who were mainly treated by "blow-hole" colostomy and ileostomy, also had no associated mortality (unpublished data).

Small Bowel Obstruction. This occurs commonly, but requires laparotomy in only 6% to 8% of patients.[34] In my own experience, ileus or obstruction was encountered in 20% of 108 patients, but only 2% required laparotomy. Adhesions, especially to the stump of a vascular pedicle, and internal volvulus constitute the major causes of obstruction. Food bolus obstruction is due to the intake of poorly digested foods, such as peanuts, popcorn, and fruit peel. It is highly likely that a predisposing condition, such as adhesions, also exists. Treatment is non-operative. After sedation of the patient, ileostomy irrigation with tap water usually breaks up the clogged material and allows it to pass. Recurrence is frequent and, on rare occasions, laparotomy is required to treat a predisposing cause.

Perineal Wound. Non-healing or delayed healing of the perineal wound is encountered more frequently after proctocolectomy for Crohn's disease than for ulcerative colitis. A common definition used is that of persistence of a sinus for longer than 6 months following surgery. Women are affected twice as often as men. There is a greater prevalence when the perineal wound is left open to drain (with suture closure of the pelvic peritoneum) than when primary closure of the perineal wound is performed. An association with steroid usage, anemia, poor nutritional state, and severity of colitis has been suggested but not proved. If the wound is managed by open drainage, about 50% of the patients will have an unhealed wound at 6 months and about 25% at 1 year.[64] Approximately 10% of all patients will require hospital admission for curettage or treatment of a persistent perineal sinus.[34] In practice, the perineal sinuses occurring after proctectomy for ulcerative colitis are rarely troublesome, as opposed to sinuses following surgery for Crohn's disease, for which sophisticated operations, such as skin grafting or placement of vascularized muscle flaps, are frequently needed. Usually, curettage or cautery with silver nitrate is sufficient for simple sinuses.

Sexual Dysfunction. Impotence, a common complication of rectal resection for cancer, is generally attributed to denervation of the sexual apparatus in an attempt to obtain wide cancer clearance. The older age of the patients who undergo this type of surgery is another factor. When proctectomy is done for inflammatory bowel disease, a disease mostly of younger patients, the surgeon attempts a more conservative type of rectal resection, hoping to avoid nerve interruption. What is also apparent is that degrees of sexual dysfunction may occur, varying from inability to sustain an erection or inability to ejaculate (or retrograde ejaculation) to impotence. Watts et al.[65] reported a 17% frequency rate of impotence in 41 patients. Burnham et al.[66] found that 5% of 128 male ileostomates were impotent, with partial impotency present in 10%. In both series, the authors noted that the risk was significantly higher in the older patients. As Goligher[28] commented, "What makes these reports on disturbances of sexual function so disappointing is that the dysfunction has arisen often despite particular efforts on the part of the surgeon to keep very close to the rectum during his pelvic and perineal dissection."

Early in the course of mobilization of the rectosigmoid, gentle anterior traction is used as the hypogastric nerves and their decussation are drawn into the operative field. Interruption here may produce subsequent retrograde ejaculation, although with sympathetic nerve injury only, erection and orgasm are still possible. The second site of vulnerability is in the area of the anterolateral rectal stalks, which must be divided close to the rectal wall, as opposed to the technique used in a cancer operation. The third area at risk is the presacral space, where breaching of Waldeyer's fascia in its superior extent exposes the fine filaments of the nerve erigentes and renders them susceptible to injury. The dissection at the promontory of the sacrum occurs in the plane between the investing layers of fascia of the rectum anteriorly and Waldeyer's fascia. Breaching that fascia, especially by the surgeon's hand, will damage these nerves. Instrument retraction allows for anterior displacement of the rectum as the surgeon gradually separates the 2 fascial layers down to the insertion of Waldeyer's fascia into the supralevator fascia. The final vulnerable area is that located anterior to the rectum, just below the peritoneal reflection. The latter is incised transversely, the dissection being carried out on the muscular layer of the rectal wall behind the fascia of Denonvilliers. The seminal vesicles are then not exposed. As the branches of the nervi erigentes intimately embrace the vesicles, injury may be avoided. Since surgeons are generally cautious with posterior and lateral dissection, it is probable that anterior dissection is more hazardous than previously thought in terms of potential nerve injury.

Proctectomy is completed by the perineal route, where dissection between the internal and external anal sphincters is carried out.[67] Essentially, only the rectum is cored out, leaving the levator muscles uninjured. In a prospective study,[41] no instance of impotence occurred when this technique was utilized.

Ileostomy Complications (Table 126–14). Ileostomy diarrhea was discussed earlier. For the person with an established ileostomy, a state of mild chronic dehydration and sodium depletion exists. Clarke et al.[68] compared ileostomy patients with a control group and found an 11% reduction in total body water and a 7% deficit in exchangeable sodium in the former; urinary excretion of water and sodium was also reduced. Patients are rarely symptomatic as a consequence of these alterations, with the exception of an increased propensity to form renal stones. In the report of Roy et al.,[69] 37 of 463 ileostomates (8%) developed urinary calculi, usually within 1

Table 126–14. COMPLICATIONS OF ILEOSTOMY*

Early	Late
Ileostomy dysfunction	Obstruction
Necrosis/gangrene	Recession
Mucosal slough	Abscess
Mucocutaneous separation	Stricture/fistula
Parastomal abscess	Hernia
Fistula	Prolapse
Bleeding	Volvulus
	Trauma
	Caput medusa
	Bleeding
	Leakage

*Excluding continent ileostomy.

to 3 years after stomal surgery. There is also an increased sensitivity to stimuli that evoke dehydration, e.g., hot weather and viral infection of the gastrointestinal tract. An increased frequency of gallstones has been observed in patients who have undergone an ileostomy. Unless there has been an extensive resection of the ileum at the time of ileostomy construction, vitamin supplements are usually not required. Vitamin B_{12} and folic acid may be needed if there is residual ileitis or if a considerable segment of ileum has been removed.

Ileostomy Dysfunction. This term is used in its broadest sense to indicate a functional abnormality of the ileostomy with respect to excessive (or sometimes abnormally low) amounts of fluid effluent. The term, first coined by Warren and McKittrick,[70] was originally used specifically to describe a profuse, watery diarrhea usually occurring within 7 days of ileostomy construction. Associated abdominal pain, distention, vomiting, and dehydration produced a picture of bowel obstruction (sometimes called "pseudo-obstruction," as there was no constipation). Turnbull and Crile[8] demonstrated the cause to be obstruction of the ileostomy at the surface level secondary to serositis of the non-everted stoma. Primary maturation of the stoma effectively eliminates this complication.

Gangrene. This is immediately recognizable and calls for urgent refashioning of the stoma. Rarely, this may be accomplished through the abdominal wall aperture, but usually the main incision will need to be opened.

Mucosal Slough. This represents a degree of ischemia short of necrosis. It varies from a small margin 1 cm or so in diameter, which is usually on the mesenteric side of the stoma or circumferential at the base of the stoma, to a major loss of mucosa. Ordinarily, no treatment is required. If a full-thickness bowel wall loss of the everted bowel edge occurs, serositis of the exposed ileum can develop. This can lead to pseudo-obstruction (the major complication of ileostomies prior to the descriptions by Brooke[10] and Turnbull[71] of primary mucocutaneous suture) and later even to ileostomy stricture.

Parastomal Abscess. It is surprising how uncommon this complication is. In the early period, one may suspect a fistula or an infected hematoma as the source. In constructing the stoma, it is important to obtain excellent hemostasis. Fat may be incised with the electrocautery, as are the anterior and posterior rectus abdominis sheaths. The muscle itself is separated but not cut. Irrigation of the subcutaneous space around the stoma will minimize the effect of any bacterial contamination. If an abscess is observed or suspected, sutures are removed from the appropriate side of the stoma and drainage is allowed. If a large abscess develops, this preferentially should be drained by making a small incision peripheral to the abscess, beyond the margin of skin encompassed by the pouching equipment, and placing a latex rubber drain into the cavity. A fistula may subsequently become manifest, which is dealt with individually.

Fistula. In the early postoperative period, a fistula usually arises from operative trauma. This is caused by failure to recognize an enterotomy (too assiduous a dissection of the mesentery from the mesenteric margin of the bowel or too deep a myotomy when 2-directional myotomy is used)[67] or by placement of "stabilizing" sutures between the anterior rectus sheath or muscle and the seromuscular layer of the bowel.

If the fistula is above the skin level to the point that pouching is still possible, no treatment is indicated. This is not generally the case, however, and revisionary surgery is required. Attempts at local repair of the fistula are usually futile, and a further segment of ileum will need to be brought out of the abdomen. This is best done either within 7 days of the initial operation or after 6 weeks have elapsed. The inflammatory reaction developing around the stomal aperture in the interim makes for a very difficult dissection.

Recession. For good or adequate ileostomy function, a "spout" of ileum needs to be present. What constitutes a well-functioning ileostomy? Aside from the critical aspect of the psychologic rehabilitation of the patient, a suitable ileostomy is one that is easily visible and accessible to the patient, one that is free from leakage problems, and one that requires a minimum of maintenance (i.e., pouch changing no more frequently than every 4 days). For hygienic reasons, we advocate pouch changing at least every 7 days, even if no leakage has occurred by then. An occasional patient with a flush stoma is able to get by without leakage for 5 to 7 days. Therefore, ileostomy recession of itself is not always a problem. Moreover, many patients who do have leakage problems because of a flush ileostomy can have resolution of this problem by appropriate stomal therapy techniques (Chapter 130). When these techniques are unavailable or ineffective, stomal revision involving the bringing out of a longer segment of ileum is required. The frequency with which revision is required was reported in 1977 as 12% by Goldblatt et al.[72] but is rarely encountered today in surgery for ulcerative colitis.

Stricture. This may occur as a late complication of ischemia of a degree short of that needed to produce stomal necrosis. Hence, stricture may follow mucosal slough (discussed earlier) as healing occurs by fibrosis. Less commonly, sepsis produced by parastomal abscess or non-absorbable suture material may cause this problem.

Parastomal Hernia. This is a common complication with colostomy but is relatively uncommon with ileostomy. Factors favoring its development include obesity, a large abdominal wall aperture in the construction of the ileostomy, placement of the stoma site outside the rectus abdominis muscle, and multiple previous incisions in the area around the stoma. When asymptomatic, no further surgery is needed for the hernia. However, the patient may complain of pain, discomfort, or difficulty in maintaining a seal around the appliance. In these situations, operative correction must be considered. Surgery involves takedown of the ileostomy and relocation to the other side of the abdomen, with repair of the hernial defect.

Prolapse. This occurs in situations similar to those favoring parastomal hernia, i.e., placement of the stoma outside the rectus sheath and construction of too large an aperture in the abdominal wall. Non-fixation of the mesentery has also been cited as a cause. Relocation of the ileostomy is required if the defect is troublesome.

Volvulus. This is preventable by obliterating the mesenteric defect through which loops of ileum may pass.

Leakage. Recession, prolapse, and hernia can predispose to early separation of the appliance from the parastomal skin. A variety of other conditions (Table 126–15) can also predispose to leakage or parastomal skin irritation. In most cases, the problem can be alleviated by taking a careful history from the patient, inspecting the stoma and equipment, and observing how the patient applies this equipment. An enterostomal therapist is an invaluable resource in managing such problems (Chapter 130).

Table 126–15. CAUSES OF LEAKAGE FROM AN ILEOSTOMY

Ileostomy recession
Poor siting of stoma
Diarrhea
Mucosal implants
Folliculitis
Allergy to tape, barriers, pouch material
Poor pouching technique
Poor equipment
Pseudo-epitheliomatous hyperplasia
Pyoderma
Psoriasis
Candidiasis
Recurrent ileitis
Trauma

References

1. Keetley CB. Quoted by Corbett, RS, 1945. (See Ref. 28.)
2. Lockhart-Mummery JP. Diseases of the Rectum and Colon. 2nd Ed. London: Bailliere, Tindall and Cox, 1934.
3. Gabriel WB. Discussion on the surgical treatment of idiopathic ulcerative colitis and its sequelae. Proc Br Soc Med 1940; 33:643.
4. Brown JY. Value of complete physiological rest of large bowel in ulcerative and obstructive lesions. Surg Gynecol Obstet 1913; 16:610.
5. McKittrick LS, Miller RH. Idiopathic ulcerative colitis: review of 149 cases with particular reference to the value of and indications for surgical treatment. Ann Surg 1935; 102:656.
6. Crile GW Jr, Turnbull RB Jr. Mechanism and prevention of ileostomy dysfunction. Ann Surg 1954; 4:459.
7. Brooke BN, Cooke WT. Ulcerative colitis. Lancet 1951; 2:463.
8. Turnbull RB Jr, Crile GW Jr. Changing trends in surgery of the colon. Am J Proctol 1952; 4:271.
9. Dragstedt LR, Dack GM, Kirsner JB. Chronic ulcerative colitis. A summary of evidence implicating bacterium necrophorum as an etiologic agent. Ann Surg 1941; 114:653.
10. Brooke BN. The management of ileostomy including its complications. Lancet 1952; 2:102.
11. Cattell RB. The surgical treatment of ulcerative colitis. Gastroenterology 1948; 10:63.
12. Ferguson LK, Stevens LW. The surgery and complications of ulcerative colitis. Gastroenterology 1948; 11:40.
13. Miller CG, Gardner CMcG, Ripstein CB. Primary resection of the colon in ulcerative colitis. J Can Med Assoc 1949; 60:584.
14. Crile GW Jr, Thomas CY Jr. The treatment of acute toxic ulcerative colitis by ileostomy and simultaneous colectomy. Gastroenterology 1951; 195:580.
15. Ravitch MM, Handelsman JC. One-stage resection of entire colon for ulcerative colitis and polypoid adenomatosis. Bull John Hopkins Hosp 1951; 88:59.
16. Kock NG. Intra-abdominal "reservoir" in patients with permanent ileostomy. Preliminary observations on a procedure resulting in fecal "continence" in five ileostomy patients. Arch Surg 1969; 99:223.
17. Lilienthal H. Extirpation of the entire colon, the upper portion of the sigmoid flexure and four inches of the ileum for hyperplastic colitis. Ann Surg 1903; 37:616.
18. Devine H. Method of colectomy for desperate cases of ulcerative colitis. Surg Gynecol Obstet 1943; 76:136.

19. Aylett SO. Ulcerative colitis: ileorectal anastomosis 1952–1968. Proc Roy Soc Med 1971; 64:967.
20. Turnbull RB Jr, Hawk WA, Weakley FL. Surgical treatment of toxic megacolon: ileostomy and colostomy to prepare patients for colectomy. Am J Surg 1971; 122:325.
21. Kock NG. Continent ileostomy. Prog Surg 1973; 12:180.
22. Ravitch MM, Sabiston DC. Anal ileostomy with preservation of the sphincter. Surg Gynecol Obstet 1948; 84:1097.
23. Parks AG, Nicholls RJ, Bellieveau P. Proctocolectomy with ileal reservoir and anal anastomosis. Br J Surg 1980; 67:533.
24. Bacon JE, Trimpi HD. The selection of an operative procedure for patients with medically intractable ulcerative colitis. Surg Gynecol Obstet 1950; 91:409.
25. Wheelock FC Jr, Warren R. Ulcerative colitis: follow-up studies. N Engl J Med 1955; 252:421.
26. VanProhaska J, Siderius N. The surgical rehabilitation of patients with chronic ulcerative colitis. Am J Surg 1962; 103:42.
27. Waugh JM, Peck D, Beahrs OH, Sauer WG. Surgical management of chronic ulcerative colitis. Arch Surg 1964; 88:556.
28. Goligher JC. Diseases of the Anus, Rectum and Colon. 4th Ed. London: Bailliere-Tindall, 1980: 689–826.
29. Lennard-Jones JE. Total left-sided distal colitis. Presented at VII World Congress of Gastroenterology, Stockholm, Sweden, June 17, 1982.
30. Fazio VW, Kodner I, Jagelman DG, Turnbull RB Jr, Weakley FL. Inflammatory bowel disease. Parenteral nutrition as primary or adjunctive treatment. Dis Colon Rectum 1976; 7:574.
31. Harford FJ Jr, Fazio VW. Total parenteral nutrition as primary therapy for inflammatory disease of the bowel. Dis Colon Rectum 1978; 8:555.
32. Zelas P, Jagelman DG. Loop ileostomy in the management of Crohn's colitis in the debilitated patient. Ann Surg 1980; 191:164.
33. Truelove SC, Willoughby CP, Lee ECG, Kettlewell MGW. Further experience in the treatment of severe attacks of ulcerative colitis. Lancet 1978; 2:1086.
34. Hawley PR, Ritchie JK. Complications of ileostomy and colostomy following excisional surgery. Clin Gastroenterol 1979; 2:403.
35. Ritchie JK. Results of surgery for inflammatory bowel disease: A further survey of one hospital region. Br Med J 1974; 1:264.
36. Goligher JC, Hoffman DC, deDombal FT. Surgical treatment of severe attacks of ulcerative colitis with special reference to the advantages of early operation. Br Med J 1970; 4:703.
37. Ritchie JK. Ulcerative colitis treated by ileostomy and excisional surgery. Fifteen years experience at St. Mark's Hospital. Br J Surg 1972; 59:345.
38. Walker TC. The Surgical Management of Ulcerative Colitis. New York: Appleton-Century-Crofts, 1969.
39. Fry PD, Atkinson KG. Current surgical approach to toxic megacolon. Surg Gynecol Obstet 1976; 143:26.
40. Klein SH, Edelman S, Kirschner PA, et al. Emergency cecostomy in ulcerative colitis with acute toxic dilatation. Surgery 1960; 47:399.
41. Fazio VW, Fletcher J, Montague D. Prospective study of the effect of resection of the rectum and male sexual function. World J Surg 1980; 4:149.
42. Goldman SL, Rombeau JL. The continent ileostomy: A collective review. Dis Colon Rectum 1978; 21:594.
43. Beart RW, Kelley K, Beahrs OH. Quoted in chapter on ulcerative colitis. *In:* Goligher JC. Surgery of the Anus, Rectum and Colon. 4th Ed. London: Bailliere-Tindall, 1980: 689–826.
44. Gelernt IM, Bauer JJ, Kreel I. The reservoir ileostomy: Early experience with 54 patients. Ann Surg 1977; 185:179.
45. Gelernt IM. Experience and late results with the continent ileostomy. *In:* Korelitz BI, ed. Inflammatory Bowel Disease—Experience and Controversy. Boston: Wright–JPSG, 1982: 207–19.
46. Jagenburg R, Dotewall G, Kewenter J, et al. Absorption studies in patients with "intra-abdominal ileostomy reservoirs" and in patients with conventional ileostomies. Gut 1971; 12:437.
47. Lee ECG, Truelove SC. Proctocolectomy for ulcerative colitis. World J Surg 1980; 4:195.
48. Watts JMcK, Hughes ESR. Ulcerative colitis and Crohn's disease: Results after colectomy and ileorectal anastomosis. Br J Surg 1977; 64:71.
49. Gallone L, Olani L. Rectal preservation in the surgical treatment of ulcerative proctocolitis. Chir Gastroenterol 1978; 12:149.
50. Korelitz BI, Dyck WP, Klion FM. Fate of the rectum and distal colon after subtotal colectomy for ulcerative colitis. Gut 1969; 10:198.
51. Grundfest SR, Fazio VW, Weiss RA, et al. The risk of cancer following colectomy and ileorectal anastomosis for extensive mucosal ulcerative colitis. Ann Surg 1981; 1:9.
52. Alexander-Williams J, Buchmann P. Criteria of assessment for suitability and results of ileorectal anastomosis. Clin Gastroenterol 1980; 2:409.
53. Jones PF, Bevan PG, Hawley PR. Ileostomy or ileorectal anastomosis for ulcerative colitis? Br Med J 1978; 1:1459.
54. Binder SE, Mullen HH, Deterling RA. Emergency and urgent operations for ulcerative colitis. Arch Surg 1975; 110:284.
55. Aylett AO. Cancer and ulcerative colitis. Br Med J 1971; 1:203.
56. Baker WN, Glass RE, Ritchie JE, et al. Cancer of the rectum following colectomy and ileorectal anastomosis for ulcerative colitis. Br J Surg 1978; 65:862.
57. Martin LW, LeCoultre C, Schulbert WK. Total colectomy and mucosal proctectomy with preservation of continence in ulcerative colitis. Ann Surg 1977; 186:477.
58. Telander RL, Perrault J. Total colectomy with rectal mucosectomy and ileoanal anastomosis for chronic ulcerative colitis in children and young adults. Arch Surg 1981; 116:623.
59. Peck DA. Rectal mucosal replacement—an update. Presented at the American Society of Colon and Rectal Surgeons 81st Annual Meeting and Exhibition, May 3, 1982, San Francisco, California.
60. Beart RW. Ileoanal anastomosis for ulcerative colitis. Presented at the American College of Surgeons 68th Annual Clinical Congress, October 29, 1982, Chicago, Illinois.
61. Parks AG, Nicholls RJ. Proctocolectomy without ileostomy for ulcerative colitis. Br Med J 1978; 2:85.
62. Flatmark A, Frethein B, Gjone E. Early colectomy in severe ulcerative colitis. Scand J Gastroenterology 1975; 10:427.
63. Truelove SC, Willoughby CP, Lee ECG, Kettlewell MGW. Further experience in the treatment of severe attacks of ulcerative colitis. Lancet 1978; 2:1086.
64. Jalan KN, Smith A, Ruckley CV, et al. Perineal wound healing in ulcerative colitis. Br J Surg 1969; 56:749.
65. Watts JMcK, deDombal FT, Goligher JC. Long-term complication and prognosis following major surgery for ulcerative colitis. Br J Surg 1966; 53:104.
66. Burnham WR, Lennard-Jones JE, Brooke BN. Sexual problems amongst married ileostomists. Gut 1977; 18:673.
67. Turnbull RB Jr, Fazio VW: Advances in the surgical technique of ulcerative colitis surgery—endoanal proctectomy and two-directional myotomy ileostomy. *In:* Nyhus L, ed. Surgery Annual. New York: Appleton-Century-Crofts, 1975: 315–29.
68. Clarke AM, Chirnside A, Hill GL, Pope G, Stewart MK. Chronic dehydration and sodium depletion in patients with established ileostomies. Lancet 1967; 2:740.
69. Roy PR, Sauer WG, Beahrs OH, Farrow GM. Experience with ileostomies. Evaluation of long-term rehabilitation in 497 patients. Am J Surg 1970; 119:77.
70. Warren R, McKittrick LS. Ileostomy for ulcerative colitis; technique, complications and management. Surg Gynecol Obstet 1951; 95:555.
71. Turnbull RB Jr. Management of the ileostomy. Am J Surg 1953; 5:617.
72. Goldblatt MS, Corman ML, Haggitt RC, Coller JA, Veidenheimer MC. Ileostomy complications requiring revision—The Lahey Clinic experience 1964–1973. Dis Colon Rectum 1977; 3:209.

Prognosis

Richard G. Farmer

Long-Term Prognosis

The long-term prognosis for patients who have ulcerative colitis has been the subject of a number of studies over the years[1–6] and is dependent on 4 factors described previously: location (extent) of disease, activity (severity), duration, and impact on the patient.

1. *Location of disease.* Ulcerative colitis affects only the colon and does not extend proximally, except for an occasional instance of "backwash ileitis." On the other hand, ulcerative colitis may involve only certain segments or the entire colon.

2. *Activity of disease.* Activity may vary from (1) acute and severe or even fulminating to (2) chronic and recurrent to (3) chronic continuous; even inactive disease may have implications for the potential development of colonic carcinoma.

3. *Duration of disease.* This relates to the length of time the various patterns of disease have been present and their nutritional and other systemic effects on the patient. Furthermore, the duration of disease may influence the effectiveness of therapy, side effects of therapy, and therapeutic response. In addition, duration of disease may be an important factor in determining the need for operation. Finally, duration of disease is an important factor in concern over development of dysplasia and/or colonic carcinoma.

4. *The overall impact of the disease on the patient.* This includes the ability of the patient to function normally in social, economic, and cultural situations. Included here are the "psychologic" factors that are sometimes considered important for patients with ulcerative colitis. Additional factors that can be considered under this heading include the family history, the effect on the patient and family, the general ability of the patient to adapt to the disease, and the overall quality of life experienced by the patient.

Ritchie and co-workers[7] described 4 questions that patients may ask regarding the prognosis in ulcerative colitis:

"Is my condition dangerous?"
"Will the inflammation spread?"
"Will I need an operation?"
"Will I develop cancer?"

Variations on these 4 questions have been reviewed from a number of centers and economic factors have been included, as well as problems associated with medications, surgery, and nutrition.[8] A Scandinavian study[9] indicated a mortality rate of 1.3% among 322 patients with ulcerative colitis followed for 1 year and noted that in the short term, the mortality rate was related to the severity of the illness and the need for operation. In another study of mortality,[10] the risk was 1.7 times that of the general population, particularly during the first year after diagnosis and the first year after surgery.

In the long term, several additional factors all become extremely important and need to be considered. These include (1) the age of onset, and thus the duration of disease; (2) the need for follow-up, (3) the importance of appropriate and cost-effective surveillance, and (4) the need for attention to psychologic and nutritional factors.

The long-term prognosis is good for 90% or more of patients with proctitis or protosigmoiditis.[7, 11–16] These patients exhibit no progression, do not need continuous therapy, and have few, if any, symptoms. In the other 10%, the inflammation extends[12, 14, 16, 17] and may involve the entire colon, and the prognosis becomes similar to that of patients with total colon disease. With regard to morbidity, for patients with proctitis or proctosigmoiditis, the disease generally resolves completely for about 75% of patients, with approximately 15% having multiple recurrences but without progression.[11] It should be noted, however, that when no proximal limit to the extent of disease can be determined by proctosigmoidoscopy, there is always a concern that inflammatory mucosal changes exist proximal to the rectal and distal sigmoid that may be too subtle to be discernible by roentgenographic study of the colon. Also worthy of comment is the assumption, often made, that mucosal inflammatory disease of the distal colon (rectum, sigmoid, and descending colon) is a variant or a lesser form of ulcerative colitis involving the entire colon. This rough equivalency, in kind if not degree, suggests common characteristics. Yet, as has been repeatedly pointed out, even though there is a common histologic substratum, distal mucosal ulcerative colitis has a far better long-term prognosis than total colon disease.

The major difficulties with the delineation of prognosis have been the need for long periods of follow-up and the imprecise demarcation of the proximal limit of disease of the colon. While our own observations of ulcerative proctosigmoiditis[11] reaffirmed that prognosis was good for the vast majority of these patients, colonoscopy was not basic to the methodology of our study. By way of comparison, Das et al.[18] studied a group of 31 patients with proctitis who underwent colonoscopy during symptomatic periods and noted that there were often microscopic abnormalities in locations more proximal to the distal 18 to 20 cm of colon that were visibly abnormal. The significance of this finding is uncertain, but it certainly emphasizes the value of colonoscopy in the evaluation of this form of ulcerative colitis and deserves further investigation.

Previous clinical experience indicates that there is little likelihood of extension of disease after a given period of time—approximately 5 years after onset of disease. If it can be shown that patients with mucosal inflammatory bowel disease can be separated on the basis of extent of disease into distinct groups having meaningful clinical differences, endoscopy and mucosal biopsy may be helpful in predicting prognosis by virtue of establishing the proximal limit of involvement.

In a study comparing the course of patients with proctosigmoiditis to those with proctitis,[13] we found that the prognosis for patients with proctitis was slightly better. The observations indicated also that even though the prognosis may be good for most patients, determination of prognosis in an individual case may be relatively difficult.

The long-term prognosis for patients with childhood onset of ulcerative colitis includes factors that are related to the age of onset and vulnerability to factors adversely affecting growth and development.[19] Michener et al.[20] reported on 316 patients with childhood-onset ulcerative colitis for whom there was a follow-up of greater than 10 years. Colectomy was required in 37%; 12% had only the single episode; 20% had an intermittent course; 52% had a chronic course with good functional status; 16% had a chronic course and were incapacitated; 5.4% died; and 3% developed cancer. Edwards and Truelove[4] also reported that most patients have a relapsing-remitting course with intervals of variable duration in which the patient may have relatively few or no symptoms.

In a review of recent date of long-term prognosis for patients with ulcerative colitis, Sales and Kirsner[21] analyzed actuarially the cumulative colectomy rates from several centers and from series recorded in the medical literature. They found that the cumulative colectomy rates ranged from 4% to 9% after 1 year of disease, from 6% to 27% after 5 years, and from 14% to 50% after 10 years of ulcerative colitis. It has been noted repeatedly that the major risk for colectomy occurs within the first few years of disease (unless colectomy is performed because of dysplasia and/or cancer). Furthermore, the most important prognostic factors correlating directly with need for surgery and also with mortality are the severity of the initial attack and the extent of the disease. Most of the deaths that occur in ulcerative colitis do so within the first 2 years of illness. Subsequently, survival curves approximately parallel those of the general population. This "early" mortality is due to severe onset of ulcerative colitis with increased risk of life-threatening complications such as massive hemorrhage, toxic dilatation of the colon, and perforation.[10]

Another subset of patients with an unfavorable prognosis are those with onset of disease after the age of 50.[5, 9, 22] Decreased survival results not only from increased mortality during the first attack of colitis, but also from debility from the acute disease and higher surgical mortality related to associated illness.

Several comparative studies have been performed on patients who have ulcerative colitis and those having Crohn's colitis. Noteworthy is the study by Lennard-Jones and colleagues,[23] in which ulcerative colitis was found to be "an illness with an acute and potentially dangerous onset but which appears to become less severe after survival for one year." This is contrast with Crohn's disease, which "tends to be a more chronic and progressive illness over several years with greater need for surgical treatment." This study indicated that ulcerative colitis was often acute and that more patients required an operation within the first year of onset of illness than did those who had Crohn's disease. However, if patients were followed for 6 years or longer, the possibility of operation among patients who had Crohn's colitis was 72% compared with 44% for patients who had ulcerative colitis. This study is in very close agreement with our results.[20] In a Danish study of 709 patients having inflammatory bowel disease, a survival rate of about 94% was found in the first year of observation compared with an expected survival rate in the general population of 99.5%, matched for sex and age.[24] After 12 years, the survival rate was about 77% for patients with both ulcerative colitis and Crohn's disease, which was about 2 to 3 times less than that in the matched population.

Other studies have compared the postoperative course of patients having ulcerative colitis and Crohn's colitis (following colectomy) with particular concern over recurrences.[24–27] For patients having ulcerative colitis, the main problem was need for ileostomy revision, but this occurred in only a small number of cases; after the first 2 years, the risk of having an ileostomy revision was low. In an English study[28] a comparison of the course following colectomy of 73 patients with Crohn's colitis and 442 patients with ulcerative colitis showed a difference in the immediate mortality of Crohn's disease (4%) and ulcerative colitis (10%). The difference was primarily because of the higher proportion of emergency operations in the latter group. The late mortality in both groups was 10%, mainly because of recurrence in Crohn's disease and the sequelae of colonic malignancy in ulcerative colitis. The hospital readmission rate was twice as high for Crohn's disease patients, as was the need for ileostomy reconstruction. Furthermore, about one-third of the patients having Crohn's disease required another operation because of recurrences. Nugent and Haggitt[29] followed patients on a long-term basis and graded the clinical status as excellent or good in 70% of those with Crohn's disease compared with 95% with ulcerative colitis, thus re-emphasizing the long-term favorable prognosis following total colectomy for patients with ulcerative colitis. Fawaz et al.,[25] from Yale, studied a group of patients of similar make-up who had total colectomy and found that the postoperative recurrence rate for patients with Crohn's disease was 38%, whereas there were no recurrences in those with ulcerative colitis. The only positive problems encountered among the patients having ulcerative colitis were those related either to sepsis at the time of surgery (often related to the severity of illness or to the emergency circumstancs under which the operation was performed) or to repair or revision of ileostomy.

Watts and Hughes,[27] in an Australian study comparing patients with ulcerative colitis and Crohn's disease treated by colectomy and ileorectal anastomosis, reported that 7% of the patients had a "satisfactory" result. They noted that "despite a high incidence of frequent loose stools and minor anorectal complications, most of the patients were satisfied with the result and would not contemplate the alternative of an ileostomy." No patient developed rectal carcinoma. It was emphasized that, provided the patient is followed carefully for the potential development of rectal carcinoma, ileorectal anastomosis can be a satisfactory alternative to ileostomy.

The results of these studies reiterate and emphasize the comments made earlier regarding questions patients ask about the overall long-term prognosis. The maximum impact of ulcerative colitis on the patient generally appears to occur earlier in the course of disease than in Crohn's colitis, and mortality is related to the severity of the disease at the time of onset, to associated sepsis, to the need for operation, and to postoperative problems.

Quality of Life

Edwards and Truelove[4] found that 69% of 101 survivors of ulcerative colitis led an entirely normal life, with another 19% having an essentially normal lifestyle except for frequent outpatient hospital visits. A more recent study from the Cleveland Clinic determined the quality of life in 308 patients with onset of ulcerative colitis in childhood and adolescence.[20] Of these patients, 21% considered their health good (normal or nearly normal functioning in comparison with their peer group; no medications on a regular basis); 72% rated their quality of life as fair (suboptimal functioning in comparison with their peer group; occasional symptoms, occasional use of medications, occasional impairment of function because of illness); and only 7% considered their health to be poor (inability to function satisfactorily, continuous use of medications, and frequent need for hospitalization).

Whether owing to improved therapeutic regimens; better understanding of the disease by physicians, patients, and their families; improved nutritional status; better surgical techniques; or improved preoperative and postoperative care, the prognosis for patients with ulcerative colitis does appear to be improving. Hendrickson and Binder[30] compared the "social prognosis" for 122 randomly selected patients with ulcerative colitis with a similar group of age- and sex-matched controls. The 2 groups were found to be similar in many aspects, including marital status, sexual problems, leisure activities, physical functioning, and economic earning capacity. They concluded, that the majority of patients with ulcerative colitis "seem to adapt themselves well to their condition and suffer few social or professional disabilities."

References

1. Banks BM, Korelitz BI, Zetzel L. The course of nonspecific ulcerative colitis. Review of twenty years' experience and late results. Gastroenterology 1957; 32:983.
2. Bargen JA, Jackman RJ, Kerr JG. Studies on the life histories of patients with chronic ulcerative colitis (thrombo-ulcerative colitis) with some suggestions for treatment. Ann Intern Med 1938; 12:339.
3. Bockus HL, Roth JLA, Buckman E, et al. Life history of nonspecific ulcerative colitis: Relation of prognosis of anatomical and clinical varities. Gastroenterologia 1956; 86:549.
4. Edwards FC, Truelove SC. The course and prognosis of ulcerative colitis. Part II. Long-term prognosis. Gut 1963; 4:309.
5. Jalan KN, Prescott RJ, Sircus W, et al. An experience of ulcerative colitis. III. Long-term outcome. Gastroenterology 1970; 59:598.
6. Watts JMcK, deDombal FT, Watkinson G, et al. Long-term prognosis of ulcerative colitis. Br Med J 1966; 1:1447.
7. Ritchie JK, Powell-Tuck J, Lennard-Jones JE. Clinical outcome of the first ten years of ulcerative colitis and proctitis. Lancet 1978; 1:1140–3.
8. Prior P, Gyde P, Allan RN. Mortality in ulcerative colitis: Methods of analysis. Gastroenterology 1982; 83:524–5.
9. Bonnevie O, Binder V, Anthonisen P, Riis P. The prognosis of ulcerative colitis. Scand J Gastroenterol 1974; 9:81–91.
10. Gyde S, Prior P, Dow MJ. Mortality in ulcerative colitis. Gastroenterology 1982; 83:36–43.
11. Farmer RG. Long-term prognosis for patients with ulcerative proctosigmoiditis (ulcerative colitis confined to the rectum and sigmoid colon). J Clin Gastroenterol 1979; 1:47–50.
12. Farmer RG, Brown CH. Ulcerative proctitis: Course and prognosis. Gastroenterology 1966; 51:219–23.
13. Farmer RG, Brown CH. Emerging concepts of proctosigmoiditis. Dis Colon Rectum 1972; 15:142–6.
14. Lennard-Jones JE, Cooper GW, Newell AC, et al. Observations on idiopathic proctitis. Gut 1962; 3:201–6.
15. Nugent FW, Veidenheimer MC, Zuberi S, et al. Clinical course of ulcerative proctosigmoiditis. Am J Dig Dis 1970; 15:321–6.
16. Powell-Tuck J, Ritchie JK, Lennard-Jones JE. Prognosis of idiopathic proctitis. Scand J Gastroenterol 1977; 12:727–32.
17. Palmer ED. The autonomy of idiopathic erosive proctitis. JAMA 1975; 232:748–9.
18. Das KM, Morecki R, Nair P, Berkowitz JM. Idiopathic proctitis: The morphology of proximal colonic mucosa and its clinical significance. Am J Dig Dis 1977; 22:524–8.
19. Korelitz BI, Gribetz D. The prognosis of ulcerative colitis with onset in childhood. II. The steroid era. Ann Intern Med 1962; 57:592.
20. Michener WM, Farmer RG, Mortimer EA. Long-term prognosis of ulcerative colitis with onset in childhood or adolescence. J Clin Gastroenterol 1979; 1:301–5.
21. Sales DJ, Kirsner JB. The prognosis of inflammatory bowel disease. Arch Intern Med 1983; Vol 143.
22. Jalan KN, Prescott RJ, Sircus W, et al. An experience of ulcerative colitis. II. Short-term outcome. Gastroenterology 1970; 59:589.
23. Lennard-Jones JE, Ritchie JK, Zohrab WJ. Proctocolitis and Crohn's disease of the colon. A comparison of the clinical course. Gut 1976; 17:477–82.
24. Storgaard L, Bischorr N, Hendriksen et al. Survival rate in Crohn's disease and ulcerative colitis. Scand J Gastroenterol 1979; 14:225–30.
25. Fawaz KA, Glotzer DJ, Goldman M, et al. Ulcerative colitis and Crohn's disease of the colon—a comparison of the long-term postoperative courses. Gastroenterology 1976; 71:372–8.
26. Vender RJ, Rickert RR, Spiro HM. The outlook after total colectomy in patients with Crohn's colitis and ulcerative colitis. J Clin Gastroenterol 1979; 1:209–17.
27. Watts JM, Hughes ESR. Ulcerative colitis and Crohn's disease: Results after colectomy and ileorectal anastomosis. Br J Surg 1977; 64:77–83.
28. Steinberg DM, Allan RN, Brooke BN, et al. Sequelae of colectomy and ileostomy: Comparison between Crohn's colitis and ulcerative colitis. Gastroenterology 1973; 68:33–9.
29. Nugent FW, Haggitt RC. Long-term follow up including cancer surveillance for patients with ulcerative colitis. Clin Gastroenterol 1980; 9:459–68.
30. Hendricksen C, Binder V. Social prognosis in patients with ulcerative colitis. Br Med J 1980; 2:581–7.

Chapter 127

Crohn's Disease

Henry D. Janowitz • Samuel Meyers • Stanley R. Hamilton • Basil C. Morson • Richard H. Marshak • Arthur E. Lindner • Daniel Maklansky • Adrian J. Greenstein*

Pathology

Stanley R. Hamilton • Basil C. Morson

The definition of Crohn's disease has widened steadily since the original description by Crohn, Ginsberg, and Oppenheimer in 1932. It is now recognized as an idiopathic inflammatory bowel disease that may have clinical manifestations in any part of the alimentary tract from the mouth to the anal region. Extraintestinal sites such as the skin, joints, liver, and eyes may also be affected. Because the etiology is as yet unknown, definition of the disease is based upon its clinical manifestations and the pathologic abnormalities producing them.

Sites Of Involvement And Gross Pathologic Appearances

Several lines of evidence indicate that Crohn's disease diffusely involves the gastrointestinal tract (see later discussion of Early Lesions of Crohn's Disease), but the gross pathologic features are mostly a manifestation of advanced involvement of one or more of its segments. The gross pathologic findings are very similar throughout the gastrointestinal tract, i.e., discontinuous ulceration, stricturing, and fistula formation. The findings in a particular patient, however, vary with diverse factors, including site, activity, duration of disease, and possibly therapy.

Small Intestine.[1] Terminal ileal involvement is extremely common. Varying lengths from the distal few centimeters contiguous with the ileocecal valve to the entire ileum may be affected. The "hose-pipe" stricture of the terminal ileum is the classic appearance (Fig. 127–1). The bowel wall is thickened and immobile with stenosis of the lumen, and the overlying mucosal surface shows ulceration. Crohn's disease can produce ulcers with a varied appearance in the jejunum and duodenum as well as the ileum. The ulcers are usually discontinuous with adjacent uninvolved mucosa. The ulceration may result in a "cobblestone" appearance (Fig. 127–2), produced by interconnecting ulcers surrounding mucosa with edematous submucosa. Fissuring ulcers with sharp crevices may penetrate deeply into the bowel wall. Extension of fissures through the wall into contiguous structures, such as other segments of bowel or pelvic organs, leads to fistulas and abscesses. Serpiginous ulcers that spread irregularly over the mucosal surface and aphthoid ulcers (tiny discrete lesions often surrounded by grossly uninvolved mucosa) are common (Fig. 127–3). Ulceration is often associated with strictures, which may be short or long, single or multiple. The peritoneal surface shows dilatation of blood vessels, adhesions, encroachment ("creeping") of mesenteric adipose tissue onto the circumference in areas underlying ulcers, and sometimes tubercles. Abnormal areas are often separated by normal areas, producing "skip" lesions.

*Deceased.

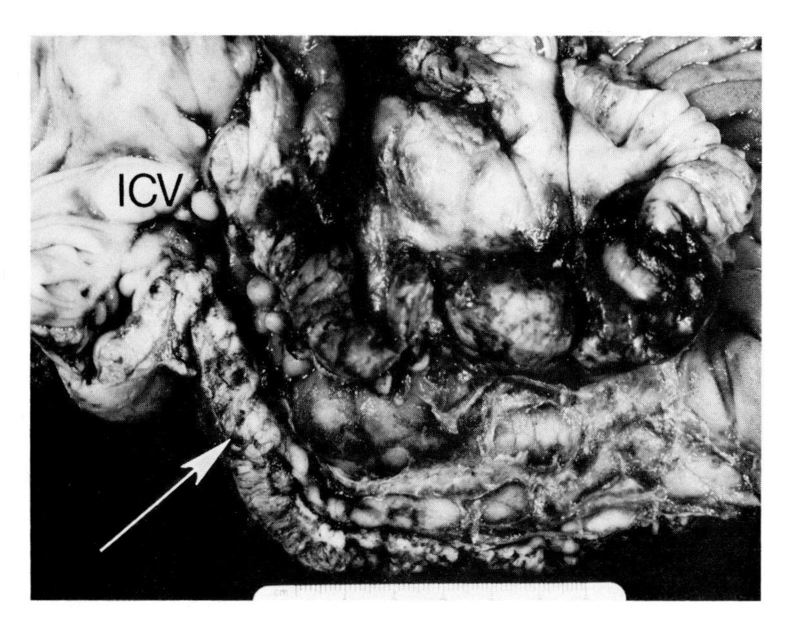

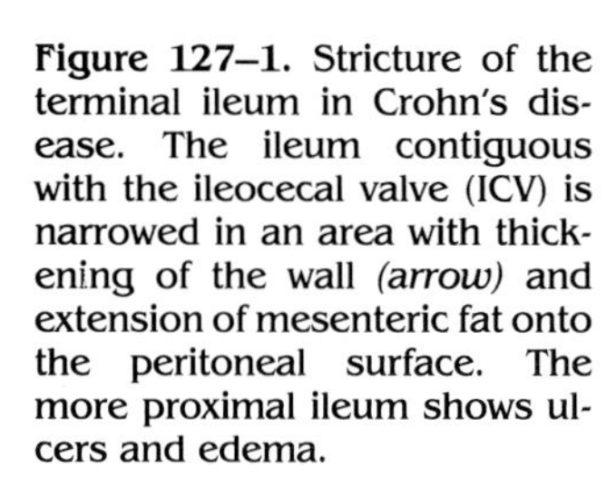

Figure 127–1. Stricture of the terminal ileum in Crohn's disease. The ileum contiguous with the ileocecal valve (ICV) is narrowed in an area with thickening of the wall *(arrow)* and extension of mesenteric fat onto the peritoneal surface. The more proximal ileum shows ulcers and edema.

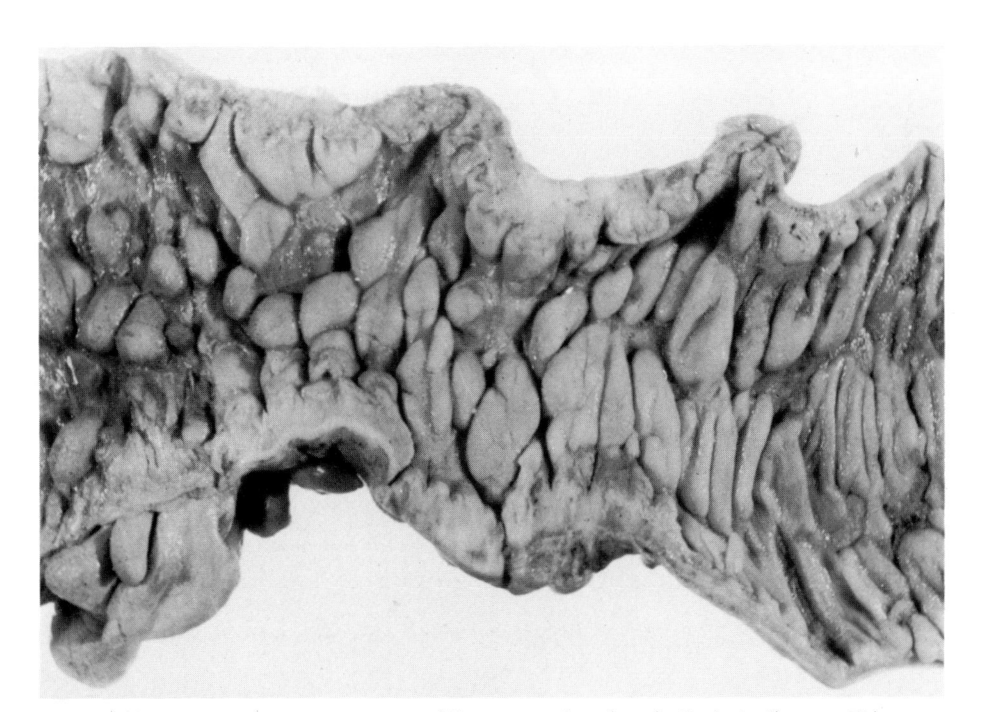

Figure 127–2. Typical cobblestone appearance of the mucosal surface in Crohn's disease. This appearance is produced by interconnecting ulcers surrounding islands of mucosa elevated by submucosal edema.

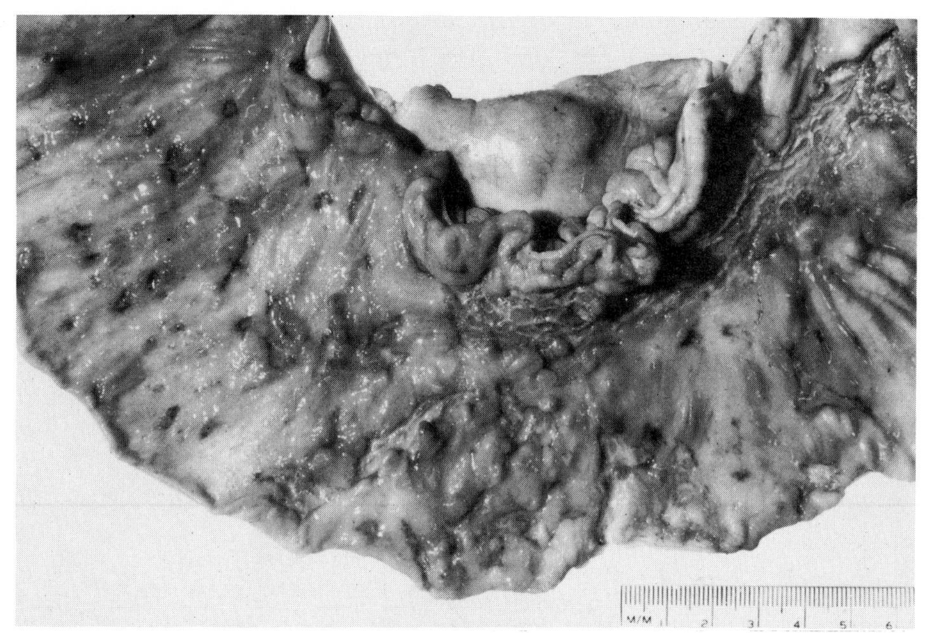

Figure 127–3. Serpiginous and aphthoid ulcers in Crohn's disease. The tiny aphthoid lesions, such as those in the mucosa on the left side of the photograph, are one of the earliest gross pathologic findings of Crohn's disease.

The regional lymph nodes are often enlarged, although the ileocecal nodes may be large even in normal persons.

Large Intestine, Appendix, and Anus.[2] Colonic involvement by Crohn's disease can occur alone or with involvement of other areas, particularly the terminal ileum ("ileocolitis"). The sites and extent of colonic involvement are highly variable. The distribution of gross abnormalities is typically discontinuous with segmental "skip" lesions (Fig. 127–4). The right colon is sometimes the site of predominant involvement, and sparing of the rectum occurs in many patients. On the other hand, Crohn's disease confined to the rectum also occurs. When involvement of the entire colon is present, at least some areas with normal mucosa usually remain.

The mucosal surface typically shows discrete ulcers surrounded by otherwise grossly uninvolved areas (Fig. 127–4). The ulcers may be serpiginous, linear and longitudinally oriented, interconnected to produce a cobblestone appearance, or aphthoid. Strictures, thickening of the wall, serosal inflammation, adhesions, and fistulas may occur in the colon, as in small bowel.

The appendix is usually involved along with another part of the gastrointestinal tract, although appendiceal involvement can be the

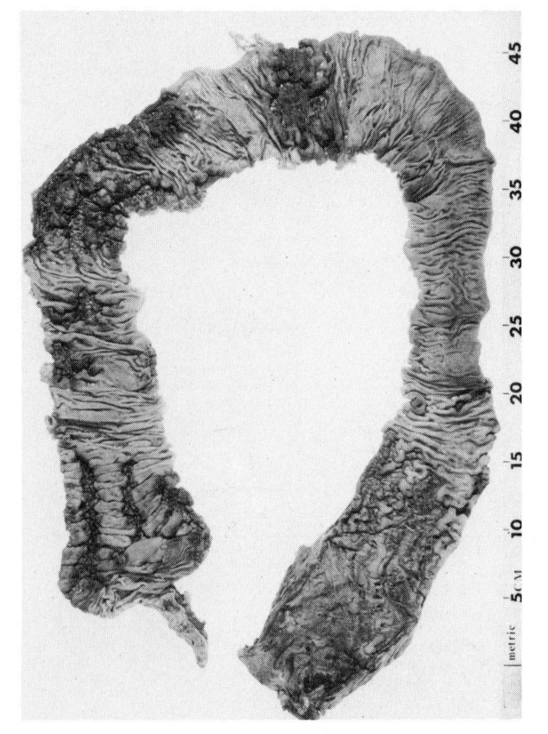

Figure 127–4. Crohn's disease of the colon and rectum, demonstrating its discontinuous nature. The colon shows patches of serpiginous ulceration (darker areas) separated by normal areas. The rectum is extensively and uniformly involved. The small intestine is normal.

presenting feature of Crohn's disease in some patients.[3]

The anal region is frequently affected.[4] Manifestations include ulcers, anorectal fistulas, and edematous skin tags (Fig. 127–5). Anal involvement may antedate by many years apparent involvement of other areas of the gastrointestinal tract.

Mouth, Esophagus, and Stomach. Ulcers in the oral cavity have been described in patients with other gastrointestinal tract involvement.[5] Esophageal manifestations include ulcers, strictures, and fistulas.[6] Involvement of the esophagus alone by Crohn's disease ("regional esophagitis") has been reported.[7]

Crohn's disease involving the stomach appears to affect the distal portion most commonly, but extensive disease resembling linitis plastica has been reported. Thickening and rigidity of the gastric wall with contraction of the lumen are frequent manifestations. Mucosal ulceration may result in a cobblestone appearance. Crohn's disease of the stomach can occur alone, but usually is found with contiguous duodenal or other small intestinal involvement.[8]

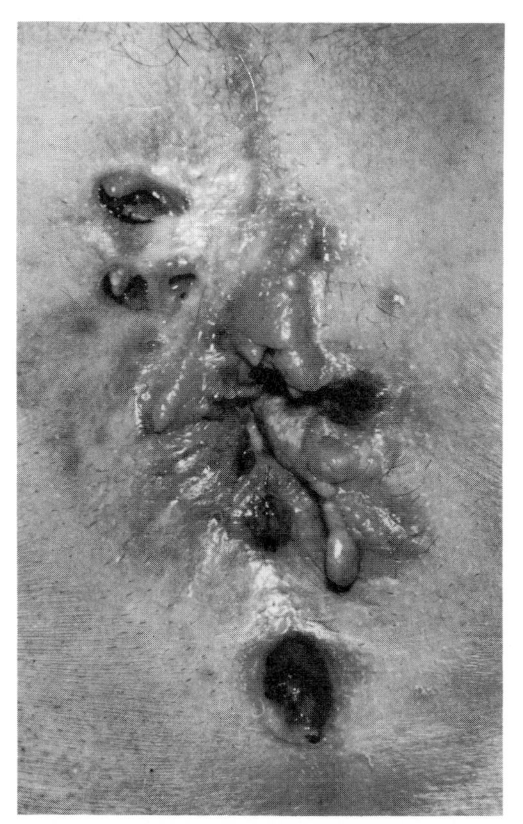

Figure 127–5. Anal involvement in Crohn's disease. Multiple fistulas and edematous skin tags are present.

Histopathology[1]

The histopathologic pattern of Crohn's disease shows substantial variability among patients, the result, in part, of the way in which the pathologist has sampled the different parts of a surgical specimen or the sites from which an endoscopist has chosen to take biopsy specimens. Optimal methods for examination of surgical specimens have been published.[1]

Granulomas, of course, are the hallmark of Crohn's disease. The granulomas are composed of a collection of epithelioid histiocytes with or without giant cells of the Langhans' type (Fig. 127–6). Hyalin and conchoidal inclusion (Schaumann) bodies identical to those in sarcoidosis and tuberculosis are occasionally seen in giant cells of Crohn's disease. Central caseous necrosis of the granulomas typically is absent. The epithelioid cell aggregates are surrounded by a variable rim of lymphocytes. Often the granulomas are so small and poorly formed that "granulomatous inflammation" is an appropriate characterization.

Granulomas are found in the majority (about 60%) of surgical specimens from patients with Crohn's disease. The number of granulomas varies greatly from one patient to another; some have very few lesions, while others have a florid granulomatous reaction. Granulomas and granulomatous inflamma-

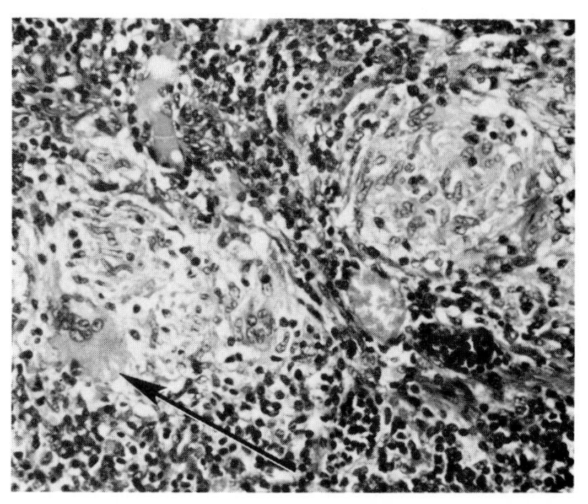

Figure 127–6. Non-caseating epitheloid cell granuloma in Crohn's disease. A multinucleated giant cell *(arrow)* is present in one granuloma. (Hematoxylin and eosin, × 280.)

tion can be found in all layers of the bowel wall, including the serosal tubercles that are seen grossly. The regional lymph nodes may contain granulomas when these lesions are present in the bowel wall. The presence of granulomas in biopsy specimens of lesions in unusual sites, such as the mouth and upper gastrointestinal tract, allows recognition of involvement by Crohn's disease.

Granulomas occur in a large number of other diseases in addition to Crohn's disease. Furthermore, granulomas may not be found in a sizeable minority of patients with this disorder. As a result, other histopathologic features are essential for the recognition of Crohn's disease. Aggregates of lymphocytes, some with germinal centers, scattered throughout the bowel wall in a transmural distribution are a characteristic feature in nearly all patients with this disease (Fig. 127–7). These aggregates are often closely related to vascular channels, particularly dilated lymphatics. In the serosa they frequently are arrayed along the outer aspect of the muscularis propria in a "rosary" formation. Much of the inflammatory infiltrate of Crohn's disease is neither lymphocytic nor granulomatous. Neutrophils and eosinophils are present in variable numbers. Plasma cells are frequent, but quantitation of IgA, IgG, and IgM plasma cells has produced inconstant results. Crypt abscesses are common in the mucosa and are characterized by acute inflammation of the epithelium with destruction leading to exudate in the crypt lumen. The mucosal inflammatory infiltrate typically has a discontinuous distribution in the lamina propria and almost always shows some variation in the intensity of inflammation in different parts of any histopathologic section.

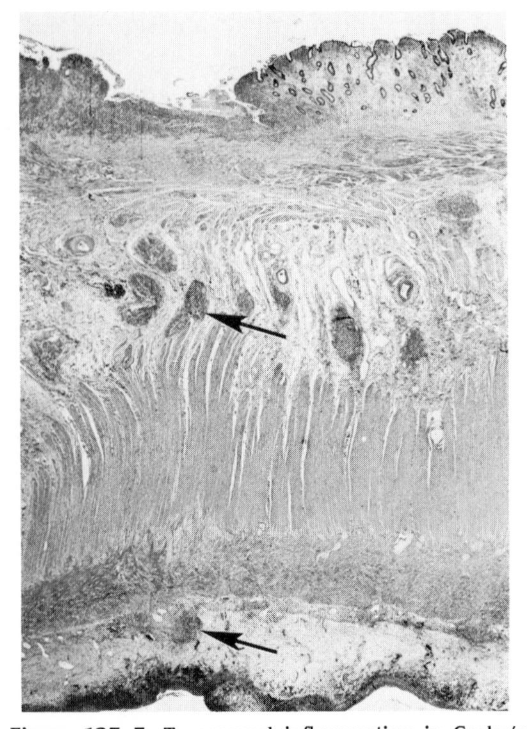

Figure 127–7. Transmural inflammation in Crohn's disease. Lymphoid aggregates are present in the submucosa and serosa *(arrows)* beneath a mucosal ulcer. Peritonitis is also present. (Hematoxylin and eosin, × 10.)

Fissuring ulceration is a distinctive but inconsistent component of the histopathology of Crohn's disease (Fig. 127–8). The crack-like fissures are localized ulcers lined by a layer of necrotic debris beneath which is a zone of granulation tissue with histiocytes and inflammatory cells. Fissures can exhibit branching; therefore, in histopathologic sections not showing communication with the lumen, the fissure may appear as an intramural abscess. Often the fissures penetrate only into the submucosa. Deep penetration leads to the formation of fistulas, but *free perforation into the peritoneal cavity is uncommon*. The mucosa surrounding fissures is often relatively uninflamed, accounting for their discrete nature. Fissures are not specific for Crohn's disease; similar lesions can be seen in fulminant ulcerative colitis (Chapter 126) and lymphomas (Chapter 112).

Aphthoid ulcers or erosions are also characteristic of Crohn's disease (Fig. 127–9) (see later discussion of Early Lesions of Crohn's Disease).

Other inconstant and non-specific features contribute to the histopathologic pattern recognizable as Crohn's disease. Pyloric gland metaplasia of small intestinal mucosa resembling the antral glands in the stomach, thickening and splaying of the fibers of the muscularis mucosae, submucosal widening due to edema and fibrosis with lymphangiectasia, peptidergic neural proliferation in the submucosal and myenteric plexus,[9] and vasculitis may all be seen. Strictures in Crohn's disease generally show granulation tissue and marked fibrosis in the submucosa.

Endoscopic Biopsy Findings.[10–17] Many of the features helpful in the recognition of Crohn's disease are gross pathologic findings or histopathologic appearances of the bowel wall. Biopsies provide a small sample of the

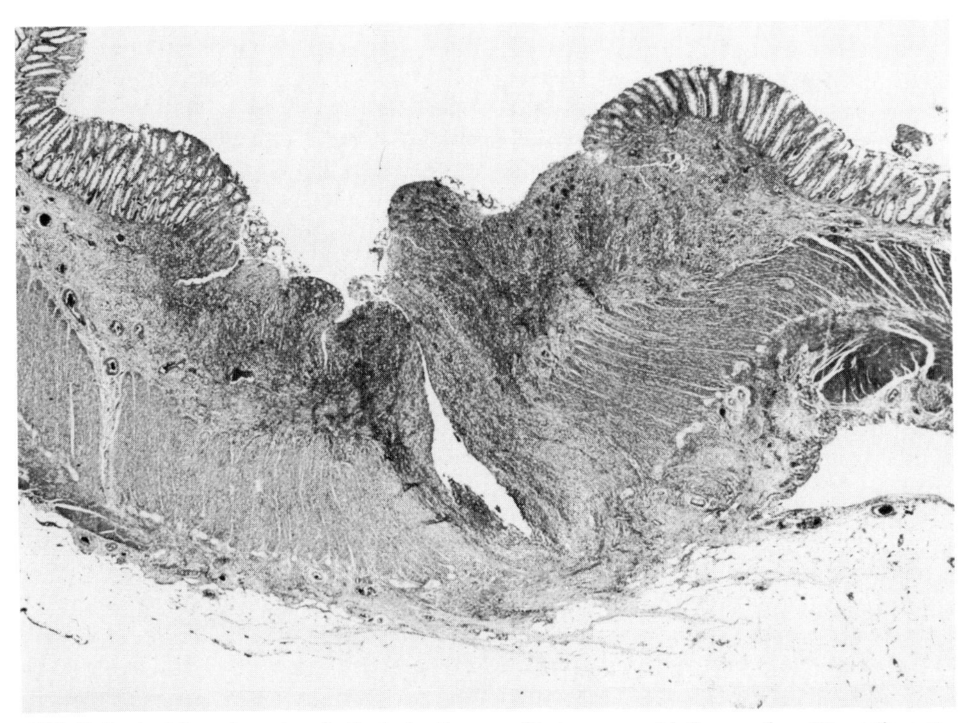

Figure 127–8. Typical fissuring ulcer in Crohn's disease with transmural inflammation. The adjacent mucosa is normal.

Figure 127–9. Aphthoid erosion over a lymphoid nodule in Crohn's disease. Surface epithelium is lost and fibrinoinflammatory exudate *(arrow)* is present in the lumen. Adjacent villi show only edema and chronic inflammation. (Hematoxylin and eosin, × 100.)

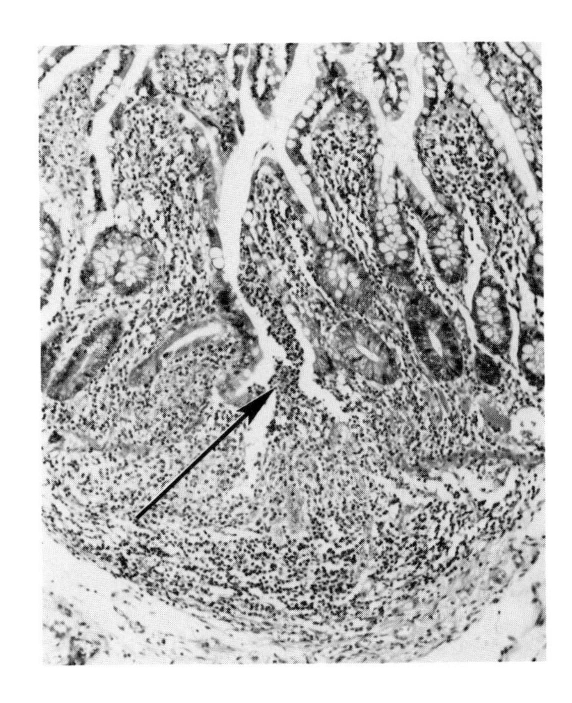

histopathologic findings in only the mucosa and superficial submucosa. Despite these limitations, biopsies are diagnostically useful.[18]

In biopsy specimens from any site, particularly the upper gastrointestinal tract and anus, characteristic non-caseating epithelioid cell granulomas are the most helpful finding for diagnosis, although these are by no means specific for Crohn's disease. The chance of discovering granulomas in biopsy specimens depends upon a number of factors, including whether or not the patient has the granulomatous type of Crohn's disease; the site, size, and number of biopsies taken; and the diligence of the tissue sectioning and histopathologic examination.[19] In rectal biopsies from patients with idiopathic inflammatory bowel disease, focal active inflammation[20] in the midst of otherwise histopathologically normal rectal mucosa (Fig. 127–10) or the absence of evidence of rectal involvement in a patient with known colitis suggests Crohn's disease.

When the sites of colonoscopic biopsies are designated, the anatomic distribution of histopathologic findings can be assessed. Active inflammation in Crohn's disease involving the colon is typically discontinuous and segmental, manifested by abnormal biopsy specimens intermixed with relatively normal samples. Right-sided predominance can also be identified. Terminal ileal biopsies obtained at colonoscopy can be particularly helpful when active inflammation is demonstrated.

The histopathologic characteristics of the inflammation are also helpful. In addition to granulomas and granulomatous inflammation, discrete ulcers that occur in otherwise uninvolved mucosa, fissuring ulcers, and aphthoid erosions or ulcers over lymphoid nodules can be identified in biopsy samples. With active crypt epithelial inflammation and crypt abscesses, epithelial mucin and crypt architecture are usually preserved, except when activity is severe. Chronic inflammation is often predominantly lymphocytic. Clustering of lymphocytes in the lamina propria, particularly around the bases of crypts, is also seen. Submucosal extension of chronic inflammation can be found as a manifestation of transmural inflammation. Disproportionate submucosal inflammation as compared with inflammation of the overlying mucosa is particularly suggestive of Crohn's disease in colorectal biopsies from patients with idiopathic inflammatory bowel disease.

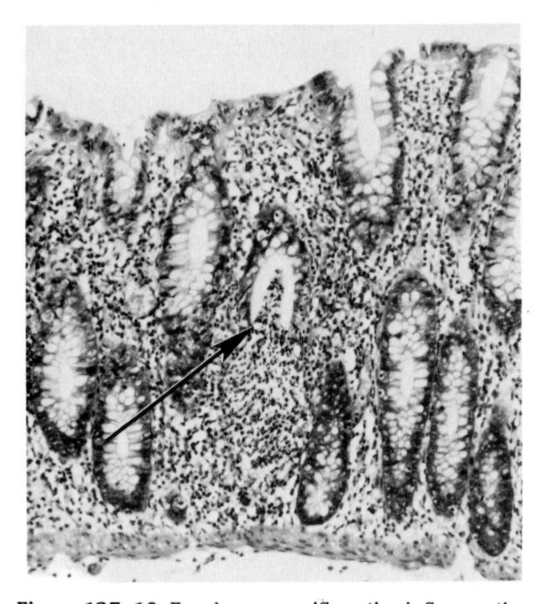

Figure 127–10. Focal non-specific active inflammation in Crohn's disease. A crypt abscess *(arrow)* with neutrophils is located in the midst of colonic mucosa with only mild chronic inflammation. No granulomas or granulomatous features are present, hence the term "non-specific active inflammation." Epithelial mucin is maintained. (Hematoxylin and eosin, × 145.)

Early Lesions of Crohn's Disease

One of the earliest gross pathologic findings of Crohn's disease is the *aphthoid ulcer*.[21] The term "aphthoid" is based on the similarity of the ulcers to aphthous ulcers of the mouth. Aphthoid ulcers may be found in grossly normal small bowel and colonic mucosa distant from obviously diseased areas. On gross examination, the ulcers are often barely visible, appearing sometimes as pinpoint hemorrhages. On scanning electron microscopy, the mucosa surrounding the small bowel ulcers shows villous abnormalities, including blunting, fusion, and epithelial bridging. In histopathologic sections, the aphthoid ulcer (Fig. 127–9) typically is located over a lymphoid nodule that may be hyperplastic. The base of the aphthoid ulcer shows exudate, and the epithelium at the margin is often proliferating, in an apparent attempt to cover the ulcer. Granulomas and granulomatous inflammation can be present in the affected lymphoid nodule. The surrounding mucosa often shows only minor abnormalities, such as edema and chronic inflammation. The underlying submucosa is often edematous. Many of the small aphthoid lesions are actually erosions that do not involve even the full thickness of the mucosa. In exceptional examples, the epithelium over the affected lymphoid nodule is intact but acutely inflamed.

The grossly normal small bowel and colonic mucosa in patients with Crohn's disease also show abnormalities on microscopic examination. Scanning electron microscopy demonstrates villous abnormalities in small bowel and increased goblet cells in the colon.[22–24] Histopathologic examination of biopsy specimens from endoscopically normal colonic mucosa shows active inflammation and granulomas in some patients.[25,26] These lesions are commonly found when histologic techniques to improve sampling of grossly normal colon from resection specimens are employed.[27] Finally, in histopathologically normal small bowel and colonic mucosa distant from evident Crohn's disease, morphometry demonstrates increased numbers of chronic inflammatory cells.[28–30] Such studies provide evidence that the mucosa of the gastrointestinal tract is diffusely abnormal in Crohn's disease.

Relationship to Pathogenesis (see Chapter 124). The features of these presumed early lesions of Crohn's disease are the basis for speculation regarding pathogenesis. The occurrence of aphthoid ulcers and erosions over lymphoid nodules is intriguing because the lymphoid nodules are covered by characteristic epithelium that transports luminal antigens for local intestinal immune response.[31] The granulomas seen in the lymphoid nodules suggest that the agent or agents responsible for Crohn's disease enter at this site. The mucosal lymphoid hyperplasia and increased chronic inflammatory cells in the lamina propria may represent evidence of mucosal immunologic response to the agents. The occurrence of non-ulcerated active inflammatory lesions and granulomas in grossly normal bowel provides additional evidence that the submucosal edema and lymphangiectasia that were thought to be early abnormalities of Crohn's disease are, in fact, secondary features. Furthermore, the presence of active inflammation and granulomas unassociated with lymphoid tissue suggests that the agents may be able to attack the mucosa directly, not only passively through the lymphoid nodules. Finally, the occurrence of granulomatous inflammation and granulomas in early lesions provides evidence that the agents are not degradable by the initial acute inflammatory response.[32] The agents, of course, remain to be defined. Another of many questions to be answered is how the heterogeneous pathologic manifestations (e.g., "ileitis" vs. "ileocolitis" vs. "colitis") occur in this disease.

Pathology of Complications

Recrudescence After Resection. The propensity of Crohn's disease to reappear after resection is well known. As discussed earlier, the mucosa of the gastrointestinal tract appears to be diffusely abnormal in Crohn's disease. As a result, the disease is seldom extirpated by resection. The pathologic features of recrudescent Crohn's disease are essentially the same as those described earlier. Recognition of recrudescence may be complicated, however, by the occurrence of inflammatory bowel disease unrelated to the underlying Crohn's disease. For example, ileitis can occur in ileostomy stomas and continent ileostomies fashioned after resection for a variety of diseases.[33, 34] Also, colitis can occur in segments of bowel from which the fecal stream has been diverted.[35] In addition, inflammatory bowel disease of other causes (e.g., infection and ischemia) can occur in patients with idiopathic inflammatory bowel disease (see later discussion of Differential Diagnosis).

Recrudescence after resection with ileostomy appears to be more common when Crohn's disease involves the ileum or the ileum and colon than when the colon alone is affected.[36] When resection and ileocolonic anastomosis are performed, "suture-line" recrudescence in the ileum proximal to the anastomotic site is common. However, the anastomotic site itself is often spared, with the histopathologic evidence of active Crohn's disease appearing a few millimeters proximal to the scar representing the anastomosis.[37] A prospective endoscopic study has shown that ileal recrudescence, which is often clinically inapparent, occurs soon after resection with ileocolonic anastomosis in a majority of patients.[38] The site of recrudescence appears to be influenced by the site of bowel resected for Crohn's disease; colonic recrudescence is usually associated with previous colonic involvement.[39]

The factors that determine clinical recrudescence after resection with anastomosis are uncertain. The relationship of granulomas in the resection specimen to subsequent recrudescence is controversial.[40–42] Aggressive surgical strategies, such as resecting long segments at points well above and below sites of evident disease and determining histopathologically uninvolved resection margins by frozen section, do not appear to improve outcome. However, there is controversy regarding these issues.[43] Medical therapy after resection also seems to have no influence.[44] Rather, the relationship of recrudescence to the length of involved bowel in the resection specimen suggests that recrudescence is an inherent characteristic of the disease in the particular patient.[43]

Fulminant Disease. The pathologic features just described are typical of chronic active Crohn's disease. In a small minority of patients, however, fulminant Crohn's disease occurs, either as a presenting event[45] or during the course of the illness. Fulminant disease can involve both the small and the large bowel. The gross pathologic features may include dilatation (hence the term "toxic megacolon" for some cases with colonic involvement), marked congestion and hemorrhage, extensive acute ulcers, and free perforation with acute peritonitis. The bowel wall is extremely friable, and muscle fiber necrosis in the muscularis propria is a usual finding in histopathologic sections (Chapter 126).

Dysplasia and Carcinoma. Small and large bowel carcinomas may develop as a complication of Crohn's disease.[46] The tumors occur in segments of bowel involved by grossly evident Crohn's disease, and many of them are accompanied by dysplasia similar to that in the colon in ulcerative colitis[47,48] (Chapters 126 and 128). Small and large bowel carcinoma have a propensity to develop in bypassed segments.[49] Detection of malignancy is complicated by the pathologic features of Crohn's disease itself, particularly stricture formation and the discontinuous distribution.

Differential Diagnosis (See also the following section of this chapter for a discussion of the clinical features in differential diagnosis.)

Inflammatory bowel disease (with the term used in a generic sense for any gastrointestinal tract disorder in which inflammation plays a role in pathogenesis) can have a large number of causes.[10] With the widespread use of gastrointestinal tract biopsies, inflammatory bowel disease due to causes for which there is specific therapy can be recognized. This recognition is essential, as only then can inappropriate and potentially harmful treatment with non-specific anti-inflammatory drugs be avoided. The pathologic features of some of the conditions that can be confused with idiopathic inflammatory bowel disease[50] are described below.

Infectious Bowel Diseases (see Chapters 118 to 121). Tuberculosis can affect any part of the gastrointestinal tract[1] and, as with Crohn's disease, most commonly involves the terminal ileum and ileocecal region. In contrast to Crohn's disease, however, tuberculosis is rare in the colon and rectum. The gross pathologic findings of intestinal tuberculosis include multiple strictures and ulcers. The ulcers in tuberculosis are often transversely oriented, and a cobblestone appearance does not occur. Acute intestinal obstruction and free perforation are more common in tuberculosis. In histologic sections from resection specimens, granulomas are a constant feature of tuberculosis but may not be found in Crohn's disease. In biopsy specimens of tuberculosis, however, sampling may lead to failure to detect granulomas. The granulomas in the 2 conditions have different features. In non-caseating tuberculosis, the granulomas are usually large and confluent, and the surrounding rim of lymphocytes is more prominent. Caseation, if present, strongly suggests tuberculosis, but central necrosis of granulomas may be seen occasionally in Crohn's disease. Hyalinization of granulomas is typical of tuberculosis and uncommon in Crohn's disease. Regional lymph node involvement by granulomas is a constant feature of tuberculosis, but is frequently absent in Crohn's disease; the presence of granulomas in regional lymph nodes but not in the bowel wall strongly suggests tuberculosis. Other features of tuberculosis that contrast with Crohn's disease are obliteration or marked reduction of the submucosa and prominent fibrosis involving the muscularis propria. Fissures and internal fistulas are not seen in tuberculosis. The deciding factor in differential diagnosis, of course, is the demonstration of acid-fast bacilli, preferably confirmed by culture, in tuberculosis, but this occasionally may be difficult or impossible.

Granulomas are also a feature of inflammatory bowel disease due to *Chlamydia trachomatis*.[51] In some cases of chlamydial proctitis, multinucleated giant cells in association with crypt abscesses are prominent in biopsies. Appropriate culture is necessary to establish the diagnosis. *Lymphogranuloma venereum*, a disorder caused by a related organism, can produce fibrous strictures and ulcers of the anorectal region as late sequelae.[52, 53] Granulomas are frequently seen, and differentiation from Crohn's disease can be difficult. Central necrosis of the granulomas and squamous metaplasia of the colonic mucosa provide evidence favoring lymphogranuloma venereum as the etiology.

Yersinial infection also produces granulomas and may be difficult to distinguish clinically from Crohn's disease.[54] The small and large bowel on gross examination usually show prominent lymphoid tissue with ulceration, mucosal congestion, and edema. In histopathologic sections, the lymphoid tissue, including regional lymph nodes, has granulomas composed of epithelioid cells and multinucleated giant cells but with characteristic central necrotic areas containing neutrophils. The presence of necrosis contrasts with Crohn's disease. Definitive diagnosis of *Yersinial* infection requires appropriate culture.

Campylobacter infections also may be confused clinically with Crohn's disease and ulcerative colitis.[55,56] The small intestine and colon have been reported to show extensive ulceration with a hemorrhagic appearance in severe cases, and perforation may occur. Histopathologically, the ulcers are non-specific and are characterized by actively inflamed granulation tissue. Features typical of Crohn's disease, including transmural lymphoid aggregates, fibrosis, strictures, fistulas, and granulomas, are absent. Thus, unless *Campylobacter* infection is superimposed on idiopathic inflammatory bowel disease, the conditions appear distinct in resection or necropsy specimens. In rectal or colonoscopic biopsies, differentiation is much more difficult. *Campylobacter* infection, like the infections caused by *Salmonella, enterotoxigenic E. coli, Clostridium difficile* that may be antibiotic-associated, *gonococcus*, and *Vibrio parahaemolyticus*, generally shows the biopsy findings of acute colitis; active inflammation and crypt abscesses occur without much crypt distortion or loss, marked chronic inflammation, or fibrosis of the lamina propria. Correct diagnosis, however, depends upon cultures in appropriate media under favorable laboratory conditions and/or toxin assay.[57–59]

In parasitic and fungal inflammatory bowel disease (Chapter 232), the causative organisms are potentially identifiable in histologic sections. In *amebiasis*, the cecum is most commonly affected, although other sites in the colon and occasionally the terminal ileum may be involved. The mucosal surface shows foci of necrosis and ulcers of varying sizes and configurations. The ulcers may be small or inapparent at endoscopy, but usually are covered with exudate. In histopathologic sections of resection and necropsy specimens, the ulcers may extend radially in the submucosa to undermine adjacent mucosa. They often show necrosis with little inflammatory reaction. These features are uncommon in Crohn's disease and ulcerative colitis, except when fulminant activity is present. In biopsy specimens, the mucosal findings may be subtle, with only low-grade active inflammation. Exudate consisting of fibrinoinflammatory debris often contains the characteristic trophozoites of *Entamoeba histolytica*, allowing morphologic definition of the correct diagnosis.[60] *Balantidium coli* produces disease similar to amebiasis and can be identified in histopathologic sections.

Heavy *Schistosoma mansoni* infection can produce inflammatory bowel disease with inflammatory polyps and occasionally fibrous strictures in the colon. In histopathologic sections, granulomas and fibrosis are common, but ova can usually be identified.[61] *Cryptosporidiosis* can produce inflammatory bowel disease involving the small and large bowel; the organisms are identifiable along the luminal surface of the epithelium.[62] *Histoplasmosis* involving the gastrointestinal tract can occasionally mimic Crohn's disease and ulcerative colitis, but the yeasts are identifiable in macrophages in histopathologic sections. *Actinomyces*, the fungus-like bacteria, have characteristic colonies in tissue sections.

In infections with *cytomegalovirus* and *herpesvirus*, characteristic inclusions may lead to recognition of the etiology. Cytomegalovirus infection, however, is often superimposed on a predisposing disease, which may include ulcerative colitis.[63] Herpes proctitis in homosexual males is often accompanied by other infections.

Ischemic Bowel Disease (see Chapter 116). In the spectrum of ischemic injury to the gastrointestinal tract, strictures of the small bowel and ischemic colitis may be difficult to differentiate from idiopathic inflammatory bowel disease. Furthermore, ischemia contributes to inflammatory bowel disease in a number of clinical settings: neonatal necrotizing enterocolitis, staphylococcal enterocolitis, chronic radiation enterocolitis, uremia, sickle cell anemia, collagen-vascular diseases, potassium-induced ulcer, and stress ulcer.[64] Characteristic features of acute ischemic bowel disease include transmural infarction in the severe forms; in less severe cases, mucosal coagulative necrosis, congestion, hemorrhage, and pseudomembrane formation with submucosal thickening by edema are seen. The findings are influenced by the anatomy of the vasculature, sites of arteriosclerotic narrowing, collateral circulation, cardiac status, and duration of hypoperfusion. The splenic flexure region is often involved in ischemic colitis. The histopathologic findings frequently include non-specific active inflammation involving crypt epithelium with crypt abscess formation that may suggest idiopathic inflammatory bowel disease. However, the presence of hemosiderin-containing macrophages indicating previous episodes of hemorrhage strongly suggests ischemic disease.[1] With resolution of an acute ischemic episode or ongoing chronic ischemia, stricture formation due to marked fibrosis of the submucosa and muscularis propria may occur. Ulceration of the mucosa with granulation tissue and scarring of the submucosa accompanied by hemosiderin-containing macrophages are often present. In contrast, hemosiderin deposition is uncommon in Crohn's disease and ulcerative colitis, unless ischemic bowel disease is also present (Tables 127–1 and 127–2).

Diverticular Disease (see Chapter 135). Diverticula of the colon are common in middle-aged and elderly patients. As a result, diverticular disease is frequently included in the differential diagnosis of Crohn's disease. Furthermore, Crohn's disease of the colon is sometimes found in association with diverticulosis, usually in the sigmoid colon. The distinction between simple diverticulitis and Crohn's disease superimposed on diverticu-

Table 127–1. COMPARISON OF CROHN'S DISEASE INVOLVING THE COLON, ULCERATIVE COLITIS, AND ISCHEMIC COLITIS: TYPICAL GROSS PATHOLOGIC ABNORMALITIES

	Crohn's Disease	Ulcerative Colitis	Ischemic Colitis
Distribution			
Continuity	Discontinuous, segmental with intervening uninvolved areas	Continuous from anus proximally	Discontinuous, segmental
Predominant site	Variable: right colon in some	Rectum with variable extent of more proximal disease	Variable: splenic flexure region in many
Rectal involvement	About half of cases; spared in others	Virtually all cases	Variable
Total colonic involvement	Rare	Sometimes	Rare
Terminal ileal involvement	Common and often extensive: ulcers, strictures	Rare and limited: dilatation and loss of plicae with "backwash"	Rare: dilatation with hemorrhage, ulcers
Anal involvement	Common: chronic deep fissure, fistula, abscess; edematous tags	Rare: acute abscess, superficial erosion, excoriation	Absent
Mucosa			
Ulcers	Discrete: fissuring—serpiginous, linear, longitudinal, interconnecting with cobblestone appearance; aphthoid—with edema	In ahaustral diffusely granular areas (but may resemble Crohn's disease in fulminant colitis)	Discrete: pseudomembrane and cobblestone appearance in acute phase
Vascularity	Prominent only in fulminant disease	Prominent with activity	Intense in acute phase, not with stricture
Inflammatory polyposis	Uncommon	Sometimes	Absent
Colonic Wall			
Spontaneous fistula	Sometimes internal or cutaneous	Rare	Absent
Stricture	Common: fibrous thickening of wall	Rare: muscular hypertrophy or malignancy	Common as late sequela: fibrosis
Shortening of length	With fibrosis	With hypertrophy of muscularis mucosae and propria	Late sequela: fibrosis
Serositis and adhesions	Common	Rare	Common
Toxic dilatation (megacolon)	Rare	Occasional	Common

Table 127–2. COMPARISON OF CROHN'S DISEASE INVOLVING THE COLON, ULCERATIVE COLITIS, AND ISCHEMIC COLITIS: TYPICAL HISTOPATHOLOGIC ABNORMALITIES

	Crohn's Disease	Ulcerative Colitis	Ischemic Colitis
Mucosa (Including Endoscopic Biopsies)			
Distal predominance	Occasional	Usual	Rare
Atrophy with crypt loss, distortion and shortfall	Sometimes	Often	Occasionally
"Follicular proctitis"	Rare	Sometimes	Absent
Vascularity	Occasional	Prominent with activity	Prominent in acute phase
Crypt abscesses	Common	Usual	Often
Diffuse chronic inflammation	Sometimes: with prominent lymphocytes in clusters	Often: with prominent plasma cells	Occasional
Focal active inflammation	Common	Occasional	Common
Ulcers	Discrete: fissuring or aphthoid	In abnormal mucosa	Discrete or in abnormal mucosa
Granulomas	Common: non-caseating epithelioid cells	Rare: foreign body reaction	Rare: foreign body reaction
Coagulative necrosis, intravascular thrombi and hemorrhage	Rare: with fulminant disease	Rare: with fulminant colitis	Common in acute phase
Goblet cell mucin depletion	Occasional	Prominent with activity	Sometimes in acute phase
Paneth cell metaplasia	Occasional	Sometimes	Rare
Hemosiderin-laden macrophages	Rare	Rare	Common as sequela of hemorrhage
Colonic Wall			
Transmural lymphoid aggregates	Usual	Occasional: with deep ulcers in fulminant colitis	Sometimes
Submucosal widening	Common: edema, lymphangiectasia, fibrosis	Rare	Common: with edema
Non-caseating granulomas	Common: bowel wall and lymph nodes	Very rare	Very rare
Neural hyperplasia	Common	Rare	Variable
Vasculitis	Sometimes	Rare: in fulminant colitis	Common: with transmural necrosis
Necrosis of muscularis propria	Rare: in fulminant disease	Rare: in fulminant colitis	Common
Fibrosis of muscularis propria	Rare	Absent	Common: with stricture

lar disease can be extremely difficult. Such distinction is important for surgical therapy, however, as postoperative complications are more common in patients with both diseases than in those with diverticular disease alone.[65,66] Radiologically, Crohn's disease in the presence of diverticular disease is suggested by fissuring ulceration or an internal fistula (other than a colovesical fistula, which may occur with simple diverticulitis). Clinically, the presence of anal lesions compatible with Crohn's disease or of active inflammatory bowel disease in biopsy specimens taken at sites other than the segment with diverticula suggests Crohn's disease. Examination of a resection specimen is sometimes needed for definitive diagnosis, but the presence of foreign body reaction around pericolic abscesses may complicate interpretation.

Exogenous Agent–Related Inflammatory Bowel Disease. A large number of exogenous agents can produce inflammatory bowel disease that can be confused with Crohn's disease and ulcerative colitis, particularly in endoscopic biopsy specimens. These agents include cytotoxic drugs such as 5-fluorouracil, heavy metals such as mercury and gold, foodstuffs and drugs to which allergy has developed, and acute ionizing radiation.[67–70] The patient's history is usually the most important factor in correct diagnosis.

Non-granulomatous Ulcerative Jejunoileitis. This "entity" is a clinically defined syndrome. The pathologic findings overlap with those of Crohn's disease of the small bowel, except that granulomas are not found.[1]

Behçet's Disease.[71, 72] Gastrointestinal tract involvement in this disorder resembles Crohn's disease. However, the multisystem nature of Behçet's disease allows its recognition.

Solitary Ulcer Syndrome.[73, 74] The occurrence of a discrete rectal ulcer in this condition may suggest Crohn's disease. Biopsy of the base of the ulcer shows non-specific inflamed granulation tissue, but the mucosa at the edge demonstrates characteristic smooth muscle proliferation from the muscularis mucosae throughout the lamina propria surrounding the crypts. The mucosa containing the prominent smooth muscle usually has elongated irregular crypts with reactive epithelial changes. Glands may be entrapped in the submucosa, producing colitis cystica profunda.

Collagenous Colitis.[75] Specimens from patients with this condition show a thick band of fibrous tissue in the lamina propria beneath the luminal surface epithelium.

Lymphoma. The clinical features of this neoplasm in the small and large bowel may simulate Crohn's disease[76] (Chapter 112). Rectal biopsies showing evidence of Crohn's disease appear to be helpful in the differential diagnosis.[77]

Ulcerative Colitis. Distinction between the 2 major forms of idiopathic inflammatory bowel disease, ulcerative colitis and Crohn's disease with colonic involvement, is a frequent problem in gastroenterology (Chapter 126). Differential diagnosis has been extensively described in the literature.[1, 10–17, 78, 79] Comparison of the pathologic features of Crohn's disease and ulcerative colitis (as well as ischemic colitis) is summarized in Tables 127–1 and 127–2. *Separation of the different types of inflammatory bowel disease often depends as much on quantitative as on qualitative differences that contribute to contrasting pathologic patterns.* The pathologic features that most reliably distinguish Crohn's disease from ulcerative colitis are shown in Table 127–3. It should be kept in mind, however, that occasional patients with both Crohn's disease and ulcerative colitis have been reported.[80]

Table 127–3. PATHOLOGIC FINDINGS THAT MOST RELIABLY FAVOR CROHN'S DISEASE INVOLVING THE COLON RATHER THAN ULCERATIVE COLITIS

1. Non-caseating epithelioid cell granulomas*
2. Transmural inflammation with lymphoid aggregates
3. Discontinous segmental involvement*
4. Right-sided predominance*
5. Rectal sparing*
6. Discrete ulcers*
7. Fissuring ulcers*
8. Aphthoid erosions or ulcers*
9. Linear ulcers
10. Active ileal inflammation*
11. Stricture due to fibrosis
12. Fistula lined by granulation tissue
13. Focal non-specific active mucosal inflammation*
14. Disproportionate submucosal inflammation*

*Detectable in colonoscopic biopsies of ileum, colon, and rectum.

Inflammatory Bowel Disease of Indeterminate Type. This term is used to indicate that a patient has inflammatory bowel disease for which the etiology or classification has not been determined. "Inflammatory bowel disease of indeterminate type" is not an entity but an expression of uncertainty regarding diagnosis. The term may be applied in 2 main clinical settings: (1) a patient presenting with inflammatory bowel disease in whom the entire range of diagnostic possibilities must be considered; and (2) a patient with idiopathic inflammatory bowel disease in whom no decision between Crohn's disease involving the colon and ulcerative colitis can be made.[81] The latter setting usually results from inconsistent combinations of the findings in Tables 127–1 to 127–3, particularly in endoscopic biopsy specimens or in patients with fulminant colitis. The classification as indeterminate is often temporary; the patient's course, as well as review of previous and subsequent biopsy or resection specimens, often results in categorization.

References

1. Morson BC, Dawson IMP. Gastrointestinal Pathology. 2nd Ed. Oxford: Blackwell, 1979.
2. Rowland R, Pounder DJ. Crohn's colitis. *In*: Sommers SC, Rosen PP, eds. Pathology Annual 1982, Part 1. Volume 17. Norwalk, Conn: Appleton-Century-Crofts, 1982: 267–90.
3. Simonowitz DA, Rusch VW, Stevenson JK. Natural history of incidental appendectomy in patients with Crohn's disease

who required subsequent bowel resection. Am J Surg 1982; 143:171–3.
4. Williams DR, Coller JA, Corman ML, Nugent FW, Vendenheimer MC. Anal complications in Crohn's disease. Dis Colon Rectum 1981; 24:22–4.
5. Scully C, Cochran KM, Russell RI, Ferguson MM, Ghouri MAK, Lee FD, MacDonald DG, McIntyre PB. Crohn's disease of the mouth—an indicator of intestinal involvement. Gut 1982; 23:198–202.
6. Haggitt RC, Meissner WA. Crohn's disease of the upper gastrointestinal tract. Am J Clin Pathol 1973; 613–2.
7. Madden JL, Ravid JM, Haddad JR. Regional esophagitis: A specific entity simulating Crohn's disease. Ann Surg 1969; 170:351–5.
8. Fielding JF, Toye DKM, Beton DC, Cooke WT. Crohn's disease of the stomach and duodenum. Gut 1970; 11:1001–6.
9. Bishop AE, Polak JM, Bryant MG, Bloom SR, Hamilton S. Abnormalities of vasoactive intestinal polypeptide–containing nerves in Crohn's disease. Gastroenterology 1980; 79:853–60.
10. Yardley JH, Donowitz M. Colo-rectal biopsy in inflammatory bowel disease. *In*: Yardley JH, Morson BC, Abell MR, eds. The Gastrointestinal Tract. International Academy of Pathology, Monograph No 18. Baltimore: Williams and Wilkins, 1977:50–94.
11. Whitehead R. Mucosal Biopsy of the Gastrointestinal Tract. 2nd Ed. Philadelphia: WB Saunders, 1979.
12. Mitros FA. The biopsy in evaluating patients with inflammatory bowel disease. Med Clin North Am 1980; 64:1037–57.
13. Surawicz CM, Meisel JL, Ylvisakev Y, Saunders DR, Rubin CE. Rectal biopsy in the diagnosis of Crohn's disease: value of multiple biopsies and serial sectioning. Gastroenterology 1981; 80:66–71.
14. Rotterdam H, Sommers SC. Biopsy Diagnosis of the Digestive Tract. New York: Raven Press, 1981.
15. Iliffe GD, Owen DA. Rectal biopsy in Crohn's disease. Dig Dis Sci 1981; 26:321–4.
16. Hamilton SR. Diagnosis and comparison of ulcerative colitis and Crohn's disease involving the colon. *In*: Norris HT, ed. Pathology of the Colon, Small Intestine, and Anus. Vol 2. New York: Churchill-Livingstone, 1983:1–19.
17. Watier A, Devroede G, Perey B, Haddad H, Madarnos P, Grand-Maison P. Small erythematous mucosal plaques: An endoscopic sign of Crohn's disease. Gut 1980; 21:835–9.
18. Frei JV, Morson BC. Medical audit of rectal biopsy diagnosis of inflammatory bowel disease. Gut 1982; 25:341–4.
19. Riddell RH. Personal communication.
20. Yardley JH, Hamilton SR. Focal nonspecific inflammation in Crohn's disease. *In*: Pena AS, Waterman IT, Booth CC, Strober W, eds. Recent Advances in Crohn's Disease. Developments in Gastroenterology, Vol 1. The Hague: Martinus Nijhoff, 1981: 62–6.
21. Rickert RR, Carter HW. The "early" ulcerative lesion of Crohn's disease: Correlative light and scanning electron microscopic studies. J Clin Gastroenterol 1980; 2:11–9.
22. Dvorak AM, Connell AB, Dickerson GR. Crohn's disease: A scanning electron microscopic study. Human Pathol 1979; 10:165–77.
23. Kaye MD, Brady AR, Whorwell PJ, Beeken WL. Scanning electron microscopy of rectal mucosa in Crohn's disease. Am J Dig Dis 1979; 24:369–75.
24. Myllarneimi H, Nickels J. Scanning electron microscopy of Crohn's disease and ulcerative colitis of the colon. Virchows Arch A Pathol Anat Histol 1980; 385:343–50.
25. Rotterdam H, Korelitz BI, Sommers SC. Microgranulomas in grossly normal rectal mucosa in Crohn's disease. Am J Clin Pathol 1977; 67:550–4.
26. Elliott PR, Williams CB, Lennard-Jones JE, Dawson AM, Bartram CI, Thomas BM, Swarbrick ET, Morson BC. Colonoscopic diagnosis of minimal change colitis in patients with a normal sigmoidoscopy and normal air-contrast barium enema. Lancet 1982; 1:650–1.
27. Hamilton SR, Bussey HJR, Boitnott JK, Morson BC. Active inflammation and granulomas in grossly uninvolved colonic mucosa of Crohn's disease resection specimens studied with *en face* histologic technique. Gastroenterology 1981; 80:1167.
28. Goodman MJ, Skinner JM, Truelove SC. Abnormalities in the apparently normal bowel mucosa in Crohn's disease. Lancet 1976; 1:275–8.
29. Dunne WT, Cooke WT, Allan RN. Enzymatic and morphometric evidence for Crohn's disease as a diffuse lesion of the gastrointestinal tract. Gut 1977; 18:290–4.
30. Sommers SC, Korelitz BI. Duodenal biopsy cell counts and histopathology in Crohn's disease. *In*: Pena AS, Neterman IT, Booth CC, Strober W, eds. Recent Advances in Crohn's Disease. Developments in Gastroenterology, Vol 1. The Hague: Martinus Nijhoff, 1981: 47–51.
31. Owen RL, Nemanic P. Antigen processing structures of the mammalian intestinal tract: a SEM study of lymphoepithelial organs. Scan Electron Microsc 1978; 2:367–78.
32. Chambers TJ. Multinucleated giant cells. J Pathol 1978; 126:125–48.
33. Knill-Jones RP, Morson B, Williams R. Prestomal ileitis: clinical and pathological findings in five cases. Q J Med 1970; 39:287–97.
34. Bonello JC, Thow GB, Manson RR. Mucosal enteritis: a complication of the continent ileostomy. Dis Colon Rectum 1981; 24:37–41.
35. Glotzer DJ, Glick ME, Goldman H. Proctitis and colitis following diversion of the fecal stream. Gastroenterology 1981; 80:433–7.
36. Glotzer DJ. Recurrence in Crohn's colitis: The numbers game. World J Surg 1980; 4:173–82.
37. Hamilton SR. Unpublished observations.
38. Rutgeerts P, Coenegrachts JL, Geboes K, Kerremans R, Vantrappen G. Prospective endoscopic follow-up of the ileocolonic anastomosis after curative resection for Crohn's disease. Acta Endosc (in press).
39. Koch TR, Cave DR, Ford H, Kirsner JB. Crohn's ileitis and ileocolitis: A study of the anatomical distribution of recurrence. Dig Dis Sci 1981; 26:528–31.
40. Glass RE, Baker NW. Role of the granuloma in recurrent Crohn's disease. Gut 1976; 17:75–7.
41. Chambers TJ, Morson BC. The granuloma in Crohn's disease. Gut 1979; 20:269–74.
42. Wolfson DM, Sachar DB, Cohen A, Goldberg J, Styczynski R, Greenstein AJ, Gelernt IM, Janowitz HP. Granulomas do not affect postoperative recurrence rates in Crohn's disease. Gastroenterology 1982; 83:405–9.
43. Hamilton SR. Pathologic features of Crohn's disease associated with recrudescence after resection. *In*: Sommers SC, Rosen PP, eds. Pathology Annual 1983. Norwalk, Conn: Appleton-Century-Crofts, 1983:191–203.
44. Wenckert A, Kristensen M, Eklund AE, Barany F, Jarnum S, Worning H, Folkenberg O, Holtz A, Bonnevie O, Riis P. The long-term prophylactic effect of salazosulphapyridine (Salazopyrin) in primarily resected patients with Crohn's disease: a controlled double-blind trial. Scand J Gastroenterol 1978; 13:161–7.
45. Jess P. Acute terminal ileitis: a review of recent literature on the relationship to Crohn's disease. Scand J Gastroenterol 1981; 16:321–4.
46. Gyde SW, Prior P, MaCartney JC, Thompson H, Waterhouse JAH, Allan RN. Malignancy in Crohn's disease. Gut 1980; 21:1024–9.
47. Craft CI, Mendelsohn G, Cooper HS, Yardley JH. Colonic "precancer" in Crohn's disease. Gastroenterology 1981; 80:578–84.
48. Simpson S, Traube J, Riddell RH. The histologic appearance of dysplasia (precarcinomatous change) in Crohn's disease of the small and large intestine. Gastroenterology 1981; 81:492–501.
49. Greenstein AJ, Sachar D, Pucillo A, Kreel I, Geller S, Janowitz HD, Aufses A. Cancer in Crohn's disease after diversionary surgery. A report of seven cases occurring in excluded bowel. Am J Surg 1978; 135:86–91.
50. Haggitt R. The differential diagnosis of idiopathic inflammatory bowel disease. *In*: Norris HT, ed. Pathology of the Colon, Small Intestine, and Anus. New York: Churchill-Livingstone, 1983:21–59.
51. Quinn TC, Goodell SE, Mkrtichian E, Schuffler MD, Wang SP, Stamm WE, Holmes KK. Chlamydia trachomatis proctitis. N Engl J Med 1981; 303:195–200.
52. Saad EA, deGouveia OF, Filho PD, Teixeira D, Pereira AA,

Erthal A. Anorecto-colonic lymphogranuloma venereum. Gastroenterologia 1962; 97:89–102.
53. Strano AJ. Lymphogranuloma venereum. *In*: Binford CH, Connor DH, eds. Pathology of Tropical and Extraordinary Diseases, Vol 1. Washington, DC: Armed Forces Institute of Pathology, 1976: 82–4.
54. VanTrappen G, Agg HO, Ponette E, Geboes K, Bertrand P. Yersinia enteritis and enterocolitis: gastrointestinal aspects. Gastroenterology 1977; 72:220–7.
55. Loss RW, Mangla JC, Pereira M. Campylobacter colitis presenting as inflammatory bowel disease with segmental colonic ulcerations. Gastroenterology 1980; 79:138–40.
56. Coffin CM, L'Heureaux P, Dehner LP. Campylobacter-associated associated enterocolitis in childhood: report of a fatal case. Am J Clin Pathol 1982; 78:117–23.
57. Giannella RA. Pathogenesis of acute bacterial diarrheal disorders. Ann Rev Med 1981; 32:341–57.
58. Day DW, Mandal BK, Morson BC. The rectal biopsy appearances in Salmonella colitis. Histopathology 1978; 2:117–31.
59. Bartlett JG. *Clostridium difficile* and inflammatory bowel disease. Gastroenterology 1981; 80:863–5.
60. Pittman FE, El-Hashimi WK, Pittman JC. Studies of human amebiasis. II. Light and electron microscopic observation of colonic mucosa and exudate in acute amebic colitis. Gastroenterology 1973; 65:588–603.
61. McCully RM, Barron CN, Cheever AW. Schistosomiasis (bilharziasis). *In*: Binford CH, Connor DH, eds. Pathology of Tropical and Extraordinary Diseases, Vol 2. Washington, DC: Armed Forces Institute of Pathology, 1976: 482–508.
62. Weinstein L, Edelstein SM, Madara JL, Falchuk KR, McManus BM, Trier JS. Intestinal cryptosporidiosis complicated by disseminated cytomegalovirus infection. Gastroenterology 1981; 81:584–91.
63. Keren DF, Milligan FD, Strandberg JD, Yardley JH. Intercurrent cytomegalovirus colitis in a patient with ulcerative colitis. Johns Hopkins Med J 1975; 136:178–82.
64. Norris HT. Ischemic bowel disease: Its spectrum. *In*: Yardley JH, Morson BC, Abell MR, eds. The Gastrointestinal Tract. International Academy of Pathology, Monograph No 18. Baltimore: Williams and Wilkins, 1977: 15–30.
65. Schmidt GT, Lennard-Jones JE, Morson BC, Young AC. Crohn's disease of the colon and its distinction from diverticulitis. Gut 1968; 9:7–16.
66. Gelb AM, Finkelstein WE. Differential diagnosis of diverticulitis and granulomatous colitis: Exacerbation of granulomatous colitis after sigmoid resection. Am J Gastroenterol 1974; 62:9–15.
67. Gelfand MD, Tepper M, Katz LA, Binder HJ, Yesner R, Floch M. Acute irradiation proctitis in man; development of eosinophilic crypt abscesses. Gastroenterology 1968; 54:401–11.
68. Rosekrans PCM, Meijer CJLM, VanderWal AM, Lindeman J. Allergic proctitis, a clinical and immunopathological entity. Gut 1980; 21:1017–23.
69. Graham CF, Gallagher K, Jones JK. Acute colitis with methyldopa. N Engl J Med 1981; 304:1044–5.
70. Lake AM, Whittington PF, Hamilton SR. Dietary protein-induced colitis in breast-fed infants. J Pediatr, 1982; 101:906–10.
71. Dilsen N, Konice M, Ovul C, eds. Behçet's Syndrome. Proceedings of an International Symposium on Behçet's Disease. New York: Elsevier North Holland, 1979.
72. Kasahara Y, Tanaka S, Nishino M, Unemura H, Shiraha S, Kuygama T. Intestinal involvement in Behçet's disease: Review of 136 surgical cases in the Japanese literature. Dis Colon Rectum 1981; 24:103–6.
73. Rutter KRP, Riddell RH. The solitary ulcer syndrome of the rectum. Clin Gastroenterol 1975; 4:505–30.
74. Feczko PJ, O'Connell DJ, Riddell RH, Frank PH. Solitary rectal ulcer syndrome: radiologic manifestations. AJR 1980; 135:499–506.
75. Guller R, Anabitarte M. Die Kollagenkolitis. Ein neues krankheitsbild oden blosse histologische abnormitat. Schweiz Med Wochenschr 1981; 111:1076–9.
76. Wen AB, Poon M, Groarke JF, Wilkerson JA. Lymphoma simulating Crohn's colitis. Dig Dis Sci 1980; 25:69–72.
77. Hyams JS, Goldman H, Katz AJ. Differentiating small bowel Crohn's disease from lymphoma: Role of rectal biopsy. Gastroenterology 1980; 79:340–3.
78. Cook MG, Dixon MF. An analysis of the reliability of detection and diagnostic value of various pathological features in Crohn's disease and ulcerative colitis. Gut 1973; 14:255–62.
79. Price AB, Morson BC. Inflammatory bowel disease: The surgical pathology of Crohn's disease and ulcerative colitis. Human Pathol 1975; 6:7–30.
80. Eyer S, Spadaccini C, Walker P, Ansel H, Schwartz M, Summer HW. Simultaneous ulcerative colitis and Crohn's disease. Am J Gastroenterol 1980; 73:345–7.
81. Price AB. Difficulties in the differential diagnosis of ulcerative colitis and Crohn's disease. *In*: Yardley JH, Morson BC, Abell MR, eds. The Gastrointestinal Tract. International Academy of Pathology, Monograph No 18. Baltimore: Williams and Wilkins, 1977: 1–14.

Clinical Features

Samuel Meyers • Henry D. Janowitz

General Features

Crohn's disease is a chronic, insidious disorder that may be manifested in a wide variety of ways, making diagnosis difficult and often delayed. The particular complex of clinical features experienced by an individual patient is determined by many factors. The severity and extent of the underlying bowel inflammation are important. These factors result in malaise, lassitude, anorexia, nausea, vomiting, weight loss, malnutrition, fever, and/or chills. In more chronic cases the inflammation leads to scarring and formation of a fixed stricture. Features of mechanical intestinal obstruction will then be superimposed upon those of the inflammation or may even predominate in the clinical picture. When the disease is active, patients usually appear ill, weak, and pale. There may be minimal to severe abdominal tenderness, which can be diffuse or located in the right lower quadrant or over areas of diseased bowel. A sense of fullness may be noted, and loops of bowel, a mass of matted mesentery, and/or an abscess may be palpable. Examination may demonstrate one or more complications, such as malnutrition, bleeding, perforation, obstruction, perianal disease, or evidence of the extraintestinal manifestations of Crohn's disease.

Influence of Disease Location

There are extensive functional and morphologic data suggesting that the entire alimentary canal is involved in every case of Crohn's disease.[1-3] Lesions seen by clinical examination represent only those locations where the disease is most advanced. The visible anatomic disease location is, however, important in determining the clinical effects of the inflammatory and scarring lesions.

Ileal or Colonic Disease. The ileum and colon are most commonly the sites of obvious Crohn's disease, accounting for up to 100% of all cases in many medical centers. Even when disease is located in other areas, there is generally concomitant disease of the ileum or colon. In unusual cases, isolated proximal bowel disease occurs alone or precedes the development of distal lesions. Representative experience reported in the medical literature,[4-6] including our patient population at the Mount Sinai Hospital, New York, is given in Table 127–4.

Many patients with disease in any of these areas share the same clinical features, including diarrhea, abdominal pain, and weight loss. Yet, location of disease is a major determinant of symptoms, clinical course, and prognosis in an individual case. Involvement of the small bowel generally has the best prognosis. Abdominal abscess and intestinal obstruction are the major hazards. Perianal fistula, internal abscess and fistula, and intestinal obstruction are the more common features in those with disease of the ileum and colon. Patients in whom colitis predominates more commonly note rectal bleeding, perianal fistula, toxic megacolon, and extraintestinal complications involving the skin and joints. The frequency of clinical manifestations according to disease location is described in a study reported from the Cleveland Clinic and shown in Table 127–5. The need for surgery is also related to the initial site of disease; 73% of patients with ileocolitis required surgery during follow-up, compared with only 51% of those with ileitis or colitis.[4]

Oral Disease. Oral lesions occur in from 6% to 20% of patients with Crohn's disease.[8] They are most frequent among patients with active colonic or ileocolonic involvement, as opposed to those with disease of the small bowel only, and are especially frequent in those who have other extraintestinal manifestations. These lesions may result in rather severe pain or may be asymptomatic and may have one of several appearances. Typical aphthous ulcers can appear anywhere in the buccal mucosa; they are superficial, single or multiple, and vary in size from 1 to 15 mm. Inflammation may result in diffuse swelling of the lips and cheeks or a cobblestone appearance of the oral mucosa. Deep linear ulcers with hyperplastic margins may appear, especially in the buccal sinuses. Indurated fissures on the midline of the lower lip

Table 127–4. INITIAL ANATOMIC SITE OF CROHN'S DISEASE

Report	Number of Patients	Disease Location: *Distal Small Bowel*	*Small Bowel and Colon*	*Colon*	*Other**
Farmer et al.[4]	615	168 (27%)	252 (41%)	166 (27%)	29 (5%)
Mekhjian et al.[5]	569	162 (28%)	314 (55%)	60 (10%)	33 (5%)
Admans et al.[6]	140	61 (44%)	30 (21%)	40 (29%)	9 (6%)
Greenstein et al.[7]	1010	383 (37%)	455 (45%)	171 (18%)	0

*Disease confined to stomach, duodenum, jejunum, appendix, or anal-rectal area.

Table 127–5. FREQUENCY OF CLINICAL FEATURES IN CROHN'S DISEASE*

Clinical Feature	Disease Location		
	Ileitis	*Ileo-colitis*	*Colitis*
Diarrhea	Virtually all patients		
Abdominal pain	65%	62%	55%
Bleeding	22%	10%	46%
Weight loss	12%	19%	22%
Perianal disease	14%	38%	36%
Internal fistulas	17%	34%	16%
Intestinal obstruction	35%	44%	17%
Megacolon	0	2%	11%

*According to data of Farmer et al.[4]

may also develop.[9] Other less specific oral lesions may be due to malnutrition, immunocompromise, or adverse drug reactions. These lesions include glossitis, macroglossia, and oral moniliasis.

Periodontal disease may occur in association with intestinal Crohn's disease. Manifestations include pain, gingival bleeding, and tooth mobility. Examination shows marginal necrosis of the teeth, disruption of the gingival architecture, gingival cratering, and tooth mobility. Roentgen examination demonstrates alveolar bone loss. Diminished neutrophil function with release of lysozyme enzyme in these patients results in resorption of alveolar bone and is postulated to be important in the etiology of the periodontal disease.[10]

Rarely, the disease involves the pharynx or even the esophagus,[11–12] resulting in pain, dysphagia, and odynophagia. The mucosa is erythematous, friable, and often nodular. In the esophagus, a stricture may result from the chronic inflammation[13]; in one case, the stricture occurred within an area of columnar epithelium (Barrett's esophagus).[14] We are aware of 2 patients whose ulceration of the mid-esophagus led to a fistula into the bronchial tree.

Gastroduodenal Disease. Gastric and duodenal Crohn's disease are uncommon, the reported frequency ranging from 0.5% to 4%.[15, 16] Involvement of the stomach results in pain, weight loss, and/or gastric outlet obstruction. There is a propensity for the antrum to be primarily involved, leading to deformity, tubular narrowing, limited distensibility, poor peristalsis, or frank obstruction. These factors combine to give the stomach an unusual but characteristic roentgenologic tubular shape with conical narrowing. The mucosa may show a cobblestone, ulcerated, or atrophic appearance. Gastric analysis occasionally reveals hypochlorhydria or achlorhydria, depending on the extent of gastric inflammation. Duodenal involvement similarly results in epigastric pain, with or without features of obstruction.[17] The mucosal inflammation results in a thickened or ulcerated appearance on roentgen examination.

The clinical behavior of gastroduodenal Crohn's disease may raise suspicion of peptic ulcer disease or even malignancy. The differential diagnosis is especially difficult when more distal Crohn's disease is not recognized or is absent. Careful evaluation, including radiography, endoscopy, and biopsy, should provide the correct diagnosis. Ulcerating Crohn's disease of the duodenum may be complicated by pancreatitis, which further confuses the clinical picture.[18]

Diffuse Small Bowel Disease. Diffuse jejunoileitis or even disease of the entire gastrointestinal tract may occur.[19, 20] The clinical consequences ordinarily correlate well with the areas of anatomic disease.[19] In addition to the usual problems related to the inflammatory and obstructive nature of Crohn's disease, consequences of diminished absorptive function and enhanced gut permeability assume clinical importance. These include anemia, vitamin and mineral deficiency, protein-losing enteropathy, hypoalbuminemia, steatorrhea, gallstones, and kidney stones.

Rectal Disease. Many clinicians regard rectal sparing as an important clinical feature of colonic Crohn's disease. This idea is not reliable, however, as *the rectum may be involved in 50% of cases and may be the only site of Crohn's disease in more than 11% of cases.*[21] Patients with rectal disease are generally older; two-thirds are over 50 years of age. Common clinical symptoms are diarrhea (79%), rectal bleeding (66%), and associated perianal disease (57%). Fibrosis and stricture formation may ensue, similar to features of Crohn's disease in other locations. These changes may result in intractable constipation.[20]

Appendiceal Disease. Involvement of the appendix in conjunction with adjacent ileal or colonic disease is common in Crohn's disease, occurring in up to 50% of cases.[22]

This is not surprising, as the appendix is developmentally similar to the colon. Isolated Crohn's disease of the appendix is much less common. These cases present clinically as acute appendicitis, with or without abscess or a cecal mass. One case with only bloody stools has been reported.[23] Generally, the true nature of the disease is not suspected, although it should be when the clinical course is protracted beyond 5 days. At surgery, the appendix appears markedly enlarged and indurated, similar to the mural thickening of typical ileal Crohn's disease.[24] Pathologic examination of the appendix confirms the diagnosis by showing acute inflammation with granuloma. Little is known of the subsequent course of patients found to have granulomatous appendicitis. Our suspicion is that their course is benign.

A controversial question has been the approach to a patient with appendicitis in whom ileitis is found at laparotomy. Most physicians favor appendectomy, since this makes evaluation of future abdominal pain easier and obviates the development of gangrenous appendicitis. The main concern in performing surgery is that a fistula will result from the appendectomy site.[25] However, evidence suggests that the risk of such fistula formation is similar to that after a simple laparotomy when the cecum is normal.[24, 26] When a fecal fistula does develop, it is the result of manipulating the small bowel and not because of the appendectomy.

Miliary Crohn's Disease

This is an unusual variant of Crohn's disease in which macroscopic miliary nodules stud the serosal surface of the small intestine.[27] The patient presents with abdominal pain, weight loss, diarrhea, fever, and other signs of intestinal inflammation. The gastrointestinal roentgen series shows abnormalities of the proximal and/or distal small bowel. Multiple nodules are visualized that often suggest a lymphoreticular neoplasm. The final diagnosis is usually not established until tissue removed at surgery is examined and the typical histologic features of Crohn's disease are seen. The etiology of this multinodular variant is unknown.

Crohn's Disease in the Elderly

The peak prevalence of Crohn's disease is prior to 35 years of age, with a subsequent decrease in frequency thereafter. Although patients older than 50 years can be affected, the diagnosis in most cases was made initially at an earlier age. Some of those over 50 years of age in whom disease develops *de novo* will in fact have ischemic bowel disease.[28] Older patients with true Crohn's disease have a clinical course with many similarities to younger patients, including presenting symptoms and systemic biochemical abnormalities.[29] However, there is a change in the disease location in the older group, with increased frequency of left colonic involvement. The duration of symptoms before diagnosis is also shorter, and various complications such as hemorrhage, operative recurrences, and medical or surgical therapeutic failures are more common. The rate of fistula formation, however, diminishes with age. The need for surgery is similar to that in the younger age group, attesting to the severity of the disease in the elderly.[29] Mortality from the disease is greater in older persons.

Crohn's Disease in Children and Adolescents

Although unusual in children, Crohn's disease has been reported as early as 4 years of age in a patient who had symptoms since age 2. The prevalence in younger groups has been increasing in recent years. Children may have any or all of the symptoms and signs seen in the adult. They may additionally suffer a delay in linear growth or sexual maturation; occasionally this is their only disease manifestation. Growth failure occurs in 20% to 30% of prepubertal patients and is more often associated with diffuse small intestinal disease than with other forms.[30] Corticosteroid exposure may explain some growth suppression but is not sufficient to explain the growth failure apparent before therapy or during periods of disease remission. Anorexia or fear of exacerbating abdominal pain and diarrhea reduces caloric intake, which is the major etiologic factor in the growth retardation of Crohn's disease.[31] Patients with even relatively stable Crohn's disease ingest only 82% or less of expected caloric intake. Combined parenteral and oral supplemental feedings providing 130% of estimated required calories will promote growth.[31] Normal endocrine status has been documented in patients with growth failure.[32]

Factors Exacerbating Crohn's Disease

A definite relationship exists between stressful life events and the onset of symptomatic disease.[33–35] Birth, death, or other situations of loss or gain of a love object, whether actual, threatened, symbolic, or fantasied, were noted to have occurred within the year preceding disease onset in 94% of one group of patients. Upper respiratory tract infection has been associated with the relapse of chronic established disease.[34] There is no clear association with other miscellaneous infections, atopy, or dietary indiscretions. A variety of enteric infections have been thought to induce relapse, including those caused by Salmonella, Shigella, Entamoeba histolytica, Campylobacter, and Giardia.[36] It has also been suggested that the intestinal microbial flora may be altered in chronic inflammatory bowel disease to favor the proliferation of *Clostridium difficile*,[37] with or without prior antibiotic exposure. The toxin synthesized by this organism further injures the mucosa and contributes to the underlying bowel disease. Studies at the Mount Sinai Hospital, however, found *C. difficile* toxin only in patients who had been exposed to antimicrobials within the preceding 2 months.[38] The presence of the toxin was not correlated with disease severity and seemed unlikely to be a significant contributory factor in Crohn's disease.

Psychologic Aspects. There appears to be a relationship between several psychologic variables or personality characteristics and Crohn's disease.[39] Whether these factors are important in the etiology, course, or exacerbation of disease or are only epiphenomena remains unknown. Dependency is the most frequently reported characteristic. Repressed rage, suppression of feelings, and anxieties are also commonly noted. Many patients are said to have a constant desire "to be rid of" events in their lives. This characteristic can be acted out through the physical symptom of diarrhea. Crohn's disease patients are often found in the middle of complex social situations, playing the role of peacemaker. Other mentioned characteristics include emotional immaturity, depression, and obsessive compulsiveness. Approximately one-third of Crohn's disease patients demonstrate appreciable psychiatric morbidity. The prevalence of the latter increases with advanced chronicity and severity of the bowel disease. There is evidence, however, that the degree and prevalence of psychiatric disturbances are similar to those in other chronic medical diseases.

Marital adjustment is similar to healthy control or irritable bowel syndrome groups.[40] Women have fewer multiple marriages and the total group with Crohn's disease is somewhat less likely to be married. Crohn's disease patients seem somewhat uninterested in sexual relationships, but have no major sexual problems.[41] Educational, vocational, and other social adjustments are not different from control groups.[40] There is very little information on how these social factors relate to disease severity, chronicity, or therapy. Most people continue to lead optimistic, useful lives. They continue to work and hope that their disease will not deteriorate. Their marital and other relationships are normal, or even better in many cases. Successful adaptation of patients to their chronic disease is found to be more closely related to their personality than to their disease.[42]

Acute Ileitis

This presents with fever, right lower quadrant or periumbilical pain, diarrhea, nausea, and vomiting. These features, as well as the laboratory data, closely simulate an attack of acute appendicitis. The acute episode usually resolves spontaneously and does not show the chronicity of typical Crohn's disease.[43] However, the acute ileitis that is destined to resolve and that which will develop into true Crohn's disease cannot be easily distinguished preoperatively. Up to 20% of patients with this acute presentation go on to develop typical Crohn's disease. An important predictive factor in these cases is the presence of some chronic, vague, subtle symptoms on careful questioning.

The most common identifiable cause of acute terminal ileitis is infection by *Yersinia enterocolitica*.[44] The appendix and the cecum can be affected as well as the colon, but this presentation rarely mimics colonic Crohn's disease. Tuberculosis, tularemia, amebiasis, actinomycosis, histoplasmosis, and infection with the larvae of the fish nematode *Anisakis* may also cause acute ileitis.

Diagnosis

Signs and Symptoms. The diagnosis of Crohn's disease is often extremely difficult. The many manifestations, often vague, may not initially suggest the proper diagnosis. The key to the proper identification is a high index of suspicion, which should be aroused by the characteristic history of chronic diarrhea, abdominal pain, anorexia, weight loss, fever, or other symptoms reflecting the underlying inflammatory and fibrotic processes. A history of perianal problems, such as fissures, fistulas, or abscesses, or extraintestinal manifestations affecting the skin, eyes, or joints increases the likelihood of Crohn's disease. A pale, thin appearance consistent with a chronic illness or the finding of an abdominal mass or tenderness, cutaneous fistulas, or other complications likewise suggests Crohn's disease. Among younger patients, evidence of retarded growth or failure of the development of secondary sex characteristics raises suspicion even higher.

Laboratory Findings. The peripheral blood count may reveal a mild to moderate anemia, characteristic of chronic illness. Deficiencies of iron, vitamin B_{12}, or folate may be contributing factors. The white blood cell count is usually normal, but may be high in the presence of a suppurative complication, either within or beyond the confines of the bowel wall. Marked thrombocytosis, with platelet counts over 1 million/mm^3 may occur. This correlates with clinical disease activity and the degree of inflammation. Thrombotic complications or bleeding can arise secondary to the elevated platelet counts.[45] The erythrocyte sedimentation rate may provide useful information regarding disease activity.[6] The majority of patients with clinical activity have a sedimentation rate over 20 mm/hour, especially those with colonic disease. Over one-third of patients with severe disease confined to the small bowel will have normal values.[6] Electrolyte and mineral abnormalities are common; hyponatremia, hypokalemia, hypocalcemia (often reflecting low serum albumin levels), and hypomagnesemia may be present.[46] Serum lysozyme activity is increased in many granulomatous diseases, such as tuberculosis and sarcoidosis. Levels have been reported to be higher among those with Crohn's disease than among either patients with ulcerative colitis or normal subjects.[47, 48] This assay, touted as useful in diagnosis and determination of disease extent, has been abandoned after reports appeared documenting its limited value.[49, 50] Serum angiotensin converting enzyme is another marker of granulomatous disease that is elevated in sarcoidosis, leprosy, Gaucher's disease, primary biliary cirrhosis, silicosis, and asbestosis. The activities in Crohn's disease, however, are either normal or reduced.[51–53] Minor abnormalities of the standard liver tests may indicate hepatic steatosis. More profound changes may indicate pericholangitis or other serious hepatic complications.

Stools should be examined for the presence of gross or occult blood. Microscopic examination with methylene blue staining shows fecal leukocytes (mainly polymorphonuclear cells) characteristic of an invasive diarrhea with disruption of the intestinal mucosa. These cells help eliminate viral, toxin-induced, or non-specific diarrheal syndromes from diagnostic consideration.[54]

The urine may contain red blood cells, especially when the disease or the complications that may ensue produce products such as crystals of urate or oxalate in the urine. Albuminuria is rare but, when present, suggests the possibility of secondary renal amyloidosis.

Since Crohn's disease affects the small bowel, the body's primary absorptive area, evidence of malabsorption is common. There is a close correlation between the length of diseased ileum and fat or vitamin B_{12} absorption.[55] When more than 90 cm of ileum is dysfunctional, tests of vitamin B_{12} absorption are abnormal and steatorrhea is marked. Carbohydrate absorption is normal except when there is more extensive small bowel disease with jejunal involvement or the presence of bacterial stasis. Absorption of other nutrients also depends on the severity and extent of bowel disease.

Radiologic Features. Once the diagnosis of Crohn's disease is suspected, confirmation is usually available by contrast roentgenograms of the bowel. When the small bowel is being evaluated, it is vital that a complete follow-through examination with careful visualization of the terminal ileum is obtained. To be emphasized is the fact that it is not uncommon to overlook severe terminal ileitis with a conventional limited upper gastrointestinal roentgen examination.

When the esophagus is affected, an esophagogram will demonstrate the lesion in the area involved by showing irregular and thickened mucosal folds. Stricturing may occur as well. Crohn's disease in the stomach has a propensity for the antrum. The inflammatory changes produce a tubular antral area with conical narrowing. The stomach distends poorly and peristalsis is diminished.

Irregular coarse folds or ulcerations may be seen or the mucosa may be atrophic. Frank stenosis with gastric obstruction can occur as well.[15] Involved small bowel appears narrowed and rigid with signs of submucosal edema. The patchy submucosal inflammation gives the mucosa a bumpy appearance, often described as "cobblestoned." This can be accentuated by longitudinal ulcerations and transverse fissures that isolate mounds of edematous mucosa and submucosa. The bowel wall thickens, producing wide separation of adjacent bowel loops. The abnormalities are asymmetric and occur as skip lesions with intervening areas of normal intestine. Narrowing of the lumen occurs owing to chronic fibrosis; if severe, signs of proximal obstruction are seen. Extensive narrowing of the terminal ileum produces the classic "string sign." Mesenteric thickening produces a large inflammatory mass over which the bowel is draped. Abscesses or fistulas may arise from the bowel and extend into the adjacent mesentery, bowel, or other viscera or even to the skin. The abnormal colon examined by barium enema will demonstrate changes similar to those in the small bowel, with inflammatory signs, ulceration, or stricture. Double contrast radiography can more easily detect the earliest changes of inflammatory bowel disease.[56] Patchy, superficial, discrete ulcers against a background of normal mucosa are characteristic. More advanced cases show contraction and cobblestone mucosa. Evidence of advanced disease may be seen in one area and early superficial ulcers in another.

Several *nuclear medicine techniques* have been used for the diagnosis and evaluation of Crohn's disease. ^{99m}Technetium diethylenetriamine penta-acetic acid (^{99m}Tc-DTPA) localizes in segments of the bowel with inflammation. The concentration of tracer is related to the clinical activity of the disease process.[57] Similar information is provided by studies using ^{67}gallium or autologous leukocytes labeled with ^{111}indium.[58, 59] While these and other radioactive tracers provide rapid, simple, atraumatic, effective techniques for identifying the site of the inflammatory process, they have not found great clinical use in our experience. Yet, they should be useful to demonstrate complications such as intra-abdominal abscesses.

Abdominal *sonography* and *computed tomography* are valuable adjunctive techniques, especially for the delineation of intra-abdominal masses and abscesses. Such complications may be definitively diagnosed, localized, and followed during therapy. Their delineation is also useful as a preoperative measure.

Recognition in the Operating Room. The proper macroscopic diagnosis during laparotomy is essential, as many acutely ill patients undergo surgery with little or no prior evaluation.[60] Once the abdominal cavity is exposed, one of the first findings may be small amounts of straw-colored or even bloody ascites. Massive ascites is unusual and suggests a diagnosis other than Crohn's disease. Serosal inflammation of the bowel results in marked erythema and a brilliant vascular display with abnormal vessels. The total bowel wall is thickened in a haphazard, asymmetric way. The mesenteric fat increases and clings to the serosal blood vessels. The fat wraps around the bowel wall and in advanced forms produces large, lipoma-like masses (Fig. 127–11). Obliteration of the mesentery bowel angle by fat and inflammatory tissue is an early sign. Segmentation and skip areas are demarcated externally by the changes on the bowel surface. Pronounced lymphadenopathy is another feature that has diagnostic value, since it is

Figure 127–11. Small bowel Crohn's disease as seen at laparotomy. The serosa is erythematous with prominent vasculature. The bowel wall is thickened with an increased in fat, arising from the mesentery. Disease is more severe toward the left.

Figure 127–12. A colonoscopic view demonstrating several pseudopolyps.

Figure 127–13. Benign stricture within an area of active Crohn's disease. The margins are smooth and the colonoscope could be passed through the stenosis.

Figure 127–14. Large discrete ulcerations typical of Crohn's disease, surrounded by normal adjacent mucosa.

Figure 127–15. Small aphthoid ulcerations with surrounding erythematous mucosa.

Figure 127–16. Multiple, variably sized protuberances of the mucosa causing a typical cobblestone pattern.

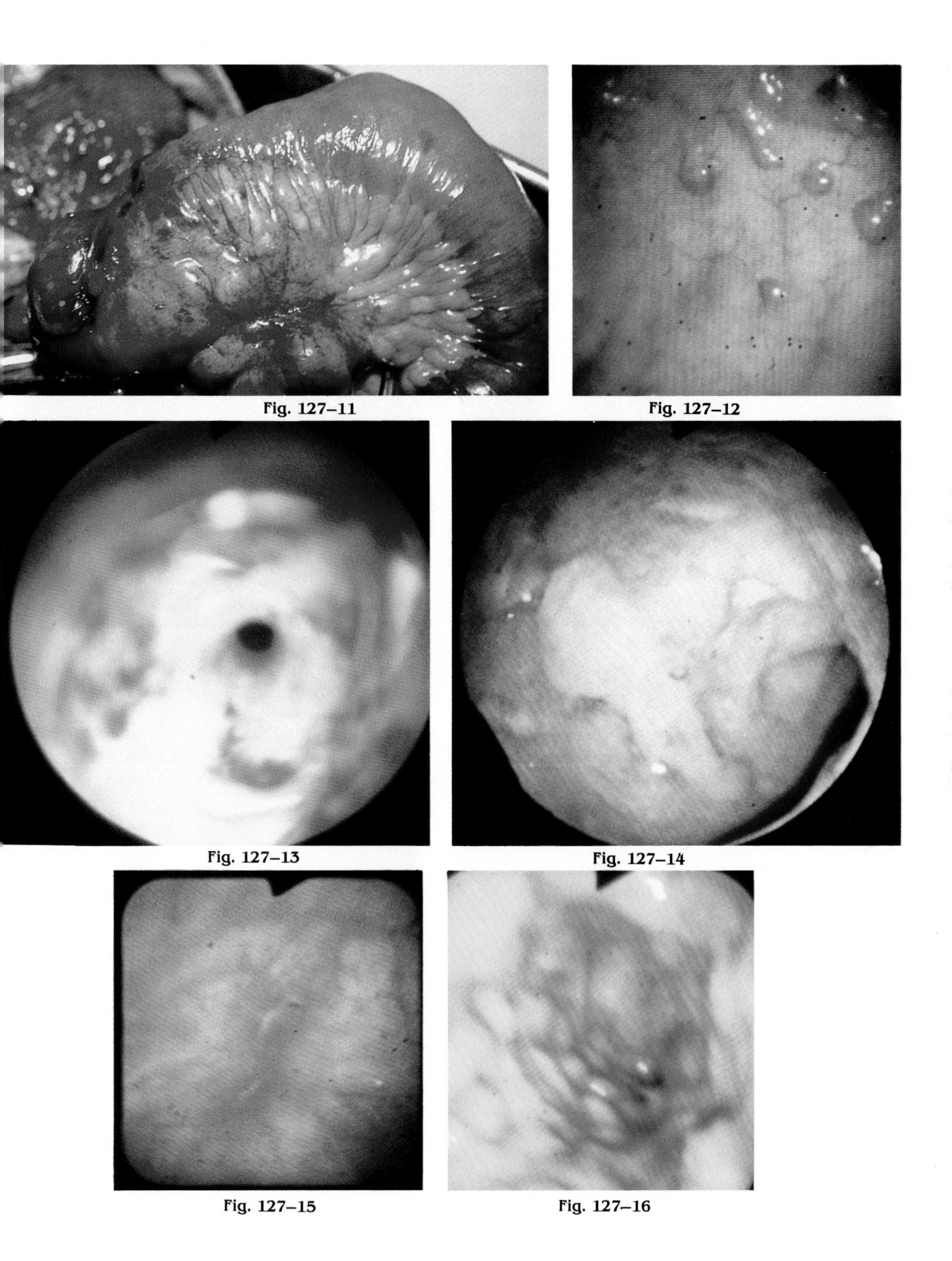

Fig. 127–11

Fig. 127–12

Fig. 127–13

Fig. 127–14

Fig. 127–15

Fig. 127–16

not present in many other bowel disorders, such as ulcerative colitis.

Endoscopy. *Proctosigmoidoscopy* is very useful to evaluate the distal sigmoid and rectal mucosa and should be performed in each case. Most patients with Crohn's disease do not require extensive colonoscopic examination. However, when adequate data are not available from clinical, radiographic, or proctosigmoidoscopic studies, colonoscopy may be important, especially with the addition of biopsy and cytology techniques.[61,62] The major indications for colonoscopy in Crohn's disease are listed in Table 127–6.

A filling defect seen on barium enema roentgenography may represent a benign or malignant polypoid lesion (Chapter 138). Benign polypoid lesions may be true polyps or pseudopolyps. Colonoscopic examination with biopsy or polypectomy will provide the diagnosis. The formation of a "pseudopolyp" begins when an island of inflamed mucosa survives the ulceration that completely surrounds it. As the previously ulcerated mucosa heals, the remnant island of mucosa grows at a different rate than the surrounding denuded mucosa. Hence, it becomes taller and projects into the lumen to assume a polypoid configuration. The overlying mucosa appears similar to colonic mucosa in other areas (Fig. 127–12) and is without malignant potential. Colonoscopic examination with biopsy or polypectomy will provide the means of distinguishing between a true polyp and a pseudopolyp. However, when multiple pseudopolyps are present, it is impossible to biopsy them all. Lesions that must be biopsied are (1) those over 1 cm in diameter, (2) those with surface friability, (3) those with a different color than other polyps, and (4) those with an irregular configuration. If polyps are pedunculated and not in a bed of ulceration, endoscopic removal by standard polypectomy technique will provide the most complete material for pathologic examination. The rare bleeding polyp should also be removed. True polyps should be treated with polypectomy, just as they would in an otherwise normal bowel.

Table 127–6. INDICATIONS FOR COLONOSCOPY IN CROHN'S DISEASE

1. Diagnosis of filling defects found on barium enema roentgenograms
2. Investigation of strictures found on roentgenograms
3. Pre- and postoperative evaluation
4. Evaluation of bowel proximal to a stoma
5. Location of bleeding source
6. Early diagnosis of malignancy

Stenotic areas of the colon may be inflammatory, fibrotic, or neoplastic. Colonoscopic techniques can help to determine the etiology. A malignancy should be suspected (1) when the stricture is so fixed that it is impossible to pass even a small-caliber endoscope through it, (2) when it is rigid with an abrupt shelf-like margin, or (3) when the tissue lining it is very friable. Even if biopsies do not confirm carcinoma, the presence of one or more of the ominous endoscopic features would favor surgery on the assumption that the stricture is malignant (Fig. 127–13).

Colonoscopy can determine the anatomic extent of Crohn's disease preoperatively, which is helpful in planning optimal surgical resection. This includes inspection and biopsy, if indicated, of the terminal ileum for evidence of small intestinal involvement in the inflammatory process.[62a] Colonoscopy is also of value in deciding the approach to patients with fistulas between the small bowel and colon. It will determine whether the fistulous communication is a manifestation of small bowel disease alone or whether the colon is also involved. When there is strong clinical suspicion of Crohn's disease despite normal proctosigmoidoscopy and roentgen findings, colonoscopy may disclose the presence of colitis. Colonoscopy can also provide a clear answer after surgical therapy when recurrent disease is suspected but questionable.

Prior surgical therapy for Crohn's disease may have left a defunctionalized distal colon. The endoscopist may then be asked to determine whether there is residual or recurrent disease in this segment. Findings typical of Crohn's disease will, of course, confirm its existence. The mucosa, however, may be finely granular, erythematous, and friable without being significantly diseased. These non-specific changes have been referred to as *diversion colitis*,[63] an inflammation that must not be confused with Crohn's disease and will reverse once intestinal continuity is restored.

Recurrence may develop proximal to an ileostomy or colostomy previously constructed during surgery for Crohn's disease. A fiberoptic instrument, easily inserted into the stoma, allows excellent visualization of the ileum for distances up to 50 cm, or the entire colon. Mucosal abnormalities may then be examined and biopsies obtained to confirm recurrence.

Colonoscopy has only limited value when there is massive rectal bleeding because of poor visualization. When performed shortly after cessation of bleeding, it may be more useful. Colonoscopy may identify a localized, severely diseased segment of bowel with large, deep, acute ulcerations, probably the source of bleeding. Colonoscopy is contraindicated in the presence of fulminant colitis, toxic megacolon, frank perforation, or peritonitis, as the complication rate in these situations is unacceptably high.

In chronic cases, use of multiple colonoscopic biopsies to search for dysplasia may increase the early diagnosis of cancer. However, the role of dysplasia as a pre-cancer sign in Crohn's colitis is less well defined than in ulcerative colitis.

Upper gastrointestinal panendoscopy is also useful. It can confirm the presence of Crohn's disease in esophageal, gastric, and duodenal areas. The macroscopic appearance, plus the ability to obtain biopsy material, adds important information not obtainable by roentgenography alone.

The single most important endoscopic feature that suggests Crohn's disease is ulceration with completely normal adjacent mucosa (Fig. 127–14). This is true whether the ulcer is small, aphthoid-like, or larger. In late stages, confluent ulcers may develop, and the mucosa becomes edematous and pale or even diffusely inflamed, similar to changes in ulcerative colitis. The earliest mucosal changes are multiple, small, well-circumscribed, raised erythematous plaques surrounded by normal mucosa.[64] Biopsy of these lesions shows focal hemorrhage in the lamina propria, rupture of the crypts, release of mucus, and frank granulomatous inflammation. The lesion may be reversible or may ulcerate, producing an aphthoid-like ulcer (Fig. 127–15). As the disease progresses, the ulcers become longitudinally linear and enlarge, ranging in size from 5 mm to 3 cm in length, 0.5 to 1 cm in width, and 1 to 5 mm in depth. The edges of the ulcers tend to be undermined and some are covered by a membrane composed of necrotic debris. Lumpy inflammatory involvement of the submucosa develops, giving the overlying mucosa a bumpy configuration called cobblestoning (Fig. 127–16). A similar appearance is less commonly due to multiple ulcerations criss-crossing the mucosa, amplifying the lumpy effect of the submucosal inflammation. Pseudopolyps and strictures are frequent results of the inflammation. Mucosal bridging is also seen. This results from ulcerations that undermine a small strip of mucosa and then heal by re-epithelization of the ulcer bed as well as the undersurface of the mucosal strip. What remains is a tube of mucosa connected at each end to non-ulcerated segments of the bowel wall.

Biopsy. A rectal biopsy can be obtained at the time of proctosigmoidoscopy, or multiple biopsies are obtainable using fiberoptic endoscopic instruments. The biopsy findings help to distinguish between Crohn's disease and ulcerative colitis, to rule out specific enteric infections, and to determine disease activity. Probably the most specific feature of Crohn's disease is the granuloma; however, *over 50% of biopsy specimens do not contain granulomas*. This feature is most likely to be demonstrated when the biopsy is obtained from the edge of an aphthous-like ulcer. Occasionally, granulomas are found in endoscopically normal mucosa.[66] Histologic evidence of inflammation may be seen in 45% and granulomas in 15% to 20% of rectal biopsies obtained from normal-appearing mucosa. The frequency of inflammation is proportional to the proximity of grossly demonstrable disease. Yet even in patients with ileitis alone, one-third will show inflammatory changes. Many pathology reports list only chronic inflammation with minimal additional description. This information adds very little to arriving at the proper diagnosis. However, when attention is directed to the colonic location of each specimen, additional information may be gained from the patchy pattern of the mucosal involvement of Crohn's disease.

Histologic examination of oral lesions shows non-caseating granulomas in up to 10% of cases and, in most cases, chronic inflammation of the lamina propria and submucosa as well. The overlying epithelium is infiltrated by lymphocytes and a few neutrophils, and may also be ulcerated. A dense perivascular infiltrate is frequently present in the submucosa, and focal collections of lymphocytes may be noted within the fibrous stroma of the minor salivary glands.[8] Chronic inflammatory changes are evident in lip biopsies in 70% of patients with seemingly uninvolved oral mucosa. Biopsy of the lip is useful, therefore, to confirm the diagnosis of Crohn's disease, but the findings do not correlate with the extent, site, or severity of the disease.[9] Esophageal biopsy may be diagnostic if granulomas are present. Their absence, however, does not rule out involvement by Crohn's disease, since transmural inflammation cannot be demonstrated by superficial mucosal biopsy. The microscopic appearance of gastric or duodenal lesions is similar to that found in more distal portions of the bowel.

Direct immunofluorescence techniques have been applied to buccal biopsies and proposed as a useful diagnostic adjunct.[67] When normal-appearing mucosa obtained from patients with Crohn's disease is incubated with autologous serum, deposited immunoglobulin may be demonstrated using a fluorescent technique. By contrast, mucosa from normal subjects or from patients with ulcerative colitis does not display this phenomenon. However, the specificity of this procedure has not been confirmed by others.[8]

Differential Diagnosis

(See also preceding section of this chapter for a discussion of the pathologic features in differential diagnosis).

Upper Gastrointestinal Crohn's Disease. Crohn's disease in this area is difficult to diagnose, in large part because it is unusual. The presence of characteristic disease in the small or large bowel would provide strong supporting evidence that the upper gastrointestinal lesion is likely to be Crohn's disease.

The esophagus can be involved in mediastinal processes of several causes that have much the same appearance as the lesions considered to be esophageal Crohn's disease.[12] Behçet's disease may be especially difficult to differentiate.[68] Among the other conditions that may cause diagnostic confusion are esophageal varices, reflux esophagitis, and carcinoma.

Gastroduodenal lesions of Crohn's disease result in ulceration or stenosis with obstruction. Numerous conditions may give rise to similar changes and thereby simulate Crohn's disease in these areas, e.g., peptic ulcer, pancreatitis, eosinophilic gastroenteritis, tuberculosis, syphilis, fungal infections, foreign body reactions, carcinoma, sarcoidosis, amyloidosis, or collagen vascular disorders.[69] Peptic ulcer disease is especially difficult to differentiate, especially since its occurrence is increased in patients with Crohn's disease.[70, 71] Indeed, it may be impossible to differentiate peptic ulcer and Crohn's disease radiologically, even in the patient with proven Crohn's disease in the small or large bowel. If the antrum and duodenum are both abnormal and display stricture, rigidity, a cobblestone appearance, or multiple punctate ulcerations, the lesion is likely to be Crohn's disease. If the descending duodenum is the only or the most severe area of duodenal involvement, Crohn's disease is also more likely. Symptomatically, severe pain favors an ulcer diathesis, whereas early obstruction favors Crohn's disease. Skip areas, a string sign, or areas of marked dilatation also make Crohn's disease more suspect. Appropriate blood studies, imaging techniques, endoscopy, biopsy, and cultures should help identify the many other problems that may be confused with inflammatory bowel disease.

Small or Large Bowel Crohn's Disease. A difficult but very common problem is to differentiate patients with Crohn's disease from those suffering from the *irritable bowel syndrome* (Chapter 134). Since the latter is so common and shares the features of altered bowel habits and abdominal pain with Crohn's disease, the disorders may be easily confused. This is compounded by the frequent omission of the small bowel during upper gastrointestinal roentgen examinations. An understanding of the insidious characteristics of Crohn's disease, awareness of its constitutional and extraintestinal manifestations and its capacity to induce growth retardation in children, and the occurrence of nocturnal bowel movements should arouse strong suspicion of this disease. A familial history of inflammatory bowel disease would reinforce this suspicion and mandate an exhaustive investigation.

Many inflammatory disorders may simulate Crohn's disease. Not every inflammatory disease in the right lower abdomen nor every lesion in the ileum or proximal colon is Crohn's disease. *Acute appendicitis* is a common problem mimicking ileitis. The clinical presentation of both may be similar. However, acute appendicitis lacks a past history of illness, in contrast to Crohn's disease in which careful questioning commonly elicits a history of 6 or more months of vague but very definite symptoms. More chronic appendiceal disorders, such as appendiceal abscess, may be even more difficult to differentiate from Crohn's disease. Right lower abdominal pain, fever, and weight loss are present. Examination may demonstrate an abdominal mass and roentgenograms may show abnormalities of the ileum and cecal tip. It is helpful if the patient can pinpoint an episode compatible with acute appendicitis, followed by milder chronic symptoms. An *appendiceal mucocele* may also simulate ileitis but is distinguished by the extensive nature of the mass and roentgen evidence of calcification. Definitive differential diagnosis of appendiceal disorders and Crohn's disease is often made only after laparotomy. In questionable acute cases, it is prudent to move promptly to laparotomy rather than risk the serious consequences of gangrene or perforation. *Cecal diverticulitis* may manifest clinical features similar to those of appendicitis and Crohn's disease and is another disorder that must be included in the differential diagnosis.

Yersinial infection must be considered in the diagnosis of ileitis.[72, 73] Fever, abdominal pain, and diarrhea due to *Yersinia* may well be considered symptoms of acute ileitis, with or without associated colitis. Yersinial infection may even be accompanied by erythema nodosum and polyarthritis. These are acute self-limited disorders but may persist for several months. Extensive study of yersinial infections has shown that while they may clinically and even radiologically resemble acute Crohn's disease, transition to typical Crohn's disease does not occur. The diagnosis of yersinial infection is confirmed by serologic tests and by culture of the organism. Radiologic changes are limited primarily to the mucosa and feature superficial ulcers. Abscesses or fistulas, stenosis, pseudodiverticula, skip lesions, and signs of mesenteric or bowel wall thickening are not observed. In the colon, the inflammatory and ulcerating changes caused by *Yersinia* may also resemble Crohn's disease. Biopsies help confirm the diagnosis, as giant cells and granulomas are not seen in yersinial infections.

Campylobacter, Salmonella, or *Shigella infection* may also cause ileocolitis with abdominal pain, fever, and diarrhea.[74] Cultures of stool should establish the diagnosis and must not be overlooked in any patient suspected of having inflammatory bowel disease. *Anisakiasis*, a roundworm infection resulting from ingestion of raw fish, produces an eosinophilic infiltration of the small bowel that radiologically resembles ileitis. The clinical picture is that of an acute self-limited ileitis.[75] *Whipworm* is another parasite that can clinically simulate Crohn's disease of the colon[76] The diagnosis of parasitic infection may demand repeated examination of the stools (see Chapter 232)..

Ileocecal tuberculosis may very closely resemble Crohn's disease in both clinical presentation and radiographic appearance[77] (Chapter 120). Hemorrhage, perforation, obstruction, fistula formation, and inanition are common in both. Even the histologic appearances may be virtually identical. Caseous necrosis with granulomatous change in the bowel wall and mesenteric lymph nodes suggests tuberculosis, but granulomas may be seen only in the lymph nodes. In Crohn's disease, caseation does not occur, and lymph node granulomas rarely are present in the absence of bowel granulomas. Identification of the acid-fast organisms by stain or culture confirms the diagnosis. A positive tuberculin test suggests tuberculosis, as does a compatible chest roentgenogram, but these studies neither confirm nor exclude bowel tuberculosis. Colonoscopy and biopsy may establish the tuberculous nature of the changes seen, but diagnosis is usually not made until laparotomy.[78] Proper diagnosis is vital, since steroid therapy for presumed Crohn's disease can be disastrous.

Histoplasmosis may also involve the ileocecal area or the colon more extensively with ulcerations and a granulomatous reaction.[79] Although the radiographic picture may be confused with Crohn's disease, a careful history, serologic studies, skin testing, and biopsy of the involved mucosa will confirm the diagnosis. *Balantidium coli infection*, which occurs in temperate climates and in institutions or areas of poor sanitation, may cause a colitis with mucosal edema, friability, and ulcers.[80] Scraping the ulcer base and examining the material for trophozoites will confirm the diagnosis.

Cytomegalovirus may infect the bowel of seriously ill or immunocompromised patients. A granular, erythematous, friable mucosa with discrete punched-out or linear ulcers occurs. Biopsy demonstrates the characteristic cellular inclusions of this disease, minimizing confusion with Crohn's disease.

Amebic colitis or ileocolitis may be impossible to distinguish from Crohn's disease, especially when obstructive features and an ameboma develop in the right lower abdomen.[81] Amebic ileitis alone is very rare. It is imperative to consider this diagnosis early, since many factors reduce the chance of finding the trophozoites in the stool. These include ingestion of kaolin- or bismuth-containing preparations, antacids, or barium. The diagnosis is confirmed by finding trophozoites in the stool or mucosal exudate or on mucosal biopsy. Staining of the biopsy specimen with periodic acid–Schiff (PAS) will increase the diagnostic yield. Serologic studies showing high or rising titers to *Entamoeba histolytica* are suggestive of amebic infection and are rarely seen in Crohn's disease.[82] *Actinomyces israelii infection* occurs in appendectomy wounds, appendiceal abscesses, or other areas of bowel and may have an appearance similar to Crohn's disease.[83] Anaerobic culture of an abscess or drainage from a fistula may demonstrate the actinomyces.

Syphilis can result in vague abdominal discomfort, tenesmus, and mucoid or bloody diarrhea. The mucosa appears granular and edematous, and discrete anal or rectal ulcers may be seen.[84] A history of anal intercourse or homosexual experiences raises suspicion of this condition. Biopsy and silver staining techniques demonstrate the spirochetes. Another venereal disease, *lymphogranuloma venereum*, may involve the rectum and resemble Crohn's disease. Disease in the genital area, prominent regional lymph nodes, and rectal stricturing suggest this diagnosis. Confirmation may be obtained by the Frei intradermal skin test and the serum complement fixation test.

Antibiotic-associated colitis also resembles Crohn's disease. The 2 disorders may be difficult to distinguish, especially in a patient with established Crohn's disease treated with sulfasalazine or other antimicrobial drugs.[38, 86] The rapid disappearance of the fecal *Clostridium difficile* toxin and clinical response to oral vancomycin therapy support the diagnosis of a post-antibiotic condition. *Gold-induced enterocolitis* is another iatrogenic condition that affects the ileum and/or colon and radiologically appears similar to Crohn's disease.

Gynecologic disease, including infection, ectopic pregnancy, cyst, or tumor, may be a problem in the differential diagnosis of Crohn's disease. A careful history and physical examination, laboratory studies, and imaging techniques should eliminate confusion. Barium contrast roentgenograms are less useful, since they may show secondary involvement of the adjacent ileum.

A variety of *neoplastic conditions* may resemble Crohn's disease. *Carcinoma* of the ileum or cecum may spread proximally to involve a long segment of the terminal ileum. The obstructive sequelae may be quite similar to those of chronic ileitis. *Carcinoid* tumor of the ileum may similarly be confused with ileitis. *Lymphomas* occur in the colon or more often in the distal small bowel and may even extend across the ileocecal valve to involve the cecum. Plasmacytomas also occur in this area, but Hodgkin's disease is rare.[87] The severity of systemic manifestations, frequent multiplicity of lesions, and presence of a mass effect or invasive nodularity on radiography all suggest lymphoma.[88] *Nodular lymphoid hyperplasia* of the bowel occurs normally in infants and children and should not be confused with Crohn's disease. There is no ulceration or thickening of the mucosal folds; only numerous tiny submucosal defects are seen, often associated with serum immunoglobulin deficits.[89] *Carcinoma metastatic to the bowel* may resemble Crohn's disease, especially when the primary tumor is silent. The origin of the tumor may be from the stomach, pancreas, colon, or breast or from a melanoma. The multiplicity of radiographic lesions and their appearance as serosal implants should make one suspect neoplasia. Final diagnosis rests on the pathologic findings.[90]

Vascular disorders often mimic Crohn's disease, especially when they occur in a younger patient with no obvious precipitating event. The spontaneous resolution of the bowel lesion over several weeks provides strong evidence against the diagnosis of Crohn's disease.[91] The etiology of the vascular lesion may be oral contraceptive pills, in women and idiopathic vasculitis, collagen vascular disease, or cryoproteinemia in the general population.[92–95] An established prior diagnosis of the primary disorder helps simplify the matter inasmuch as vasculitis or cryoproteinemia may be a secondary complication of Crohn's disease.[94,95] *Radiation enteritis*, also a type of vascular injury, may mimic Crohn's disease in some patients. The history of prior radiotherapy should properly suggest the diagnosis.

A variety of other disorders must also be considered. Most of these are of uncertain etiology. Although *celiac disease* should be easily differentiated, a possibly related disorder known as *chronic non-granulomatous ulcerative jejunoileitis* presents a more difficult problem. This process is characterized by multiple chronic benign ulcers of the small bowel, most often of the jejunum. Abdominal pain, fever, diarrhea, and often progression to intestinal stricture occur. Atrophic jejunitis or malabsorption often precedes the ulceration by many years.[96] However, the characteristic pathologic findings of granulomatous bowel disease are lacking. The predominance of malabsorption, protein-losing enteropathy, dysgammaglobulinemia, and villous atrophy points away from a diagnosis of Crohn's disease.

The *ulcerative jejunitis of Zollinger-Ellison syndrome* can resemble Crohn's disease. The lack of inflammatory manifestations, predominant involvement of the proximal bowel, marked secretion, and elevated serum gastrin levels serve to identify the disorder.

Eosinophilic gastroenteritis may involve the bowel in a manner resembling Crohn's disease.[97] The correct diagnosis is suggested by peripheral eosinophilia and the almost universal involvement of the gastric antrum and proximal small bowel. Confirmation depends on biopsy. *Amyloidosis* is another infiltrative disorder that may be confused with Crohn's disease. A helpful differential feature suggesting amyloidosis is the more nodular and infiltrative radiologic pattern in this disorder. Biopsy with specific staining confirms the diagnosis.

Behçet's disease is a chronic relapsing complex of oral and genital ulcerations and ocular inflammation. Colitis may occur and differentiation from Crohn's colitis may be difficult.[98] These disorders have extensive overlap in clinical manifestations, both intestinal and extraintestinal. Rectovaginal fistulas may even occur in both diseases. The laboratory provides little help in their differentiation. The frequent combination of complications in the central nervous system and the genital involvement should suggest Behçet's disease.

Solitary ulcer of the rectum is another process of unknown etiology that results in one or more ulcers in the rectal mucosa. These occur most often on the anterior aspect of the rectal wall. Patients usually remain asymptomatic, although they may experience rectal bleeding. Examination of the colon by barium enema or colonoscopy should easily separate this condition from Crohn's colitis.[99]

Hermansky-Pudlak syndrome is a triad of albinism, platelet dysfunction with bleeding, and accumulation of ceroid-like pigment in many tissues. It may be complicated by transmural granulomatous colitis.[100] A family history consistent with autosomal recessive inheritance and the typical features of the syndrome clearly suggest the diagnosis. The approach to treatment of this type of colitis is similar to that used in a patient with Crohn's colitis. It is vital to recognize the syndrome because of the ever present danger of bleeding, especially when drugs are used that inhibit platelet aggregation.

Differentiation of Crohn's Disease and Ulcerative Colitis. Lockhart-Mummery and Morson[101] in 1960 emphasized the entity of "Crohn's disease" isolated to the colon. This pattern has many similarities to that of ulcerative colitis, and their distinction may cause confusion. The separation, however, is of practical importance inasmuch as differences exist in the prognosis and medical or surgical therapy.

The epidemiologic and demographic features are similar and do not help in differential diagnosis. Clinical manifestations are also very similar except that major perirectal abscess and fistula formation are considered characteristic of Crohn's disease. When a patient suspected of having ulcerative colitis develops these significant perianal complications, the diagnostic label is changed to Crohn's disease, and the initial diagnosis is considered to be an error. Minor perianal complications or rectovaginal fistulas may occur in either disorder. Early and consistent rectal bleeding is more characteristic of ulcerative colitis but may occur on occasion in Crohn's disease as well.

Involvement of the rectal mucosa is characteristic of ulcerative colitis (seen in 98% of cases at the time of diagnosis). By contrast, the rectum is spared in at least 50% of the cases of Crohn's disease.[102] This difference in area involved, however, is not diagnostic. Many patients with Crohn's colitis have rectal disease, either grossly or on biopsy. Furthermore, even definite ulcerative colitis may on occasion have rectal sparing. This is more common in chronic disease or after periods of therapy with corticosteroid enemas. If a disorder has the features of ulcerative colitis for many years and then the rectum improves, the diagnosis should not be changed to Crohn's disease. Again, confusion may arise, since 20% of ulcerative colitis patients have inflammation extending across the ileocecal valve to the terminal ileum (so-called *backwash ileitis*). The ileitis associated with ulcerative colitis causes dilatation of the ileum rather than contraction as in Crohn's disease, does not develop a fistula, and is not accompanied by an inflammatory mass.[103] Barium enema examination, other than for demonstrating disease location, may also fail to clearly distinguish these disorders. The following are features that would suggest Crohn's disease: localized skip lesions, asymmetric haustral markings, cobblestone mucosa, disorganized mucosal folds, deep ulcers, internal fistulas, thickened ileocecal valve, and pseudodiverticula.[103]

Endoscopy may provide further clues in the differential diagnosis.[103, 104] Features of Crohn's colitis include normal rectum; patchy, asymmetric disease; cobblestoning of the mucosa; lack of friability; normal vascular pattern, even in areas of diseased bowel; ulcerations in otherwise normal mucosa; and serpiginous ulcerations that may course for several centimeters longitudinally along the bowel wall. Biopsies may provide further information, even when they show only nonspecific acute and/or chronic inflammation. Patchy abnormalities interspersed with normal mucosa suggest Crohn's disease, as does normal mucosa between ulcers. The presence of granulomas confirms the diagnosis.[104] Specific cell types obtained in proctosigmoidoscopic biopsies may be helpful.[105] In a minimally inflamed or normal mucosa, the lamina propria of Crohn's disease contains more macrophages than does that of ulcerative colitis; the latter has more mast cells, plasma cells, eosinophils, and neutrophils. Mucosal epithelial cell count reveals no significant differences in the 2 disorders.

At the time of laparotomy, several findings point to Crohn's colitis: predominantly right colonic disease, transmural inflammation, increase in mesenteric fat wrapping around the bowel, miliary tubercles on the serosa, and small bowel involvement.

Crohn's disease and ulcerative colitis have been reported to occur in the same patient.[106] It is unclear whether this is a coincidence or evidence that the 2 diseases represent different ends of the same spectrum.

Indeterminate Colitis. An appreciable number (approximately 15%) of the cases of idiopathic colitis cannot presently be classified as either ulcerative or Crohn's colitis. They may represent new diseases that remain to be classified.[107] This form of colitis is more common among women and generally has an acute onset with abdominal pain, diarrhea, and rectal bleeding. Medical therapy has been of limited value, with most patients requiring surgery. Colectomy specimens show extensive areas of ulceration with intervening normal mucosa, often with rectal sparing. The ulcers vary in size from 0.5 to 6.0 cm and are confined to the mucosa. The submucosa is only superficially involved up to the muscularis propria. In areas of deep ulceration, scattered non-aggregated inflammatory cells can be demonstrated through the full thickness of the bowel wall. Increased vascularity is present at the base of the ulcer. Fissuring that extends into the muscularis propria may be seen. More specific lymphoid aggregates, crypt abscesses, or granulomas are not seen.

Crohn's Disease Versus Diverticulitis. Since Crohn's disease may occur in the older patient, it is not surprising that inflammation may appear in an area containing diverticula.[108] Diverticulosis is more common in men, but this combined pattern is more common in women. In this setting, active Crohn's colitis masquerades as diverticulitis. Distinction is important, since medical and surgical management differs.

Hallmarks of Crohn's disease include chronic illness with anemia, weight loss, extraintestinal manifestations, perianal complications, rectal bleeding, or fistulas. These may occur as well in diverticulitis. Barium enema examination showing deep, narrow spurs of barium representing the fissuring of Crohn's disease may be differentiated from the typical appearance of diverticula. Involvement of the bowel at a distance from the diverticula or recurrence after prior surgical resection should suggest an associated condition. A long longitudinal intramural sinus tract parallel to the bowel lumen on roentgenography had been viewed as pathognomonic for Crohn's disease, but may also be found in diverticulitis alone.[109]

Colonoscopy is contraindicated in the face

of suspected diverticulitis, but proctosigmoidoscopy may be useful. Mucosal granularity, friability, and edema or pus in the rectosigmoid lumen favor Crohn's colitis. Such findings occur in 90% of patients with Crohn's disease[108] and in 20% with diverticulitis alone.[107] Rectal biopsy may demonstrate suggestive inflammatory features or the more specific granuloma.

Clinical Disease Activity Indices

There is no uniform measurement of disease activity available. This hampers the physician caring for the patient as well as the investigator studying the course or therapy of Crohn's disease. Several clinical and laboratory criteria have been proposed to assess this problem.

An early detailed index of disease activity was proposed by the National Cooperative Crohn's Disease Study Group.[110] The index was composed of 8 selected variables: number of stools, abdominal pain, general wellbeing, need for opiates or related antimotility drugs, abdominal mass, hematocrit, body weight, and several symptoms and findings related to Crohn's disease. Each of these factors was assigned a value, multiplied by a specific factor, and then expressed as the Crohn's Disease Activity Index (CDAI). The index requires the patient to keep a diary for at least 1 week and is so cumbersome a pocket calculator was suggested for calculation. Its reliance on subjective symptoms and non-specific signs makes it subject to patient or physician variability. Nor does it allow proper assessment of the patient who has had resection of diseased bowel or who has an ileostomy.

A number of alternate indices have been proposed that rely on clinical and/or laboratory values. Among the latter criteria are the sedimentation rate, serum mucoprotein level, $alpha_1$-antitrypsin concentration, haptoglobin determination, white blood cell count, and platelet count.[110–120] Van Hees et al.[118] include a factor to allow for prior surgical resection. A simple and reliable activity index that we have found useful is that proposed by Harvey and Bradshaw.[119] This is based on clinical criteria and is applicable to a single outpatient visit. Laboratory criteria of inflammatory activity are complementary but not mandatory. Severity of the disease and activity of inflammation have been separated in still another index.[121] Activity is measured by several clinical and laboratory parameters, while disease severity is evaluated by measures of the quality of life.

Prognosis

The syndrome of acute ileitis is a benign, self-limited inflammation that generally appears in younger people. Complete recovery follows a single attack and recurrence is rare.

Established cases of Crohn's disease have a chronic, recurrent course, and no specific therapy is available. This diagnosis is a life sentence of illness, but not necessarily of "sickness." It is one characterized by exacerbations and remissions of clinical activity and even of radiographic appearance.[122] The chronic nature is the one feature above all others that distinguishes the prognosis of Crohn's disease from that of other bowel disorders and even of ulcerative colitis. The latter, despite the havoc it causes, is curable by proctocolectomy. Crohn's disease surgery, no matter how radical, cannot guarantee cure. During the course of the illness, patients exhibit a wide variety of symptoms that depend in large part on the anatomic extent of the disease. In excess of 90% of patients exhibit the triad of diarrhea, abdominal pain, and weight loss. These may combine with nutritional, septic, or other complications to produce serious disability. Social and economic consequences are highly significant for the patients and their family. These problems are compounded by the abnormalities that invariably result from chronic illness. Particularly important is the secondary gain that may be obtained by maintaining the "sick role" behavior. Adverse effects of therapy may be significant and add further to disability. In children, the problems of retarded linear growth and sexual maturation are superimposed on all the others that have been noted.

No treatment strategy is generally agreed upon. Medical therapy is useful in the short-term treatment of disease exacerbations, but there is no evidence that the natural history of the disease is altered.[122] The prognosis after medical therapy is best when disease is restricted to the colon. Over 10% of these patients achieve full clinical remission, with only 3% progressing to chronic invalidism. The rate of surgery when disease is limited to the colon is relatively low. Even so, it becomes necessary in more than 50% of the cases. At the other end of the spectrum are the patients with diffuse small and large bowel disease. Less than 1% achieve full clinical remission with medical therapy.[123]

Over two-thirds of all patients with Crohn's disease will require an operation if they are followed over 10 or more years.[124–126] Those requiring surgery do so for specific complications or for failure of medical therapy. Common surgical indications in ileocolitis are fistulas, intestinal obstruction, and perianal disease. Intestinal obstruction is the most frequent surgical indication for patients with gastroduodenal or small bowel disease. Those with colitis are more likely to have chronic intractable disease requiring surgery. Operation may be required as well in these patients for toxic megacolon, perianal disease, and internal fistulas.

A problem in dealing with the question of surgical therapy has been the inexorable trend for recurrence.[127] Thus, not only must the patient and his or her physician consider the mortality and morbidity of the surgical procedure and the possible need for a colostomy or ileostomy, but also the likely prospect of disease recurrence. Recurrent disease may or may not respond to medical therapy, and up to 50% of the patients will require another operation. The anatomic disease location is important in these considerations.[128] Ileitis and ileocolitis more often require initial surgery and are marked by a higher recurrence rate. Furthermore, if the original indication for surgery was an internal fistula in the ileocecal region, the patient is at the highest risk for subsequent recurrence and need for yet another operation.

The prognosis also depends to a great extent on the spread of the lesions. This may occur in up to 25% of patients, usually in an aboral direction.[129] Lesions may spread to involve areas adjacent to the original site, or there may be disappearance of the initial lesions with simultaneous appearance of fresh lesions distally. Spread commonly occurs during periods of clinical exacerbation, but may be noted during quiescent times.

The quality of life experienced by the patient must be an important consideration in the long-term prognosis. This aspect is generally quite impaired.[130] The Cleveland Clinic group has described 522 young patients who were studied over a 10-year period. Only 23% considered their lives to be good, 67% were functioning at a suboptimal level, and 6% described their state of health as poor; 2.4% died during the study period. Medical and surgical groups were mixed in this study. At the Mount Sinai Hospital, we studied only those patients who underwent surgery, with an 8-year mean follow-up thereafter.[131] All of the patients had considerable difficulty preoperatively because of their illness, which was described as severe in most. Sixty-seven per cent reported overall good functioning with no trouble related to their illness at the time of the final postoperative interview. The presence of an ileostomy or recurrence of disease, often requiring several subsequent operations, impaired their functional capacity, yet surgery clearly improved their lives. Other reports in which surgery was a frequent therapeutic modality have noted similar good results.[125] The risk of *carcinoma* complicating Crohn's disease must be considered as a factor in determining the quality of life and long-term prognosis.[132]

The mortality rate among patients with Crohn's disease is about twice that of the general population. Moreover, there has been no improvement in recent years despite supposedly better medical care.[133] Steroid therapy may increase late-appearing mortality.[134] During the initial attacks of disease, the risk of death is least in younger patients, mortality being rare among patients less than 20 years old. In one report, mortality was zero in patients under 20 years of age, 1.9% in those 20 to 39 years old, 5.3% in those 40 to 59 years old, and 14.8% in those over 60 years of age.[123] The mortality is higher among women than among men. In chronic established disease, the greatest risk to life is in the younger patient of both sexes.

Risk falls as the time from diagnosis increases. Patients first diagnosed after they are 45 years old and followed 15 or more years have about the same risk of dying as an individual in the general population.[134] Even though the disease behaves similarly at all ages, there is a real difference in the overall mortality risk.[130, 133–135] There is a small but definite excess death risk from tumors of the gastrointestinal tract and from suicides in women among all groups with Crohn's disease.[134–136] However, most of the mortality among patients with Crohn's disease is attributable to the disease or to associated gastrointestinal complications.[134]

References

1. Goodman MJ, Skinner JM, Truelove SC. Abnormalities in the apparently normal bowel mucosa in Crohn's disease. Lancet 1976; 1:275–8.
2. Dvorak AM, Connell AB, Dickersin GR. Crohn's disease:

A scanning electron microscope study. Hum Pathol 1979; 10:165–76.
3. Korelitz BI, Waye JD, Kreuning J, Saminers SC, Fein HD, Beeber J, Gelberg BJ. Crohn's disease in endoscopic biopsies of the gastric antrum and duodenum. Am J Gastroenterol 1981; 76:103–9.
4. Farmer RG, Hawk WA, Turnbull RB Jr. Clinical patterns in Crohn's disease: A statistical study of 615 cases. Gastroenterology 1975; 68:627–35.
5. Mekhjian HS, Switz DM, Melnyk CS, Rankin GB, Brooks RK. Clinical features and natural history of Crohn's disease. Gastroenterology 1979; 77:898–906.
6. Admans H, Worwell PJ, Wright R. Diagnosis of Crohn's disease. Dig Dis Sci 1980; 25:911–5.
7. Greenstein AJ, Dicker A, Meyers S, Aufses AH Jr. Periileostomy fistulae in Crohn's disease. Ann Surg 1983; 197:179–82.
8. Basu MK, Asquith P. Oral manifestations of inflammatory bowel disease. Clin Gastroenterol 1980; 9:307–21.
9. Basu MK, Asquith P, Thompson RA, Cooke WT. Oral manifestations of Crohn's disease. Gut 1975; 16:249–54.
10. Lamster I, Sonis S, Hannigan A, Kolodkin A. An association between Crohn's disease, periodontal disease and enhanced neutrophil function. J Periodontal 1978; 49:475–9.
11. Croft CB, Wildinson AR. Ulceration of the mouth, pharynx and larynx in Crohn's disease of the intestine. Br J Surg 1972; 59:249–59.
12. Miller LJ, Thistle JL, Payne WS, Gaffey TA, O'Duffy JD. Crohn's disease involving the esophagus and colon. Mayo Clin Proc 1977; 52:35–8.
13. Dyer NH, Cook PL, Kemp-Harper RA. Oesophageal stricture associated with Crohn's disease. Gut 1969; 10:549–54.
14. Lee CS, Mangla JC, Lee SSC. Crohn's disease in Barrett's esophagus. Am J Gastroenterol 1978; 69:646–54.
15. Farman J, Faegenburg D, Dallemand S, Chen CK. Crohn's disease of the stomach: The "Ram's Horn" sign. AJR 1975; 123:242–51.
16. Johnson OA, Hoskins DW, Todd J, Thorbjarnarson B. Crohn's disease of the stomach. Gastroenterology 1966; 50:571–7.
17. Frandsen PJ, Jarnum S, Malmstrom J. Crohn's disease of the duodenum. Scand J Gastroenterol 1980; 15:683–8.
18. Legge DA, Hoffman HN, Carlson HC. Pancreatitis as a complication of regional enteritis of the duodenum. Gastroenterology 1971; 61:834–7.
19. Swan CHJ, Cooke WT. Treatment and prognosis in diffuse jejuno-ileitis Gut 1971; 12:864.
20. Colon AR, Klein LH. "Universal" Crohn's disease. South Med J 1979; 72:1476–7.
21. Williams NS, Macfie J, Celestin R. Anorectal Crohn's disease. Br J Surg 1979; 66:743–8.
22. Nugent FW. Crohn's disease of the appendix. Am J Gastroenterol 1976: 65:83.
23. Brown WK, Peters RW. Crohn's disease of the appendix presenting as lower intestinal hemorrhage and cecal mass. Am J Gastroenterol 1976; 65:349–52.
24. Yang SS, Gibson P, McCaughey RS, Arcari FA, Bernstein J. Primary Crohn's disease of the appendix. Ann Surg 1979; 189:334–9.
25. Jacobson S. Crohn's disease of the appendix, manifested as acute appendicitis with postoperative fistula. Am J Gastroenterol 1979; 71:592–7.
26. Kovalcik P, Simstein L, Weiss M, Mullern J. The dilemma of Crohn's disease: Crohn's disease and appendectomy. Dis Colon Rectum 1977; 20:377–80.
27. Werlin SL, Blicklich M. Miliary Crohn's disease. Am J Gastroenterol 1981; 75:48–51.
28. Brandt L, Boley S, Goldberg L, Mitsudo S, Berman A. Colitis in the elderly. Am J Gastroenterol 1981; 76:239–45.
29. Rusch V, Simonwitz. Crohn's disease in the older patient. Surg Gynecol Obstet 1980; 150:184–6.
30. Gryboski J, Hillemeier C. Inflammatory bowel disease in children. Med Clin North Am 1980; 64:1185–1202.
31. Kelts DG, Grand RJ, Shen G, Watkins JB, Werlin SL, Boecme C. Nutritional basis of growth failure in children and adolescents with Crohn's disease. Gastroenterology 1979; 76:720–7.
32. Kirschner BS, Voinchet O, Rosenbery IH. Growth retardation in inflammatory bowel disease. Gastroenterology 1978; 75:503–11.
33. Hislop IG. Onset setting in inflammatory bowel disease. Med J Austral 1974; 1:981–4.
34. Mee AS, Jewel DP. Factors inducing relapse in inflammatory bowel disease. Br Med J 1978; 2:801–2.
35. Gerbert B. Psychological aspects of Crohn's disease. J Behav Med 1980; 3:41–58.
36. Goodman JM, Pearson KW, McGhie D, Dutt S, Deodhar SG. Campylobacter and *Giardia lamblia* causing exacerbation of inflammatory bowel disease. Lancet 1980; 2:1247 (Letter).
37. Trnka YM, LaMont JT, Peppercorn MA. Association of *C. difficile* toxin with relapse of chronic inflammatory bowel disease. Gastroenterology 1981; 80:693–6.
38. Meyers S, Mayer L, Bottone E, Desmond E, Janowitz HD. Occurrence of *Clostridium difficile* toxin during the course of inflammatory bowel disease. Gastroenterology 1981; 80:697–700.
39. Latiner PR. Crohn's disease: A review of the psychological and social outcome. Psychol Med 1978; 8:649–56.
40. Monk M, Mendeloff AI, Siegel CI, Lilienfeld A. An epidemiological study of ulcerative colitis and regional enteritis among adults in Baltimore. III. Psychological and possible stress precipitating factors. J Chronic Dis 1970; 22:565–78.
41. Ford CV, Glober GA, Castelnuovo-Tedesco P. A psychiatric study of patients with regional enteritis. JAMA 1969; 208:311-5.
42. Gazzard BG, Price HL, Libby GW, Dawson AM. The social toll of Crohn's disease. Br Med J 1978; 2:1117-9.
43. Morain CO. Acute ileitis. Br Med J 1981; 283:1075.
44. Mayer L, Greenstein AJ. Acute yersinial ileitis: A distinct entity. Am J Gastroenterol 1976; 65:548–51.
45. Morowitz DA, Allen LW, Kirsner JB. Thrombocytosis in chronic inflammatory bowel disease. Ann Intern Med 1975; 135:686–90.
46. Beeken WL. Remediable defects in Crohn's disease. A prospective study of 63 patients. Arch Intern Med 1975; 135:686–90.
47. Falchuk KR, Perrotto JL, Isselbacher KJ. Serum lysozyme in Crohn's disease and ulcerative colitis. N Engl J Med 1975; 293:395–7.
48. Falchuk KR, Perrotto JL, Isselbacher KJ. Serum lysozyme in Crohn's disease: A useful index of disease activity. Gastroenterology 1975; 69:893–6.
49. Peeters TL, Vantrappen G, Gebses K. Serum lysozyme levels in Crohn's disease and ulcerative colitis. Gut 1976; 17:300–5.
50. Dranfield MW, Langman MJS. Serum lysozyme in inflammatory bowel disease. Gut 1975; 16:985–7.
51. Silverstein E, Fierst SM, Simmon MR, Weinstock JV, Friedland J. Angiotensin-converting enzyme in Crohn's disease and ulcerative colitis. Am Soc Clin Pathol 1981; 75:175–8.
52. Numez-Gornes JF, Tewksburg DA. Serum angiotensin-converting enzyme in Crohn's disease. Am J Gastroenterol 1981; 75:383–5.
53. Weaver LJ, Simmonwsitz D, Driscoll R, Solliday N. Serum angiotensin converting enzyme in patients with Crohn's disease. J Surg Res 1980; 29:475–8.
54. Harris JC, DuPont HL, Hornick RB. Fecal leukocytes in diarrheal illness. Ann Intern Med 1972; 76:697–703.
55. Gerson CD, Cohen N, Janowitz HD. Small intestinal absorptive function in regional enteritis. Gastroenterology 1973; 64:907–12.
56. Laufer I, Mullens JE, Hamilton J. Correlation of endoscopy and double-contrast radiography in the early stages of ulcerative and granulomatous colitis. Radiology 1976; 118:1–5.
57. Kadir S, Strauss HW. Evaluation of inflammatory bowel disease with ^{99m}Tc-DTPA. Radiology 1979; 130:443–6.
58. Joseph U, Ohingran SG, Johnson PC. Gallium-67 imaging and Crohn's disease. J Nucl Med 1979; 20:903–4 (Letter).
59. Segal A, Ensel J, Munrs JM, Sarner M. Indium-111 target leukocytes in the diagnosis of inflammatory bowel disease. Lancet 1981; 2:230–2.
60. Weakley FL. Crohn's disease: Recognition in the operating room. Dis Colon Rectum 1975; 18:198–9.
61. The Role of Colonoscopy in Patients with Inflammatory

Bowel Disease: Guidelines for Clinical Application. Elmwood, MA: American Society for Gastrointestinal Endoscopy, 1982.
62. Waye JD. Endoscopy in inflammatory bowel disease. Clin Gastroenterol 1980; 9:279–96.
62a. Schuman BM. Ileoscopy—if forgotten it will be foresaken. Gastrointest Endosc 1984; 30:213–4.
63. Glotzer DJ, Glick ME, Goldman H. Proctitis and colitis following diversion of the fecal stream. Gastroenterology 1981; 80:438–41.
64. Watier A, Devroede G, Perey B, Haddad H, Madarnas P, Grand-Maison P. Small erythematous mucosal plaques: An endoscopic sign of Crohn's disease. Gut 1980; 21:835–9.
65. Chambers TJ, Morson BC. Large bowel biopsy in the differential diagnosis of inflammatory bowel disease. Invest Cell Pathol 1980; 3:159–73.
66. Korelitz BI, Sommers SC. Rectal biopsy in patients with Crohn's disease: Normal mucosa on sigmoidoscopic examination. JAMA 1977; 237:2742–4.
67. Walker JEG. Possible diagnostic test for Crohn's disease by use of buccal mucosa. Lancet 1978; 2:759–60.
68. Lockhart JM, McIntyre W, Caperton EM. Esophageal ulceration in Behçet's syndrome. Ann Intern Med 1976; 84:572–3 (Letter).
69. Bragby RJ, Rogers JV Jr, Hobbs C. Crohn's disease of the esophagus, stomach and duodenum: A review with emphasis on the radiographic findings. South Med J 1972; 65:515–23.
70. Fieding JF, Cooke WT. Peptic ulceration in Crohn's disease. Gut 1970; 11:998–1000.
71. Haggitt RC, Meissner WA. Crohn's disease of the upper gastrointestinal tract. Am J Clin Pathol 1973; 59:613–22.
72. Vantrappen G, Agg HO, Ponette E, Geboes K, Bertrand PH. Yersinia enteritis and enterocolitis: Gastroenterological aspects. Gastroenterology 1977; 72:220–7.
73. Carlson MG, Sternby NH. A case of human infection with Pasteurella pseudotuberculosis X. Acta Pathol Microbiol Scand 1964; 62:128–32.
74. Lambert JR, Tischler ME, Karmali MA, Newman A. Campylobacter ileocolitis: An inflammatory bowel disease. Can Med Assoc J 1979; 119:329–31.
75. Richman RH, Lewicki AM. Right ileocolitis secondary to anisakiasis. 1973; 119:329–31.
76. Sandler M. Whipworm infestation in the colon and rectum simulating Crohn's colitis. Lancet 1981; 1:210 (Letter).
77. Abrams JS, Holden WD. Tuberculosis of the gastrointestinal tract. Arch Surg 1964; 89:282–93.
78. Breiter JR, Hajjar JJ. Segmental tuberculosis of the colon: Diagnosis by colonoscopy. Am J Gastroenterol 1981; 76:369–73.
79. Weidd RF, Haskell BF. Anorectal manifestations of histoplasmosis. Am J Surg 1952: 84:541–4.
80. Baskerville L, Ahmed Y, Ramchand S. Balantidium colitis: Report of a case. Am J Dig Dis 1970; 15:727–31.
81. Tucker PC, Webster PD, Kilpatrick ZM. Amebic colitis mistaken for inflammatory bowel disease. Arch Intern Med 1975; 135:681–5.
82. Pittman FE, El-Hashimi WK, Pittman JC. Studies of human amebiasis. I. Clinical and laboratory findings in eight cases of acute amebic colitis. Gastroenterology 1973; 65:581–7.
83. Brewer NS, Spencer RJ, Nichols DR. Primary anorectal actinomycosis. JAMA 1974; 228:1397–400.
84. Akdamar K, Martin RJ, Ichinose H. Syphilitic proctitis. Am J Dig Dis 1977; 22:701–4.
85. Abrams AJ. Lymphogranuloma venereum. JAMA 1968; 205:199–202.
86. Pokorney BH, Nichols TW Jr. Pseudomembranous colitis: A complication of sulfasalazine therapy in a patient with Crohn's colitis. Am J Gastroenterol 1981; 76:374–6.
87. Kristin H, Farren-Brown G. Primary lymphomas of the gastrointestinal tract. I. Plasma cell tumors. Histopathology 1977; 1:53–6.
88. Hyams JS, Goldman H, Katz AJ. Differentiating small bowel Crohn's disease from lymphoma: Role of rectal biopsy. Gastroenterology 1980; 79:340–3.
89. Marshak RH, Maklansky D, Lindner AE, Wolf BS. Lymphosarcoma of the large bowel. Mt Sinai J Med 1976; 43:392–408.
90. Koos L, Field RE. Metastatic carcinoma of breast simulating Crohn's disease. Int Surg 1980; 65:359–62.
91. Marshak RH, Lindner AE. Ischemic bowel disease: A problem in differential diagnosis. Hosp Pract 1971; 6:124–34.
92. Kilpatrick ZM, Silverman JF, Betancourt E, Farman J, Lawson JP. Vascular occlusion of the colon and oral contraceptives. N Engl J Med 1968; 278:438–40.
93. Kurlander DJ, Kirsner JB. The association of chronic "nonspecific" inflammatory bowel disease with lupus erythematosus. Ann Intern Med 1964; 60:799–813.
94. Reza MJ, Roth BE, Pops MA, Goldberg LS. Intestinal vasculitis in essential, mixed cryoglobulinemia. Ann Intern Med 1974; 81:632–4.
95. Mayer L, Meyers S, Janowitz HD. Cryoproteinemia in the cutaneous gangrene of Crohn's disease: A report of two cases. J Clin Gastroenterol 1981; 3:17–21.
96. Armstrong BK, Ammon RK, Finlay-Jones LR, Joske RA, Vivian AB. A further case of chronic ulcerative enteritis. Gut 1973; 14:649–52.
97. Haberkern CM, Chriotie DL, Haas JE, Eosinophilic gastroenteritis presenting as ileocolitis. Gastroenterology 1978; 74:896–9.
98. O'Duffy JD, Carney A, Deodhan S. Behçet's disease: Report of 10 cases, 3 with new manifestations Ann Intern Med 1971; 75:561–70.
99. Madigan MR, Morson BC. Solitary ulcer of the rectum. Gut 1969; 10:871–81.
100. Schinella RA, Greco A, Cobert BL, Denmark LW, Cox RP. Hermansky-Pudlak syndrome with granulomatous colitis. Ann Intern Med 1980; 92:20–3.
101. Lockhart-Mummery HE, Morson BC. Crohn's disease (regional enteritis) of the large intestine and its distinction from ulcerative colitis. Gut 1960; 1:87–105.
102. Kirsner JB. Problems in the differentiation of ulcerative colitis and Crohn's disease of the colon: The need for repeated diagnostic evaluation. Gastroenterology 1975; 68:187–91.
103. Bance M, Rossini FP, Ferrari A, Roatta L, Gilli E, Cirillo R. The role of colonoscopy in the differential diagnosis between idiopathic ulcerative colitis and Crohn's disease of the colon. Am J Gastroenterol 1975; 65:539–45.
104. Waye JD. The role of colonoscopy in the differential diagnosis of inflammatory bowel disease. Gastrointest Endosc 1977; 23:150–4.
105. Korelitz BI, Sommers SC. Differential diagnosis of ulcerative and granulomatous colitis by sigmoidoscopy, rectal biopsy and cell counts of rectal mucosa. Am J Gastroenterol 1974; 61:460–9.
106. Eyer S, Spadaccini CI, Walker P, Ansel H, Schwartz M, Sumner HW. Simultaneous ulcerative colitis and Crohn's disease. Am J Gastroenterol 1980; 73:345–9.
107. Lee KS, Medline A. Indeterminate colitis in the spectrum of inflammatory bowel disease. Arch Pathol Lab Med 1979; 103:173–6.
108. Berman IR, Cormon ML, Coller JA, Veidenheim MC. Late onset Crohn's disease in patients with colonic diverticulitis. Dis Colon Rectum 1979; 22:524–9.
109. Marshak RH, Janowitz HD, Present DH. Granulomatous colitis in association with diverticula. N Engl J Med 1970; 283:1080–4.
110. Best WR, Beckel JM, Singleton JW, Kern F. Development of a Crohn's disease activity index. National Cooperative Crohn's Disease Study Group. Gastroenterology 1976; 70:439–44.
111. Week B, Jarnum S. Serum concentration of 19 serum proteins in Crohn's disease and ulcerative colitis. Gut 1971; 12:297–302.
112. Talstad I, Gjone E. The disease activity of ulcerative colitis and Crohn's disease. Scand J Gastroenterol 1976; 11:403–8.
113. Von Tongeren JH, Eekhout AL. Criteria to assess the severity of Crohn's disease and the effect of treatment. *In:* Pena AS, Booth CC, eds. The Management of Crohn's Disease. Amsterdam: Excerpta Medica, 1976: 153–8.
114. Allan R, Steinberg DM, Williams JA, Cooke WT. Crohn's

disease involving the colon. Gastroenterology 1977; 73:723–32.
115. Fiasse R, Lurhuma AZ, Cambiaso CL, Masson PL, Dive C. Circulating immune complexes and disease activity in Crohn's disease. Gut 1978; 19:611–7.
116. Descos L, Andre C, Beorchia S, Vincent C, Revillard JP. Serum levels of B_2-microglobulin: A new marker of activity in Crohn's disease. N Engl J Med 1979; 301:440–1 (Letter).
117. André C, André F, Drughet M, Descos L. Etude comparative des index d'activite clinique, inflammatoire et immunitaire dans les enterocolutes cryptoginetiques. Gastroenterol Clin Biol 1979; 3:77.
118. Van Hees PAM, Van Elteren PH, Van Lier HJJ, Van Tongeren JHM. An index of inflammatory activity in patients with Crohn's disease. Gut 1980; 21:279–86.
119. Harvey RF, Bradshaw JM. A simple index of Crohn's disease activity. Lancet 1980; 1:514.
120. Andre C, Descos L, Landais P, Fermanian J. Assessment of appropriate laboratory measurements to supplement the Crohn's disease activity index. Gut 1981; 22:571–4.
121. Maratka Z. Crohn's disease activity indexes: Need for distinguishing activity from severity. Hepato-Gastroenterol 1981; 28:187–8.
122. Mekhjian HS, Switz DM, Melnyk CS, Rankin GB, Brooks RK. Clinical features and natural history of Crohn's disease. Gastroenterology 1979; 77:898–906.
123. DeCombal FT, Burton IL, Clamp SE, Goligher JC. Short-term course and prognosis of Crohn's disease. Gut 1974; 15:435–43.
124. Truelove SC, Pena AS. Course and prognosis of Crohn's disease. Gut 1976; 17:192–201.
125. Cooke WT, Mallas E, Prior P, Allan RN. Crohn's disease: Course, treatment and long-term prognosis. Q J Med 1980; 195:363–84.
126. Farmer RG. Factors in the long-term prognosis of patients with inflammatory bowel disease. Am J Gastroenterol 1981; 75:97–103.
127. Greenstein AJ, Sachar DB, Pasternack BS, Janowitz HD. Reoperation and recurrence in Crohn's colitis and ileocolitis: Crude and cumulative rates. N Engl J Med 1975; 293:685–90.
128. Farmer RD. Clinical features and natural history of inflammatory bowel disease. Med Clin North Am 1980; 64:1103–15.
129. Brahme F, Wenckert A. Spread of lesions in Crohn's disease of the colon. Gut 1970; 11:576–84.
130. Farmer RG, Michener WM. Prognosis of Crohn's disease with onset in childhood or adolescence. Dig Dis Sci 1979; 24:752–7.
131. Meyers S, Walfish JS, Sachar DB, Greenstein AJ, Hill AG, Janowitz HD. Quality of life after surgery for Crohn's disease: A psychosocial survey. Gastroenterology 1980; 78:1–6.
132. Weedon DD, Shorter RG, Ilshup DM, Huizenga KA, Taylor WT. Crohn's disease and cancer. N Engl J Med 1973; 289:1099–103.
133. Storgaard L, Bischoff N, Henriksen FW, Fischerman K, Jarnum S. Survival rate in Crohn's disease and ulcerative colitis. Scand J Gastroenterol 1979; 14:225–30.
134. Prior P, Gyde S, Cooke WT, Waterhouse JAH, Allan RN. Mortality in Crohn's disease. Gastroenterology 1981; 80:307–12.
135. Mayberry JF, Newcombe RG, Rhodes J. Mortality in Crohn's disease, Q J Med 1980; 193:63–8.

Extraintestinal Manifestations

Samuel Meyers • Henry D. Janowitz

Several complications of Crohn's disease occur in areas remote from the gastrointestinal tract. Patients who develop one extraintestinal manifestation are at an increased risk of developing others. While the occurrence of combinations of such manifestations suggests a common pathogenetic mechanism, the exact cause of these complications remains to be determined. An immune mechanism has been suspected for at least some of them, a possibility supported by the demonstration of polyarthritis and circulating immune complexes in Crohn's disease patients and in morbidly obese patients after an intestinal bypass operation.[1–3] Perhaps antigenic material enters from the gut lumen and initiates the immune processes.

Studies at the Mount Sinai Hospital, New York,[4] and confirmed elsewhere,[5] suggest that extraintestinal complications can be subdivided into 2 main groups, depending upon their association with either small or large bowel Crohn's disease. There is also a smaller, less specific third group. The first group, the "colitis"-related manifestations, comprises those complications that involve the joints, skin, mouth, or eyes and are closely associated with the underlying gut inflammation. They often respond to medical or surgical treatment aimed at the bowel disease. In the Mount Sinai Hospital experience,[4] the joints were involved in 22% of the entire series of 700 patients, the skin in 13%, the mouth in 4%, and the eyes in 4%. The frequency of manifestations in these structures among patients with colitis was 39%, 23%, 11%, and 13%, respectively, as compared with 14%, 9%, 3%, and 1% respectively among those with ileitis. The second group, the extraintestinal complications more related to small bowel inflammatory disease, included malabsorption, gallstones, kidney stones, and obstructive uropathy (these manifestations are closely related to the extent and location of the bowel disease and are discussed in the section on Complications). The final group of less specific extraintestinal complications were less common. They consisted of peptic ulcer (10%), osteoporosis (3%), and amyloidosis (1%) (see section on Complications). One-third or more of all patients had more than one complication appearing together or separately at some point during their illness. Still other, more unusual abnormalities (discussed in this section) are those affecting the lungs, blood or blood vessels, and nervous system.

Joints

Peripheral Arthritis. This complication appears in up to 20% of patients suffering from Crohn's disease.[4-6] Multiple joints are involved in an asymmetric distribution, with the lower limbs more often affected than the upper limbs. In order of frequency, the knees, hips, and ankles are most commonly involved. Occasionally, only a single joint is affected. Small joints of the hands or feet are less commonly inflamed. Simple arthralgia may be the only complaint, but true synovitis is common, with the joint becoming erythematous, edematous, painful, and tender. The joint fluid has features compatible with an inflammatory process but is sterile. Septic arthritis, however, may occur, usually in the hip, where there may be contiguous spread from an adjacent psoas abscess or from an intestinal fistula.[7] Rheumatoid factor is absent in both the blood and the joint fluid.

The arthritis most commonly appears with the first attack of the bowel disease or within the first year of illness. Acute attacks usually accompany flares of the underlying inflammatory bowel disease, and the severity of the arthritis generally reflects the activity of the Crohn's disease. Once the latter is in remission, an exacerbation of the joint symptoms often heralds recurrence of active bowel disease. Infrequently, the arthritis precedes the initial onset of the inflammatory bowel disease and seems independent of its course.[6,8]

Some patients have been described with arthritis associated with radiologic changes that included erosive joint damage.[9] Granulomatous inflammation may involve the synovium or adjacent bone in both the erosive and the non-erosive forms of arthritis.[9] Granulomatous myositis has also been reported.[10]

The peripheral arthritis runs a self-limited course, subsiding spontaneously over 6 to 12 weeks. Rarely, this acute stage merges into a more chronic active stage. Permanent joint deformity, however, is of a low order of frequency. Non-steroidal anti-inflammatory agents provide symptomatic relief, but therapy is aimed primarily at the underlying bowel disease.

Ankylosing Spondylitis. This extraintestinal manifestation appears in approximately 20% of Crohn's disease patients when carefully looked for with radiography, but in only half of these patients is the spondylitis symptomatic.[4-6] Spondylitis is more common than expected among women with Crohn's disease. It is also more common among blood relatives of patients with Crohn's disease, having been reported in 8.3% of first-degree relatives and 19% of second-degree relatives.[5] The HLA phenotype B27 may have some role in this genetic linkage, since it is increased in frequency among Crohn's disease subjects with spondylitis. This HLA phenotype is present in up to 75% of such patients, an occurrence rate similar to the 85% to 95% association of HLA-B27 with idiopathic spondylitis.[11]

The pathogenesis of spondylitis associated with Crohn's disease is probably similar to that of the idiopathic variety and is linked in some way to the HLA-B27 gene locus. There must also be a non-HLA-linked genetic predisposition to inflammatory bowel disease that confers susceptibility to spondylitis.[12] This alternative mechanism would explain the lesser frequency of HLA-B27 in the spondylitis of Crohn's disease than in the idiopathic variety. HLA-B27 occurs among patients with Crohn's disease complicated by peripheral arthritis with a frequency similar to that in the general population.

Spondylitis may be detected before the intestinal disease is recognized. Exacerbations of both diseases often occur independently.[13] There is also little or no correlation of the spondylitis with the extent, duration, or severity of the Crohn's disease or following its surgical resection.

The initial symptom is a mild backache of gradual onset. Morning stiffness and nocturnal pain over the lower back are also common. The pain is aggravated by exertion or bending. Arthralgias of the shoulders and hips are often associated findings. Tenderness over the bony prominences of the spine and sacroiliac joint is found on examination. Periodic recurrences are common and unpredictable. Symptoms of each episode may last for months. Flexion contractures and an impaired range of motion may develop, but these occur considerably less often than with idiopathic ankylosing spondylitis.

Symptomatic therapy is all that can be offered to the patient. Analgesic or anti-inflammatory medications combined with simple muscle exercise may provide some relief. Medical or surgical therapy directed at the underlying Crohn's disease has little effect on the spondylitis.

Osteoarthropathy. Osteoarthropathy with periosteal new bone formation is associated with Crohn's disease but is quite rare.[14] Patients complain of pain in large joints. Radiographic examination discloses periosteal new bone formation without evidence of joint abnormalities. This complication may occur concomitantly with spondylitis and/or finger clubbing.

Skin

Erythema Nodosum. The most common cutaneous lesion in Crohn's disease, erythema nodosum, is seen in 15% of patients.[4] These lesions appear as light red nodules, round or oval in shape, which are tender and usually occur on the anterior aspects of the lower extremities. The lesions correlate well as a rule with clinical disease activity, but may precede an acute exacerbation of the inflammation in the bowel. Peripheral arthritis may often occur in conjunction with the erythema nodosum. Therapy that improves the bowel disease is also helpful for this skin manifestation.

Pyoderma Gangrenosum. This complication occurred in 1% of 498 patients with Crohn's disease that we reported previously.[4] In our updated group of 1010 patients, the same 1% prevalence rate was found.[15] Pyoderma gangrenosum begins as an erythematous plaque, papule, or vesicle that soon develops into a destructive burrowing ulcer with irregular edges and ragged purple-red margins.[16] The ulcer most commonly appears on the lower extremities. Despite extensive bacteriologic and immunologic studies, the etiology remains obscure and the pathologic changes are non-specific.[17,18] There does seem to be a relationship to trauma, which often precipitates the cutaneous lesion in the absence of clinical exacerbation of the bowel disease.[19]

Aside from the obvious cosmetic disfigurement, pain and superimposed infection are the chief clinical complaints. Pain may also occur at the site of future skin lesions and antedate any visible changes. In its most advanced form, the spreading ulceration leads to necrosis and loss of the limb. Local therapy, including cleansing and debridement, is essential. Antibiotics, either local or systemic, may be useful when infection is proved or suspected. It has been assumed that control of the underlying bowel disease will succeed in arresting the pyoderma.[20, 21] Sulfasalazine, steroids, immunostimulant and immunosuppressive drugs, and surgery have indeed been accompanied by healing of the cutaneous lesions. However, there are several reports documenting the failure of pyoderma gangrenosum to heal following definitive removal of all diseased bowel, and others have described its appearance years after surgery.[22, 23]

We have identified 2 subgroups of patients with pyoderma gangrenosum and Crohn's disease[15]: (1) those with very active bowel disease in whom the skin lesions are more related to the bowel activity, and (2) patients with quiescent bowel disease in whom the 2 disorders are apt to have divergent clinical courses. In the group with active bowel activity, surgical resection of all diseased bowel is followed by prompt skin healing, whereas those with mild bowel activity do not experience such prompt healing. Surgery in the latter group, however, may make further medical therapy more effective, and healing may occur within 1 year.

Epidermolysis Bullosa Acquisita. This rare complication is marked by cutaneous blisters that tend to be localized to the extremities[24] and may heal with atrophic scars. The nails may be normal or dystrophic, and mouth lesions are variable.

Erythema Multiforme/Stevens-Johnson Syndrome. Erythema multiforme is characterized by its distinctive target lesion and diagnostic sequence of pathologic changes. When it involves mucosal surfaces and internal organs and is accompanied by constitutional symptoms, it is called the *Stevens-Johnson syndrome*. This is uncommonly reported as a complication of Crohn's disease, being seen in only 1 of the 498 patients reported from our institution.[4] The erythema multiforme may be related not to the bowel disease but to the drugs (such as antibiotics or corticosteroids) used in its therapy.

Mouth

Aphthous ulcerations occur but are relatively infrequent (seen in 4% of our patients with Crohn's disease).[4] They are characterized by painful, single or multiple ulcerations of the oral mucosa that appear on the floor of the mouth, gums, upper and lower lip, palate, and uvula. The typical ulcer is less than 0.5 cm in diameter, is shallow, has a regular border and a yellow-gray covering membrane, and is surrounded by a narrow, discrete, erythematous margin. The histopathologic features are that of a non-specific chronic ulcerative process. This complication either precedes or coincides with an exacerbation of the intestinal disease. Certain patients seem especially predisposed, with every flare of their bowel disease being regularly heralded by a crop of mouth ulcers.

Numerous therapeutic regimens have been aimed at these lesions, but treatment remains chiefly symptomatic and supportive. Several local agents are useful, including tetracycline suspension and steroid ointments. Prompt control of the active Crohn's disease helps resolve these oral lesions.

Eyes

A wide variety of ocular lesions may occur among patients with Crohn's disease and result in discomfort or disturbed vision. Although a systematic ophthalmologic study of all patients at our hospital has not been performed, 4% have been noted to have some form of eye disease.[4] At other institutions where more thorough examinations were performed, the prevalence rate was similarly low.[25] Some lesions, such as congenital cataracts or blepharitis, are undoubtedly incidental to the bowel disease. Other eye lesions, such as steroid-induced cataract or maculopathy associated with total parenteral nutrition,[26] are perhaps related not to the disease but to its treatment. Nevertheless, in many cases the eye disease is a genuine complication of the bowel inflammation.

Uveitis. A non-granulomatous anterior uveitis occurs as an extraintestinal complication of Crohn's disease. This is the most common eye lesion, occurring in 2.4% of all patients with the disease.[25] Symptoms include blurred vision, eye pain, photophobia, and headache. Blindness may be the final result but is uncommon. Asymptomatic transient uveitis may also appear, emphasizing the wide range of the clinical nature of the uveitis.[27] Slit lamp examination will disclose flare and cells in the anterior chamber, posterior synechiae, keratic precipitates, atrophy of the iris, and deposits of pigment on the lens. The lesion most commonly appears during an exacerbation of the bowel inflammation, but may also occur during quiescent periods or may even precede the diagnosis of the bowel disease. Therapy aimed at the underlying Crohn's disease (when active) may, but does not always, reduce the activity of the ocular lesion.[25] Local corticosteroids may provide symptomatic benefit.

Corneal Lesions. Corneal infiltrates or ulcers form part of the spectrum of eye lesions in Crohn's disease.[28, 29] These abnormalities have been reported in 1.2% of a large group of patients.[25] The infiltrates seem to be of 2 types: (1) an epithelial or subepithelial infiltration seen in the anterior cornea as small, gray, pale dots; and (2) a deep lamellar, nebulous, subepithelial infiltrate or scarring. Perhaps the first type represents an acute inflammatory phase and the scarring is secondary. Peripheral corneal ulcers have also been noted. Vision is not affected by the infiltrates or ulcers, since they spare the central cornea. Mild irritative symptoms may be bothersome. The corneal lesions generally reflect the activity of the bowel disease and improve with therapy aimed at the bowel.[30] These extraintestinal lesions, however, do occur in some patients with quiescent bowel disease and usually clear with topical steroid therapy.

Miscellaneous. Several other lesions appear uncommonly in the eyes of patients with Crohn's disease. Blepharitis, episcleritis, cataracts, conjunctivitis, and posterior segment lesions each occur in less than 1% of the patients.[25] As noted earlier, several of the lesions are not due directly to the bowel disease process. In our experience, episcleritis has been especially closely related to the bowel disease activity. It often heralds exacerbation and resolves with systemic therapy that concomitantly improves the gut.

Liver

A wide spectrum of hepatic dysfunction has been reported in association with Crohn's disease. Nearly all patients have some hepatic abnormality. While over two-thirds of the changes are more than minor abnormalities, serious, life-threatening liver disease or even clinically apparent abnormalities are unusual.[31] An elevated serum alkaline phosphatase activity is of value in detecting hepatic lesions of Crohn's disease. Other "liver function tests" (Chapter 30) are not useful; the serum bilirubin and aminotransferase determinations are too insensitive and the serum protein and sulfobromophthalein excretion tests too non-specific.[32, 33] It is very difficult to decide on the exact prevalence rate of liver involvement from reports in the literature, since the criteria for the definition of the liver disease and the type of liver biopsy vary from study to study. Also, the liver status among all patients with Crohn's disease is unknown. No large population of patients has been routinely studied by liver biopsy, nor is such a study likely to be made because of the ethical issues involved.

Pericholangitis. This lesion is present in over two-thirds of all patients with Crohn's disease in whom a liver biopsy is performed.[31] However, only one-third of these patients have clinical or laboratory evidence of liver disease.[34] The hepatic inflammation is initially related to the portal veins but later involves the entire portal tract. It is patchy in distribution and is composed mainly of round cells. In addition, there is a local intralobular inflammatory cell infiltration in 20% of cases, often related to areas of minor focal hepatic cell necrosis. Once the inflammation subsides, it may be replaced by periductular fibrosis; rarely, this progresses to bridging portal cirrhosis. The fibrosis is most extensive among patients with disease of the terminal ileum, especially when associated with total colonic involvement.[31]

The pathogenesis of the pericholangitis is unknown. A prominent hypothesis is that toxic substances pass through the wall of the diseased bowel into the portal system and subsequently damage the liver. Bacterial products and/or bile acids, such as lithocholic acid, have been postulated as the potential toxic substances.[32] The severity of the inflammatory cell infiltration correlates with the severity of the intestinal disease; laboratory abnormalities return toward normal after surgical resection in more than 50% of cases. These data support at least some direct connection between the pericholangitis and the bowel disease.[33] Medical therapy for Crohn's disease has little influence on the pericholangitis.

Steatosis. Fatty infiltration of the liver occurs in over one-third of all patients with Crohn's disease.[31] The fat is seen as large droplets within the hepatic parenchymal cells. Inflammation is minimal or absent, portal fibrosis is minimal or moderate, and Mallory bodies are not present. There is little association with nutritional status but good correlation with the overall bowel disease severity. Extensive fatty infiltration is found in seriously ill patients and resolves with recovery.[32]

Cirrhosis. This potentially severe complication is encountered in less than 1% of patients with Crohn's disease.[33] It is most common among those patients with colonic involvement, and it becomes more pronounced with time.[31,33] These associations provide an explanation for the observation that colectomy arrests the progression of the liver disease.[35] Cirrhosis is probably a late sequela of pericholangitis.

Hepatitis. This inflammatory complication would be expected among Crohn's disease patients because of the frequent parenteral injections and blood product transfusions that they receive. Actually, hepatitis occurs uncommonly. It seems to play no part in the prevalence of serious liver complications of Crohn's disease.[32]

Sclerosing Cholangitis (see Chapter 164). This is a well-recognized hepatic complication of ulcerative colitis, but is rare in Crohn's disease.[33,35,36] Its pathogenesis and relationship to pericholangitis are uncertain. An association is suggested by the apparent progression from pericholangitis to sclerosing cholangitis in a few patients and by the appearance of pericholangitis in the liver of some patients with sclerosing cholangitis. Cholangiograms of the sclerotic ducts show diffuse, irregular narrowing of the ductal lumen. Pathologic examination shows fibrotic thickening of the duct wall with an associated mononuclear cell inflammatory infiltrate. Primarily extrahepatic ducts are involved, although intrahepatic ducts and even the gallbladder wall may be affected. The hepatic parenchyma may be normal or show pericholangitis, cholestasis, or cirrhosis. The patients have right upper quadrant or epigastric abdominal pain, nausea, vomiting, fever, jaundice, or pruritus. In time, the complications of cirrhosis and portal hypertension predominate. There is no correlation between the sclerosing cholangitis and the underlying bowel disease and no improvement with medical or surgical therapy aimed primarily at the bowel. Bile duct cancer may rarely complicate sclerosing cholangitis associated with ulcerative colitis (Chapter 126), but does not seem to occur in Crohn's disease.

Miscellaneous. Patients with Crohn's disease can develop hepatic granuloma, abscess, or amyloid.[31] The incidence of amyloidosis discovered at necropsy was 29.4% in a small series of cases at the Mount Sinai Hospital.[37] Also very common is hepatic sinusoidal and central vein dilatation, which is seen in liver biopsy in over 80% of Crohn's disease patients.[38] There is no correlation between the presence or degree of the dilatation and the site, clinical activity, or course of Crohn's disease.

Lungs

Abnormalities of pulmonary function occur in patients with diseases associated with circulating immune complexes, such as systemic lupus erythematosus.[39, 40] The finding of immune complexes in Crohn's disease suggests that similar pulmonary abnormalities may occur. This question becomes even more important since sulfasalazine has been reported to cause pulmonary abnormalities.[41]

Hyperinflation of the lungs occurs during an attack of Crohn's disease.[42] This is manifested by an increased functional reserve capacity that returns to normal as the disease activity diminishes in the bowel. Pulmonary volumes and airway resistances are otherwise normal. Pulmonary diffusion capacity has been reported as diminished in Crohn's disease patients.[43,44] This abnormality is not related to bowel disease activity or extent. There is also no relation to sulfasalazine, steroids, or other medications. The mechanisms of these abnormalities are unclear. The pulmonary changes are ordinarily clinically silent and do not seem to contribute to overall disease morbidity.

Upper airway obstruction has been reported in 2 patients with Crohn's disease.[45] The obstruction was due in one patient to decreased motion of the arytenoids and edema over the cricoarytenoid joint. This joint was affected by Crohn's disease or an associated arthritic process. The second patient had edema of the laryngeal area due to an extensive localized inflammatory process. The bowel disease was inactive in both patients, yet high-dose steroid therapy relieved their obstructed airways.

Blood

Hemostatic Alterations. In the majority of patients with Crohn's disease, the blood is in a hypercoagulable state. This probably contributes to thromboembolism, an occasional complication[46, 47] that may affect the cerebral venous or arterial circulation, the thoracoepigastric veins, the ileofemoral veins, the femoral arteries, or the pulmonary veins.[47–49] The platelet count and fibrinogen levels are increased in these patients, and antithrombin III activity is decreased, all of which contribute to the hypercoagulable state.[50] Other abnormalities include increased levels of the coagulation factors V, VIII, and IX; increased platelet turnover rates; and qualitative platelet abnormalities, suggesting their constant activation.[46, 47, 51] The prothrombin and thrombin times are normal, as is the bleeding time. Partial thromboplastin time is normal or shortened.

The mechanisms of the hemostatic changes are unknown. Endotoxin or other substances may reach the circulation through increased permeability of the diseased bowel to bacteria or other products. Endotoxin derived from the gut bacteria, if it contacts monocytes, can release clotting factors and help initiate the coagulation abnormalities.[52] The relationship between the hemostatic alterations and the diseased bowel is further strengthened by its correlation with the clinical activity[46] of the Crohn's disease. The hypercoagulable state, when complicated by thromboembolism, results in considerable morbidity and even in mortality. Therapy with heparin and/or antiplatelet drugs is rational and often necessary. Such therapy, however, is dangerous in view of the risk of cerebral and/or intestinal bleeding. Therapy should be directed at control of the underlying bowel disease in addition to measures aimed at treating the thromboembolic state. Prompt therapy for the Crohn's disease should reverse the hemostatic alterations and prevent ensuing complications.

Cryoproteinemia. *Cryoglobulinemia* may occur in the patient with Crohn's disease, although studies in our hospital suggest that this is rare.[53] We have seen one patient with quiescent Crohn's disease in whom cryoglobulinemia was complicated by cutaneous gangrene, Raynaud's phenomenon, arthralgias, nephritis, and thromboembolism.[54, 55] The pathogenesis of the cryoglobulin formation is unclear; perhaps it is provoked by antigens gaining access to the circulation through the diseased bowel. Once formed, the cryoglobulins cause symptoms by vascular obstruction and/or inflammation. The diagnosis of Crohn's disease may be difficult and suspect in these patients, since essential cryoglobulinemia itself may be associated with an ileocolitis very similar to Crohn's disease.[56]

Cryofibrinogenemia occurs in the majority of patients with Crohn's disease. Its presence has little or no correlation with the clinical disease activity, and its pathogenesis is unknown.[53] We have treated one patient who developed cutaneous gangrene secondary to cryofibrinogens; his bowel disease was clinically quiescent.[55]

The therapeutic approach to patients with cryoproteinemia is difficult to determine in view of the paucity of available data. Whether this disease aspect should be aggressively diagnosed and treated in all patients or only in those with specific complications is unknown. Steroids, plasmapheresis, immunosuppressives, penicillamine, and hydrochloroquine have been successful in cases of cryoproteinemia of diverse causes. However, they were frequently used along with therapy aimed at the underlying disorder. Anticoagulation seemed useful in our one patient with cryofibrinogenemia and gangrene.[55]

Blood Vessels

Vascular changes are universal in Crohn's disease.[57] These lesions are non-specific and are present in the arteries and veins of the bowel wall and adjacent mesentery. The arterial alterations are characterized by medial hypertrophy and concentric fibroelastic subintimal proliferation. The veins are thickened owing to hypertrophy of the fibroelastic, fibrohyaline, and fibromuscular tissue. More specific inflammatory lesions of the blood vessels may also occur.

Small vessel leukocytoclastic vasculitis has been reported in muscle.[58] Since this type of vasculitis is known to be immunologically mediated, it may also be so in Crohn's disease. The finding of deposits of complement components and of fibrinogen in the affected blood vessels supports a role for immune complexes in the pathogenesis of this vasculitis.[58]

Medium-sized blood vessels may be involved in an inflammatory process producing a cutaneous *polyarteritis nodosa*.[59, 60] This is characterized clinically by livedo reticularis, painful subcutaneous nodules, and cutaneous ulcerations. Polyarthritis, myalgias, and peripheral neuropathy may also be present. Histologic examination of the involved areas shows a panarteritis. The inflammation may result in complete obliteration of the vessel or only mild fibrinoid deposits in the intima. Peripheral nerve and muscle arteries may be affected, but systemic vasculitis is rare. A giant cell arteritis of the bowel wall has been reported in which the vascular lesions closely resembled typical giant cell arteritis of the temporal artery.[61]

Other vascular disorders have also been noted in association with Crohn's disease, including systemic lupus erythematosus, progressive systemic sclerosis, and pleuropericarditis.[61–64] These, however, are rare occurrences. Perhaps immune complex deposition or other immunologic phenomena are the common threads tying these disorders together. The demonstration of circulating immune complexes in Crohn's disease is an important clue.[1]

The vascular disorders do not correlate well with the clinical activity of the Crohn's disease. They may undergo spontaneous remission or require therapy with steroids. There is no relationship between the timing of bowel surgery and the course of the skin lesions.

Large vessels may also be the site of inflammatory complications. These lesions have presented as occlusive vascular disease or typical Takayasu's disease with associated large vessel aneurysms.[65,66] Takayasu's disease is marked by an inflammatory lesion that extends through all layers of the involved arteries. The aorta and its major branches are commonly affected. The etiology of this vasculitis is unknown, but again an immune mechanism has been suggested. The presence of circulating antibody to the aorta or colonic mucosa in patients with Takayasu's disease or inflammatory bowel disease, respectively, supports this hypothesis.[67, 68]

Nervous System

We have noted a variety of neurologic complications in 30 of our patients with Crohn's disease who were seen over a 10-year period.[69] Abnormalities were seen in both the central and the peripheral nervous system. These included neuropathy, myopathy, seizures, focal central nervous system defects, confusional episodes, meningitis, syncope, and extrapyramidal and migraine syndromes. Cerebral glioma and multiple sclerosis each appeared in one patient. The mechanism and the association of these complications to the bowel disease are unknown. There was no relationship to the use of steroid therapy.

References

1. Doe WF, Booth CC, Brown DL. Evidence for complement-binding immune complexes in adult celiac disease, Crohn's disease and ulcerative colitis. Lancet 1973; 1:402–3.
2. Wands JR, LaMont JT, Manne E, Isselbacher KJ. Arthritis associated with intestinal-bypass procedure for morbid obesity. Complement activation and characterization of circulating cryoproteins. N Engl J Med 1976; 294:121–4.
3. Shagrin JW, Frame B, Duncan H. Polyarthritis in obese patients with intestinal bypass. Ann Intern Med 1971; 75:377–80.
4. Greenstein AJ, Janowitz HD, Sachar DB. The extra-intestinal complications of Crohn's disease and ulcerative colitis: A study of 700 patients. Medicine 1976; 55:401–12.
5. Rankin GB, Watts HD, Melnyk CS, Kelley ML Jr. National Cooperative Crohn's Disease Study: Extraintestinal manifestations and perianal complications. Gastroenterology 1979; 77:914–20.
6. Haslock I, Wright V. The musculo-skeletal complications of Crohn's disease. Medicine (Baltimore) 1973; 52:217–25.
7. London D, Fitton JM. Acute septic arthritis complicating Crohn's disease. Br J Surg 1970; 57:536–7.
8. Fernandez-Herlihy L. The articular manifestations of chronic ulcerative colitis. An analysis of 555 cases. N Engl J Med 1959; 261:259–63.
9. Tomlinson IW, Jayson MI. Erosive Crohn's arthritis. J R Soc Med 1981; 74:540–2.
10. Menard DB, Haddad H, Blain JG, Beaudry R, Devraede G, Masse S. Granulomatous myositis and myopathy associated with Crohn's colitis. N Engl J Med 1976; 295:818–9.
11. Morris RI, Metzger AL, Bluestone R, Terasaki PI. HLA-B27—A useful discrimination in the arthropathies of inflammatory bowel disease. N Engl J Med 1974; 290:1117–9.
12. Enlow RW, Bias WB, Arnett FC. The spondylitis of inflammatory bowel disease. Evidence for non-HLA linked axial arthropathy. Arthritis Rheumatol 1980; 23:1359–65.
13. McBride JA, King MJ, Baikie AG, Cream GP, Sircus W. Ankylosing spondylitis and chronic inflammatory diseases of the intestine. Br Med J 1963; 2:438–6.
14. Farman J, Effman EL, Grinja V. Crohn's disease and periosteal new bone formation. Gastroenterology 1971; 61:513–22.
15. Talansky AL, Meyers S, Greenstein AJ, Janowitz HD. Does surgical intervention cure the pyoderma gangrenosum of inflammatory bowel disease? J Clin Gastroenterol 1983; 5:207–10.
16. Callen JP. Pyoderma gangrenosum. *In*: Callen JP, ed. Cutaneous Aspects of Internal Disease. Chicago: Year Book Medical Publishers, 1981: 161–72.
17. Holt PJ, Davies MG, Saunders KC, Nuki G. Pyoderma gangrenosum: Clinical and laboratory findings in 15 patients with special reference to polyarthritis. Medicine 1980; 59:114–33.
18. Shore RN. New look at pyoderma gangrenosum. Cutis 1977; 20:209–13, 217–9.
19. Finkel SI, Janowitz HD. Trauma and the pyoderma gangrenosum of inflammatory bowel disease. Gut 1981; 22:410–2.
20. Edwards FC, Truelove SC. The course and prognosis of ulcerative colitis. Part III. Complications. Gut 1964; 5:1–22.
21. Corbett RS. Recent advances in the surgical treatment of chronic ulcerative colitis. Ann R Coll Surg Engl 1952; 10:21–32.
22. Johnson ML, Wilson HTH. Skin lesions in ulcerative colitis. Gut 1969; 10:255–63.
23. Cook TJ, Lorincz AL. Pyoderma gangrenosum appearing ten years after colectomy and apparent cure of chronic ulcerative colitis. Arch Dermatol 1962; 86:105–6.
24. Cheesbrough MJ, Kinmont PDC. Epidermolysis bullosa acquisita and Crohn's disease. Br J Dermatol 1978; 99(Suppl 16):53–4.
25. Hopkins DJ, Horan E, Burton IL, Clamp SE, DeDombal FT, Goligher JC. Ocular disorders in a series of 332 patients with Crohn's disease. Br J Opthalmol 1974; 58:732–7.
26. Yassur Y, Snir M, Melamed S, Ben-Sira I. Bilateral maculopathy simulating "cherry-red spot" in a patient with Crohn's disease. Br J Ophthalmol 1981; 65:184–8.
27. Daum F, Gould HB, Gold D, Dinari G, Friedman AH, Zucker P, Cohen MI. Asymptomatic transient uveitis in children with inflammatory bowel disease. Am J Dis Child 1979; 133:170–1.
28. Schulman MF, Sugar A. Peripheral corneal infiltrates in inflammatory bowel disease. Ann Ophthalmol 1981; 13:109–11.
29. Knox DL, Snip RC, Stark WJ. The keratopathy of Crohn's disease. Am J Ophthalmol 1980; 90:862–5.
30. Ellis PP, Gentry JH. Ocular complications of ulcerative colitis. Am J Ophthalmol 1964; 58:779–85.
31. Eade MN, Cooke WT, Williams JA. Liver disease in Crohn's disease. A study of 100 consecutive patients. Scand J Gastroenterol 1971; 6:199–204.
32. Eade MN, Cooke WT, Brooke BN, Thompson H. Liver disease in Crohn's colitis. A study of 21 consecutive patients having colectomy. Ann Intern Med 1971; 74:518–28.
33. Dew MJ, Thompson H, Allan RN. The spectrum of hepatic dysfunction in inflammatory bowel disease. Q J Med 1979; 48:113–35.
34. Cohen S, Kaplan M, Gottlieb L, Patterson J. Liver disease and gallstones in regional enteritis. Gastroenterology 1971; 60:237–45.
35. Atkinson AJ, Carroll WW. Sclerosing cholangitis. Association with regional enteritis. JAMA 1964; 188:183–4.
36. Sparberg M, Cottschalk A, Kirsner JB. Liver abscess complicating regional enteritis. Report of two cases. Gastroenterology 1965; 49:548–59.
37. Werther JL, Shapira A, Rubinstein O, Janowitz HD. Amyloidosis in regional enteritis. A report of five cases. Am J Med 1960; 29:416–23.
38. Capron JP, Lemay JL, Gontier MF, Dupas JL, Capron-Chivrac C, Lorriaux A. Hepatic sinusoidal dilation in Crohn's disease. Scand J Gastroenterol 1979; 14:987–99.
39. Estes D, Christian CL. The natural history of systemic lupus erythematosus by prospective analysis. Medicine 1971; 50:85–95.
40. Zubler RH, Lambert PH. Immune complexes in clinical

investigation. *In*: Thompson RA, ed. Recent Advances in Immunology. London: Churchill Livingstone, 1977: 126–47.
41. Jones GR, Malone DNS. Sulphasalazine-induced lung disease. Thorax 1972; 27:713–7.
42. Pasquis P, Colin R, Denis P, Baptiste P, Galmiche JP, Hecketsweiter P. Transient pulmonary impairment during attacks of Crohn's disease. Respiration 1981; 41:56–9.
43. Johnson NM, Mee AS, Jewell DP, Clarke SW. Pulmonary function in inflammatory bowel disease. Digestion 1978; 18:416–8.
44. Eade OE, Smith CL, Alexander JR, Whorwell PJ. Pulmonary function in patients with inflammatory bowel disease. Am J Gastroenterol 1980; 73:154–6.
45. Kelly JH, Montgomery WW, Goodman ML, Mulvaney TJ. Upper airway obstruction associated with regional enteritis. Ann Otol Rhinol Laryngol 1979; 88:95–9.
46. Lake AM, Stauffer JQ, Stuart MJ. Hemostatic alterations in inflammatory bowel disease: Response to therapy. Am J Dig Dis 1978; 23:897–902.
47. Mori K, Watanabe H, Hiwatashi N, Sugai K, Goto Y. Studies on blood coagulation in ulcerative colitis and Crohn's disease. Tohoku J Exp Med 1980; 132:93–101.
48. Schneiderman JH, Sharpe JA, Sutton DMC. Cerebral and retinal vascular complications of inflammatory bowel disease. Ann Neurol 1979; 5:331–7.
49. Sigsbee B, Rottenberg DA. Sagittal sinus thrombosis as a complication of regional enteritis. Ann Neurol 1978; 3:450–2.
50. Lam A, Borda IT, Inwood MJ, Thomson S. Coagulation studies in ulcerative colitis and Crohn's disease. Gastroenterology 1975; 168:245–51.
51. Talstad I, Rootwelt K, Gjone E. Thrombocytosis in ulcerative colitis and Crohn's disease. Scand J Gastroenterol 1973; 8:135–8.
52. Juhlin L, Krause U, Shelly WB. Endotoxin-induced microclots in ulcerative colitis and Crohn's disease. Scand J Gastroenterol 1980; 15:311–4.
53. Cohen L, Meyers S. Personal communications.
54. Altman A, Meyers S, Sachar DB, Janowitz HD. Crohn's ileocolitis, cutaneous gangrene and cryoglobulinemia. Mt Sinai J Med 1979; 46:293–6.
55. Mayer L, Meyers S, Janowitz HD. Cryoproteinemia in the cutaneous gangrene of Crohn's disease. J Clin Gastroenterol 1981; 3(Suppl 1):17–21.
56. Reza MJ, Roth BE, Pops MA, Goldberg LS. Intestinal vasculitis in essential, mixed cryoglobulinemia. Ann Intern Med 1974; 81:632–4.
57. Morson BC, Dawson IMP. Gastrointestinal Pathology. Philadelphia: JB Lippincott, 1974.
58. Gilliam JH III, Challa VR, Agudelo CA, Albertson DA, Huntley CC. Vasculitis involving muscle associated with Crohn's colitis. Gastroenterology 1981; 81:787–90.
59. Verbov J, Stansfeld AG. Cutaneous polyarteritis nodosa and Crohn's disease. Trans St Johns Hosp Dermatol 1972; 58:261–8.
60. Solley GO, Winkelmann RK, Rovelstad RA. Correlation between regional enterocolitis and cutaneous polyarteritis nodosa. Two case reports and review of the literature. Gastroenterology 1975; 69:235–9.
61. Teja K, Crum CP, Friedman C. Giant cell arteritis and Crohn's disease: An unreported association. Gastroenterology 1980; 78:796–802.
62. Shafer RB, Gregory DH. Systemic lupus erythematosus, presenting as regional ileitis. Minn Med 1970; 53:789–92.
63. Shaps RS, Stoopler M. Systemic sclerosis and regional enteritis occurring simultaneously. Am J Gastroenterol 1976; 65:552–6.
64. Goodman MJ, Moir DJ, Holt JM, Truelove SC. Pericarditis associated with ulcerative colitis and Crohn's disease. Am J Dig Dis 1976; 21:98–102.
65. Owyand C, Miller LJ, Lie JT, Fleming CR. Takayasu's arteritis in Crohn's disease. Gastroenterology 1979; 76:825–8.
66. Silverstein A, Present DM. Cerebrovascular occlusions in relatively young patients with regional enteritis. JAMA 1971; 215:976–7.
67. Lagercrantz R, Hammerstrom S, Perlman P, Gustafsson BE. Immunological studies in ulcerative colitis. IV. Origin of autoantibodies. J Exp Med 1968; 128:1339–52.
68. Ito I, Saito Y, Nonaka Y. Immunological aspects of aortitis syndrome. Jap Circ J 1975; 39:459–62.
69. Gendelman S, Present D, Janowitz HD. Neurological complications of inflammatory bowel disease. Gastroenterology 1982; 82:1065 (Abstract).

Roentgen Features

Richard H. Marshak • Arthur E. Lindner • Daniel Maklansky

Stomach And Duodenum

Roentgen Features. The roentgen findings are similar in the stomach and duodenum.[1] In general, they follow the pattern described for Crohn's disease of the small bowel[2] and the colon[3] (discussed later). In our experience, gastroduodenal Crohn's disease is uncommon, but some authors[4] have found it to be more frequent.

Stenosis is such a prominent feature that we have divided the gastroduodenal roentgen findings into *non-stenotic* and *stenotic* phases of the disease.

Non-Stenotic Phase. The earliest findings of this phase are tiny aphthous ulcerations (Fig. 127–17). These aphthae are best demonstrated early in the examination with the double contrast technique using small amounts of dense barium and air. As in the small bowel and colon, the gastroduodenal aphthae probably progress to thickening and blunting of the folds, larger ulcerations, a cobblestone pattern, denudation of the mucosa, fibrosis, and ultimately stricture formation. This sequence, however, has been difficult to demonstrate in the stomach and duodenum, although individual examples of each of these alterations may be seen. Thus far we have not seen such lesions progress to the more typical features of Crohn's disease.

The early tiny ulcerations of the stomach have the same appearance as that of erosive gastritis and, in the absence of biopsy proof, an unequivocal diagnosis of Crohn's disease cannot be made. The other features of Crohn's disease can be relied on more confidently to identify this disorder in the stomach and duodenum. Among these features are thickened folds in the duodenum, cobblestoning (Figs. 127–18 and 127–19), and stenosis. In almost all patients with gastroduodenal Crohn's disease, lesions are present elsewhere in the gastrointestinal tract as well, and this facilitates identification of the nature and basis of the changes in the stomach and duodenum.

Stenotic Phase. In the stenotic form of

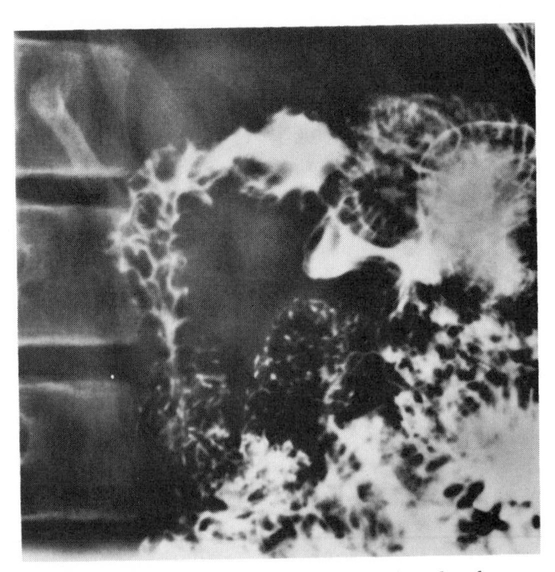

Figure 127–18. Crohn's disease of the duodenum. There is cobblestoning of the second portion of the duodenum due to transverse and linear ulcerations. The folds are thickened and edematous.

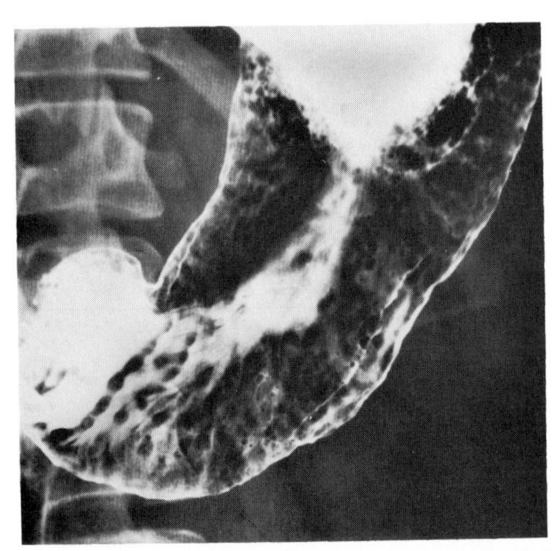

Figure 127–17. Crohn's disease of the stomach. Multiple small aphthous ulcers are seen in the distal half of the stomach. The minute ulcers are surrounded by a halo of radiolucent edematous mucosa.

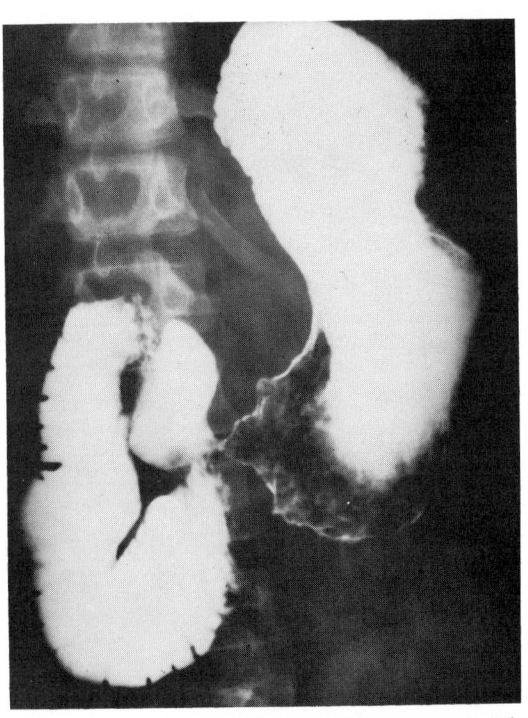

Figure 127–19. Crohn's disease of the stomach. Minimal cobblestoning is seen, associated with a moderate degree of stenosis.

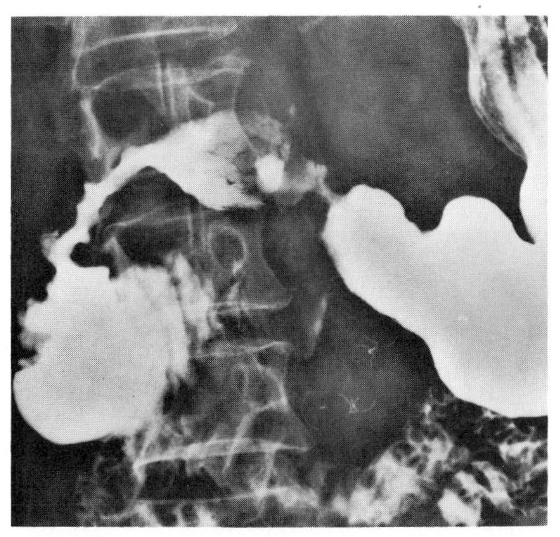

Figure 127–20. Crohn's disease of the duodenal bulb. An ulcer is present at the base of the bulb. The second portion of the duodenum is narrowed and rigid with pseudodiverticula caused by eccentric skip lesions.

Crohn's disease of the stomach and duodenum (Figs. 127–19 and 127–20), the most significant abnormality is narrowing of the antrum, associated with rigidity. The contours are smooth and ulceration is rarely seen. The pyloric channel appears obliterated, but the concentrically situated lumen often is patulous and continuous with the duodenal bulb. This appearance has been likened by Farman et al.[5] to a "ram's horn." Associated narrowing and rigidity of the duodenal bulb and the second portion of the duodenum are frequently seen. The stenosis may be severe and pseudodiverticula may be displayed. Despite the narrowing, some degree of patency tends to be maintained.

Sinus tracts and fistulas are rarely observed to originate in the stomach and first portion of the duodenum, but they have been reported in the second portion. Fistulas of the stomach in Crohn's disease usually derive from the small bowel or colon. No mass is seen, and no evidence of extrinsic pressure on the stomach or duodenum is found. The third portion of the duodenum may also be involved; sometimes the lesion progresses distally to involve the ligament of Treitz and the proximal jejunum.

When the stomach and duodenum are both involved, the appearance has been described as having a "pseudo-Billroth I" configuration.[6] It is of interest that in none of the cases that we have observed has the proximal half of the stomach been implicated, nor have we observed a documented case of Crohn's disease involving the esophagus.

Differential Diagnosis. The most important differential diagnosis is *scirrhous carcinoma of the stomach.* The smooth borders of the antrum, the continuation of the lesion into the duodenum, the patulous pyloric channel, and the lack of ulceration in Crohn's disease distinguish this disorder from scirrhous carcinoma. Primary *carcinoma of the duodenum,* which must also be considered in the differential diagnosis, exhibits a rigid, angulated, eccentric lumen with overhanging edges.

Small Intestine

Technique. The small intestine is examined with 16 to 24 oz of a barium-water mixture. Use of smaller amounts of contrast material may cause incomplete filling of loops and simulate a small bowel abnormality. With large volumes, however, many intestinal loops are visualized in continuity, and the relationship of one segment to another can be evaluated. Fluoroscopy with multiple compression films is essential during the study.

Classification. Some investigators have divided the roentgen findings into acute, subacute, and chronic stages. However, the classic form of Crohn's disease of the small bowel (regional enteritis) is a low-grade inflammatory process with episodes of acute exacerbation, and it has been difficult to identify clear-cut roentgen patterns that correspond to the clinical activity of the disease. Acute regional enteritis may well occur, but usually it is impossible to determine the precise onset of the disease even on clinical grounds. What is described as acute regional enteritis may simply be a more acute phase of the chronic illness.

From the radiologic standpoint, cases may be conveniently divided into *stenotic* and *nonstenotic* types. It should be noted, however, that it is impossible to classify cases from the roentgen appearance of the gut as "early" or "late," inasmuch as patients may have disease in the small bowel for many years without stenosis. Nor can cases be classified as "active" or "inactive" from the roentgen appearance, since patients with long segments of stenotic and probably fibrotic intestine may at times show considerable clinical activity manifested by findings such as fever, abdominal pain, and leukocytosis.

Proximal and distal extension of the disease process is rarely seen during serial roentgen examinations over a period of many years. The maximum length of the involved segment is usually determined by the initial roentgen studies. This is not true, however, after bypass procedures or resections, when longitudinal spread is common.

Non-Stenotic Phase. The roentgen findings[2] closely parallel the pathologic features. Early changes are blunting, flattening, thickening, distortion, and straightening of the valvulae conniventes with or without associated aphthoid ulcers. The folds are arranged in a fairly regular, symmetric, parallel fashion; they appear to be rigid and are perpendicular to the long axis of the intestine. With time, the folds become thicker, irregular, indistinct, and partially fused (Figs. 127–21 and 127–22). The lumen and contour become irregular. Occasionally, the irregularity of contour and of the valvulae conniventes is seen early, without distinct blunting or thickening of the folds. These early changes are due to submucosal and mucosal thickening and the occasional presence of aphthae.

Aphthae are difficult to recognize in the small bowel; they are best seen in the distal ileum. These tiny ulcers, surrounded by a radiolucent halo, may be maximally visualized with the use of compression. As in the mouth, the aphthae in the small intestine may spontaneously disappear and are not pathognomonic for Crohn's disease. In all likelihood, the tiny ulcers enlarge, coalesce, and become the longitudinal and transverse ulcers that produce a cobblestone configuration.

A *thickened fold pattern* is more commonly found in the jejunum, probably because the valvulae conniventes are more prominent in this region. *Ulceration* continues at the expense of the intervening islands of mucosa, producing an irregular network of interlacing streaks of barium. The appearance at this stage has no uniformity or symmetry, and the mucosal pattern is hazy and reticulated. Denudation of the mucosa is usually incomplete, leaving behind islands of inflamed mucosa (inflammatory polyps) that produce multiple smooth defects of varying size (Fig. 127–23). Their prominence is increased by narrowing of the bowel lumen, owing to

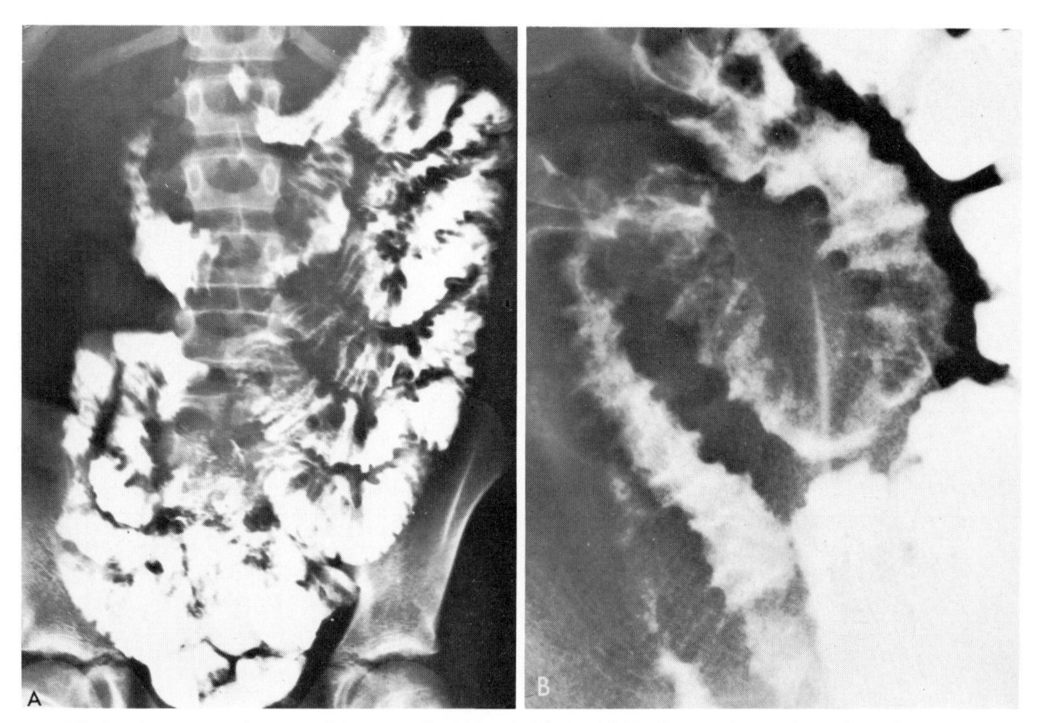

Figure 127–21. Non-stenotic type of Crohn's disease. *A,* Slight thickening and blunting of the folds are present with moderate irregularity of the contour of the bowel. Numerous small defects are noted which, in some areas, appear to be submucosal. There is a slight rigidity of the bowel. *B,* Early non-stenotic type of Crohn's disease in a young man with a 10-day history. The folds are thickened and blunted in the distal ileum with moderate separation of the loops of bowel.

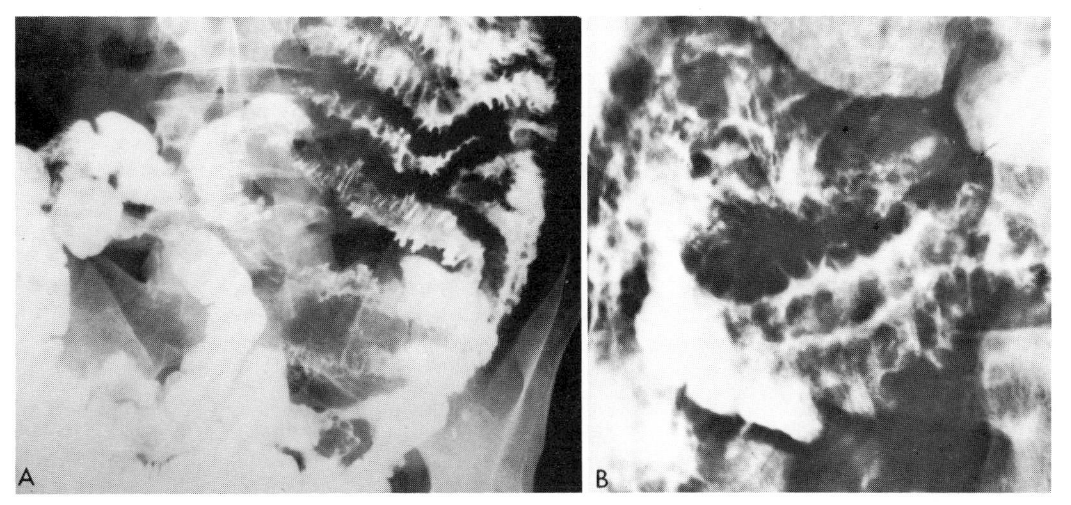

Figure 127–22. Non-stenotic type of Crohn's disease. *A,* The mucosal folds are thickened, blunted, and in some areas fused. The contour of the lumen is irregular. There is some rigidity and separation of the loops of intestine, which also appear straightened or uncoiled. *B,* There is marked thickening of the loops of bowel associated with longitudinal streaks of barium, indicating ulceration. The contour is irregular with some rigidity and separation of the loops of intestine.

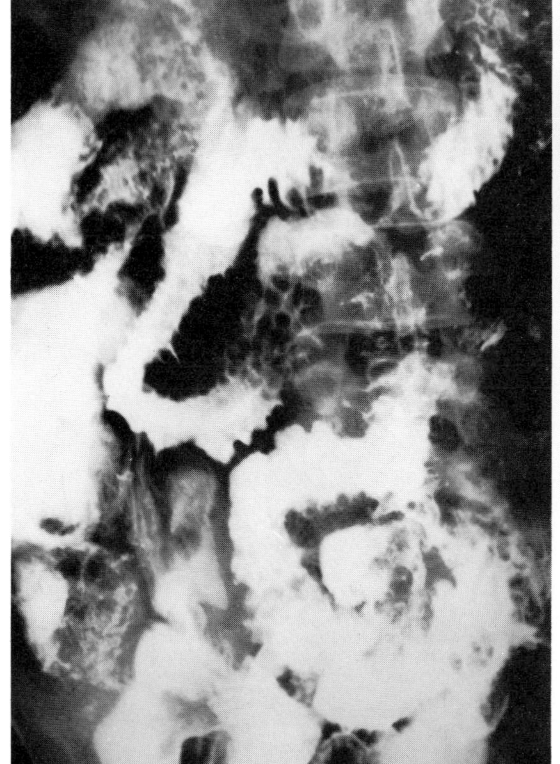

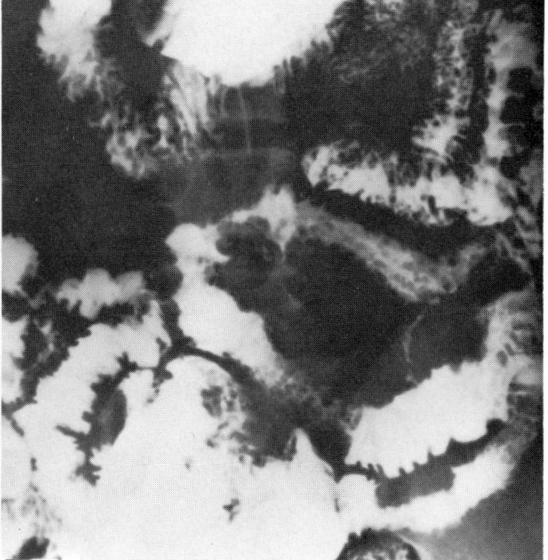

Figure 127–23. Non-stenotic type of Crohn's disease. A fistulous communication is demonstrated between the involved segments of bowel.

cicatricial contraction that begins at this stage. Finally, the roentgenologic image appears of a uniform, rigid, cast-like tube filled with barium and showing no mucous membrane pattern. This appearance is similar to that of ulcerative colitis and represents the stage at which scarring and regeneration of an atrophic mucosa are progressing (Fig. 127–24). As scarring proceeds, the transition to the stenotic phase occurs.

Coincident with changes in the mucosa, other characteristic roentgen features appear. The bowel lumen reveals varying degrees of narrowing. Early in the disease, the submucosal thickening and associated spasm are responsible for the narrowing of the lumen. Later, as fibrosis occurs, narrowing is more marked and leads finally to the stenotic stage. In the early phases, rigidity of contour and of mucosal pattern is incomplete. Some flexibility or dynamic activity is evident from the change in contour and in mucosal pattern during successive roentgenograms. Later, the roentgen appearance is fixed and unvarying. Pliability is also lost. Furthermore, early in the disease, the normal serpentine or coiled pattern of the loops of small intestine disappears. The diseased segments are straightened and rigid. This finding is probably due to loss of flexibility in the intestinal wall and mesentery, as well as to longitudinal shortening due to spasm.

Not infrequently, the loops of intestine appear to surround a mass. Although this may be due to an abscess resulting from perforation, more often it is caused by an indurated mesentery associated with a marked increase in mesenteric fat and enlarged lymph nodes. The silhouette of the intestine may be hazy. This is because the intestine is diffusely ulcerated and contains exudate and excessive secretions, and barium does not adhere to the walls. Despite the increase in intestinal content, the barium mixture remains fluid and homogeneous. Neither agglutination, clumping, nor formation of masses of barium is found in regional enteritis, in contrast to the findings in the sprue pattern. Segmentation, as is characteristic of sprue, is not observed. When unequivocal segmentation occurs, the diagnosis of regional enteritis should be suspect.

Skip areas, segments of normal intestine intervening between diseased segments, represent another characteristic feature. The length of the skip area may vary from a few inches to several feet. The extent of involvement on a roentgenogram may be quite accurately determined in most cases because the transition from areas of disease to areas

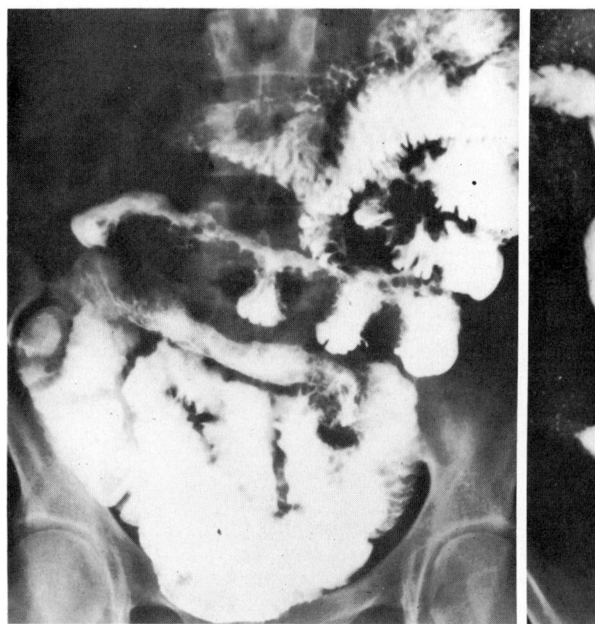

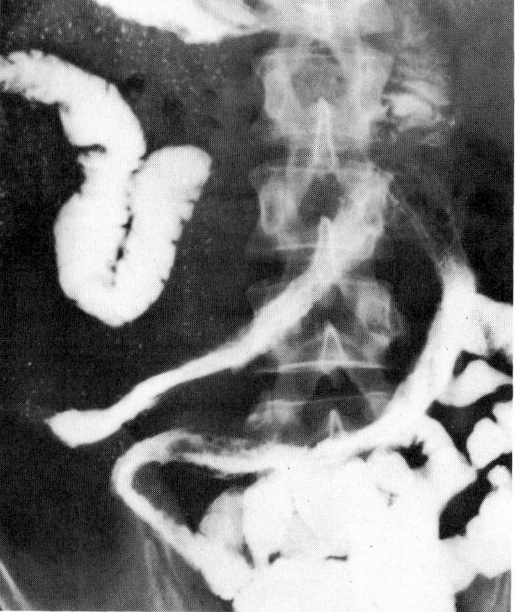

Figure 127–24. Non-stenotic type of Crohn's disease. There is rigidity and separation of the loops of intestine with numerous small filling defects due to inflammatory polyps and eccentric skip areas.

of normal intestine is fairly abrupt. In some instances, marked spasm and irritability may be seen in intrinsically normal small bowel because of proximity to diseased segments. Hence, several examinations may be necessary before it can be accurately determined that these spastic and irritable loops of bowel are not involved with regional enteritis. This assessment is important for both the surgeon and the radiologist when planning a resection.

Outpouchings of the bowel lumen between the thickened folds (Fig. 127–25) occur in some cases, creating the suggestion of large diverticula. This appearance is unusual in that it seems to affect one side of the intestine and not the other. Such pseudodiverticula represent small eccentric skip areas and are highly characteristic of regional enteritis. They may also be seen in the late stages of ischemia of the bowel.

Stenotic Phase. In this stage, many of the rigid loops described in the preceding discussion become constricted to a remarkable degree. These stenotic segments resemble rigid pipestems (Figs. 127–26 and 127–27) as a consequence of marked thickening and contraction of the wall of the small intestine. Stenosis may extend only through 1 or 2 cm, or it may involve long segments of the gut. With severe narrowing, *dilatation* of the proximal intestine may be marked. In many instances it is difficult to state whether or not intrinsic disease is present in a dilated area. Very often, disease is present when a loop of dilated intestine exists between 2 points of constriction. On the other hand, when there is a single area of constriction with proximal dilatation, disease may not be present in the dilated segment. However, because of the retained secretions, secondary inflammatory changes, tension ulcers, and muscular hypertrophy, the appearance of the dilated loops may be confused with the alterations seen in regional enteritis. This distinction is of great importance when surgery is being considered, as many patients have been denied operative intervention because the surgeon believed that the entire intestine was involved. Extreme dilatation of long segments of the intestine is rarely associated with intrinsic granulomatous disease.

Many of the roentgenographic phenomena observed in the non-stenotic phase of the disease are again noted in the stenotic stage. The mucosal pattern may be cobblestoned, reticulated, or cast-like. Small filling defects and inflammatory polyps are distributed irregularly throughout the diseased segments. Skip areas and wide spacing between the

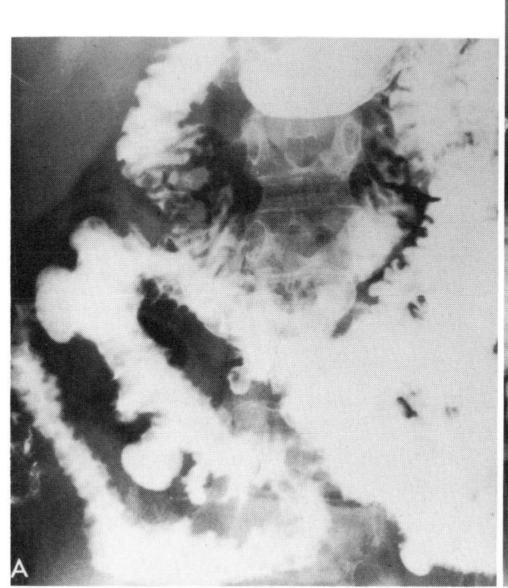

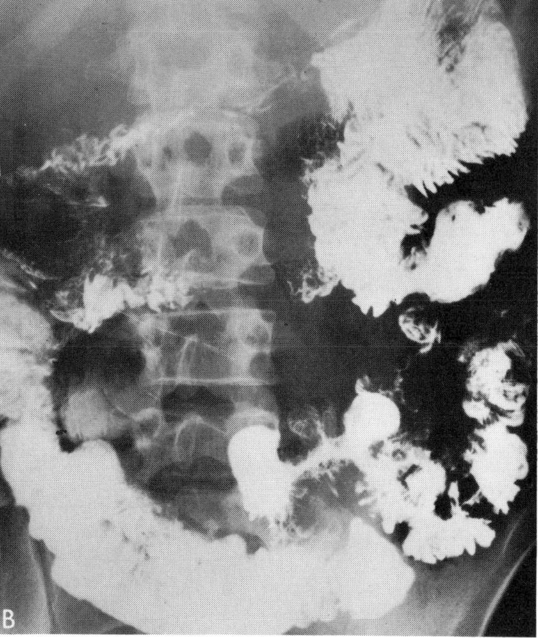

Figure 127–25. Non-stenotic type of Crohn's disease. Marked narrowing of the bowel lumen associated with pseudodiverticula.

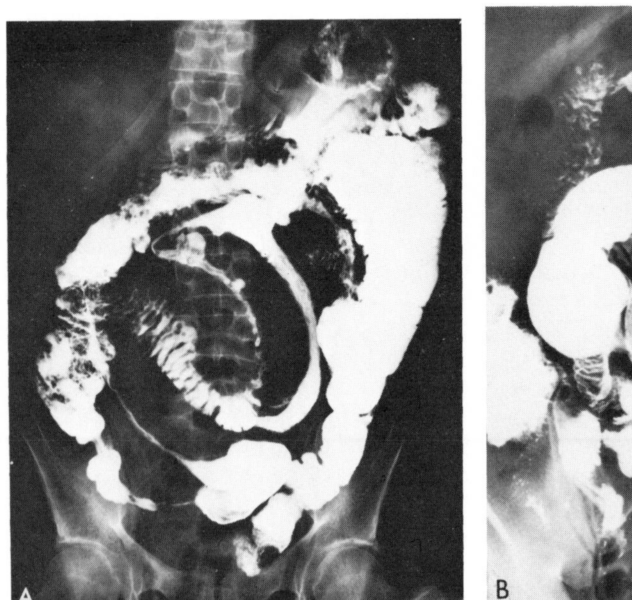

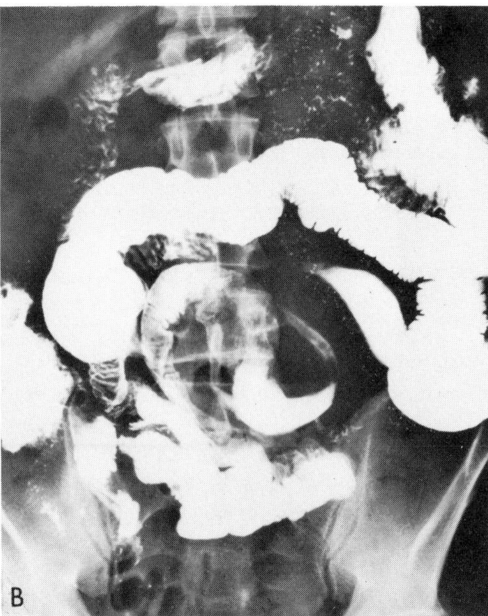

Figure 127–26. Early stenotic type of Crohn's disease. *A,* The mucosa is ulcerated and inflammatory polyps are present. The loop is rigid, narrowed, and surrounds an inflammatory mass. There is slight proximal dilatation. *B,* Long, rigid, narrowed segments are noted in the distal jejunum and proximal ileum with proximal dilatation.

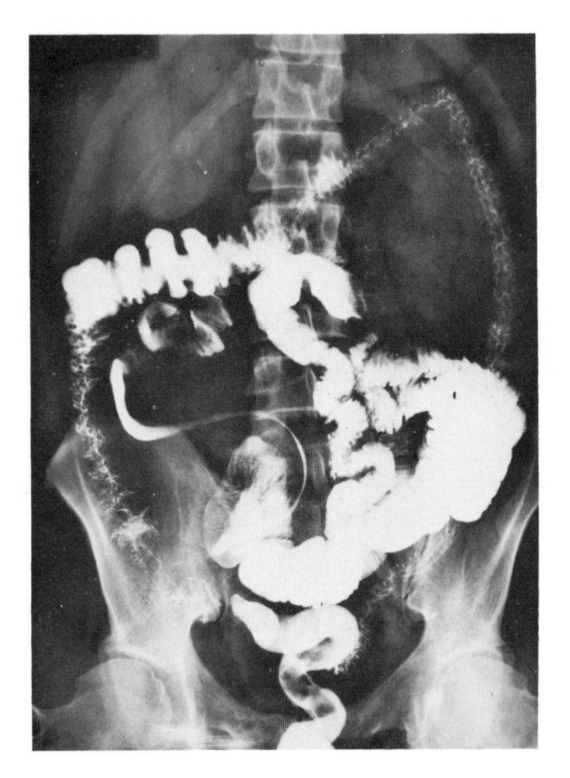

Figure 127–27. Stenotic type of Crohn's disease. The entire ileum is involved with marked stenosis.

segments of intestine are more striking. The loops are rigid and maintain a constant position from film to film, and the diseased intestinal segments seem to encircle an inflammatory mass. *Fistulas,* usually involving the distal ileum and adjacent loops of intestine, may be seen. Occasionally, these are difficult to demonstrate, especially when dilated loops of intestine produce overlapping. The fistulas may extend to and penetrate the abdominal wall.

In general, the roentgen findings in regional enteritis are as described. However, there are certain characteristics that are peculiar to the area of involvement in the small bowel, and these merit special note.

Site Of Small Bowel Involvement

Ileitis. The most frequent site of involvement of the small bowel with regional enteritis is the *terminal ileum.* Depending on the degree of inflammation, this segment exhibits varying roentgen alterations. Early in the disease, there may be only slight disturbance in peristaltic activity manifested by minimal flattening of the contours or irregular pseudodiverticular contractions and no limitation in distensibility. Slight spiculation of the contours may be identified, with minimal thickening and irregularity of the mucosal folds (Fig. 127–28). As ulceration proceeds, there is more spasm and irritability and more coarsening and thickening of the folds.

The final development is the so-called *string sign.* This sign has come to be identified as a pathognomonic roentgen manifestation of regional enteritis, most frequently noted in the terminal portion of the ileum. It has been described as a thin linear shadow, suggesting a frayed cotton string in appearance (Fig. 127–29*A*). The cause of the string sign is incomplete filling due to irritability and spasm associated with marked ulceration. It may be seen in both the non-stenotic and the stenotic phases of this disease. Repeated spot films will demonstrate that some distensibility is still present in this segment (Fig. 127–29*B*). The bowel proximal to the string sign may or may not be dilated, depending on the stage of the disease. In the non-stenotic phase, the proximal intestinal lumen is generally not dilated despite the marked narrowing associated with the string sign. This points up the importance of spasm in producing the characteristic appearance. The spasm is usually inconstant, but when it is persistent, temporary proximal dilatation may occur with signs of obstruction. In the stenotic phase there is constant proximal dilatation, which may be accentuated by spasm secondary to ulceration. Despite the narrow-

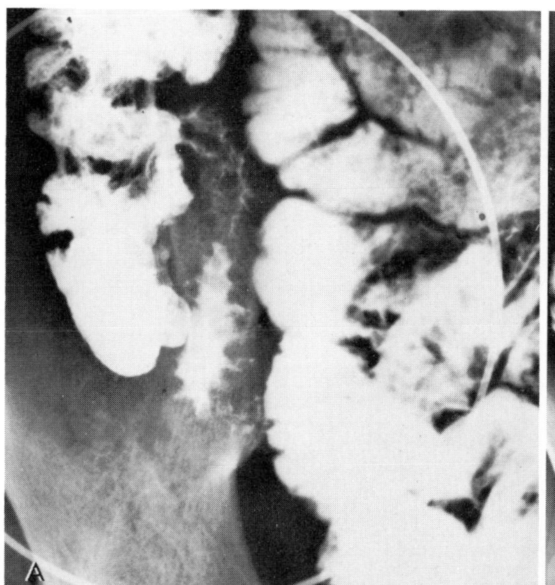

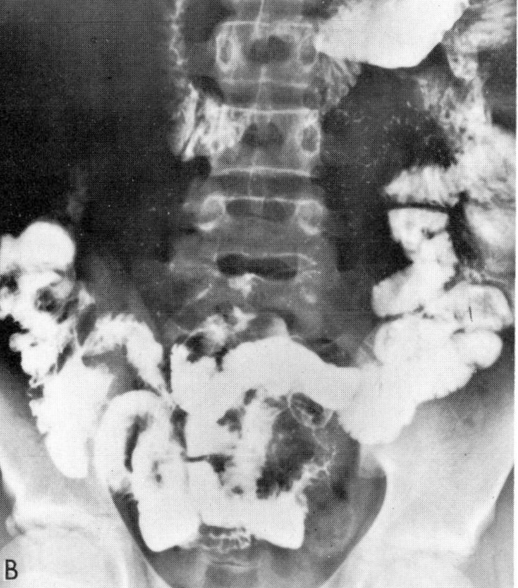

Figure 127–28. *A,* Minimal changes involving the terminal ileum, characterized by spasm and irritability and slight thickening and irregularity of the mucosal folds. *B,* Slightly more marked involvement of the distal 2 feet of ileum in a 15-year-old boy. There is ulceration of the mucosa with thickening and blunting of the folds.

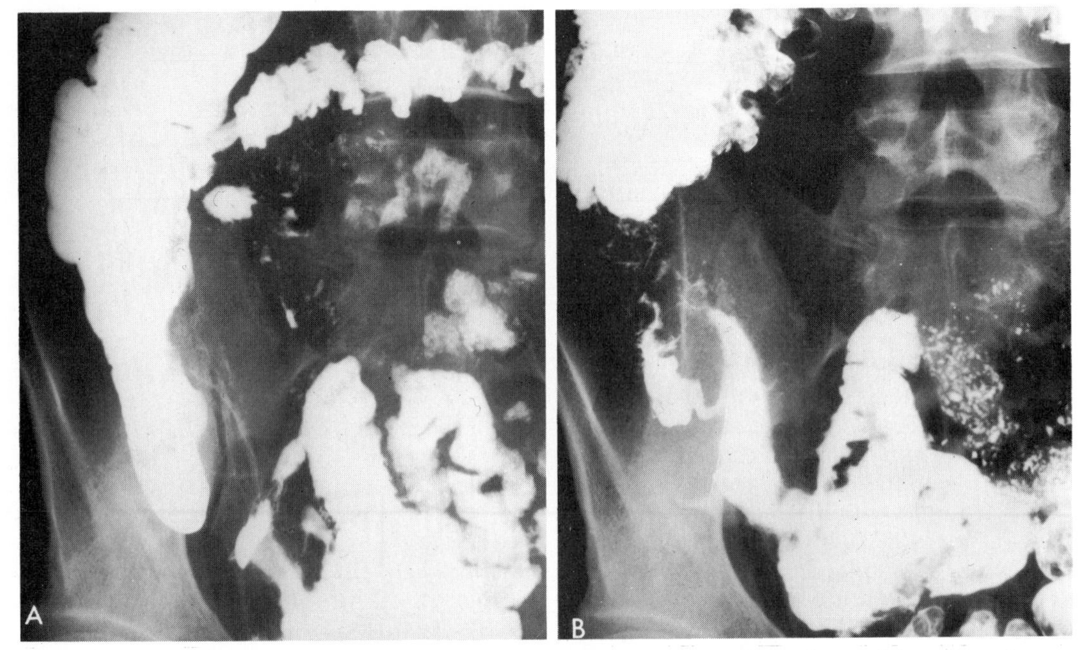

Figure 127–29. *A,* "String sign" in Crohn's disease. *B,* Same patient a few minutes later. There is more distensibility of the distal ileum. The cecum and ascending colon are more constricted. The findings in the ileum are due to marked ulceration and secondary spasm. The narrowing and rigidity of the cecum and ascending colon are due to a fistula from the distal portion of the terminal ileum (found at operation).

ing, complete intestinal obstruction is uncommon. It is important to realize that the string sign does not always indicate marked fibrosis and stenosis.

Because of the marked ulceration, fistulas, and perforation (Fig. 127–30), thickening of the mesentery and separation of the loops of bowel are more frequent in the distal ileum than in the remainder of the small bowel.

Deformities of the cecum and ascending colon are not unusual with involvement of the terminal ileum. These changes may vary from a gentle concavity in the mesial aspect of the cecum at the ileocecal region to marked narrowing of the cecum. This is an important sign, particularly if, at the time of the first barium enema examination, the terminal ileum cannot be filled because of marked

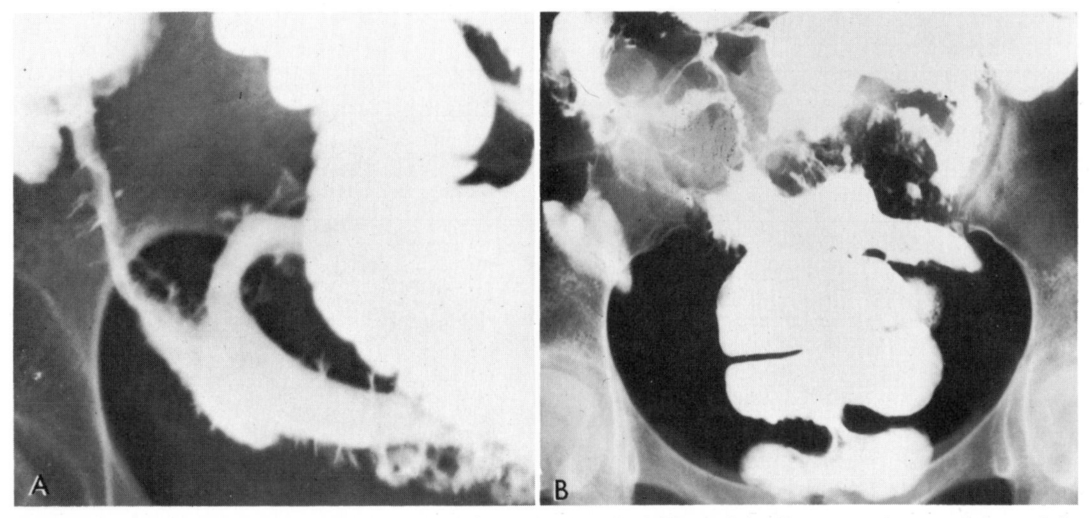

Figure 127–30. *A,* Numerous fistulas extend from the terminal ileum into the mesentery and toward the bladder. *B,* Numerous fistulas extend from the terminal ileum into the lower sigmoid.

spasm and irritability. The presence of this sign is very suggestive of regional enteritis, and re-examination for filling of the terminal ileum is important.

Deformity of the mesial aspect of the cecum is most often due to pressure on the colon by the thickened terminal ileum with its inflamed mesentery and by the heavy pad of mesenteric fat. In some cases, it is due to fistulas or intramural sinus tracts arising from the terminal ileum and extending into the right side of the colon.

Jejunoileitis. The distal half of jejunum and proximal half of ileum are involved in similar fashion. Skip areas are frequent and large inflammatory polyps may be noted. Ulceration is not as marked as in the terminal ileum, and fistula formation is less frequent. Because of the extent of involvement, operative intervention is often postponed, thereby allowing long follow-up observations to be made of the natural course of the disease. Transition from the non-stenotic to the stenotic stage can be observed to occur over an interval of 4 to 16 years in the average case.

It is of interest that many of the patients with such extensive involvement of the intestinal tract are able to maintain an adequate nutritional status despite the extent of disease and despite numerous episodes of partial intestinal obstruction.

Jejunitis. When the initial manifestations are mainly or exclusively in the jejunum, the roentgenographic pattern in some respects differs from that of disease localized in the ileum. Almost all of our patients with jejunitis have had longstanding disease, but early cases of jejunitis are now being recognized.

In distal ileitis, the roentgenographic picture is dominated by the appearance of diseased segments of bowel *per se*. In jejunitis, on the other hand, the sequelae of the diseased stenotic segments, i.e., markedly dilated, chronically obstructed loops, are the striking findings (Fig. 127–31). Retention of food and secretions and the inflammatory reaction that frequently develops in these chronically obstructed loops produce roentgenographic features that are characteristic of prolonged obstruction. It is often impossible in this situation to determine roentgenologically whether intrinsic involvement is present or whether changes are produced by the longstanding obstruction. The diameter of the doubly obstructed loops may attain the proportions of a markedly distended colon.

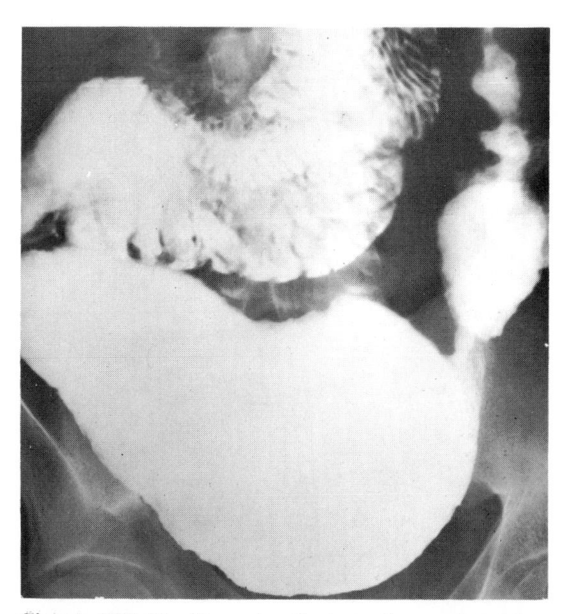

Figure 127–31. Stenosing Crohn's disease involving the jejunum. There is a huge dilated loop of jejunum in continuity with several strictured segments. At operation the disease was confined to the jejunum and multiple areas of stenosis were found.

In most instances the stenotic segments are easily visualized (Figs. 127–32 to 127–34). When numerous overlapping dilated intestinal loops are present, however, a single short stricture may be difficult to delineate.

Although stenotic segments indicate a considerable degree of fibrosis, narrowing may be enhanced by superimposed edema and spasm resulting from inflammation. The contours of the narrowed segments are usually smooth. The lumen is concentrically located. The mucosa may be cast-like or may reveal numerous pseudopolyps and ulcerations. The stenotic segments are rigid, may be single or multiple, and vary in length. If only a single area of constriction is present, a more or less uniform dilatation of the proximal bowel may be seen. The presence of skip lesions may result in a "hammock type" or "sausage link type" of deformity. When obstruction occurs near the ligament of Treitz, duodenal and even gastric dilatation may be evident. Ulceration, perforation, and their sequelae are much less common in jejunitis than in ileitis.

Recurrent Regional Enteritis. Recurrent disease is common following operation. The recurrence occurs most often during the first 2 years, but many years may elapse before new involvement is seen. Many patients with

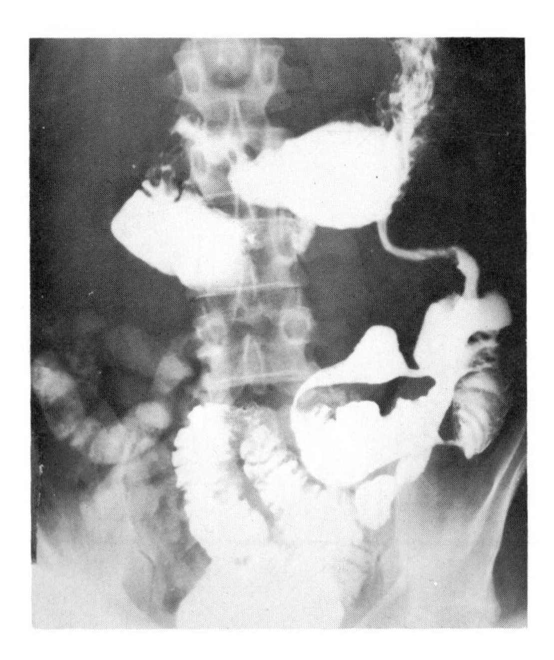

Figure 127–32. Starting at the ligament of Treitz, alternating areas of constriction and dilatation of the upper jejunum are seen. The duodenum is dilated. There is marked rigidity and uncoiling of the bowel loops with effacement of the mucosal folds. Diagnosis: stenosing jejunitis.

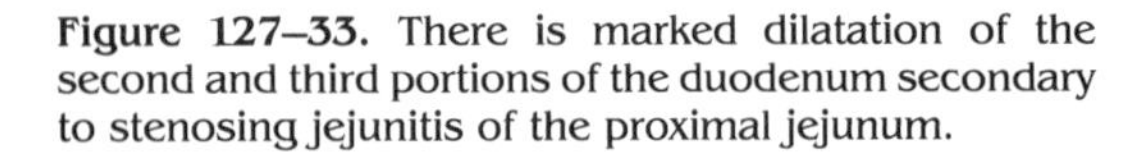

Figure 127–33. There is marked dilatation of the second and third portions of the duodenum secondary to stenosing jejunitis of the proximal jejunum.

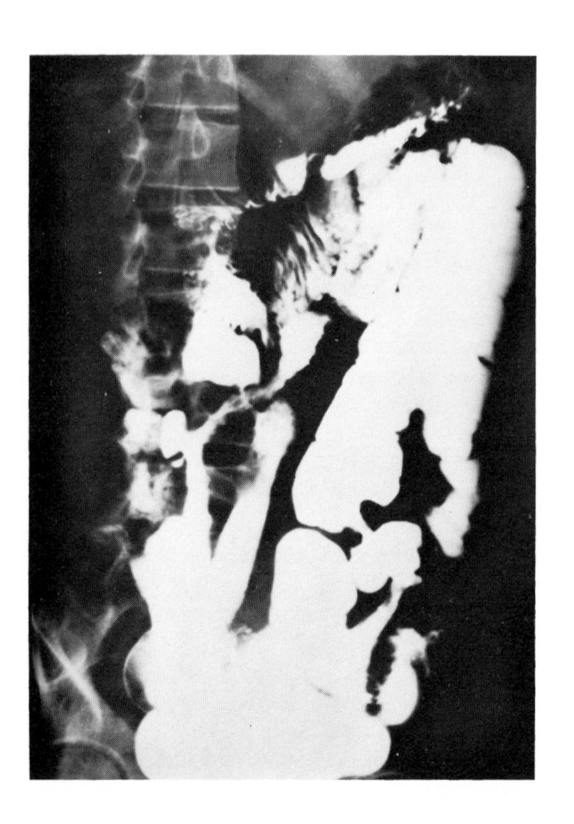

Figure 127–34. Alternating areas of stenosis and dilatation. These are best identified on the lateral or marked oblique projection. Diagnosis: stenosing jejunitis.

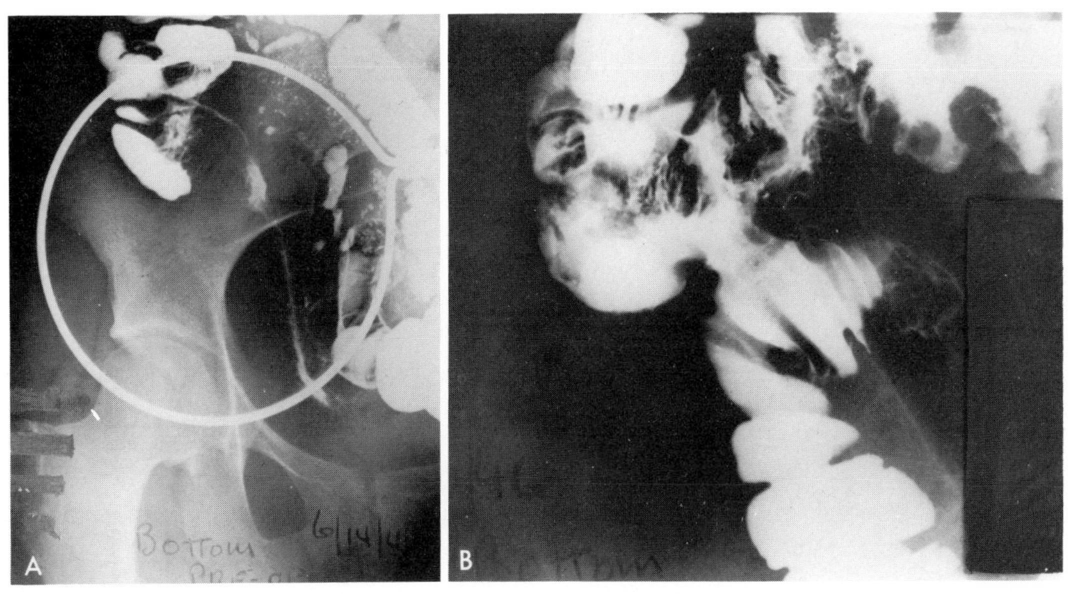

Figure 127–35. *A,* Original terminal ileitis in a 22-year-old woman. *B,* Barium enema 6 weeks after resection and proximal ileotransverse colostomy.

early recurrent lesions are asymptomatic for long periods of time.

In general, recurrent lesions resemble the original process roentgenologically. The earliest roentgen findings are thickening and blunting of the folds progressing from the non-stenotic to the stenotic phase. Fistula formation appears less often. The length of the original lesions has no effect on the recurrence rate. A remarkable feature is that the recurrences are almost always at the site of the anastomosis (Figs. 127–35 to 127–37). Extension into the colon also occurs postoperatively.

Healing. Roentgenologic demonstrations of improvement without operation are uncommon in our experience. However, remarkable changes have been observed occasionally, both spontaneously and following therapy, indicating that healing may occur

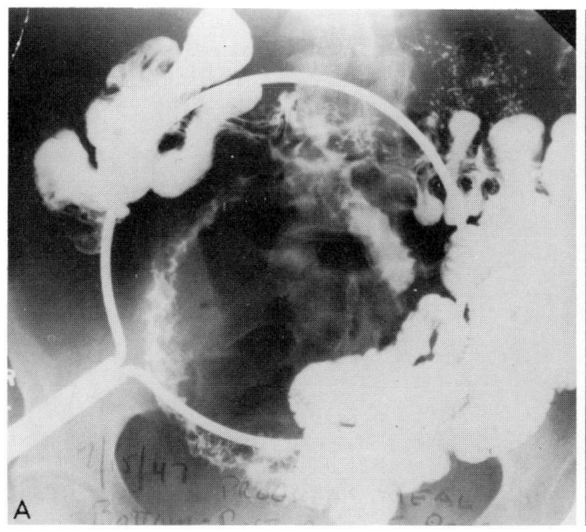

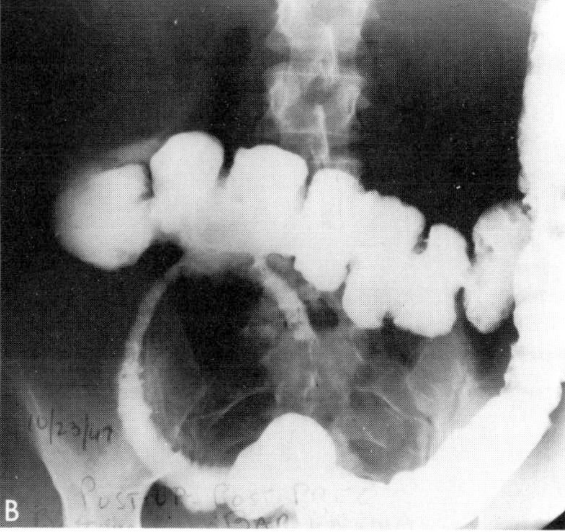

Figure 127–36. Case shown in Figure 127–35. *A,* One year later, showing nodular rigid terminal ileum characteristic of recurrent terminal ileitis. *B,* Three months later there is increased shortening, narrowing, and rigidity of the involved segment.

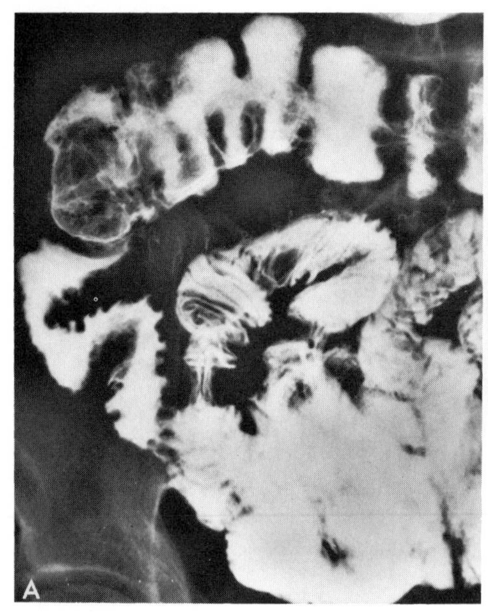

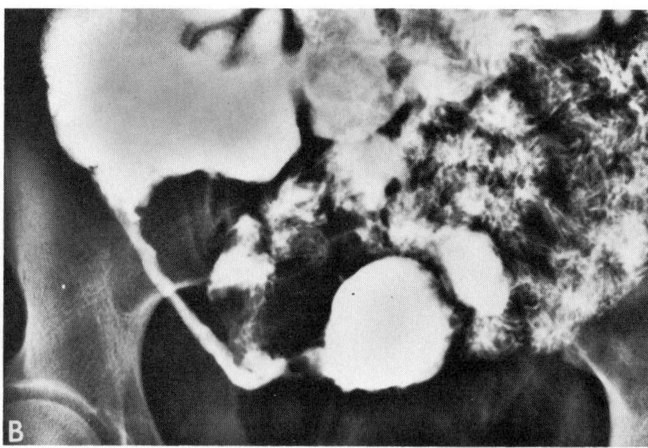

Figure 127–37. Recurrent ileitis. *A,* Six months after ileo-ascending colostomy, the new terminal ileum demonstrates spasm, irritability, blunting of folds, and early pseudodiverticula formation. *B,* Same patient 2 years later. Progression has occurred to the stenotic phase with narrowing and shortening of the terminal ileum.

(Fig. 127–38). The course of the disease is continuous in the great majority of patients, although many years may elapse before stenosis supervenes. It should be pointed out that secondary changes may occur in patients who are clinically improved, notably stenosing lesions and permanent loss of the normal small intestinal structure. These changes are due to healing with scar formation.

Carcinoma. Adenocarcinoma of the small bowel may develop in association with long-standing regional enteritis or in surgically excluded loops. The diagnosis of superimposed carcinoma is difficult to establish preoperatively because the presence of multiple strictures with intervening segments of dilated bowel obscures the associated malignancy on small bowel examination, and the

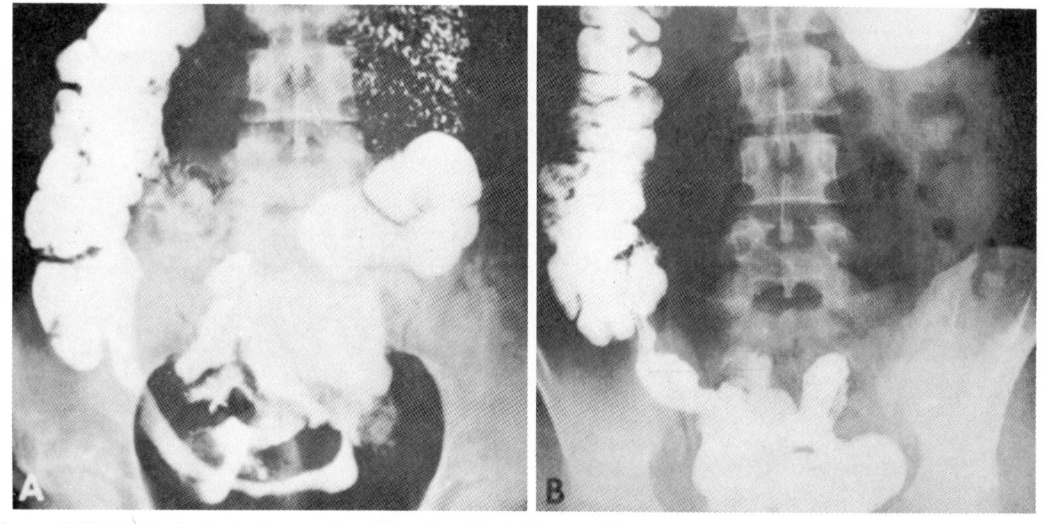

Figure 127–38. *A,* Crohn's disease involving the distal 45 cm of ileum. *B,* Six months later. There is a marked resolution of the appearance of the lesion. Despite the apparent healing of the mucosal ulcerations, this patient's disease progressed to fibrosis and partial intestinal obstruction requiring surgical intervention.

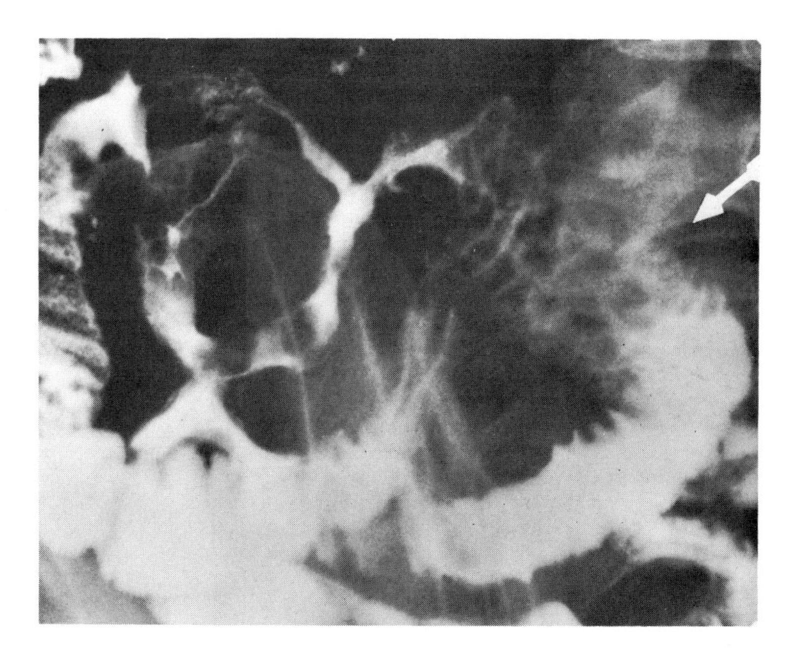

Figure 127–39. Endo-exo-enteric lymphoma of the distal ileum. The normal bowel lumen is replaced by many intercommunicating tortuous tracts through the tumor. The arrow points to the nodular mucosal pattern proximal to the mass. The lumen of this segment is not narrowed. This film was interpreted as Crohn's disease, but 3 months later a mass appeared in the neck that proved on biopsy to be lymphosarcoma. The fistulas represented multiple intercommunicating tortuous tracts through the tumor mass.

clinical features of the carcinoma resemble those of obstructing inflammatory disease.

Differential Diagnosis. The roentgen alterations in regional enteritis are sufficiently characteristic that differential diagnosis is not difficult in most instances. The following diseases, however, may on occasion simulate the roentgen findings of Crohn's disease of the small intestine:

Lymphoma (see Chapter 112). This disorder can simulate the non-stenotic phase of regional enteritis.[7] Thickening and blunting of the folds, irregularity of the contour, ulceration, intraluminal nodules, and fistulas are features that are common to both (Figs. 127–39 and 127–40). More inflammation occurs in regional enteritis, producing spasm and narrowing of the bowel lumen and associated cobblestoning. Irregular nodules that can be identified as tumors are uncommon with regional enteritis, but are a frequent finding in lymphoma. Although narrowing of the bowel lumen can be seen in lymphoma as a result of tumor encroachment, the bowel as a rule is of normal caliber or is dilated. Ulcerations in lymphoma are usually discrete or multiple and do not have the cobblestone configuration seen in regional enteritis. Separation of the loops of bowel in regional enteritis is also more marked than in lymphoma.

Hodgkin's Disease. This disease can produce all the roentgen alterations just described for lymphoma plus marked fibrosis of the bowel with constriction of the lumen. The features that distinguish this disease from a single stenotic lesion of regional enteritis are the eccentric lumen, the presence of a tumor nodule, and the absence of chronic intestinal obstruction in the former. In regional enteritis, multiple areas of stenosis are more frequent, and the proximal dilated loops of bowel are usually longer, with evi-

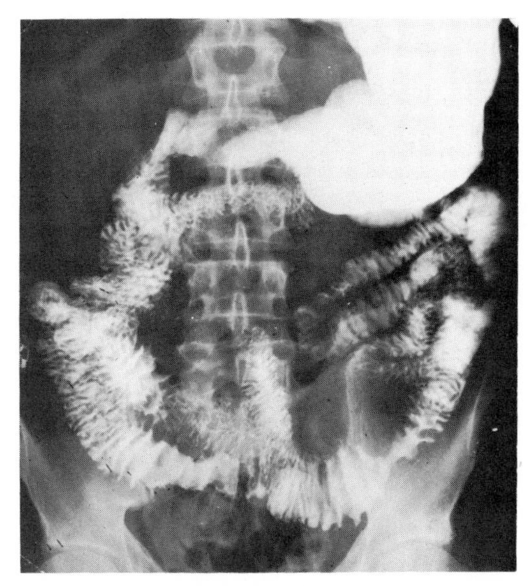

Figure 127–40. Lymphoma of the distal jejunum simulating the non-stenotic phase of Crohn's disease.

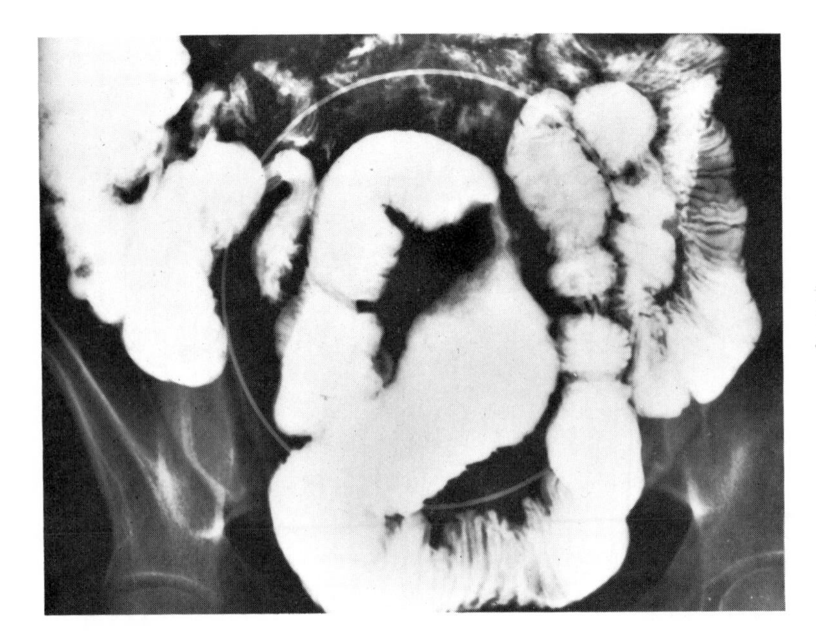

Figure 127–41. Segmental infarction of the ileum producing an area of stenosis.

dence of considerable secretion and chronic obstruction. In addition, cobblestoning is commonly present.

Ischemia of the Small Intestine (see Chapter 116). An ischemic small bowel may show fairly rapid progressive changes leading to stricture formation. An individual segment may completely simulate a stenotic segment in regional enteritis, but evidence of chronic proximal intestinal obstruction is less marked, and the history is usually characteristic (Figs. 127–41 and 127–42). Chronic ischemia may be especially difficult to distinguish from Crohn's disease in the elderly.

Malabsorption Syndrome. Although the clinical features of both regional enteritis and the malabsorption syndrome may be similar (Chapter 101), the roentgen features are entirely different (Chapter 102). In the sprue-like states, stenosis is rare and evidence of an inflammatory process is either minimal or completely absent. Dilatation, segmentation, and increased secretions are the prominent roentgen features in celiac sprue.

Nodular Lymphoid Hyperplasia. The normal terminal ileum in children contains sufficient lymphoid tissue to produce small filling defects within the lumen. These are usually symmetric and fairly sharply demarcated with no evidence of an inflammatory process. This is also a normal finding in adolescents and tends to disappear (Fig. 127–43). When the process is diffuse in the small bowel, nodular lymphoid hyperplasia may be related to immunodeficiency states.[8]

Tuberculosis (see Chapter 120). Tuberculosis can completely simulate the findings of regional enteritis,[9] but in the former there is usually more marked involvement of the colon than of the terminal ileum. The defect tends to have more irregular contours. The mucosal markings are also coarser owing to the large, irregular ulcerations frequently

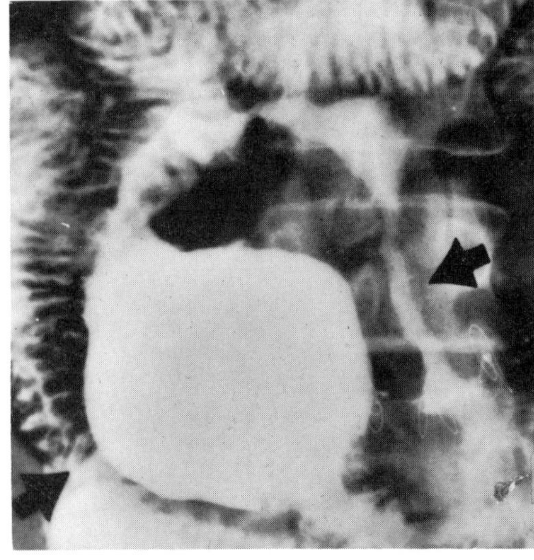

Figure 127–42. Infarction of the small bowel secondary to a strangulated incisional hernia. There is a striking resemblance to Crohn's disease.

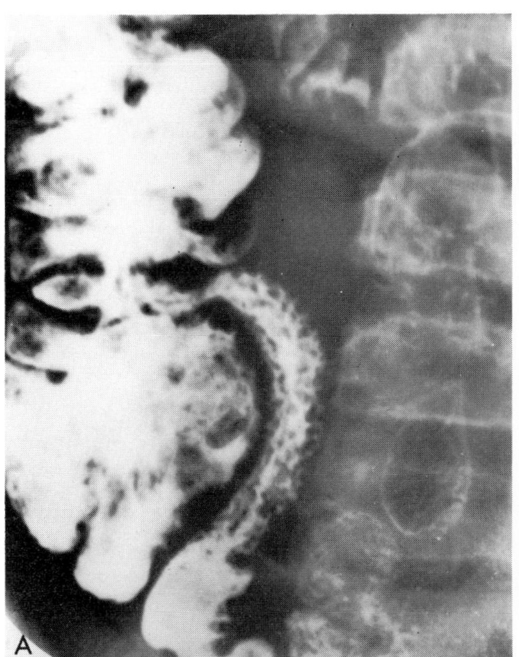

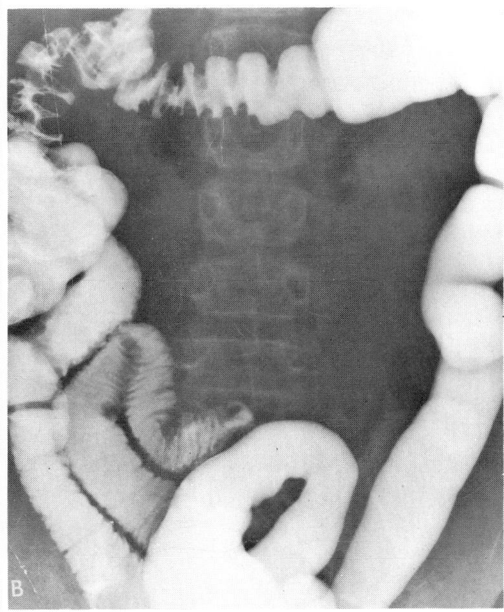

Figure 127–43. Nodular lymphoid hyperplasia. Numerous small and fairly sharply demarcated radiolucent filling defects are seen in an asymptomatic young woman. This is a normal finding in adolescents and young adults.

seen in tuberculosis. Tuberculosis of the small intestine is not necessarily associated with involvement of the lungs, and this can make the problem of differential diagnosis all the more difficult.

Amebiasis (see Chapter 232). Amebiasis involving the small bowel is rarely observed in the United States. A cone-shaped appearance of the cecum is often mentioned as a pathognomonic radiographic feature of amebiasis, but we have seen this configuration much more often with regional enteritis, appendicitis, and Crohn's disease of the colon.

Carcinoid Tumors (see Chapter 113). These tumors involve long segments of the small bowel, with muscle hypertrophy and fibrosis. The changes resemble those of regional enteritis. Tumor nodules can usually be identified, however, and their presence permits differentiation from inflammatory disease. Sometimes the distinction cannot be made radiologically, and the carcinoid tumor is an unexpected finding at laparotomy or in the pathology laboratory.

Yersinia Enterocolitis (see Chapter 118). Acute infections with *Yersinia* can cause spasm, irritability, and thickening and blunting of the folds in the terminal ileum resembling the changes seen in the non-stenotic phase of regional enteritis. Aphthoid ulcerations may develop, but large ulcerations and cobblestoning are not seen.

Carcinoma of the Cecum. When carcinoma of the right colon extends into the terminal ileum, the resultant narrowing and rigidity may simulate regional enteritis. However, the roentgen features of carcinoma of the colon are always present (Chapter 139) and serve to distinguish this disease.

Colon

Technique. Our technique for barium enema examination is similar for the various types of inflammatory bowel disease. Because diarrhea is usually moderately severe, we prefer to avoid laxatives. Many patients use antidiarrheal agents, and at times constipation may occur, accompanied by large numbers of fecoliths. In such individuals, gentle cleansing with laxatives is necessary. In the typical patient, however, who has multiple bowel discharges during the day, we suggest the following: a liquid diet for 2 days, followed by tap water enemas until the returns are clear. Many patients have difficulty retaining barium, and administration of glucagon is helpful for muscle relaxation just prior to the examination. In fulminant or very active disease, of course, barium enema examination should be deferred until symptoms have subsided.

The roentgenologic method employed should be the one that best demonstrates the changes in inflammatory bowel disease. Presently, 2 basic methods are used for performing barium enema examinations (Chapter 33): (1) The conventional method of filling the colon with barium sulfate mixtures and utilizing high kilo-voltage and multiple compression spot films. The barium-water mixture must not be too dilute and should contain a suitable suspending agent. Evacuation films are regularly obtained. (2) The double contrast technique using high density barium to coat the bowel, followed by immediate injection of air to produce high quality air contrast films. Multiple projections are employed, including films taken with the patient upright and in the lateral decubitus position.

Both of these methods are excellent. The double contrast method is superior for the detection of tiny or aphthoid ulcers, but a good evacuation film cannot be obtained. All the other roentgen alterations can be well identified with either method. Air contrast examination is being increasingly utilized for the detection of minimal inflammatory disease. Except for the demonstration of the aphthoid ulcers, either method is satisfactory for the early diagnosis of inflammatory disease.

Roentgen Features. One of the striking radiologic features of Crohn's disease of the colon is the frequency of concomitant and similar disease in the small bowel. Indeed, 85% of the patients we have studied with this form of disease in the colon have the disease as well in the ileum; in 15%, the disease is confined to the large bowel. The most frequent distribution that we have seen in Crohn's colitis is involvement of the terminal ileum and the colon to the splenic flexure or to the sigmoid with sparing of the rectum. Universal involvement of the colon, including the rectum, is noted in 10% to 15% of patients.

The radiologic features characteristic of Crohn's colitis are basically the same as those seen in the small bowel in patients with regional enteritis. These are listed in Table 127–7.

Table 127–7. ROENTGEN FINDINGS IN CROHN'S DISEASE OF THE COLON

1. Tiny discrete superficial ulcers (aphthoid ulcers) usually associated with small radiolucent nodules
2. Segmental distribution, more disease on the right than on the left
3. Universal distribution in colon, almost always associated with involvement of the terminal ileum
4. Nodular irregular pattern after evacuation
5. Edematous mucosa
6. Punched out ulcers, small or large, smooth or irregular
7. Longitudinal and transverse ulcerations
8. Combination of transverse and longitudinal ulcerations with cobblestoning
9. Strictures
10. Irregularity of contour with asymmetric involvement and pseudodiverticula
11. Skip lesions
12. Fistulas, frequent in the ileum but considerably less common in the colon
13. Intramural abscesses

The early roentgen findings are minute ulcerations (aphthoid ulcers). With air contrast and high density barium, the aphthoid ulcers appear as small central barium densities, each surrounded by a radiolucent halo. On the single contrast study, they appear as diminutive specks within the lumen, tiny spicules projecting from the contours of the bowel, or minute ulcers within irregular nodules (Figs. 127–44 to 127–46). The nodules are secondary to lymphoid hyperplasia and obstructive lymphedema. In some cases, miniscule nodular lymphoid defects are seen distal to the main lesion on air contrast studies. These aggregates of lymphoid tissue are the most frequent sites of aphthoid ulcers (Fig. 127–47).

As mentioned earlier, aphthoid ulcers alone are not specific for Crohn's disease. They may be identified in the early stage of any acute inflammatory disease, including infection with *Yersinia, Entamoeba histolytica,* herpes virus, and *Salmonella,* as well as gonococcal proctitis, shigellosis, and tuberculosis.

Other early roentgen alterations include thickening of the haustral septae, slight rigidity, and increased secretions (Figs. 127–48 to 127–51). These alterations may be diffuse, confined to a short segment, or seen in the form of multiple lesions with normal intervening bowel (skip lesions).

The mucosal pattern after evacuation is helpful in demonstrating thickening or nodularity of the mucosa. Adequate post-evacu-

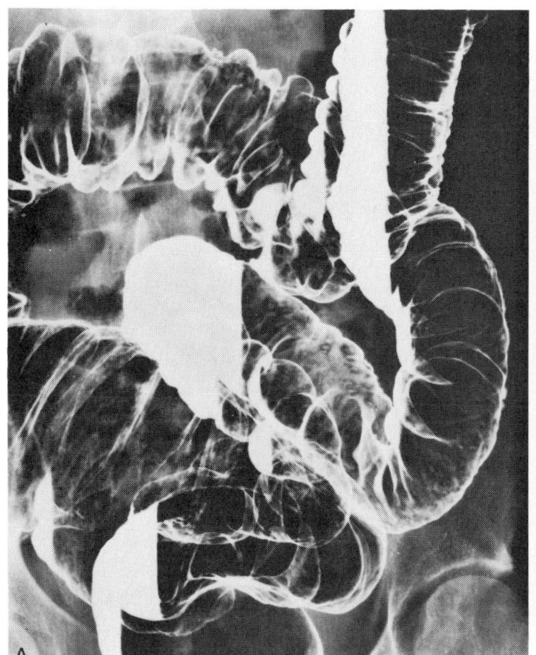

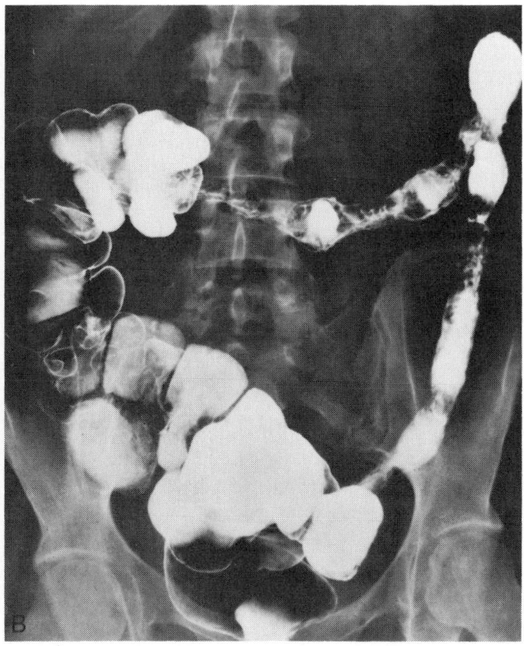

Figure 127–44. *A,* Crohn's colitis. Aphthous ulcers in the sigmoid are demonstrated on air contrast studies. The ulcers appear as flecks of barium surrounded by radiolucent halos. There are minimal alterations in the haustral pattern of the transverse colon. *B,* Same patient as shown in *A* 1 year later. There has been considerable progression with narrowing, rigidity, cobblestoning, and skip lesions. Such rapid change from aphthous ulcers to moderately severe Crohn's disease is unusual.

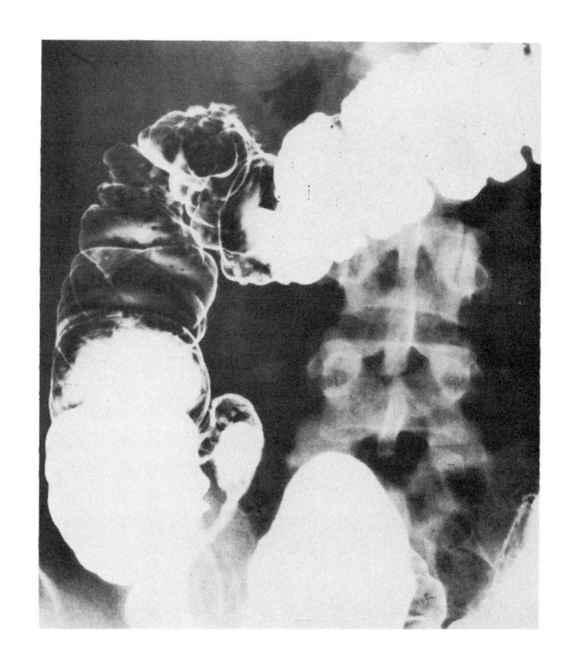

Figure 127–45. Crohn's colitis. Aphthous ulcers in the ascending colon and punched out ulcers in the hepatic flexure. The terminal ileum is also involved. (Courtesy of Dr. I. Laufer.)

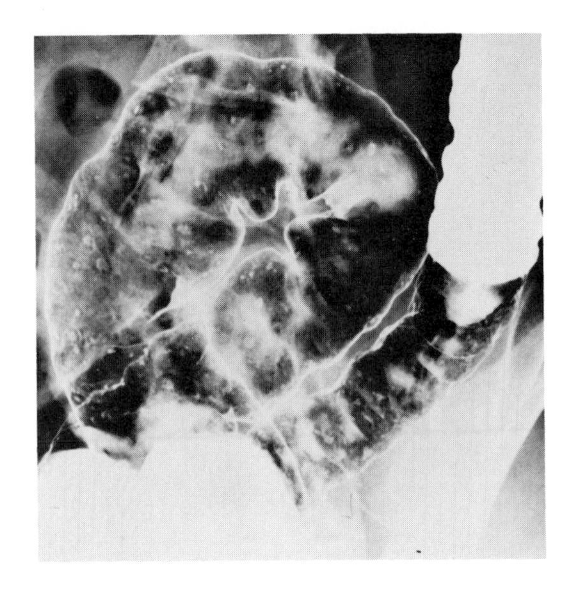

Figure 127–46. Aphthous ulcers in the sigmoid. (Courtesy of Dr. C. Bartram.)

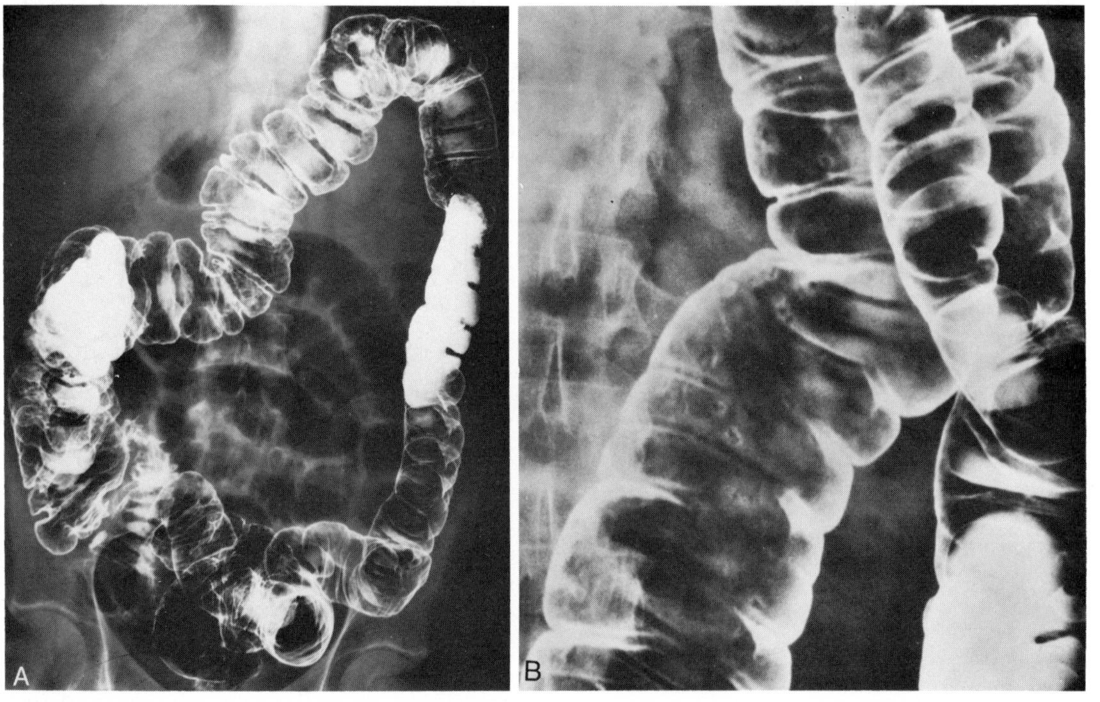

Figure 127–47. Ileocolitis. *A,* Air contrast study showing moderately severe changes involving the terminal ileum. Numerous small nodular defects are present in the ascending and transverse colon. At surgery some of the nodules were found to be associated with aphthous ulcers. *B,* Spot film of same patient taken over distal transverse colon showing nodular defects.

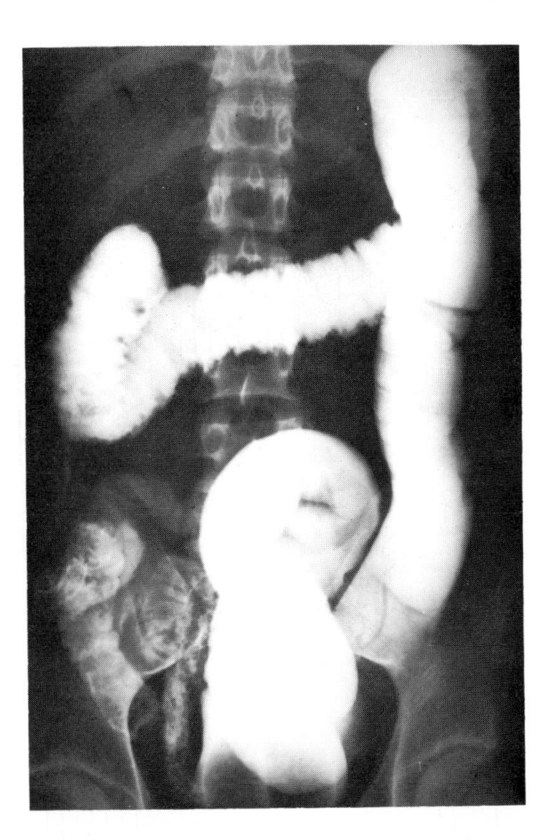

Figure 127–48. Crohn's disease of the colon. There are numerous small irregular nodular defects along the contour of the transverse colon associated with minimal rigidity. The cecum and ascending colon are spastic and irritable.

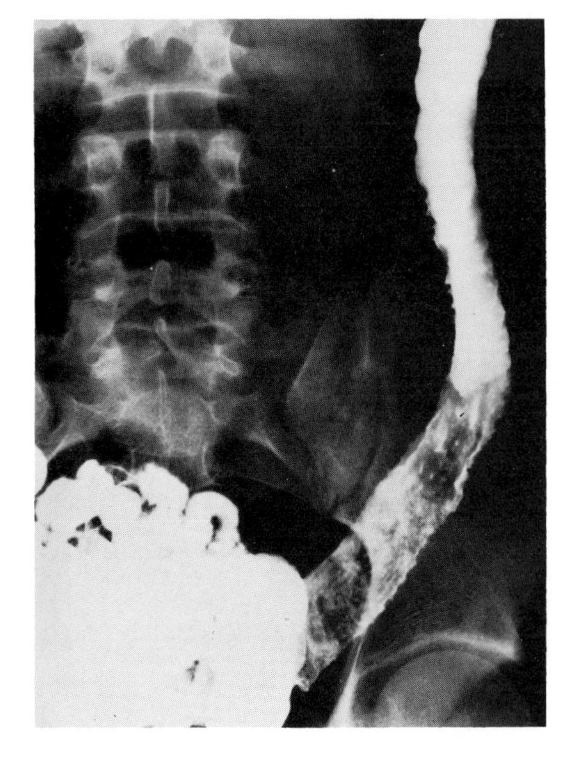

Figure 127–49. Crohn's disease of the colon. There are numerous small ulcerations within the lumen and along the contours of the bowel in the region of the distal descending colon. There is also slight narrowing and rigidity.

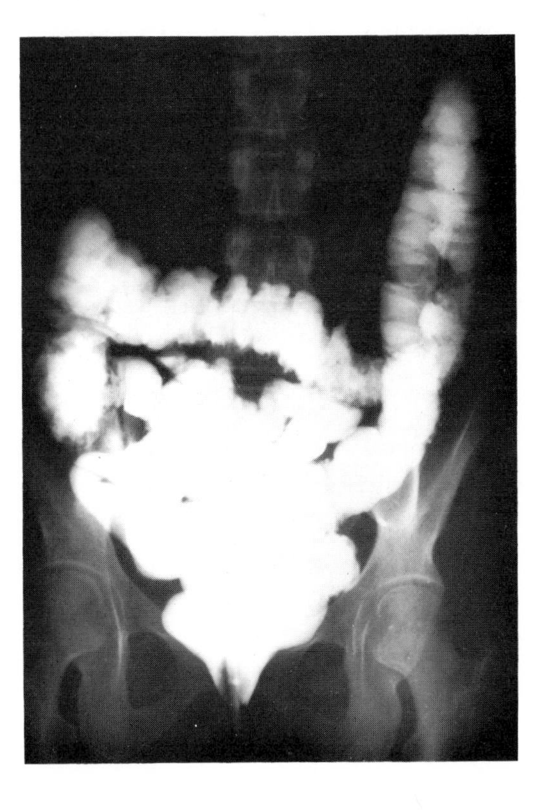

Figure 127–50. Crohn's disease of the colon. There is involvement of the colon from the cecum to the splenic flexure characterized by irregularity of the contour with multiple small nodular defects. The findings are most marked in the distal transverse colon, where there is rigidity and lack of distensibility.

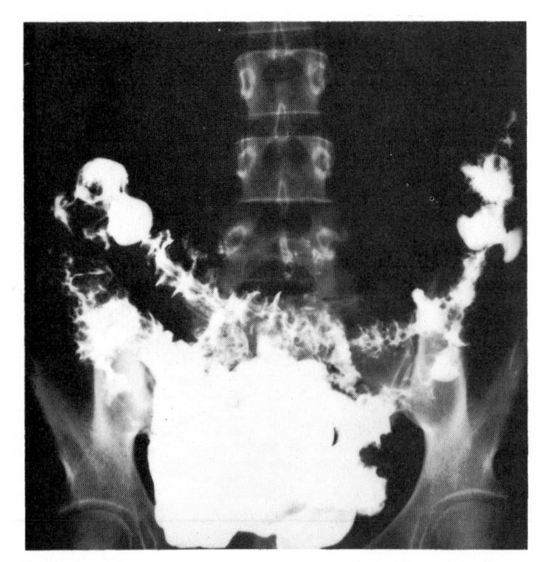

Figure 127–51. Evacuation film of patient in Figure 127–50. The mucosal pattern has an irregular nodular appearance. Small skip lesions indicated by pseudodiverticula are identified. Involvement of the left side of the colon, not appreciated in Figure 127–50, is well demonstrated on this film, showing the value of an evacuation film in Crohn's colitis.

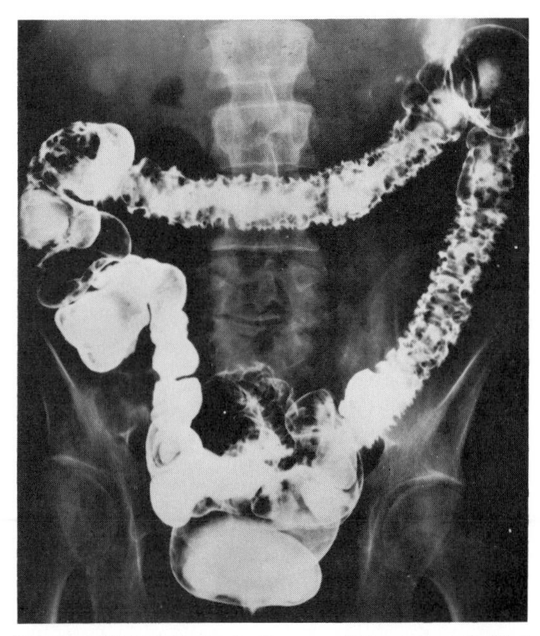

Figure 127–52. Crohn's disease of the colon. Multiple ulcerations are associated with a moderate degree of narrowing and rigidity. The terminal ileum and rectum are normal.

ation films cannot be obtained after air contrast studies. Also of value is a film to follow the barium through the colon as part of the small bowel examination. This film may detect early changes not recognized in the filled colon or on air contrast studies.

On occasion, ulcerations are suggested by straightening or rigidity of a segment of bowel associated with pseudodiverticula on the opposite wall (Figs. 127–50 and 127–51). Pseudodiverticula are created by involvement of one wall of a segment of bowel but not the opposite wall. Ulceration produces spasm and contractions, but the opposite uninvolved wall becomes folded, creating the appearance of diverticula (eccentric skip lesions).

The minute aphthae grow larger and become irregular punched-out ulcers (Fig. 127–52) that combine to produce longitudinal and transverse *fissures*. The inflamed mucosa between the longitudinal and transverse fissures produces a cobblestone pattern (Fig. 127–53). Cobblestoning does not always indicate ulcerations; it may also represent barium caught between edematous mucosal folds, compartmentalized by underlying fibrosis.

Deep "collar button" ulcers are seen as often in Crohn's colitis as in ulcerative coli-

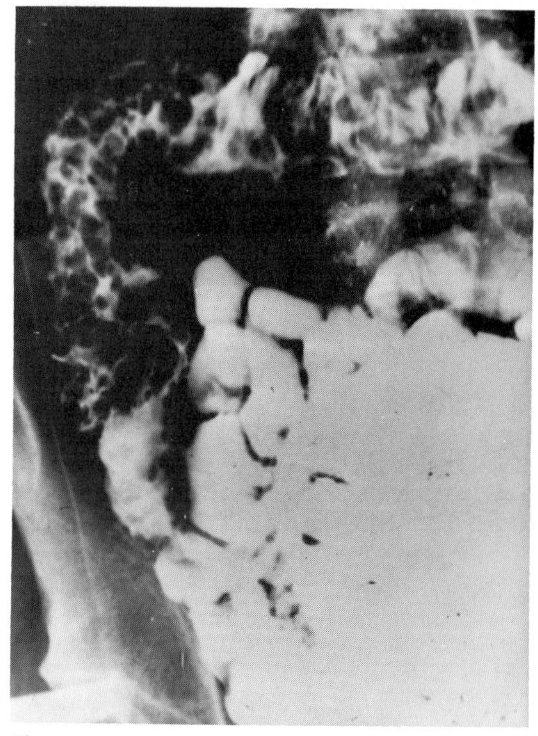

Figure 127–53. Ileocolitis. There is cobblestoning produced by longitudinal and transverse ulcerations with narrowing and rigidity of the colon. The findings in the colon and ileum are identical.

tis. They may also be found in ischemia of the colon and in amebiasis. Ulcers may penetrate beyond the contour of the bowel and appear in profile as numerous long spicules perpendicular to the long axis of the bowel. Localized abscesses may occur, producing rounded sac-like structures simulating diverticula. When a fissure penetrates into an adjacent loop, a *fistula* is formed (Figs. 127–54 and 127–55). In the later stages of the disease, the entire mucosa may be sloughed because of diffuse ulcerations.

In those cases in which the bowel is diffusely and symmetrically involved and there are no typical features of Crohn's disease, differentiation from ulcerative colitis may be impossible. This is especially so in the absence of character changes in the small intestine (Fig. 127–56). Diagnosis is also difficult and challenging when only the rectum and sigmoid or the left colon is involved. These cases can be distinguished from ulcerative colitis only if radiologic features characteristic of Crohn's disease are present within the area of involvement (Fig. 127–57).

In some patients, large, irregular, nodular contour defects with hazy margins are seen (Fig. 127–58). These lesions primarily reflect mucosal and submucosal edema associated with ulcerations. Large inflammatory polyps may also be identified. When multiple, these may simulate a neoplasm or cause obstruction (Fig. 127–59). Skip lesions may be identified at all stages of the disease. Thickening of the bowel produces irregular stenotic segments and strictures. Rarely is Crohn's colitis seen as a single stricture of the colon. When this stricture is eccentric and associated with suggestions of overhanging edges, differentiation from carcinoma may be impossible. In most cases, however, there is further evidence of involvement of the bowel in the form of skip lesions, strictures, or other identifying features of Crohn's disease.

Ileocolitis. The radiologic features of ileocolitis are a combination of those of Crohn's disease of the colon and regional enteritis (Fig. 127–53). The characteristic findings of regional enteritis are not affected by the presence of concomitant inflammatory disease in the colon. In most cases, the inflammatory process in the small bowel is confined to the terminal ileum, but at times long segments of small bowel are involved. Characteristically, the involvement of the colon is in continuity with the disease of the ileum.

Ileocolitis must be distinguished from *backwash ileitis* associated with ulcerative colitis. In backwash ileitis, narrowing of the intestinal lumen is usually minimal and the length of ileum involved is small. Sinus tracts, skip areas, and fistulas are not seen. The mucosa is only slightly altered, with minimal thickening of the folds. In a rare case, differentiation is impossible.

Carcinoma of the Colon. Ulcerative colitis is considered potentially a premalignant lesion because of the predisposition for carcinoma to develop in bowel involved with this disease (Chapter 126). Colonic carcinoma may also arise in patients with Crohn's colitis, but the occurrence rate is much lower. When carcinoma of the colon does appear, even though it has the typical roentgen features of malignancy (Chapter 139), it is difficult to isolate from adjoining severe inflammatory disease.

Toxic Dilatation. The colon affected by Crohn's disease would appear to be unlikely to develop severe dilatation and threatened perforation because the chronic inflammation is transmural and tends to thicken the wall. Yet, in more active and early forms of the disease, before fibrosis has become a conspicuous feature, moderate degrees of dilatation may occur. In such instances, deep abscesses and sinus tracts are frequently associated features, and the findings have usually been confined to the transverse colon. We have not had occasion to observe in any of our patients with Crohn's disease of the colon the markedly distended colon seen in patients with toxic dilatation complicating ulcerative colitis.

Recurrences and Linear Extension of Disease. Crohn's disease of the colon may progressively display more severe inflammatory changes within the area involved. Minimal radiologic alterations are often subtle and easy to overlook but become readily identified on subsequent examinations. Observers may differ in evaluating a segment as normal or minimally diseased. This circumstance may be responsible for reports of "spread" of Crohn's disease into an apparently normal segment of bowel; the putative "spread" may represent worsening of a mild inflammatory process rather than the advent of disease in a previously uninvolved area. It is well known that Crohn's disease in the colon or small bowel may recur following surgery. Linear extension of the disease in the absence

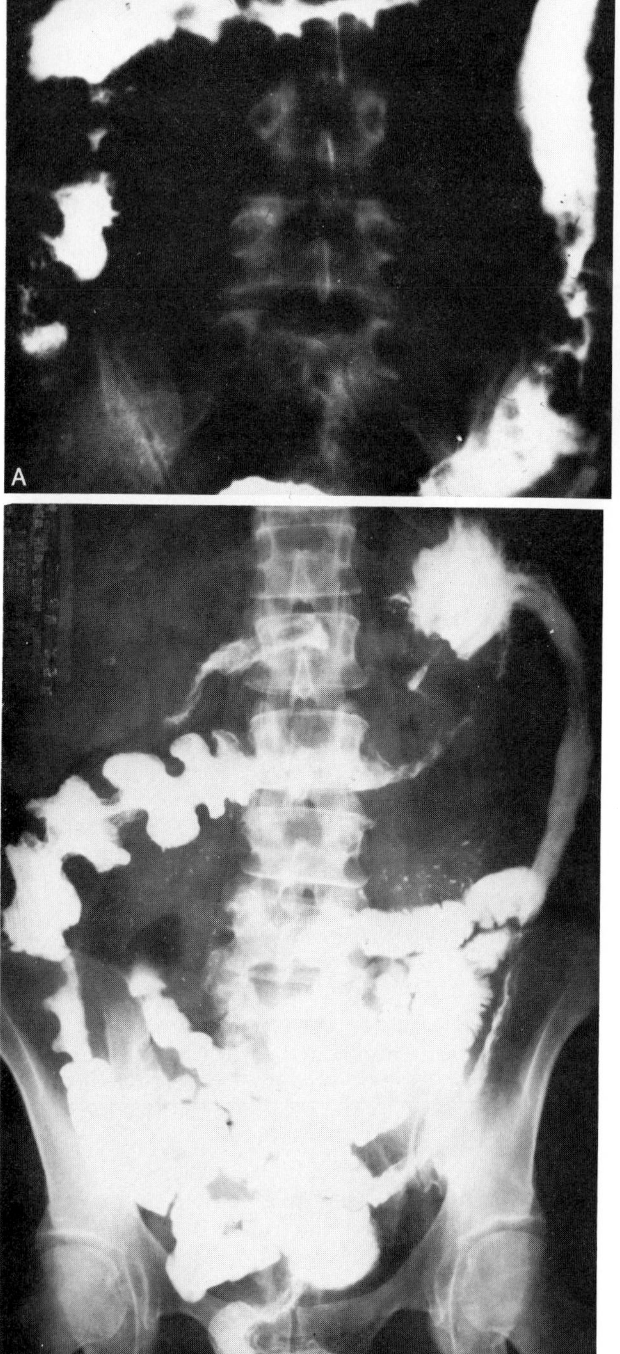

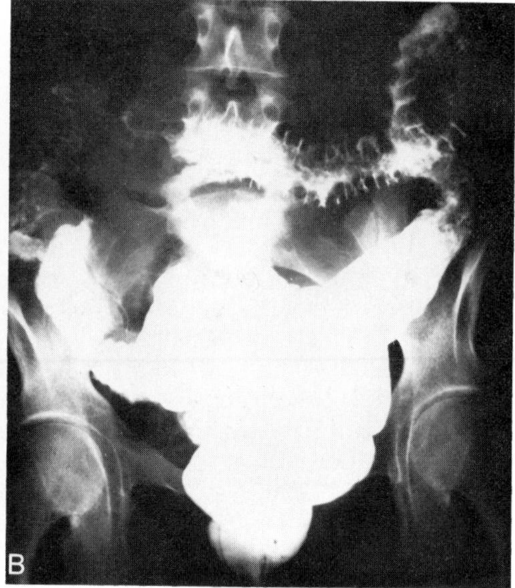

Figure 127–54. Crohn's disease of the colon. *A,* There are longitudinal ulcerations and transverse ulcerations in the transverse colon. *B,* A film taken 6 months later showing extensive ulceration of the colon from the cecum to the mid-descending colon. Marked transverse ulcerations are present in the transverse colon. The terminal ileum is also involved. The rectum, sigmoid, and lower descending colon are normal. *C,* Two years after the original study. There is more extensive involvement of the colon with a fistulous communication between the splenic flexure and the stomach. The distal transverse colon is ulcerated with gross irregularity of the contours.

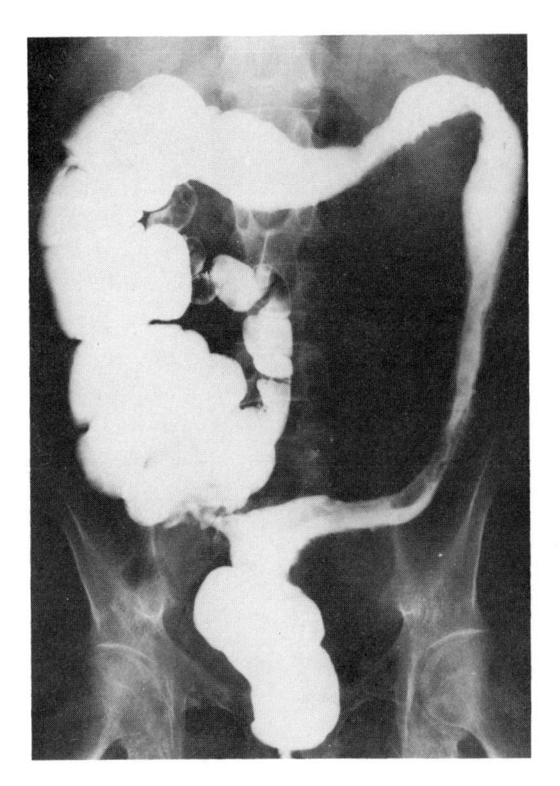

Figure 127–55. Crohn's disease of the colon. There is a fistulous communication between the distal ileum, cecum, and sigmoid.

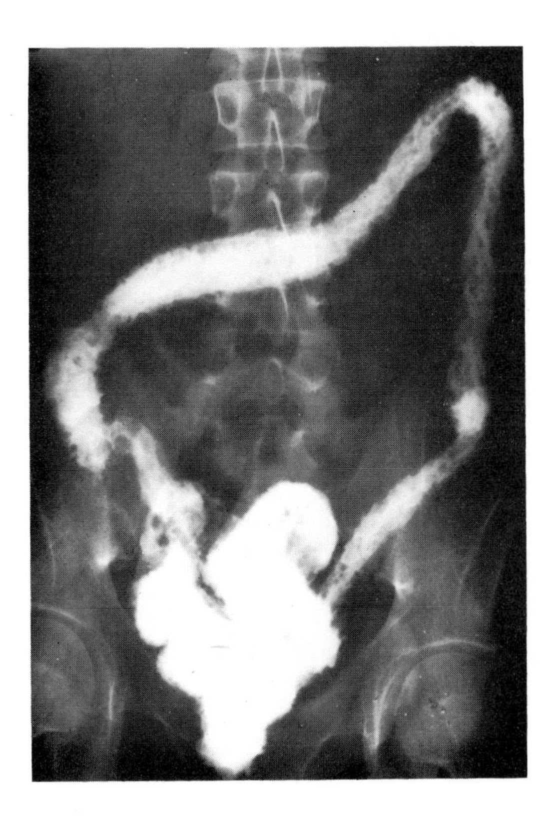

Figure 127–56. Ileocolitis. There is a moderate degree of narrowing and rigidity of the entire colon with ulcerations of the mucosa and numerous small inflammatory polyps. This type of diffuse involvement is more commonly seen in ulcerative colitis, but it can also be identified in Crohn's disease. In this patient the involvement of the terminal ileum with typical regional enteritis enables the radiologist to make a diagnosis of Crohn's disease affecting both the ileum and the colon (ileocolitis).

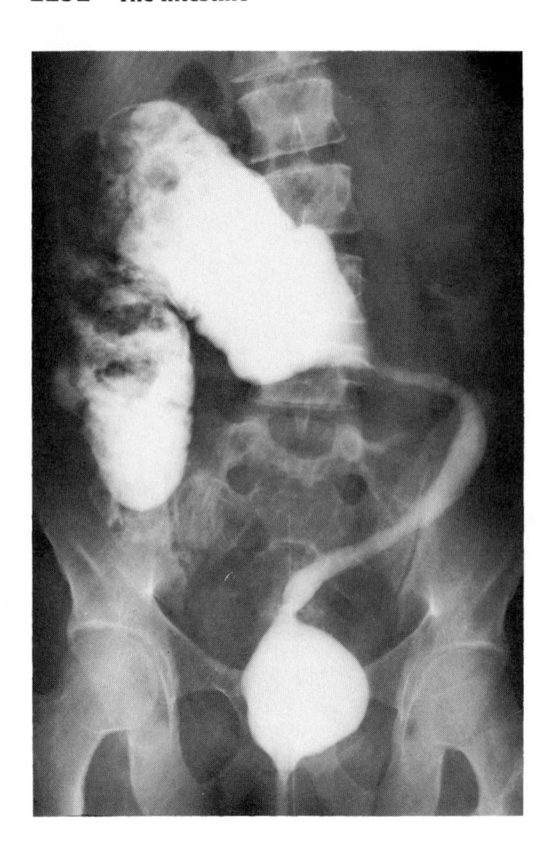

Figure 127–57. Crohn's disease of the colon. There is predominantly left-sided involvement in association with shortening, narrowing, and stricture of the descending colon, sigmoid, and rectum. Note that the splenic flexure has been markedly depressed.

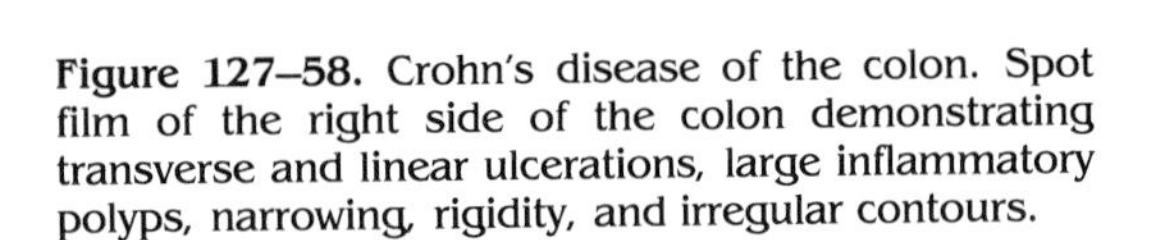

Figure 127–58. Crohn's disease of the colon. Spot film of the right side of the colon demonstrating transverse and linear ulcerations, large inflammatory polyps, narrowing, rigidity, and irregular contours.

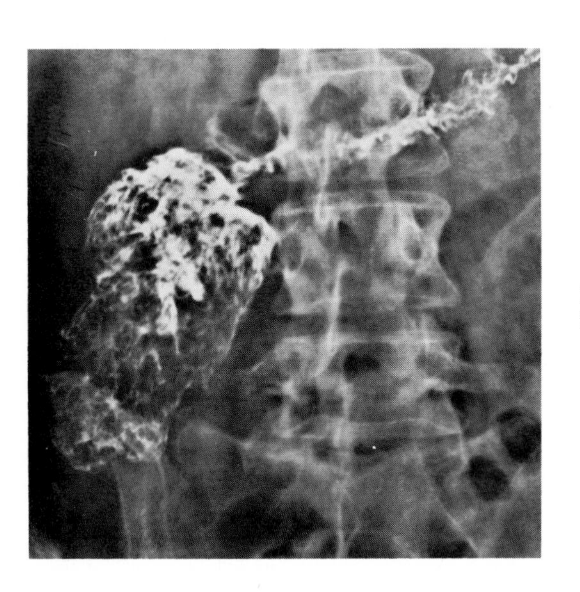

Figure 127–59. Crohn's disease of the colon. Massed inflammatory polyps on right side of colon.

of surgery is uncommon in our experience, although it does occur. Presumably normal areas between skip lesions may become severely and diffusely ulcerated in a short period of time.

Reversibility. Reversibility may be observed on occasion in serial examinations of patients with Crohn's disease of the colon. This change has usually followed a course of therapy with steroids or sometimes with antibiotics in a patient with active acute disease. We have noted dramatic instances of this type of radiologic recovery. Submucosal edema may disappear, and the colon may assume an appearance indistinguishable from that of a normal colon. Unlike ulcerative colitis, in which even the chronic changes of a shortened colon sometimes return to normal, complete resolution in the more chronic cases of Crohn's colitis has not been observed.

Inflammatory Disease of Stomas. Because ileostomy and colectomy are performed for both ulcerative colitis and Crohn's disease of the colon, the appearance postoperatively of inflammatory disease in the ileum proximal to the ileostomy stoma is important. Such "prestomal ileitis" is of 2 varieties: (1) ileitis secondary to obstruction of the stoma related to narrowing or retraction of the ileostomy (*ileostomy dysfunction*) (Chapter 130), and (2) ileitis due to extension of the Crohn's disease process.

Ileostomy dysfunction may be seen following surgery for both forms of colitis and is related to the technique of construction of the ileostomy and to local mechanical complications (Chapter 130). In our own series of cases, prestomal ileitis of the Crohn's variety has been seen with increasing frequency in patients with preoperative disease in both the ileum and the colon. We have seen this complication less commonly in those patients in whom the disease was confined to the colon prior to operation.

The radiologic findings in ileostomy dysfunction and granulomatous or transmural prestomal ileitis differ. In ileostomy dysfunction, the ileum is dilated, and secretion is abundant. The folds are slightly thickened, and ulcerations are minimal and difficult to identify. When prestomal ileitis of the Crohn's disease variety develops, however, the radiologic findings are identical to those of regional enteritis (Fig. 127–60).

Crohn's Disease of the Colon and Diverticulitis. Diverticulitis may be confused with Crohn's colitis, especially when the disease is confined to the sigmoid colon. Since both Crohn's disease and diverticular disease occur in middle-aged and elderly patients, the 2 disorders may coexist.

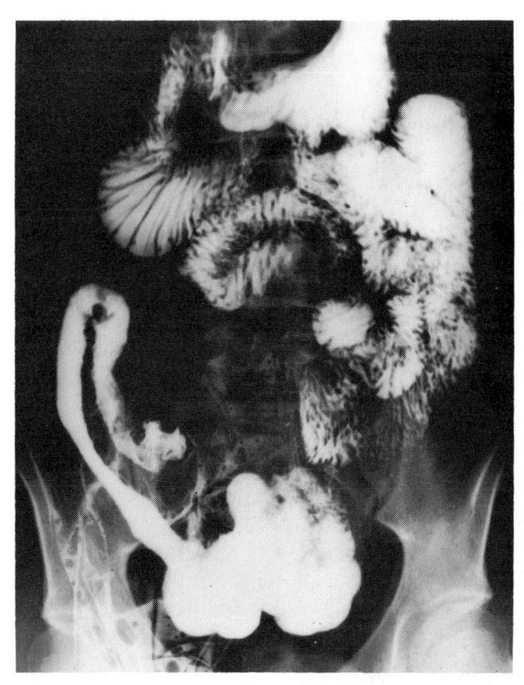

Figure 127–60. Recurrent disease at the ileostomy site following resection of colon for Crohn's colitis. There is recurrent ileitis involving the distal 30 to 45 cm of ileum proximal to the stoma characterized by narrowing, rigidity, and ulceration of the mucosa.

In Crohn's disease of the colon the involved segment tends to be long, usually 10 cm or longer, whereas in diverticulitis the segment is often short, perhaps 3 to 6 cm in length. However, the involved segment in diverticulitis can become more extensive[10]; a tract longer than 10 cm may be observed as a result of multiple perforations of diverticula or of communicating diverticulitis. When Crohn's colitis develops in a patient with diverticula, the transverse fissures penetrate easily through the mucosa of the diverticulum, producing diverticulitis.[11]

The abscesses of Crohn's colitis often have a triangular shape, but at times they may be difficult to distinguish from coexistent diverticula. In contrast to the cobblestone appearance of the mucosa in Crohn's disease of the colon, the abscess developing from a perforated diverticulum usually creates an extramural defect or an arcuate configuration of the folds that stretch over the abscess. The transverse fissures and mucosal edema of

Crohn's colitis also help to distinguish this entity from diverticulitis.

Differential Diagnosis

Amebiasis. In the acute stage, amebiasis resembles ulcerative colitis. In the chronic phase, especially when the rectum is spared, it may simulate Crohn's colitis.[12] Features typical of Crohn's disease, such as cobblestoning, strictures, or fistulas, are uncommon, and the small bowel is not usually involved in amebiasis. In milder cases with only distortion of the haustral markings, narrowing, and rigidity, differentiation is difficult. The so-called "cone-shaped cecum," sometimes described in amebiasis, may occur in any right lower quadrant inflammatory process and is not diagnostic.

Tuberculosis. It is impossible to differentiate tuberculosis from Crohn's ileocolitis on the basis of roentgen features alone. The problem in distinguishing between the 2 disorders is compounded by the fact that patients with intestinal tuberculosis may have a normal chest roentgenogram.

Ischemic Colitis. Ischemic colitis is differentiated from Crohn's colitis by the characteristic acute episode of abdominal pain and bleeding and by the rapid progression of the radiologic findings from a stage of inflammatory edema, with thumbprinting, segmental disease, spasm, irritability, and increased secretion, to resolution or stenosis. This sequence of events rarely requires more than 6 weeks. If the patient is examined radiologically at any particular phase of this process, the appearance may suggest inflammatory disease. Pseudosacculations are common residua of ischemic disease.

Scirrhous Carcinoma. Long segments of colon, usually the sigmoid colon, may be involved with carcinoma in a linitis plastica or scirrhous presentation. The differential diagnosis from a single segment of Crohn's colitis may be difficult. In carcinoma, however, nodularity is prominent and the inflammatory mucosal alterations seen with Crohn's colitis are not usually present.

References

1. Marshak RH, Lindner AE, Maklansky D. Radiology of the Stomach. Philadelphia: WB Saunders, 1983: 75–90.
2. Marshak RH, Lindner AE. Radiology of the Small Intestine. 2nd Ed. Philadelphia: WB Saunders, 1976: 179–245.
3. Marshak RH, Lindner AE, Maklansky D. Radiology of the Colon. Philadelphia: WB Saunders, 1980: 120–88.
4. Laufer I. Double Contrast Gastrointestinal Radiology with Endoscopic Correlation. Philadelphia: WB Saunders, 1980: 357.
5. Farman J, Faegenburg D, Dallemand S, Chen CK. Crohn's disease (regional enteritis) of the stomach: The "ram's horn" sign. AJR 1975; 123:242–51.
6. Nelson SW. Some interesting and unusual manifestations of Crohn's disease (regional enteritis) of the stomach, duodenum and small intestine. AJR 1969; 107:86–101.
7. Marshak RH, Lindner AE, Maklansky D. Lymphoreticular disorders of the gastrointestinal tract: roentgenographic features. Gastrointest Radiol 1979; 4:103–20.
8. Marshak RH, Lindner AE, Maklansky D. Immunoglobulin disorders of the small bowel. Radiol Clin North Am 1976; 14:477–91.
9. Theoni RF, Margulis AR. Gastrointestinal tuberculosis. Seminars Roentgenol 1979; 14:283–94.
10. Marshak RH, Lindner AE, Pochaczevsky R, Maklansky D. Longitudinal sinus tracts in granulomatous colitis and diverticulitis. Seminars Roentgenol 1978; 11:101–10.
11. Meyers M, Alonson DR, Morson BS. Pathogenesis of diverticulitis complicating granulomatous colitis. Gastroenterology 1978; 74:24–31.
12. Tucker PC, Webster FD, Kilpatrick ZM. Amebic colitis mistaken for inflammatory bowel disease. Arch Intern Med 1975; 135:681–5.

Complications

Samuel Meyers • Henry D. Janowitz

A wide variety of complications may occur during the course of Crohn's disease. These may develop directly as a result of the local bowel inflammatory process, arise secondary to nutrient absorptive defects, or be generated by the action of other unknown factors. The complications may herald the diagnosis of Crohn's disease or occur at any time after the disease has been clinically recognized. They may vary in severity from barely perceptible to extreme, even dominating the entire clinical picture. The subject of malignancy engrafted on Crohn's disease and complicating this disorder is discussed in Chapter 128.

Massive Hemorrhage. Gastrointestinal bleeding occurs in up to 65% of cases.[1,2] It may be the initial manifestation, but this is not common. The amount of bleeding varies from massive and life threatening to only occult fecal bleeding.[3] Colonic involvement is most commonly associated with bleeding, but it also occurs with disease confined to the small bowel. Gryboski and Spiro[2] demonstrated the importance of the anatomic location of disease. Six per cent of their patients with ileitis had bleeding as their initial symptom, while 33% with ileocolitis noted such bleeding. Farmer et al.[4] reported that 10% of their patients with small bowel disease noted rectal bleeding during the course of their disease as compared with 22% with ileocolitis and 46% with colitis. Among our patients at the Mount Sinai Hospital in New York, overt rectal bleeding occurred in 53% of those with colitis, 30% with ileocolitis, and 4% with ileitis. Massive bleeding is usually a single event, but recurrent episodes can occur and low-grade bleeding may be chronic.[5] When hematemesis occurs alone or with rectal bleeding in a patient with Crohn's disease, upper gastrointestinal tract involvement by the disease should be suspected.

Crohn's disease is characteristically associated with multiple deep ulcerations, often extending to the submucosa or deeper. It is less surprising, therefore, that bleeding should occur than that it does not occur more often. Perhaps edema of the bowel wall or cicatrization surrounding the ulcers prevents erosion into large blood vessels.

Management of bleeding in patients with Crohn's disease is basically similar to that for gastrointestinal bleeding of other causes (Chapters 6 and 69). We would note here only that parenteral corticosteroid therapy has been useful in our experience to control the massive bleeding of Crohn's disease. Also, should surgery become mandatory because of persistent hemorrhage, resection of the diseased segment is the preferred procedure when this is possible.[3]

Free Perforation. The terminal ileum is most frequently the site of perforation, probably because it is the most common site of disease involvement. Perforation may also occur in other areas of the small or large bowel.[6] The perforation may occur as the sole complication or be associated with toxic megacolon or distal intestinal obstruction.[6–9] Steroid therapy has been implicated as a contributory factor, but this has not been definitely substantiated.[6–9]

Free perforation is uncommon in Crohn's disease because the inflammatory process affects the entire bowel wall. Involvement of the serosa leads to adhesions that provide tracts for fistulas and favor localized perforation with abscess formation. Perforation is more likely in acute early disease, when ulcers penetrate deeply through the bowel wall and the wall is not yet well thickened and protected.[10]

The chronically ill patient and the patient on steroid therapy may have minimal findings, and the only suggestion of this catastrophe may be an abrupt overall clinical deterioration. Survival depends upon prompt surgical intervention in addition to the usual supportive medical measures (Chapter 69).

Toxic Megacolon. Toxic megacolon is an emergency life-threatening complication of Crohn's colitis or ileocolitis. It may occur during the course of the inflammatory bowel disease or more frequently as the initial manifestation.[11] Approximately 6% of *all* patients with Crohn's disease exhibit this complication. Among those in whom the colon is involved, the frequency of this complication is even greater.

So-called toxic megacolon was discussed in some detail in Chapter 69 as a complication of ulcerative colitis. Suffice it here to stress that (1) patients may develop toxicity without megacolon or have megacolon without severe systemic toxicity; (2) the etiology of the megacolon is unclear; (3) antidiarrheal agents, opiates, belladonna alkaloids, and barium enema studies are viewed as potentially capable of precipitating dilatation;[11] and (4) steroids have been implicated in causation, but without convincing evidence.[13]

When a patient with established Crohn's disease presents with toxic megacolon, it would be assumed, and properly so, that the two were related to each other. However, if a patient being seen for the first time is found to have a dilated colonic segment, associated non-specific inflammatory bowel disease cannot be assumed. Other conditions such as amebiasis, bacillary colitis, ischemic colitis, pseudomembranous colitis, volvulus, diverticulitis, or colonic obstruction due to carcinoma may be attended by toxic megacolon. The diagnosis of inflammatory bowel disease would be suspected if there is a history of altered bowel habits, with or without abdominal pain or bloody stools. Perianal disease would strongly suggest Crohn's disease.

Also worthy of note is that the distribution of colonic gas in toxic megacolon is largely governed by the influence of gravity and the anatomic position of the colon in the peritoneal cavity.[14] Preferential distention of the transverse colon is the result of its anterior position and the convention that most plain films are taken of patients in the supine position. Colonic gas in toxic megacolon will move freely when the position of the patient is changed. The absence or disturbance of the haustral pattern is an important feature demonstrating disease in the dilated segment. Examination of the gas/mucosal outline may give valuable information about the type and extent of the colitis.

Proctoscopy is helpful by showing features useful in the diagnosis of the underlying colitis. More commonly, however, only a non-specific inflammatory pattern is seen in the rectal mucosa. Even in this circumstance, proctoscopy is useful, as it facilitates collection of stool for the identification of parasitic or other infective organisms. However, more invasive diagnostic procedures, such as proctosigmoidoscopy, colonoscopy, or barium enema, carry a risk of colonic perforation and are contraindicated. Rectal biopsy may be dangerous and provides little additional information. The pathologic features of the resected specimen of acute colitis with megacolon are very similar in both ulcerative and Crohn's colitis.[15] Hence, it is not uncommon for the surgeon and pathologist alike to be uncertain of the diagnosis even when examining the gross or microscopic specimens.

There is no uniformly accepted therapy, but we stress the close cooperation of medical and surgical teams.[16] Conventional medical measures include careful observation of the vital signs and correction of fluid and electrolyte balance and hemoglobin deficits. Twice daily abdominal examinations and daily radiographs are essential to search for perforation. Since toxic megacolon is often accompanied by a small bowel paralytic ileus, nasogastric or long intestinal tube decompression is reasonable. Broad-spectrum antibiotics to control aerobic and anaerobic organisms are rational, as the permeability of the colon to invasion by colonic bacteria is impaired. Steroid therapy is usually included in the medical program despite lack of evidence that steroids are efficacious. They are, of course, mandatory for those patients already or recently treated with these agents to prevent the adrenal dysfunction that may occur with the stress of severe illness. Medical therapy is often helpful, but if this is prolonged in a patient who is clearly not responding, impressive morbidity occurs, mostly within the first 10 days. Colectomy is suggested for those patients who do not respond to therapy after 24, 48, or 72 hours. This approach minimizes the incidence of colonic perforation, which is associated with an 80% mortality rate, and decreases overall mortality to less than 6%. Colon decompressing procedures may be a temporizing maneuver in the extremely ill, moribund patient with severe peritoneal infection. More than 75% of our patients at the Mount Sinai Hospital respond well to medical measures, but most of them ultimately require surgery for continuing symptoms or relapses.[17]

Acute toxic dilatation limited to the ileum has been reported to occur in Crohn's disease.[18] The clinical features are similar to toxic megacolon, but the disorder more often responds to conservative medical therapy.

Pseudopolyposis. Pseudopolyps form as extensive ulceration destroys the mucosa, leaving only scattered mucosal islands. These develop the appearance of polypoid structures because of edema and inflammation and may even contain granulomas.[19] The mucosa may then heal, leaving these mucosal tags ("pseudopolyps") surrounded by relatively normal tissue. In this situation the pseudopolyps may be the only evidence of the previous extent of the inflammation. One or a few pseudopolyps may be present or the mucosa may be diffusely studded with small pseudopolyps. These polypoid extensions may fuse or bridge with each other and are capable of elongating into giant masses. The prevalence of these lesions is higher among patients with severe disease and extensive colonic involvement.[20] They may form during the course of Crohn's disease or with the initial attack of colitis and then become more common with chronic disease. On occasion, the pseudopolyps disappear as the disease becomes chronic.

No specific symptoms suggest the presence of pseudopolyps. They are ordinarily discovered incidentally during roentgen or endoscopic examination. Colonic obstruction and/or intussusception may occur with giant pseudopolyps.[21, 22] These polypoid lesions are not premalignant and colon carcinoma is not more common in patients with such lesions.

Pseudopolyps that attain giant size in a localized area of the colon may simulate carcinoma. The presence of other roentgen features of Crohn's disease is helpful in arriving at the proper diagnosis, but is not completely reassuring in view of the increased frequency of cancer of the colon in Crohn's disease.[22] Colitis cystica profunda can simulate the lesion and can even coexist with it.[23]

Identification of pseudopolyps should be possible by colonoscopy with biopsy.[20,21] When multiple pseudopolyps are present, it is not practical to biopsy or remove each polyp. It is wise, however, to biopsy lesions over 1 cm in diameter and those that differ in color from the others. Removal or biopsy should also be considered when the surface of the lesion is irregular and/or friable. Although polypectomy provides more tissue for pathologic examination, an attempt to extirpate the lesion(s) should not be made if the adjacent mucosa is inflamed. The pseudopolyp itself does not require any specific therapy unless obstruction occurs.

Strictures. Strictures result from the transmural nature of the inflammation of Crohn's disease and the attendant fibrosis and scarring. Thus, strictures may be primarily inflammatory or fibrotic and are part of the natural progression of the disease. As the bowel lumen narrows, symptoms of obstruction eventually occur. The nature of these symptoms depends upon the level of the stricture. Gastroduodenal or proximal small bowel obstruction results in frequent vomiting without significant abdominal distention. Distal small bowel obstruction is more common, since the ileum is the most frequent site of intestinal involvement. Stricture in this site is characterized by abdominal colicky pain and various degrees of abdominal distention. Bloating, nausea, and anorexia are common. Vomiting is infrequent but does occur later and may be feculent.

Colonic strictures may also cause obstruction, but distinction between benign stricture and cancer producing narrowing of the colon cannot always be made.[24] Colonoscopic examination is helpful in distinguishing benign from malignant strictures but may be misleading because (1) some strictures demonstrated on roentgenography are distensible by air insufflation and (2) the spherical aberration produced by modern instrument optics makes small changes in colonic diameter difficult to appreciate. Most strictures can be detected and successfully negotiated for complete examination with a standard or pediatric endoscope. If the stricture is rigid, has shelf-like edges, or is impossible to negotiate with the colonoscope, malignancy is suspected. Multiple biopsies should be taken from the edges and lumen of the stricture. Brush cytology is an important adjunct to the biopsies.

Intestinal obstruction due to strictures generally improves with medical therapy. Nasogastric tube decompression as well as restoration of fluid and electrolyte balance is essential. Parenteral antibiotics and/or corticosteroids may be necessary for the underlying Crohn's disease. This approach allows the inflammatory component of the stricture to resolve and the obstruction to lessen. Fibrotic strictures or those with a high index of suspicion for malignancy require surgical intervention.

Abscess and Fistula. Deeply burrowing fissures are frequently found in histologic sections of the bowel wall in Crohn's disease. These fissures form the basic pathologic feature responsible for the intramural subserosal tracking seen on barium roentgenograms and the peri-intestinal abscesses that are so common. Increased intraluminal pressure above a fibrosed bowel segment promotes more extensive fissuring. Reduced tissue vitamin C levels may interfere with collagen formation and be another promoting factor.[25] The fissures may travel beyond the bowel wall to form either an internal fistulous communication with adjacent adherent viscera or an external fistula between diseased bowel and skin. Some fistulas end blindly to form abscesses in the adjacent mesentery or retroperitoneal tissues or within the peritoneal cavity. In our hospital, fistulas are most often associated with ileal Crohn's disease and communication is most often between the ileum and the sigmoid colon, the cecum, another segment of ileum, or the skin. Ileovesical and ileorectal fistulas are less frequently seen. Ileovaginal fistulas are uncommon in the absence of a prior hysterectomy. Fistulas arising from colonic disease include colocolic and colovaginal types, the latter due to the close proximity of the sigmoid colon and rectum to the vagina.[26] Unusual varieties of fistulas may be found, including gastrocolic and ileoduodenal. Fistulous extension has even been observed to the spleen with associated splenic rupture.[27]

In our hospital, the prevalence rates of fistulas are 32% for internal and 13% for external types.[26] The true frequency of internal fistulas may be underestimated, since they can be extremely difficult to recognize radiologically and even at surgery. The pathologist may also have difficulty untangling matted loops of bowel to demonstrate an internal fistula.

Symptoms of an enteroenteric fistula are non-specific. If the fistula results in bypass of large segments of bowel, maldigestion or the blind loop syndrome due to bacterial overgrowth may be exhibited. Fistulous formation should be suspected if a flare-up of symptoms of Crohn's disease is associated with the development of persistent abdominal pain or an area of abdominal tenderness. The finding of a mass provides additional evidence for such a fistula. Some fistulas allow decompression of an obstructed or infected segment and thereby actually result in improvement of the clinical situation. Only when the fistula extends to other organs are more specific symptoms present. Fistulas to the bladder may result in dysuria, pneumaturia, fecaluria, or recurrent urinary tract infection. Rectovaginal fistula is characterized by the passage of pus, stool, or gas through the vagina with dyspareunia. The last complaint may also be described when there is simply juxtaposition of an inflamed ileum to the uterus and posterior fornix without any fistulous formation.

Internal fistulas penetrating into the adjacent peritoneal cavity or retroperitoneal area usually result in an abscess. These may occur in close proximity to the diseased bowel or in more distant sites, such as the liver.[28] Abscesses may occur at any time during the course of Crohn's disease, but are most common in the patient with postoperative disease recurrence. In a rare case, an abscess appears many years after surgery.[29] Abdominal pain, tenderness, and a mass associated with recurrent spiking fevers are the cardinal manifestations.

A *plain roentgenogram* of the abdomen or a *contrast intestinal film* may be suggestive when a mass effect is seen displacing adjacent viscera. *Ultrasonography* may suggest the presence of the abscess but may also be confusing, inasmuch as an intra-abdominal abscess can have an echo pattern very similar to fluid- or feces-filled bowel loops. The number of false-positive results can be reduced by repeating the examination in 24 to 48 hours. A *computed tomogram* or *gallium scan* may provide confirmatory evidence of an abscess.

A fistula may subside spontaneously, but more often it persists until the primary source of disease is eradicated. Retroperitoneal abscesses produce features very similar to appendicitis. Important clues to this diagnosis in a patient with Crohn's disease are difficulty in walking, and flexion of the hip and pain radiating down the thigh on the ipsilateral side.

External fistulas usually follow surgery, whether for Crohn's disease or other reasons, and arise from areas of active bowel disease. The tract of the fistula follows the path of least resistance, i.e., as provided by a prior incisional scar. Thus, the opening at the skin is usually in the scar site. Spontaneous fistulas may also form from diseased bowel and burrow along a persistent urachal remnant to open at the umbilicus.[30] An enterocutaneous fistula appears at the skin surface as a visible reddened, palpable mass with local tenderness and heat. It subsequently becomes fluctuant and discharges pus, often followed by gas and feces.

The mere presence of a fistula does not mandate therapy. Complications related to the fistula, such as the blind loop syndrome, high output through an external fistula, or associated infection, require therapy. Medical measures, including use of elemental diets, total parenteral nutrition, antibiotics, and immunosuppressive drugs, are discussed later in this chapter. Corticosteroids should not be used because they retard fistula closure and favor abscess formation. Surgical intervention generally is required for incision and drainage of an abscess, bypass of the affected area, or resection of the diseased segment of bowel. Occasionally, only diversion of the fecal stream and drainage of the infected area can be tolerated by the critically ill patient. Diversion or bypass procedures often reduce fistula flow and infection. However, only resection of the diseased segment regularly results in resolution of the problem.

Perianal Complications. Perianal lesions occur in up to 94% of all patients with Crohn's disease. The frequency of occurrence and detection varies with their classification and the care of the examination. Despite a wide variation in reports of their prevalence,

Table 127–8. FREQUENCY OF PERIANAL LESIONS RELATED TO THE SITE OF INTESTINAL CROHN'S DISEASE

Representative Reported Series	Small Bowel		Small and Large Bowel		Large Bowel		Overall
	*n**	%†	*n*	%	*n*	%	%
Fielding[31]	118	76	35	94	14	92	80
Williams et al.[38]	127	14	—	—	115	52	22
Homan et al.[39]	69	22	22	26	73	50	28

*n = Number of patients within each group.
†% = Percentage of the patients within each group with perianal lesions.

most agree they are more common in Crohn's colitis than ileitis. The more distal the extent of the disease, the more likely are perianal complications (Table 127–8).[31–40] They may occur at any time during the course of the disease and occasionally are the first manifestation, involvement of other areas occurring years later or perhaps not at all.[32] In such instances, of course, other causes for similar lesions must be considered before concluding that the lesion represents isolated anorectal Crohn's disease.

Skin Lesions. The skin in the perianal area may be macerated with superficial erosions caused by scratching by the patient. The skin becomes edematous and has a corrugated appearance. Deep ulcerations with subcutaneous infection may occur, causing severe pain. Skin tags are common and represent edematous, corrugated perianal skin.

Involvement of the genital skin by Crohn's disease occurs rarely. Young adults, primarily women, are affected. There is cutaneous ulceration in the perineum, vulva, penis, or scrotum, which may occur with or without direct extension from the gut. The histopathologic appearance is typical of Crohn's disease, even with the presence of granuloma.[41]

Anal Canal Lesions. Fissures, ulcers, or stenosis may occur as complications in the anal canal. The fissures are often multiple and are usually situated at either side of the midline. Although nearly always painless, they are tender to palpation. Ulcers cavitate deeply into or through the anal sphincter muscles and may extend above the dentate line into the rectum. Pain is usually experienced during defecation. Incontinence is rare. Longstanding fissures or ulcers may result in induration and stenosis of the anal canal.

Fistula and Abscess. These complications arise from the deep penetrating ulcers. If these ulcers end blindly in the perirectal area, complex abscesses may result. An abscess may drain spontaneously to the perianal skin and result in a fistula. When the abscess drains well, few symptoms occur.[37] If drainage is impaired, tissue tension rises and results in pain that is exacerbated by walking, sitting, or defecation. Signs of persistent infection also appear in these circumstances. Examination of the poorly draining fistula will reveal an area of induration, swelling, and erythema in close relationship to the anus. Digital rectal examination is painful and areas of induration may be palpable. If an ischiorectal abscess is present, the patient is likely to be febrile, appear ill, and feel weak.

Hemorrhoids. This problem is infrequent in Crohn's disease as a cause for anorectal symptoms. Noteworthy as well is the high complication rate following surgical therapy for hemorrhoids in patients with Crohn's disease.[42] Surgical morbidity occurs in approximately 40% of patients and includes anal pain or fistulas. Excision of the rectum is eventually required in some cases.

Therapy. Although perianal complications of Crohn's disease may seem serious and disabling, they usually run a benign course and tend to resolve spontaneously.[36,37] In some cases, to be sure, the course is less benign, with recurrent infection, pain, and general disability. The more distal the location of the intestinal lesion, the poorer the prognosis. If the disease includes the large bowel and the rectum or just the rectum, the chance of spontaneous cure is poor.[35]

There have been no well-controlled trials evaluating medical therapy specifically for perianal disease. Sitz baths, local hygiene, and cortisone creams (the last used when necessary to reduce inflammation) are generally sufficient to provide relief. Most lesions become quiescent with such local management, provided the Crohn's disease elsewhere in the gut is also treated.[40] Elemental diets and total parenteral nutrition may bring about apparent healing, although in our experience, once the patient resumes regular feedings, the perianal complications worsen. Supplemental nutrition, however, may be important in preparing the depleted patient for surgery. Metronidazole appears to have much promise as a means of improving or even curing this complication.[34] However, further study and evaluation are needed. Other antimicrobials are also often used to control local infection and provide significant relief.

Surgery is indicated when continued pain occurs from a poorly draining fistula or abscess or if there is stenosis of the anus. A local procedure to provide adequate drainage or anal dilatation will usually solve the problem. The extent of the surgery is controversial, but the maintenance of anal continence must be of concern. Diversion of the fecal stream may provide temporary relief in advanced cases prior to more definitive surgery. In patients with multiple fistulas and involvement of the rectum by disease, surgical prognosis is poor and rectal excision may be required.

Malnutrition. Poor nutrition among Crohn's disease patients is common and is generally multifactorial in origin. The etiology includes oral food deprivation, malabsorption, exaggerated catabolism, and protein loss from the gut.

Food deprivation is the result of anorexia, nausea, vomiting, and abdominal pain. Several studies have documented reduced caloric intake among patients with Crohn's disease. Dietary restriction, either self-imposed or advised by physicians, may contribute to the poor intake. Ingestion of folic acid and vitamins C and D is also generally reduced,[25, 45] while protein and zinc intake is maintained.[46, 47]

Malabsorption of nutrients may be related to small bowel inflammation and/or surgical bowel resection. Inflammation alone, even when diffusely involving the small bowel, does not generally interfere to any appreciable degree with the absorption of nutrients.[48] Several substances, however, including iron and nicotinic acid, may be poorly absorbed even in the absence of extensive small bowel disease.[49] Reduced absorption is consistently demonstrated only after resection of the small bowel, and even then the amount of bowel removed is a factor. Resection of 30 cm of distal ileum results in bile acid malabsorption. Resection of 60 cm results additionally in impairment of vitamin B_{12} absorption. With resections over 90 cm, substantial reduction in fat absorption occurs. Thus, malabsorption becomes clinically important only in patients with a markedly shortened bowel.[50] Extensive proximal bowel resection is rare in Crohn's disease, and jejunal function remains normal with distal resections.

Bacterial overgrowth in the small bowel, developing with or without predisposing strictures or fistulas,[51] contributes to poor absorption. Sulfasalazine interferes with absorption of folate and increases its requirement, thereby adding to malnutrition.[52] Folate malabsorption can also result directly from Crohn's disease. The mechanism underlying this defect is unclear; gross jejunal disease *per se* does not seem the sole factor.[53] A low lactose diet is frequently suggested for Crohn's disease patients because of the presumed high frequency of lactose malabsorption and its consequent symptoms, especially when the small bowel is diffusely involved. The prevalence of this defect, however, is the same as that of a control population when differences in ethnic background are considered.[54] Since milk products are good nutritional sources, lactose malabsorption should be documented before a strict lactose-free diet is suggested. The use of lactose-free formulas or the addition of commercially available yeast lactase (Lact-Aid) to milk will alleviate symptoms.

The *catabolic effect* of chronic inflammation and steroid therapy further adds to malnutrition. This is evidenced by the greater than normal caloric requirements of Crohn's disease patients.[43] All calculations of nutritional needs for these patients must take this factor into account. Intestinal *protein loss,* a common occurrence and an important contributor to malnutrition, correlates best with the extent of the mucosal inflammation.[55]

Clinical manifestations of inadequate nutrition include multiple vitamin and mineral deficiencies (vitamins B, C, and D, folic acid, zinc, iron, calcium, and magnesium[25, 44, 45, 47, 49, 56]) and protein-calorie malnutrition. Deficiencies in immunocompetance occur as a result of the protein-calorie malnutrition.[57] Zinc deficiency has recently been emphasized. This is an essential trace element required for both RNA and DNA synthesis as well as for the function of a variety of zinc-dependent enzymes. Zinc is absorbed mainly from the small bowel. Over 40% of Crohn's disease patients have reduced serum zinc levels and occasional patients have clinical manifestations of zinc deficiency.[47] In geographic areas of high oral zinc intake, serum levels are likely to be within the normal range, but are still lower than in healthy subjects.[58] There are no specific laboratory tests to clearly document tissue zinc deficiency. Serum levels do not accurately reflect the actual zinc status, but a low serum level, especially when combined with physiologic indicators of deficiency (such as taste impairment), would suggest actual tissue zinc reduction. Clinical consequences may include hypogonadism, growth retardation, taste sensation abnormalities, acrodermatitis enteropathica, poor wound healing, impaired immunity, and night blindness. Growth and maturation retardation are important clinical consequences of malnutrition.[43] Important effects on inflammation, fistula formation, and the response to therapy are also suggested, but are not yet clarified.[25]

The therapy for malnutrition may take a number of forms in addition to the management of the underlying Crohn's disease. Correction of specific deficiency syndromes is essential. Other clinical features that also clearly require nutritional therapy are growth retardation in adolescents and severe malabsorption in patients with diffuse small bowel disease or resection. Medical therapy primarily aimed at eradicating or suppressing active inflammation helps correct the nutritional disturbances. Appetite and food intake are increased, catabolism is diminished, and the loss of nutrients due to poor absorption or gut leakage is reduced.

Urologic Complications

Ureteral Obstruction. This may occur as a result of an inflammatory process in the peritoneal or retroperitoneal areas.[59] Complaints suggesting this complication include flank or anterior thigh pain, difficulty in hip extension and walking, and fever. Ureteral obstruction may also occur insidiously without associated symptoms. Urinary complaints are often absent and studies of the urine likewise are usually normal. Sterile pyuria is seen, as a clue, in 20% of patients.

Gastrointestinal contrast roentgenograms show an inflammatory mass, most commonly arising from the terminal ileum. There is a high rate of associated ileosigmoidal fistulization. An IV pyelogram will confirm the presence of ureteral obstruction, usually in the right lower third of the ureter because of the Crohn's disease in the terminal ileum. Proximal left ureteral involvement is rare but implies jejunal disease. Distal involvement of the left ureter is more common with Crohn's disease of the descending colon.

Successful therapy directed at the underlying bowel disease results in resolution of the ureteral complication. Medical therapy with antibiotics or steroids may solve the problem, although surgical intervention will usually be necessary, with resection of diseased bowel being the suggested procedure. Some surgeons state that ureterolysis must be performed to free the ureter from its fibrous encasement.[60] Our experience proves that this is not necessary and may even be harmful.

Enterovesical Fistula. This complication is rather unusual, occurring in only 2% of patients with Crohn's disease.[61] Inflammation in the adjacent bowel, usually the ileum, irritates the bladder, and this is reflected by urinary frequency and dysuria. In more advanced cases, frank fistula formation occurs. The ensuing fistula may communicate directly or indirectly with an intervening abscess cavity arising from the bowel wall. Pneumaturia, fecaluria, passage of urine through the rectum, and persistent cystitis or pyelonephritis indicate the presence of a fistula. Symptoms of the bowel disease of variable severity are superimposed. Once the fistula forms and drainage is established, the urinary complaints often dominate the clinical picture.

An IV pyelogram or retrograde cystogram often fails to identify the fistulous tract, although a filling defect may be noted in the bladder. A barium enema study will more often demonstrate the fistula, owing to the higher pressure generated during this procedure. At cystoscopy, the bladder wall shows inflammation, edema, or pseudotumor on the posterolateral wall. Cystitis cystica and glandularis has been reported on biopsy, but more often non-specific inflammation is noted.[62]

The presence of the fistula alone does not necessarily mandate therapy, but active treatment is usually required because of recurrent bowel or bladder symptoms. Medical therapy is directed at reduction of the bowel inflammation and urinary tract infection. Surgical management consists of bowel resection, excision and closure of the fistula, and, if needed, partial bladder resection. In patients with multiple fistulas and obstruction, a temporary proximal bowel diversion may be wise in order to allow safer definitive surgery at a later day.

Calculous Disease. Urinary tract calculi are considerably more common among Crohn's disease patients than in the general population. The pathogenesis of the calculi may involve either an increase in the urinary concentration of crystalloids constituting the stones or a physicochemical change in the urine or walls of the urinary tract, favoring precipitation of these crystalloids. Obstruction, urinary tract infection, dehydration, and excretion of an acid urine are contributory factors.[63] The calculi are usually composed of uric acid, calcium oxalate, or magnesium ammonium phosphate. Crystals may not form discrete stones, but instead may be deposited in the renal parenchyma, resulting in acute reversible renal failure.[64]

Formation of *uric acid stones* is favored by exacerbations in the bowel disease or diarrhea. These factors combine to enhance uric acid production and urinary urate concentration. Metabolic acidosis with acidotic urine reduces solubility of uric acid in the urine and further favors stone formation. Urate synthesis can be reduced by allopurinol therapy, which alleviates the risk of stone formation. Adequate hydration, therapy for the bowel inflammation, and alkalization of the urine, when necessary, are important in the prophylactic therapy of uric acid calculi.

Formation of *calcium oxalate stones* is favored by the presence of steatorrhea and factors that increase urinary calcium levels, such as recumbency and steroid therapy. The primary hypothesis advanced to explain these oxalate stones is that unabsorbed fatty acids combine with calcium in the gut lumen. This prevents the formation of insoluble calcium oxalate and allows oxalate to remain in solution and thus available for absorption.[65] Unabsorbed fatty acids and bile salts may also contribute by enhancing the permeability of the gut to oxalate.[66] The colon provides the site for free oxalate absorption.[65] Therapy is aimed at reducing dietary oxalate and reducing its absorption.[66] A low oxalate diet is useful, but is very difficult to maintain in the usual out-patient setting. Foods high in oxalate are chocolate, kidney, liver, citrus fruit peels, rhubarb, beets, carrots, celery, greens, parsley, beans (snap, green, wax), and cola beverages,[67] but not all the dietary sources of oxalate are known. A low fat diet, supplemented with medium chain triglycerides as a caloric source, will reduce steatorrhea and thereby make less oxalate available for absorption. Oral cholestyramine or calcium supplements will bind gut oxalate and reduce the amount available for absorption. Other cations, such as aluminum, may also be used to bind oxalate; aluminum is readily available in antacid preparations. Cholestyramine also binds bile acids, reducing their detrimental effect on colonic permeability (Chapter 108).

The increased prevalence of urinary tract infection due to urea-splitting microbes is important in the pathogenesis of calculous complications. The action of these organisms encourages formation of magnesium ammonium phosphate stones. Adequate hydration and prompt, complete antibiotic therapy for infections are vital to the prevention of this type of calculus.

Renal Amyloidosis. Amyloidosis is frequently noted at necropsy. It may also develop during life and cause insidious uremia and eventually death. Among our patients at the Mount Sinai Hospital in New York, renal amyloid has been found in 29.4% of patients with Crohn's disease at necropsy, but in only 1% during life.[68, 69] It primarily occurs with ileitis, but there is little correlation between the risk of amyloidosis and the duration, extent, and suppurative complications of Crohn's disease.[68, 70] The diagnosis is suggested by the clinical picture of a slowly progressive deterioration of renal function with or without the classic picture of the nephrotic syndrome. The onset may be from 1 to over 15 years after the diagnosis of Crohn's disease.[71] The diagnosis is established by demonstrating amyloid material in a renal biopsy specimen. Attempts to treat renal amyloidosis, either surgically by removal of the diseased bowel or medically with steroids or immunosuppressants, have met with little success.[71] A rare patient, however, may improve.[72] The use of colchicine is being explored, and there is some suggestion that steroids may be helpful in treating amyloidosis, but a direct clinical relationship with steroid therapy has not been documented.[72] The role of hemodialysis or renal transplantation is undefined but may be useful.

Cholelithiasis. Gallstones are present in up to one-third of Crohn's disease patients with ileitis. This frequency is at least 3 times that of the general population.[73–76] Ileal disease or resection results in malabsorption of bile salts and reduction in their body pool. This allows for supersaturation of the bile with cholesterol and resultant stone formation.[77] The reduction in the bile acid pool is not related to the extent of radiologically demonstrable bowel lesions, but does correlate well with clinical activity of disease. The bile acid pool may also be diminished in Crohn's colitis. Indeed, there may be functional defects of the terminal ileum conducive to bile acid malabsorption even though the roentgen appearance of this segment of gut is normal.[78] Gallstone ileus with intestinal obstruction has been noted with terminal ileal Crohn's disease.[76]

Finger Clubbing. This physical sign is present in 37% to 58% of Crohn's disease patients.[79, 80] The hyponychial angle, a reliable marker of clubbing, correlates well with bowel disease activity and the degree of fibrosis seen in resected specimens. *This sign tends to regress after surgical resection of all visible Crohn's disease.* Clubbing is most common when the areas of the gut innervated by the vagus are diseased, but the exact pathogenesis of the clubbing is unknown. It has been suggested that disease activity and fibrosis are important stimuli in the afferent pathway of a finger clubbing reflex mediated by the vagus nerve.[80] Several autonomic pathways or other factors may also play a role.

Enterolithiasis. Patients with Crohn's disease of the terminal ileum with fibrosis may develop an ileal stricture with obstruction proximal to it. The chemical and physical environment in the obstructed area is conducive to the formation of calcified enteroliths.[81] These may contribute to intestinal obstruction or perforation, but are more commonly asymptomatic. Since both enteroliths and gallstones may be associated with intestinal obstruction, differentiation between these 2 complications must occasionally be made. A history of cholelithiasis, air in the biliary tree, or the demonstration of an intestinal-biliary fistula and the presence of an opaque stone in the gut would favor the diagnosis of gallstone ileus.

Metastatic Crohn's Disease. Typical pathologic findings of Crohn's disease, consisting of non-caseating granulomas and a chronic inflammatory infiltrate, may be seen in skin lesions that generally spread outward in a contiguous fashion from the perineum toward the genital area or from a diseased stoma.[41] Non-contiguous disease of the skin is termed metastatic Crohn's disease and is a rare complication.[82] It usually appears in the buttocks or umbilicus or in areas where there is skin apposition within flexures, such as the submammary, retroauricular, or anterior abdominal wall skin fold regions.[82, 83] Granulomatous inflammation may occur not only in the skin but also in subcutaneous tissue.[85] Therapy is aimed at the underlying Crohn's disease, since the skin lesions respond as the gut inflammation resolves.

References

1. Rubin M, Herrington JL, Schneider R. Regional enteritis with major gastrointestinal hemorrhage as the initial manifestation. Arch Intern Med 1980; 140:217–9.
2. Gryboski JD, Spiro HM. Prognosis in children with Crohn's disease. Gastroenterology 1978; 74:807–17.
3. Greenstein AJ, Kark AE, Dreiling DA. Crohn's disease of the colon. II. Controversial aspects of hemorrhage, anemia, and rectal involvement of granulomatous disease involving the colon. Am J Gastroenterol 1975; 63:40–8.
4. Farmer RG, Hawk WA, Turnbull RB. Clinical patterns in Crohn's disease: a statistical study of 615 cases. Gastroenterology 1975; 68:627–35.
5. Sparberg M, Kirsner JB. Recurrent hemorrhage in regional enteritis: Report of 3 cases. Am J Dig Dis 1966; 8:652–7.
6. Tugwell P, Southcott D, Walmesley P. Free perforation of the colon in Crohn's disease. Br J Clin Pract 1972; 26:44–5.
7. Javett SL, Brooke BN. Acute dilatation of the colon in Crohn's disease. Lancet 1970; 2:126–8.
8. Shahmanesh M, Wilkan BJ. Perforated Crohn's disease. Lancet 1970; 2:363–4 (Letter).
9. Nasr K, Morowitz DA, Anderson JGD, Kirsner JB. Free perforation in regional enteritis. Gut 1969; 10:206–8.
10. Lockhart-Mummary HE, Morson BC. Crohn's disease of the large intestine. Gut 1964; 5:493–509.
11. Whorwell PJ, Isaacson P. Toxic dilatation of the colon in Crohn's disease. Lancet 1981; 2:1134–6.
12. Turnbull RB, Hawk WA, Weakley FL. Surgical treatment of toxic megacolon: ileostomy and colostomy to prepare patients for colectomy. Am J Surg 1971; 122:325–31.
13. Meyers S, Janowitz HD. The place of steroids in the therapy of toxic megacolon. Gastroenterology 1978; 75:729–31.
14. Kramer P, Wittenberg J. Colonic gas distribution in toxic megacolon. Gastroenterology 1981; 80:430–7.
15. Fazio VW. Toxic megacolon in ulcerative colitis and Crohn's colitis. Clin Gastroenterol 1980; 9:389–407.
16. Meyers S, Janowitz HD. The management of toxic megacolon. J Clin Gastroenterol 1979; 1:345–7.
17. Greenstein AJ, Kark AE, Dreiling DA. Crohn's disease of the colon. III. Toxic dilatation of the colon in Crohn's disease. Am J Gastroenterol 1975; 40:117–28.
18. Greene L, Kresch L, Held B. Acute toxic dilatation limited to the ileum in Crohn's disease. Am J Dig Dis 1972; 17:439–46.
19. Buchanan WM, Fyfe AHB. Giant pseudopolyposis in granulomatous colitis. Am J Pathol 1979; 127:51–4.
20. DiFebo G, Cappello IP. Unusual case of colonic sub-obstruction by giant pseudopolyposis in Crohn's colitis. Endoscopy 1981; 13:90–2.

21. Katz S, Rosenberg RF, Katzka I. Giant pseudopolyps in Crohn's colitis. Am J Gastroenterol 1981; 76:267–71.
22. Weedon DD, Shorter RG, Ilstrup DM, Huizenga KA, Taylor WF. Crohn's disease and cancer. N Engl J Med 1973; 289:1099–103.
23. Henrichs HR, Goldman H. Localized giant pseudopolyps of the colon. JAMA 1968; 205:248–9.
24. Mandelstam P, Kwaan HM, Jenevein EP, Rush BF. Problems in the diagnosis and management of colonic strictures in chronic ileocolitis: Report of a case. Gastroenterology 1965; 49:560–8.
25. Gerson CD, Fabry EM. Ascorbic acid deficiency and fistula formation in regional enteritis. Gastroenterology 1974; 67:428–33.
26. Greenstein AJ, Kark AE, Dreiling DA. Crohn's disease of the colon. I. Fistula in Crohn's disease of the colon, classification, presenting features and management in 63 patients. Am J Gastroenterol 1974; 62:419–29.
27. Nichols TW, Wright FM, Pyeatte JC, O'Connell JP. Spontaneous rupture of the spleen: An unusual complication of Crohn's disease. Am J Gastroenterol 1981; 75:226–8.
28. Nelson A, Frank HD, Taubin HL. Liver abscess: A complication of regional enteritis. Am J Gastroenterol 1979; 72:282–4.
29. Steinberg DM, Cooke WT, Alexander-Williams J. Abscess and fistula in Crohn's disease. Gut 1973; 14:865–9.
30. Davidson ED. Crohn's disease with spontaneous cutaneous-urachovesicoenteric fistula. Dig Dis Sci 1980; 25:460–3.
31. Fielding JF. Perianal lesions in Crohn's disease. J R Coll Surg Edinb 1972; 17:32–7.
32. Baker WNW, Milton-Thompson GJ. The anal lesion as the sole presenting symptom of intestinal Crohn's disease. Gut 1971; 12:865 (Abstract).
33. Lockhart-Mummery HE. Crohn's disease: Anal lesions. Dis Colon Rectum 1975; 18:200–2.
34. Brandt LJ, Bernstein LH, Boley SJ, Frank MS. Metronidazole therapy for perineal Crohn's disease: A follow-up study. Gastroenterology 1982; 83:383–7.
35. Bergstand O, Ewerth S, Hellers G, Holmstrom B, Ullman J, Wallberg P. Outcome following treatment of anal fistulae in Crohn's disease. Acta Chir Scand 1980; 500 (Suppl):43–4.
36. Buchman P, Alexander-Williams J. Classification of perianal Crohn's disease. Clin Gastroenterol 1980; 9:323–30.
37. Buchman P, Keighley MRB, Allan RN, Thompson H, Alexander-Williams J. Natural history of perianal disease. Ten year follow-up: A plea for conservation. Am J Surg 1980; 140:642–4.
38. Williams DR, Coller JA, Corman ML, Nugent W, Veidenheimer MC. Anal complications in Crohn's disease. Dis Colon Rectum 1981; 24:22–4.
39. Homan WP, Tang CK, Thorbjarnarson B. Anal lesions complicating Crohn's disease. Arch Surg 1976; 111:1333–5.
40. Marks CG, Ritchie JK, Lockhart-Mummery HE. Anal fistulas in Crohn's disease. Br J Surg 1981; 68:525–7.
41. Cockburn AG, Krolikowski J, Balogh K, Roth RA. Crohn's disease of penile and scrotal skin. Urology 1980; 15:596–8.
42. Jeffery PJ, Ritchie JK, Parks AG. Treatment of hemorrhoids in patients with inflammatory bowel disease. Lancet 1977; 1:1084–5.
43. Kirschner BS, Klich JR, Kalman SS, DeFavaro MV, Rosenberg I. Reversal of growth retardation in Crohn's disease with therapy emphasizing oral nutritional restitution. Gastroenterology 1981; 80:10–15.
44. Hoffbrand AV, Stewart JS, Bloth CC, Mollin DL. Folate deficiency in Crohn's disease: Incidence, pathogenesis and treatment. Br Med J 1968; 2:71–5.
45. Compston JE, Creamer B. Plasma levels and intestinal absorption of 25-hydroxyvitamin D in patients with small bowel resection. Gut 1977; 18:171–5.
46. Kasper M, Sommer M. Dietary fiber and nutrient intake in Crohn's disease. Am J Clin Nutr 1979; 32:1891–1901.
47. McClain C, Soutor C, Zieve L. Zinc deficiency: A complication of Crohn's disease. Gastroenterology 1980; 78:272–9.
48. Farivar S, Fromm H, Schindler D, McJunckin B, Schmidt FW. Tests of bile-acid and vitamin B_{12} metabolism in ileal Crohn's disease. Am J Clin Pathol 1980; 73:69–74.
49. Pollack S, Enat R, Haim S, Zinder O, Barzilai D. Pellagra as the presenting manifestation of Crohn's disease. Gastroenterology 1982; 82:948–52.
50. Gerson CD, Cohen N, Janowitz HD. Small intestinal absorptive function in regional enteritis. Gastroenterology 1973; 64:907–12.
51. Rutgeerts P, Ghoos Y, Vantrappen G, Eyssen H. Ileal dysfunction and bacterial overgrowth in patients with Crohn's disease. Eur J Clin Invest 1981; 11:199–206.
52. Franklin JL, Rosenberg IH. Impaired folic acid absorption in inflammatory bowel disease: effects of salicylazosulfapyridine (Azulfidine). Gastroenterology 1973; 64:517–25.
53. Elsborg L, Larsen L. Folate deficiency in chronic inflammatory bowel diseases. Scand J Gastroenterol 1979; 14:1019–24.
54. Kirschner BS, DeFavaro MV, Jensen W. Lactose malabsorption in children and adolescents with inflammatory bowel disease. Gastroenterology 1981; 81:829–32.
55. Beeken WL, Busch JH, Sylvester DL. Intestinal protein loss in Crohn's disease. Gastroenterology 1972; 62:207–15.
56. Howdle PD, Bone I, Losowsky MS. Hypocalemic chorea secondary to malabsorption. Postgrad Med J 1979; 55:560–3.
57. Law DK, Dudrick SJ, Abdov NI. Immunocompetence of patients with protein-calorie malnutrition. Ann Intern Med 1973; 79:545–50.
58. Timny E, Horwitz C, Graff E, Rozen P, Gilat T. Serum zinc and taste acuity in Tel-Aviv patients with inflammatory bowel disease. Am J Gastroenterol 1982; 77:101–4.
59. Present BH, Rabinowitz JG, Banks PA, Janowitz HD. Obstructive hydronephrosis: A frequent but seldom recognized complication of granulomatous disease of the bowel. N Engl J Med 1969; 280:523–8.
60. Block GE, Enker WE, Kirsner JB. Significance and treatment of occult uropathy complicating Crohn's disease. Ann Surg 1973; 178:322–32.
61. Badlani G, Sutton AP, Abrams HJ, Buchbinder M, Levin L. Enterovesical fistulas in Crohn's disease. Urology 1980; 16:599–600.
62. Schujman E, Delpre G, Kadish U. Cystitis cystica and glandularis: An unusual complication of terminal ileitis. A case report with discussion of its significance. Am J Proctol Gastroenterol Colon Rectal Surg 1981; 32:10–11,24.
63. Grossman MS, Nugent FW. Urolithiasis as a complication of chronic diarrheal disease. Am J Dig Dis 1967; 12:491–8.
64. Mandell I, Krauss E, Millan JC. Oxalate-induced acute renal failure in Crohn's disease. Am J Med 1980; 69:628–32.
65. Dobbins JW, Binder HJ. Importance of the colon in enteric hyperoxaluria. N Engl J Med 1977; 296:298–301.
66. Earnest DL. Perspectives on incidence, etiology, and treatment of enteric hyperoxaluria. Am J Clin Nutr 1977; 30:72–5.
67. Grills NJ, Bosscher MV. Manual of Nutrition and Diet Therapy. New York: Macmillan, 1981.
68. Werther JL, Shapira A, Rubinstein O, Janowitz HD. Amyloidosis in regional enteritis: A report of five cases. Am J Med 1960; 29:416–23.
69. Greenstein AJ, Janowitz HD, Sachar DB. The extra-intestinal complications of Crohn's disease and ulcerative colitis. Medicine 1976; 55:401–12.
70. Mir-Madjlessi SH, Brown CH, William AH. Amyloidosis associated with Crohn's disease. Am J Gastroenterol 1972; 58:563–77.
71. Rashid H, Blake D, Gokal R, Gooptu D, Kerr DNS. The association of renal amyloidosis with regional enteritis (Crohn's disease): Report of two cases and review of the literature. Clin Nephrol 1980; 14:154–7.
72. Verbank J, Lameire N, Praet M, Ringoir S, Elevaut A, Barbier F. Renal amyloidosis as complication of Crohn's disease. Acta Clin Belg 1979; 34:1–13.
73. Heaton KW, Read AD. Gall stones in patients with disorders of the terminal ileum and disturbed bile salt metabolism. Br Med J 1969; 3:494–6.
74. Cohen S, Kaplan M, Gottlieb L, Patterson J. Liver disease

and gallstones in regional enteritis. Gastroenterology 1971; 60:237–45.
75. Baker AL, Kaplan M, Norton RA, Patterson J. Gallstones in inflammatory bowel disease. Am J Dig Dis 1974; 19:109–12.
76. Highman L, Jagelman DG. Gallstone ileus complicating terminal ileal Crohn's disease. Br J Surg 1981; 68:201–2.
77. Dowling IH, Bell GD, White J. Lithogenic bile in patients with ileal dysfunction. Gut 1972; 13:415–20.
78. Rutgeerts P, Ghoos Y, Vantrappen G. Bile acids studies in patients with Crohn's colitis. Gut 1979; 20:1072–7.
79. Fielding JF, Cooke WT. Finger clubbing and regional enteritis. Gut 1971; 12:442–4.
80. Kitis G, Thompson H, Allan RN. Finger clubbing in inflammatory bowel disease: Its prevalence and pathogenesis. Br Med J 1979; 2:825–8.
81. Zeit RM. Enterolithiasis associated with ileal perforation in Crohn's disease. Am J Gastroenterol 1979; 72:662–4.
82. Phillips RKS, Glazer G. Metastatic Crohn's disease of the umbilicus. Br Med J 1981; 283:887.
83. Scott OLJ. Granuloma of the groin and perineum secondary to chronic proctocolitis. Proc R Soc Med 1961; 54:1019.
84. Parks AG, Morson BC, Pegum JS. Crohn's disease with cutaneous involvement. Proc R Soc Med 1965; 58:241–2.
85. Lieberman TR, Greene JF. Transient subcutaneous granulomatosis of the upper extremities in Crohn's disease. Am J Gastroenterol 1979; 72:89–90.

Medical Management

Samuel Meyers • Henry D. Janowitz

There is no specific medical cure for Crohn's disease at this time and probably none will become available until the etiology of this complex, multifaceted disorder is finally unraveled. Nevertheless, medical therapy may provide considerable comfort and prolong life. There are 3 main objectives of a medical program: (1) to reduce the bowel inflammation, (2) to correct nutritional disturbances, and (3) to provide symptomatic relief for the intestinal and extraintestinal manifestations. This chapter section focuses on the several pharmacologic agents and other measures currently in use to try to achieve these goals.

Sulfasalazine. The efficacy of this widely used drug is supported by the findings of several small clinical studies as well as more recent controlled trials. A Scandinavian multicenter trial compared sulfasalazine (3 g daily) with a placebo.[1] Sulfasalazine therapy was not superior to a placebo in 12 patients with disease relapse after prior surgical resection. However, symptomatic improvement was detected in a second group without prior surgery. The treatment period continued for only 1 month, perhaps too short a time to demonstrate adequately the full effect of sulfasalazine therapy. The National Cooperative Crohn's Disease Study (NCCDS) compared sulfasalazine (1 g/kg of body weight) with a placebo, each given for 17 weeks.[2] Sulfasalazine resulted in superior symptomatic improvement for those patients with colonic involvement, but was not effective against disease confined to the small bowel. If the patients were receiving prednisone at entry into the study, they were unlikely to respond to sulfasalazine. The NCCDS used the so-called Crohn's Disease Activity Index to determine drug response rates. This index, however, is largely determined by subjective feelings of the patients and by variables not necessarily related to gut inflammatory activity, such as diarrhea in patients after an ileal resection. Interpretation of the data, therefore, is clouded. Sulfasalazine, 4 to 6 g daily, was superior to a placebo when measured by another activity index more closely reflecting the inflammatory activity. Both small and large bowel disease responded equally well.[3] Sulfasalazine has not been shown to prevent relapse in patients after surgical resection or in those with quiescent disease,[2, 4] although a trend favoring therapy has been noted.[5]

In our own experience, sulfasalazine has been useful in the treatment of both small and large bowel Crohn's disease and for disease recurrence after previous surgical resection. This has especially been the case in those patients with mild to moderate disease activity. We use this drug alone as the first line agent or in combination with corticosteroids or other drugs. Very often, the addition of sulfasalazine to the therapeutic program allows corticosteroids to be given in a lower dose for a shorter period of time.

Sulfasalazine therapy should be initiated slowly and given with meals to minimize dyspepsia, which is a common adverse effect. We start with 500 mg the first day and add one 500 mg tablet each day until a daily total of 2 to 4 g is achieved, divided into 3 or 4 doses. Those patients who complain of persistent dyspepsia may tolerate an enteric-coated tablet better, and children may prefer the suspension. Therapy is continued for as long as the patient remains symptomatic. Once a clinical remission is achieved, the amount of corticosteroids, if used in combination with sulfasalazine, is gradually reduced. When the corticosteroid has been discontinued, the patient is retained on sulfasalazine and if the clinical condition remains good for several weeks, sulfasalazine is also stopped.

Sulfasalazine is split by gut bacteria in the colon into sulfapyridine and 5-aminosalicylic acid (patients with Crohn's disease often have an increase in their small bowel microbial population and can split sulfasalazine in this site as well as in the colon). Both moieties are then absorbed. The 5-aminosalicylic acid blood levels are very low, suggesting poor absorption or a very fast first pass metabolism in the liver or intestine. Sulfapyridine blood levels are considerably higher. Absorbed metabolites are primarily conjugated in the liver to their corresponding acetylated forms.[6–8] The acetylation rate of sulfapyridine being genetically controlled.[9–10] The side effects of sulfasalazine are related to the serum sulfapyridine levels. Thus, they occur more often after larger doses of sulfasalazine or when the patient is a slow acetylator.[8, 11–13] The evidence at hand strongly suggests that 5-aminosalicylic acid is the active moiety, with the sulfapyridine having little or no therapeutic activity.[14–16]

The adverse effects of sulfasalazine were evaluated prospectively by the NCCDS.[17] The most frequent were gastric intolerance and headache. The dyspepsia was sufficiently severe in 4% of the patients to cause drug withdrawal or dose reduction. Interestingly, none of the side effects occurred significantly more frequently among those taking sulfasalazine than among those taking a placebo.

The mode of action of sulfasalazine, specifically the 5-aminosalicylic acid component, is a matter of dispute. The inhibition of prostaglandin synthesis has been considered important.[18–22] However, other more specific inhibitors of prostaglandin synthesis have not been successful in the therapy of inflammatory bowel disease.[23] Some favor the idea that it is not the synthesis that is affected, but the metabolism of prostaglandins.[24] Still others postulate an action of sulfasalazine or its components on the phagocytic process and polymorphonuclear cell function.[25] Despite these controversies, most agree that the 5-aminosalicylic acid acts locally on the bowel. Newer preparations composed of 5-aminosalicylic acid alone are being developed. These should allow optimal therapy without the side effects of sulfasalazine.

Corticosteroids. These agents are widely used for the treatment of active symptomatic Crohn's disease, and early uncontrolled clinical studies support their use. Good initial symptomatic response was obtained in 75% to 90% of patients treated with 30 mg/day of prednisone or its equivalent.[26, 27] Fever, pain, and diarrhea subsided, appetite and well-being improved, and, in most cases, the hematocrit, sedimentation rate, or serum orosomucoid levels returned toward normal. These favorable clinical responses were not necessarily associated with improvement in the radiologic appearance. It was concluded that steroid therapy produced short-term benefits, but probably would not alter the long-term course of the disease.

Only one controlled, prospective, double-blind study of steroid therapy has been reported to date. The NCCDS confirmed the overall results of the earlier data and provided much new information.[2] Prednisone

(0.25 to 0.75 mg/kg of body weight) was especially effective for active disease involving the small bowel. Prednisone was not superior to a placebo when the disease was confined to the colon. The number of such patients (34) was small, however, and this may have allowed a beneficial effect to be overlooked in the latter group. Sulfasalazine therapy at entry to the study seemed to blunt the response to prednisone.

We use corticosteroids for the therapy of either small or large bowel Crohn's disease. However, we are careful not to initiate such therapy in the presence of suppurative complications (see preceding section on Complications), a situation in which we find antibiotics more useful. Therapy is initiated with 45 to 60 mg/day of prednisone, given in 3 or 4 divided doses. This high dose is continued for approximately 10 to 14 days and is then tapered at the rate of 5 mg every 7 to 10 days. The reduction should be made from the evening dose. As lower doses are achieved, more is administered in the morning to help minimize the side effects. If there is a relapse in disease activity, the steroid dose must be raised again. Once disease control is achieved, the tapering process is resumed. The inability to withdraw steroid therapy completely within 1 year is a relative indication for surgery. Prolonged use of alternate-day steroid doses or immunosuppressive drug therapy may be other options in selected cases.

The absorption of oral corticosteroids is adequate, even in the presence of severe involvement of the bowel with Crohn's disease.[27] In very ill patients or in those not able to tolerate oral therapy, parenteral corticoids are used, optimally IV hydrocortisone or adrenocorticotropic hormone (ACTH). There are no studies that help decide which of these agents is superior, but some guidance may be obtained from studies performed in severe ulcerative colitis. We have found hydrocortisone superior for patients who had previously been receiving corticosteroids continuously and ACTH superior for those who had not been on such therapy.[28] Intravenous therapy is administered as a continuous infusion of either 100 mg of hydrocortisone or 40 units of ACTH mixed with 500 ml of 5% dextrose and water. This mixture is infused over each 8-hour period (daily dose of 300 mg of hydrocortisone or 120 of units ACTH) for 7 to 14 days. Once optimal benefit is achieved, IV treatment is discontinued and prednisone is given orally at a dose of 45 to 60 mg/day, as previously outlined.

The role of prophylactic steroid therapy in both quiescent disease and after surgical resection has been examined in several trials. A range of therapeutic programs was represented in these trials: 7.5 mg of prednisone daily for 3 years,[29] a dose decreasing from 15 mg to 5 mg of prednisone/day combined with sulfasalazine for 33 weeks and followed for 3 years,[30] and 1 to 4 mg of prednisone/kg of body weight for 2 years.[2] In each study, prednisone-treated subjects fared no better than those taking a placebo. In fact, there was a trend suggesting that steroid-treated patients did worse. No appreciable toxicity was attributed to the therapy at doses of 7.5 mg of prednisone daily or less.[29, 30] However, 20% of the subjects in the NCCDS who received higher doses required dose reduction or withdrawal because of side effects.[2] Clearly, prophylactic steroid therapy is not indicated in Crohn's disease.

The withdrawal of corticosteroids once remission is obtained is desirable but is often a problem. Clinical experience suggests that as the dose is reduced, recrudescence of symptoms occurs within a year in at least one-third of the patients.[26] The NCCDS found that withdrawal of prednisone in quiescent disease was not associated with more relapses than occurred with the continuance of this agent. However, if the bowel disease was active, prednisone withdrawal caused the condition to deteriorate.[2] Once the optimal therapeutic benefit has been obtained and the patient is in clinical remission, withdrawal often may be successfully accomplished.

The toxicity of steroid therapy at the doses used to suppress active Crohn's disease is appreciable. Also, use of these substances is thought to increase the overall mortality rate as well as the need for surgery.[26] The NCCDS provided important information regarding the frequency and severity of steroid side effects during the therapy for Crohn's disease.[17] Contrary to earlier clinical reports, complications such as perianal disease, intra-abdominal abscess, peritonitis, bowel perforation, and fistulas were not increased. On the other hand, a large number of adverse effects were noted. Changes of minor importance, such as facial mooning, acne, and ecchymosis, occurred in 47%, 30%, and 17%, respectively, of the patients receiving larger doses of prednisone. When a lower dose of prednisone was evaluated, the cumulative prevalence rates of these changes were less; facial mooning occurred in 25%, ecchymosis in 16%, and acne in 19%, rates similar to the placebo group. More serious side effects were noted among 32% of those on higher doses and 26% of those on lower doses. Very severe side effects occurred in 18% and 25%, respectively. The high rate in those on a low dose was thought to be attributable most likely to the long duration of such therapy. Peptic ulcer, hypertension, and severe emotional disturbances were the most frequently seen major side effects. These complications generally responded to withdrawal or reduction of the prednisone dose and specific therapy for the complication, but were life-threatening problems. Interestingly, the severe complications occurred with a similar frequency in the placebo group. Thus, although the relationship of these complications to steroid therapy is suspected, it is not proved. No patient in this study suffered more than one major adverse effect, in contrast to some previous reports.[26] The NCCDS observed steroid toxicity sufficient to cause withdrawal from the study in 18% of the patients receiving therapeutic doses for 17 weeks, a rate considerably higher than the 6% withdrawal rate after placebo therapy.

Since prednisone and sulfasalazine are both effective single agents for the therapy of active symptomatic Crohn's disease, the logical extension would seem to be to use both. The NCCDS indeed compared this combination with prednisone alone or a placebo and found that the combination was less effective than prednisone or placebo alone.[31] Sulfasalazine also showed no steroid-sparing effect. Despite the negative findings of this impressive investigation, most clinicians continue to combine these agents and feel this is useful. Perhaps they are right, or perhaps they are only frustrated by the lack of proven therapeutic alternatives. Clearly, more study of this important area is awaited.

Immunosuppressive Agents. *Azathioprine* was popularized for the therapy of Crohn's disease in 1969.[33] Since that time, immunosuppressive agents have been the subject of intense controversy, still unresolved. In 1971, a controlled trial was reported that consisted of 16 Crohn's disease patients.[33] Therapy given at entry to the study was continued with the addition of azathioprine, 4 mg/kg of body weight, for 10 days and 2 mg/kg thereafter for 2 months. Some subjects seemed to improve after azathioprine was added, but striking improvement was unusual and no definite benefit over a placebo could be identified. Klein et al.[34] then conducted a study of 27 patients who received either a placebo or azathioprine (3 mg/kg of body weight) for 4 months. During the subsequent 4 months, the therapy for the 2 groups was reversed. Some patients continued using corticosteroids throughout the study. Again, there was no significant difference in efficacy between azathioprine and a placebo. No steroid-sparing effect could be demonstrated in these reports. Others, however, have suggested that azathioprine allows a reduction in the steroid dose without worsening the symptoms in some patients who require prolonged steroid therapy.[35, 36] The NCCDS evaluated azathioprine at a dose of 2.5 mg/kg of body weight for 17 weeks.[2] Azathioprine-treated groups fared no better than those receiving placebo. This study was unique, as no other therapy was administered, thus allowing evaluation of azathioprine as a single agent.

Some have suggested a role of azathioprine in the prevention of relapse of medically or surgically controlled bowel disease. A higher relapse rate after azathioprine withdrawal than when it was continued supports this position.[37] The data from the NCCDS, however, provided negative evidence.[2] It should be noted, however, that there were important differences between these studies that may help to explain the discrepancy. The former investigation consisted of a select group of patients who were in remission attributed to azathioprine;[37] they had already demonstrated their ability to respond to this drug. It should be no surprise that withdrawal of therapy was attended by relapse in these patients. Also, higher doses of azathioprine were given to these patients, and more of them had colonic disease than did the patients in the NCCDS.[2]

Other workers have evaluated the role of *6-mercaptopurine* in Crohn's disease.[38] This study compared 6-mercaptopurine (1.5 mg/kg of body weight) with a placebo for 1 year, followed by a cross-over of therapy for a second year. Conventional medications were used as needed. Significant improvement occurred with 6-mercaptopurine therapy. Over two-thirds of the patients receiving this drug responded favorably, with either elimination of symptoms, reduction in steroid requirements, or improvement in fistulas.

Azathioprine is metabolized to 6-mercaptopurine, which is the active agent. Several factors may explain the difference between the more favorable effects reported for 6-mercaptopurine as compared with the results of the NCCDS for azathioprine. One may be the time of the study period. Response to 6-mercaptopurine was not seen in many patients for over 4 months; the NCCDS was terminated at 17 weeks. The random tapering of steroid therapy in over one-third of the patients could have biased the NCCDS against azathioprine. If the Crohn's disease was suppressed by the steroids, the process would be likely to exacerbate with withdrawal or diminution of steroids, thereby prejudicing any beneficial effect of the slower acting azathioprine. The NCCDS also used a lower dose of medication. Despite these considerations, most clinicians agree that immunosuppressive agents have, at best, a limited role in the therapy of Crohn's disease and are not effective as single agents.

Patients who require prolonged use of corticosteroids to maintain disease control should be considered for surgery. If they refuse or are not eligible for this approach, because of either associated medical conditions or the diffuse nature of their Crohn's disease, the use of the immunosuppressive drugs may be considered. In these circumstances, the rationale is to utilize the steroid-sparing action of these agents. Our experience is greater with azathioprine, which we employ in daily doses of 2 to 3 mg/kg of body weight for several months or occasionally even for years. Close observation, frequent blood counts, and the advice of a hematologist experienced with these drugs all help reduce their potential adverse effects.

Nausea, vomiting, headache, infection, leukopenia, arthralgias, and hypersensitivity reactions are frequent adverse effects of azathioprine. Of these, leukopenia seemed particularly associated with therapy in the NCCDS.[17] Bone marrow depression is a well-known dose-dependent risk of this drug. Total white blood cell counts of less than 4000/μl were seen in 15% of the patients in the NCCDS.[17] Present et al.[38] in their study of 6-mercaptopurine, found that all of their patients had mild leukopenia and 2 developed very low counts of 300/mm^3 and 1200/mm^3, respectively. In the NCCDS, 16% of the patients were withdrawn because of adverse effects of azathioprine; 30% of these patients developed pancreatitis, which subsided when the drug was discontinued.[17, 39] The overall prevalence of pancreatitis among the 113 patients receiving azathioprine in the NCCDS was 4.4%;[39] all cases developed within the first 21 days of therapy. A similar percentage of patients (10%) treated with 6-mercaptopurine were withdrawn because of adverse effects; pancreatitis occurred in one patient.[38]

Hepatotoxicity may be a possible long-term effect of immunosuppressive therapy, but the most concern centers around the potential cancer risk. The risk of malignancy (particularly of non-Hodgkin's lymphoma) for patients receiving azathioprine is greatest among those taking this drug after a renal transplantation.[40] The risk for those using azathioprine for other reasons still is about 10 times that in the general population. There are no similar data for 6-mercaptopurine, but it seems reasonable to consider the 2 drugs as equivalent in this respect until epidemiologic studies indicate otherwise. Concern is heightened by use of immunosuppressive drugs in Crohn's disease patients, who already have an increased propensity for malignancy.

Antibiotics. When bacterial overgrowth occurs in the small bowel secondary to a stricture or an intestinal anastomotic operation, a broad-spectrum antibiotic is useful. Most physicians would not question the use of antibiotics for clear-cut suppurative complications of Crohn's disease, such as an intra-abdominal abscess. The administration of antibiotics to treat uncomplicated, more active Crohn's disease may, however, be debated. Use of a variety of antibiotics (ampicillin, sulfonamides, cephalosporins, tetracycline, or paromomycin) is not without its advocates. In the absence of controlled trials, justification for these drugs is lacking. We often find them helpful, especially when there is any evidence of a suppurative component such as fever or abdominal tenderness. One clinical report supports their use.[41] Ampicillin, tetracycline, clindamycin, cephalothin, or erythromycin was used continuously in 44 patients. Symptomatic improvement occurred in 41 (93%) who were treated for 6 months or longer. Radiographic follow-up demonstrated improvement in 57% of those for whom post-therapy films were available. These changes occurred within weeks in some patients and over a period of years in others. Patients with perianal fistulas or recurrence after surgery accounted for the therapeutic failures.

Metronidazole has received a great deal of attention since Ursing and Kamme[42] reported on its use in 5 patients with Crohn's disease. Four of the 5 improved after 4 weeks of treatment; in 3 patients, corticosteroids and sulfasalazine could be withdrawn. In one of the patients, response was slow and 4 months of treatment were necessary before improvement was noted. Another uncontrolled trial also supports the beneficial action of metronidazole.[43] Two controlled studies comparing metronidazole with a placebo, however, failed to confirm the earlier clinical experience.[44, 45] These controlled trials did note that metronidazole seemed most effective in patients with colonic Crohn's disease.

A randomized, double-blind trial conducted in Sweden compared metronidazole (0.8 g/day) with sulfasalazine (3 g/day).[46] No difference in efficacy was noted between these 2 drugs when clinical criteria of disease activity were measured. On the other hand, reduction of the serum orosomucoid level, an index of bowel inflammatory activity, was more pronounced in the metronidazole group. Also, those patients with active disease despite sulfasalazine therapy improved clinically when switched to metronidazole. Such improvement was not seen when patients treated with metronidazole were switched to sulfasalazine; in fact, the serum concentration of orosomucoid increased in this group. It was concluded that metronidazole is slightly more effective than sulfasalazine, both drugs being more efficacious for colonic than for small bowel Crohn's disease. In our experience, low doses of metronidazole are well tolerated and may represent a valuable therapeutic option. The drug would seem especially useful for those patients who are allergic, intolerant, or unresponsive to sulfasalazine.

The initial observations on metronidazole led to more extensive study of its use in perineal Crohn's disease. Bernstein et al.[47] used this drug (20 mg/kg of body weight) in 21 consecutive patients with chronic, unremitting perineal disease. There was improvement in 20 patients and complete healing in 10 of 18 patients maintained on therapy. A subsequent report[48] included 26 patients, 17 of whom were also included in the first study. All patients initially showed a good clinical response to the drug, with 10 experiencing complete healing. Gradual reduction in dosage or drug discontinuation was not successful in most cases; metronidazole was successfully discontinued in only 28% of those in whom cessation of therapy was attempted. Those patients in whom the drug was gradually discontinued seemed to have a better chance of healing than those in whom therapy was stopped abruptly. When dosage reduction was associated with disease exacerbation, a prompt response was achieved with reinstitution of full dosage. The effect of therapy persisted for long periods, the preparation continuing to be effective for periods as long as 36 months. Among 15 patients observed for at least 12 months, only one suffered disease exacerbation while on full dosage. One other patient treated for 8 months had an increase in disease activity while on full dosage.

Metronidazole is generally well tolerated. Reactions include minor gastrointestinal disturbances, metallic taste, glossitis, furry tongue, urticaria, vaginal and urethral burning, dark urine, and reversible neutropenia. A disulfiram-like reaction may occur in response to alcohol ingestion. Nervous system side effects include headache, ataxia, vertigo, encephalopathy, seizures, and peripheral neuropathy. Paresthesias occur in 50% of patients and develop approximately 6 months after the initiation of drug therapy. They are dose-related and disappear after dose reduction; they may be prolonged, however, even after discontinuation of the drug.

Despite the exciting data reported, the studies have not been controlled, double-blind investigations using a placebo and thus are open to criticism. We use metronidazole in the management of perineal complications of Crohn's disease. Although we have observed some benefit, our results are not as glowing as those reported. We prescribe 20 mg/kg of body weight and continue therapy until healing occurs or significant adverse effects necessitate dose reduction or discontinuation. A potential problem with widespread metronidazole therapy is the finding in experimental studies showing the drug to be carcinogenic in rodents[49] and mutagenic in bacteria.[50] However, there have been no reported cases in which cancer has been attributed to metronidazole in humans,[51] nor does the drug induce chromosomal aberrations.[52]

The mechanism of antimicrobial action of the drug in Crohn's disease is unknown. To the extent that infectious complications contribute to a particular case, reduction in the number of bacteria would be useful. Reduction or elimination of bacterial overgrowth in the small bowel should improve absorption. Microbial reduction in the gut may also remove a potential source of antigen, which could be of significance in the pathogenesis of the disease. Metronidazole also suppresses cell-mediated immunity, especially granuloma formation, and this action may be important.[53]

Immunostimulants. Cell-mediated immunity is impaired in many patients with Crohn's disease.[54] This has suggested the use of immunostimulants as therapeutic modalities. Oral administration of *bacillus Calmette-Guérin* (BCG) has been used to stimulate the immune response. However, controlled trials show no benefit of this agent in the therapy of Crohn's disease.[55, 56] *Levamisole*[57] and *transfer factor*[58] are other agents capable of stimulating immunity, but controlled trials also show no evidence of therapeutic efficacy for them in Crohn's disease. Levamisole, however, may have a role in maintaining a remission attained by other forms of medical treatment,[59] although this form of maintenance therapy, has not yet been subjected to a controlled trial. *Interferon* has an important action against virus infections, mainly because it inhibits viral replication by individual cells. It also is associated with immune stimulatory activity. A preliminary clinical trial in 5 patients suggested that interferon may have a role in the therapy of Crohn's disease, as improvement was noted in 4 of the 5 patients.[60] The role of interferon in disease pathogenesis and therapy awaits further study.

Disodium Cromoglycate. This drug has been suggested as possibly being beneficial in ulcerative colitis. In Crohn's disease, however, controlled trials have shown no benefit over a placebo.[61, 62]

Plasmapheresis. This technique was employed in a clinical study of 6 patients with Crohn's disease.[63] The symptoms in one patient were controlled by this procedure alone, and the steroid requirements were reduced in 5 others. Clinical relapses could be managed in these patients by plasmapheresis without increasing the steroid dose. A reduction in circulating soluble immune complexes may be the basis for the benefit of this form of treatment. Further study is clearly indicated.

Vitamin A. This vitamin has been noted to improve clinical symptoms as well the impaired intestinal permeability in one patient with Crohn's disease.[64] The known effect of vitamin A in supporting normal intestinal epithelium and mucus production may explain its supposed beneficial action.[65] Here again, more study is necessary to define the role of this preparation in Crohn's disease.

Fluid, Electrolytes, and Minerals. Replacement of fluid and electrolytes is often mandatory to correct losses from hemorrhage, vomiting, diarrhea, or gram-negative sepsis. Depletion of potassium is often exacerbated by steroid therapy. Magnesium depletion may also become a problem because of diarrhea and malabsorption, especially during prolonged IV therapy. Suggestive symptoms include nervousness, irritability, paresthesias, muscular weakness, and mental confusion. Hypocalcemia may occur secondary to malabsorption and/or associated magnesium deficiency and must be promptly corrected. Acid-base balance may also be altered in Crohn's disease patients because of the same factors affecting fluid and electrolyte balance. This too should be looked for and corrected as necessary.

Hematologic and Coagulation Factors. Anemia may occur as a result of blood loss, malabsorption of iron, folic acid, and vitamin B_{12}, poor diet, marrow depression due to the toxic illness, or hemolysis due to the disease *per se* or its treatment. Correction of the anemia is important to the life and well-being of the patient. We have also found that the other facets of the medical program, such as the response to corticosteroids, are more effective once anemia has been corrected. Proper therapy consists of replacement of the deficient factors and blood transfusion when required. Oral iron preparations are often necessary, but are poorly tolerated by many patients. Parenteral iron may provide an alternative, but has its own adverse effects, which must be considered.

Coagulation disturbances occur rarely in Crohn's disease as a consequence of coagulation factor deficiency from complicating hepatic disease or vitamin K malabsorption.

Factor replacement and/or parenteral vitamin K is essential in these situations.

Protein Products. Hypoproteinemia is commonly due to the malnutrition and/or protein loss through the diseased gut. Albumin or amino acid replacement therapy is not helpful for the patient with protein-losing enteropathy, as administered protein is rapidly lost through the leaky gut. Steroid therapy quickly improves the protein loss and is the preferred therapy for this complication.

Antidiarrheal Agents. These medications relieve the rectal urgency and frequent bowel movements and help reduce abdominal crampy pain. Diphenoxylate, loperamide, codeine, paregoric, and deodorized tincture of opium are all used for these purposes. These drugs may be useful in mild or moderately severe cases of Crohn's disease, but should be avoided in more severe cases, in which they may precipitate toxic megacolon. Even when used, they provide only limited and temporary benefit. The diarrheal symptoms are best resolved by aiming therapy at the reduction in the inflammation within the gastrointestinal tract. Hydrophilic mucilloids, such as psyllium fiber, may provide form to the stools. They often make the patient with loose stools more comfortable, provided there is no component of intestinal obstruction.

Tranquilizers. Careful interview by a concerned physician often identifies psychosocial factors that are important in the exacerbation or perpetuation of disease. Intervention by the physician, family, social worker, or psychiatrist in these cases is useful and is a vital aspect of any treatment program. The adjunctive use of tranquilizers or antidepressant medications may provide added benefit in selected cases.

Anticholinergic Agents. These drugs may help reduce postprandial pain and diarrhea. They should be avoided in more severe attacks, in which they may contribute to the development of toxic megacolon. When there is evidence of small bowel obstruction, they are also best avoided.

Analgesics. We prefer to avoid these drugs whenever possible. Propoxyphene or acetaminophen has little value for the abdominal pain of Crohn's disease. Aspirin is especially to be avoided because it increases the tendency for bleeding. Opiates may increase bowel spasm; thus, after providing initial relief, even more pain may follow. Opiates are also implicated as a contributory factor in the development of toxic megacolon. The best therapy for the abdominal pain of Crohn's disease is suppression of the inflammatory state. Very severe or persistent pain may signal complications, such as perforation, abscess, or biliary or renal colic. This should not be masked by analgesics; rather, specific treatment should be administered after the correct diagnosis has been established.

Diet. Most experienced physicians agree that diet plays little role in the management of Crohn's disease. There is no evidence that what the patient eats affects the symptoms or the long-term course of the disease. By trial and error, patients gradually find out which foods are well tolerated and which ones aggravate the diarrhea or precipitate bouts of intestinal obstruction.

All agree that the diet should be well balanced and provide sufficient proteins, vitamins, minerals, and calories to maintain good health, but special diets are employed only in certain circumstances. When the bowel is stenotic, the elimination of roughage often reduces the risk of partial or complete intestinal obstruction. A low residue diet also helps reduce diarrhea in more severe active cases. If there is evidence of lactose intolerance, confirmed by a lactose tolerance test (Chapter 104), a low lactose diet should be given. Such a diet should not be routinely prescribed, since milk products are important sources of minerals, vitamins, and protein. The prevalence of lactose deficiency among patients with Crohn's disease is similar to that in the general population. When the small bowel is extensively diseased or has been previously resected, a low fat diet decreases diarrhea and improves absorption. The optimal diet should contain 50% to 75% of the total fat in the form of medium-chain triglycerides.

Patients admitted to the hospital with severe Crohn's disease are often placed on total bowel rest with no food allowed by mouth. This avoidance of oral intake may reduce symptoms of obstruction, or allow patients to improve symptomatically as a result of decreased mechanical, physical, and chemical activities of the bowel. The practice of proscribing eating, however, encourages nutritional depletion, and this is detrimental to both the general medical condition and the gut function. Thus, bowel rest should only be temporary and limited to severely ill patients who are unable to tolerate oral feedings.

Preliminary data have been reported suggesting that a fiber-rich, unrefined carbohydrate diet is beneficial for Crohn's disease.[66] This type of diet combined with conventional medical therapy had a favorable effect on the course of the disease. There was a reduced need for hospitalization and surgery, without leading to intestinal obstruction. Controlled, prospective dietary studies are now being performed, especially in the United Kingdom.

Nutritional Supplementation. If the patient can tolerate oral feedings, this route is preferable to provide basic and supplemental nutrition. Oral elemental or polymeric defined formula diets can supplement food intake or provide the total nutritional source. These formulas are absorbed in the upper small bowel and therefore allow for relative bowel rest while maintaining adequate nutritional balance.[67–69] They may be ingested by the patient or administered through an indwelling feeding tube. More severely ill patients or those with intestinal obstruction will not be able to tolerate enteral feedings. Nutrient solutions can then be given by peripheral or central venous routes. Solutions containing vitamins, minerals, protein, carbohydrate, or fat are available.

Parenteral nutrition allows correction of malnutrition and provides adequate nutrition during periods of bowel rest. It would appear reasonable to suppose that if total parenteral nutritional support can achieve restoration of nutritional balance while allowing total bowel rest, it might well play a role in the primary therapy of Crohn's disease. A number of investigations have shown that patients with both fistulous and non-fistulous Crohn's disease enter remission after a period of total parenteral nutrition and total bowel rest.[70] The reduction in disease activity may allow these patients to avoid surgery temporarily or even for sustained periods.[71, 72] Weight gain and a positive nitrogen balance have also been documented in these patients. While long remissions have been observed, this is unusual. Most patients will relapse once the parenteral nutrition is discontinued and oral feedings are again introduced. Sustained closure of fistulas after parenteral nutrition is also not the rule. Earlier enthusiasm for this approach may have been engendered by the response of fistulas in patients who did not have inflammatory bowel disease. Furthermore, the unpredictable chronic nature of Crohn's disease must always raise serious questions about the validity of uncontrolled, enthusiastic reports of short-term benefit. One controlled, prospective study of parenteral nutrition sounded a discouraging note, concluding that there was no primary therapeutic effect.[73] A possible role of parenteral nutrition in the therapeutic program, however, is not excluded by this study. Only 36 patients were included, patients with ulcerative colitis and Crohn's disease were mixed together, and the control group was not strictly comparable with the study group. Further intensive study in this area is required.

Among patients being considered for surgery, preoperative nutritional supplementation would appear to be advisable if protein-calorie malnutrition is present. While there are few data on the effect of such treatment in Crohn's disease, there is evidence from other surgical experience (as in gastrointestinal cancer) of fewer complications after surgery when protein-calorie malnutrition was corrected.[74]

Growth arrest and delayed sexual maturation may complicate childhood-onset Crohn's disease. The ability of both oral nutritional supplementation and parenteral alimentation to reverse these complications, even when other medical therapy has failed, has been impressive.[75–78] Oral nutritional supplementation can dramatically improve growth and maturation without resorting to prolonged hospitalization for parenteral alimentation or to surgical intervention in the absence of other primary indications for surgery.[78] Children will demonstrate catch-up growth and achievement of pre-illness height percentile. Whether nutritional restitution will overcome the suppressive effects of daily doses of corticosteroids remains unanswered.

While protein and other nutrients are important, caloric intake appears to be the most important determinant of growth. The relative efficacy of oral versus parenteral nutritional supplementation is unknown, but the nearly identical changes in growth velocity achieved by either technique suggests that their efficacy is similar.[76, 79] In general, the relatively inexpensive and non-invasive oral approach is preferred, but the age of the child may play a role in the selection. With advanced skeletal age, the more controlled and rapid restitution of nutritional status by parenteral methods may make this the logical choice. Parenteral alimentation is otherwise reserved for the nutritional support of patients who either fail to respond to oral supplementation or who require absolute and total bowel rest.

Parenteral nutrition or oral supplements can be safely provided at home.[77, 80] For the patient who has a short bowel as a result of extensive disease or following major intestinal resection, home nutritional support may provide long periods of good health until adaptive responses in the intestine permit oral maintenance. In rare cases, therapy for an indefinite period is necessary.

Therapeutic Approach To The Patient. The careful clinical studies performed in patients with Crohn's disease provide an important framework on which to base therapy. Certainly, further work will be necessary to define more carefully which treatment to select and to answer additional questions. Pending these studies, much of the therapeutic program is an art acquired through experience.

The first step in choosing therapy is to make a global assessment of the disease activity in the individual patient. There is no uniform method of measuring disease activity. A simple and reliable activity index we have found useful is that proposed by Harvey and Bradshaw.[81] This is based on clinical criteria and is applicable to a single outpatient visit. Five items are considered: general well-being (0 = very well, 1 = slightly below par, 2 = poor, 3 = very poor, 4 = terrible); abdominal pain (0 = none, 1 = mild, 2 = moderate, 3 = severe); number of liquid stools per day; abdominal mass (0 = none, 1 = dubious, 2 = definite, 3 = definite and tender); complications (arthralgias, uveitis, erythema nodosum, aphthous ulcers, pyoderma grangrenosum, anal fissure, new fistula, abscess—score 1 per item). Disease activity is considered mild to moderate when the index score is 1 to 5 and severe when over 5. We will briefly review the general approach to the patient with Crohn's disease.

Patients with Mild to Moderate Disease Activity. Ambulatory patients with mild to moderate disease activity should be given sulfasalazine as initial therapy. The dose is slowly increased to a level of 2 to 4 g/day or occasionally higher. Since approximately 60% of patients will achieve a good response within 6 weeks,[2] this time period seems reasonable before judging the effect of this drug. If successful, therapy is continued until a full clinical remission is secured. Those who fail to respond will require the addition of steroids. Prednisone, 45 to 60 mg/day in divided doses, should be given to these patients. The dose is continued for 7 to 14 days and then tapered over approximately 2 months as symptoms improve. The continuation of high doses of prednisone for prolonged periods is not advisable. While there is no evidence that the combination of sulfasalazine with the prednisone conveys added benefit, it is our practice to use them together, especially while the prednisone dose is being slowly tapered.

Patients presenting with fever, abdominal pain or tenderness, and/or evidence of a suppurative complication often benefit from antibiotic therapy. These agents can be used alone or with sulfasalazine. This approach may obviate the need for steroids, especially in those patients intolerant to or not responding to sulfasalazine. Antibiotics are especially useful to relieve the symptoms due to bacterial stasis, which commonly occurs in the patient with small bowel strictures or previous resection. A variety of preparations, including antidiarrheals, anticholinergics, and analgesics, may be of symptomatic benefit. During the period of active disease, we advise avoidance of fresh fruits and vegetables in the diet. This helps reduce diarrhea and episodes of intestinal obstruction. A trial of avoidance of lactose-containing milk products may be worthwhile during this active stage. Proper nutritional balance and adequate rest are both important, but strict bed rest is not necessary.

Patients with Severe Disease Activity. These patients generally require hospitalization. We prescribe oral feedings if they are tolerated, but patients more severely ill will require bowel rest with nothing by mouth or even with nasogastric suction. Intravenous fluid and electrolyte therapy will be required to ensure adequate replacement. If a full diet cannot be reinstituted within 10 to 14 days, total parenteral nutrition should be considered. If the patient is febrile or there is any suspicion of a suppurative complication, broad-spectrum antibiotics should be instituted. Sulfasalazine can be used in these patients, but we generally avoid this drug because the onset of its action is slow and it may be poorly tolerated. Corticosteroids will usually be necessary, but should not be used if there is a definite abscess. An oral dose of 40 to 60 mg/day of prednisone or its IV equivalent is used. ACTH (120 units) or hydrocortisone (300 mg daily) may be used as parenteral corticoid therapy. The former may be preferred for the patient not already on steroid therapy.

Intravenous therapy is administered as a continuous infusion for 7 to 14 days. Once the maximal benefit is achieved, therapy is continued with 45 to 60 mg/day of oral prednisone, in the manner described for mild or moderate disease activity. Antibiotics, sulfasalazine, and corticosteroids may be used alone or in any combination. Those patients who do not improve promptly with vigorous medical therapy should be considered for surgery (see section on Complications for detailed discussion of the therapy of specific complications).

Patients with Crohn's Disease in Remission. Once clinical activity has subsided, attempts to withdraw steroid therapy must be made. If successful, sulfasalazine and other drugs are also discontinued. The patient in remission requires no therapy. Neither sulfasalazine, steroids, nor immunosuppressive drugs have been conclusively proved to be useful in the prevention of later disease exacerbation. Unfortunately, many patients treated with steroids are not able to be withdrawn from these drugs without a flare-up of their disease. Continued therapy may be required to suppress chronic symptoms. We consider surgical intervention preferable to long-term steroid side effects. Azathioprine or 6-mercaptopurine may be useful adjuncts and allow steroid withdrawal, but have potentially serious side effects. We feel that these agents will find their major use in older patients in whom the fear of late malignancy is less or in those whose disease is not amenable to surgery. Antibiotics administered over months or years may also have a beneficial adjunctive role.

Upper Gastrointestinal Tract Disease. Local steroid preparations are useful for Crohn's disease involving the mouth. Disease of the stomach and duodenum may require systemic steroid therapy. Sulfasalazine can be very effective, but may have an irritant action upon the already diseased bowel. A low residue or liquid diet may be required if the disease has resulted in pyloric or duodenal stenosis. If obstruction is not promptly responsive to medical therapy, surgical bypass of the diseased area will provide palliation, although there is a real threat of recurrence of the disease or involvement of previously apparently unaffected segments. The upper gastrointestinal tract disease will generally be accompanied by disease in more distal areas. The therapy is guided by the principles previously discussed, with all diseased areas responding similarly.[82]

References

1. Anthonisen P, Barany F, Folkenborg O, Holtz A, Jarnum S, Kristensen M, Rilis P, Walan A, Worning H. The clinical effect of salazosulphapyridine (Salazopyrin®) in Crohn's disease. Scand J Gastroenterol 1974; 9:549–54.
2. Summer RW, Switz DM, Sessions JT, Becktel JM, Best WR, Kern F, Singleton JW. National Cooperative Crohn's Disease Study: Results of drug treatment. Gastroenterology 1979; 77:847–69.
3. Van Vees PAM, Van Lier HJJ, Van Elteren PH, Driesseor WMM, Van Hogezand RA, Ten Velde GPM, Bakker JH, Van Tongeren JHM. Effect of sulphasalazine in patients with active Crohn's disease: A controlled double-blind study. Gut 1981; 22:404–9.
4. Multicenter Trial. Sulphasalazine in asymptomatic Crohn's disease. Gut 1977; 18:69–72.
5. Wenckert A, Kristensen M, Eklund AE, Barany F, Jarnum S, Worning H, Folkenborg O, Holtz A, Bonnevie O, Riis P. The long-term prophylactic effect of salazosulphapyridine (Salazopyrin®) in primarily resected patients with Crohn's disease: A controlled double-blind trial. Scand J Gastroenterol 1978; 13:161–7.
6. Schroder H, Campbell DES. Absorption, metabolism and excretion of salicylazosulfapyridine in man. Clin Pharmacol Ther 1972; 13:539–51.
7. Peppercorn MA, Goldman P. Distribution studies of salicylazosulfapyridine and its metabolites. Gastroenterology 1973; 64:240–5.
8. Das KM, Eastwood MA, McManus JPA, Sircus W. The metabolism of salicylazosulphapyridine in ulcerative colitis. I. The relationship between metabolites and the response to treatment in inpatients. Gut 1973; 14:631–6.
9. Evans DAP, White TA. Human acetylation polymorphism. J Lab Clin Med 1964; 63:394–403.
10. Das KM, Eastwood MA. Acetylation polymorphism of sulfapyridine and its constancy in patients with inflammatory bowel disease. Gastroenterology 1974; 66:681 (Abstract).
11. Das KM, Dubin R. Clinical pharmacokinetics of sulphasalazine. Clin Pharmacokinet 1976; 1:406–25.
12. Fisher C, Klotz U. Is plasma level monitoring of sulfasalazine indicated in the treatment of Crohn's disease or ulcerative colitis? Ther Drug Monitor 1980; 2:153–8.
13. Das KM, Eastwood MA, McManus JPA, Sircus W. Adverse reactions during salicylazosulfapyridine therapy and the relation with drug metabolism and acetylator phenotype. N Engl J Med 1973; 289:491–5.
14. Khan AKA, Piris J, Truelove SC. An experiment to determine the active therapeutic moiety of sulfasalazine. Lancet 1977; 2:892–5.
15. Van Vees PAM, Van Tongeren JHM, Bakker JH, Van Lier HJJ. Active therapeutic moiety of sulphasalazine. Lancet 1978; 1:277.
16. Klotz U, Maier K, Fisher C, Heinkel K. Therapeutic efficacy of sulfasalazine and its metabolites in patients with ulcerative colitis and Crohn's disease. N Engl J Med 1980; 303:1499–1502.
17. Singleton JW, Law DH, Kelley ML, Mekhjian HS, Sturdevant RAL. National Cooperative Crohn's Disease Study:

Adverse reactions to study drugs. Gastroenterology 1979; 77:870–82.
18. Gould SR. Prostaglandins, ulcerative colitis, and sulfasalazine. Lancet 1975; 2:988.
19. Gould SR. Assay of prostaglandin-like substances in feces and their measurement in ulcerative colitis. Prostaglandins 1976; 11:489–97.
20. Sharon P, Ligumoky M, Rachmilewitz D, Zor U. Role of prostaglandins in ulcerative colitis: Enhanced production during active disease and inhibition by sulfasalazine. Gastroenterology 1978; 75:638–40.
21. Harris DW, Smith PR, Swan CHJ. Determination of prostaglandin synthetase activity in rectal biopsy material and its significance in colonic disease. Gut 1978; 19:875–7.
22. Smith PR, Dawson DJ, Swan CHJ. Prostaglandin synthetase activity in acute ulcerative colitis: Effects of treatment with sulfasalazine, codeine phosphate and prednisolone. Gut 1978; 20:802–5.
23. Campieri M, Lanfranchi GA, Bozzocchi G. Salicylate other than 5-aminosalicylic acid ineffective in ulcerative colitis. Lancet 1978; 2:993.
24. Hoult JRS, Moore PK. Effects of sulfasalazine and its metabolites on prostaglandin synthesis, inactivation and actions on smooth muscle. Br J Pharmacol 1980; 68:719–30.
25. Molin L, Stendahl O. The effect of sulfasalazine and its active components on human polymorphonuclear leukocyte function in relation to ulcerative colitis. Acta Med Scand 1979; 206:451–7.
26. Sparberg M, Kirsner JB. Long-term corticosteroid therapy for regional enteritis: An analysis of 58 courses in 54 patients. Am J Dig Dis 1966; 11:865–80.
27. Tanner AR, Halliday JW, Powel LW. Serum prednisolone levels in Crohn's disease or celiac disease following oral prednisolone administration. Digestion 1981; 21:310–15.
28. Meyers S, Sachar DB, Goldberg JD, Janowitz HD. A randomized double-blind comparison of corticotropin (ACTH) and hydrocortisone (HC) in the treatment of severe ulcerative colitis. Gastroenterology 1983; 85:351–7.
29. Smith RC, Rhodes J, Heatley RV, Hughes LE, Crosby DL, Rees BI, Jonks H, Evans KT, Lawrie BW. Low dose steroids and clinical relapse in Crohn's disease: A controlled trial. Gut 1978; 19:606–10.
30. Bergman L, Krause U. Postoperative treatment with corticosteroids and salazosulphapyridine (Salazopyrin) after radical resection for Crohn's disease. Scand J Gastroenterol 1976; 11:651–6.
31. Singleton JW, Summer RW, Kern F, Becktel JM, Best WR, Hansen RN, Winship DH. A trial of sulfasalazine as adjunctive therapy in Crohn's disease. Gastroenterology 1979; 77:887–97.
32. Brooke BN, Hoffman DC, Swarbrack ET. Azathioprine for Crohn's disease. Lancet 1969; 2:612–4.
33. Rhodes J, Bainton D, Beck P, Campbell H. Controlled trial of azathioprine in Crohn's disease. Lancet 1971; 2:1273–6.
34. Klein M, Binder HJ, Mitchell M, Aaronson R, Spiro H. Treatment of Crohn's disease with azathioprine: A controlled evaluation. Gastroenterology 1974; 66:916–22.
35. Rosenberg JL, Levin B, Wall AJ, Kirsner JB. A controlled trial of azathioprine in Crohn's disease. Am J Dig Dis 1975; 20:721–6.
36. Willoughby JMT, Kumar PJ, Beckett J, Dawson AM. Controlled trial of azathioprine in Crohn's disease. Lancet 1971; 2:944–7.
37. O'Donoghue DP, Dawson AM, Powell-Tuck J, Bown RL, Lennard-Jones JE. Double-blind withdrawal trial of azathioprine as maintenance treatment for Crohn's disease. Lancet 1978; 2:955–7.
38. Present DH, Korelitz BI, Wisch N, Glass JL, Sachar DB, Pasternack BS. Treatment of Crohn's disease with 6-mercaptopurine: A long-term randomized double-blind study. N Engl J Med 1980; 302:981–7.
39. Sturdevant RAL, Singleton JW, Deren JJ, Law DH, McCleery JL. Azathioprine-related pancreatitis in patients with Crohn's disease. Gastroenterology 1979; 77:883–6.
40. Kinlen LJ, Sheil AGR, Peto J, Doll R. Collaborative United Kingdom-Australasian study of cancer in patients treated with immunosuppressive drugs. Br Med J 1979; 2:1461–6.
41. Moss AA, Carbone JV, Kressel HY. Radiologic and clinical assessment of broad-spectrum antibiotic therapy in Crohn's disease. AJR 1978; 131:787–90.
42. Ursing B, Kamme C. Metronidazole for Crohn's disease. Lancet 1975; 1:775–7.
43. Kasper H, Sommer H, Kuhn HA. Therapy of Crohn's disease with metronidazole: An uncontrolled trial. Acta Hepato-Gastroenterol 1979; 26:217–21.
44. Allan R, Cooke WT. Evaluation of metronidazole in the management of Crohn's disease. Gut 1977; 18:A422 (Abstract).
45. Blichfeldt P, Blomhoff JP, Gjone M, Gjone E. Metronidazole in Crohn's disease: A double blind cross-over clinical trial. Scand J Gastroenterol 1978; 13:123–7.
46. Ursing B, Alm T, Barany F, Bergelin I, Ganrot-Norlin K, Hoevels J, Huitfeldt B, Jarnerot G, Krause U, Krook A, Lindostrom B, Nordle O, Rosen A. A comparative study of metronidazole and sulfasalazine for active Crohn's disease: The Cooperative Crohn's Disease Study in Sweden. II. Result. Gastroenterology 1982; 83:550–62.
47. Bernstein LH, Frank MS, Brandt LJ, Boley SJ. Healing of perineal Crohn's disease with metronidazole. Gastroenterology 1980; 79:357–65.
48. Brandt LJ, Bernstein LH, Boley SJ, Frank MS. Metronidazole therapy for perineal Crohn's disease: A follow-up study. Gastroenterology 1982; 83:383–7.
49. Rustia M, Shubik P. Induction of lung tumors and malignant lymphomas in mice by metronidazole. J Nat Cancer Inst 1972; 48:721–9.
50. Speck WT, Stein AB, Rosenkranz HS. Mutagenicity of metronidazole: Presence of several active metabolites in human urine. J Nat Cancer Inst 1976; 56:283–4.
51. Beard CM, Noller KL, O'Fallon WM, Kurland LT, Dockerty MD. Lack of evidence for cancer due to use of metronidazole. N Engl J Med 1979; 301:519–22.
52. Mitelman F, Stombeck B, Ursing B. No cytogenetic effect of metronidazole. Lancet 1980; 1:1249–50 (Letter).
53. Grove DI, Mahmond AAF, Warren KS. Suppression of cell-mediated immunity by metronidazole. Clin Res 1976; 24(Suppl):285 (Abstract).
54. Meyers S, Sachar DB, Taub RN, Janowitz HD. Dinitrochlorobenzene (DNCB) in inflammatory bowel disease: Family and post-operative studies. Gut 1978; 19:249–52.
55. Burnham WR, Lennard-Jones JE, Hecketsweilles P, Colin R, Geffroy Y. Oral BCG vaccine in Crohn's disease. Gut 1979; 20:299–33.
56. Rahban S, Sherman JH, Opelz G, Conley DR, Panish JF, Marks JW, Terasaki PI, Schoenfield LJ. BCG treatment of Crohn's disease. Am J Gastroenterol 1979; 71:196–201.
57. Wesdorp E, Schellekens PTA, Weening RS, Meuwissen SGM, Tytgat GN. Levamisole in Crohn's disease: A double-blind controlled trial. Digestion 1978; 18:186–91.
58. Vicary FR, Chambers JD, Dhillon P. Double blind trial of the use of transfer factor in the treatment of Crohn's disease. Gut 1979; 20:408–13.
59. Segal AW, Levi AJ, Loewi G. Levamisole in the treatment of Crohn's disease. Lancet 1977; 2:382–4.
60. Vantrappen G, Coremans G, Billiau A, DeSomer P. Treatment of Crohn's disease with interferon: A preliminary clinical trial. Acta Clin Belg 1980; 35:238–42.
61. Williams SE, Grundman MJ, Baker RD, Turnberg LA. A controlled trial of disodium cromoglycate in the treatment of Crohn's disease. Digestion 1980; 20:395–8.
62. Binder V, Elsborg L, Greibe J, Hendriksen C, Lene HØJ Jensen BK, Kristensen E, Madsen RJ, Marner B, Riis P, Willumsen L. Disodium cromoglycate in the treatment of ulcerative colitis and Crohn's disease. Gut 1981; 22:55–60.
63. Holdstock GE, Fisher JA, Hamblin TJ, Loehry C. Plasmapheresis in Crohn's disease. Digestion 1979; 19:197–201.
64. Skogh M, Sundquist T, Tagesson C. Vitamin A in Crohn's disease. Lancet 1980; 1:766 (Letter).
65. Dvorak AM. Vitamin A in Crohn's disease. Lancet 1980; 1:1303–4.

66. Heaton KW, Thornthon JR, Emmet PM. Treatment of Crohn's disease with an unrefined-carbohydrate, fiber-rich diet. Br Med J 1979; 2:764–6.
67. O'Morain C. Elemental diets in the treatment of Crohn's disease. Proc Nutr Soc 1979; 38:403–7.
68. O'Morain C, Segal AW, Levi AJ. Elemental diets in treatment of acute Crohn's disease. Br Med J 1980; 2:1173–5.
69. Logan RFA, Gillon J, Ferrington C, Ferguson A. Reduction of gastrointestinal protein loss by elemental diet in Crohn's disease of the small bowel. Gut 1981; 22:383–7.
70. Driscoll RH, Rosenberg IH. Total parenteral nutrition in inflammatory bowel disease. Med Clin North Am 1978; 62:185–201.
71. Axelsson C, Jarnum S. Assessment of the therapeutic value of an elemental diet in chronic inflammatory bowel disease. Scand J Gastroenterol 1977; 12:89–95.
72. Elson CO, Layden TJ, Nemchaustky BA, Rosenberg JL, Rosenberg IH. An evaluation of total parenteral nutrition in the management of inflammatory bowel disease. Dig Dis Sci 1980; 25:42–7.
73. Dickinson RJ, Ashton MG, Axon ATR, Smith RC, Yeung CK, Hill GL. Controlled trial of intravenous hyperalimentation and total bowel rest as an adjunct to the routine therapy of acute colitis. Gastroenterology 1980; 79:1199–1204.
74. Muller JM, Brenner U, Dienst C, Pichlmaier H. Preoperative parenteral feeding in patients with gastrointestinal cancer. Lancet 1982; 1:68–71.
75. Layden T, Rosenberg JL, Nemchausky B, Elson C, Rosenberg IH. Reversal of growth arrest in adolescents with Crohn's disease after parenteral alimentation. Gastroenterology 1976; 70:1017–21.
76. Kelts DG, Grand RJ, Shen G. Nutritional basis of growth failure in children and adolescents with Crohn's disease. Gastroenterology 1979; 76:720–7.
77. Strobel CT, Byrne WJ, Ament ME. Home parenteral nutrition in children with Crohn's disease: An effective management alternative. Gastroenterology 1979; 77:272–9.
78. Morin CL, Roulet M, Roy CC, Weber A. Continuous elemental enteral alimentation in children with Crohn's disease and growth failure. Gastroenterology 1980; 79:1205–10.
79. Kirschner BS, Klich JR, Kalman SS, DeFavoro MV, Rosenberg IH. Reversal of growth retardation in Crohn's disease with therapy emphasizing oral nutritional restitution. Gastroenterology 1981; 80:10–15.
80. Main ANH, Morgan RJ, Hall MJ, Russell RI, Shenkin A, Fell GS. Home enteral tube feeding with a liquid diet in the long-term management of inflammatory bowel disease and intestinal failure. Scot Med J 1980; 25:312–4.
81. Harvey RF, Bradshaw JM. A simple index of Crohn's disease activity. Lancet 1980; 1:514.
82. Fitzgibbons TJ, Green G, Silberman H, Eliasoph J, Halls JM, Yellin AE. Management of Crohn's disease involving the duodenum including duodenal cutaneous fistula. Arch Surg 1980; 115:1022–8.

Surgical Management

Adrian J. Greenstein

Historical Perspectives

The first successful surgically treated series of a granulomatous disease of the intestine is attributed to T. Kennedy Dalziel.[1] In 1913, in an address to the 81st Annual Meeting of the British Medical Association, he reported 9 patients with chronic intestinal disease operated upon between 1901 and 1913. The patients presented with crampy abdominal pain, watery or bloody diarrhea, and weight loss, and most cases culminated in subacute obstruction. At laparotomy, localized or widespread thickening of the small and/or large intestine was found. Dalziel successfully resected the proximal jejunum, midileum, ileocecal region (3 cases), and transverse and sigmoid colon in 7 separate procedures—a truly remarkable accomplishment. Two patients were unresectable and incurable because of widespread disease. The description, in 1923, by Moschowitz and Wilensky[2] at the Mount Sinai Hospital in New York of non-specific intestinal granulomas associated with external fistula following small bowel resection led to the classic paper by Crohn et al.[3] published in 1932. Figure 127–61 shows the sequence of 18 operations carried out by A. A. Berg at the Mount Sinai Hospital. This culminated in the 14 resected specimens that formed the basis for the clinicopathologic description by Crohn. In 1933, Ginzburg and Oppenheimer[4] published the report of their surgical experi-

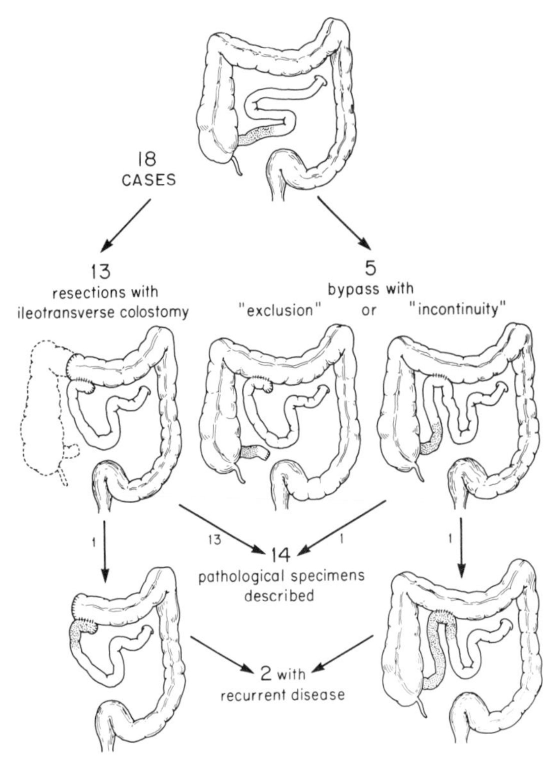

Figure 127–61. The sequence of operative procedures and postoperative recurrences among the original 18 cases of granulomatous disease, from which 14 pathologic specimens were derived and studied in the classic 1932 paper of Drs. Crohn, Ginzburg, and Oppenheimer.

ence with the disease, which they presented at the 1932 meeting of the American Gastroenterological Association.

The earliest resections resulted in external fistulas in some instances and were followed by the development of recurrent disease in others. As a result, Berg constructed an ileotransverse colostomy through normal proximal small bowel, successfully bypassing the diseased segment (Fig. 127–61). This was carried out first in continuity by simple side-to-side enteroenterostomy. Subsequently, bypass with exclusion was perfected by transecting the normal small bowel proximal to the diseased segment and closing the distal side prior to construction of the ileotransverse colostomy. Because of the sequence of preferred procedures at the Mount Sinai Hospital, Garlock,[5] in 1951, found a higher recurrence rate of disease among patients who had had small bowel resection and hence a longer duration of follow-up, (46%) than that following the various bypass procedures (23%).

Crohn and associates[3] recognized the problem of recurrent disease in their classic paper, when they described recurrences in 2 of the 17 survivors among the original 18 operated patients. They attributed this problem to spread from the distal diseased segment in one patient with an ileotransverse colostomy-in-continuity and to incomplete removal of the diseased segment in the other. As a consequence, the concept of radical resection developed, culminating in the suggestion that 60 cm of proximal normal bowel be removed in an attempt to eradicate or cure the disease by surgical resection.[6] This concept is believed to be fallacious today because it is now believed that the disease may involve the digestive tract from mouth to anus, even if in an occult form.[7–14]

Overall View of Surgical Treatment

The medical therapy for Crohn's disease controls symptoms in most patients for variable periods of time, but at the cost of the side effects of the drugs that are prescribed. Because of the high recurrence rates,[15–18] surgery for regional enteritis and ileocolitis is usually delayed until complications such as hemorrhage, obstruction, or perforation supervene.[19] In Crohn's disease confined to the colon, however, intractability to medical management is the most frequent indication for operative intervention.[19–21] Studies on Crohn's disease reported from the United States,[22] England,[23,24] and Scandinavia[25] have demonstrated that if patients are followed for a sufficiently long period of time, over 90% will eventually require surgery. Surgical treatment results in good palliation for variable periods of time and a mean disease-free interval of approximately 5.8 years.[15] During interoperative periods, most of the patients have excellent palliation[22,26] and are relatively asymptomatic for as much as 90% of the time.[27]

Indications for Surgery

In 1976, Farmer, et al.[20] demonstrated highly significant differences in the indications for surgery among patients with ileal, ileocolic, and pure colonic disease. Thus, in patients with disease confined to the small intestine, the primary indications were intestinal obstruction in more than half the cases, followed by abscess and fistula in one-third. In disease involving both the small and the large bowel, the primary indications were fistula and abscess, followed by obstruction and perianal disease. In Crohn's colitis, the surgical indications were more diverse, poor response to medical therapy being a common indication, followed by internal fistula, abscess, toxic megacolon, and perianal disease. Similar but not identical results have been reported by Allan et al. in Birmingham, England,[28] and Greenstein et al. in New York.[29] Table 127–9 shows a comparison of the different indications in the 3 series, including unpublished data for regional enteritis from a small series of 93 patients undergoing surgery from the Mount Sinai Hospital. There has been a considerable change in the anatomic distribution of Crohn's disease over the past 50 years (Table 127–10) and hence a corresponding change in the indications for surgery. In fact, the early era of hope for cure by relatively early surgery was tempered by the gloomy reports regarding recurrence and prognosis from the Mayo Clinic in 1954 and the Mount Sinai Hospital in 1958.[30,31] Following these reports, surgery for a while was used only as a last resort in many hospitals, leading on occasion to disaster. Only now are we beginning to attempt to approach the fundamental problem of the indications for surgery more rationally, balancing the good and the harmful effects of drugs against the unavoidable sequel of recurrence following increasingly safe surgery. Nevertheless, there are still today wide differences of opinion: Cooke et al.[23] feel that there is little place for prolonged use of steroids and is positive about early surgery; Glotzer and Silen[32] state that the most effective operations for Crohn's disease are performed for intractability, despite the suggestion by some that indications for operation in small intestinal Crohn's disease tend to be specific; and Korelitz[33] believes that "in Crohn's disease intractability and fistula are no longer valid indications for surgery."

Failure of Medical Management. "Medical intractability" is an important reason for operating on patients with Crohn's disease, particularly those in whom the disease is predominantly or exclusively in the colon. Operative intervention may be necessitated by: (1) persistent symptoms, especially weight loss, fever, and toxicity; (2) complications of steroid therapy, such as overt Cushing's syndrome, osteoporosis with vertebral collapse, diabetes, and psychosis; (3) side effects of sulfasalazine or prolonged antibiotic therapy; and (4) in children, failure to thrive despite adequate drug therapy.

In general, the health of the patient is the key to the decision. When the dangers and problems of drug therapy outweigh its advantages, and when the patient is unable to function socially and lead a normal life, no matter how imprecise the indication is, surgery is mandatory. The one exception may be the patient with extensive ileojejunitis or multiple skip areas. In most cases, such patients are not surgical candidates, although limited procedures, such as multiple bypasses in patients with multiple strictures, have been suggested.[34, 35]

Complications. Complications that may occur in patients with Crohn's disease are specifically considered in another section of this chapter. Only passing reference will be made here, therefore, to those that justify or may require surgical management.

Obstruction. Intestinal obstruction is a common surgical indication in ileitis or ileocolitis (Fig. 127–62). There almost invariably is an excellent response to nasogastric intubation and large doses of steroids. However, the attacks recur in almost all instances. Hence, the development of a second episode or the subsequent progressive deterioration in the health of the patient constitutes an important indication for surgical intervention.

Perforation. Perforations may be divided into 3 basic types, depending upon the rapidity with which they develop and upon the degree of adherence to surrounding structures: (1) acute type with free perforation, (2) subacute perforation with abscess formation (Fig. 127–63); and (3) chronic perforation with fistula formation (Fig. 127–64).

Free perforation of the small bowel is a relatively infrequent complication of Crohn's disease[36] and colonic perforation is even more uncommon.[37, 38] In the small intestine, the ileum is usually involved but the jejunum may also be affected.[39] Free perforation has even been recorded in an excluded segment of small bowel.[40]

There were 15 cases of generalized peritonitis from free perforation of the bowel and 6 cases originating in a ruptured abscess among 1010 patients with Crohn's disease

Table 127–9. COMPARISON OF INDICATIONS FOR SURGERY IN CROHN'S DISEASE

	Ileocolitis			Crohn's Colitis			Regional Enteritis	
	Farmer et al.[20]	*Greenstein et al.*[29]	*Allan et al.*[28]	*Farmer et al.*[20]	*Greenstein et al.*[29]	*Allan et al.*[28]	*Farmer et al.*[20]	*Greenstein**
Number of patients	225	199	53	127	51	112	130	93
Obstructive symptoms	35	32	50	12	10	17	55†	50
Abdominal abscess or fistula	44†	36	26	23	36	10	32	27
Intractability	7	17	23	26†	20	53	8	17
Perianal disease	12	4	0	19†	9	13	5	0
Acute hemorrhage	0	2	2	0	1	7	0	3
Toxic megacolon	2	1	0	20†	8	0	0	0

*Unpublished data.
†Significantly increased.

Table 127–10. COMPARISON OF THE ANATOMIC DISTRIBUTION OF LESIONS OF CROHN'S DISEASE IN DIFFERENT CENTERS

	Shapiro (1939)[200] (Review)		Weedon et al. (1973)[122] Mayo Clinic (1919–1965)		Truelove & Pena (1973)[160] Radcliffe Infirmary Oxford (1938–1970)		Farmer et al. (1975)[23] Cleveland Clinic (1966–1973)		Greenstein (1982)* Mount Sinai Hospital (1960–1982)	
	No. of Cases	*(%)*	*No. of Cases*	*(%)*	*No. of Cases*	*(%)*	*No. of Cases*	*(%)*	*No. of Cases*	*(%)*
Small intestine	333	72.2	93	21	67	30.3	176	28.6	369	37
Small and large intestine	106	23.0	262	58	92	41.6	252	41.0	453	45
Large intestine	22	4.8	94	21	57	25.8	166	27.0	178	18
Other sites (stomach, mouth, duodenum, etc.)	0	0.0	0	0	5	2.3	21	3.4		
Total	461	100	449	100	221	100	615	100	1000	100

*Unpublished data.

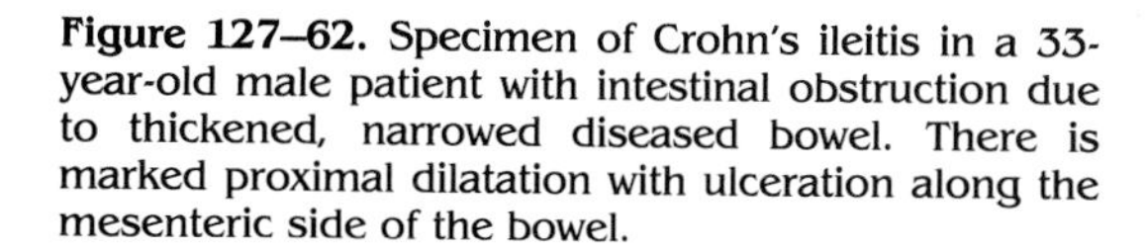
Figure 127–62. Specimen of Crohn's ileitis in a 33-year-old male patient with intestinal obstruction due to thickened, narrowed diseased bowel. There is marked proximal dilatation with ulceration along the mesenteric side of the bowel.

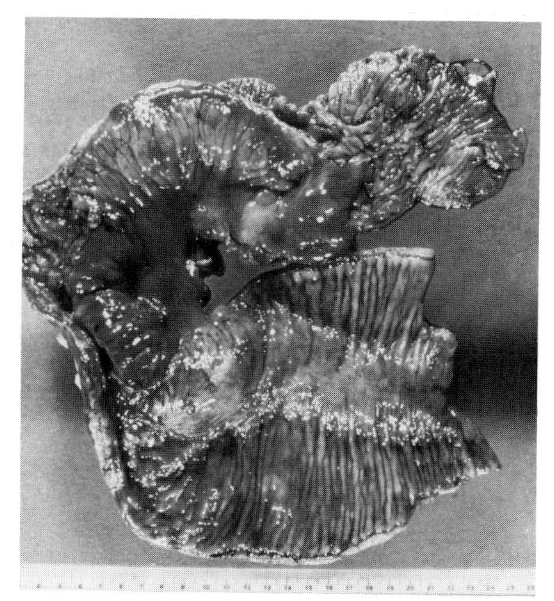

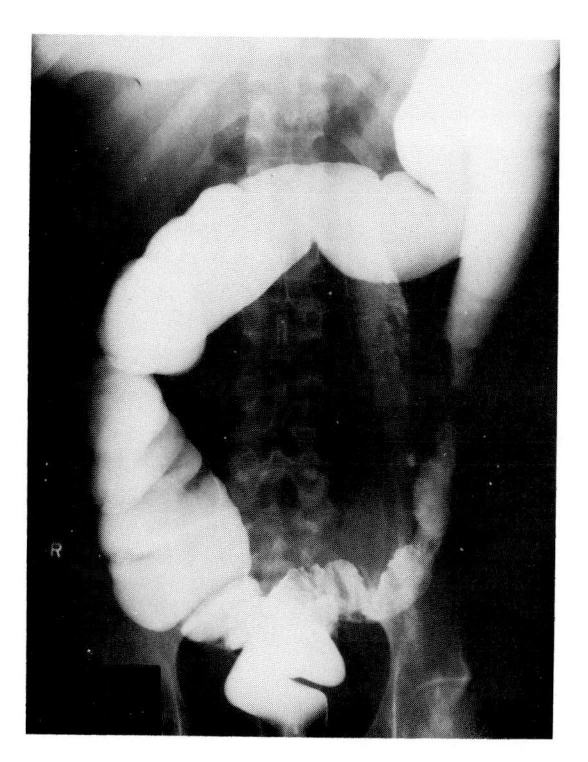

Figure 127–63. Granulomatous colitis in a 27-year-old patient, most severe in the descending colon with perforation and psoas abscess. The psoas sheath outlining the psoas muscle is clearly delineated by barium to the left of the vertebral bodies.

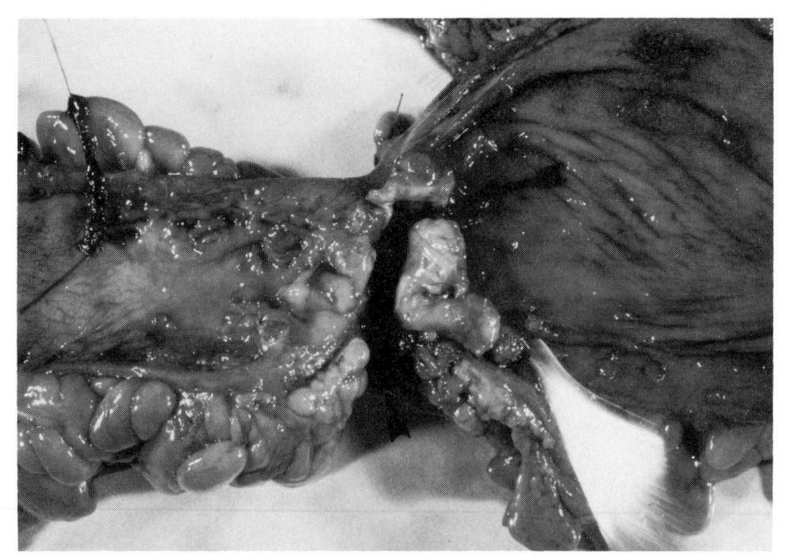

Figure 127–64. Site of a jejunocolonic fistula in a 24-year-old female patient with universal Crohn's colitis and narrowing of the descending colon. This was treated by colectomy and ileostomy with wedge resection and closure of the jejunum.

admitted over a 20-year period to the Mount Sinai Hospital in New York.[41] Of the 15 patients with free perforation, the perforation interestingly originated in the colon in 10.

Free perforation of the bowel with generalized peritonitis is rare because the thickened fibrotic bowel with serositis usually adheres to adjacent organs. However, peritonitis may also result from intraperitoneal rupture of an abscess when the area of inflammation is not adequately walled off by adjacent adherent viscera or omentum. Immediate surgery following rapid resuscitation is mandatory if a successful result is to be achieved. Although simple closure has been suggested, the mortality following this form of limited surgery is considerable.

Resection of the perforated diseased segment is clearly the preferred form of treatment. In the presence of any suggestion of active peritonitis or delay in treatment, exteriorization of both ends of bowel with copious irrigation of the peritoneal cavity "to extinction" and insertion of multiple drains is the safest form of treatment. With ruptured abscess, proximal diversion and drainage or resection and drainage are alternative methods of surgical treatment. Our experience at the Mount Sinai Hospital with exteriorization and proximal diverting ileostomy has been gratifying. The mortality was exceptionally low (1 of 19 patients)[41–43] and there were no deaths, surprisingly, in the 15 patients with free perforation.[41]

Intra-abdominal Abscess. Formation of an abscess is a frequent complication of Crohn's disease.[44] It is generally considered a subacute form of perforation of the bowel occurring either between the leaves of mesentery or between the serosal surface of bowel and adjacent viscera. Percutaneous drainage of such abscesses is unlikely to result in long-term resolution of the problem in Crohn's disease because the feeding focus, i.e., the fistulous tract from the bowel, persists even though the pus has been evacuated. Drainage, however, may reduce toxicity and allow elective and controlled surgery to be carried out later by excision of the diseased segment of bowel without gross contamination.

Intra-abdominal abscesses may be divided anatomically into enteroparietal (Fig. 127–65), intraloop, and intramesenteric types.[45] The enteroparietal abscesses are most effectively and simply treated by primary incision and drainage, followed at a second stage by resection of the resulting enterocutaneous fistula and diseased bowel. Deep abscesses in the mesentery or pelvis or between loops of bowel constitute a more difficult problem. If spontaneous drainage into the bladder or colon does not occur during antibiotic therapy, laparotomy, drainage of the abscess, and proximal diversion or exteriorization will

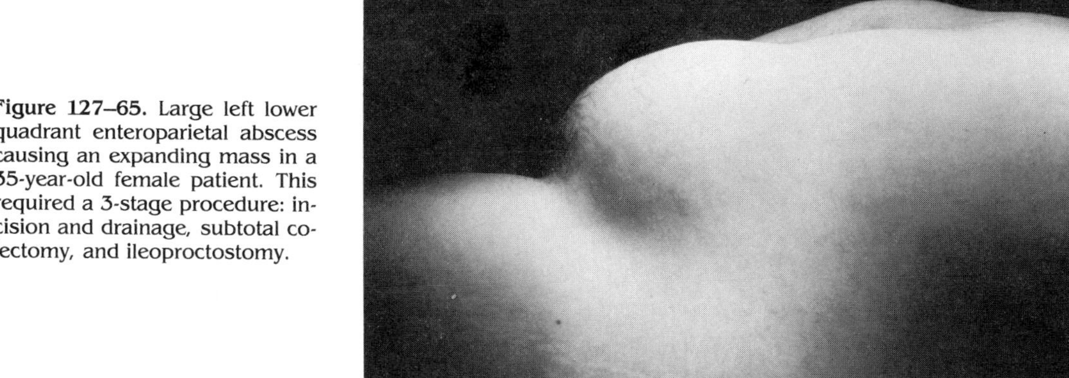

Figure 127–65. Large left lower quadrant enteroparietal abscess causing an expanding mass in a 35-year-old female patient. This required a 3-stage procedure: incision and drainage, subtotal colectomy, and ileoproctostomy.

be necessary. By contrast with the salutary results achieved in acute free perforation,[41] the mortality rate for inadequately drained abscesses present before surgery[29, 44] has been considerable in our series of cases at the Mount Sinai Hospital.

Fistula. Three major types of fistulas occur in Crohn's disease: *internal, external,* and *perianal.*[46]

INTERNAL FISTULAS. These are epithelial-lined tracts lying between 2 epithelial lined-organs that result from direct penetration of the fissure-ulcers of Crohn's disease into an adjacent organ or from rupture of a perienteric abscess into an adjacent organ. The most common internal fistulas are *enteroenteric, enterovesical,* and *rectovaginal.* The enteroenteric fistulas include jejunoileal, ileoileal, ileocecal, ileosigmoid (Fig. 127–66), and colocolonic types (Fig. 127–67). Enterovesical fistulas originate in the ileum or colon, or both. Rectovaginal fistulas are a form of perianal fistula.

Internal fistulas are relative indications for surgery. Broe et al.[47] studied the natural history of 24 of 64 patients with *enteroenteric fistulas* who were not operated upon immediately. Ten patients were operated upon within 1 year for intestinal obstruction, enterovesical fistula, or failure to respond to medical management; 8 others required operation after 1 to 9 years of non-operative treatment. In only 6 of the original 64 patients (9%) was surgery unnecessary; in 2 patients the fistulas could no longer be demonstrated radiologically, and 4 patients were studied more than 5 years after the original radiologic demonstration of the fistulas. Thus, the results of treatment of patients with fistulas by elemental diet,[48] hyperalimentation,[49] and immunosuppressive drugs,[33, 50, 51] even when successful, appear in most instances to be temporary. Enteroenteric fistulas remain a relative indication for surgery, with most patients ultimately coming to resection be-

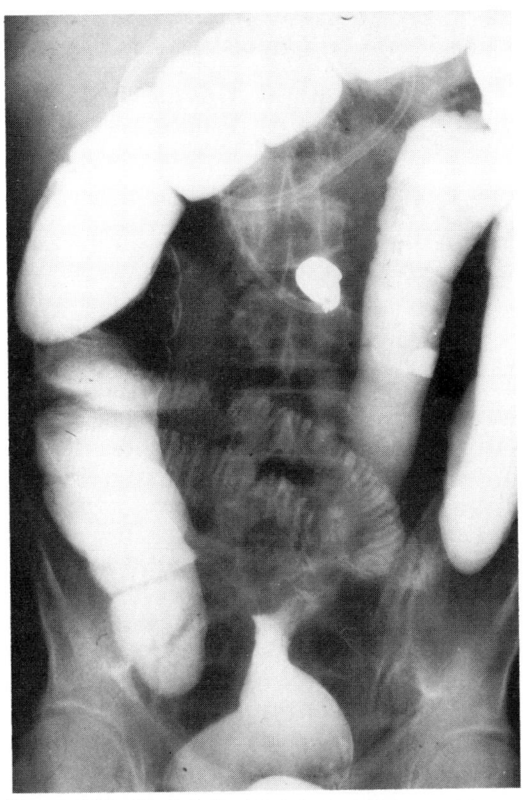

Figure 127–66. Coloileal fistula in a 52-year-old male patient with Crohn's ileocolitis of 20 years' duration. This required ileocolic and sigmoid resection plus diverting ileostomy. The ileostomy was closed 6 months later.

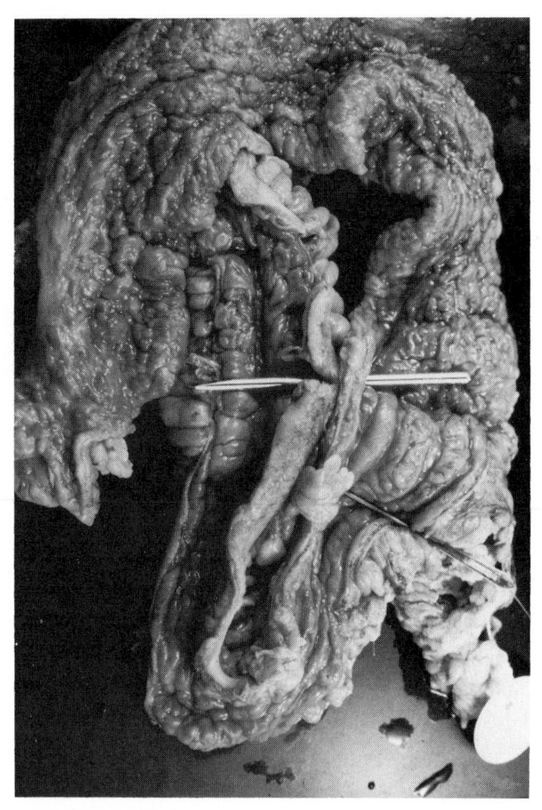

Figure 127–67. Colocolonic fistula in a 32-year-old female patient with granuomatous colitis sparing the rectum. This was treated by abdominal colectomy with ileosigmoidostomy.

cause of the underlying severity of the penetrating intestinal disease.

Ileocecal fistulas, or fistulas from the ileum to the right colon, are seldom a problem in the absence of intra-abdominal abscess, as only a short length of bowel is bypassed by the fistula. Should surgery become necessary for progressive obstructing intestinal disease or the development of an abscess, resection of the right colon will encompass the area of the fistula and surrounding inflammatory tissue so that a simple ileotransverse colostomy can be constructed. The author favors an end-to-side ileocolostomy, but others prefer the side-to-side and still others prefer the end-to-end types of anastomosis. Our preference avoids the discrepancy of bowel size often found in the end-to-end anastomosis, and this procedure may delay the obstruction due to recurrent anastomotic disease in the presence of a narrow ileum. It also eliminates the possibility of a blind loop in the side-to-side anastomosis, a possible development even when a small blind end is left.

Ileosigmoid fistulas usually result from ileal disease. In the absence of colonic disease, Garlock[52] recommended detachment of the ileum, resection of the diseased ileocolic segment, and simple closure of the colon. Fazio et al.,[53] however, advocate ileocolic resection plus segmental sigmoid resection, with or without a temporary Turnbull ileostomy. If the disease is present on both the ileal and the colonic sides of the fistula, there is little controversy; ileocolic resection plus sigmoid resection with 2 separate anastomoses will be required. In this case, particularly if the ileum is joined with a moderately diseased rectum, a diverting proximal loop ileostomy may be advisable.[54] If the disease is primarily colonic, subtotal colectomy or segmental colectomy with ileoproctostomy and limited small bowel resection may be possible. Occasionally, extensive colonic disease may make total proctocolectomy and ileostomy the procedure of choice.

The same general principles apply to *enterovesical fistulas*. These occur much more commonly in men, because of the anatomic location of the uterus in women. Although pneumaturia, dysuria, hematuria, and fecaluria are distressing symptoms, immediate surgery is not mandatory, as septicemia rarely develops from the fistula itself. When septicemia does occur, it usually results from an ileo-colo-vesical abscess lying within the pelvis that is not adequately drained through the bladder or colon. Nevertheless, such a fistula generally indicates serious penetrating bowel disease, and most patients come to surgery for associated problems of the severe intestinal disease or for repeated septic episodes due to accumulation of pus adjacent to the bladder. Hence, many view the presence of an enterovesical fistula as an absolute indication for surgery.[32, 47] and surgical resection as the preferred form of procedure.[46] Surgical treatment involves resection of the involved segment of ileum or colon, or both, and disconnection of the bladder fistula, with or without closure of the opening. In a series of 38 patients with enterovesical fistulas, (5.6% of 683 patients with Crohn's disease studied at the Mount Sinai Hospital) 6 patients were treated conservatively for periods of 2 to 6 years and all except 2 eventually required surgical resection. All other patients[30] were operated upon early. None developed a recurrent bladder fistula, although a number did develop recurrent disease.[55]

ENTEROCUTANEOUS FISTULAS. Simple incision and drainage of an intra-abdominal abscess without concomitant diversion will result in an enterocutaneous fistula in a high percentage of patients, as the feeding focus remains in-situ.[44] External fistulas usually penetrate through to the skin level at the site of a previous abdominal incision. Occasionally, colocutaneous fistulas present as spontaneous coloumbilical fistulas through the relatively thin fascial layer of the umbilicus or periumbilical region.[36, 56] External fistulas communicating with bowel usually originate in the ileum or colon and rarely cause the skin excoriation and discomfort characteristic of high small bowel fistulas. They usually discharge pus or mucus intermittently and require one or several dressing changes daily. Although they may be tolerated for long periods of time, they seldom heal spontaneously. Even reports of their closure following prolonged intravenous alimentation, oral elemental diet, 6-mercaptopurine, or metronidazole (Flagyl) are not too sanguine about the long-term outlook, as most fistulas recur after discontinuing medical therapy.[33, 57] Most patients ultimately need to undergo resection of the diseased bowel together with the fistulous tract and subsequently do well thereafter. Fistulas originating at a suture line will heal in the same way as other suture line fistulas in the absence of actual overt disease at the anastomosis, distal obstruction, foreign body, or carcinoma.

PERI-ILEOSTOMY FISTULAS. Greenstein et al.[58] described 15 cases of parastomal fistulas among 1010 patients with Crohn's disease, a prevalence of 1.8%; all patients had recurrent Crohn's disease proximal to the stoma. Peri-ileostomy fistulas represent a particularly unpleasant form of external fistula, having the combined problems of persistent drainage from an ileocutaneous fistula and the concomitant difficulty of maintaining the seal of an appliance. The latter problem results in severe skin excoriation. When such fistulas are preceded by a parastomal abscess or when multiple fistulas are present, the skin surface is usually grossly irregular, and transposition of the stoma to the left lower quadrant of the abdomen may be necessary following resection of the diseased segment of ileum proximal to the stoma. This may be done through a formal laparotomy incision or by the direct stoma-to-stoma technique.[58]

Carcinomas may present as ileocutaneous[49, 59] or ileovesical fistulas,[60] particularly when they develop in bypassed loops of bowel.[60] Palliative resection should be attempted in such cases, but no cure has been reported and death usually ensues within a few months to a year.

PERIANAL FISTULAS AND ABSCESSES. Anorectal abscesses and fistulas are common complications of Crohn's disease, being most frequent in distal colonic disease, least frequent in ileal disease, and of intermediate frequency in the ileocolonic form of the disease.[61] The perianal lesions may precede the onset of the intestinal disease by as long as 20 years. The extensive excavation attained by some perianal fistulas and abscesses results from reluctance to treat them actively for fear of aggravating the local condition. This problem should be seen less often with early local drainage and fistulotomy[62, 63] and with use of the Parks' internal sphincterectomy.[64, 65] The latter procedure partially resects and divides the internal sphincter, removes the area of local fibrosis, and allows the abscess to drain internally. Although complete healing will not be achieved in many instances, especially if the active intestinal disease is not controlled, this conservative form of treatment leads to a satisfactory clinical result in the majority of patients.[62,63]

Occasionally, pronounced perianal disease is associated with severe distal Crohn's colitis, fecal incontinence, and/or anorectal stricture with obstruction.[66] Total proctocolectomy and ileostomy is the only solution to this intractable problem. Fecal diversion alone does not result in healing of extensive perianal disease.[32, 67, 68] Rarely, perianal fistulas originate in the upper rectum or a loop of ileum with perirectal tracking of the fistula. Correction of the proximal disease with ileal resection is the solution to this unusual high fistula of ileal origin. Proctocolectomy may be necessary for high rectal fistulas if the perianal abscess and fistula are incapacitating or track to the buttocks or hip joints and if the colonic disease is extensive and severe.

Obstructive Uropathy. Hydronephrosis and hydroureter may occur in Crohn's disease as the result of periureteral inflammation and fibrosis or oxalate or uric acid calculi. The treatment of the calculous form of obstruction is quite simply removal of the obstructing stone, whether by conservative watchful waiting, percutaneous nephrostomy, or surgical intervention. The management of "cicatricial periureteric fibrosis involving the anterior retroperitoneal spaces"[69] is more controversial. Although Goldman and Glickman,[70] in 1962, described a patient seen at the Mount Sinai Hospital with ureteric obstruction requiring nephrectomy, no case of nephrectomy for this problem has been reported since that time. Present et al., in 1969,[71] described 11 patients in whom treatment resulted in resolution of the ureteric obstruction without extensive ureterolysis. Ureterolysis was recommended in 1973 by Block et al.,[69] who described 27 ileocolitis patients with hydronephrosis and/or hydroureter who were treated by resection and ureterolysis without any urinary tract complications. However, most operations mobilizing the right or descending colon of necessity partially liberate the underlying ureter during the course of dissection. We have not encountered any renal damage in over 40 patients with hydroureter and/or hydronephrosis, and almost complete resolution occurred in all those studied with IV pyelography following intestinal resection. Hence, we feel that extensive ureterolysis is unnecessary. In a cautionary note, Altemeier[72] warns that there is danger of damaging not only the ureter by the procedure but also the femoral nerve, which is not easily identifiable in the dense scar tissue.

Multiple Strictures with Extensive Jejunoileitis (Figs. 127–68 and 127–69). This problem is one of the most difficult in an already complex disease. Surgery certainly should be deferred as long as possible. If the strictured segments are confined to a relatively localized segment of 30% to 50% of jejunoileum, resection and anastomosis of that segment is possible. However, progressive stricturing in discontinuous disease with dilation of multiple intervening loops results in development of the stagnant loop syndrome with malabsorption. Ultimately, obstruction of one or more loops develops. In this widespread form of disease, limited resection,

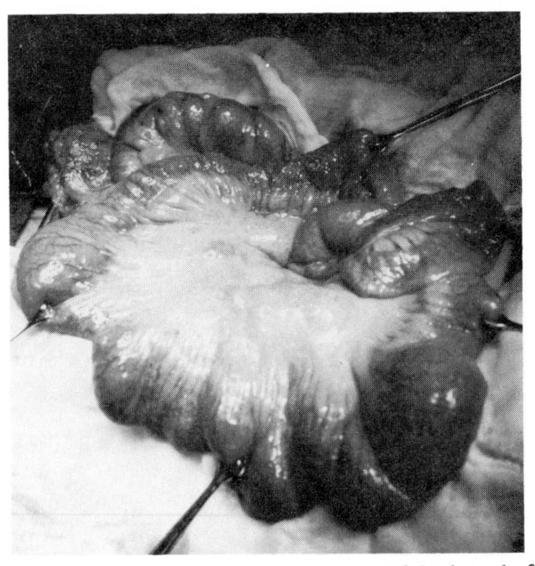

Figure 127–68. Operative appearance of the bowel of a 24-year-old female patient with multiple strictures and stenosis involving 100 cm of distal jejunum and proximal ileum. This was treated by primary resection and anastomosis with an excellent result because of an entirely normal distal small bowel.

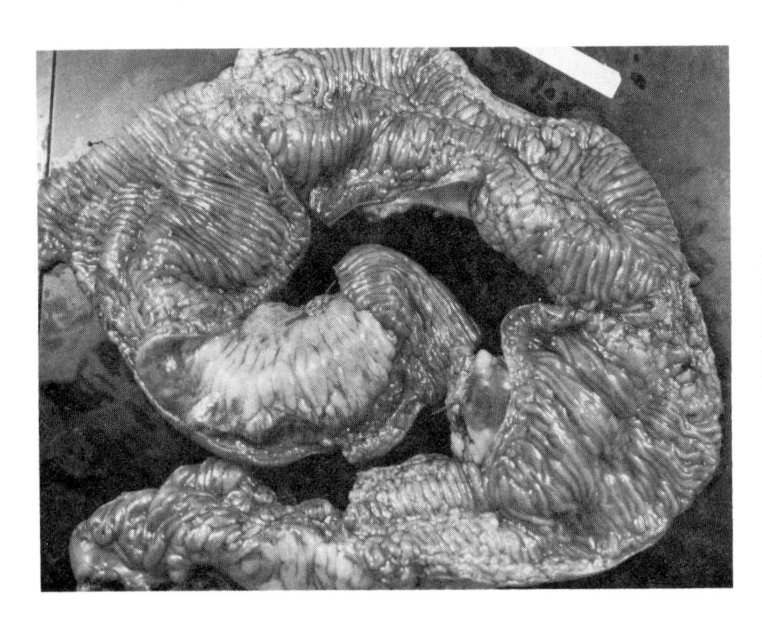

Figure 127–69. The surgical specimen of the same 24-year-old female patient as in Figure 127–68 showing cobblestoning and multiple areas of narrowing with dilatation between the strictured areas.

bypass, or enteroplasty has been recommended by Alexander-Williams[34] and Lee[35] (Fig. 127–70). We have carried out limited resection and anastomosis when possible. In cases of multiple strictures with extremely short bowel, we have occasionally reluctantly carried out several resections, particularly of the most stenotic areas, and employed side-to-side enteroanastomosis in other areas to bypass the extremely narrowed areas. Our short-term results over a period of 1 to 4 years have been excellent. The prospects of multiple bypassed segments remaining in-situ, however, is disconcerting in view of the occurrence of cancers in bypassed segments of small bowel.[59, 73] Nevertheless, by use of this limited type of surgery, extensive small bowel resection may be deferred for a number of years, thus avoiding a severe short bowel syndrome (Chapter 108).

Carcinoma. Carcinoma of the small or large bowel is being recognized with increasing frequency in Crohn's disease[59, 60, 73–75] (Chapter 128). As of 1980, there were 48 reported cases of small bowel cancer in Crohn's disease (Fig. 127–71), 19 occurring in bypassed segments, and 34 cases of large bowel cancer, 20 occurring in proximal bowel.[74] Although about one-third of the cases of carcinoma of the small bowel develop within the first decade of the disease,[76] the majority develop after the disease has existed for a long time (a mean of 17 years,[76] with a mean of 28 years for cancers in excluded loops[60]).

The observed occurrence rate of cancer in patients with Crohn's disease is considerably higher than the expected rate in the general population,[77] and the relative cancer risk is greater in the later years of life. The prognosis with intestinal cancer complicating Crohn's disease is extremely poor, especially for small bowel cancers.[74]

Some unsuspected cases are detected following resection, but most are already disseminated at the time of surgical exploration and radical extirpation is usually futile. Most deaths occur within 1 year, particularly in cancers occurring in excluded loops, because diagnosis is not made until late in the course.[60] For this reason, patients with excluded loops should have removal of such loops whenever possible, and this should always be done when subsequent exploration is necessary for recurrent disease. Resection rather than bypass is preferred whenever possible. In suitable patients, this may take the form of a radical cancer operation. A small number of long-term survivors have

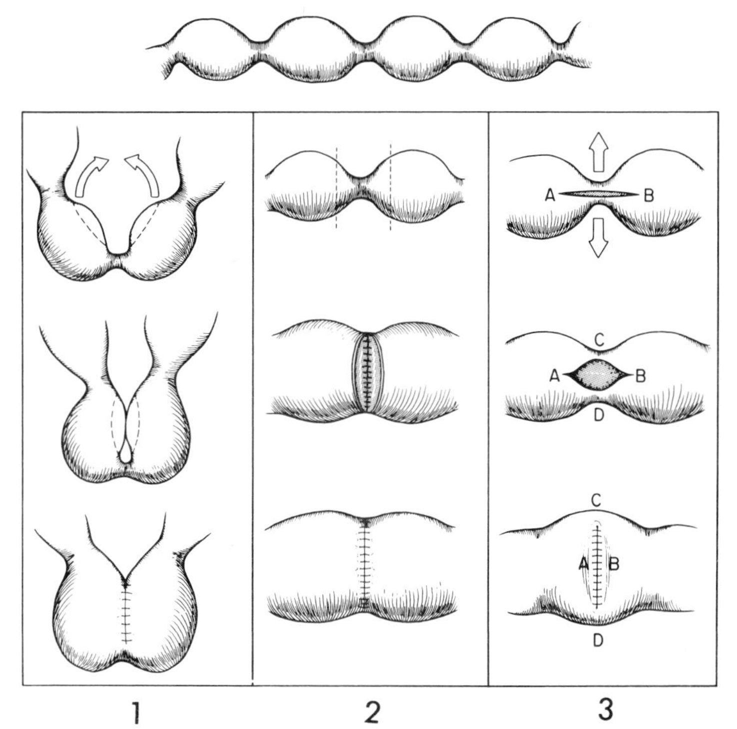

Figure 127–70. Three methods of treating patients with multiple strictures as recommended by Lee et al.[35] and Alexander-Williams.[34] *1,* Side-to-side anastomosis. *2,* Limited resection and anastomosis. *3,* "Enteroplasty."

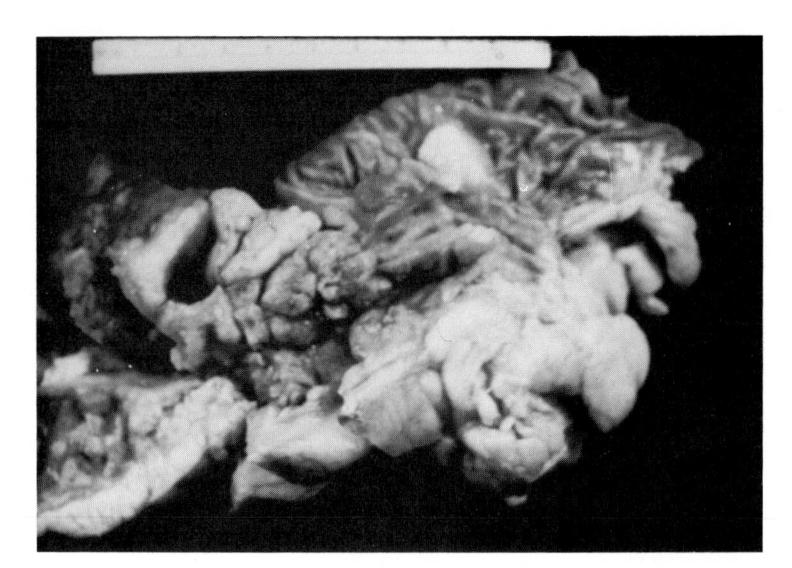

Figure 127–71. Carcinoma of small bowel occurring in Crohn's disease involving the small bowel.

been reported for in-continuity small bowel adenocarcinoma and more commonly for colorectal cancer.[59, 73–75]

Massive Hemorrhage. Rectal bleeding is common in Crohn's disease, but massive hemorrhage is relatively infrequent overall.[79] Marked bleeding, however, is the major reason for emergency colectomy in 11% to 60% of cases of fulminant disease.[80, 81] A definite indication for surgery is persistent hemorrhage originating in diseased bowel and requiring blood transfusions of 1000 to 2000 ml daily over 3 days, usually in association with diarrhea, toxemia, and weight loss. Viewed somewhat differently, pronounced bleeding is the major indication for surgery in only about 1% to 2% of patients with Crohn's disease.[78, 79] Massive hemorrhage may also originate in peptic, steroid, or stress-induced ulcers in these seriously ill patients, and a thorough study should be made to rule out such causes.

In a series of 53 patients with inflammatory bowel disease coming to emergency surgery reported by Block et al.,[80] 23 had major hemorrhage, and in 14 of these the hemorrhage occurred in association with toxic megacolon. The mortality was 12.5% following subtotal colectomy; no deaths followed proctocolectomy. Considering that rectal hemorrhage may persist or develop following abdominal colectomy[79] and early reoperation will therefore be required, proctocolectomy is the procedure of choice for universal and left-sided colitis involving the rectum.[80]

Toxic Megacolon. Toxic dilatation of the colon is being noted with increasing frequency in Crohn's disease of the colon.[38, 82, 83] Most early series of toxic megacolon in ulcerative colitis undoubtedly included some patients with unrecognized Crohn's disease.

The initial treatment of toxic dilatation, in the absence of perforation, should be medical. Worsening of the clinical condition, with increasing tachycardia, development of abdominal tenderness, a rising white blood cell count, progressive colonic dilatation, and "toxemia" would indicate the need for surgical intervention. Katzka et al.[84] report 13 of 19 patients treated successfully by medical means, and Present et al.[85] report only 2 deaths among 16 medically treated patients. However, the overall mortality rate in 604 cases collected from the medical literature by Strauss et al.[86] was 27% (43 of 160 patients), a rate somewhat greater than the 19% mortality rate in the 444 surgically treated patients. The keystone to successful management is avoidance of colonic perforation; 8 of the 9 patients with perforation in the series collected by Strauss and associates[86] died. Therefore, if medical treatment is not successful within 72 hours, the patient should be operated upon. Colectomy is the accepted operative procedure, most surgeons doing an abdominal colectomy with preservation of the rectum and construction of a mucous fistula. Goligher et al.[87] have had excellent results with early surgery. Flatmark et al.[88] had only one death in 10 patients subjected to proctocolectomy and no deaths in 62 patients undergoing subtotal colectomy. Block et al.[80] also favor subtotal colectomy over proctocolectomy because of the lower mortality rate.

An alternative, more limited procedure has been suggested by Turnbull et al.,[83] i.e., diverting loop ileostomy with single or multiple decompressing colostomies. This form of "conservative surgery" is particularly valuable for patients with sealed perforation, as complete mobilization of the compromised colon, with possible rupture and contamination, is avoided. Turnbull and his co-workers reported only one death among 42 patients, but 38 patients required subsequent definitive surgery: subtotal colectomy or proctocolectomy (30 patients) or ileorectal anastomosis (8 patients). This would suggest that the colon can seldom be preserved after this procedure, and the technique has not gained wide acceptance.

The earlier procedure of emergency cecostomy suggested by Klein et al.[89] is rarely used today. A diverting ileostomy alone has occasionally been used successfully in Crohn's colitis.[38] The introduction of a long catheter through the terminal ileum enables decompression of the colon before subtotal colectomy and should be carried out as a routine procedure to avoid contamination from areas of sealed perforation.

Surgical Indications in Ileocolitis and Crohn's Colitis. As pointed out by Farmer et al.[20, 21] the indications for surgery in disease affecting primarily the colon differ from those in small bowel disease. The indications are similar in many respects to those for ulcerative colitis, except for the problem of postoperative recurrence. The latter, as noted by Goligher,[90] leads to some caution in resorting to surgery. Furthermore, the cancer risk in Crohn's disease involving the colon appears to be less than that in ulcerative colitis[77] (Chapter 128). Thus, the finding of dysplasia in universal Crohn's disease should all the more be followed by repeated colonoscopy and careful surveillance.

Acute Exacerbation of Colitis or Fulminating Disease. Medical treatment should be tried in all patients with fulminating disease, with failure to respond considered an indication for surgical intervention. The primary indications for laparotomy and colon resection in these patients are massive hemorrhage, toxic colonic dilatation, and acute perforation of the colon. According to deDombal et al.[91] and Watts et al.,[92] the natural history of the first referred attack of Crohn's colitis is completely different from that of ulcerative colitis, with radical operative surgery required more frequently and with a lower remission rate for Crohn's colitis. In a series of 415 patients studied by deDombal et al.,[78] early surgery in the seriously ill patient reduced the postoperative mortality from 10% to 2.9% over the 3 decades from 1939 to 1968.

Surgical Procedures

The surgery of Crohn's disease has evolved through several phases. Early radical resection was born of the hope of cure. Early complications resulted in the more limited bypass or diversionary procedure of Berg (Fig. 127–61), but disillusionment supervened in the 1950s with appreciation of the high recurrence rates. This led to delay in operating and excessive delay, in turn, led to high complication and mortality rates. However, Goligher in Leeds practiced early surgery.[87] A cautious approach has progressively evolved in which drugs are used judiciously, followed by limited surgery for selected indications when possible but interrupted by early surgery for fulminating disease when necessary.

The basic types of operative procedures utilized in Crohn's disease are diversionary,[42] or "split" ileostomy,[93, 94] or bypass;[3, 5, 60] resection with reconstruction of continuity,[30, 95] occasionally with concomitant proximal diverting ileostomy,[55] abdominal or total colectomy with ileostomy,[80, 90, 95, 96] and various more limited "combined procedures" for multiple strictures.[34, 35] Because of the extensive longitudinal nature of the disease throughout the gastrointestinal tract, the wide resection margins of earlier years have been replaced by more limited 4 to 10 cm margins. This more conservative approach should reduce the frequency of the short bowel syndrome. Bypass is employed only when resection is not feasible.

In general, all resection procedures require mobilization of the affected segment of bowel along the appropriate lines of embryologic adherence. The diseased bowel with adjacent mesentery is resected, taking only as much mesentery as is necessary to achieve a good anatomic approximation of the bowel ends and an adequate closure of the mesentery. A

2-layer end-to-side anastomosis is our preference, but side-to-side or end-to-end anastomoses, especially with dilated obstructed bowel, have been used successfully.

Resection with reconstruction of continuity is the most frequently performed operation for Crohn's disease and includes small bowel resection, ileocolic resection, right hemicolectomy, left colectomy, and subtotal colectomy with ileosigmoid or ileorectal anastomosis. Abdominal colectomy and ileoproctostomy is more frequently possible in Crohn's colitis or ileocolitis than in ulcerative colitis because of the common occurrence of rectal sparing in the former.

Ileostomy. Ileostomy, first described by Brown in 1913, [97] has its proponents as a diversionary procedure in Crohn's disease (Fig. 127–72), particularly in the presence of severe disease in an extremely ill patient with fulminating disease. It has been used as a temporary "split ileostomy" by Oberhelman et al.[93] and subsequently by Lee,[94] with relatively poor results.

Temporary ileostomy in Crohn's colitis to establish fecal diversion has been recommended by Aufses and co-workers,[42, 43] and McIlrath,[98] and Burman et al.[68] have also reported successful diversion utilizing ileostomy or colostomy. Zelas and Jagelman[99] found that diverting ileostomy resulted in subjective and objective improvement in 91% of 79 patients with severe debilitating Crohn's disease. However, approximately one-third of the patients relapsed and 4 of the 79 patients (5.1%) died. Even though their patients were particularly ill and debilitated, Zelas and Jagelman recommended, based on their experience, that early definitive resection be done. This form of management should be reserved for the seriously ill patient as defined by the criteria originally suggested for ulcerative colitis patients by Truelove and Witts[100] and Truelove and Jewell,[101] i.e., 6 or more bowel movements per day, continuous or severe abdominal pain and tenderness, macroscopic blood in the stools, mean pulse rate of 90/minute, temperature of 37.8°C (100°F), hemoglobin 70% of normal, and weight loss of 14 pounds or more. In view of the high relapse rate (as high as 49% in some series[68, 94, 99, 102] definitive resection is advisable between 3 months and 3 years following ileostomy.

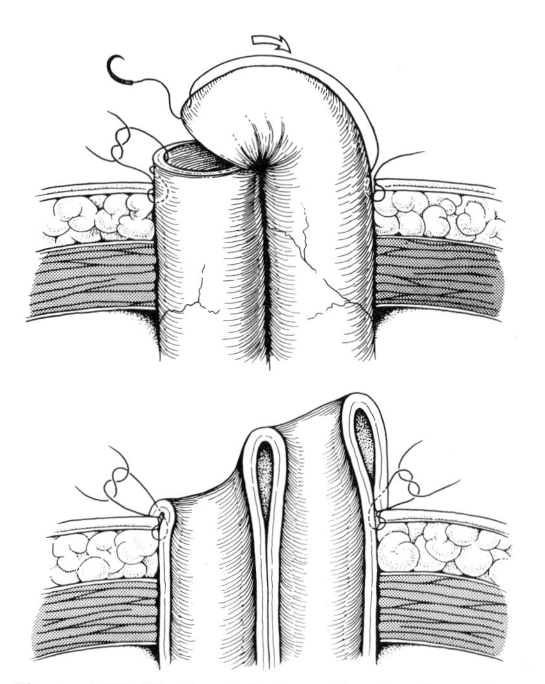

Figure 127–72. Turnbull type diverting loop ileostomy. Requires 90° rotation in a clockwise direction of the axis of the small bowel, as well as 180° rotation of the cut segment, as shown.

Resection. Small bowel resection, solitary or multiple, may be carried out for segmental jejunoileal disease. However, several authors recommend side-to-side enteroenterostomy or various forms of "enteroplasty" (Fig. 127–70, Panel 3) to limit removal of large segments of bowel in patients with multiple "skip" areas.[34, 35] This form of surgery should be restricted to patients with extensive jejunoileitis or short bowel syndrome, a very small proportion of the total number of patients coming to surgical excision. There is always the long-term cancer risk in the retained severely diseased segments. While this risk is low, this non-resectional procedure should be used with discretion until its value has been fully established and compared with multiple limited resections.

Ileocolic Resection. Ileocolic resection is the most common operation carried out for Crohn's disease in view of the predilection of this disease for the terminal ileum. Probably no more than 4 to 8 cm on either side of the overtly diseased bowel should be resected utilizing ileoascending or ileotransverse colostomy. End-to-end anastomosis is safe with obstructed dilated proximal bowel; end-to-side anastomosis is useful in all cases with a gross disparity in lumen; side-to-side anastomosis has also been suggested (Fig. 127–73).

Subtotal Colectomy (Fig. 127–74). Subtotal

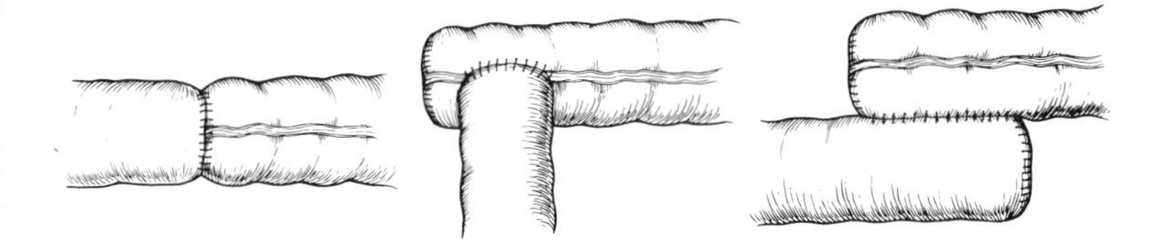

Figure 127–73. Three methods of reapproximating the small bowel, as recommended by various authors: end-to-end, end-to-side, and side-to-side. Each method has its value, depending on the relative size of proximal and distal bowel.

colectomy is frequently carried out with ileosigmoidostomy (Fig. 127–75) or with ileoproctostomy because of the prevalence of rectal sparing in Crohn's disease. Reoperation rates are high in all series following this form of reconstruction.[96, 103, 104]

Segmental Colon Resection. Segmental colonic resection is carried out only occasionally, as colonic disease is usually quite extensive. When possible, a segmental resection, usually sigmoid, is carried out with end-to-end anastomosis. This may be part of a combined procedure with ileocolic resection for ileosigmoid fistula when the colon is intrinsically diseased. We resect the colon only when it is diseased or is so adherent to the ileal mass that it cannot be closed safely.[55]

Total Proctocolectomy. Total proctocolectomy with end ileostomy (Fig. 127–76) is a particularly effective procedure in the management of Crohn's disease confined to, or predominantly involving, the colon and rectum. It is being carried out more frequently at present as a one-stage procedure, both for Crohn's disease and for ulcerative colitis[105] and is believed by most surgeons to result in a lower rate of disease recurrence in the neoterminal ileum than almost any other surgical procedure. The key to successful proctocolectomy is the rectal dissection because the postoperative problems of this procedure center on the question of the development of a non-healing perineal wound or perineal sinus and the possibility of complete or partial impotence.

Impotence, which occurs in as many as one-third of the patients,[106, 107] can be reduced to a minimum by an understanding of the 4 critical areas where damage to autonomic nerves is possible: (1) the hypogastric nerves

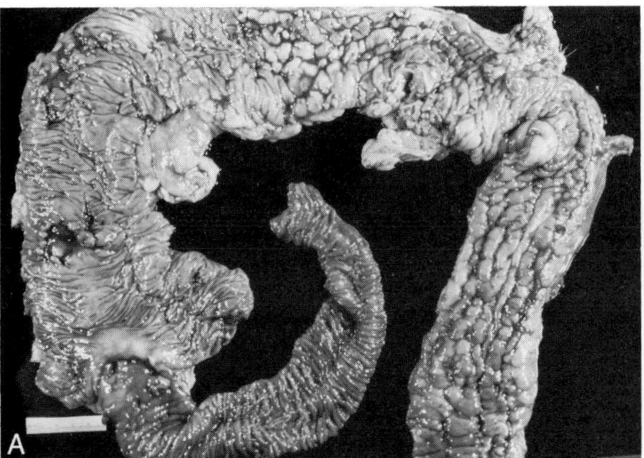

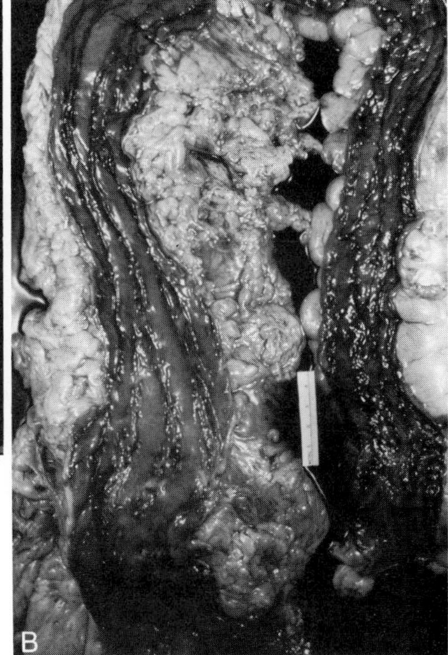

Figure 127–74. *A,* Subtotal colectomy specimen of a 41-year-old female patient presenting with massive hemorrhage superimposed on active ileocolitis of 9 years' duration. The distal ileum shows ulceration. The ascending colon shows a large geographic ulcer, which was the source of the hemorrhage. The transverse colon shows cobblestoning, and the descending colon shows cobblestoning plus longitudinal ulceration. *B,* Subtotal colectomy specimen showing the longitudinal ulceration of Crohn's colitis.

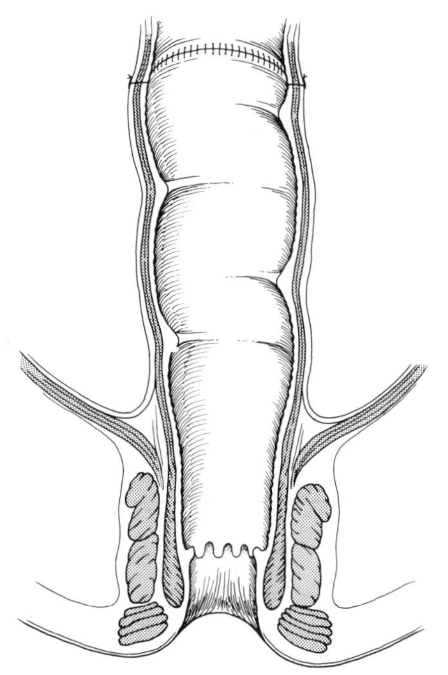

Figure 127–75. Diagrammatic representation of an ileosigmoidostomy.

over the sacral promontory, (2) the anterolateral stalks, (3) the presacral space, and (4) the plane anterior to the rectum below the peritoneal reflexion.[108, 109] Damage to the hypogastric nerves results in retrograde ejaculation. Damage to the nervi erigentes lower down causes partial or complete impotence. Particular care should be devoted to the perineal dissection. "Perimuscular dissection," described by Lee and Dowling,[110] or preferably "intermuscular dissection," described by Lyttle and Parks[109] (Fig. 127–77), are the preferred techniques. These dissections are carried out in a plane close to the internal sphincter muscle or between the muscle layers in the plane of embryologic fusion between the somatic and autonomic nervous systems.

Delayed wound healing and development of a late perineal sinus may be reduced to a minimum, albeit not entirely prevented,[108] (1) by preserving the muscles below and reapproximating the layers anatomically, (2) by conserving as much as possible of the pelvic peritoneal floor in order to create a deep pelvic pouch, and (3) by introducing a lateral sump catheter into the perineal wound with continuous irrigation in an uncontaminated wound.[111]

In the presence of a chronic untreated perineal sinus (one of the most frustrating of surgical problems), various methods of achieving complete healing have been advised. Anderson and Turnbull[112] prefer skin grafting; Silen and Glotzer[113] advise resection of the coccyx and lower sacrum; and Baek et al.[114] recommend transposition of a gracilis myocutaneous flap.

Other Procedures. The standard ileostomy used in patients with Crohn's disease, referred to earlier in this section, is a permanent end-type of ileostomy. Kock[115, 116] described and applied a so-called *continent ileostomy* ("Kock pouch"), which does not require an exposed and open end of small bowel. In his early series he created this

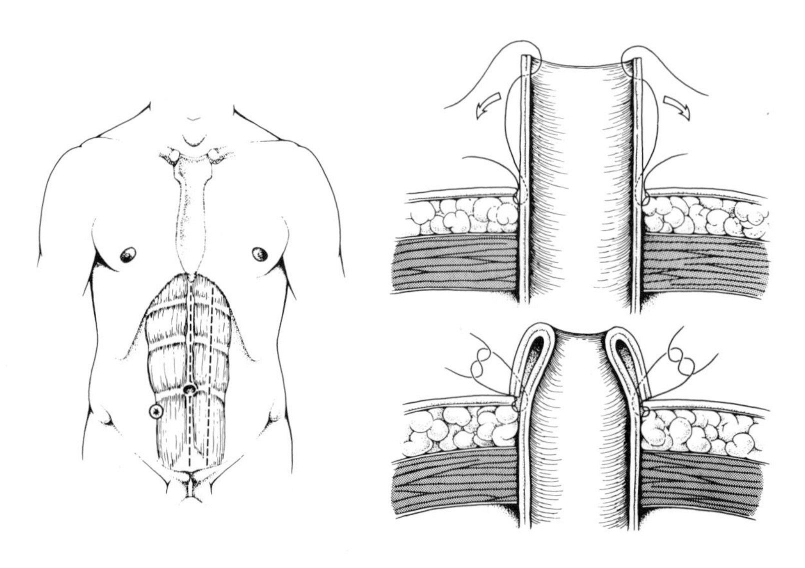

Figure 127–76. Usual left paramedian incision for colectomy and ileostomy. Typical everting Brooke ileostomy shown on left side. Some surgeons (Sir Allan Parks, personal communication) prefer a midline incision so that a subsequent transposition to an unspoiled field in the left lower quadrant can be done if necessary.

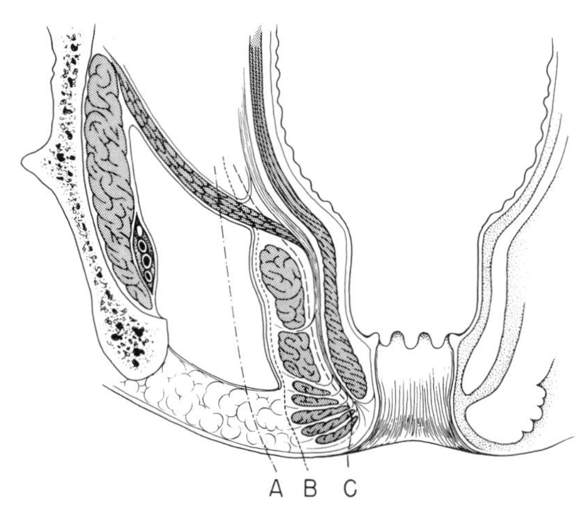

Figure 127–77. Lines of dissection for a standard *(A)*, perimuscular *(B)*, and intermuscular *(C)* dissection of the rectum. Anatomy after Oh and Kark.[117]

pouch in 39 patients with Crohn's disease, with success in 28.[116] With time, however, he found it necessary to remove the pouch in a higher percentage of patients with Crohn's disease than with ulcerative colitis because of recurrent disease within and proximal to the pouch and inflammation within the pouch. The general practice today is to confine the use of the continent pouch exclusively to patients with ulcerative colitis.

A more recent innovation is the use of *ileoanal-pull-through*, with or without a pelvic pouch. These procedures preserve the outer layers of the distal rectum, maintain intestinal continuity, and retain the anal sphincter mechanism.[117] Variations of J- and S-shaped pouches have been described by several authors.[118–121] These procedures at the present time are likewise limited to patients with ulcerative colitis.

Postoperative Mortality

Postoperative mortality may be divided into early and late groups.[29] The *early mortality* group, occurring in the immediate postoperative period, usually results from leaking anastomoses or from sepsis due to cardiopulmonary complications[90] or inadequately drained abscesses.[44] *Late mortality* may be the consequence of recurrent disease with perforating complications, short bowel syndrome, or cancer developing either in bowel in continuity or in excluded loops.[29, 122] The overall operative mortality rate varies from 2.5% to 6.5%[20, 78, 90, 123–126] Goligher,[90] who reported a 6.5% mortality rate, noted that the mortality for elective procedures as reported in most series was approximately one-tenth of that found in his patients undergoing urgent or emergency ileostomy and colectomy. There were 10 deaths in 34 patients (29%) undergoing emergency surgery, compared with 9 deaths in 292 patients (3%) undergoing elective surgery. Mortality in his series was due to peritonitis and septicemia in 11 patients and to cardiopulmonary complications in 5. One patient died of an anastomotic leak, while 2 others survived such a leak. In the series of Greenstein et al.,[29] there were 8 early deaths among 250 patients (3.2%), all due to preoperative abscesses in which the sepsis was not controlled by the operative procedure. Eight late deaths were due to cancer in 6 patients (a higher occurrence rate than in most series, probably a result of the referral pattern at the Mount Sinai Hospital) and recurrent disease in 2 patients. Although a leaking anastomosis is usually the most lethal postoperative complication, all 4 patients with anastomotic leaks in our series survived following prompt diversionary surgery.

Most deaths are due to the intestinal disease itself.[29, 127] Other factors contributing to mortality later in the course of Crohn's disease include cancer,[122, 127, 128] hemorrhage and pulmonary embolism,[129] malignant hypertension in steroid-treated patients,[127] suicide,[125, 127] and myocardial infarction.[127]

Postoperative Complications

The reported prevalence of *wound infection* ranges from none, when the wound is left entirely open, to as high as 38%,[130] with the usual rate being about 3% to 7%.[29, 131, 132] Wound infection can be virtually eliminated in the elective case by a combination of mechanical measures and antibiotic administration: thorough mechanical cleansing, preoperative oral neomycin-erythromycin[132] and/or systemic antibiotics in the perioperative period, local antibiotics in the wound, and packing between the sutures or open drainage. Wound disruption has been reported in from 1.2% to 4.6% of patients with inflammatory bowel disease[29, 78, 133] and may be lethal, particularly if associated with underlying intra-abdominal abscess. The frequency of this serious complication can be reduced by careful abdominal wound closure and prevention of wound infection.

Postoperative *sepsis* resulting from *peritonitis* and *intra-abdominal abscess* is the single most lethal complication in the postoperative period. In 3 separate series from London,[131] Leeds,[133] and New York[29] the mortality rate from this complication ranged from 3.2% to 4%. The most frequent causes of postoperative intra-abdominal sepsis are inadequately drained intra-abdominal abscess, anastomotic disruption, and leakage from a retained rectal stump. These dangers may be avoided by adequate drainage, meticulous technique in suturing the anastomosis utilizing an area of relatively normal bowel, and the use of a sigmoid mucous fistula. Other unexpected causes of sepsis, such as perforated ulcer and internal herniation with gangrene, may be more difficult to predict and prevent. Localization of abscess to subphrenic, pelvic, intramesenteric, or intraloop areas of bowel requires specific sonographic determination. Precise local drainage should then be accomplished as soon as possible.

Allsop and Lee[134] correlated mortality and morbidity with certain specific factors: contamination, operation performed (sepsis rate for proctocolectomy of 59% versus 11% for split ileostomy), the presence of a preoperative stoma, pathologic diagnosis (perineal wounds healed more slowly in Crohn's disease than in ulcerative colitis), and site of drain. The organisms are usually of intestinal origin—Bacteroides, Aerobacter, and anaerobic streptococci. Immediate drainage, with concomitant administration of antibiotics is mandatory—usually IV cefazolin or cefoxitin, with clindamycin and/or gentamicin or tobramycin. Percutaneous catheter drainage under sonographic control, utilizing CT scan or ultrasound to localize the abscess and real time ultrasonography or fluoroscopy to introduce the catheter, has been suggested by Gerzof et al.[135] and others. It still remains to be proved that this method of drainage will reduce mortality. However, failure of drainage to result in immediate resolution of the septic process, with complete disappearance of the abscess on CT scan, should indicate need for surgical intervention without delay. Block[136] supports the concept of radical surgical debridement proposed by Hudspeth in 1975,[137] but this approach is seldom used.

Late *wound hernia* has been reported in 1.3% to 3.9% of cases,[78, 131] usually following a previous wound infection. These hernias require surgical repair utilizing non-absorbable sutures and occasionally a Marlex mesh.

Ileostomy Complications

At the Mount Sinai Hospital, 210 of 1010 patients with Crohn's disease required an ileostomy to control their disease.[58] The Brooke ileostomy (Fig. 127–66),[138] with complete eversion of small bowel, is the usual type used in Crohn's disease. The Turnbull type, with mucosal eversion only, is utilized occasionally in ulcerative colitis, but is probably less suitable for Crohn's disease in which aphthous ulceration extends beyond the resection margins. Post-ileostomy complications, such as *serositis, stenosis,* and *skin excoriation* with *ileostomy dysfunction,* occurred in as many as 61% of patients in the 1950s.[139] These problems have become relatively rare, being reported currently in only about 2% of patients.[29] Other ileostomy complications seen occasionally include *prolapse,* para-ileostomy *hernia,* and, at times, *gangrene.*[29, 131, 140] Goligher et al.[90] evaluated the inconvenience of an ileostomy and found that 68% of patients with primary ileostomies had absolutely no problems, 24% had occasional skin soreness, and 8% had many problems with leakage and profuse output. Following subsequent resections, 17% of the patients fell into the last category.

Peri-ileostomy ileocutaneous fistula is a particularly distressing problem that occurred in 15 of our group of 210 ileostomy patients.[58] All patients had recurrent disease from 4 to 30 cm in length, and fistulas were multiple in 13 of the 15 patients. In addition to the usual problems of recurrent disease, such as intestinal obstruction and hemorrhage, these patients had major difficulties maintaining the seal of an appliance. All patients required surgical resection of the diseased bowel and reconstruction of their ileostomy; 10 required transposition to the left side of the abdomen.

Postoperative Recurrence

Crohn et al.,[3] in their initial paper in 1932 on regional ileitis, noted that recurrent disease occurred in 2 of their 14 patients. In the years that followed, it became evident that the most common postoperative sequel of Crohn's disease is recurrent ileitis, most frequently affecting the neoterminal ileum just proximal to or at the anastomosis. Occasionally, the colon distally, or even the rectum farther down the intestinal tract, becomes diseased. It also became apparent that reoperations were required more frequently in patients who had bypass procedures than those who had resections, although for many years this fact was in doubt. Because of this and because of the various complications of a bypassed loop, such as late development of abscess, occasional rupture of an excluded distal segment,[40] and the possibility of cancer developing in excluded loops,[59, 60] surgeons returned to resection procedures. It came next to be the belief that the more radical the resection, the greater the likelihood of cure.[25, 141–144] This idea of radical resection, however, has been disputed.[18, 145]

Many factors influence the postoperative recurrence rate. Important among the surgical considerations are the type of operation performed (bypass versus resection, or complete versus staged procedures), the length of bowel involved, the presence of microscopic or macroscopic disease at the resection margins, and the amount of normal-appearing bowel removed.

It is generally accepted that the rate of postoperative recurrence is high in Crohn's disease involving only or mainly the small bowel.[24, 30, 146–148] The question of recurrence in Crohn's colitis in which the disease is confined to the large bowel remains controversial.[149–152] There is considerable variation, however, in reported recurrence rates for all types of inflammatory bowel disease, reflecting the differences in patient populations, referral patterns, ways of defining recurrent disease, methods of calculating recurrence rates, operative procedures, and lengths of follow-up.

Diagnosis of Recurrent Crohn's Disease. The diagnosis of primary and recurrent Crohn's disease in the symptomatic patient has classically been established by radiologic methods (Fig. 127–78).[153] Sites of recurrence may be seen endoscopically, provided they are within reach of the colonoscope from below or the gastroduodenoscope or a special enteroscope from above.[154] With these instruments, biopsies can be taken and on rare occasions granulomas demonstrated, confirming the presence of active Crohn's disease. The final pathologic proof will be obtained at laparotomy in those patients coming to surgical resection.

Definition of Recurrent Disease. Many patients are seen postoperatively who have severe diarrhea, crampy abdominal pains, and other symptoms suggestive of active Crohn's disease. However, not all of them prove to have Crohn's disease. Lennard-Jones and Stalder[148] divided recurrences into (1) recurrence of clinical symptoms without evidence of new disease, (2) recurrent symptoms with radiologic and/or histologic proof of disease, and (3) recurrent disease requiring further surgery. Recurrence was clearly less in the second category and least in the surgical group. Many of the discrepancies in the literature with regard to recurrence rates reflect the differing definitions of disease recurrence.

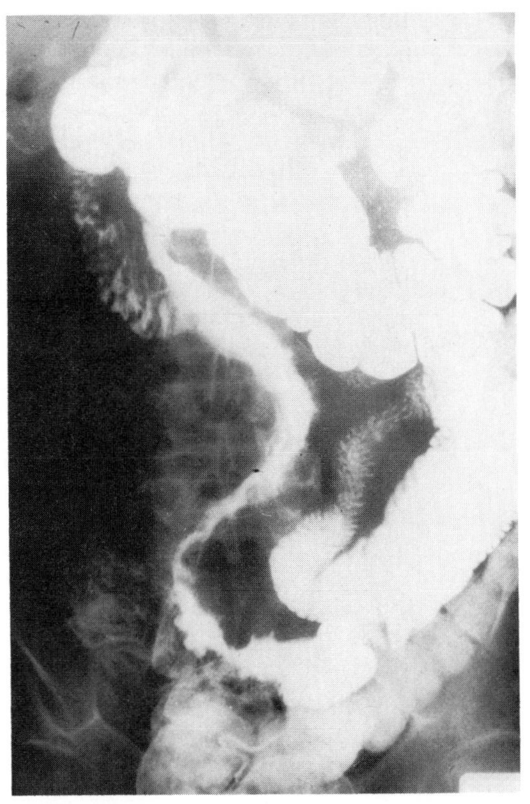

Figure 127–78. Recurrent Crohn's ileocolitis in distal 1 foot of neoterminal ileum proximal to an ileotransverse colostomy. This required secondary ileocolic resection and ileotransverse colostomy and was followed by hypocalcemia and hypokaluria treated by electrolyte replacement.

DeDombal et al.[146] noted that in many instances residual disease was left *in situ* at the time of surgery, occasionally following incomplete or staged resection and always following bypass procedures. This clearly represents *residual disease* and in the presence of recurrent symptoms should be categorized as recrudescent rather than truly recurrent disease. Furthermore, these authors observed that some postoperative symptoms were the direct result of the surgical resection itself. For example, excessive passage of bile salts into the colon as a result of resection of a large segment of terminal ileum may result in a choleretic type of diarrhea with excessive loss of water and electrolytes into the colon (Chapter 108). This form of diarrhea requires treatment other than surgery. Lee et al.[18, 35, 156] have suggested the following simple classification: (1) *Recurrence*, the appearance of objective signs—defined radiologically, endoscopically, or pathologically—of Crohn's disease in the bowel of a patient who has previously had a resection for macroscopically diseased tissue; and (2) *relapse*, the appearance of the clinical features of Crohn's disease after a symptom-free interval in patients with known disease, provided that other non-related causes of these symptoms have been excluded.

The problem of postoperative recurrence in Crohn's disease is colored by the fact that most of the patients hospitalized for this disease ultimately require operation whether the disease is in the small or the large bowel.[15, 22, 23, 30, 157] Mekhjian et al.[22] drew actuarial curves showing that approximately 60% of patients with Crohn's disease required surgery by 10 years from onset of disease, 70% by 20 years, and 85% by 30 years. The overall frequency of primary operation thus steadily increases with time the longer the period of follow-up.

Methods of Estimating Recurrence. Many of the early discrepancies reported in the literature reflect the fact that the earliest reports estimated overall recurrence rates in a *crude* fashion, simply noting the number of recurrences occurring in the number of patients in the total group studied. In 1967, Lennard-Jones and Stalder[148] utilized *actuarial* methods incorporating the data obtained with progressive passage of time into an actuarial life table. In 1975, Greenstein et al.[15] examined several different factors influencing recurrence as calculated actuarially and confirmed many of the earlier findings (Fig. 127–79). Sachar et al.[158] and Wolfson et al.,[159] using multivariate analysis, have observed that the critical question is not only which factors influence recurrence rates, but which factors do so independently of other confounding influences.

Recurrence rates calculated by actuarial methods for varying durations of time are listed in Table 127–11. As shown, the 5-year recurrence rates vary considerably from 19% for disease involving the colon to as high as

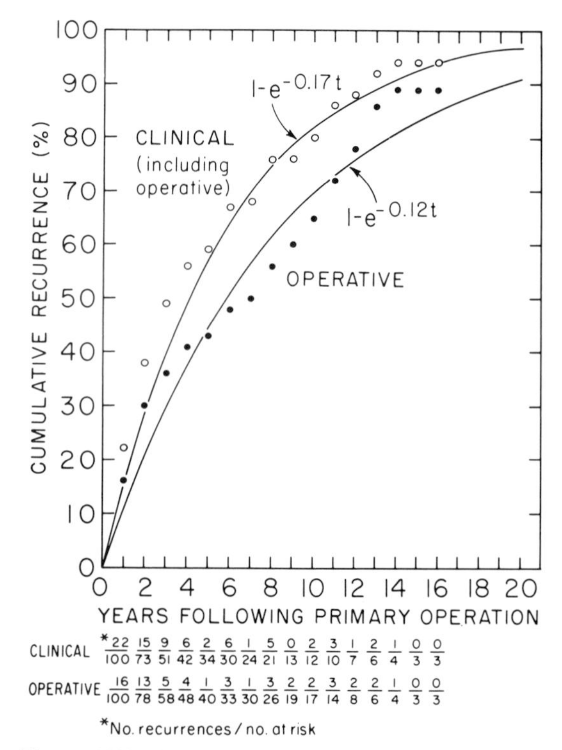

Figure 127–79. Cumulative operative and clinical recurrence rates following bypass or resection and reanastomosis in Crohn's (ileo) colitis. (From Greenstein AJ et al. N Engl J Med 1975; 293:685–90. Reprinted by permisson of the New England Journal of Medicine.)

43%; the 10-year recurrence rates from 19% in colon disease to 65%; and the 15-year recurrence rates from 23% to 86%. However, all series studied actuarially show a steady increase in the recurrence rates with passage of time, this being a major and dominant factor in these rates.

Factors Influencing Recurrence. Age appears to have a definite influence on the tendency to recurrence. In all reports on the subject, the recurrence rate has been consistently greater in younger age groups.[15, 17, 23, 30, 124, 147, 157, 158] Thus, Goligher[157] found that recurrence rates in patients with Crohn's colitis or ileocolitis decreased from 25% at age 10 to 19 years at the time of operation to 13.6% in the 20- to 29-year-old age group, 10.7% in the 30- to 49-year-old age group, and 8.3% in the 50- to 79-year age group.

This influence of age remains valid even when actuarial methods are used to correct for variations in follow-up intervals.[15, 124, 157] Sachar et al.,[158] however, while noting that age has an influence on actuarially calculated

Table 127–11. RECURRENCE RATES CALCULATED BY ACTUARIAL METHODS (PERCENTAGE)

Site of Disease	Duration of Follow-up (Years)			
	5	*10*	*15*	*20*
Small Bowel				
Greenstein (unpublished data)	37	57	69	
Hellers (1979)[16]	30	50	60	
deDombal (1971)[146]	27	40	43	
Alexander-Williams (1972)[45a]	25	42	Res.	
	60	90	Bypass	
Goligher (1972)[24]	40	62	70	
Sachar (1982)[158]	50	60	70	
Himal (1981)[201]	25	40	42	
Colon				
Hellers (1979)[16]	20	35		
Greenstein (1976)[15]	37	37		
deDombal (1971)[146]	17	20	22	
Lock (1981)[17]	10	20	28	
Goligher (1972)[24]	21	29	40	
Sachar (1982)[158]	42	42		
Himal (1981)[201]	35	55		
Goligher (1978)[202]	8.5	16	36.8	
Ileocolitis				
Hellers (1979)[16]	30	50	55	
Greenstein (1976)[15]	50	74	91	
Mixed Sites and Various Procedures				
Karesan (1981)[142]	27	35	45	
McDermott (1980)[203]	80	88		
Cooke (1980)[23]	38	56	66	75
Greenstein (1976)[15]	50	70	88	88
Lennard-Jones (1967)[148]	23	51		
Proctocolectomy and Ileostomy				
Vender (1979)[163]	25	45		
deDombal (1971)[78]	8	8		
Lock (1981)[17]	10	25	27	
Colectomy Plus Ileorectal Anastomosis				
Hellers (1979)[16]	50	70		
Alexander-Williams (1980)[204]	28	35	42	65
*Second Operation**				
Lennard-Jones (1967)[148]	67			
Greenstein (1976)[15]	60	80		
McDermott (1980)[203]	73			
Lock (1981)[17]	30	45	50	
Hellers (1979)[16]	45	60		
Cooke (1980)[23]	34	49	67	75

*Mixtures of regional enteritis, ileocolitis, and Crohn's colitis.

recurrence rates, reported that the more important influence demonstrated by multivariate analysis appeared to be the preoperative duration of disease.

As regards *sex*, most authors find no difference in recurrence rates between men and women,[147, 158] although a considerably poorer prognosis in women has been noted by some.[78, 160]

The *anatomic site* of involvement helps to determine the likelihood of recurrence. High recurrence rates, both crude and actuarial, have been reported for most series of patients with regional ileitis following resection, with recurrence rates ranging from 42% to 86% at 15 years.[15, 16, 24, 78, 158] Even higher rates follow bypass, and little controversy surrounds recurrence in small bowel disease. The question of recurrence in Crohn's colitis in which the disease is initially confined to the colon, however, has engendered argument. Most observers believe that patients with disease confined to the colon have a lower rate of recurrence than those in whom the terminal ileum is involved.[15, 17, 78, 152, 161] Goligher,[157] however, found that patients with Crohn's colitis followed for as long as 10 to 18 years had a recurrence rate of 37% and at 15 to 18 years had a recurrence rate of 40%, thus demonstrating progressive increase in rate of recurrence with increasing length of follow-up. Glotzer,[149] after examining the data in various reports, attributed the discrepancy in recurrence rates in Crohn's colitis to variations in the base population and to incorrect classification between ulcerative colitis and Crohn's colitis.

Ritchie,[162] following patients with ileostomy after total proctocolectomy, found a 23% cumulative recurrence rate at 18 years but no subsequent increase up to 25 years. Hellers[16] found a 25% recurrence rate at 5 years and 40% at 10 years following total proctocolectomy and ileostomy carried out in 103 patients for large bowel disease. Steinberg and associates,[124] using actuarial methods, found an identical rate of recurrence regardless of whether the terminal ileum was involved. Similarly, Goligher[157] found no difference in recurrence regardless of whether the small bowel was involved if a total proctocolectomy and ileostomy had been carried out for Crohn's colitis or ileocolitis. Vender et al.[163] found a considerable difference in the recurrence rates of Crohn's colitis when the ileum was involved (48% with ileal involvement, 18% without). When both large and small bowel were clearly involved, deDombal et al.[146] found a recurrence rate of 46%, similar to that for small bowel disease alone. However, with the disease confined to the large bowel, the recurrence rate was 10%. Nugent et al.[152] found that involvement of the distal small bowel, if relatively localized, did not increase the tendency to recurrence after proctocolectomy and ileostomy. Lock et al.[17] reported that at 11 years the reoperation rate was 46% (±9%) in patients with ileal involvement and 23% (±5%) in those without it. The question of the association of ileal involvement with a higher recurrence rate is therefore still not established.

There is agreement that recurrence following subtotal colectomy and ileorectal or ileosigmoid anastomosis is high.[104, 105, 152, 155, 164, 165] The recurrence rate in patients with anastomotic procedures was 61% in Goligher's[157] series, 75% in the series of Fawaz et al.,[96] and 66% in the series of Veidenheimer et al.[166] These figures are not very different from the recurrence rates of 50% at 10 years and 80% at 14 years after resection and reanastomosis, as reported by Greenstein et al.[15] Fawaz et al.[96] also noted a 75% incidence of recurrence with reconstructive large bowel procedures in Crohn's disease involving the colon, and others show recurrences from 40% to 100%.[146, 167, 168] The data for recurrence after reanastomosis, therefore, are not in dispute.

The propensity of the segments of the gut to develop evidence of disease after an operative procedure has bearing on the problem of postoperative recurrence. Most authors report recurrences in the neoterminal ileum just proximal to the suture line in patients with anastomosis or in the most distal ileum following ileostomy. Koch et al.[169] found that the site of recurrence was determined by the site of primary disease. In ileitis, 100% of recurrences involved the proximal gut, 30% were both proximal and distal, and none was exclusively distal. Recurrences in ileocolitis patients developed proximally in 19%, distally in 19%, and both proximally and distally in 62%. Thus, disease initially confined to the terminal ileum may subsequently progress to involve the colon following resection and reanastomosis. Of 68 surgically treated cases of inflammatory bowel disease sparing the rectum, Korelitz[164] found distal spread to the rectum in 43 (39%), proximal spread in 39 (35%), proximal and distal spread in 16 (14%), and no spread in 16 (14%). In ileocolitis or colitis, therefore, distal recurrence is as common as proximal recurrence, whereas in ileitis, proximal recurrence is considerably more common.

There appears to be a clear inverse relationship between recurrence and *preoperative duration of the disease*: the shorter the duration, the higher the recurrence rate.[30, 146, 158, 163] Indeed, Sachar et al.[158] found the preoperative duration of disease to be the most important single factor influencing postoperative recurrence rates when age, sex, anatomic location, operative procedure, and preoperative duration of disease were considered separately and collectively. The proposition that *each surgical procedure is followed by an increased tendency to reoperation* has been examined by a number of investigators[14, 17, 30, 148] and remains investigational. In the National Crohn's Disease Study, Mekhjian et al.[22] showed an actuarially calculated increased rate of reoperation that was greater after the second resection than after the first for the total series. Hellers[16] noted a similar phenomenon of higher actuarially calculated recurrence rates 10 years after a second operation than after the first. However, Cooke et al.[23] and Allan et al.[28] showed the reoperation rate to be similar after each operative procedure. There is a considerable difference of opinion among surgeons regarding the *amount of apparently normal bowel* that should be resected beyond the obviously diseased segment. Lengths of variable extent has been suggested.[6, 28, 142–144] However, the findings of a study by Pennington et al.[145] did not support the concept of radical bowel resection. These observers found no difference in recurrence rates whether there was disease at the resection margin or not. Lee et al.[18] also reported that there was no significant difference in the times or frequencies of recurrence among 24 patients with active inflammation up to the limit of resection and a similar number studied with no disease at the resection margin. Their surgical recommendation, therefore, is simply to carry out "plasty" procedures (see Panel 3 in Fig. 127–70) on patients with multiple areas of recurrent disease. They claim satisfactory results, with preservation of as much bowel as possible using these non-resectional techniques.

Several authors have noted that there is an *increased risk of* recurrence in patients *with extensive involvement* of bowel.[30, 44a, 55, 147, 170] Van Patter et al.[30] noted that recurrence rates were higher only when more than 50 cm of bowel was involved. However, Atwell et al.[170] found a 38% recurrence rate with less than 7.5 cm of resected bowel compared with 67% if over 30 cm was diseased. None of these findings was verified actuarially nor were corrections made for other confounding variables.

The belief that the *presence of macroscopic or microscopic disease at the resection margins*, as may be shown by examination of a frozen section during operation, is a factor adversely affecting recurrence[142, 146] is being increasingly challenged.[18, 145] Lee et al.[18] found that it was difficult for the pathologists to obtain histologic sections of sufficient quality for adequate assessment. The majority of surgeons use the macroscopic appearance of the bowel as noted from the serosal aspect and the degree of ulceration on opening the bowel following removal of the specimen as clues to an adequate resection margin. Most surgeons resect the diseased tissue and take out between 5 and 10 cm of adjacent normal bowel.

There is difference of opinion regarding the significance of *enlarged lymph nodes* and the virtue of removing them.[53, 147] Most surgeons feel that the prognosis is not affected by either the extent of lymph node involvement or the completeness of resection of the mesentery.

Glass and Baker[171] and Chambers and Morson[172] reported that *granulomas* are associated with fewer recurrences, but most reported studies have failed to demonstrate any association of granulomas with recurrence rates.[30, 145, 159, 173, 174]

Although Ritchie and Lockhart-Mummery[123] reported an increased recurrence rate in patients with *staged operative procedures*, this finding is disputed by Steinberg et al.,[124] who found no such difference.

Cooke et al.[23] found that the number of operations was greater in patients who received *steroids*. However, patients who have required and received steroid therapy are not in most respects clinically comparable to those who have not.

Various attempts have been made to use drug therapy to reduce postoperative recurrence in Crohn's disease. Smith et al.[175] and Summers et al.[176] failed to show any significant reduction in recurrence with use of postoperative steroids in controlled studies. The use of sulfasalazine prophylactically was shown by Wenkert and associates[230] to have a slight but insignificant advantage for treated patients, and no effect was found in the National Crohn's Cooperative Study.[176]

Ultimate Outcome

The ultimate objective of the treatment of Crohn's disease is a physiologically well patient, who is able to lead a normal life, work regularly, and interact socially in his or her ordinary environment. Allan et al.[28] reported a good quality of life following surgery. Goligher[157] found that 73% of his patients fitted this favorable definition; 19% were able to manage most, but not all, activities, while 8% were considerably restricted. Meyers et al.[26] found in a psychosocial survey that 92% of the patients were satisfied with their surgical outcome, and only 8% would not chose surgery again. Disease recurrence and the presence of an ileostomy were significantly unfavorable influences, yet patients still reported substantial improvement as compared with their preoperative status.

Acute Ileitis

Acute ileitis is often discovered in the course of an emergency operation for abdominal symptoms and signs simulating appendicitis. Acute terminal ileitis usually resolves spontaneously.[174] Progression to chronic regional enteritis has been claimed to be as low as zero[177] and as high as 28%,[91] with most reports setting the frequency at 10% to 20%.[178, 179]

Yersinia pseudotuberculosis, a gram-negative coccus, has been cultured from a mesenteric lymph node[180] and *Yersinia pseudotuberculosis* or *enterocolitica* has been recovered from the stools of patients with acute ileitis.[179, 181, 182] Positive titers greater than 1:80 for this organism are considered significant.[179, 180] Sjostrom[179] cultured *Yersinia enterocolitica* from the stools of 21 of 29 patients with acute terminal ileitis. None of the patients went on to develop symptoms of Crohn's disease. Thus, the detection of *Yersinia* organisms in a patient with acute ileitis who was operated upon for suspected acute appendicitis makes it unlikely that the patient has true Crohn's disease. The standard procedure at laparotomy in such instances is appendectomy, provided that the underlying cecum is not severely inflamed. When disease is localized to the appendix, *appendectomy* alone is a satisfactory form of treatment. With contiguous disease in the cecum, ileum, and ascending colon, an *ileocolectomy*, including the appendix, should be carried out if there is no perforation or gangrene. If an abscess is present, adequate *drainage* is mandatory and resection may be deferred to a later date if necessary. It is surprising that despite a considerable proportion of patients with contiguous disease, no fistula originating at the operative site has been reported.

Crohn's Disease of the Mouth, Epiglottis, and Aryepiglottic Folds

Involvement of the mouth in Crohn's disease occurs in approximately 6% to 20% of cases.[183–186, 188] The lesions are found more commonly in patients with Crohn's disease involving the colon[188] and may precede the development of symptomatic intestinal disease.[187] Tracheostomy may be necessary if severe laryngeal obstruction develops that is not adequately controlled by steroids, as it was in the patient of Wilder et al.[189]

Crohn's Disease of the Esophagus

Three patients with benign strictures of the esophagus secondary to transmural disease with the histologic features of Crohn's disease were described by Madden et al.[190] Failure to respond to esophageal bougienage led to esophagocardiectomy and intrapleural esophagogastrostomy.

Crohn's Disease of the Stomach and Duodenum

Crohn's disease limited to the stomach is rare and occurs usually in conjunction with associated disease of the adjacent duodenum.[191–193] Crohn's disease of the duodenum is more common, occurring in 0.5% to 7% of cases.[194]

The ideal treatment, when possible, is posterior gastroenterostomy. However, gastrectomy may be necessary to control bleeding or for extensive gastric involvement. If a vagotomy is performed, it is probably advisable to elect a parietal cell or selective vagotomy, preserving the nerve supply of the distal bowel so that the diarrhea of Crohn's disease is not increased. Because of the risk of fistula formation, pyloroplasty should be avoided if possible.

Surgical Aspects of Extraintestinal Manifestations of Crohn's Disease

The extraintestinal manifestations of Crohn's disease are discussed in detail in another section of this chapter. Few studies have been carried out on the effect of surgery on the natural history of these extraintestinal manifestations. There is one report that colectomy may lead to regression of hepatic and renal amyloidosis.[195] Most of the extraintestinal manifestations that are exacerbated during active disease improve with colectomy. However, uveitis and sacroiliitis are not influenced by colectomy. Although the effect of colectomy in liver disease is uncertain, and advanced cirrhosis is certainly not influenced by colectomy, early liver disease may be improved and progression to cirrhosis might be prevented by this procedure.[196, 197] Sclerosing cholangitis (Chapter

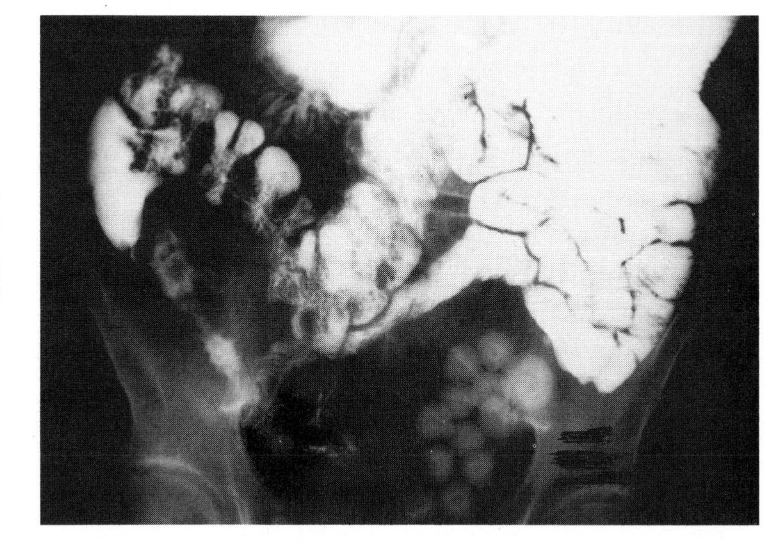

Figure 127–80. Recurrent ileocolitis in a 67-year-old man with ileocoitis of 15 years' duration, showing 12 large urinary calculi (lower left pelvis) associated with occasional minor urinary infection.

164) occurs in association with inflammatory bowel disease, but there seems to be no relationship to activity of disease and many cases do not even appear until long after colectomy.[198] Pyoderma gangrenosum associated with very active colitis improves rapidly following colectomy, but if its severity is out of proportion to a relatively inactive and mild colitis, it appears to respond to colectomy only slowly if at all.[199]

Gallstones in inflammatory bowel disease are frequently asymptomatic. As in ordinary gallstone disease, the indications for cholecystectomy are clear if the stones become symptomatic or if acute cholecystitis supervenes. The more difficult question is whether or not to perform incidental cholecystectomy for asymptomatic stones during the course of elective bowel surgery for Crohn's disease. Many surgeons will not do a concomitant cholecystectomy when carrying out an ileal, colonic, or ileocolonic resection because of the danger of infective complications. However, cholecystectomy may be advisable on occasion in the presence of obvious chronic inflammation in the gallbladder found at the time of an uncomplicated bowel resection. If carried out meticulously with careful hemostasis and with adequate drainage of the gallbladder bed, additional complications are unlikely.

Renal stones occur fairly often in patients with ileocolic resections or ileostomies. The former group develop oxalate stones as a result of hypoxaluria, and the latter usually develop calcium urate stones due to a combination of factors, including tissue breakdown from chronic debilitating disease, bed rest, and episodes of dehydration. Nephrectomy, nephrostomy, and nephroureterolithotomy, as well as removal of bladder stones (Fig. 127–80), may be necessary at times, especially in the patient with a long duration of disease and frequent and repeated resections. On occasion, percutaneous nephrostomy and dilatation of ureteral strictures may be required for stricturing disease of the distal ileum related to periureteral fibrosis. This was necessary in one patient of ours among more than 40 who developed hydronephrosis during the course of their disease.

References

1. Dalziel TK. Chronic intestinal enteritis. Br Med J 1913; 2:1068–70.
2. Moschowitz E, Wilensky AD. Non-specific granulomata of the intestine. Am J Med Sci 1923; 166:48–64.
3. Crohn BB, Ginzburg L, Oppenheimer GD. Regional ileitis; a pathologic and clinical entity. JAMA 1932; 99:1323–9.
4. Ginzburg L, Oppenheimer GD. Non-specific granulomata of the intestines (inflammatory tumors and strictures of the bowel). Ann Surg 1933; 98:1046–62.
5. Garlock JH, Crohn BB, Klein SH, Yarnis H. An appraisal of the long term results of surgical treatment of regional ileitis. Gastroenterology 1951; 19:414–23.
6. Colp R, Dreiling DA. Persistent or recurrent proximal ileitis following surgery. Arch Surg 1952; 64:28–46.
7. Ferguson R, Allan RN, Cooke WT. A study of the cellular infiltrate of the proximal jejunal mucosa in ulcerative colitis and Crohn's disease. Gut 1975; 15:205–8.
8. Crucioli V. Rectal biopsy in Crohn's disease. Rendic Gastroenterol 1972; 4:73–80.
9. Allan R, Steinberg DM, Dixon K, Cooke WT. Changes in bidirectional sodium flux across the intestinal mucosa in Crohn's disease. Gut 1975; 15:201–4.
10. Dunne WT, Allan R, Cooke WT. Enzymatic and quantitative histological evidence for Crohn's disease as a diffuse

lesion of the gastrointestinal tract. Gut 1976; 17:399. (Abstract).
11. Bersack SR, Howe JS, Rehak EM. A unique case with roentgenologic evidence of regional enteritis of long duration and histologic evidence of diffuse adenocarcinoma. Gastroenterology 1958; 34:703–10.
12. Clemmensen T, Johansen A. A case of Crohn's disease of the colon associated with adenocarcinoma extending from cardia to anus. Acta Path Microbiologica Scand 1972; 80:5–8.
13. Flemming KA, Pollock AC. A case of "Crohn's carcinoma". Gut 1975; 16:533–7.
14. Keighley MRB, Thompson H, Alexander-Williams J. Multifocal carcinoma and Crohn's disease. Surgery 1975; 78:534–7.
15. Greenstein AJ, Sachar DB, Pasternak BS, Janowitz HD. Reoperation and recurrence in Crohn's colitis and ileocolitis: Crude and cumulative rates. N Engl J Med 1975; 293:685–90.
16. Hellers G. Crohn's disease in Stockholm County 1955–1974. A study of epidemiology, results of surgical treatment and long-term prognosis. Acta Chir Scand 1979; 409 (Suppl):830.
17. Lock MR, Fazio VW, Farmer RG, Jagelman DG, Lavery IC, Weakley FL. Proximal recurrence and the fate of the rectum following excisional surgery for Crohn's disease of the large bowel. Ann Surg 1981; 194:754–60.
18. Lee ECG, Papaioannou N. Recurrences following surgery for Crohn's disease. Clinics Gastroenterol 1980; 9:419–38.
19. Janowitz HD. Problems in Crohn's disease: Evaluation of the results of surgical treatment. J Chron Dis 1975; 28:63–6.
20. Farmer RG, Hawk WA, Turnbull RB. Indications for surgery in Crohn's disease. Analysis of 500 cases. Gastroenterology 1976; 71:245–50.
21. Farmer RG, Hawk WA, Turnbull RB. Clinical patterns in Crohn's disease: A statistical study of 615 cases. Gastroenterology 1975; 68:627–35.
22. Mekhjian HS, Switz DM, Watts HD, Deren JJ, Katon RM, Berman FM. National cooperative Crohn's disease study: factors determining recurrence of Crohn's disease after surgery. Gastroenterology 1979; 77:907–13.
23. Cooke WT, Mallas E, Prior R, Allan RN. Crohn's disease: Course, treatment and long-term prognosis. Q J Med 1980; 195:363–84.
24. Goligher JC, DeDombal FT, Burton I. Crohn's disease with special reference to surgical management. Progr Surg 1972; 10:1–23.
25. Krause U, Bergman L, Norlen BJ. Crohn's disease. A clinical study based on 186 patients. Scand J Gastroenterol 1971; 6:97–108.
26. Meyers S, Walfish JS, Sachar DB, Greenstein AJ, Hill AG, Janowitz HD. Quality of life after surgery for Crohn's disease: A psychosocial survey. Gastroenterology 1980; 78:1–6.
27. Steyn JP, Kyle J. Quality of life after surgery for Crohn's disease. J Roy Coll Surg (Edin) 1982; 27:22–5.
28. Allan R, Steinberg DM, Williams JA, Cooke WT. Crohn's disease involving the colon: An audit of clinical management. Gastroenterology 1977; 73:723–32.
29. Greenstein AJ, Meyers S, Sher L, Heimann T, Aufses AH Jr. Surgery and its sequelae in Crohn's colitis and ileocolitis. Arch Surg 1981; 116:285–8.
30. Van Patter WN, Bargen JA, Dockerty MB, Feldman WH, Mayo CW, Waugh JM. Regional enteritis. Gastroenterology 1954; 26:347–450.
31. Crohn BB, Yarnis H. Regional enteritis. 2nd Ed. New York: Grune and Stratton, 1958.
32. Glotzer DJ, Silen W. Indications for operation. *In*: Kirsner JB, Shorter RG, eds. Inflammatory Bowel Disease. Philadelphia: Lea & Febiger, 1980: 488–517.
33. Korelitz BI. Therapy of inflammatory bowel disease including the use of immunosuppressive agents. Clin Gastroenterol 1980; 8:331–50.
34. Alexander-Williams J. New directions for future research 1982. *In*: Rachmilewitz D, ed. Inflammatory Bowel Disease. The Hague: Nijoff 1982: 306–7.
35. Lee ECG. Aspects of treatment. Minimal surgery for chronic obstruction in patients with extensive or univeral Crohn's disease. Ann Roy Coll Surg Eng 1982; 64:229–33.
36. Greenstein AJ, Kark AE, Dreiling DA. Crohn's disease of the colon. I. Fistula in Crohn's disease of the colon, classification, presenting features and management in 63 patients. Am J Gastroenterol 1974; 62:419–27.
37. Orda R, Goldwaser B, Wiznitzer T. Free perforation of the colon in Crohn's disease. Report of a case and review of the literature. Dis Colon Rectum 1982; 25:145–7.
38. Greenstein AJ, Kark AE, Dreiling DA. Crohn's disease of the colon. III. Toxic dilatation of the colon in Crohn's colitis. Am J Gastroenterol 1975; 63:117–28.
39. Menguy R. Surgical management of free perforation of the small intestine in regional enteritis. Ann Surg 1972; 175:178–89.
40. Waye JD, Lithgow C. Small bowel perforation in regional enteritis. Gastroenterology 1967; 53:625–9.
41. Greenstein AJ, Mann DJ, Aufses AH. Free perforation in inflammatory bowel disease. Am J Surg 1984; 147:788–92.
42. Aufses AH, Jr. Kreel I. Ileostomy for granulomatous ileocolitis. Ann Surg 1971; 173:91–6.
43. Slater G, Kreel I, Aufses AH Jr. Temporary loop ileostomy in the treatment of Crohn's disease. Ann Surg 1978; 188:706–9.
44. Greenstein AJ, Sachar DB, Greenstein RJ, Janowitz HD, Aufses AH, Jr. Intraabdominal abscess in Crohn's (Ileo) colitis. Am J Surg 1982; 143:727–30.
44a. Schofield PF. The natural history and treatment of Crohn's disease. Ann Roy Coll Surg (Eng.) 1965; 36:258–79.
45. Nagler SM, Poticha SM. Intraabdominal abscess in regional enteritis. Am J Surg 1979; 137:350–4.
45a. Alexander-Williams, J. Surgery and the management of Crohn's disease. Clin Gastroenterol 1972; 1:469–91.
46. Kyle J. Crohn's Disease. New York: Appleton-Century-Crofts, 1972: 127.
47. Broe PJ, Bayless TM, Cameron JL. Crohn's disease: Are enteroenteral fistulae an indication for surgery: Surgery 1982; 91:249–53.
48. Bury KD, Stephens RD, Randall HT. Use of a chemically refined liquid elemental diet for nutritional management of fistulas of the alimentary tract. Am J Surg 1971; 121:174–83.
49. Fischer JE, Foster GS, Abel AN, Abbott WM, Ryan JA. Hyperalimentation as primary therapy for inflammatory bowel disease. Am J Surg 1973; 125:165–75.
50. Brooke BN, Javett SL, Davison OW. Further experience with azathioprine for Crohn's disease. Lancet 1970; 2:1050–3.
51. Javett SL. Azathiaprine in Crohn's disease. Clin Gastroenterol 1972; 1:507–20.
52. Garlock JH. Surgery of the Alimentary Tract. New York: Appleton-Century-Crofts, 1967: 271–6.
53. Fazio VW, Wilk I, Turnbull RB Jr. The dilemma of Crohn's disease: Ileosigmoidal fistula complicating Crohn's disease. Dis Colon Rectum 1977; 20:381–6.
54. Heimann T, Greenstein AJ, Aufses AH Jr. The management of ileosigmoid fistula. Am J Gastroenterol 1979; 72:21–4.
55. Greenstein AJ, Sachar DB, Tzakis A, Sher L, Heimann T, Aufses AH, Jr. Enterovesical fistulae occurring during the course of Crohn's disease. (In preparation).
56. Hiley PC, Cohen N, Present DH. Spontaneous umbilical fistula in granulomatous (Crohn's) disease of the bowel. Gastroenterology 1971; 60:103–7.
57. Sachar DB, Present DH. Immunotherapy in inflammatory bowel disease. Med Clin North Am 1978; 62:172–83.
58. Greenstein AJ, Dicker A, Meyers S, Aufses AH Jr. Periileostomy fistulae in Crohn's disease. Ann Surg 1983; 197:179–82.
59. Lightdale CJ, Steinberg SS, Posner G, Sherlock P. Carcinoma complicating Crohn's disease: Report of seven cases and review of the literature. Am J Med 1975; 59:262–8.
60. Greenstein AJ, Sachar DB, Pucillo A, Kreel I, Geller S, Janowitz HD, Aufses AH Jr. Cancer in Crohn's disease after diversionary surgery. A report of 7 carcinomas occurring in excluded bowel. Am J Surg 1978; 135:86–90.
61. Buchmann P, Alexander-Williams J. Classification of perianal disease. Clin Gastroenterol 1980; 9:323–30.
62. Sohn N, Korelitz BI, Weinstein MA. Anorectal Crohn's

disease: Definitive surgery for fistulas and recurrent abscesses. Am J Surg 1980; 139:394–7.
63. Buchmann P, Keighley MRB, Allan RN, Thompson H, Alexander-Williams J. Natural history of perianal Crohn's disease. Ten year follow-up: a plea for conservation. Am J Surg 1980; 140:642–4.
64. Parks AG. Pathogenesis and treatment of fistulae in ano. Br Med J 1961; 1:462–9.
65. Goligher JC, Ellis M, Pissidis AG. A critique of anal glandular infections and the aetiology and treatment of idiopathic anorectal abscesses and fistulas. Br J Surg 1967; 54:977–83.
66. Greenstein AJ, Sachar DB, Kark AE. Stricture of the anorectum in Crohn's disease involving the colon. Ann Surg 1975; 181:207–12.
67. Lockhart-Mummery HE. Anal lesions of Crohn's disease. Clin Gastroenterol 1972; 1:377–82.
68. Burman JH, Thompson H, Cooke WT, Alexander-Williams J. The effect of diversion of intestinal contents on the progress of Crohn's disease of the large bowel. Gut 1971; 12:11–15.
69. Block GE, Enker WE, Kirsner JB. Significance and treatment of occult obstructive uropathy complicating Crohn's disease. Ann Surg 1973; 187:322–32.
70. Goldman HJ, Glickman SI. Ureteric obstruction in regional enteritis. J Urol 1962; 88:616–20.
71. Present DH, Rabinowitz JG, Banks PA. Obstructive hydronephrosis: a frequent but seldom recognized complication of granulomatous disease of the bowel. N Engl J Med 1969; 280:523–8.
72. Altemeier WA. In discussion of paper by Block GE, Enker WE, Kirsner JB. Significance and treatment of occult obstructive uropathy complicating Crohn's disease. Ann Surg 1973; 178:331.
73. Frank JD, Shorey BA. Adenocarcinoma of the small bowel as a complicating of Crohn's disease. Gut 1973; 14:120–4.
74. Greenstein AJ, Sachar DB, Smith H, Janowitz HD, Aufses AH Jr. Patterns of neoplasia in Crohn's disease and ulcerative colitis. Cancer 1980; 46:403–7.
75. Weedon DD, Shorter RG, Ilstrup DM, Huizenga KA, Taylor WF. Crohn's disease and cancer. N Engl J Med 1973; 289:1099–103.
76. Fresko D, Lazarus SS, Dotan J, Reingold M. Early presentation of carcinoma of the small bowel in Crohn's disease ("Crohn's carcinoma"). Case reports and review of the literature. Gastroenterology 1982; 82:783–9.
77. Greenstein AJ, Sachar DB, Smith H, Janowitz HD, Aufses AH Jr. A comparison of cancer risk in Crohn's disease and ulcerative colitis. Cancer 1981; 48:2742–5.
78. deDombal FT, Burton I, Goligher JC. The early and late results of surgical treatment for Crohn's disease. Br J Surg 1971; 58:805–16.
79. Greenstein AJ, Kark AE, Dreiling DA. Crohn's disease of the colon. II. Controversial aspect of hemorrhage, anemia and rectal involvement in granulomatous disease involving the colon. Am J Gastroenterol 1975; 63:40–8.
80. Block GE, Moossa AR, Simonowitz D, Hassan SZ. Emergency colectomy for inflammatory bowel disease. Surgery 1977; 82:531–6.
81. Lumb G, Protheroe RHB, Ramsay GS. Ulcerative colitis with toxic dilatation of the colon. Br J Surg 1955; 43: 182–8.
82. Buzzard AJ, Baker WNW, Needham PRG, Warren RE. Acute toxic dilatation of the colon in Crohn's colitis. Gut 1974; 15:416–20.
83. Turnbull RB, Hawk WA, Weakley FL. Ileostomy and colostomy to prepare patients for colectomy. Am J Surg 1971; 122:325–31.
84. Katzka I, Katz S, Morris E. Management of toxic megacolon: The significance of early recognition in medical management. J Clin Gastroenterol 1979; 1:307–11.
85. Present DH, Wolfson D, Gelernt IM, Rubin PH, Bauer J, Chapman ML. The medical management of toxic megacolon: technique of decompression with favorable long term follow up. Gastroenterology 1981; 80:1255(Abstract).
86. Strauss RJ, Flint GW, Platt N, Levin L, Wise L. The surgical management of toxic dilatation of the colon: A report of 28 cases and a review of the literature. Ann Surg 1976; 184:682–8.
87. Goligher JC, Hoffman DC, deDombal FT. Surgical treatment of severe attacks of ulcerative colitis, with special reference to the advantages of early operation. Br Med J 1970; 4:703–6.
88. Flatmark A, Fretheim B, Gjone E. Early colectomy in severe ulcerative colitis. Scand J Gastroenterol 1975; 10:427–31.
89. Klein SH, Edelman S, Kirsner JB, et al. Emergency cecostomy in ulcerative colitis with acute toxic dilation. Surgery 1960; 47:399–407.
90. Goligher JC, Duthie HL, Nixon HH. Surgery of the anus, rectum and colon. *In*: Crohn's Disease (Granulomatous Enteritis). 4th Ed. London: Bailliere Tindall, 1980: 827–57.
91. deDombal FT, Burton IL, Clamp SE, Goligher JC. Short-term course and prognosis of Crohn's disease. Gut 1974; 15:435–43.
92. Watts JM, deDombal FT, Watkinson G, Goligher JC. The early course of ulcerative colitis. Gut 1966; 7:16–29.
93. Oberhelman HA, Kohatsu S, Taylor KB, Kivel RM. Diverting ileostomy in the surgical management of Crohn's disease of the colon. Am J Surg 1968; 115:231–40.
94. Lee ECG. Results of split ileostomy in Crohn's colitis. *In*: Weterman IT, Pena AS, Booth CC, eds.The Management of Crohn's Disease. Amsterdam: Excerpta Medica, 1976.
95. Alexander-Williams JA. The place of surgery in Crohn's disease. Gut 1971; 12:739–49.
96. Fawaz KA, Glotzer DJ, Goldman H, Dickersin GR, Gross W, Patterson JF. Ulcerative colitis and Crohn's disease of the colon—a comparison of the long-term postoperative courses. Gastroenterology 1976; 71:372–8.
97. Brown JY. Value of complete physiological rest of large bowel in treatment of certain ulcerations and obstructive lesions of this organ. Surg Gynecol Obstet 1913; 16:610–3.
98. McIlrath D. Diverting ileostomy or colostomy in the management of Crohn's disease of the colon. Arch Surg 1971; 103:308–10.
99. Zelas P, Jagelman DG. Loop ileostomy in the management of Crohn's colitis in the debilitated patient. Ann Surg 1980; 191:164–8.
100. Truelove SC, Witts LJ. Cortisone in ulcerative colitis. Final report on a therapeutic trial. Br Med J 1955; 2:1041–8.
101. Truelove SC, Jewell DP. Intensive intravenous regimen for severe attacks of ulcerative colitis. Lancet 1974; 1:1067–70.
102. Oberhelman HA Jr. The effect of intestinal diversion by ileostomy on Crohn's disease of the colon. *In*: Weterman IT, Pena AS, Booth CC, eds. The Management of Crohn's Disease. Amsterdam: Excerpta Medica 1976: 216.
103. Weterman IT, Pena AS. The long-term prognosis of ileorectal anastomosis and proctocolectomy in Crohn's disease. Scand J Gastroenterol 1976; 11:185–91.
104. Flint G, Strauss R, Platt N, Wise L. Ileorectal anastomosis in patients with Crohn's disease of the colon. Gut 1977; 18:236–9.
105. Lee ECG, Truelove SC. Proctocolectomy for ulcerative colitis. World J Surg 1980; 4:195–201.
106. Burnham WR, Lennard-Jones JE, Brooke BN. Sexual problems among married ileostomists. Gut 1976; 18:673–7.
107. Fazio VW, Fletcher J, Montague D. Prospective study of the effect of resection of the rectum on male sexual function. World J Surg 1980; 4:149–52.
108. Fazio VW, Turnbull RB. Ulcerative colitis and Crohn's disease of the colon. A review of surgical options. Med Clin North Am 1980; 64:1135–59.
109. Lyttle JA, Parks AG. Intersphincteric excision of the rectum. Br J Surg 1977; 64:413–6.
110. Lee ECG, Dowling BL. Perimuscular excision of the rectum for Crohn's disease and ulcerative colitis. Br J Surg 1972; 59:29–32.
111. Waits JO, Dozois RR, Kelly KA. Primary closure and continuous irrigation of the perineal wound after proctectomy. Mayo Clinic Proc 1982; 57:185–8.
112. Anderson R, Turnbull RB. Grafting the unhealed perineal wound after coloproctectomy for Crohn's disease. Arch Surg 1976; 111:335–8.
113. Silen W, Glotzer D. The prevention and treatment of the persistent perineal sinus. Surgery 1974; 75:535–42.
114. Baek S, Greenstein A, McElhinney AJ, Aufses AH Jr. The gracilis myocutaneous flap for persistent perineal sinus after proctocolectomy. Surg Gynecol Obstet 1981; 153:713–6.

115. Goligher JC, Goteborg MD. The quest for continence in the surgical treatment of ulcerative colitis. *In*: Jordan GL, ed. Advances in Surgery. Vol. 14. Chicago: Year Book Medical Publishers, 1980: 53–83.
116. Kock NG, Darle N, Hulten L, Kewenter J. The conventional ileostomy. Curr Prob Surg 1977; 14:6–52.
117. Oh C, Kark AE. Anatomy of the external anal sphincter. Br J Surg 1972; 59:717–23.
118. Martin L, LeCoultre C, Schubert WK. Total colectomy and mucosal proctectomy with preservation of continence in ulcerative colitis. Ann Surg 1977; 186:477–80.
119. Fonkalsrud EW. Endorectal ileal pullthrough with lateral ileal reservoir for benign colorectal disease. Ann Surg 1981; 194:761–6.
120. Utsunomiya J, Iwama T, Imajo M, Matsuo S, Sawai S, Yaegashi K, Hirayama R. Total colectomy, mucosal proctectomy, and ileoanal anastomosis. Dis Colon Rectum 1980; 23:459–66.
121. Parks AG, Nicholls RJ, Belliveau P. Proctocolectomy with ileal reservoir and anal anastomosis. Br J Surg 1980; 67:533–8.
122. Weedon DD, Shorter RG, Ilstrup DM, Huizenga KA, Taylor WF. Crohn's disease and cancer. N Engl J Med 1973; 289:1099–103.
123. Ritchie JK, Lockhart-Mummery HE. Non-restorative surgery in the treatment of Crohn's disease of the large bowel. Gut 1973; 14:263–9.
124. Steinberg DM, Allan RN, Thompson H, Brooke BN, Alexander-Williams J, Cooke WT. Excisional surgery with ileostomy for Crohn's colitis with particular reference to factors affecting recurrence. Gut 1974; 15:845–51.
125. Allan R, Steinberg DM, Alexander-Williams J, Cooke WT. Crohn's disease involving the colon: An audit of clinical management. Gastroenterology 1977; 73:723–32.
126. Young S, Smity IS, O'Connor J, Bell JR, Gillespie G. Results of surgery for Crohn's disease in the Glasgow region, 1961–1970. Br J Surg 1975; 62:528–34.
127. Prior P, Fielding JF, Waterhouse JA, Cooke WT. Mortality in Crohn's disease. Lancet 1970; 1:1135–7.
128. Greenstein AJ, Sachar DB, Smith H, Janowitz HD, Aufses AH Jr. A comparison of cancer risk in Crohn's disease and ulcerative colitis. Cancer 1981; 48:2742–5.
129. Block GE. Empiric caval interruption in operations for inflammatory bowel disease. Curr Surg 1978; 35:297–8.
130. Barker K, Graham N, Mason M, et al. The relative significance of preoperative oral antibiotics, mechanical bowel preparation, and preoperative peritoneal contamination in the avoidance of sepsis after radical surgery for ulcerative colitis and Crohn's disease of the large bowel. Br J Surg 1971; 58:270–3.
131. Ritchie JK. Ileostomy and excisional surgery for chronic inflammatory disease of the colon: a survey of one hospital region. Gut 1971; 12:528–40.
132. Condon RE. Rational use of prophylactic antibiotics in gastrointestinal surgery. Surg Clin North Am 1975; 55:1309–18.
133. Watts J McK, deDombal FT, Goligher JC. Long-term complications and prognosis following major surgery for ulcerative colitis. Br J Surg 1966; 53:1014–23.
134. Allsop JR, Lee ECG. Factors which influenced postoperative complications in patients with ulcerative colitis or Crohn's disease of the colon on corticosteroids. Gut 1978; 19:729–34.
135. Gerzof SG, Spira R, Robbins AH. Percutaneous abscess drainage. Semin Roentgenol 1981; 16:62–71.
136. Block GE. Current concepts. Surgical management of Crohn's colitis. N Engl J Med 1980; 302:1068–70.
137. Hudspeth AS. Radical surgical debridement in the treatment of advanced generalized bacterial peritonitis. Arch Surg 1970; 110:1233–400.
138. Brooke BN. The management of an ileostomy including its complications. Lancet 1952; 2:102–4.
139. Warren R, McKittrick LS. Ileostomy for ulcerative colitis. Surg Gynecol Obstet 1951; 93:555–67.
140. Block GE, Giuliano A. Complications of the surgical treatment of ulcerative colitis and Crohn's disease. *In*: Kirsner JB, Shorter RG, eds. Inflammatory Bowel Disease. Philadelphia: Lea & Febiger, 1980: 577–604.
141. Wallensten S. Results of surgical treatment in Sweden. *In*: Regional Enteritis. Stockholm: Scandia International Symposium Nordiska, Bokhandelns Forlag, 1971, 177–94.
142. Karesen R, Serch-Hanssen A, Thoresen BO, Hertzberg J. Crohn's disease: Long-term results of surgical treatment. Scand J Gastroenterol 1981; 16:57–64.
143. Krause U. Post-operative complications and early course of the surgical treatment of Crohn's disease. Acta Chir Scand 1978; 144:163–74.
144. Nygaard K, Fausa O. Crohn's disease. Recurrence after surgical treatment. Scand J Gastroenterol 1977; 12:577–84.
145. Pennington L, Hamilton SR, Bayless TM, Cameron JL. Surgical management of Crohn's disease. Influence of disease at margin of resection. Ann Surg 1980; 192:311–8.
146. deDombal FT, Burton IL, Goligher JC. Recurrence of Crohn's disease after primary excisional surgery. Gut 1971; 12:519–27.
147. Stahlgren LH, Ferguson LK. The results of surgical treatment of chronic regional enteritis. JAMA 1961; 175:986–9.
148. Lennard-Jones JE, Stalder GA. Prognosis after resection of chronic regional ileitis. Gut 1967; 8:332–6.
149. Glotzer DJ. Recurrence in Crohn's colitis: The numbers game. World J Surg 1980; 4:173–80.
150. Greenstein AJ, Sachar DB. Invited commentary. Recurrence in Crohn's colitis. World J Surg 1980; 4:180–2.
151. Korelitz BI, Present DH, Alpert LI, Marshak RH, Janowitz HD. Recurrent regional ileitis after ileostomy and colectomy for granulomatous colitis. N Engl J Med 1972; 287:110–4.
152. Nugent FW, Veidenheimer MC, Meissner WA, Haggitt RC. Prognosis after colonic resection for Crohn's disease of the colon. Gastroenterology 1973; 65:398–402.
153. Marshak RH, Lindner AE. Radiology of the Small Intestine. 2nd Ed. Philadelphia: WB Saunders, 1976: 179–300.
154. Waye JD. Endoscopy in inflammatory bowel disease. Clin Gastroenterol 1980; 9:279–96.
155. Lindner AE, Marshak RH, Wolf BS, Janowitz HD. Granulomatous colitis. A clinical study. N Engl J Med 1963; 269:379–85.
156. Lee ECG: Discussion and conclusions. *In*: Lee ECG, ed. Crohn's Workshop. A Global Assessment of Crohn's Disease. London: Heyden, 1981: 170.
157. Goligher JC. The outcome of excisional operations for primary and recurrent Crohn's disease of the large intestine. Surg Gynecol Obstet 1979; 148:1–8.
158. Sachar DB, Wolfson DM, Greenstein AJ, Goldberg J, Styczynski R, Janowitz HD. Risk factors for postoperative recurrence of Crohn's disease. Gastroenterology 1983; 85:917–21.
159. Wolfson DM, Sachar DB, Cohen A, Goldberg J, Styczynski R, Greenstein AJ, Gelernt IM, Janowitz HD. Do granulomas affect postoperative recurrence rates in Crohn's disease? Gastroenterology 1982; 83:405–9.
160. Truelove SC, Pena AS. Course and prognosis of Crohn's disease. Gut 1976; 17:192–201.
161. Glotzer DJ, Stone PA, Patterson JF. Prognosis after surgical treatment of granulomatous colitis. N Engl J Med 1967; 277:273–9.
162. Ritchie JK. A current assessment of Crohn's disease in Britain—an analysis of epidemiological studies and the experience of St. Mark's Hospital, London. *In*: Lee ECG, ed. Crohn's Workshop. A Global Assessment of Crohn's Disease. London: Heyden, 1981: 59.
163. Vender RJ, Rickert RR, Spiro HM. The outlook after total colectomy in patients with Crohn's colitis and ulcerative colitis. J Clin Gastroenterol 1979; 1:209–17.
164. Korelitz BI. Clinical course, late results and pathological nature of inflammatory disease of the colon initially sparing the rectum. Gut 1967; 8:281–90.
165. Steinberg DM, Allan RN, Cooke WT, Williams JA. The place of ileorectal anastomosis in Crohn's disease. Aust NZ J Surg 1976; 46:49–54.
166. Veidenheimer MC, Nugent FW, Haggitt RC. Ulcerative colitis or Crohn's colitis: Is differentiation necessary? Surg Clin North Am 1976; 56:721–6.
167. Burman JH, Cooke WT, Alexander-Williams J. The fate of ileorectal anastomosis in Crohn's disease. Gut 1971; 12:432–6.
168. Korelitz BI, Gribetz D, Kopel FB. Granulomatous colitis in

children: a study of 25 cases and comparisons with ulcerative colitis. Pediatrics 1968; 42:446–57.
169. Koch TR, Cave DR, Kirsner JB. Anatomical patterns of post surgical recurrence of Crohn's ileitis and ileocolitis. Gastroenterology 1980; 78:1197 (Abstract).
170. Atwell JD, Duthie HL, Goligher JC. The outcome of Crohn's disease. Br J Surg 1965; 52:966–72.
171. Glass RE, Baker NW. Role of the granuloma in recurrent Crohn's disease. Gut 1976; 17:75–7.
172. Chambers TJ, Morson BC. The granuloma in Crohn's disease. Gut 1979; 20:269–74.
173. Wilson JAP, Burkhardt RT, Kumar N, et al. Relationship of granulomas in clinical parameters in Crohn's disease. Gastroenterology 1980; 78:1291 (Abstract).
174. Assarsson N, Raf L. Incidence of granuloma in Crohn's disease. Acta Chir Scand 1974; 140:249–51.
175. Smith RC, Rhodes J, Heatley RV, et al. Low-dose corticosteroids and clinical relapse in Crohn's disease: A controlled trial. Gut 1978; 19:606–19.
176. Summers RW, Switz DM, Sessions JT, Becktel JM, Best WR, Kern F Jr, Singleton JW. National cooperative Crohn's disease study: Results of drug treatment. Gastroenterology 1979; 77:847–69.
177. Thomasson B, Havia T. Is acute terminal ileitis a precursor of Crohn's disease? Acta Chir Scand 1973; 139:192–3.
178. Gump F, Lepore M, Barker H. A revised concept of acute regional enteritis. Ann Surg 1967; 166:942–6.
179. Sjostrom B. Acute terminal ileitis and its relation to Crohn's disease. *In*: Engel A, Larson T, eds. Regional Enteritis. Stockholm: Scandia International Symposium, Nordika Bokhandels Forlag, 1971: 73–6.
180. Knapp W, Masshoff W. Zur Atologie der Abszedierenden Reticulozytaren Lymphadenitis. Dtsch Med Wochenschr 1954; 79:1266–71.
181. Carlsson M, Ryd H, Sternby N. A case of human infection with pasteurella pseudotuberculosis Y. Acta Pathol Microbiol Scand 1964; 62:128–32.
182. Mayer L, Greenstein AJ. Acute yersinial ileitis: A distinct entity. Am J Gastroenterol 1976; 65:548–51.
183. Basu MK, Asquith P, Thompson RA, Cooke WT. Oral manifestations of Crohn's disease. Gut 1975; 16:249–54.
184. Dudeney TP, Todd IP. Crohn's disease of the mouth. Proc Roy Soc Med 1969; 62:1237.
185. Issa MA. Crohn's disease of the mouth. Br Dent J 1971; 130:247–8.
186. Kyle J. Crohn's Disease. New York: Appleton-Century-Crofts, 1972: 19.
187. Bishop RP, Brewster AC, Antonioli DA. Crohn's disease of the mouth. Gastroenterology 1972; 62:302–6.
188. Greenstein AJ, Janowitz HD, Sachar DB. The extraintestinal complications of Crohn's disease and ulcerative colitis: a study of 700 cases. Medicine 1976; 55:401–12.
189. Wilder WM, Slagle GW, Hand AM, Watkins WJ. Crohn's disease of the epiglottis, aryepiglottic folds, anus, and rectum. J Clin Gastroenterol 1980; 2:87–91.
190. Madden JL, Ravid JM, Haddad JR. Regional esophagitis: A specific entity simulating Crohn's disease. Ann Surg 1969; 170:351–67.
191. Johnson OA, Hoskins DW, Todd J, Thorbjarnarson B. Crohn's disease of the stomach. Arch Surg 1966; 50:571–7.
192. Marshak RH, Maklansky D, Kurzban JD, Lindner AE. Crohn's disease of the stomach and duodenum. Am J Gastroenterol 1982; 77:340–3.
193. Krause J, Schneider R. Pernicious anemia caused by Crohn's disease of the stomach. Am J Gastroenterol 1979; 71:202–5.
194. Miller EM, Moss AA, Kressel HY. Duodenal involvement with Crohn's disease: A spectrum of radiographic abnormality. Am J Gastroenterol 1979; 71:107–16.
195. Fitcher JH. Amyloidosis and granulomatous ileocolitis. N Engl J Med 1975; 292:352.
196. Eade MN, Cooke WT, Brooke BN, Thompson H. Liver disease in Crohn's colitis. A study of 21 consecutive patients having colectomy. Ann Intern Med 1971; 74:518–28.
197. Cooperman AM, Judd ES. The role of colectomy in hepatic disease accompanying ulcerative and granulomatous colitis. Mayo Clin Proc 1972; 47:36–8.
198. Sivak MV Jr, Farmer RG, Lalli AF. Sclerosing cholangitis: Its increasing frequency of recognition and association with inflammatory bowel disease. J Clin Gastroenterol 1981; 3:261–6.
199. Talansky AL, Meyers S, Greenstein AJ, Janowitz HD. Does intestinal resection heal the pyoderma gangrenosum of inflammatory bowel disease. J Clin Gastroenterol 1983; 3:207–10.
200. Shapiro R. Regional ileitis: a summary of the literature. Am J Med Sci 1939; 198:269–92.
201. Himal HS, Belliveau P. Prognosis after surgical treatment for granulomatous enteritis and colitis. Am J Surg 1981; 142:347–9.
202. Goligher JC. Current status of surgical treatment for ulcerative colitis and Crohn's disease of the large bowel. Can J Surg 1978; 21:28–38.
203. McDermott FT, Hughes ESR, Milne BJ, Price AB. Results of operative management of Crohn's disease: A series of 50 patients managed by one surgeon. Dis Colon Rectum 1980; 23:492–7.
204. Alexander-Williams J, Buchmann P. Criteria of assessment for suitability and results of ileorectal anastomosis. Clin Gastroenterol 1980; 9:409–17.

Chapter 128

Inflammatory Bowel Disease and Cancer

Burton I. Korelitz

Ulcerative Colitis

Just as other organ systems affected by prolonged inflammation are at risk of developing neoplastic degeneration, so too is the colon involved with ulcerative colitis. There are 3 features of this specific carcinoma that differ from other neoplasms and create a challenging situation both diagnostically and therapeutically: (1) *The tumor is often multicentric in origin.*[1–3] This must in some way be attributable to the characteristic alternating inflammation and healing at multiple sites in the rectum and colon. Perhaps damaged but still vital mucosal cells are buried during the regeneration process and provide the nidus for neoplastic development. (2) *The tumor does not always allow reasonably easy diagnosis*[4,5] (Table 128–1). This is so because clinically, endoscopically, and radiologically there are 2 diseases occurring simultaneously. The colon involved with longstanding ulcerative colitis is usually shortened and narrowed, while the mucosa remains the site of active inflammation or has become atrophic. The early neoplasm, therefore, may not be surrounded by an area of normal mucosal relief and haustral pattern, the distortion of which leads to early recognition of carcinoma in the bowel not associated with ulcerative colitis. (3) *The carcinoma almost always occurs many years after the ulcerative colitis activity has waned,* a situation that provides a problem in patient compliance as well as a challenge in management[6–15] (Table 128–2).

Influence of Improved Management on Risk of Carcinoma. The most severe clinical manifestations of ulcerative colitis occur during the first 2 years of disease. Though the patient is susceptible to recurrences for a lifetime thereafter, recurrences statistically are less frequent and of less severity with time. Therefore, the proportion of patients needing colectomy for symptoms of the primary disease reaches its peak in the early years of the illness. Based on early studies, the frequency of surgical correction after 10 to 25 years of the disease was 14% to 66%,[15] the larger figures representing studies of patients with an onset in childhood. In effect, many of the most seriously involved colons were removed before they had the opportunity to develop a carcinoma, even though many carcinomas were found in the surgical specimens.

The medical management of ulcerative colitis has distinctly improved. With greater utilization of newer therapies the need for surgical intervention has been eliminated in some patients or postponed in others. Thus, a greater number of colons susceptible to carcinoma remain viable.

In large series of patients with ulcerative colitis followed over many years, the frequency of complicating carcinoma of the rectum or colon has averaged about 6% (Table 128–3).[8–10, 13, 15–21] When patients of all ages of onset are compared with other special groups including (1) those with onset in childhood (in whom the risk is markedly increased), (2)

Table 128–1. DIFFERENCES BETWEEN CARCINOMA OF COLON WITH AND WITHOUT ULCERATIVE COLITIS (UC)*

	Without UC	With UC
Ratio of frequency	1	10–30
Lesion identified by radiologist	99%	70%
Overhanging edges (by roentgenography)	+ + +	+
Stricture (by roentgenography)	+	+ + +
Recognition as carcinoma by radiologist	95%	40%
Combined clinical and pathologic accuracy	95%	57%
Multiple synchronous carcinomas	+	+ + + +
Average age at onset of carcinoma (years)	58	37
Distribution of sites of carcinoma	+ +	+ + + +
Mucoid type carcinoma	+	+ + +
Dysplasia	0	+ + +

*Modified from Korelitz et al.[4]

those who required colectomy for the primary bowel disease (in whom the risk is lower but still high), and (3) those assessed by the use of actuarial methods of analysis (showing the increased risk according to duration of disease), some sense of proportion is achieved as to the scope of the overall problem of carcinoma. Differing opinions of the true risk of cancer continue to appear.[21a, 21b]

Factors in Disposition to Carcinoma

Duration of Ulcerative Colitis. It has been well documented that the risk of carcinoma increases exponentially after 10 years of disease[8–15] (Tables 128–2 and 128–3). Among young patients followed for long periods of time, 5% will develop a carcinoma within 15 years and 10% within 25 years of onset of ulcerative colitis.[9] Using actuarial methods, the risk increases.[13, 22, 23] However, since reports of highest incidence come from centers that serve wide areas and/or attract the sickest patients,[13, 24] these issues, and perhaps many others, must be viewed in proper perspective. Though most carcinomas are diagnosed after 10 years or more of disease, programs for early diagnosis must consider the exceptional cases with early onset. I have observed a 17-year-old girl who underwent abdomino-perineal resection 5 years after the onset of ulcerative colitis and in whose extirpated bowel a carcinoma was found.[9]

Early Age of Onset. There is no proof that onset of ulcerative colitis in the first 2 decades of life carries a more specific risk of carcinoma as opposed to a later onset with the same duration. Devroede et al.[13] suggested that children whose disease began at ages 5 to 9 years might be particularly vulnerable. Perhaps the greater severity of disease with onset in childhood also has a role.

Severity of Initial Inflammation. There is no evidence that this is a predisposing factor. Nevertheless, the carcinoma must be based on earlier inflammation and I agree with others that this issue remains unresolved. In at least 16% of children who undergo colectomy for ulcerative colitis, a carcinoma is discovered in the surgical specimen when

Table 128–2. NATURAL HISTORY OF THE CARCINOMA (CA) OF THE COLON COMPLICATING ULCERATIVE COLITIS (UC)

	Age of Onset of UC		Age at Diagnosis of CA		Time from Diagnosis of UC Until Diagnosis of CA	
Reference	*Mean*	*Range*	*Mean*	*Range*	*Mean (Years)*	*Range (Years)*
11	All	—	—	—	21	9–40
	<20	—	—	—	16	—
	>20	—	—	—	25	—
12	24	10–50	44	26–62	21	8–40
10	—	—	41	20–72	—	—
8	10.5	—	<31	—	14	7–20
9	11.5	1–15	—	17–40	—	5–25
7	—	—	—	—	10.2	—

Table 128–3. CARCINOMA (CA) OF COLON AND RECTUM COMPLICATING ULCERATIVE COLITIS (UC)*

Reference	Total UC (No.)	CA		Cumulative Risk	
		(No.)	*(%)*	*Yrs of UC*	*%CA*
16	226	9	3.7	12	36.0†
17	245	9	3.7	—	—
10	624	22	3.5	20	12.6
18	637	15	4.6	—	—
21	—	—	—	20	5
19	95	6	6.3	—	—
8	401	40	10.0	—	—
9	85	8	9.5	—	—
13	396	52	13.0	20	23.0
				35	43.0
20	24	—	—	15–22	29.1
				25	16.5

*Age groups: All children.
†Operated cases.
Modified from Korelitz.[15]

active incapacitating disease is the most common indication for surgery.[9] Therefore, until there is an objective way for measuring severity and duration of inflammation and applying these to double-blind evaluation, the severity of the initial process must still be considered as possibly contributing to the pathogenesis.

Chronicity of Inflammation. The reasoning here is the same as with the severity of the initial inflammation. Inasmuch as surgically removed specimens have provided the highest yield of carcinomas[25] and colectomy is performed mostly for complications of chronic inflammation, it would seem that there should be a relationship between chronicity and disposition to cancer development.

Extent of Disease. It has been well documented that carcinoma most often occurs in the colon that is universally involved with ulcerative colitis.[4, 14, 22] *Universal* often is used to refer to roentgenologically demonstrable involvement of the colon from the rectum as far proximal as the hepatic flexure, since the wide cecum and ascending colon are not always conducive to sufficiently precise radiologic examination. Therefore, current disease, just as residual damage from previous involvement, can be missed. Even a grossly normal appearance of the right colon at colonoscopy does not rule out earlier involvement in this area.

Lack of universal involvement, conversely, is no protection against carcinoma. An increased risk has been noted when ulcerative colitis is limited to the left colon, though the time until development of the carcinoma is considerably longer.[23] This in itself should again raise consideration of the severity and chronicity of inflammation as contributing factors. No cases of carcinoma have been reported when the ulcerative colitis is limited to the rectal segment (proctitis) or the rectum and sigmoid (proctosigmoiditis).

Drug Treatment. There is no evidence that treatment with sulfasalazine, ACTH, corticosteroids, or immunosuppressives has increased the risk of carcinoma of the rectum or colon. The only 2 cases of carcinoma reported after treatment with an immunosuppressive occurred after ulcerative colitis of 13 and 14 years' duration,[26, 27] at a time when naturally occurring carcinoma is expected.

Diagnostic Radiation. Since radiation has been implicated as a causative factor in other carcinomas, its contributory role in neoplasms associated with ulcerative colitis is often mentioned. This is a valid concern since barium enema radiologic examinations are performed with some regularity in patients with ulcerative colitis, a disease that attacks mostly young people. Nevertheless, the role of radiation remains speculative since there are no objective data. If colonoscopy eventually reduces the need for barium enema studies, data might then be provided.

Natural History of Carcinoma Complicating Ulcerative Colitis. The risk of development of carcinoma apparently increases significantly after 10 years in the patient with universal disease, but the secure period of freedom from risk is not absolute. Most commonly, the carcinoma is diagnosed 14 to 17 years after the onset of ulcerative colitis. The most representative course is one of exacerbations and remissions of blood per rectum for 5 to 8 years, followed by apparent remission with normal-appearing rectal mucosa seen on proctosigmoidoscopy. Since ulcerative colitis is essentially a disease of young people, the remission often occurs during college years or at times of adjustment to marriage or to a career. If rectal bleeding resumes at 25 to 35 years of age, the patient assumes that the ulcerative colitis has recurred. In fact, however, the symptom could be a manifestation of carcinoma. If the bleeding is minor or transient, a visit to the gastroenterologist is apt to be postponed. Even if the colon is re-evaluated in a limited manner, such as proctosigmoidoscopy and/or barium enema examination, an early carcinoma in ulcerative colitis may be missed because it is so often flat and lacking the characteristic features. The yield has increased with the aid of colonoscopy and air-contrast barium enema examination.

The example of a 37-year-old woman who presented with metastases from a carcinoma of the transverse colon 22 years after the onset of ulcerative colitis, and after approximately 18 years of remission, accentuates the problem. Patient—and perhaps physician—denial contributes to the difficulties inherent in management.[4]

Whereas carcinomas of the colon unrelated to ulcerative colitis are more likely to occur in the rectum and distal left colon,[28] carcinomas associated with ulcerative colitis are more evenly divided among all segments of the colon. This is as would be expected if the universal distribution of the underlying disease process is a predisposing factor.

Pathology of Complicating Carcinoma. In almost all cases of malignant neoplasm complicating ulcerative colitis, the lesion is a carcinoma. Lymphomas occur rarely.[29] The carcinomas in about half the cases have the usual cauliflower-like, raised, ulcerated, or napkin ring appearances[30] (Fig. 128–1*A*). In the other cases the carcinoma commonly arises from a flat mucosa and can easily be missed radiologically[5], or develops in a stricture (Fig. 128–1*B*). Similarly, on proctosigmoidoscopy or colonoscopy the carcinomatous lesion may appear like the usual carcinoma or adenomatous or villous polyp unassociated with ulcerative colitis, or it may be characterized by a patch of granularity, smoothness, paleness, atrophy, fibrosis, or friability—or combinations of these. In the presence of pseudopolyps, an area with features that differ from the surrounding polypoid elevations warrants special attention. Microscopically, the lesion is a poorly differentiated mucinous or adenocarcinoma; about half are Dukes classification type C or D.[1,30] Scirrhous or signet ring cell carcinomas also occur, but are less common.[30] The tumor is often multicentric in origin.[1–3]. Survival rates are generally considered to be poorer than with ordinary colon cancer,[31] but reports to the contrary have been made.[32]

Management of Risk Factors

Total Proctocolectomy. When surgery is indicated in the course of ulcerative colitis, the operation of choice is total proctocolectomy, which eliminates the risk of carcinoma. Until just a few years ago, elective proctocolectomy was recommended for universal ulcerative colitis of 10 years or more duration. This proposal was unacceptable to most patients and physicians, however, because the ulcerative colitis had often been quiescent for extended periods. The introduction of surveillance programs to search for premalignant and malignant lesions has moderated, if not eliminated, the controversy that the recommendation of prophylactic proctocolectomy generated. At present, if a patient with ulcerative colitis of more than 10 years' duration has other indications for surgery that are borderline, the risk of carcinoma would serve to tip the balance in favor of colonic resection.

Subtotal colectomy does not eliminate the risk of carcinoma; the retained rectal segment, whether diverted[17,32a] or anastomosed to the ileum,[33] may be the site of development of a neoplasm. Whether the current surgical procedure involving anastomosis of the ileum to a sleeve of rectal muscle will eliminate the risk will require long follow-up; theoretically, it should do so if the mucosal surface of the retained rectal segment can be entirely stripped.

Gross Lesions. Several defects in the colon of ulcerative colitis patients may be revealed radiologically or endoscopically that require consideration of carcinoma.

PSEUDOPOLYPS. These inflammatory polyps of varied size and shape result from alternating inflammation and healing. They are neither malignant nor premalignant lesions. Nevertheless, the polyps can individually or

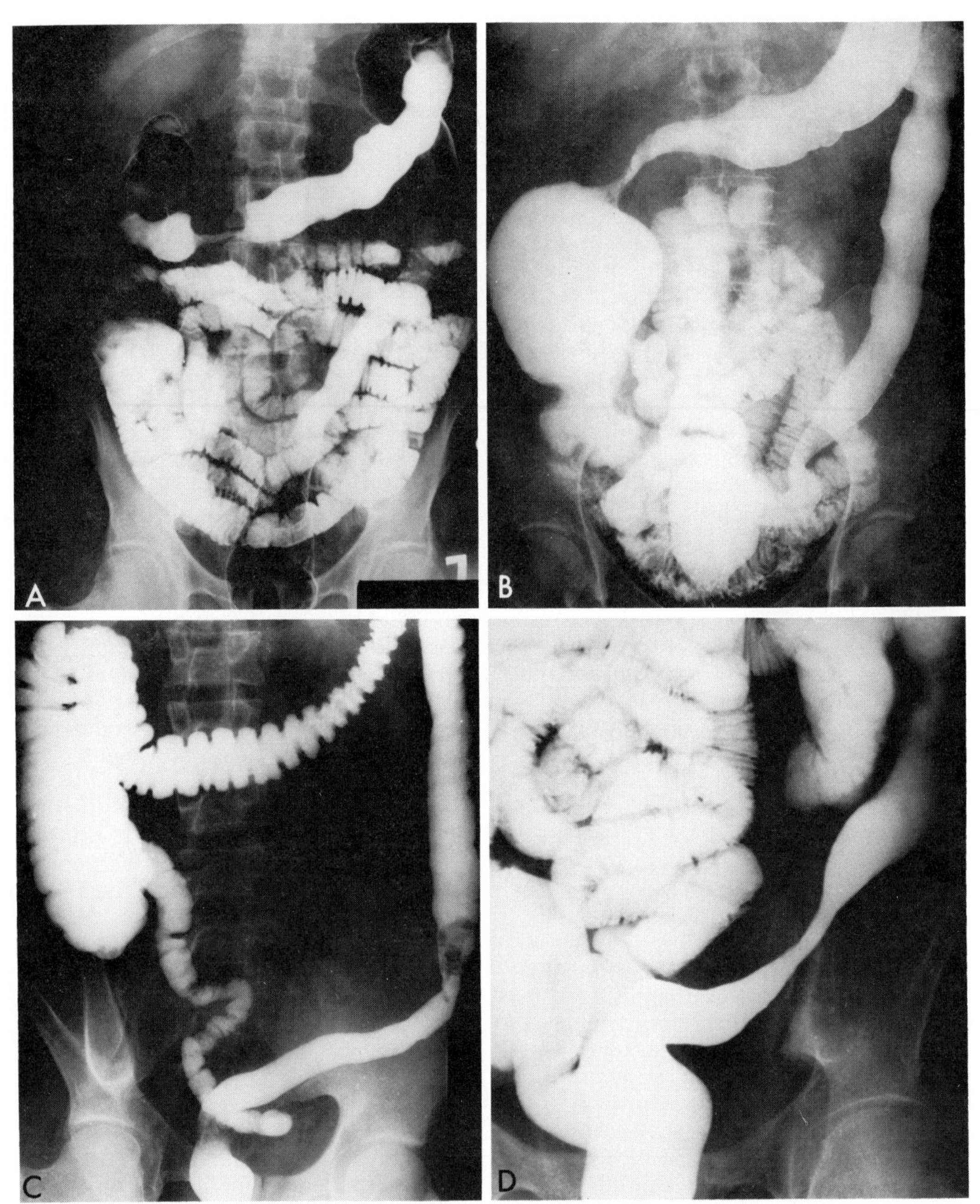

Figure 128–1. *A,* Barium enema study showing carcinoma of the transverse colon with "napkin-ring" appearance complicating ulcerative colitis of 25 years' duration. Rectal biopsy showed moderate dysplasia. *B,* Barium enema study showing stricture of the proximal transverse colon after ulcerative colitis of 25 years' duration. While the distal margin showed a tapering effect, the proximal margin suggested more of an "apple-core" lesion. Biopsies from the stricture showed mild dysplasia. The resected specimen disclosed adenocarcinoma proximal to the stricture. *C,* Barium enema study showing filling defects at the junction of the sigmoid and descending colons, raising consideration of carcinoma. On colonoscopy, the defects proved to be a collection of large pseudopolyps. *D,* Barium enema study showing benign stricture of the sigmoid colon after ulcerative colitis of 30 years' duration. Both ends of the stricture are smoothly tapered. The resected colon revealed no indication of either dysplasia or carcinoma.

collectively become so large (giant pseudopolyps) that they give the appearance of a mass while raising consideration of a carcinoma (Fig. 128–1C). In the rare situation when biopsies fail to exclude an underlying neoplasm satisfactorily, colectomy may be necessary.

In almost all instances, the physician experienced in endoscopy can recognize the benign pseudopolyp despite its varied size and shape by its texture and smooth configuration. However, when most of the colonic surface is distorted by these pseudopolyps, an underlying lesion can be missed by the most experienced endoscopist. More than the usual number of biopsies should be taken in such instances. Biopsies are also particularly warranted when the following are encountered: a pseudopolyp with an irregular surface, a polyp differing in color from its neighboring polyps, a polypoid lesion that is friable, or a pseudopolyp that is greater than 1 cm in size.[34]

ADENOMATOUS POLYPS. True polyps are far less frequent than pseudopolyps in the colon involved with ulcerative colitis, but they do occur. It is doubtful that an adenomatous polyp precedes all carcinomas in patients with ulcerative colitis or, indeed, that it predisposes to a carcinoma any more frequently than in the general population. Nevertheless, adenomatous polyps found in the colon of the ulcerative colitis patient should be removed.

STRICTURES. Strictures develop fairly often in the course of chronic inflammation of ulcerative colitis, with resultant narrowing, shortening, and imbalance of elasticity of the colonic muscle.[35] However, the ulcerative colitis colon tends to obscure the landmarks by which conventional carcinoma is recognized (Chapter 139), any stricture in patients with this disease *must be considered malignant* until proved otherwise. In fact, about one-third of the strictures mask a carcinoma.

The stricture is usually smooth and tapered at both ends (Fig. 128–1*D*). It may only be long enough to be recognizable as a stricture, or it may extend as far as 30 cm. If any part of the stricture exhibits roentgen features suggestive of a carcinoma, (Fig. 128–1*B*) colectomy is indicated. Otherwise the suspicious lesion should be carefully calculated by endoscopy and biopsy. The proctosigmoidoscope or colonoscope must be passed through the stricture and biopsy specimens taken from the proximal and distal edges, as well as from the stricture itself. Should the margins of the stricture be irregular, should there be an abrupt diminution in caliber, or should friability be a feature, the likelihood of carcinoma increases.

If the conventional instruments cannot be passed through the stricture, an attempt should be made with endoscopes of narrower caliber (pediatric instruments). If biopsy specimens cannot be obtained in this way, an attempt should be made to pass a brush through the stricture to obtain cells for cytologic study. Narrowness of the stricture to this extent in itself increases the index of suspicion. When the stricture cannot be adequately evaluated utilizing these methods, colectomy must be considered, even though the patient is asymptomatic and the odds favor that the stricture is benign. This is one of those situations in the management of ulcerative colitis where all objective findings and knowledge of the disease must be shared with the patient and the decision made on a partnership basis.

CONVENTIONAL CARCINOMA. Whenever cancer related to ulcerative colitis is discussed, emphasis is usually placed on lack of conventional features and multicentric origin. Yet, in perhaps one-third or more of cases the lesion has most or all of the same features seen radiologically or endoscopically in carcinoma unrelated to ulcerative colitis[30] (Fig. 128–1*A*).

DYSPLASIA-ASSOCIATED LESIONS OR MASS (DALM). This terminology was introduced to represent all gross mucosal abnormalities found in ulcerative colitis patients (by conventional barium enema study or double-contrast examination or endoscopy) that on biopsy reveal premalignant changes.[36] In 112 patients with longstanding ulcerative colitis, DALM was found in 12, including a single polyp in 5, multiple polyps in 5, and plaque-like lesions in 2. A carcinoma of the colon was eventually disclosed in 7 of these 12 patients, whereas only 1 carcinoma was found in 27 patients in whom dysplasia was found in biopsies taken at random as part of a surveillance program. Lesions, therefore, must be carefully sought at endoscopy with special attention paid to slightly elevated segments of colonic mucosa with deviant texture.

Dysplasia. Dysplasia in patients with ulcerative colitis[37,38] is thoroughly described in the Pathology section of Chapter 126. The value of recognizing dysplasia as a premalignant lesion in ulcerative colitis has also been summarized by Dobbins.[39] He found dysplasia in 88% of the colons removed from patients with ulcerative colitis of greater than 10 years' duration when the colons also harbored a carcinoma. In contrast, dysplasia was present in 13% of the colons without a carcinoma removed from patients with ulcerative colitis. The usefulness of the finding of dysplasia for purposes of surveillance remains to be determined and poses many questions:[4, 40] (1) Can dysplasia be classified so that its diagnosis and gradation can be recognized and this information exchanged by pathologists everywhere? (2) Can dysplasia be diagnosed in the presence of inflammation, or is it limited to periods or segments of inactivity? (3) Does dysplasia always signify a premalignant state, or is it reversible? (4) If the dysplasia is premalignant, by how long does it precede the development of malignancy? (5) Can lack of dysplasia be utilized to permit the asymptomatic patient with ulcerative colitis of long duration to retain his colon without risk.

The classification of dysplasia includes subdivision into degrees,[42] examples of which are shown in Figures 128–2 to 128–4. For purposes of prognosis and further simplification, the major categories of dysplasia are currently referred to as "high-grade" and "low-grade."

Inflammation can simulate dysplasia so that the finding of dysplasia has greatest value when the underlying ulcerative colitis is inactive. Dysplasia may also be reversible inasmuch as multiple repeat biopsies taken from the same area where dysplasia was originally found have been normal. This phenomenon is less likely to occur, however, when the dysplasia is classified closer to the severe spectrum than to the mild. Determination of the period of time that dysplasia precedes the development of carcinoma is particularly difficult. Based on those cases in which carcinoma had been preceded by dysplasia, a working "prodromal period" would be approximately 4 years.[11] Unfortunately, however, carcinoma may be found in one area of the colon at the same time that dysplasia is found (see Fig. 128–1*A*). Furthermore, carcinoma may be found without either preceding or coincident dysplasia. Had these cases been included in a prospective study, perhaps the dysplasia might have been recognized before the carcinoma.

Surveillance. In principle, recognition of dysplasia as a premalignant lesion should serve as a basis for a program of surveillance. This would allow the ulcerative colitis patient at risk for the development of carcinoma to retain his colon so long as no other indication for colectomy existed. At the same time, it would carry the tacit understanding that the discovery of severe dysplasia would lead to colectomy. These concepts have introduced considerable controversy as to the best means of finding the dysplasia, the frequency with which it should be sought, and the accuracy of the findings once obtained. The concept

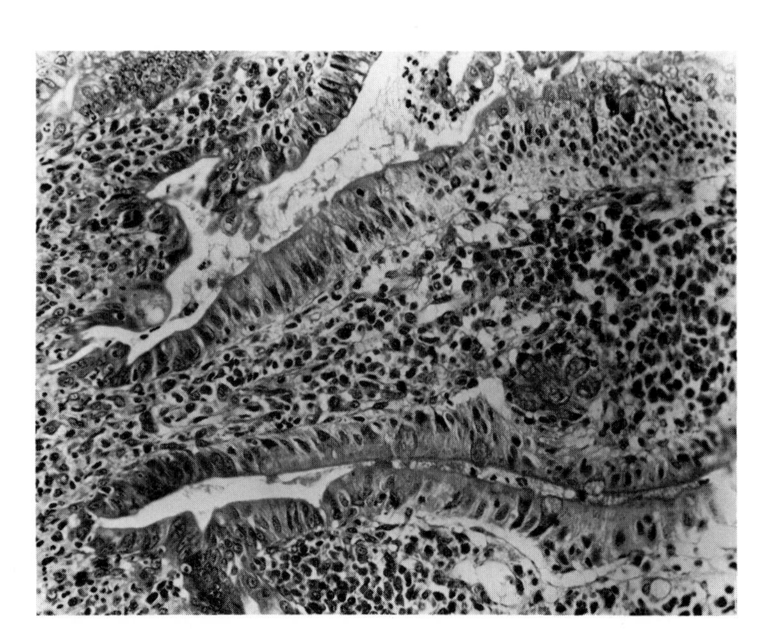

Figure 128–2. Slight dysplasia in ulcerative colitis with crowding and layering of crypt epithelium. (Hematoxylin and eosin, × 400.)

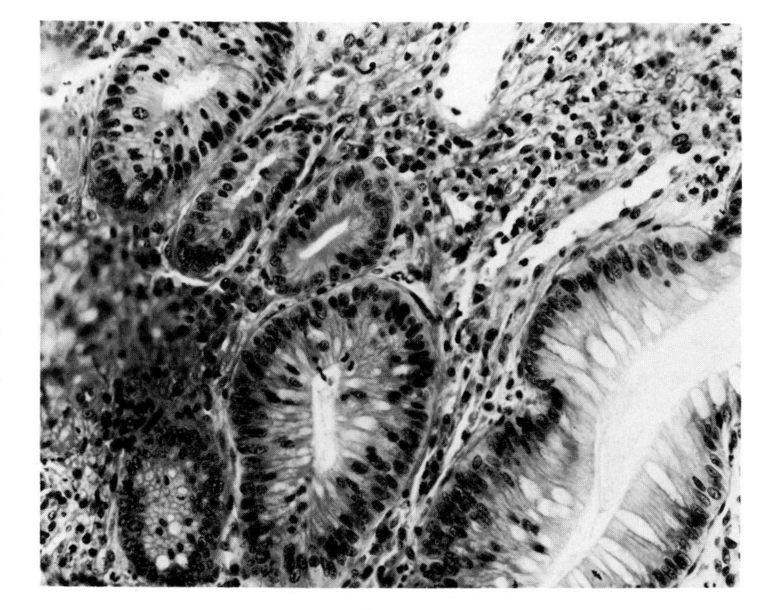

Figure 128–3. Moderate dysplasia in ulcerative colitis. Considerable crowding, stratification, and irregular arrangement of nuclei. (Hematoxylin and eosin, × 296.) (From Rotterdam H, Sommers C. Biopsy Diagnosis of the Digestive Tract. New York: Raven Press, 1981. Reproduced with permission.)

of surveillance emphasizes utilization of colonoscopy of the entire colon and multiple biopsies. The true value of both of these measures, however, remains theoretical until the results of long-term prospective studies become known. The issue of whether scattered biopsies of representative mucosa yielding tiny bits of tissue are accurate has not yet been adequately scrutinized. The yield of dysplasia has been much greater to date from rectal biopsies, but this must be tempered by the facts that the rectum has been the segment longest involved with the inflammatory process, the greater size and depth of rectal biopsy specimens, and the influence of multiple samples taken within a short segment of tissue. Also to be borne in mind is that surveillance studies do not always distinguish between biopsies taken from overt or suspicious lesions encountered at endoscopy and those taken from sites of apparently inactive ulcerative colitis.

Detection Procedures

RECTAL BIOPSY. Cooke and Goligher[3] found that dysplasia was present in some part of the large intestine in 15 of 19 surgical specimens of carcinoma from patients with ulcer-

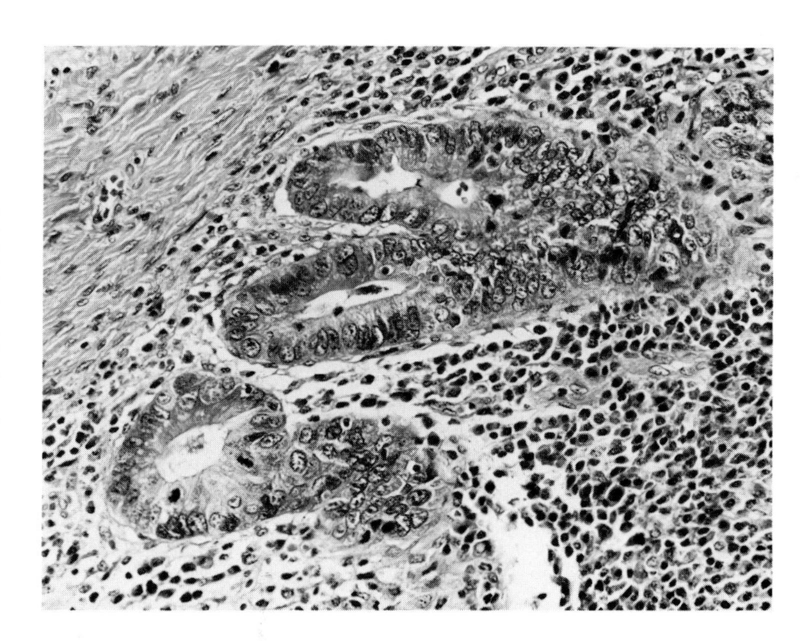

Figure 128–4. Severe dysplasia in ulcerative colitis. Considerable variation in nuclear size and staining. Most nuclei and nucleoli are enlarged. (Hematoxylin and eosin, × 173.) (From Rotterdam H, Sommers C. Biopsy Diagnosis of the Digestive Tract. New York: Raven Press, 1981. Reproduced with permission.)

ative colitis. The distribution of the dysplasia was patchy and frequently spared the rectum. The authors concluded from these observations that negative rectal biopsies were of no value in that they could miss even an established carcinoma situated more proximally in the colon. However, Cooke and Goligher did not actually perform rectal biopsies preoperatively; dysplasia in the rectal segment might have been found if multiple biopsies had been done. Proctosigmoidoscopy and rectal biopsy must still be considered, therefore, as having a potentially significant role as screening procedures, all the more so because of their relative simplicity as compared with colonoscopy and multiple biopsies.

On the negative side, there are many instances when dysplasia has not been found even close to an established carcinoma proximal to the rectum as well as not being found in the rectal mucosa on biopsy. Kewenter et al.[24] reported many instances of more proximally situated carcinoma as well as dysplasia without having found dysplasia on rectal biopsy. They do not clarify the method of taking the biopsies or the number of biopsies taken, however. Further, they do not specify how many of the biopsies taken at colonoscopy that showed dysplasia were obtained from specific lesions, suspicious areas, or uninvolved areas near the existing carcinoma or were merely multiple samplings of grossly uninvolved areas. The study of Kewenter et al. emphasizes the most recent colonoscopic biopsy findings; no information is provided on earlier surveillance procedures (when the yield should have been lower). For comparative purposes in evaluating colonoscopic and rectal biopsies as prophylactic surveillance procedures, both the duration of the disease and how many previous examinations were made should be noted.

Morson and Pang[38] first suggested rectal biopsy as a method of finding dysplasia. They reported on 148 patients with ulcerative colitis who had rectal biopsies. Of these, 54 later had colectomies and 16 (29%) were found to have dysplasia in the surgical specimen as well as in the biopsy; cancer was found in 5 of the 16. Myrvold et al.[43] found dysplasia in 18 of 47 patients with operated ulcerative colitis, including 7 who had rectal biopsies showing dysplasia. All 5 patients in whom a carcinoma was found had demonstrable dysplasia on rectal biopsy. Nugent et al.[12] described 8 patients with dysplasia on colonoscopy, in all of whom dysplasia was noted in the rectal biopsy specimen as well; 6 of the 8 were operated on and 2 had carcinoma. Riddell and Morson[44] observed 15 patients with carcinoma of the colon of whom 13 had rectal biopsies showing dysplasia. Of 22 patients showing dysplasia in the resected colon, 21 also had dysplasia on rectal biopsy. Therefore, if carcinoma was present, there was a 92% chance that it might have been foreseen by finding dysplasia on rectal biopsy. Riddell and Morson emphasized multiple biopsies because of the small foci of dysplasia seen in some instances. Fochios et al.[45] found many instances of dysplasia on rectal biopsy in which (1) no dysplasia was found more proximally on colonoscopic biopsies, and (2) the original dysplasia disappeared on repeated biopsies. Theoretically, the rectal segment in ulcerative colitis should be the one longest involved with the disease process and perhaps also the segment most severely affected. If multiple rectal biopsies were made in a studied search for dysplasia in ulcerative colitis, perhaps the yield of dysplasia, which may disappear and recur in its less severe form, would be increased.

COLONOSCOPY AND COLONIC BIOPSY. Colonoscopy, theoretically, should be the most dependable arm of a surveillance program because of its access to all segments of the colon. Its shortcomings include the small size of the biopsy specimens and the random sampling; there often is no specific lesion to biopsy and the pathologist is unable to clearly document dysplasia in the presence of inflammation. The results of studies of colonoscopic surveillance to date have been mostly retrospective, and these suffer from the fact that they include many patients with ulcerative colitis of very long duration who are examined for the first time when the yield is likely to be unrepresentatively high. The results of prospective studies are only now beginning to appear.

Lennard-Jones et al.[21] reported finding dysplasia in 13 of 229 colonoscopic biopsies; 7 patients were operated on and carcinoma was found in 5 (4 of which were Dukes classification A). Nugent et al.[12] described their experience with 36 patients with ulcerative colitis (average duration, 16 years) in which colonoscopic biopsies showed dysplasia in 8; 6 of the 8 had colectomies, which revealed carcinoma in 2 of the 6. Granqvist et al.[47] reported on 150 patients judged to have total colitis (duration greater than 10 years in 100) with dysplasia present in 12; cancer was found in one patient at a later date. Dickinson et al.[48] noted dysplasia in 9 of 43 cases ("longstanding") of colitis extending at least as far as the splenic flexure; in 2 of the 9 patients the dysplasia was severe; they were operated on and carcinoma was found in one. Williams[49] performed 231 colonoscopic examinations in 197 patients with total ulcerative colitis of 10 to 35 years' duration and uncovered dysplasia in 10%; carcinoma was found in half of those undergoing colectomy. Fuson et al.[50] make a clear distinction between the yields from surveillance observations and from diagnostic colonoscopic examinations. Their survey disclosed 11 cancers, 7 by means of biopsies of specific lesions and 4 by general surveillance. Seven patients underwent colectomy because dysplasia had been found on colonoscopic biopsy, and 5 of the 7 had cancer. Waye et al.[51] reported on the results of 238 colonoscopic studies in 188 patients similarly divided into diagnostic and surveillance groups. When specific lesions were biopsied in 125, dysplasia was found in 10; 3 were operated on, and one had a carcinoma (in a stricture). Another 6 patients had carcinoma without associated dysplasia. Therefore, in only 1 of 7 cases was carcinoma discovered because of dysplasia in the diagnostic group. Colonoscopy was performed for surveillance in 63 patients with universal disease of greater than 8 years' duration; 5 (8%) had dysplasia—one already had cancer at another site and 4 were followed for 3 years thereafter without any indication of cancer.

My personal experience now extends to more than 100 colonoscopic studies performed either as part of a surveillance program or for surveillance combined with the need to gather information about extent or severity. Dysplasia (mild or moderate) has been noted only 3 times. One patient had colectomy done as a consequence, and no cancer was found. In the other 2, dysplasia could not be verified on follow-up colonoscopy.

BARIUM ENEMA EXAMINATION. Enthusiasm for barium enema examination as a surveillance measure has dwindled because of its ability to detect only gross lesions, albeit with a high yield of carcinoma, and the attendant radiation exposure. However, advancement in the quality of roentgen study of the colon through use of air contrast methods has identified small, flat lesions that serve to direct the colonoscopist to specific sites where the yield of dysplasia and carcinomas is likely to be higher.[52] Furthermore, it is evident that not all carcinomas complicating ulcerative colitis are preceded by dysplasia and the barium enema study must still be relied on to recognize this group. In addition, some patients will not accept repeated colonoscopic examinations but are willing to tolerate the barium enema study with which they became familiar in the earlier phases of their illness. Against the use of serial roentgen examinations in a surveillance program is the as yet undetermined risk of provoking neoplastic changes by cumulative radiation to a colon already predisposed to carcinoma.

OTHER DIAGNOSTIC PROCEDURES. Ideally, measurement of serial carcinoembryonic antigen (CEA) levels should serve as an early indicator of premalignant or malignant degeneration.[53] Unfortunately, the CEA level has been shown to correlate with activity of the ulcerative colitis and possibly with the extent of disease so that its role in the detection of malignant changes is very limited.[54]

Brushing or lavaging the colonic mucosa during endoscopy for specimens to be examined cytologically for premalignant epithelial lesions has had a meaningful yield only in the hands of investigators well versed in these methods.[55,56]

Potential roles for thymidine uptake, specificity of immunoperoxidase staining reactions of biopsy specimens, or other indicators such as special stains to highlight zones of dysplasia are needed.[57–59]

Surveillance Program. While we await the long-term results of prospective studies using colonoscopy with multiple biopsies for the detection of dysplasia and while we accumulate experience in the management of the patient with dysplasia once it is found, some working program of surveillance is necessary. My current program for surveillance, based on consideration of all reported experience as well as my own, is shown in Table 128–4. As indicated, I favor colonoscopy biennially after 8 years of the disease; others[60, 61] advocate it on an annual basis.

The natural course of ulcerative colitis, however, does not lend itself to a program limited to surveillance. If there is constant or recurrent ulcerative colitis activity after the last colonoscopy, an earlier repeat examination or a barium enema is indicated. In patients who remain asymptomatic, there is as yet no evidence that the yield increases on

Table 128–4. PROGRAM FOR DETECTION OF CARCINOMA COMPLICATING ULCERATIVE COLITIS

1. Proctosigmoidoscopy and rectal biopsy
   a. Annually until 10 years
   b. Semi-annually after 10 years
2. Barium enema examination
   a. Biennially until 10 years*
   b. Annually after 10 years*
3. Colonoscopy and multiple biopsies
   a. Biennially after 8 years*
4. Colonic washings for cytologic study after 10 years (when available)

*More often if recurrent symptoms; less often if disease is quiescent and no suspicious lesions are found on previous examinations. (Modified from Korelitz BI. Inflammatory Bowel Disease, Experience and Controversy. Littleton, Massachusetts, and Bristol, England: John Wright • PSG, Inc., 1982: 175–8.)

an annual program compared with a biennial program. Furthermore, proctosigmoidoscopy with multiple biopsies has fully justified itself as an integral part of the surveillance program, and when no gross lesion has been demonstrated by barium enema or by the colonoscopy, it remains to be determined whether the yield of dysplasia is any less significant by this method. As already mentioned, the patient accustomed to proctosigmoidoscopy from the earlier years of ulcerative colitis is more apt to accept this procedure and therefore adopt a more cooperative attitude toward the surveillance program.

Management of Patient with Ulcerative Colitis and Dysplasia. Of definite concern is the management of the patient once dysplasia has been found by whatever method. If the dysplasia is of high grade, its severity agreed upon by highly experienced gastrointestinal pathologists, and its presence confirmed by repeat examination, colectomy is indicated. If the dysplasia is of low grade but was found in association with a mass lesion, colectomy must be considered. If the low-grade dysplasia is independent of any mass or other lesion and there are no other clinical indications for colectomy, the management decision may await a follow-up examination. This should be performed at some time within the next 6 to 12 months. When proctosigmoidoscopy or colonoscopy or both are done again at that time, biopsies should be taken at closer intervals. If the dysplasia is found once more but is still of low grade, a partnership decision must be made with the patient. If the dysplasia is no longer found, the surveillance program should continue as before.

Prognosis with Complicating Carcinoma. Despite the concentration on dysplasia and surveillance, carcinoma in ulcerative colitis is seen infrequently by gastroenterologists who have followed their patients closely and who recommend colectomy when other indications exist. In my own experience, carcinoma has been confined to patients who consulted me for the first time after years without surveillance or, in some cases, even without follow-up. In these patients, the lesion was always disclosed by barium enema examination.

Based on early studies (Table 128–5), carcinoma accounts for 20% to 50% of the mortality rate in ulcerative colitis.[15] If current efforts to perfect a surveillance program are successful, these figures should be reduced dramatically.

Crohn's Disease

Among the 10% of patients with Crohn's disease in whom the extent of involvement as revealed by roentgenography is limited to the colon, resolution of its differentiation from ulcerative colitis always carried the fringe benefit of freedom from risk of complicating carcinoma (Chapter 127). In the past, Crohn's disease in all of its subdivisions was not considered a premalignant pathologic process. Even with the early reports of carcinoma complicating regional ileitis[62] and regional jejunitis,[63] and acknowledgment that predisposing granulomatous inflammation of the small bowel increased the risk of superimposed carcinoma 10-fold, there was little concern, since carcinoma of the small bowel was so rare (3/100,000 patients) that even with this increased vulnerability it remained highly uncommon.

Table 128–5. ROLE OF CARCINOMA (CA) IN PROGNOSIS OF ULCERATIVE COLITIS*

Age Group	Reference Number	Death Due to CA
All ages	17	33%
	18	31%
	10	20%
Children	8	41%
	9	50%

*Survivors of early years of ulcerative colitis. (Modified from Korelitz.[15])

Carcinoma of the colon complicating granulomatous colitis was first reported in 1948.[64] Since Crohn's disease of the colon as a pathologic entity was not popularized until 1960,[65] attention was not drawn to its association with carcinoma of the colon until the report of Weedon et al.[66] These observers found a 20-fold increase in risk of cancer in patients who had the onset of their disease in childhood (2.2%) and therefore had a potentially long duration of the disease after onset. The average age at the time of diagnosis of cancer is about 46 years, younger than in the general population. Most of the carcinomas have been found in the right colon,[67–69] but many have also been disclosed in the rectum,[68, 69] the rectal stump after diversionary surgery,[70] and the anus.[71] In most cases, the carcinoma is found at a site of previous involvement with Crohn's disease, but there are many exceptions.

Currently it would seem that the risk of carcinoma in patients with Crohn's disease of the colon, although greater than in the population in general, is far less than that expected in universal ulcerative colitis but similar in magnitude to that found in left-sided ulcerative colitis.[72]

There are theoretical reasons to consider Crohn's disease still more vulnerable to complicating carcinoma than ulcerative colitis. Crohn's disease, too, is a disease of young people, but its activity does not diminish as in ulcerative colitis.[15] Crohn's disease is prone to recurrent bursts of activity for a lifetime. Furthermore, following surgical resection, extension to the next proximal segment is anticipated. Despite the lack of enthusiasm for surgery in Crohn's disease because of this phenomenon, surgical resections have been performed for incapacitating complications more often than in ulcerative colitis. It is perhaps because of these resections of the most diseased segments, which are performed relatively early in the course, that the risk of carcinoma is less than in ulcerative colitis.

There is also some evidence of a genetic predisposition to intestinal carcinoma in patients with Crohn's disease. In an epidemiologic study, 3.4% of patients with Crohn's disease had a mother or father with bowel carcinoma, including 8 involving the colon and one of the small bowel.[73]

Risk of Carcinoma. The prevalence of carcinoma of the intestinal tract in Crohn's disease has been reported to be 0.45%.[69] No figures based on actuarial methods are available. To date, approximately 100 instances of carcinoma in Crohn's disease have been reported. The average duration from the diagnosis of Crohn's disease to the diagnosis of the carcinoma is 15.5 years,[69] although a carcinoma has been found at the time of the first attack of ileitis.[74] Based on the cases accumulated to the present time, the following observations seem warranted:

1. The risk of carcinoma increases with the duration of Crohn's disease, similar to the situation in ulcerative colitis.[74]

2. The risk of carcinoma is particularly high (as high as 31%[74]) in loops of bowel involved with Crohn's disease that have been surgically bypassed.[75,76] In almost all instances the carcinoma arose in a segment of small bowel involved with ileitis; its origin in bypassed colon, whether or not involved in the original inflammatory process, could not always be excluded. The average period of time from the original diagnosis of Crohn's disease and from creation of the bypass until the discovery of carcinoma was 27 and 13 years, respectively.[76]

3. There are a sufficient number of reports of carcinoma occurring at the sites of Crohn's disease strictures to warrant special attention.[69] Presumably these have not been strictures caused by the carcinoma, since in almost all instances it is inferred that the stricture long preceded the carcinoma. One of the most common sites of carcinoma occurring in a Crohn's disease stricture is the rectum.

4. There are also a sufficient number of reports of carcinomas found at sites of persistent fistulization to warrant concern of specific predisposition at these locations.[69,70] Since a fistula often occurs in association with a stricture, these 2 situations might be related in regard to the carcinoma.

5. The relationship between carcinoma of the small bowel and ileitis is statistically significant.[77,78] Although rare, carcinoma of the small bowel in the general population occurs more often in the jejunum and at an older age, while that following ileitis occurs in the ileum and at a younger age.

6. Carcinoma of the rectum and colon in Crohn's disease usually occurs at a site of previous involvement with the inflammatory process[66, 67]; this cannot always be verified, however, and in some instances it occurs in segments of colon or rectum that are clearly uninvolved.[68]

7. There are many reports of neoplasms complicating Crohn's disease occurring at sites far distant in the gastrointestinal tract[68, 78] and in extraintestinal organs.[68, 69] Whether the frequency of these neoplasms that do not occur at the site of earlier granulomatous inflammation is statistically significant has not yet been determined.

Since the neoplasm in Crohn's disease is so difficult to diagnose, the first recognized manifestations often are those related to spread of the tumor. These include rapid deterioration in general condition, weight loss, anemia, fatigue, and perhaps a palpable mass. In 39 of 58 cases of carcinoma in the small bowel collected from the literature, the indication for the surgery that led to disclosure of the carcinoma was intestinal obstruction. Similarly, in 10 of 29 cases of carcinoma of the colon reviewed,[78a] the indication for surgery was a fistula, while in another 3 it was an obstruction. There are many reports of multifocal involvement.[69, 79, 80] Lymphomas have also been reported to occur at sites of bowel involved with Crohn's disease.[81, 82]

A 5-year mortality rate of 82% has been reported for carcinoma complicating Crohn's disease[68] and a mean survival time of 7.8 months.[83]

Therapeutic Implications of the Risk of Carcinoma. Since the risk of carcinoma in Crohn's disease appears to be small, surgical resection is indicated only for the inflammatory disease and its complications, and not for prophylaxis for malignancy (Chapter 127). Rarely is the cancer diagnosed preoperatively; much more often it is found in the surgical specimen after resection for obstruction or some other reason.

The Bypassed Loop. In the early days of surgical management following the original description of regional ileitis, a bypass procedure leaving the involved segment *in situ* was commonplace. Although this operation has been discarded in favor of resection, bypasses established many years ago present a problem in management that is controversial.[84] Among the problems is the propensity of the bypassed bowel to develop carcinoma and its inaccessibility to roentgenologic and endoscopic examination. This and other problems are considered in the section on "Surgical Management of Crohn's Disease" (Chapter 127).

Strictures. Narrowing in the small bowel in Crohn's disease cannot usually be reached endoscopically. If the narrowed segment is not responsible for obstruction, it is not *per se* an indication for surgery despite concern for an underlying carcinoma. This pertains as well to strictures in the colon that cannot be reached and biopsied by means of colonoscopy. Those strictures that can be reached with the colonoscope should be examined and biopsies obtained from within the stricture and from adjoining areas. If the findings are negative, re-examinations should *arbitrarily* be conducted every 2 years so long as the patient is asymptomatic. Symptoms such as progressive obstruction, recurrence of mucoid diarrhea, or rectal bleeding would warrant earlier examination. Rectal strictures are the most accessible and can be re-examined more often. If strictures cannot be entered with the endoscope, a brush should be advanced through the lumen to obtain cells for cytologic study. Barium roentgenography suggesting a neoplasm or malignant change in a Crohn's disease stricture should serve as an indication for resection.

Fistulas. These complications are sufficiently common in Crohn's disease as to rarely in themselves suggest an underlying carcinoma. When exudative output from enteroenteric or abdominal wall fistula is not reduced at all by drug therapy (especially by 6-mercaptopurine) or by total parenteral nutrition, and particularly when the fistula occurs just proximal to a bowel stricture, an underlying carcinoma should be considered. Again, if barium roentgenography suggests a carcinoma in the bowel or neoplastic changes in a stricture at the source of the fistula, this would provide an indication for resection.

Surveillance. The view has been advanced that the risk of carcinoma in Crohn's disease is sufficiently low that there is no practical value in conducting a surveillance program for early lesions. Nevertheless, dysplasia of the same premalignant variety as seen in the patients with longstanding ulcerative colitis has been noted in one-third of the cases of small bowel carcinoma complicating Crohn's disease.[85,86] At Lenox Hill Hospital, transient dysplasia has been seen in rectal biopsies of normal-appearing mucosa, in rectal biopsies of mucosa adjoining strictures, and in a surgical specimen of mucosa adjoining a carcinoma complicating Crohn's disease of the colon. Therefore, some surveillance seems warranted, whether the lesser risk will prevail or whether, with sufficient follow-up, carcinoma will prove to be as frequent as in ulcerative colitis.

Because deformity of the colon due to the inflammatory process of Crohn's disease is likely to be more marked than in ulcerative colitis, surveillance will depend more on colonoscopy than on the barium enema. Arbitrarily, colonoscopy might be performed every 3 years after 10 years of disease (regardless of the extent of involvement) when the Crohn's disease is inactive; annually if the patient is symptomatic. In some instances, the opportunity to enter and biopsy the terminal ileum could prove to be a fringe benefit. Sonography may also have a contributory role in a surveillance program in Crohn's disease.

Extra-intestinal Cancer

There is nothing about IBD that protects the patient from developing cancer in structures other than the gut. In this regard, the patient with IBD probably differs little from other persons. One clear exception, however, is biliary tract cancer, particularly cancer of the bile ducts (Chapter 199). Accumulated data indicate that this relatively uncommon form of cancer occurs more often in those with ulcerative colitis than in the population at large.[87] Predisposition to bile duct cancer might be related to the fact that patients with ulcerative colitis are more liable to develop sclerosing cholangitis (Chapter 164). In many cases, however, the bile duct cancer appears to have evolved independently and in the absence of preceding cholangitis.[88]

Cancer as it affects various structures of the digestive system is fully covered in those chapters dealing with these subjects and needs no further discussion here. Likewise, detailed reviews of sclerosing cholangitis and of bile duct cancer can be found in Chapters 164 and 199, respectively.

References

1. Shands WC, Dockerty MD, Bargen JA. Adenocarcinoma of the large intestine associated with chronic ulcerative colitis; clinical and pathological features of 73 cases. Surg Gynecol Obstet 1952; 94:302–19.
2. Morson BC. Cancer in ulcerative colitis. Gut 1966; 7:426–36.
3. Cooke MG, Goligher J. Carcinoma and epithelial dysplasia complicating ulcerative colitis. Gastroenterology 1975; 68:1127–36.
4. Korelitz BI, Pearlmutter N, Sommers SC, Waye JD, Shapiro S, Sohn N, Hoffman I, Fein H, Wechsler RL. Carcinoma complicating ulcerative colitis. Dig Dis Sci 1980; 24:216–27.
5. Fennessy JJ, Sparberg MB, Kirsner JB. Radiological findings in carcinoma of the colon complicating chronic ulcerative colitis. Gut 1968; 9:388–97.
6. Gleckler WJ, Brown CH. Carcinoma of the colon complicating chronic ulcerative colitis. Gastroenterology 1950; 14:458–64.
7. Weckesser EC, Chinn AB. Carcinoma of the colon complicating ulcerative colitis. JAMA 1953; 152:905–8.
8. Michener WM, Gage RP, Sauer WG, Stickler GB. The prognosis of chronic ulcerative colitis in children. N Engl J Med 1961; 265:1075–9.
9. Korelitz BI, Gribetz D, Danziger I. The prognosis of ulcerative colitis with onset in childhood. I. The pre-steroid era. Ann Intern Med 1962; 57:582–91.
10. Edwards FC, Truelove SC. The course and prognosis of ulcerative colitis. IV. Carcinoma of the colon. Gut 1964; 5:15–22.
11. Diamond MP, Yardley JH, Bayless TM, Roberts J. Colon carcinoma and severe epithelial dysplasia in patients with ulcerative colitis. Gastroenterology 1978; 74:1120.
12. Nugent FW, Haggitt RC, Colcher H, Kutteruf GC. Malignant potential of chronic ulcerative colitis. Gastroenterology 1979; 76:1–5.
13. Devroede GJ, Taylor WF, Sauer WG, Jackman RJ, Stickler GB. Cancer risk and life expectancy in children with ulcerative colitis. N Engl J Med 1971; 285: 17–21.
14. Butt JH, Lennard-Jones JE, Ritchie JK. A practical approach to the cancer risk in inflammatory bowel disease. Med Clin North Am 1980; 64:1203–20.
15. Korelitz BI. Prognosis in inflammatory bowel disease—a North American View. *In*: Kirsner JB, Shorter RG, eds. Inflammatory Bowel Disease. 2nd Ed. Philadelphia: Lea & Febiger, 1980: 645–60.
16. Lyons AS, Garlock JH. Relationship of chronic ulcerative colitis to carcinoma. Gastroenterology 1951; 18:170–8.
17. Banks B, Korelitz BI, Zetzel L. The course of non-specific ulcerative colitis: Review of twenty years experience and late results. Gastroenterology 1957; 32:983–1012.
18. MacDougall IPM. The cancer risk in ulcerative colitis. Lancet 1964; 2:655–8.
19. Jackman RJ, Bargen JA, Helmholz HF. Life histories of ninety-five children with ulcerative colitis. Am J Dis Child 1940; 59:459–67.
20. Rosenquist H, Ohrling H, Lagercrantz R, Edling N. Ulcerative colitis and carcinoma coli. Lancet 1959; 1:906–8.
21. Lennard-Jones JE, Morson BC, Ritchie JK, Shove DC, Williams CB. Cancer in colitis: Assessment of the individual risk by clinical and histological criteria. Gastroenterology 1977; 73:1280–9.
21a. Katzka I, Brody RS, Morris E, Katz S. Assessment of colorectal cancer risk in patients with ulcerative colitis: Experience from a private practice. Gastroenterology 1983; 85:22–9.
21b. Yardley JH, Ransohoff DF, Riddell RH, Goldman H. Cancer in inflammatory bowel disease: How serious is the problem and what should be done about it? (Editorial). Gastroenterology 1983; 85:197–9.
22. Devroede GS, Taylor WF. On calculating cancer risk and survival of ulcerative colitis patients with the life table method. Gastroenterology 1976; 71:505–9.
23. Greenstein AJ, Sachar DB, Smith H, Pucillo A, Papatestas AE, Kreel I, Geller SA, Janowitz HD, Aufses AH Jr. Cancer in universal and left-sided ulcerative colitis: Factors determining risk. Gastroenterology 1979; 77:290–4.
24. Kewenter J, Hulten L, Ahren C. The occurrence of severe epithelial dysplasia and its bearing on treatment of long-standing ulcerative colitis. Ann Surg 1981; 195:209–13.
25. Sloan WP, Bargen JA, Gage RP. Life histories of patients with ulcerative colitis. Gastroenterology 1950; 16:25–38.
26. Patterson JF, Norton RA, Schwartz RS. Azathioprine treatment of ulcerative colitis, granulomatous colitis and regional enteritis. Dig Dis Sci 1971; 16:327–32.
27. Theodor E, Niv Y, Bat L. Imuran in the treatment of ulcerative colitis. Am J Gastroenterol 1981; 76:262–6.
28. Welch CE, Burke JF. Carcinoma of the colon and rectum. N Engl J Med 1962; 266:211–9.

29. Wagonfeld JB, Platz CE, Fishman FL, Sigley RK, Kirsner JB. Multicentric colonic lymphoma complicating ulcerative colitis. Dig Dis Sci 1977; 22:502–8.
30. Rotterdam H, Sommers SC. Biopsy Diagnosis of the Digestive Tract. New York: Raven Press, 1981.
31. Devroede GJ, Dockerty MB, Sauer WG, Jackman RJ, Stickler GB. Cancer of the colon in patients with ulcerative colitis since childhood. Can J Surg 1972; 15:369–74.
32. Thorlakson RH. Carcinoma of the colon and rectum associated with chronic ulcerative colitis. Surg Gynecol Obstet 1956; 130:41–50.
32a. Korelitz BI, Dyck P, Klion FM. Fate of the rectum and distal colon after subtotal colectomy for ulcerative colitis. Gut 1969; 10:198–201.
33. Aylett SO. Cancer and ulcerative colitis. Br Med J 1971; 2:203–5.
34. Waye JD. Where has colonoscopy had its greatest value in the management of inflammatory bowel disease? *In*: Korelitz BI, ed. Inflammatory Bowel Disease, Experience and Controversy. Littleton, Massachusetts, and Bristol, England: John Wright · PSG Inc., 1982: 87–90.
35. Marshak RH, Bloch C, Wolf BS. The roentgen findings in strictures of the colon associated with ulcerative and granulomatous colitis. AJR 1963; 90:709–16.
36. Blackstone MO, Riddell RH, Rogers BHG, Levin B. Dysplasia associated lesion or mass (DALM) detected by colonoscopy in long-standing ulcerative colitis: An indication for colectomy. Gastroenterology 1981; 80:366–74.
37. Dawson IMP, Pryse-Davies J. The development of carcinoma of the large intestine in ulcerative colitis. Br J Surg 1959; 47:113–28.
38. Morson BC, Pang LSC. Rectal biopsy as an aid to cancer control in ulcerative colitis. Gut 1957; 8:423–34.
39. Dobbins WO III. Current status of the precancer lesion in ulcerative colitis. Gastroenterology 1977; 73:1431–3.
40. Sommers SC. The problems arising in diagnosis of dysplasia as a premalignant lesion in ulcerative colitis. *In*: Korelitz BI, ed. Inflammatory Bowel Disease, Experience and Controversy. Littleton, Massachusetts, and Bristol, England: John Wright · PSG Inc., 1982: 161–74.
41. Proceedings of the Pathology Conference, National Foundation for Ileitis and Colitis, Inc. Tarrytown, New York, October 29–30, 1977.
42. Riddell RH, Goldman H, Ransohoff DF, Appelman HD, Fenoglio CM, Haggitt RC, Ahren C, Correa P, Hamilton SR, Morson BC, Sommers SC, Yardley JH. Dysplasia in inflammatory bowel disease: Standard classification with provisional clinical application. Hum Pathol 1983; 14:931–68.
43. Myrvold HE, Kock NG, Ahren C. Rectal biopsy and precancer in ulcerative colitis. Gut 1974; 15:301–4.
44. Riddell RH, Morson BC. Value of sigmoidoscopy and biopsy in detection of carcinoma and premalignant change in ulcerative colitis. Gut 1979; 20:575–80.
45. Fochios SE, Kapadia L, Sommers SC, Korelitz BI. The role of rectal biopsy in surveillance for carcinoma of the rectum and colon complicating ulcerative colitis. Am J Gastroenterol 1980; 74:81.
46. Korelitz BI. A surveillance program for carcinoma of the rectum and colon in patients with ulcerative colitis: The role of rectal biopsies performed at sigmoidoscopy. Second International Symposium on Colo-Rectal Cancer. Washington, DC, March, 1981.
47. Granqvist S, Granberg-Ohman I, Sundelin P. Colonoscopic biopsies and cytological examination in chronic ulcerative colitis. Scand J Gastroenterol 1980; 15:283–8.
48. Dickinson RJ, Dixon MF, Axon ATR. Colonoscopy and the detection of dysplasia in patients with long-standing ulcerative colitis. Lancet 1980; 2:620.
49. Williams CB. Colonoscopy and precancer in chronic ulcerative colitis. Second International Symposium on Colo-Rectal Cancer. Washington, DC, March, 1981.
50. Fuson JA, Farmer RG, Hawk WA, Sullivan BH. Endoscopic surveillance for cancer in chronic ulcerative colitis. Second International Symposium on Colo-Rectal Cancer. Washington, DC, March, 1981.
51. Waye JD, Braunfeld S, Geller S. Dysplasia and ulcerative colitis: A colonoscopy study. Gastroenterology 1982; 82(Pt 2):1208.
52. Frank PH, Riddell RH, Feczko PJ, Levin B. Radiological detection of colonic dysplasia (precarcinoma) in chronic ulcerative colitis. Gastroenterology 1975; 3:209–19.
53. Rule AH, Goleski-Reilly C, Sachar DB, Vande Voorde J, Janowitz HD. Circulating carcinoembyronic antigen (CEA): Relationship to clinical studies of patients with inflammatory bowel disease. Gut 1972; 14:880–4.
54. Gardner RC, Feinerman AE, Kantrowitz PA, Gootblatt S, Lowenstein MS, Zamcheck N. Serial carcinoembryonic antigen (CEA) blood levels in patients with ulcerative colitis. Dig Dis Sci 1978; 23(2):129–33.
55. Granqvist S, Gabrielsson N, Sundelin P, Thorgeirsson T. Precancerous lesions in the mucosa in ulcerative colitis: A radiographic, endoscopic and histopathologic study. Scand J Gastroenterol 1980; 15:289–96.
56. Katzka I, Platt N, Haydn EO, Bassett E. Carcinoma in chronic ulcerative colitis. Diagnostic role of segmental colonic lavage. Dig Dis Sci 1977; 22:355–64.
57. Fenoglio CM, Haggett RC, Hamilton SR, Lumb G, Pascal RR, Riddell RH. Colonic dysplasia (a symposium). Pathol Ann 1981; 1:181–213.
58. Sherlock P. Future thrusts in the detection of cancer in inflammatory bowel disease. Second International Symposium on Colo-Rectal Cancer. Washingtion, DC, March, 1981.
59. Yardley JH, Bayless TM, Diamond TM. Cancer in ulcerative colitis. Gastroenterology 1979; 76:221–4.
60. Sachar DB, Greenstein AJ. Cancer in ulcerative colitis: Good news and bad news. Ann Intern Med 1981; 95:642–4.
61. Levin B, Riddell RH, Kirsner JB. Management of precancerous lesionsf jejunum occurring in a case of regional enteritis. Surgery 1956; 39:347–51.
62. Ginzburg L, Schneider KM, Dreizin DH, Levinson C. Carcinoma of jejunum occurring in a case of regional enteritis. Surgery 1956; 39:347–51.
63. Kornfeld P, Ginzburg L, Adlersberg D. Adenocarcinoma occurring in regional jejunitis. Am J Med 1957; 23:493.
64. Warren S, Sommers SC. Cicatrizing enteritis (regional ileitis) as a pathologic entity. Am J Pathol 1948; 24:475–510.
65. Lockhart-Mummery HE, Morson BC. Crohn's disease (regional enteritis) of the large intestine and its distinction from ulcerative colitis. Gut 1960; 1:87–105.
66. Weedon DD, Shorter RG, Ilstrup DM, Huizenga KA, Taylor WT. Crohn's disease and cancer. N Engl J Med 1973; 289:1099–103.
67. Lightdale CJ, Sternberg SS, Posner G, Sherlock P. Carcinoma complicating Crohn's disease: Report of seven cases and review of the literature. Am J Med 1975; 59(2):262–8.
68. Greenstein AJ, Sachar DB, Smith H, Janowitz HD, Aufses AH Jr. Patterns of neoplasia in Crohn's disease and ulcerative colitis. Cancer 1980; 46:403–7.
69. Korelitz BI. Carcinoma of the intestinal tract in Crohn's disease: Results of a survey conducted by the National Foundation for Ileitis and Colitis. Am J Gastroenterol 1983; 78:44–6.
70. Traube J, Simpson S, Riddell RH, Path MRC, Levin B, Kirsner JB. Crohn's disease and adenocarcinoma of the bowel. Dig Dis Sci 1980; 25:939–44.
71. Daly JJ, Madrazo A. Anal Crohn's disease with carcinoma in situ. Dig Dis Sci 1980; 24:464–6.
72. Greenstein AJ, Sachar DB, Smith H, Janowitz HD, Aufses AH Jr. A comparison of cancer risk in Crohn's disease and ulcerative colitis. Cancer 1981; 48:2742–5.
73. Korelitz BI. From Crohn to Crohn's disease: 1979. An epidemiologic study in New York City. Mt Sinai J Med 1979; 46:533–40.
74. Fresko D, Lazarus SS, Doton J, Reingold M. Early presentation of carcinoma of the small bowel in Crohn's disease ("Crohn's carcinoma"): Case reports and review of the literature. Gastroenterology 1982; 82:783–9.
75. Brown N, Weinstein VA, Janowitz HD. Carcinoma of the ileum 25 years after bypass for regional enteritis: A case report. Mt Sinai J Med 1971; 37:675–7.
76. Greenstein AJ, Sachar D, Pucillo A. Cancer in Crohn's disease after diversionary surgery. Am J Surg 1978; 135:86–90.
77. Darke SG, Parks AG, Grogono JL, Pollock DJ. Adenocarcinoma and Crohn's disease. Br J Surg 1973; 60:169–75.
78. Gyde SN, Prior P, Macartney JC, Thompson H, Waterhouse

JAH, Allan RN. Malignancy in Crohn's disease. Gut 1980; 21:1024–9.
78a. Cooper DJ, Weinstein MA, Korelitz BI. Complications of Crohn's disease predisposing to dysplasia and cancer of the intestinal tract: Consideration of a surveillance program. J Clin Gastroenterol 1984; in press.
79. Keighley MRB, Thompson H, Alexander-Williams J. Multifocal colonic carcinoma and Crohn's disease. Surgery 1975; 78(4):534–7.
80. Castellano TJ, Frank MS, Brandt LS, Mahadevia P. Metachronous carcinoma complicating Crohn's disease. Arch Intern Med 1981; 141:1074–5.
81. Codling BW, Keighley MRB, Slaney G. Hodgkin's disease complicating Crohn's colitis. Surgery 1977; 82(5):625–8.
82. Collins WJ. Malignant lymphoma complicating regional enteritis: Case report and review of the literature. Am J Gastroenterol 1977; 68(2):177–81.
83. Hoffman JP, Taft DA, Wheelis RF, Walker JH. Adenocarcinoma in regional enteritis of the small intestine. Arch Surg 1977; 112:606–11.
84. Collected letters. Small bowel cancer and Crohn's disease. Correspondence Society of Surgeons 1982; 5:1–7.
85. Craft CF, Mendelsohn G, Cooper HS, Yardley JH. Colonic "precancer" in Crohn's disease. Gastroenterology 1981; 80:578–84.
86. Simpson S, Traube J, Riddell RH. The histologic appearance of dysplasia (precarcinomatous change) in Crohn's disease of the small and large intestine. Gastroenterology 1981; 81:492–501.
87. Ritchie JK, Allan RN, Macartney J, Thompson H, Hawley PR, Cooke WT. Biliary tract carcinoma associated with ulcerative colitis. Q J Med 1974; 43:263–79.
88. Converse CF, Reagan JW, DeCosse JJ. Ulcerative colitis and carcinoma of the bile ducts. Am J Surg 1971; 121:39–45.

Chapter 129

Inflammatory Bowel Disease and Reproduction

Tuvia Gilat • Yoram Bujanover

The reciprocal relationship between inflammatory bowel disease (IBD) and the human reproductive process is now better understood and documented. Large-scale studies performed during the last decade have substantiated some previously held medical opinions and refuted others. It is also possible that the clinical situation has changed somewhat and that recent findings reflect a better level of medical care.

Fertility

Female Fertility in Ulcerative Colitis. Most recent studies have found the fertility of women with ulcerative colitis (UC) to be within the normal range (Table 129–1). Fertility, defined as the percentage of women able to conceive, is approximately 90%, about the same as that of the healthy population in several study areas.[2–4] Criteria had to be standardized to make the various studies comparable. Thus, only married women having UC during their reproductive years (15 to 44) were included in the analyses. Excluded were women who were unable to conceive because of hysterectomy or other reasons, who were unwilling to conceive, or who had completed their family prior to the onset of UC. Some investigators compared the number of pregnancies per woman in patients with UC with the healthy population of the area and found the numbers to be quite similar.[3,4] Studies conducted during earlier decades, such as those by de Dombal et al.[1] and Banks et al.[5] had found a reduced fertility of 31% to 42%. This may relate to less rigorous selection of patients, shorter follow-up, or less effective medical therapy.

Fertility in women was found to be reduced following total colectomy and ileostomy.[6,7] This was less marked after ileorectal anastomosis and was thought to be related to the local effects of proctectomy, such as tubal obstruction and damage to the vagina.

Female Fertility in Crohn's Disease. The findings of studies of fertility in Crohn's disease (CD) are shown in Table 129–1. While some investigators found a near normal fertility, most studies investigating large numbers of patients have concluded that fertility in women with CD is reduced to the 60% range. Among the suggested causes are in-

Table 129–1. FERTILITY IN WOMEN WITH ULCERATIVE COLITIS AND CROHN'S DISEASE

References	No. of Women	% Fertile
	Ulcerative Colitis	
de Dombal et al.,1965[1]	229	31
Webb and Sedlack, 1974[2]	61	90
Ganchrow and Benjamin, 1975[3]	34	88
Willoughby and Truelove, 1980[4]	129	92
	Crohn's Disease	
Crohn et al., 1956[13]	85	62
Fielding and Cooke, 1970[8]	77	68
de Dombal et al., 1972[12]	86	47
Norton and Patterson, 1972[14]	20	90
Ganchrow and Benjamin, 1975[3]	17	94
Homan and Thorbjarnarson, 1976[9]	78	33

flammatory damage to the pelvic organs, including tubal obstruction, fistulas, pelvic inflammatory mass, and abscess.[8–10]

In the more extensive studies in which fertility was found to be reduced, the average number of pregnancies per woman was also found to be somewhat diminished in comparison with the healthy population of the area.[9,11] There is some controversy as to whether fertility is reduced more in women with colonic CD than in women with CD of the small bowel. Some investigators found such a difference,[8] while others did not.[9,12] The study by de Dombal et al.[12] reported that fertility rose after surgery for CD, reaching almost normal levels.

Male Fertility in Inflammatory Bowel Disease. Investigation of infertility in married couples who both had IBD sometimes showed normal fertility in the wife and impaired fertility in the husband. The number, motility, and morphology of the spermatozoa were found to be abnormal. This does not seem to be related to the IBD but rather to sulfasalazine therapy (discussed later).

Proctectomy may interfere with sexual function and ejaculation and reduce fertility.[6]

Effect of Inflammatory Bowel Disease on Pregnancy

Ulcerative Colitis. The outcome of pregnancy in patients with UC was found to be similar to that in the healthy population (Table 129–2). The major parameters used to assess the outcome of pregnancy are: (1) *The percentage of normal live births.* This has been about 80% in most studies, corresponding closely to the expected percentage in the normal population of the various study areas. (2) *The percentage of spontaneous abortions.* In most studies this was found to be close to 10%, again similar to the expected rate in normal subjects. (3) *The percentage of therapeutic abortions.* This is a more arbitrary and subjective parameter that reflects both temporal and geographic variations in medical opinion and judgment. Some abortions are performed on social and not medical grounds. Currently, *therapeutic abortion is not recommended for medical reasons associated with IBD except in the most severe circumstances.* In support of this position are the basically normal course of pregnancy in patients with UC and the dubious benefits of therapeutic abortion to the health of the mother and the course of UC. Both exacerbation of UC and maternal mortality have been reported following therapeutic abortion.[11,15]

The frequency of various complications of pregnancy, such as toxemia, placenta previa, abruptio placentae, and retained placenta, is given in only some of the studies. In general, complications are within the 2% to 3% range, similar to the frequency rate in the general population.[2,3] The percentage of cesarean sections varies markedly in reported series and may reflect differences in obstetric approach and judgment. Maternal mortality is minimal

Table 129–2. OUTCOME OF PREGNANCY IN PATIENTS WITH ULCERATIVE COLITIS AND CROHN'S DISEASE

References	No. of Pregnancies	Normal Live Births (%)	Spontan. Abortion (%)	Cesarean Section (%)	Complications* (%)	Maternal Mortality (%)
			Ulcerative Colitis			
de Dombal et al., 1965[1]	107	83.0	6.0	1.0	—	1.38
McEwan, 1972[15]	50	90.0	8.0	8.0	—	0
Webb and Sedlack, 1974[2]	79	78.5	16.5	5.0	2.5	—
Ganchrow and Benjamin, 1975[3]	138	81.8	—	—	2.1	0
Mörl et al., 1977[11]	20	70.0	20.0	—	—	—
Levy et al., 1981[16]	60	85.0	11.6	—	—	0
Willoughby and Truelove, 1980[4]	216	78.8	10.6	—	—	0
Mogadam et al., 1981[17]	309	97.4	0.6	—	—	—
			Crohn's Disease			
Fielding and Cooke, 1970[8]	98	83.7	13.3	—	—	—
de Dombal et al., 1972[12]	60	88.3	5.0	0	6.8	1.7
Norton and Patterson, 1972[14]	19	84.2	10.5	—	—	—
Ganchrow and Benjamin, 1975[3]	51	78.2	—	—	1.4	0
Homan and Thorbjarnarson, 1976[9]	42	78.0	17.0	6.2	—	0
Mogadam et al., 1981[17]	222	93.2	2.7	—	—	—

*Complications: Placenta previa, abruptio placentae, retained placenta. *Key:* — = Not reported, 0 = no cases.

Table 129–3. FETAL OUTCOME IN PREGNANCIES OF WOMEN WITH INFLAMMATORY BOWEL DISEASES

References	No. of Pregnancies	Still Birth (%)	Prematurity (%)	Congenital Anomalies (%)
			Ulcerative Colitis	
de Dombal et al., 1965[1]	107	2.0	—	3.0
McEwan, 1972[15]	50	2.0	—	0
Webb and Sedlack, 1974[2]	79	1.2	1.2	2.5
Levy et al., 1981[16]	60	0	1.6	0
Willoughby and Truelove, 1980[4]	216	0.9	—	2.3
			Crohn's Disease	
Fielding and Cooke, 1970[8]	98	2.0	4.1	0
de Dombal et al., 1972[12]	60	5.0	0	1.7
Norton and Patterson, 1972[14]	19	0	—	—
Homan and Thorbjarnarson, 1976[9]	42	2.3	2.3	2.3
			Inflammatory Bowel Disease	
Mogadam et al., 1981[17]	531	0.75	0.94	0.75

and well within the normal range (Table 129–2).

The outcome of pregnancy in relation to the fetus is shown in Table 129–3. The percentages of stillbirths and prematurity are within the normal range. Concern has been expressed about an increased frequency of congenital abnormalities related to the UC or to its medical treatment.[4] However, this has not been borne out by the data.

All the foregoing figures relate to overall data for pregnant patients with UC as compared with pregnant women in the healthy population. Willoughby and Truelove,[4] however, compared the outcome of pregnancy in patients with UC whose disease was quiescent throughout the pregnancy with those who had active disease during all or part of the pregnancy. Although the differences were not great, patients whose disease was quiescent fared better. The live birth rate was 70% in patients with active disease and 80% in patients with quiescent disease. The small proportion of patients with severe disease during pregnancy had an even smaller chance of a normal outcome.

The majority of patients conceive during remission of disease, a feature noted in most studies (Table 129–4).

Crohn's Disease. CD, as a rule, has no deleterious effect on pregnancy. Using the same parameters as for UC, the outcome of pregnancy appears to be well within the normal range (see Tables 129–2 and 129–3). The percentages of normal live births, spontaneous abortions, complications of pregnancy, and fetal problems are similar to those found in UC patients and in the healthy

Table 129–4. CONCEPTION RELATED TO ACTIVITY OF DISEASE IN PATIENTS WITH ULCERATIVE COLITIS AND CROHN'S DISEASE

References	No. of Pregnancies	Conception During Remission (%)	Conception During Activity (%)
		Ulcerative Colitis	
de Dombal et al., 1965[1]	86	96.5	3.5
Willoughby and Truelove, 1980[4]	184	70.0	30.0
Levy et al., 1981[16]	60	81.6	18.4
Mogadam et al., 1981[18]	178	39.0	61.0*
		Crohn's Disease	
de Dombal et al., 1972[12]	56	60.7	39.3
Homan and Thorbjarnarson, 1976[9]	42	76.0	24.0
Mogadam et al., 1981[18]	146	49.0	51.0†

*37% had mild, 20% had moderate, and only 4% had severe activity.
†37% had mild, 12% had moderate, and only 2% had severe activity.

population. Norton and Patterson[14] studied 18 women and compared the outcome of 40 pregnancies before the onset of CD with 19 pregnancies after onset of the disease. The percentages of normal deliveries were 85% before and 84% after onset. The percentages of spontaneous abortions were 12.5% before and 10.5% after, and the percentages of stillbirths were 2.5% before and zero after onset of disease.

Mogadam et al.[17] carried out a survey of pregnancy in IBD using questionnaires sent to members of the American Gastroenterological Association and the American College of Gastroenterology. Replies were obtained from almost 50%, from which the outcome of 531 pregnancies could be evaluated. It was concluded that IBD, treated or not, does not affect the outcome of pregnancy. Patients with very severe CD, however, might be an exception. Their complication rate was higher than in patients with mild IBD, but still well within the range found in the general population.

Occasionally, surgery for IBD has to be performed during pregnancy. The numbers reported are small and relate mostly to colonic surgery for severe colitis. The results were not good, with high fetal and appreciable maternal mortality.[15]

In summary, it would seem from these considerations that: (1) a woman with IBD can expect an uneventful course and normal outcome of her pregnancy, particularly if she conceived during remission and if the disease is inactive or moderately active during pregnancy; (2) the chances for a normal course and outcome are diminished but still good if there is severe disease during pregnancy; (3) intensive medical therapy with sulfasalazine and steroids is advisable to induce remission prior to conception or during pregnancy; and (4) surgery for IBD is undesirable during pregnancy.

Effect of Pregnancy on Inflammatory Bowel Disease

UC and CD react similarly to pregnancy. *Pregnancy has no deleterious effect on the course of either form of IBD.* Indeed, a slight beneficial effect cannot be excluded. Most women conceive during remission of the disease (see Table 129–4) and most of them continue to be in remission throughout pregnancy (Table 129–5).

When conception occurs during active disease, most patients continue to have moderately active disease throughout pregnancy. In roughly equal proportions, disease activity in these patients improves or worsens (Table 129–6).

In the survey of Mogadam et al.,[18] which included 324 patients with IBD, 75% of those with quiescent or mild disease at conception had the same disease course during pregnancy, and only 26% had a moderate or severe course. Of the patients with moderate or severe disease at conception, only 49% had quiescent or mild disease during pregnancy, while 51% had moderate or severe disease.

The disease may be active or may be reactivated during any one of the trimesters of pregnancy.[18] Most investigators have noted a slightly higher frequency of disease activity during the first trimester (Table 129–7). There is considerable controversy as to whether recurrence of disease is particularly frequent during the 3 months of the puerperium (postpartum period) (Table 129–7). Several investigators found very high attack rates during

Table 129–5. EFFECT OF PREGNANCY ON INFLAMMATORY BOWEL DISEASES (CONCEPTION DURING REMISSION)

References	Disease*	No. of Pregnancies	Remission During Pregnancy (%)	Activity During Pregnancy (%)
de Dombal et al., 1965[1]	UC	80	67.0	33.0
McEwan, 1972[15]	UC	25	84.0	16.0
Willoughby and Truelove, 1980[4]	UC	129	69.7	30.3
Homan and Thorbjarnarson, 1976[9]	CD	32	91.0	9.0
Mogadam et al., 1981[18]	IBD	142	56.0	44.0†

*UC = ulcerative colitis, CD = Crohn's disease, IBD = inflammatory bowel disease.
†19% had mild, 16% mderate, and only 8% had severe disease.

Table 129–6. EFFECT OF PREGNANCY ON INFLAMMATORY BOWEL DISEASES (CONCEPTION DURING ACTIVITY)

			Activity of Disease During Pregnancy		
References	**Disease***	**No. of Pregnancies**	*Unchanged (%)*	*Improved (%)*	*Worsened (%)*
de Dombal et al., 1965[1]	UC	3	33.0	66.0	—
McEwan, 1972[15]	UC	22	19.0	36.0	45.0
Ganchrow and Benjamin, 1975[3]	UC	34	29.0	15.0	56.0
Willoughby and Truelove, 1980[4]	UC	55	27.0	40.0	33.0
Mogadam et al., 1981[18]†	UC	178	41.0	27.0	31.0
Fielding and Cooke, 1970[8]	CD	98	58.5	28.4	13.1
de Dombal et al., 1972[12]†	CD	60	73.3	15.0	10.0
Mogadam et al., 1981[18]†	CD	146	47.0	25.0	29.0

*UC = ulcerative colitis, CD = Crohn's disease.
†Includes patients with both active and inactive disease at conception.

the postpartum period and considered women to be particularly vulnerable at this time.[1,5,12] It was suggested by de Dombal et al.[1] that high serum cortisol levels during pregnancy affected the course of IBD favorably, while the precipitous fall of serum cortisol in the postpartum period caused the high relapse rate. It has been pointed out, however, that the high cortisol levels are a response to high progesterone levels that compete for tissue-binding sites. In effect, these are the "normal" levels required during pregnancy to maintain adequate biologic activity.[18] It was also thought that disease occurring during the puerperium was apt to be more severe.[1,8] However, other more recent studies have not found a higher frequency of recurrence during the puerperium. Nor was the disease in the postpartum period more severe than usual.[4,13]

In a survey of 317 patients made in the United States by Mogadam et al.,[18] disease activity in the postpartum period was unchanged in 55%, improved in 29%, and worsened in 15%. A comparison of disease activity at term and postpartum revealed a similar picture; the majority of patients were unchanged, while a higher proportion improved than deteriorated. Only 13% of the patients with quiescent or mild disease at term had moderate to severe disease postpartum, in contrast to 53% of the patients with active disease at term.

The differences in observations reported by the various investigators may be due to geographic or temporal variations in the course of the disease or, more likely, they reflect a better level of medical control of IBD in recent years.

It has been reported that when the onset of UC or CD occurs during pregnancy or the puerperium, it frequently is severe. Both fetal and maternal mortality were encountered, and it has been suggested that surgery and/or therapeutic abortion be considered.[19] Recent studies, however, do not support this view. Willoughby and Truelove[4] described 16 patients with UC that began during preg-

Table 129–7. TIMING OF DISEASE ACTIVITY DURING PREGNANCY IN INFLAMMATORY BOWEL DISEASES

			Disease Activity During			
References	**Disease***	**No. of Pregnancies**	*1st Trimester (%)*	*2nd Trimester (%)*	*3rd Trimester (%)*	*Puerperium (%)*
de Dombal et al., 1965[1]	UC	44	25.0	16.0	16.0	43.0
Ganchrow and Benjamin, 1975[3]	UC	12	33.3	8.3	25.0	33.3
Willoughby and Truelove, 1980[4]	UC	39	46.0	18.0	20.0	15.0
de Dombal et al., 1972[12]†	CD	60	33.3	24.1	27.3	60.3

*UC = ulcerative colitis, CD = Crohn's disease.
†These authors give percentage of *all* patients with active disease at each period.

nancy, usually in the first or second trimester. The attacks were adequately controlled by medical therapy in all cases. There was no maternal mortality, and 14 of the 16 patients had live normal births. Nine patients in their series developed UC during the puerperium; 8 of these attacks were mild and one was of moderate severity.

The probability of the disease becoming active during the 12 months of pregnancy and the puerperium as compared with years of disease without pregnancy has been calculated. In a series of 80 pregnancies in patients with UC, de Dombal et al.[1] recorded an attack of colitis in 33% of the 80 patient years; in 69% there was remission throughout. Collected data from several reports established that colitis became active in 44% of 393 patient years during pregnancy. By contrast, a control group of non-pregnant women of similar age with UC experienced an attack of colitis in 47% of 438 patient years. Similar data have been recorded by others, both in UC and in CD.[2,14] The effect of successive pregnancies on the disease course has also been evaluated in a small number of patients.[15] No consistent effect was noted.

It seems, therefore, that a woman with IBD should have no fear of becoming pregnant, inasmuch as the natural course of the disease is not affected by pregnancy. Thus, there is no reason to discourage desired conception.

Gynecologic and Obstetric Problems Associated with Inflammatory Bowel Disease

There are very few gynecologic and obstetric complications associated with UC, and this includes patients who have undergone surgery for the disease. Even patients with total colectomy and ileostomy usually have an uncomplicated pregnancy and delivery.

Stretching and bulging of an ileostomy with associated discomfort have been reported during pregnancy. More seriously, intestinal obstruction associated with ileostomy may complicate pregnancy or delivery.[7] Diagnosis is sometimes delayed because a complication of pregnancy is erroneously suspected.

Patients with CD may have gynecologic complications, sometimes even before diagnosis of the disease. Abscesses, infections, ulcers, and fistulas may involve the internal pelvic organs and also the vulvovaginal and perineal regions. Some patients present with an acute abdomen, and pelvic inflammatory disease or an ovarian cyst may be suspected preoperatively. Donaldson,[10] on analyzing the records of 431 female patients with CD, found 103 to have various gynecologic manifestations. Symptomatology was confusing in some of these patients and appeared to be primarily gynecologic, the diagnosis of CD becoming established only at laparotomy or after further investigation. Donaldson also found, however, that the disease had no unfavorable effect on pregnancy. Saegesser[20] found genital complications in 16.8% of 119 adults (61 men and 58 women) operated on for CD.

Effect of Drugs

Concern was expressed in previous decades that drugs used in the treatment of IBD during pregnancy might be harmful to the fetus or newborn. The effects of sulfasalazine and corticosteroids caused particular worry. In recent years, however, more basic data have accumulated establishing the safety of these 2 drugs during pregnancy.

Sulfasalazine

Effect on Fertility. As previously noted, no female infertility has been found in association with sulfasalazine. Fertility in patients with UC is normal in treated and untreated women alike, whereas in women with CD, reduced fertility is attributed to the disease and not to its therapy.

A detrimental effect of sulfasalazine on male fertility has recently been described. Malchow[21] collected 17 cases from the literature of men with IBD who were treated with sulfasalazine and showed reversible infertility. Married couples who were infertile were examined, with no abnormality demonstrated in the wife. The number, motility, and morphology of spermatozoa in the husband were abnormal, as was the volume of semen. Within 3 months after discontinuation of sulfasalazine, the abnormalities improved and most couples became fertile.

These initial observations have recently been extended.[22-25] Toovey et al.[22] studied 28 men, aged 22 to 49, with IBD. The 4 patients who did not receive sulfasalazine had no abnormalities of their semen; the 7 patients receiving sulfasalazine for less than 2 months had markedly reduced sperm motility without significant changes in sperm density and morphology. Of the 18 patients receiving sulfasalazine (2 to 4 g/day) for more than 2 months, none had normal sperm motility, only 2 had normal (low normal) sperm density, and only 6 had normal sperm morphology. After 2 months without sulfasalazine, sperm density and motility started to improve but morphology remained abnormal. Eight previously infertile patients achieved impregnation a mean 2½ months after sulfasalazine withdrawal. Birnie et al.[23] found sperm abnormalities in 86% of 21 men taking sulfasalazine; oligospermia was present in 72%. Schramm et al.[24] found sperm abnormalities in 26 of 29 patients with CD, at least 19 of whom were taking sulfasalazine. Thus, after many decades of use, a major new side effect of sulfasalazine therapy has come to light. Men in their reproductive years taking sulfasalazine for more than 2 months must now be considered at high risk of developing sperm abnormalities and, probably, infertility. This effect seems to be transient, but more permanent damage cannot be excluded without additional observations.

The mechanism of this effect of sulfasalazine has not been definitely established. A direct toxic effect of sulfapyridine, similar to that reported for other sulfonamides, is suspected.[22]

Effect on Pregnancy. Mogadam et al.[17] compared 287 pregnancies in patients with IBD during which sulfasalazine and/or steroids were used with 244 pregnancies in untreated patients with IBD. The outcome of pregnancy in patients with UC was similar in the treated and untreated groups. Patients with CD treated with sulfasalazine also had no more complications than did the untreated group. The complications of pregnancy in both treated and untreated patients with IBD were less frequent than expected from data based on the general population. Similar data for patients with UC treated with and without sulfasalazine were reported by Willoughby and Truelove.[4]

Effect on the Fetus. Sulfasalazine is poorly absorbed in the small bowel and is split by bacteria, mostly in the colon, to sulfapyridine and 5-aminosalicylic acid. There are no data to support any teratogenic effect of sulfapyridine or other sulfonamides, nor has fetal damage been associated with this drug.[26,27] In experimental animals, high doses of acetylsalicylic acid, producing blood levels in the 200 μg/ml range, may be teratogenic. The effect, however, is dose-dependent.

The suggestion has been advanced that mothers of malformed infants take more aspirin during pregnancy than mothers of normal babies,[28] but this was not confirmed in subsequent large-scale epidemiologic surveys.[29] The blood levels of aspirin in these pregnant women, as well as levels in the umbilical cord blood, were in the 10 to 30 μg/ml range, whereas the salicylate levels of patients treated with sulfasalazine are in the 1 μg/ml range (Table 129–8). No teratogenic effect or other harmful effects to the fetus have been demonstrated in patients with IBD treated with sulfasalazine.[14,26,30,31] Most investigators, therefore, now recommend using sulfasalazine during pregnancy according to the same criteria as in non-pregnant patients with IBD.

Table 129–8. TERATOGENICITY OF ACETYLSALICYCLIC ACID (ASA)

References	Dosage of ASA (mg/kg)	Serum Concentration of ASA (μg/ml)	Recipients	Teratogenic Effect
Wilson et al., 1977[42]	100	128–169	Rats	No
	150	185–238	Rats	Yes
Robertson et al., 1979[43]	500–600	—	Rabbits	Yes
	< 200	—	Rabbits	No
Robertson et al., 1979[44]	400	—	Dogs	Yes
	100	—	Dogs	No
Wilson et al., 1977[42]	100	116–159	Rhesus monkeys	No
	150	169–197	Rhesus monkeys	No
Turner and Collins, 1975[28]	Regular intake	10–50	Pregnant women	No*
Palmisano and Cassady, 1969[45]	Regular intake	12–100†	Pregnant women	No
Das et al., 1973[46]	Sulfasalazine	1 ± 0.9	Patients with IBD	—‡

*Not excluded with certainty.
†Umbilical cord blood.
‡Not explored.

Effect on Lactation. It is known that sulfonamides may precipitate kernicterus in the newborn by displacing bilirubin from albumin.[32] It was feared that sulfasalazine might have similar results when given to lactating mothers. Hence, the manufacturers recommended that treatment be stopped during the last month of pregnancy and while breastfeeding. It was recently found, however, that only negligible amounts of sulfasalazine pass into human milk, but its metabolite, sulfapyridine, is secreted into the milk, attaining 40% of its concentration in serum.[33] It has been calculated that if a lactating mother is taking 2 g of sulfasalazine per day, the infant would be receiving 3 mg/kg of sulfapyridine. This is a very small amount, especially since sulfapyridine has a very poor bilirubin displacing capacity.[33]

In large series of patients, pathologic jaundice of the newborn was not found to be more frequent in the offspring of mothers treated with sulfasalazine.[4,17] Nor was kernicterus reported in association with this drug.[17,33] Treatment of the nursing mother with sulfasalazine, does not therefore, appear to present any danger to the healthy newborn.

Steroids. Until recently, obstetricians were loath to use steroids in pregnant women for several reasons. In animal studies, large doses of steroids given early in pregnancy produce an increased number of fetal abnormalities, such as cleft palate, islet cell degeneration, and stillborn fetuses. However, several studies of women who have been treated with steroids during pregnancy for various reasons have not shown any difference in frequency of fetal malformations or injury.[34] Cortisol secretion in newborns whose mothers had been treated with steroids was also normal.[35]

Concern has been expressed that women treated with steroids before delivery would have a higher rate of underweight newborns. This finding has been disputed.[36,37] In the study of Mogadam et al.,[17] the proportion of fetal complications in mothers with UC receiving steroids was the same as in mothers not receiving steroids. The proportion of underweight infants born to IBD patients receiving steroids during pregnancy was also considerably less than would be expected in the general population. In the study of patients with UC conducted by Willoughby and Truelove,[4] the prevalence rate of low-birth-weight babies was the same for mothers who received steroids during pregnancy as for mothers who were not treated with steroids.

In general, the modern approach favors the use of sulfasalazine and steroids as needed prior to and during pregnancy. This is based on 3 main arguments: (1) Women are more likely to conceive and have an uneventful pregnancy if their disease is in remission; (2) mothers and babies fare better when the disease is not active or severe during pregnancy; and (3) no danger to the mother or fetus from the use of corticosteroids and sulfasalazine has been demonstrated.

Metronidazole. In view of the demonstration by the Cooperative Crohn's Disease Study in Sweden that metronidazole is an effective drug in CD,[38] the use of this drug in IBD will undoubtedly rise. To date, there are no large-scale studies on the use of this drug in pregnancy, particularly not in patients with IBD. In several small-scale studies of women treated with metronidazole for various reasons, during pregnancy, no increased teratogenic risk has been demonstrated, irrespective of the trimester of exposure.[39,40] An early report of chromosomal aberrations following treatment with metronidazole has not been confirmed by the same authors in a large-scale controlled study.[41]

The manufacturer warns that metronidazole should be avoided during pregnancy. Until larger-scale studies become available, this is probably the most prudent course to follow.

Azathioprine and 6-Mercaptopurine. The usefulness of the immunosuppressive agents azathioprine and its metabolite, 6-mercaptopurine, in IBD is still controversial. Cytotoxic agents in general have been shown to have a damaging effect on the reproductive capacity in humans.[47,48] Leb et al.[49] have demonstrated the transplacental passage of azathioprine. Severe congenital malformations in offspring of pregnant animals, such as mice, receiving azathioprine have been reported.[47] However, teratogenicity has not been reported in humans,[50,51] with the exception of one report of a newborn infant with congenital pulmonary stenosis.[51] It was suggested, but not fully proved, that azathioprine taken by kidney transplant patients during pregnancy caused prematurity and low birth weight as well as lymphopenia and low serum immunoglobulin levels in the newborn.[30,50] These effects were transient. We are not aware of any reports on patients with

IBD taking azathioprine or 6-mercaptopurine during pregnancy.

On the basis of current limited knowledge of their effects, it would seem prudent to recommend withdrawal of both agents before intended or during pregnancy.

In summary, the drug treatment of pregnant and nursing women with IBD, or women trying to conceive, should consist basically of sulfasalazine and steroids. The indications and dosage are the same as for the nonpregnant patient. A man with IBD should discontinue sulfasalazine for at least 2 months before attempting impregnation. Metronidazole, azathioprine, and 6-mercaptopurine should all be avoided before conception and during pregnancy.

References

1. de Dombal FT, Watts JM, Watkinson G, Goligher JC. Ulcerative colitis and pregnancy. Lancet 1965; 2:599–602.
2. Webb MJ, Sedlack RE. Ulcerative colitis in pregnancy. Med Clin North Am 1974; 58:823–7.
3. Ganchrow MI, Benjamin H. Inflammatory colorectal disease and pregnancy. Dis Colon Rectum 1975; 18:706–9.
4. Willoughby CP, Truelove SC. Ulcerative colitis and pregnancy. Gut 1980; 21:469–74.
5. Banks BM, Korelitz BI, Zetzel L. The course of nonspecific ulcerative colitis: Review of twenty years experience and late results. Gastroenterology 1957; 32:983–1012.
6. Grüner OPN, Naas R, Fretheim B. Marital status and sexual adjustment after colectomy. Scand J Gastroenterol 1977; 12:193–7.
7. Hudson CN. Ileostomy in pregnancy. Proc Roy Soc Med 1972; 65:281–3.
8. Fielding JF, Cooke WT. Pregnancy and Crohn's disease. Br Med J 1970; 2:76–7.
9. Homan WP, Thorbjarnarson B. Crohn's disease and pregnancy. Arch Surg 1976; 111:545–7.
10. Donaldson LB. Crohn's disease: Its gynecologic aspect. Am J Obstet Gynecol 1975; 131:196–202.
11. Mörl M, Rottler H, Hartwich G. Schwangerschaftsverlauf bei colitis ulcerosa und morbus Crohn. Dtsch Med Woenschr 1977; 102:387–91.
12. de Dombal FT, Burton IL, Goligher JC. Crohn's disease and pregnancy. Br Med J 1972; 2:550–3.
13. Crohn BB, Yarnis H, Korelitz BI. Regional enteritis complicating pregnancy. Gastroenterology 1956; 31:615–28.
14. Norton RA, Patterson JF. Pregnancy and regional enteritis. Obstet Gynecol 1972; 40:711–2.
15. McEwan HP. Ulcerative colitis in pregnancy. Proc Roy Soc Med 1972; 65:279–81.
16. Levy N, Roisman I, Teodor I. Ulcerative colitis in pregnancy in Israel. Dis Colon Rectum 1981; 24:351–4.
17. Mogadam M, Dobbins WO, Korelitz BI, Ahmed SW. Pregnancy in inflammatory bowel disease: Effect of sulfasalazine and corticosteroids on fetal outcome. Gastroenterology 1981; 80:72–6.
18. Mogadam M, Korelitz BI, Ahmed SW, Dobbins WO, Baiocco PJ. The course of inflammatory bowel disease during pregnancy and postpartum. Am J Gastroenterol 1981; 75:265–9.
19. Martimbeau PW, Welch JS, Weiland LH. Crohn's disease and pregnancy. Am J Obstet Gynecol 1975; 122:746–9.
20. Saegesser F. Complications urogenitales de la maladie de Crohn. Helv Chir Acta 1979; 46:727–30.
21. Malchow H. Effects of sulphasalazine on fertility. Z Gastroenterol 1981; 19(Suppl):20–2.
22. Toovey S, Hudson E, Hendry WF, Levi AJ. Sulphasalazine and male infertility: Reversibility and possible mechanism. Gut 1981; 22:445–51.
23. Birnie GG, McLeod TIF, Watkinson G. Incidence of sulphasalazine-induced male infertility. Gut 22; 452–5.
24. Schramm P, Ewe K, Karbach V. Spermiogramm untersuchungen bei morbus Crohn patienten. Andrologia 1981; 13:352–8.
25. Freeman JG, Reece VAC, Venables CW. Sulphasalazine and spermatogenesis. Digestion 1982; 23:68–71.
26. Fahrländer H. The use of azulfidine/salazopyrine during pregnancy. Z Gastroenterol 1981; 19:23–5.
27. Fahrländer H. Salazosulfapyridin in der schwangerschaft? Dtsch Med Wochenschr 1980; 105:1729–31.
28. Turner G, Collins E. Fetal effects of regular salicylate ingestion in pregnancy. Lancet 1975; 2:338–9.
29. Slone D, Heinonen OP, Kaufman DW, Siskind V, Monson RR, Shapiro S. Aspirin and congenital malformations. Lancet 1976; 1:1373–5.
30. Lennard-Jones JE, Powel-Tuck J. Drug treatment of inflammatory bowel disease. Clin Gastroenterol 1979; 8:187–217.
31. Azad Khan AK, Truelove SC. Placental and mammary transfer of sulphasalazine. Br Med J 1979; 2:1553.
32. Järnerot G. Mammary and placental transfer of sulphasalazine and sulphapyridine and the influence of the vacant amount of high affinity bilirubin binding site on albumin. Z Gastroenterol 1981; 19(Suppl):26–7.
33. Järnerot G, Into-Malmberg MB. Sulphasalazine treatment during breast feeding. Scand J Gastroenterol 1979; 14:869–71.
34. Heinomen OP. Birth Defects and Drugs in Pregnancy. Littleton, Massachusetts: Publishing Sciences Group, 1977.
35. Kenny FM, Preeyasombat C, Spaulding JJ, Migeon CJ. Cortisol production rate in infants born of steroid-treated mothers and diabetic mothers. Pediatrics 1966; 37:960–6.
36. Bongiovanni AM, McPadden AJ. Steroids during pregnancy and possible fetal consequences. Fertil Steril 1960; 11:181–6.
37. Warrell DW, Taylor R. Outcome for the foetus of mothers receiving prednisolone during pregnancy. Lancet 1960; 1:117–8.
38. Ursing B, Alm T, Bárány F, Bergelin I, Ganrot-Norlin K, Hoevels J, Huitfeldt B, Järnerot G, Krause U, Krook A, Nordle O, Rosen A. A comparative study of metronidazole and sulfasalazine for active Crohn's disease. The Cooperative Crohn's Disease Study in Sweden (CCDSS). Gastroenterology 1982; 83:550–62.
39. Petterson WF, Stourch JE, Ryder CD. Metronidazole in pregnancy. Am J Gynecol 1966; 94:343–9.
40. Goldman P. Metronidazole. N Engl J Med 1980; 303:1212–7.
41. Mitelman F, Strombeck B, Ursing B. No cytogenetic effect of metronidazole. Lancet 1980; 1:1249–56.
42. Wilson JG, Ritter EJ, Scott WJ, Fradkin R. Comparative distribution of embryotoxicity of acetylsalicylic acid in pregnant rats and rhesus monkeys. Toxicol Appl Pharmacol 1977; 41:67–78.
43. Robertson R, Minsker D, Bokelman D. Teratogenicity of acetylsalicylic acid in the rabbit. Teratology 1979; 19:43A–4A.
44. Robertson R, Delwin HA, Bokelman D. Aspirin: Teratogenic evaluation in the dog. Teratology 1979; 20:313–7.
45. Palmisano PA, Cassady G. Salicylate exposure in the perinate. JAMA 1969; 209:556–8.
46. Das KM, Eastwood MA, McManus JPA, Sircus W. The metabolism of salicylazosulphapyridine in ulcerative colitis. I. The relationship between metabolites and the response to treatment in inpatients. Gut 1973; 14:631–41.
47. Reimers TJ, Sluss PM. 6-Mercaptopurine treatment of pregnant mice: Effects on second and third generations. Science 1978; 201:65–7.
48. Steckman ML. Treatment of chronic disease with 6-mercaptopurine: What effects on fertility? N Engl J Med 1980; 303:817.
49. Leb DE, Weisskopf B, Kanovitz BS. Chromosome aberrations in the child of a kidney transplant recipient. Arch Intern Med 1971; 128:441–4.
50. Price HV, Salman JR, Laurence KM, Langmaid H. Immunosuppressive drugs and the foetus. Transplantation 1976; 21:294–8.
51. Jacob ET, Grunstein S, Shapira Z, Berant M, Better OS, Boner G. Successful pregnancy in a recipient of a cadaver kidney allograft. Isr J Med Sci 1974; 10:206–12.

Chapter 130

Stomal Function and Care

Bryan N. Brooke • Katherine F. Jeter

Colostomy

Permanent colostomy most commonly results from abdominoperineal excision of the rectum undertaken for cancer, in which the proximal end of the divided sigmoid is brought to the surface in the left iliac fossa and secured by mucosa to skin sutures. It is the most satisfactory form of colostomy, for the excreta are formed, evacuation can either be controlled by intelligent anticipation or induced by lavage, and the stoma is of a discrete size.

More proximal colostomy, such as transverse or loop colostomy, is indicated only as a temporary procedure. Such a colostomy is usually created to relieve cancerous obstruction before an elective procedure for removal of the growth, to obtain fecal deflection following large bowel trauma, or to treat an infant with a congenital anomaly such as Hirschsprung's disease or anorectal dysplasia. Rarely, in advanced terminal abdominal cancer, a loop colostomy may be the only means whereby obstruction can be relieved.

When colostomy is undertaken in emergency situations, certain guidelines should be borne in mind:

1. A transverse colostomy is bulky, messy, and troublesome to manage; it should be avoided if possible.

2. If a loop has to be formed, the time-honored support for the spur by a glass rod, or even a softer material such as rubber or plastic, has no place today. Apart from the discomfort the support causes and the problem posed as to when it can be safely removed, it impedes the application of an appliance. In its place, the skin at the colostomy site should be incised at the outset on 2 sides of a triangle, leaving the base intact. The apex of skin thus formed can be passed through the mesentery of the large bowel loop as it is drawn through the abdominal wall, each incision accommodating one limb of the loop. Except for the removal of cutaneous sutures, the skin bridge remains undisturbed until the colostomy is closed or removed.

3. A temporary colostomy to relieve large bowel obstruction due to cancer should be placed as close to the lesion as possible without disturbing the growth. It may thereby be excised with the growth, permitting the second operation to be the final one. Apart from reducing the conventional 3-stage procedure (colostomy, excision of the cancer, and closure of the colostomy) to 2 operations, this technique has the added advantage of allowing complete freedom of maneuver for the elective excision. This is not possible when the colostomy is maintained for subsequent closure.

Colostomy may also be performed for the emergencies of diverticular disease (perforation, acute diverticulitis, and obstruction), although these complications do not constitute absolute indications.[1] It should be borne in mind that preliminary fecal deflection has no place in the treatment of pericolic abscess, which persists despite a colostomy and will respond only to resection of the diverticular area.

Cecostomy is still favored by some surgeons as a temporary safety vent to "cover" large bowel resection and anastomosis; however, little evidence can be adduced in support of this view. It has no place in the relief of obstruction occurring, for example, at the hepatic flexure; this is better achieved by either ileotransversostomy or ileostomy, which provides what cecostomy can never do—a stoma controllable by an appliance.

A satisfactory continent colostomy has yet to be developed. The Erlangen magnetic device introduced by Feustel and Hennig[2] has not fulfilled its early promise. Infection has proved a problem at the site of implantation of the magnetic ring; scarring at the stoma site leads too readily to a failure of alignment between ring and cap; and discomfort prevents the cap's being worn in the recumbent position at night.[3]

Preparing the Patient. Beyond the routine preparatory measures undertaken for all preoperative patients, those scheduled for colostomy require more attentive and careful instruction and counsel. Many people have little understanding of how their gastrointestinal tract normally functions and how evacuation occurs. Moreover, the elderly tend to have fixed ideas about how many bowel movements they should have each day or week and what form they should take. Compounding the impact of a major operation are the social and emotional consequences of colostomy. Time has not eroded the unconscious meaning attached to feces and the taboos associated with certain bodily orifices.[4]

When a temporary transverse colostomy is required, it is well to prepare patients regardless of the limited length of time they may have to live with the stoma; what may seem a brief period to a physician is likely to appear indefinite to the patient burdened with colostomy care. Patients who are told that they will have a "temporary" colostomy tend to resist learning to care for it and refuse to resume activities of daily living until closure has been accomplished. This is particularly unfortunate if it later becomes apparent that restoration of bowel continuity is not feasible. So it is advisable to term the procedure a "resting" colostomy and to encourage the patient and his family to become proficient in all aspects of care.

Patients requiring a colostomy in the descending or sigmoid colon with removal of the rectum will have to be prepared for several postoperative sequelae. The colostomy will be controlled either by an adherent pouch or by irrigation (which obviates the need for an appliance). Additionally, the perineal wound will need scrupulous attention for weeks or months after proctectomy; we do not favor sitz baths because of evidence indicating that these increase secondary infection. It is better for patients to be prepared for the necessity for perineal dressings than to learn about such requirements after operation when they are weak, anxious, and easily confused.

It is not unusual for the diagnosis of cancer to be so overwhelming that all other information is rejected or misconstrued. Important as it is to prepare patients adequately for colostomy by instruction and demonstration, it is no less crucial that this should be timely and appropriate to age, educational level, socioeconomic and occupational status, and religious or cultural background. When, for example, religious law requires a Moslem to kneel on the floor 5 times daily with a clean body, colostomy care for that patient must be arranged accordingly.

Diet. Apart from exigencies arising from the stoma itself (the need to control flatus, odor, and fluidity), there is no more reason for dietary control or restriction by a patient after a colostomy than before. Accepting the precept that the alimentary response to foods varies greatly from individual to individual, there are nevertheless some common features, and suggestions can be made to ease patients' individual problems based on this general experience.

The brassicas, onions, and beans may be responsible for excessive flatus, and green vegetables, fish, and onions are more likely to cause odor than are other dietary items. Fruit, in particular, may cause the consistency of the stools to become fluid, as may greens, but less frequently so. Juices can have a loosening effect. Alcohol may act likewise, especially beer, which may also be a cause of flatus. It has been asserted that chlorophyll compounds can control odor, but there is no scientific basis for this nor evidence to substantiate the claim.

Colostomy control is facilitated by knowledge and manipulation of dietary effects, more so when evacuation is regulated by the natural method, although it is also important in conjunction with the washout routine.

The Enterostomal Therapist (ET). Nurses

have often had to assume responsibility for instruction in stoma care, sometimes with inadequate experience. In 1958, Turnbull of the Cleveland Clinic conceived a new discipline, later termed *"enterostomal therapy."* Since then, a growing number of nurses have been working exclusively with stoma patients, serving as clinical specialists in the hospital and the outside community. *Enterostomal therapists* (ETs), or stoma care nurses as they are called in some European countries, combine nursing, counseling, and educational training.

Before operation it is usually the ET nurse's task to mark on the abdomen the best site for the stoma (Fig. 130–1). This provides an opportunity to explain the appearance and function of the exposed colon to the patient.

Most ET nurses work closely with "ostomy" associations and arrange with them to have a trained volunteer of similar age, sex, and interests make a preoperative visit to the patient. Contact with an individual who has survived a similar ordeal and returned to normal life is singularly reassuring; the appropriate arrangements should be made for all except those for whom a colostomy is a brief palliative measure in terminal disease or in an emergency situation, when a visit can be made subsequently. It is important to include family members in ostomy preparation, since an informed spouse or relative can facilitate rehabilitation.[5]

Educational programs for stoma therapists now include sex counseling because of the possibility of impotence as a consequence of rectal excision. Whether this needs to be mentioned to the patient, however, is debatable and controversial, since the mere suggestion of the possibility of impotence to a susceptible man can in itself cause this undesired effect. So-called defensive medicine, i.e., practiced primarily to protect the physician from charges of malpractice, has not yet become so widespread (in the United Kingdom at least) as to require that a warning about this be given routinely to all patients about to undergo proctectomy. It should, however, be considered in each case and the decision made by the surgeon, who may protect himself medicolegally by writing in the case notes his reasons why the patient has not been informed. In all other respects, both men and women usually welcome an invitation to discuss the physical and psychologic effects of colostomy on sexual function.

Preparation for colostomy is a complex process calling for planning and coordination between the medical and nursing team and the patient and his or her family. A well-prepared patient is likely to have a smoother recovery in the early postoperative phase and return to full activity more effectively in the extended period.

Control by Natural Evacuation. Regularity of daily routine provides the essential basis

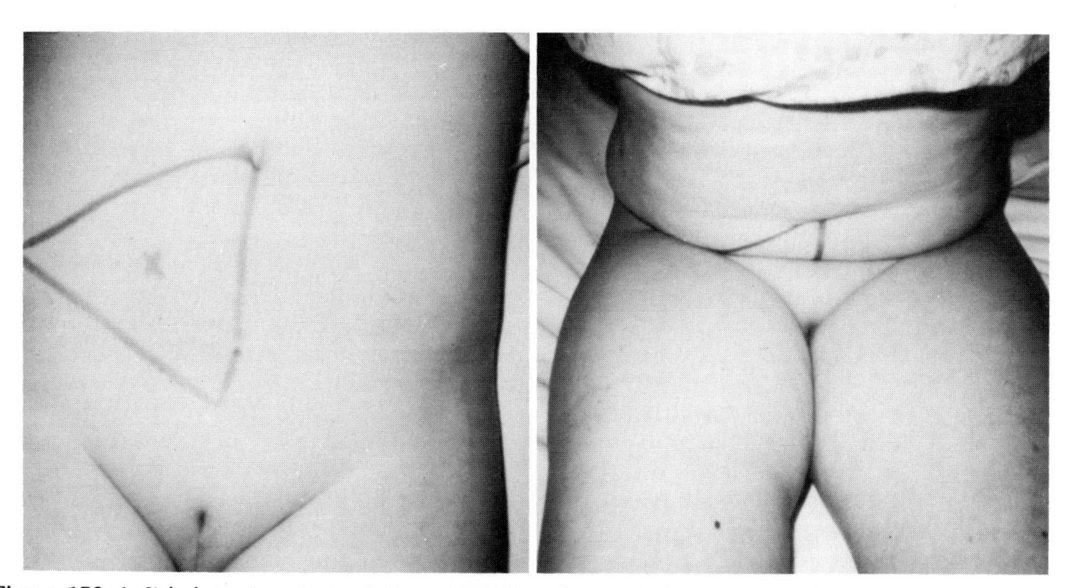

Figure 130–1. It is important to mark the stoma site preoperatively, examining the patient in all postures. What appears to be the optimal site when the patient is supine *(left)* actually disappears in abdominal creases when the patient sits up *(right)*.

for this method, the object of which is the anticipation of a natural bowel movement at a predicted time. The patient is advised to go to bed at approximately the same time each night and rise at a regular time each morning; more important, meals should be taken at regular intervals and at the same time from day to day. This allows mass action of the gastrocolic reflex at anticipated times, once or twice a day, by means of the regular ingestion of food. In order to obtain bowel action at the convenient and conventional time of rising in the morning, the mass action can be initiated by taking a cup of tea or coffee on waking. Many patients nevertheless find that further small actions may occur after meals later in the day, particularly after an evening meal.

The colostomate is also advised to observe the reactions of his alimentary system to specific items of diet; an intelligent patient can then learn to adjust the consistency of the stool to avoid constipation or looseness. In addition, bulking agents, such as coarse bran, methyl cellulose, and psyllium seeds, can be prescribed to improve consistency and reduce odor, while codeine phosphate, diphenoxylate (Lomotil), and loperamide (Imodium) may be used to reduce intestinal activity, if required. For the colostomate who is also depressed because of gut overactivity, the tricyclic antidepressants such as amitriptyline (Elavil) and imipramine (Tofranil) are particularly useful; they have anticholinergic properties as well and thus reduce colonic motility.

Essential to the success of this method is proper and careful instruction followed by continued surveillance. If regularity of bowel action is not obtained after a reasonable trial by the patient following return to normal daily life and activity, the technique should be abandoned without hesitation in favor of the washout routine.

Control by Irrigation. The loss of anal control presents a daunting psychologic hurdle. Some patients with a left iliac colostomy will regain their presurgical bowel habits by simply studying their diet in order to avoid foods with a laxative effect and those that produce excess flatus. However, many patients are not confident that dietary moderation will be sufficient to keep them free from odor, embarrassing flatulence, or inopportune bowel action.

Colostomy irrigation has gained universal popularity in the United States as the method of management. Complete evacuation of the colon on a daily or triweekly or biweekly basis will afford security against unpredictable bowel action and minimize the passage of gas. With a few exceptions, irrigation has generally been in disfavor in the United Kingdom, partly on account of the time required by the method and partly because of fear of bowel perforation. The fear, however, is misplaced since this complication has been a late and rare event; it probably is non-existent with modern methods, particularly with the use of the conical nozzle. The natural method is sometimes less successful than was previously appreciated, so that there is now a renewal of interest in and recourse to irrigation in the United Kingdom. Meanwhile, irrigation is being used more selectively in the United States. At the Sydney Hospital, Australia, this dilemma is overcome by postponing the choice until several weeks after the patient has returned home, when he has regained strength and his natural bowel function.[6]

When considering candidates for colostomy irrigation, the following criteria are important:

1. The patient should have a sufficient length of large bowel to produce formed stool.
2. The preoperative bowel habit should have been regular.
3. The patient should not be receiving radiotherapy, chemotherapy, or immunotherapy, which cause gastrointestinal dysfunction, or be suffering from residual effects of anti-tumor therapy.
4. The patient should be prepared to adhere to a time-consuming regimen, be intelligent enough to perform the manipulation safely, and be physically able to carry out the task.
5. Bathroom facilities with running water, which can be used in privacy without causing inconvenience to other household members, are necessary.
6. Instruction and correction during the early postoperative period are important to ultimate success.

An irrigation guaranteed to evacuate the bowel completely, and so assure the patient of being stool-free until the next scheduled washout in 2 to 3 days, can be carried out in the following manner:

1. The patient sits on the toilet or, if the

perineal wound is uncomfortable, on a chair with a cushion or rubber ring, facing the commode. An irrigation sleeve is placed around the stoma, with the end directed to the toilet bowel.

2. The irrigating bag is filled with 1 liter of lukewarm tap water; the tubing is cleared of air by running water through it.

3. An irrigating cone or soft flexible catheter fitted with a nipple or special shield to prevent water from returning is introduced into the stoma. A regulating clamp on the tubing from the water bag is important to maintain a gentle water flow.

4. Water is instilled very slowly under minimal pressure to avoid stimulating a premature peristaltic response or causing cramps. This usually requires 10 to 15 minutes during which the cone or shield is held firmly against the stoma to prevent backflow and incomplete filling.

5. Once the reservoir is empty, the cone or shield should be held in place for a minute or so.

6. The cone is removed to allow evacuation to proceed. Usually, patients prefer to sit on the toilet with the sleeve in the bowl for 15 to 20 minutes. During the final 10 to 20 minutes, as bowel action slows, they may choose to close the end of the sleeve and go about household or toilet chores.

7. When the irrigation is finished (patients quickly identify the feeling of completion as they did for preoperative bowel movements), the peristomal area should be cleansed thoroughly and a security pouch or gauze square secured about the stoma.

8. The irrigating bag, tubing, and sleeve are washed and stored for the next use.

Generally, patients are most successful when they adhere to a fairly rigid routine, performing the irrigation at the same time and same daily interval. While postoperative teaching may begin with daily washouts, it rarely is necessary or advisable to continue daily enemas past the sixth postoperative week. Once patients understand that, in contrast to natural bowel movement, they are *completely* cleansing the bowel, they will realize that the colon probably will not transport feces from its right side to the stomal orifice in 24 hours (unless they consume a high-fiber diet). This knowledge alleviates the compulsion to have a daily movement.

It is advisable to give patients written instructions and to have a visiting nurse come to the home to monitor the first irrigations and so ensure that anxiety and postoperative fatigue do not lead to improper or inappropriate technique.

Finally, patients ought to be informed that under normal circumstances irrigation is an elective procedure and that social, occupational, and recreational schedules may be kept in spite of it. An array of odor-proof colostomy appliances with flatus valves and filters are available for those who are unable or unwilling to devote several hours per week to mechanical emptying.

Appliances and Management. The type of appliance and the form of skin care are selected according to the type and construction of the stoma.

Loop Colostomy. Despite the advantages of a skin bridge, the loop of bowel, even in this day and age, may be held up by a rod, rubber tubing, a plastic bridge, or a butterfly specifically designed for the purpose. When a rod and rubber tubing are in place, a skin barrier must be positioned snugly around the stoma *under* the rod (Fig. 130–2). A pouch is then brought up over the rod and made to adhere to the skin barrier and surrounding skin. For an experienced ET nurse, this procedure is time-consuming but not especially difficult. For the novice or nurse generalist, it poses a frustrating challenge that usually results in the skin's being exposed to fecal

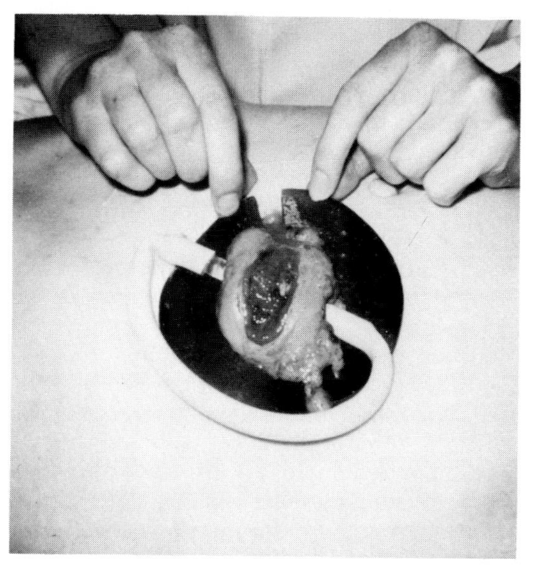

Figure 130–2. Skin barrier for a transverse loop colostomy supported by a rod; a karaya or pectin wafer is brought around and under the bowel in horseshoe fashion.

contact, with subsequent leakage and skin maceration. Sets containing a bridge or butterfly, with a skin barrier and pouch, for application in the operating suite may be more convenient and conducive to obtaining a leakproof seal with minimal "creative tailoring."

It is important to protect peristomal skin inasmuch as feces from the transverse colon contains sufficient enzymes to denude the epidermis in a short time. Plastic films (in the form of wipes, roll-ons, or sprays) may be used. Otherwise, a karaya or pectin wafer is indicated; some ET nurses use both in combination. Where there are creases, scars from previous procedures, or skin folds, a pectin wafer and paste will probably be required to compensate for the irregular surface in order to achieve a leakproof seal. When the appliance is changed, it is important to remove the residue of the skin barrier, clean and dry the skin thoroughly, and reapply the protective product.

Pouches should be odor-proof and drainable. When closed-end pouches are used with a transverse colostomy, they will require changing 2 to 4 times daily; besides being time-consuming and expensive, the frequent removal and reapplication potentiate skin breakdown. There are several types of deodorants for colostomy appliances, among them powders, drops, and sprays. Modern products have eliminated the need for earlier used potions that created odors more offensive than the ones they masked.

Once the rod is removed and the patient is prepared for hospital discharge, appliance selection is based upon the patient's acceptance of the ostomy, fecal output, stoma location, manual dexterity, physical impairments, and—in some situations—availability and cost. Common to all systems should be a skin barrier that fits the stoma in order to prevent feces from eroding surrounding skin or leaking (Fig. 130–3). Before discharge, patients should be able to demonstrate proficiency in the care of their stoma and be given a list of ostomy suppliers where they can replenish their equipment.

Some patients with a transverse colostomy prefer to change their appliance daily; others wear one pouch for several days and flush it with water periodically.

End Colostomy. Whether or not a colostomy in the descending colon is to be irrigated, it does require an appliance in the immediate postoperative phase. After preoperative bowel preparation, surgical intrusion, and IV and liquid diets, the colostomy will pour out liquid stool and copious flatus. A drainable stoma bag at this stage, with a gas filter, will permit easy emptying and facilitate observation of the quantity and nature of stool.

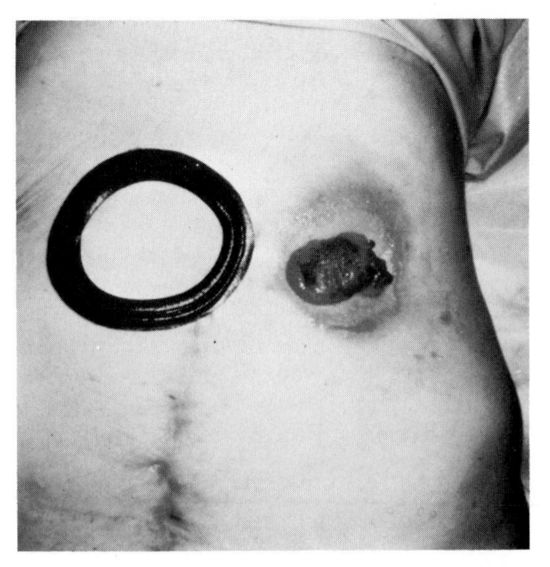

Figure 130–3. It is important to remeasure the stoma as postoperative edema subsides; otherwise skin exposed to stool may become painfully inflamed.

The stoma should be measured and a pouch with an opening ⅛ inch larger than the stoma margin ordered; as postoperative edema subsides, the appliance aperture will need to be reduced. If the correct-sized opening is temporarily unavailable, the exposed skin can be covered with a karaya or pectin wafer.

Most new colostomy patients now enjoy the convenience of disposable pouches that are sealed to the skin with a karaya washer, Stomahesive wafer, or similar pectin product. These new methods have eliminated most skin problems caused by adhesive allergy or abrasion, have simplified training, and have contributed to the patient's early acceptance of the colostomy.

When patients resume regular activity and meals and the stools become formed, they may choose to wear a closed-end pouch. If the colostomy is regulated by irrigation, they may choose a small security cap to protect the stoma, filter flatus, and absorb mucus.

Medication and diet alter the color, consistency, and amount of stool, information that should be included in the written material given to home-going patients. Since patients may not remember details, a ready reference when predictable changes do occur will prevent unnecessary alarm.

Rehabilitation. The protracted process of rehabilitation after colostomy may require as much as a year. Flatus control, irrigation or appliance security, return to full recreational and vocational participation, and physical well-being are components of the process.

When ostomates were asked "If you were going into the hospital tomorrow to have the same operation, what would you like to see changed?" 81% said they would remedy the psychologic and educational neglect they suffered, 35% wished they had received more preoperative counseling and information, and 21% cited the nursing staff's insufficient knowledge of a stoma.[7]

Colostomy patients may be assured that

1. Flatus can be kept to a minimum by dietary discretion, regular meals to avoid an empty stomach, and avoidance of habits that cause air-swallowing.
2. Clothing need not be altered. A moderately snug belt or waistband will not injure a stoma. Women can continue to wear light girdles and pantyhose.
3. Swimming and bathing are permissible. Most colostomates take showers or baths without an appliance to give the peristomal skin a thorough cleansing. It is advisable, however, to wear an appliance over the stoma when swimming in salt or fresh water.
4. No special diet is required. Foods that were well tolerated before operation may be eaten after surgery. Nuts and difficult-to-digest foods should be masticated more completely.

Equally important in the counsel and education of colostomy patients are these warnings:

1. Cancer patients and colostomates have suffered job discrimination.[8] It is important to ascertain that any adverse decision in this respect is not the result of lack of information and to have access to legal advice when discrimination does occur.
2. It is not unusual for friends and neighbors to be embarrassed by the thought of a colostomy; their response may be avoidance.
3. Efficient though modern stoma management may be, few patients escape the occasional embarrassment of noisy flatulence or soiling from a leaking appliance. Such events must be taken in stride and be borne with fortitude.

A colostomy is compatible with any lifestyle when the stoma is appropriately sited and properly constructed, appliances are chosen carefully, irrigation is recommended selectively, and the patient and family are educated judiciously.

Complications. *Ischemia* may affect the colostomy in the immediate postoperative period to a greater or lesser degree; if "die back" of the mucosa is slight, nothing further may develop. In addition to the risk of acute cellulitis of the abdominal wall, more considerable loss, as by retraction of the colon from the skin incision, may lead to a disabling stricture's developing within the ensuing 3 months. Stricture can be avoided by immediate revision of the stoma. It may also be allowed to develop, to be excised at a later date together with mobilization of the colon in order to deliver more bowel for suture to the skin without tension. Otherwise, the development of a stricture at skin level is uncommon when mucosa has been sutured to skin.

Prolapse more commonly involves a transverse loop colostomy and rarely a permanent end stoma. Since the transverse loop colostomy is ordinarily temporary, prolapse can usually be managed until closure is undertaken (which may be expedited because of this complication). For prolapse at a permanent end stoma, it is more effective to approach the colon transabdominally so as to fix the colonic mesentery after excision of the redundent bowel. The less radical maneuver of simple removal of the excess bowel at the stoma site is too frequently followed by further prolapse.

Hernia may involve the colostomy in one of 3 ways: (1) diffusely so that the stoma lies at the apex of a bulge, causing disfigurement rather than disability; or (2) by interstitial or (3) parastomal herniation, both of which tend to cause obstructive episodes necessitating revision or repair. If repair of the diffuse bulge is undertaken, it is doomed to failure unless the stoma is resited.

Small bowel obstruction due to internal herniation in a patent paracolic gutter requires emergency laparotomy. The colon itself may be obstructed by hard scybala and a narrowed conduit through the abdominal wall or by recurrent growth. *Colonic perforation*

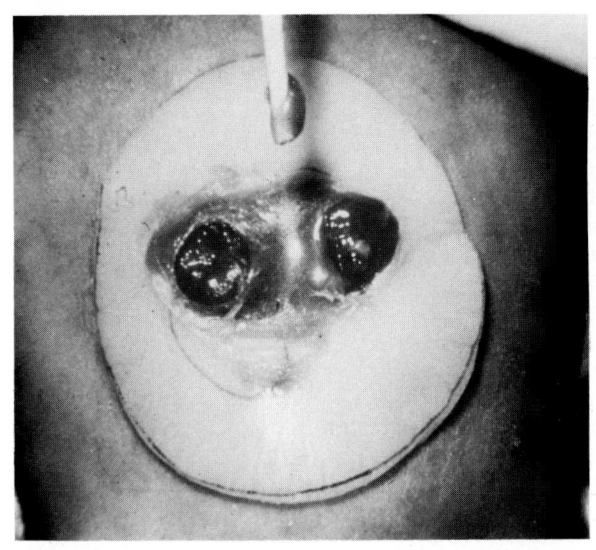

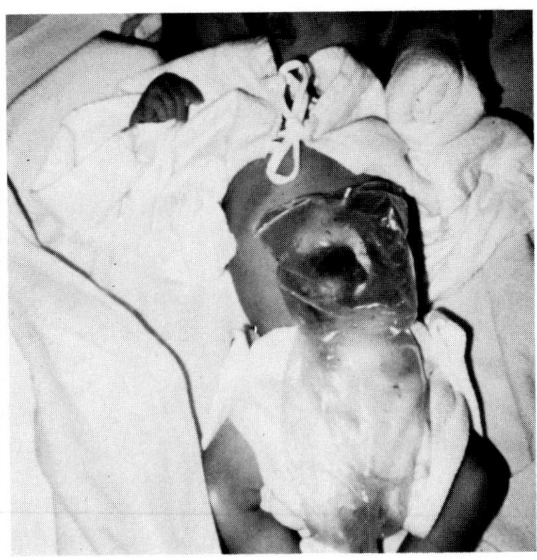

Figure 130–4. Pouching procedure in infant with fecal diversion. A pectin wafer is placed on the skin with an opening cut for both stomas, and exposed skin is covered with a paste of karaya or pectin amalgam *(left)*. A small pouch of odor-proof plastic wrap is applied over the pectin wafer so that no adhesive is in contact with the infant's skin *(right)*. The pouch is drained frequently to prevent it from overfilling.

during washout was a rare but serious complication, the risk of which has now almost been eliminated by the introduction of the conical "nozzle." A *stitch abscess* beside the stoma is a rare late development that may, even more rarely, result in a *fistula*. The most common cause of colostomy fistula today is recurrence affecting the stoma after fecal deflection for large bowel or anorectal Crohn's disease.

Pericolostomy skin complications are uncommon. Excoriation may develop if the colostomy excretion is persistently fluid. A pectin amalgam, Stomahesive, may be used as a therapeutic dressing as well as a protective skin barrier. Its hydrophilic properties cause it to adhere as well to moist as to dry skin. Even open, weeping lesions will respond favorably when the affected area is thoroughly cleansed with soap, rinsed with clear water, patted dry, and covered with a Stomahesive wafer. Unless the patient experiences pain underneath the wafer or fever, there is no reason to remove the pectin covering for 3 to 5 days; significant healing should then have occurred underneath. Karaya powder and karaya wafers continue to be used effectively to treat minor irritation.

Problems in Infants. Infants who require colostomy pose a nursing challenge; their small abdominal surface and incessant activity combine to create problems in management. In some centers a paste of karaya powder and zinc oxide is spread generously around the stoma and no appliance is used. If the stoma is low enough, one diaper may be applied in the usual fashion. If the stoma is high, a diaper may be wrapped around the abdomen for the stool and another applied in the usual manner for urine. Otherwise, small pouches of multilaminate plastic (Fig. 130–4) are preferred, for it is easier to keep a new incision clean, manage all other support systems, and present an appealing baby to anxious parents when an appliance is used. Once in place, it is important to cover the pouch with a diaper or shirt to prevent the baby from pulling it off.

It is wise to assess the parents' attitudes and intelligence carefully and involve them in the development of a colostomy care routine that will be most feasible in their home environment.

Ileostomy

Ileostomy is a relatively recent innovation brought about by the invention of the first successful adherent appliance in 1944 by Koenig, aided and abetted by his surgeon Strauss.[8a] This achievement established surgery for ulcerative colitis; it enabled the diseased colon to be removed with creation of an end stoma. Within 10 years, what is now the conventional eversion stoma had been developed,[9] and the criteria regarding siting in the right iliac fossa and length of ileum to be exposed for satisfactory application of the appliance had been established.

With the recognition that Crohn's disease can affect the large bowel, this condition has become an indication for ileostomy on 2 counts: (1) a standard divided loop or end ileostomy may become necessary to deflect the fecal stream from a severely or acutely diseased colon; and (2) a divided loop ileostomy may be employed for diversion and to enable the topical application of steroids through the distal opening ("split" ileostomy).[10]

Total removal of the large bowel necessitating permanent ileostomy is commonly undertaken for ulcerative colitis and sometimes for Crohn's disease of the colon. Though permanence is not envisaged for the ileostomy required simply for fecal deflection in Crohn's disease, the stoma undertaken in these circumstances often becomes so. The intent behind the "split" ileostomy is ultimate restoration of bowel continuity, even after a period of years.

Permanent ileostomy is sometimes required in familial polyposis coli when the rectum is so involved as to necessitate proctocolectomy rather than colectomy and ileorectal anastomosis; a permanent stoma is also required when malignancy or premalignant polyps affect several sites in the large intestine.

Attempts to obtain a continent device have proved more successful with ileum than with colon. In 1969 Kock[11] reported the use of an ileal reservoir for an ileostomy as an adaptation of the technique he had originally devised to replace the urinary bladder. The stoma of the continent ileostomy lies flush with the skin in the right iliac fossa; the subjacent reservoir is emptied through this stoma by catheter passed 2 or 3 times daily, assisted by gentle massage of the abdominal wall around the stoma.

A further development of the continent stoma has been the application by Parks and Nicholls[12] of the ileal reservoir to ileoanal anastomosis, thus using the anal sphincters to achieve continence with restoration of intestinal continuity.

Preparing the Patient. The preparation of a patient for ileostomy differs from that for colostomy patients. Patients with inflammatory bowel disease are younger (most often between the ages of 15 and 35 years) and are in the midst of the years of decision regarding marriage, occupation, and social and recreational activities. For many, ileostomy will bring to an end years of chronic disease; for the ulcerative colitis patient it promises a cure but for patients with Crohn's disease there may be recurrence in remaining portions of the alimentary tract. There are 4 critical principles of preparation for ileostomy:

1. *Emotional support.* The creation of an ileostomy disturbs the body image at a time when there are many psychosocial issues at stake. Females may wonder if they will be sexually attractive and if they can become pregnant, carry a baby to term, and be delivered vaginally or by cesarean section. Males are likely to fear loss of potency and desirability. For some patients, ileostomy represents failure of medical therapy and "5 to 7 wasted years of suffering"; for others, the cure of their disease will create new potential and responsibility that may be more fearful than exciting. Parent-child relationships, fortified during the dependency of illness, will be interrupted—an adjustment for the entire family.

2. *Stoma site selection.* Since the hours in the operating room will be followed by years of life with an ileostomy, the site and configuration of the stoma are prime determinants of the quality of that life. It is crucial that the patient's occupational and recreational interests be considered along with anatomic and physiologic requirements. It is best to examine patients in all postures (see Fig. 130–1) and, except in emergency circumstances, give them an opportunity to wear a trial appliance to determine optimal location. Time and thought given to this will ensure that the patient's rehabilitation is not impeded by leaking, uncomfortable appliances.

3. *Introduction to ileostomy care.* Some preoperative training in stoma care will eliminate unnecessary concern and facilitate postoperative independence. When patients are introduced to the products and accessories, they see that "the bag" is not a huge, conspicuous apparatus but a small, odor-proof, rustle-free device. Several simple reassuring demonstrations to patients and family members will minimize fear and misconceptions.

4. *Presentation of a rehabilitated ileostomate of*

the same sex and of similar age and interests. No amount of surgical or nursing wisdom supplants the importance of a volunteer visitor from an ostomy association. The sight of a clean, healthy individual without a "bulging bag," body odor, or a sense of shame is often the turning point in a patient's acceptance of an impending or newly created ileostomy. Ostomy self-help groups have improved their effectiveness in recent years by screening and training prospective volunteer visitors within their associations. The mutual aid of ostomy associations provided by their visiting programs, publications, and scheduled meetings is an important facet of rehabilitation.[13, 14]

Frequently, an ET nurse becomes the catalyst for the preparatory activities that lead to ileostomy. Without such a specialist, it falls to the surgeon or a designated staff nurse to orchestrate the components of pre- and postoperative education, counseling, and training.

Physiology and Metabolic Abnormalities. Excretion from an established stoma is stimulated by taking food and so may be anticipated within 20 to 30 minutes after starting a meal. Most ileostomates find that activity is minimal from 1½ to 2 hours after eating. This interval may provide an opportunity to change an appliance, if need be, although regular care is usually undertaken on rising in the morning when excretion is also minimal. Some individuals restrict food intake at the end of the day and avoid meals or drinks for 2 hours before going to bed so as to avoid having the pouch fill during the night and becoming dislodged.

Daily output varies between 200 and 500 ml in volume, the stool consistency being semisolid at the lower end of the range. High volume fluid loss of approximately 1 to 2 liters or more daily in the immediate postoperative period, leading to the serious condition of ileostomy dysfunction,[15] was found to be due to exposure of ileal serosa[16] and has been virtually eliminated by eversion of the stoma.[9]

An ileostomy begins to function with an output at first lower than usual and then gradually increasing to the levels of the established stoma.[17] This is an important observation since in the ulcerative colitis patient the occurrence of a higher output in the postoperative period indicates either intra-abdominal sepsis or partial obstruction and is often the first indication of these complications. A higher output may be expected in a patient with Crohn's disease. Hill et al.[18] have shown ileostomy output to be related to body weight: 70-kg "normal" man will excrete 500 to 600 ml, and a daily output greater than this should be regarded as abnormal.

Output may increase with the ingestion of certain foods, such as the brassicas,[19] or if more than 15 g of salt is ingested daily[20]; any excess water drunk is excreted in the urine. Conversely, a reduction in output cannot be manipulated by dietary means alone, other than by a "salt-free" diet. Diphenoxylate (Lomotil), loperamide (Imodium), and codeine phosphate reduce output, codeine being the most effective; psyllium seed preparations thicken the effluent but increase the volume of excreta.[21]

Sodium concentration in ileostomy excreta is 115 mg/liter; under ordinary circumstances the daily loss of 50 to 60 mMol is readily overcome. Trouble arises with ileostomy diarrhea, when sodium loss becomes excessive, less easily restored in the absence of the colon, and associated with dehydration. It is important, therefore, that the ileostomate be aware of the need to ingest extra salt and fluid when stomal output rises and following excessive sweating. If vomiting occurs, potassium depletion may develop; the normal daily need for this electrolyte can be met by a glass of orange juice. Magnesium deficiency only becomes a problem in longstanding ileostomy diarrhea, as in Crohn's disease. Nitrogen loss in the excreta of patients with a normal small intestine is no greater than in patients with an intact colon, nor does steatorrhea occur in these circumstances.

Weight gain is usual and may even continue to an abnormal degree, thus creating a new health problem. Similarly, vitamin deficiency is not a problem except for vitamin B_{12} in Crohn's disease or when the terminal ileum has been resected or effectively reduced by the formation of a continent pouch.

Gallstone formation in ileostomy patients is related to the amount of ileum lost to function; Hill et al.[22] demonstrated a higher than normal frequency of gallstones, although neither Goligher et al.[23] nor Ritchie[24] was able to show an increase in frequency of cholecystectomy in patients followed for long periods. In a group of 2270 women followed by Rang[25] for 10 years after ileostomy and colectomy,

180 (5.7%) underwent cholecstectomy for gallstones, while an additional 32 (1.4%) were found to have gallstones. Hence, 7% of these 2270 women were known to have developed gallstones—less than one-third of the frequency Hill et al.[22] found in their 108 patients of both sexes, and lower than the expected frequency for women (9.7%) presented by Hill and co-workers.

A patient with a healthy ileostomy has a slightly increased risk of forming *renal uric acid and calcium stones*, a risk increased by loss of ileal function by either resection or disease. Of the 2270 women studied by Rang,[25] 116 (5.1%) developed renal stones or colic,[25] an occurrence rate almost half that published in another study by Hill et al.[26]

Complications. *Mechanical complications* at an eversion ileostomy, mostly preventable by careful technique when the stoma is instituted, usually call for operative correction. Fixation of the mesentery across the paraileal gutter obliterates a site of internal herniation and thus eliminates one cause of obstruction. It also anchors the intestine so that prolapse cannot occur, although the complementary complication of recession is not entirely avoided thereby.

Acute recession can develop within 24 hours of operation owing to insufficient protection of the newly everted ileum from pressure of bedclothes and the appliance. A cotton-wool ring splint around the stoma within the pouch will prevent pressure from the plastic appliance, while a bed cradle keeps the weight of the bedclothes away. The condition can be corrected by inserting a small-delta Duval forceps through the flush stoma, grasping the ileum, and withdrawing it once more; all of which can be achieved without anesthesia. To ensure fixation, the Duval forceps should be retained across one side of the apex with light pressure for 24 hours and can be incorporated within the appliance.

Chronic recession occurring at any time subsequently is at present the most common mechanical complication. It presents in 2 ways: (1) The ileum subsides freely into the abdomen. This is usually due to detachment of the mesenteric fixation and can be corrected only by laparotomy and refixation. (2) The ileum recedes intermittently. This occurs more often into the interstices of the abdominal wall than into the abdomen proper.

The diagnosis of the interstitial condition is readily made with the patient supine; pressure around the flush stoma will cause it to evert. Operative revision in this circumstance can be confined to the stoma site. The mucocutaneous junction is opened, the ileum unraveled, the interstitial pocket closed, and, as eversion is restored, circumferential serosal sutures of catgut are inserted between the outgoing and returning layers of ileum to induce adherence. This is easier to perform if the returning layer is cut along its antimesenteric border. The fixation of the 2 layers is enhanced if this incision remains unsutured so that a triangle of outgoing serosa remains exposed with its apex at the stoma apex and its base at skin level.

Excision of the excess ileum has no place in the surgical cure of *prolapse*, except occasionally when the ileum has been so damaged by edema and ulceration that a limited area must be removed. Correction of prolapse ordinarily requires reattachment of the mesentery at formal laparotomy.

The opening through the abdominal wall to accommodate the emerging ileum calls for good judgment as regards size; otherwise, stomal, parastomal, or interstitial herniation may develop. On the average, the opening should accommodate the tips of 2 fingers, but clearly factors such as obesity (which is occasionally encountered in ulcerative colitis patients) must affect this. Repair of stomal hernia is less satisfactory than for the parastomal or interstitial forms and may require resiting of the stoma.

Fistula development is most often due to Crohn's disease. The stoma is occasionally lacerated when the facepiece of the appliance is displaced either during strenuous activity or by the thigh's flexing against a stoma that has been placed too low. Sometimes the development of a stitch abscess leads to fistula. Stomal fistulas of whatever cause do not heal spontaneously; surgical revision is then required.

Stomal ulceration may result from pressure against the inner surface of the pouch. The cause usually is recognizable from the site of the ulcers at the apex or on the anterior aspect of the stoma, or as being due to Crohn's disease.

Except in Crohn's disease, *stenosis* is now rare, being virtually eliminated by immediate mucosa-to-skin suture undertaken at eversion.

The frequency of *operative revision* necessary to maintain an efficient stoma is difficult to establish owing to a paucity of published reports. For ulcerative colitis, in the experience of one of us (B.N.B.), it has been 2%. Of 464 ulcerative colitis patients treated in Birmingham, England, 308 survivors were followed over a mean period of 20 years after operation; of these, 48 required ileostomy revision (70 operations).[27] The probability of revision is 4 times higher during the first postoperative year in a patient with Crohn's disease; for patients with either Crohn's disease or ulcerative colitis, revision is more likely in the first 4 postoperative years and remains lower thereafter.[28]

Continent Ileostomy. The most common complication arises from failure of the nipple valve necessary to maintain fecal retention. Extrusion of the nipple tends to occur as the reservoir enlarges, allowing its contents to increase in volume and so drag the whole pouch away from the abdominal wall. In the experience of most surgeons, *revision* to correct the resulting incontinence is necessary in 30% of patients after about 18 months.

Due to the extensive suturing required for the formation of the intestinal reservoir, there is an immediate postoperative risk of leakage and peritonitis. The operation carries an inherent mortality of up to 3% over and above that of panproctocolectomy.

Later complications include the inelegantly termed condition of *"pouchitis,"* an inflammatory state involving mucosa and sometimes the whole thickness of the intestinal wall, both of which may be destroyed. This may be a "stercoral" phenomenon, for the continent stoma relies upon obstruction for its effectiveness. The inflammatory state is a late complication, becoming manifest at around 5 years postoperatively, and is sometimes associated with stenosis. Conversion to an eversion ileostomy is required.

Vitamin B_{12} deficiency is known to develop in some patients at a late stage because of loss of mucosal function in the terminal ileum, and individual cases of megaloblastic anemia are encountered.

Appliances and Management. The ileostomy appliance selected for use in the hospital during the early postoperative period will differ from the one the patient uses in the home. In the immediate postoperative phase, the appropriate collection device selected should meet the following criteria: (1) allow visualization of the stoma; (2) be drainable; (3) be made of odor-resistant material, such as multilaminate plastic (Saran wrap); (4) have a skin barrier as an integral component or be compatible with the use of a skin barrier; (5) be available with a variety of apertures or permit cutting to specification for exact stomal fit; and (6) permit lateral positioning while the patient is recumbent to facilitate emptying.

It may be necessary, particularly when the nursing staff is unfamiliar with ostomy care, to arrange to have the bag emptied every 2 to 3 hours. When appliances overfill, they leak and jeopardize the new incision and the integrity of the peristomal skin.

Selection of an appliance for use after hospital discharge has been complicated by advances in appliance design; there are 1-piece, 2-piece, and multi-piece systems and reusable, throw-away, and combination assemblies. The patient's interest in the care of his stoma, his level of intelligence, his occupational and recreational requirements, and economic status all have to be taken into consideration. A fine point, not easily dismissed, is where and how patients will dispose of discardable ostomy bags.

Few ileostomy patients want to change their appliance once a day, but some fastidious people do. Most would like to put on an opaque, odor-resistant, inconspicuous throw-away pouch and leave it in place for 5 to 7 days, emptying it 4 to 6 times daily between changes.

Once the selection has been made, it is advisable to set aside several days to train the patient before discharge from the hospital. However, skin will not tolerate repeated removal and reapplication of appliances for the sake of achieving proficiency. During the first 6 postoperative months, edema of the stoma will decrease and it is important for patients to modify their procedures or their appliances so that peristomal skin is not exposed to the enzyme-containing fecal output. Included in their instructional literature should be the signs and symptoms of complications that may occur, such as prolapse, herniation, and obstruction, and the action to be taken should these develop.

Peristomal excoriation secondary to allergy, abrasion, fecal contact, or pressure potentiates a vicious circle of appliances that will not adhere and increasing maceration because of leakage. Since the development of Stomahesive wafers, the plight of the ileostomate with weeping, painful irritation has been eased. The pectin wafer will adhere to broken, oozing surfaces and a pouch can then be applied to the Stomahesive covering. The skin will heal within 1 week if no longer exposed to further irritants.

The development of karaya and pectin amalgam pastes, squeezed from a tube, has facilitated the accommodation of an appliance to the most irregular abdominal surface and around a retracted or sunken stoma. These pastes can be used on excoriated skin, but the alcohol content causes temporary discomfort.

Patients who have had an ileostomy for many years and who use skin cements or double-sided adhesive discs will not escape transient skin breakdown. Often they are more willing to tolerate their superficial discomfort than to change their familiar procedure in order to restore the skin surface. A compromise may be achieved by applying a Stomahesive wafer to the skin while continuing with their application routine; the use of ointments and creams is of little value in these circumstances. Any topical treatment must provide for the continuous use of an adherent collection device.

Rehabilitation. Rehabilitation is complete when patients are as healthy, or healthier—physically and mentally—than they were preoperatively, and when they are in full control of their appliance rather than controlled by it. The culmination of the rehabilitative process is the product of a combined approach to pre- and postoperative education and counseling.

In the early postoperative period "the honeymoon phenomenon" may account for patients' enthusiasm for their ostomy and disregard for social and occupational consequences, release from the debilitating effects of inflammatory bowel disease being the positive event. This transient exuberance usually gives way to normal concern before reasonable appreciation of the benefits of an ileostomy is achieved.

Experience with ostomy associations and research groups indicates that few inconveniences are experienced by ileostomates in their pursuit of a satisfying life. They work in all fields, marry, divorce, and remarry in the same way as do individuals in the population at large; many women have given birth. Meticulous attention to the details of proctectomy for benign disease will preserve the potency of men.

Critical to ileostomy acceptance is comfortable, reliable, and affordable appliance management. While the initial selection of an appliance is likely to be made in the hospital by the ET nurse, the patient's best source of information for the day-to-day aspects of stoma care is an ostomy association. Whether the question is what to do with the pouch during intercourse, how to reduce flatus, or which appliance is best suited to a tennis player in the tropics, the most reliable answer lies with an ostomate who has found a solution through personal trial and error.

The diagnosis, treatment, and surgical eradication of inflammatory bowel disease are of supreme importance, but once the colon has been removed and an appliance is required, patients want more than medical management alone can provide.[7]

Sexual Problems Associated with Colostomy and Ileostomy

Sexual problems fall into the categories of organic and psychologic disability; organic disability is the result of either the original disease or the operation to correct it.

Organic Disability. The institution of a stoma *per se* is not a cause of impotence or infertility. *Impotence* arises from excision of the rectum during which either parasympathetic nerves (the nervi erigentes) responsible for erection, or sympathetic fibers (passing beneath the presacral nerve) responsible for ejaculation, are damaged. Although the sensory component through the pudendal nerve can be damaged, this has happened only through naturally occurring accidents and has not yet been recorded as a surgical accident resulting from rectal excision; however, this is conceivable in complete pelvic exenteration, in which loss of motor function would then predominate. Impotence, complete or partial, is more common after rectal excision for cancer because of the wider clearance needed than for inflammatory bowel disease. Nevertheless, the literature is singularly lacking regarding prevalence figures following rectal excision for cancer.

Of 100 men with ulcerative colitis specifically studied after protocolectomy in Birmingham, 11 had sexual impairment; the impairment amounted to total impotence in 6 of the patients, but 2 of them had diabetes.[29] In a later study undertaken by the Ileostomy Association of Great Britain and Ireland[30] of patients operated upon in different centers, impotence was complete in 6 of 118 (5%) men, and 28 (24%) had partial dysfunction. It was observed that the frequency of impotence increased with age at the time of operation. It should be borne in mind that impotence cannot be ascribed to organic damage with certainty unless confirmed by penile plethysmography. Evidence has been forthcoming to indicate that function may return in cases of indubitable organic origin (such as after total cystectomy, when all motor pathways are severed); apparently regeneration can sometimes take place in the pelvic autonomic nerves in 3 to 4 years.

Conversely, the Ileostomy Association study disclosed that the proportion of 165 women experiencing orgasm and pleasurable sensation increased following rectal excision. This was despite the fact that pelvic scarring, albeit temporary, was a cause of dyspareunia in some.

Infertility. *Infertility* was noted by Daly and Brooke[29] in the patients they observed in Birmingham, although it has yet to be determined whether this was due to the effects of pelvic inflammatory disease or the disturbance of a pelvic operation. Fertility has been determined in 2133 women born before 1944 who had colectomy and ileostomy performed for ulcerative colitis before 1970; 729 (33.5%) had no children.[25] In the United Kingdom population at large, infertility ranged between 10% and 16% in women born between 1920 and 1950.[31] Both groups inevitably embrace all causes of failure to conceive, including voluntary infertility, so the difference in frequency is a significant implication of the effect of the disease or the pelvic operation. This would seem all the more so since adoption rates appeared to be high in the stoma group. Of the latter group, only 1246 (57.3%) achieved their first pregnancy by the age of 30, as opposed to 70% to 80% in the control group referred to earlier.

The direct effect of a stoma on sexual function is confined to psychologic revulsion and inhibition; only 10 of the 376 ileostomates in the Ileostomy Association study[30] found the presence of the stoma to be a cause of difficulty at intercourse. Over 85% made the appropriate mental adjustment and were able to overcome their aversion to shyness about their own stoma. The spouses seldom saw their partners as less attractive because of the presence of the stoma; only 9% of wives and 6% of husbands were thus affected.

Pregnancy. This is hardly a circumstance to be considered in relation to colostomy, since the vast majority of women are beyond child-bearing age by the time colostomy is performed. Ileostomy, *per contra*, is a stoma of young people, and, fortunately, it constitutes no bar to pregnancy.

During pregnancy, an ileostomy patient suffering hyperemesis will have greater difficulty in controlling electrolyte balance, and IV therapy may be required. Iron therapy may cause ileostomy diarrhea. The stoma itself may be affected, occasionally becoming edematous or prolapsed. A change of appliance is also sometimes necessary as the abdominal contour alters.

Through the auspices of the Ileostomy Association of Great Britain and Ireland, a study was undertaken by Hudson[32] of 89 pregnancies in 75 women. Of these, 84 went to term; there were 3 miscarriages and 2 terminations for unspecified reasons. Episodes of obstruction were not uncommon during pregnancy. Normal delivery *per vaginam* was achieved in all but 17 pregnancies; cesarean section was undertaken only once for reasons related to the stoma (prolapse in that instance). The presence of a stoma provided no hazard for mother or infant.

References

1. Hughes LE. Complications of diverticular disease: Inflammation, obstruction and bleeding. Clin Gastroenterol 1975; 4:147–69.
2. Feustel H, Hennig G. Kontinente Kolostomie durch magnetverschluss. Deutsch Med Wochenschr 1975; 100:1063–4.
3. Alexander-Williams J, Amery AH, Devlin HB, Goligher JC, Heald RJ, Parks AG, Porter N, Thomson JPS, Todd IP. Magnetic continent colostomy device. Br Med J 1972; 1:1269–70.
4. Kubie L. The fantasy of dirt. Psychoanal Q 1937; 6:388–425.
5. Mikolon S. Psychosocial issues in ostomy management. *In*: Broadwell DC, Jackson BS, eds. Principles of Ostomy Care. St. Louis: CV Mosby, 1982:438–42.
6. Stuart M. Personal communication, 1982.
7. Achterberg J, Lawlis GF, Carlton A, Smith P. The psychological road to recovery. Ostomy Q 1979; 16(3):19–20,22,30.
8. Kumbula T. Cancer patients suffer job bias, study finds. Ostomy Q 1977; 14(2):45.

8a. Strauss AA, Strauss SF. Surgical treatment of ulcerative colitis. Surg Clin North Am 1944; 24:211–24.

9. Brooke BN. The management of an ileostomy, including its complications. Lancet 1952; 2:102–4.
10. Truelove SC, Ellis H, Webster CU. Place of double barrelled ileostomy in ulcerative colitis and Crohn's disease of the colon: A preliminary report. Br Med J 1965; 1:150–3.
11. Kock NG. Intra-abdominal reservoir in patients with permanent ileostomy. Arch Surg 1969; 99:223–31.
12. Parks AG, Nicholls RJ. Proctocolectomy without ileostomy for ulcerative colitis. Br Med J 1978; 2:85–8.

13. Gartner A, Riessman F. Self-help in the Human Services. San Francisco: Jossey-Bass, 1977.
14. Trainor MA. Acceptance of ostomy and the visitor role in a self-help group for ostomy patients. PhD thesis. The Catholic University of America, Washington DC, 1980.
15. Warren R, McKittrick LS. Ileostomy for ulcerative colitis; technique, complications and management. Surg Gynecol Obstet 1951; 93:555–67.
16. Crile G, Turnbull RB. Mechanism and prevention of ileostomy dysfunction. Ann Surg 1954; 140:459–66.
17. Hill GL. Ileostomy. Surgery, Physiology and Management. New York: Grune and Stratton, 1976.
18. Hill GL, Millward SF, King RF, Smith RC. Normal ileostomy output: close relation to body size. Br Med J 1979; 2:831–2.
19. Kramer P, Kearney MM, Inglefinger FJ. The effect of foods and water loading on the ileal excreta of ileostomized human subjects. Gastroenterology 1962; 42:535–45.
20. Kramer P. The effects of varying sodium loads on the ileal excreta of human ileostomized subjects. J Clin Invest 1966; 45:1710–18.
21. Newton CR. The effect of codeine phosphate, Lomotil and Isogel on ileostomy function. Gut 1973; 14:424–5.
22. Hill GL, Mair WSJ, Goligher JC. Gallstones after ileostomy and ileal resection. Gut 1975; 16:932–6.
23. Goligher JC, de Dombal FT, Watts J McK, Watkinson G. Ulcerative Colitis. Baltimore: Williams and Wilkins, 1968.
24. Ritchie JK. Ulcerative colitis treated by ileostomy and excisional surgery. Fifteen years experience at St. Mark's Hospital. Br J Surg 1972; 59:345–51.
25. Rang E. Personal communication, 1982.
26. Bambach CP, Robertson WG, Peacock M, Hill GL. Effect of intestinal surgery on the risk of urinary stone formation. Gut 1981; 22:257–63.
27. Dew MJ. Bile acids and the liver in inflammatory bowel disease. M.D. thesis. University of Birmingham, 1980.
28. Fawaz KA, Glotzer DJ, Goldman H, Dickersin GR, Gross W, Patterson JF. Ulcerative colitis and Crohn's disease of the colon—a comparison of the long term post-operative courses. Gastroenterology 1976; 71:372–8.
29. Daly DW, Brooke BN. Ileostomy and excision of the large intestine for ulcerative colitis. Lancet 1967; 2:62–4.
30. Burnham WR, Lennard-Jones JE, Brooke BN. Sexual problems among married ileostomists. Gut 1977; 18:673–7.
31. Thompson J. The age at which child bearing starts: a generation perspective. Office of Population Control Statistics; Population Trends (MK) 1980: 21.
32. Hudson CN. Ileostomy in pregnancy. Proc R Soc Med 1972; 65:281–3.

Chapter 131

Anatomy of the Colon

William S. Haubrich

Embryologically and functionally the colon is divisible into 2 parts. That portion proximal to the middle of the transverse colon, in common with the small intestine, springs from the embryonal midgut and receives its blood supply from the superior mesenteric artery. With the small intestine it shares an important absorptive function. The distal half of the colon is derived from the hindgut and receives its blood supply, for the most part, from the inferior mesenteric artery and its branches. The left half of the colon is essentially a storage unit, having little, if any, digestive or absorptive function.

Size of the Colon

In animals, variations in the relative size of the colon depend, in part, upon the dietary habits of the species. Herbivorous animals generally have large colons with commodious cecal pouches which permit bacterial digestion of cellulose fibers that constitute the bulk of vegetable diets. In carnivores the colon is comparatively short. Although man is omnivorous, his colon resembles more that of the carnivore than that of the herbivore. Perhaps there is a lesson in this for the person having an unusually long and capacious colon who may complain of constipation while subsisting on a meat and starch diet and whose elimination might be facilitated by a high-residue vegetable diet (Fig. 131–1).

By careful intubation studies in living human subjects, Blankenhorn et al.[1] determined the ratios of nose-anus length to body height and found them to vary between 2.54 and 3.69 m. In these subjects the colon length was estimated to be from 91 to 125 cm. It is apparent that the length of the intestine varies considerably, not only according to body size but also among normal individuals of the same size.

The caliber of the colon progressively diminishes distally from a maximum diameter at the cecum (about 8.5 cm) to a minimum diameter at the sigmoid segment (about 2.5 cm). This fact, together with the increased inspissation of feces, accounts for the frequency with which small annular cancers can obstruct the distal colon.

Parts of the Colon and Their Attachments

In sequence, the segments of the colon customarily are designated as the cecum, the ascending colon, the hepatic (right) flexure, the transverse colon, the splenic (left) flexure, the descending colon, the sigmoid colon, and the rectum (Fig. 131–2). Often clinicians and surgeons refer to that portion of the large intestine proximal to the middle of the trans-

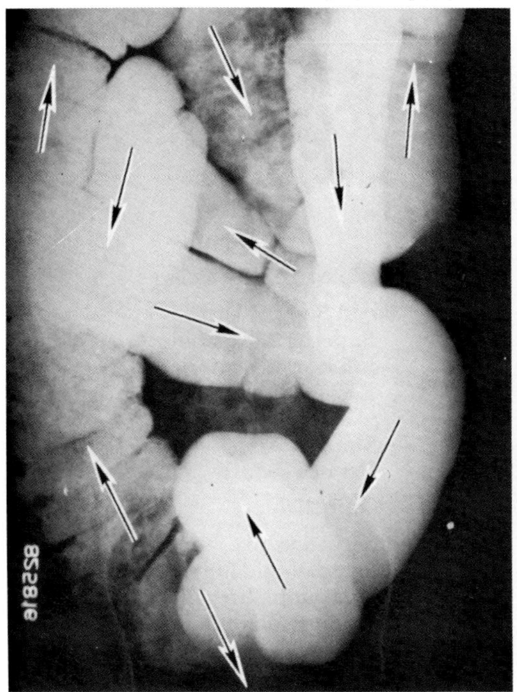

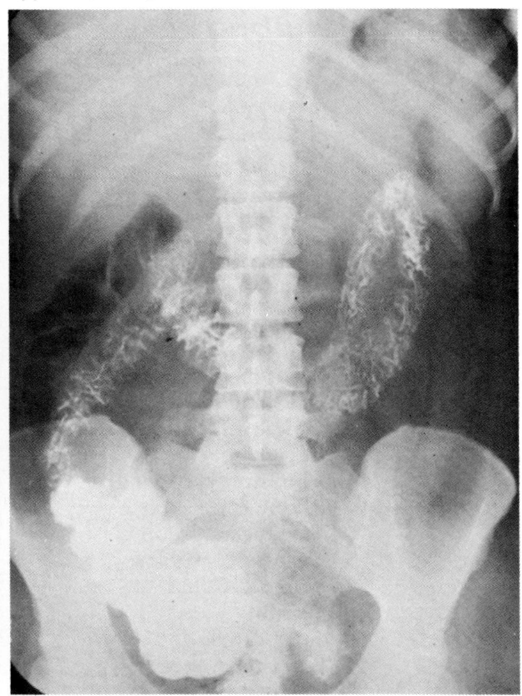

Figure 131–1. Barium enema radiographs outlining the colon in a healthy 26-year-old woman who complained of constipation. The arrows in the barium-filled colon *(left)* indicate the tortuous course of this remarkably redundant colon, an example of the anomaly of dolichocolon. In the postevacuation film *(right)* taken at the same examination, note how efficiently the colon has contracted.

verse segment collectively as the "right colon," whereas the distal portion becomes the "left colon."

The approximate position of the normal colon as it relates to the surface anatomy of the anterior abdominal wall is illustrated in Figure 131–3.

Ileocecal Junction. The entrance of the small intestine into the colon is situated only about 15 cm diagonally from the ligament of Treitz, and the proximal jejunum and terminal ileum are parallel, albeit their polarity is opposite. Hence, the terminal ileum comes up to the right in its approach to the posterior medial wall of the colon. The terminal several centimeters of ileum may be fused to the medial wall of the cecum and, thus, normally appear fixed in radiographs.[2] The terminal ileum further may be fixed by a triangular or quadrilateral membrane attaching the antimesenteric border of the distal ileum to the parietal peritoneum covering the right iliac fossa *(Lane's membrane).* As it enters the colon, the lumen of the ileum is directed horizontally or even slightly downward, giving in radiographs the configuration of a bird's neck, head, and beak (Fig. 131–4).

In the opened cecum, the ileal entrance appears as a mouth with semilunar lips. The upper lip protrudes more (1.5 cm) than the lower lip (0.5 cm). Unfortunately, the actual ileal orifice is seldom seen through the forward-viewing tip of the colonoscope; the endoscopic landmark is the prominent, fixed fold on the medial wall representing the upper lip of the ileocecal junction. The angles of the mouth taper off as the frenula (plural of the Latin *frenulum,* "bridle"), which form transverse folds demarcating the cecum and ascending colon. In the 55% of specimens he considered typical, Buirge[3, 4] observed that increased intracecal tension rendered the frenula taut and closed the lips of the orifice. As such, the ileocecal junction could qualify as a competent "valve." Still, in many subjects (90% according to Fleischner and Bernstein[2]), a barium suspension given by enema refluxes in varying amounts into the terminal ileum. It is worth noting that often the reflux of barium is seen only, or in greater

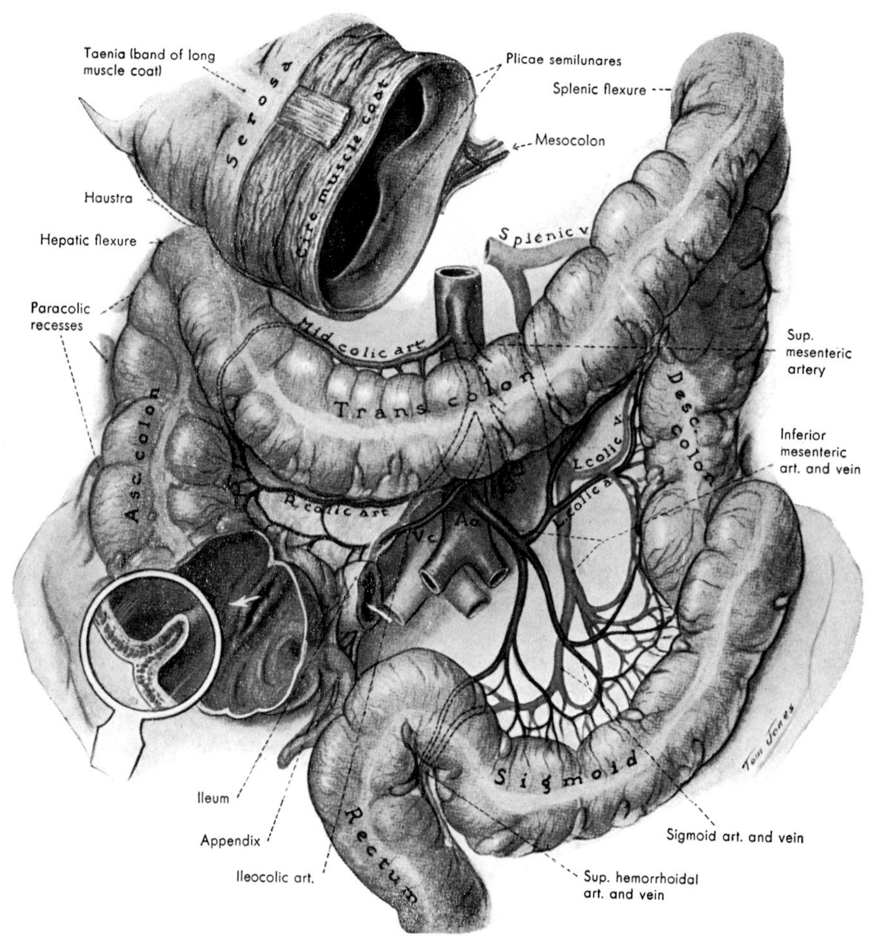

Figure 131–2. The position of the colon is shown as it usually appears in anteroposterior barium radiographs. The anterior wall of the cecum is removed to show the entrance of the ileum and the characteristic folds. Above is an enlarged cutaway section of the transverse segment showing the muscular coats and the semilunar folds separating the haustra.

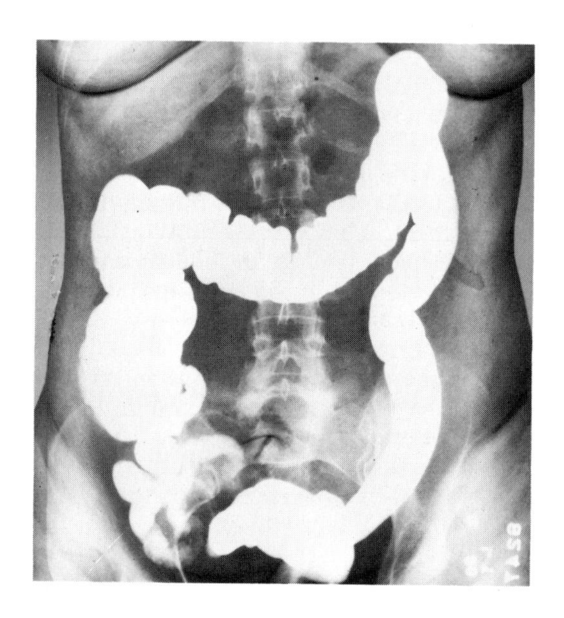

Figure 131–3. Radiograph of the barium-filled colon superimposed on a photograph of the anterior abdomen, both taken of the same normal subject in the supine position. This illustrates only the approximate relation of the colon to surface anatomy, and account must be made for appreciable individual variations.

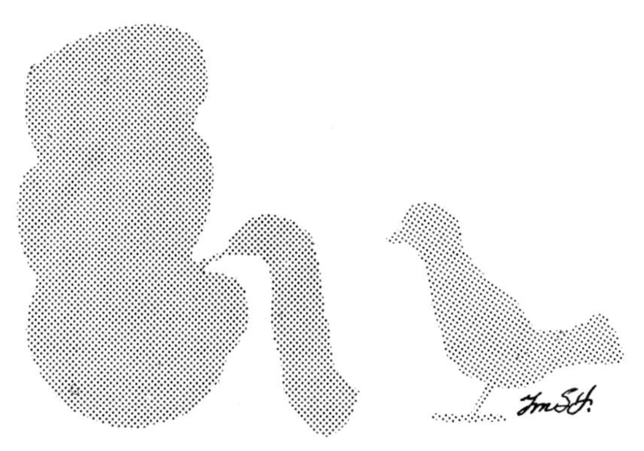

Figure 131–4. The barium outline of the terminal ileum entering the cecum resembles the profile of a bird.

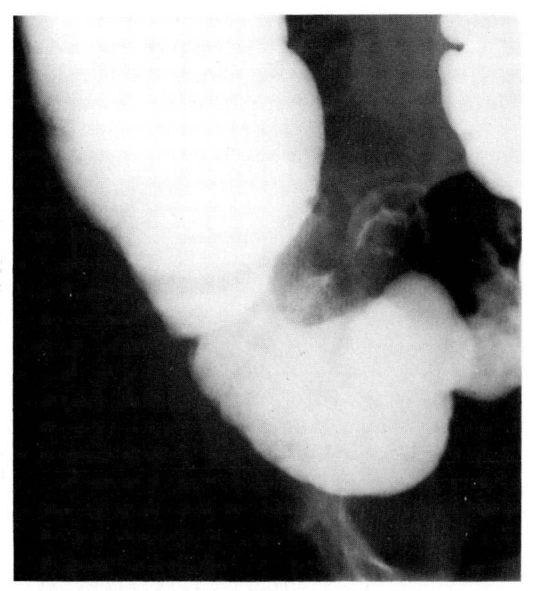

Figure 131–5. An unusually prominent ileal protrusion as seen in the barium enema examination of an asymptomatic 45-year-old woman. By its smooth outline and characteristic situation, such a configuration is not apt to be confused with an abnormal filling defect in the cecum.

amount, in postevacuation films rather than in views of the filled colon. It is now generally recognized that ileal reflux is a normal phenomenon and not significant of any particular disease or disorder.

Competency or incompetency at the ileocecal junction is a matter of importance only in the case of obstruction in the colon beyond the cecum. If there exists a competent "valve," then gas and fluid accumulating in the colon have no egress by reflux and cannot be aspirated through the small intestine. This constitutes a "closed-loop" colon obstruction, a precarious condition which can lead to perforation, usually at the cecum.

If the ileocecal junction is only occasionally a valve, is it ever a sphincter? The lips of the ileal orifice protruding into the cecum often appear thicker than the wall of either the ileum or the colon (Fig. 131–5). In children, the protuberance may appear larger because of abundant lymphoid tissue in the ileal wall. Ulin et al.[5] describe the ileal protrusion as a muscular papilla. Anatomic dissection in the cadaver, however, usually fails to disclose any well-developed sphincteric muscle. Through a fistula in a living cecum, Buirge[4] observed no tonic contraction at the ileal orifice such as one might expect in a true sphincter. He did note that prodding the mucosa or attempting to stretch the orifice elicited a marked muscular contraction. The observation that chyme is delivered into the cecum in small spurts, rather than continuously, suggests that some control on the movement of chyme is exerted at the ileocecal junction. It is of clinical significance that the patient deprived of his ileocecal "valve," as following an ileo-ascending colostomy, often experiences protracted diarrhea that suggests defective motor control. Another factor may be contamination of the small intestine by coliform bacterial flora to which the intact ileocecal orifice is presumed to be a partial barrier. This may also account for the "backwash ileitis" often seen with chronic ulcerative pancolitis.

Cecum. The pouch of colon below the entrance of the small intestine derives its name from the Latin *caecus,* "blind." The cecum usually is wider (about 8.5 cm) than it is long (about 6.5 cm). If rotation of the intestine has been complete, the cecum normally nestles in the right iliac fossa when the body is supine. It may slide over the brim of the true pelvis when the body is upright. If the colon is unusually redundant, the cecum may extend toward the midline. In the event of incomplete intestinal rotation, the cecum may remain in the right upper abdominal quadrant or even in the left side of the peritoneal cavity.

In its development, the cecum begins as a conical pouch with the appendix at its apex, and it appears as such in the newborn. With maturity, the 2 large haustra on either side of the anterior taenia enlarge unequally, the growth of the lateral sac exceeding that of the medial sac. Hence, the cecum assumes an eccentric shape with the base of the appendix eventually along its medial aspect. Still, the base of the appendix can be located by tracing the convergence of the taeniae.

Because the cecum is actually an outpouching from the antimesenteric border of the gut rather than a segment in continuity, the cecum can claim no true mesentery. Its peritoneal attachment posteriorly is normally variable. Among 125 specimens, Wolfer et al.[6] found the cecum fused to the posterior parietes in 5.6%, adherent over a third or more of its posterior surface in 11.2%, and with little or no membranous attachment in the remainder. The range of normal mobility of the cecum has made attractive, in some quarters, the supposition that discomforting symptoms may arise from peregrinations of the cecum. It is true that actual volvulus of the cecum is a recognized, although fortunately rare, entity. Also, a cecal "bascule" has been described[7] in which the unattached cecum folds over the ascending colon anteriorly to produce a "flap-valve" obstruction. Nevertheless, cecopexy as a remedy for functional bowel disorders is an ill-conceived maneuver. Hollinshead[8] makes the valid point that the term *"mobile cecum"* should be applied only in those unusual instances in which the ascending colon has a loose mesenteric attachment to the right posterior peritoneal wall.

Vermiform Appendix. This wormlike structure was originally at the cecal apex. Because of the eccentric growth of the cecum, the base of the appendix arises from the posterior medial aspect of the fully developed cecum about 2.5 cm below the ileocecal junction. The appendix is a blind tube averaging 0.8 cm in its outside diameter; its length averages 8.5 cm but varies from 2.5 to 22.5 cm in different subjects. The anatomic location of the appendix is not reliably indicated by the familiar McBurney's point (5 cm medial to the superior anterior iliac spine on a line extending to the umbilicus), which represents only the usual focus of acute tenderness in appendicitis. As noted by Hollinshead,[8] the base of the appendix is almost always retrocecal. The tip of the appendix may be found in any position within the abdomen which the location of the cecum and length of the appendix and its peritoneal attachment will allow (Fig. 131–6). Commonly the attachment to the posterior wall

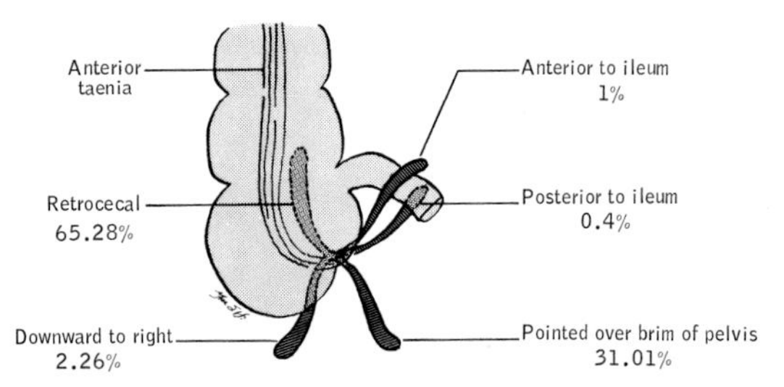

Figure 131–6. The frequencies of the various positions of the appendix as determined by Wakeley[9] in a review of 10,000 specimens. In a later survey, Maisel[10] found only 26.7% retrocecal and 58% pointed toward the pelvis.

takes the form of a triangular fold of peritoneum known as the mesoappendix or mesenteriole. This fold is resorbed in the case of the retrocecal appendix, which then adheres to the colon or to the posterior abdominal wall.

Ascending Colon. From the ileocecal junction, the colon ascends on the right in front of the quadratus lumborum and transversus abdominis muscles to a level overlying the lower pole of the right kidney, a distance of about 20 cm. Superiorly is the undersurface of the right liver lobe lateral to the gallbladder, and here the colon angulates acutely medially and downward, forming the hepatic (right) flexure. Wolfer et al.[6] identified a semblance of a mesentery to the ascending colon in only 5% of 125 subjects. The ascending colon is retroperitoneally fixed to the posterior abdominal wall in the great majority of persons. Occasionally, reference is made to filmy adhesions extending from the right abdominal wall at the anterior taenia of the ascending colon as *Jackson's membrane.* These vascular adhesions may obscure the right colic gutter and hamper surgical mobilization of the right colon.

A peritoneal fold extending downward from the hepatorenal ligament may provide support to the hepatic flexure. A further extension is continuous with the posterior layer of the omental bursa. Nevertheless, the hepatic flexure is by no means fixed, but rather descends appreciably with the liver at each inspiration. A deep breath may render a tumor in this segment accessible to palpation.

Transverse Colon. This longest (40 to 50 cm) and often most mobile segment of the colon is festooned across the anterior abdomen between the hepatic and splenic flex-

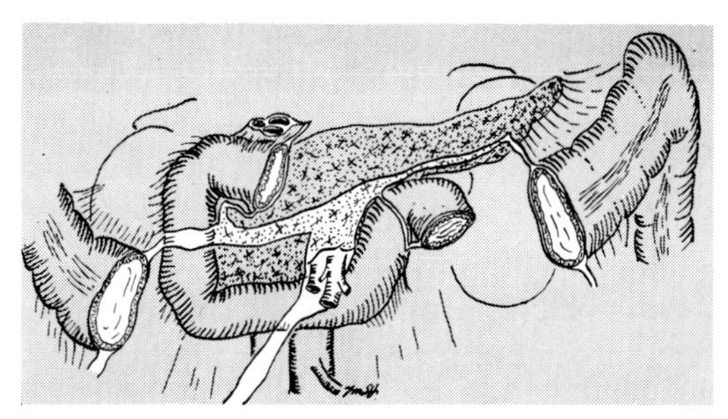

Figure 131–7. The posterior attachment of the transverse mesocolon. The oblique space extending from the roots of the mesenteric vessels represents the attachment of the mesentery supporting the small intestine.

ures. Its most dependent midportion reaches a variable level. In recumbent subjects of a normal habitus, it descends usually to the iliac crests; in the upright position it may dip into the pelvis. In the upright position in those of an asthenic habitus, the midportion may rest on the floor of the pelvis. Because of its anterior situation, it is seldom displaced by retroperitoneal masses.

The transverse colon is almost wholly developed between layers of the transverse mesocolon, which derived as a transverse fold from the posterior perioneum overlying the duodenum and the pancreas (Fig. 131–7). Of course, what appears as a single fold in the adult represents a fusion between the dorsal mesogastrium and the original mesentery of the colon. The upper layer of this fused fold is continuous posteriorly with the wall of the lesser peritoneal sac, and the lower layer, inferior to the colon, forms a wall of the greater omentum (Fig. 131–8).

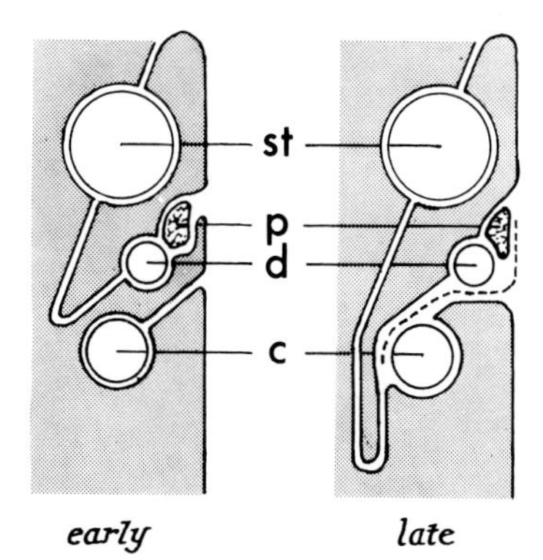

Figure 131–8. The development of the transverse mesocolon and the greater omentum (st = stomach, p = pancreas, d = duodenum, c = colon).

In the transverse colon the haustra are more prominent than in other segments of the colon. According to Pace,[11] the situation of the *haustra* (Latin *haustor,* "that which draws water, as a bucket") may be determined by taenial fibers which branch off into the circular muscle coat, by separate thin sheets of circule muscle containing dense collagen bundles, or by submucosal collections of elastic fibers.

The colon is firmly attached high in the left hypochondrium to the undersurface of the diaphragm at the level of the tength and eleventh ribs by the *phrenicocolic ligament,* which also serves to support the spleen (hence, it is also known as the *sustentaculum lienis*). The angle formed at the splenic flexure is not in the frontal plane but rather in the sagittal plane, where the distal transverse colon lies in front of the proximal descending colon; thus, in anteroposterior radiographs, the 2 limbs are superimposed. To see them separately usually requires a lateral projection[12] (Fig. 131–9).

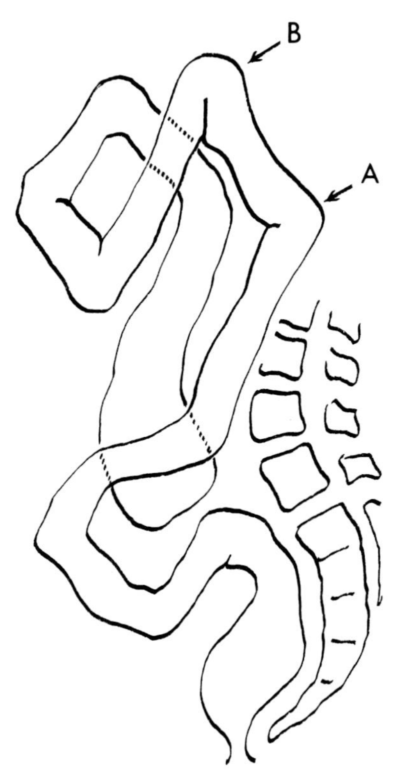

Figure 131–9. In the lateral projection of the colon, the transverse segment lies anterior to the ascending and descending segments. The anatomic splenic flexure (A) is fixed while the radiographic splenic flexure (B) may move. (Redrawn from Whalen and Riemenschneider.[12])

For most persons, the splenic flexure is the least dependent portion of the colon and its most acute angulation. These facts form an anatomic basis for the *"splenic flexure syndrome"* (Chapter 134). In those instances in which the attachment of the hepatic flexure is higher than that of the splenic flexure, precisely the same symptoms are referred to the right hydrochondrium.

Descending Colon. In its descent from the acute angle at the splenic flexure, the colon passes the lateral border of the left kidney, turns somewhat medially, and descends in the groove between the psoas and the quadratus lumborum muscles. The length of this course averages about 30 cm. The junction of the descending colon with the sigmoid segment is not demarcated intrinsically, but the level of the adjacent pelvic brim serves as a convenient, if arbitrary, landmark.

The descending colon is usually applied closely to the posterior abdominal wall, and only the anterior two-thirds of its circumference is covered by peritoneum.

The lumen of the distal descending colon is the narrowest in the large intestine; hence, the proclivity for obstruction by even small encircling growths. At the same time, it is in this segment that the muscle coat is the heaviest, and often it is in the left lower abdominal quadrant that spasm in an irritable colon can be the most distressing. Through a thin abdominal wall, even without appreciable bowel spasm, the lower descending colon is frequently palpable.

Sigmoid Colon. From the point where the descending colon reaches the pelvic brim to the beginning of the rectum, at the peritoneal reflection, the colon often forms a redundant Σ; hence, its designation as the sigmoid segment. It may be short or long, from 15 to 50 cm. Almost always it has a generous mesentery (pelvic mesocolon), which permits much mobility and variation in its course. Occasionally, a long sigmoid colon segment rises high in the abdomen, even to the level of the splenic flexure (Chapter 87). Because of its long mesentery, the sigmoid segment is the commonest site of volvulus. The serosal surface of the sigmoid colon is readily recognized by the numerous, fat-laden *appendices epiploicae.*

It is difficult to discern the individual loops of the tortuous sigmoid segment in the ordinary anteroposterior projections of a barium enema examination. Therefore, the sigmoid colon is best viewed in lateral or oblique projections. Because the sigmoid segment is a frequent site of cancer in the colon, utmost care must be taken to scrutinize separately each redundant loop.

The mucosa of the distal third of the sigmoid colon, together with the rectum, is within the range of the ordinary 25-cm sigmoidoscope (Chapter 42). The sinuous sigmoid segment is the most difficult portion to negotiate with the fiberoptic colonoscope.

Rectum. Belying its name (from the Latin, "straight"), the rectum's course is curved, and its lumen is zigzag. Apparently the designation as "rectum" came from its relatively straight course in certain quadripeds that were the objects of dissection by early anatomists. Viewed from the abdominal cavity, the rectum begins where the pelvic mesocolon ends. Viewed through the sigmoidoscope, the rectum begins at the acute angle where the corrugated mucosa of the sigmoid colon becomes the smooth mucosa of the rectum. These points are at about the level of the third sacral vertebra.

The posterior rectal wall follows the curve of the sacral concavity. The lumen of the rectum is fusiform; its midportion often is called the *rectal ampulla.* The lumen is indented by 3 variably prominent crescentic folds, usually 2 on the left and 1 on the right (Fig. 131–10). These shelflike folds are known

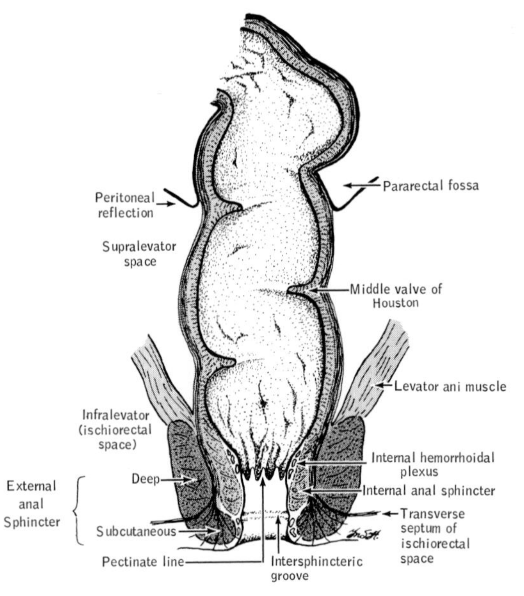

Figure 131–10. Longitudinal section of the rectum and anal canal.

as the superior, middle, and inferior *valves of Houston* and serve as convenient landmarks for designating the levels of lesions seen in the rectal mucosa. The middle valve usually is the most prominent and often can be demonstrated at barium enema examination.[13]

An index finger of average length (about 8 cm) can be inserted almost to the level of the superior valve of Houston. By instructing the patient to "bear down," the examiner often can feel an additional 2 to 3 cm of rectum slide over his fingertip, thus increasing by almost one-third the range of his digital examination. With the fingertip in the uppermost rectum, one may palpate loops of ileum or sigmoid colon lying in the pararectal fossa. Anteriorly is the rectouterine recess in the female *(pouch of Douglas)* or the retrovesical recess in the male, which can be the site of Blumer's shelf, a sign of metastatic neoplasia. As the finger is withdrawn in the male, it passes over the retrovesical and retroprostatic spaces on either side of the seminal vesicles and, in the midline, the prostate and proximal urethra. Anteriorly, in the female, one feels the uterine cervix and the posterior vaginal wall. Lateral to the rectum are the bony ischial walls of the pelvis, the levator ani muscles, and the ischiorectal spaces. Posteriorly, the finger passes over the fascialined presacral space as one feels the pelvic hollow of the sacrum and the coccyx.

Anal Canal. The floor of the pelvis is a funnel-shaped fibromuscular diaphragm in which apertures permit the passage of tubular structures, viz., the rectum, the urethra, and in the female the vagina. The pelvic diaphragm consists chiefly of the 3 more or less distinct components of the *levator ani muscle* (the pubococcygeus and the ileococcygeus portions); posteriorly it is completed by the smaller coccygeus muscle. Anteriorly and laterally the levator ani muscle arises from the pubis, the obturator fascia, and the ischium. The more medial fibers, arising anteriorly, join from either side behind the lower rectum, forming a loop which is aptly described as the "puborectal sling" (Fig. 131–11). Within this sling the lower rectum turns somewhat posteriorly.

The course of the anal canal is short (3 cm) but heavily guarded by musculature which is uniquely an interrelated complex of both involuntary and striated muscle components. This important segment has been the subject of recent, intensive study by Shafik,[14–16] an Egyptian proctologist.

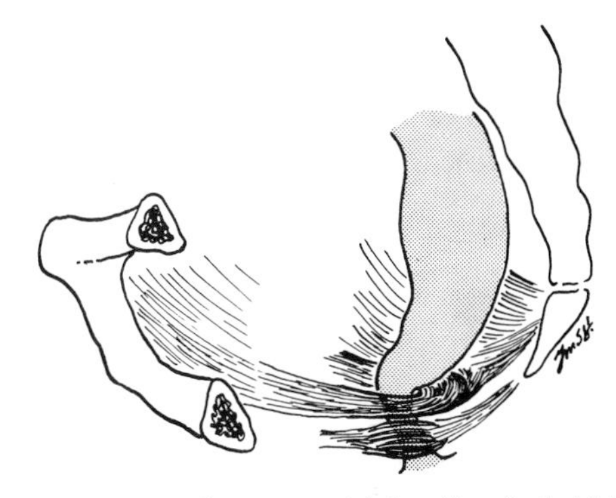

Figure 131–11. The anorectal junction is held in a muscular sling formed by the fibers of the puborectalis portion of the levator ani muscle. Just below this is the external sphincter muscle.

The internal sphincter of the anal canal is actually a continuation of the circular smooth muscle of the rectum; it extends to within 1 cm of the anal orifice. According to Goligher,[17] its fibers are grouped in discrete, imbricated bands (Fig. 131–12). The *external sphincter* forms a collar around the anal canal; above, its fibers mingle with those of the levator ani muscle. It is attached posteriorly

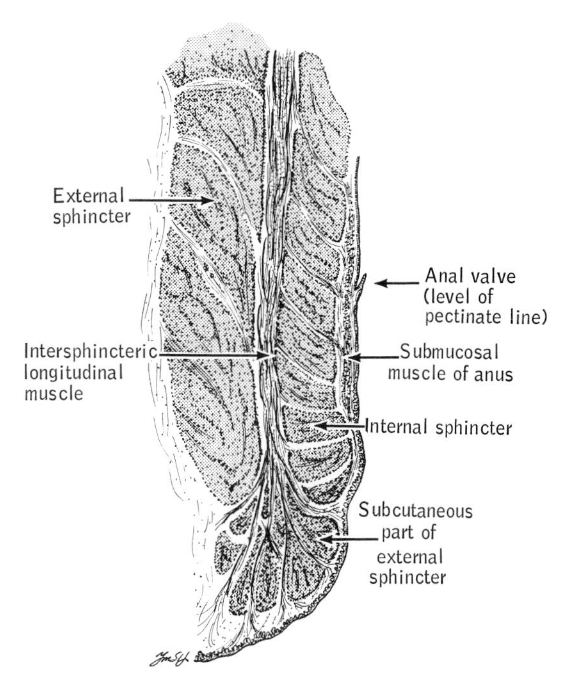

Figure 131–12. Longitudinal section through the muscles in the wall of the anal canal. (From photomicrographs by Goligher.[17])

to the coccyx and anteriorly to the perineal body. The internal and external sphincters are separated by a thin layer of elastic fibers and longitudinal muscle which is an extension of the outer longitudinal muscle coat of the rectum. Below, these fibers fan out to penetrate the subcutaneous portion of the external anal sphincter and insert into the skin surrounding the anus. The subcutaneous portion of the external sphincter and the lower margin of the internal sphincter are distinct. The separation of the sphincters can sometimes be seen at the anus as the "white line of Hilton" and usually can be palpated as the intersphincteric groove (Fig. 131–13).

Just as the dressmaker sometimes solves the problem of bringing a full skirt to a narrow waist by constructing pleats, so the mucosa of the rectal ampulla is gathered into folds as it enters the narrow anal canal. These longitudinal folds comprise the rectal *columns of Morgagni* which terminate as the *anal papillae.* The papillae occasionally appear as elongated epithelial tags and may resemble neoplastic polyps, which they are not. A narrow membrane connecting the papillae forms the anal valves. To some observers the row of papillae has resembled a comb (hence, "*pectinate*" line); to others, a set of teeth (hence, "*dentale*" line). Between the longitudinal folds are the rectal sinuses, which descend as small anal crypts behind the valve-like membrane (Fig. 131–14). These sinuses can be the seat of infection and may be implicated in the formation of anal fistulas.[16] The middle third of the anal canal, between the anal papillae and the intersphincteric groove is sometimes called the pecten ("comb"). The lowermost margin of the anal canal is the anal verge.

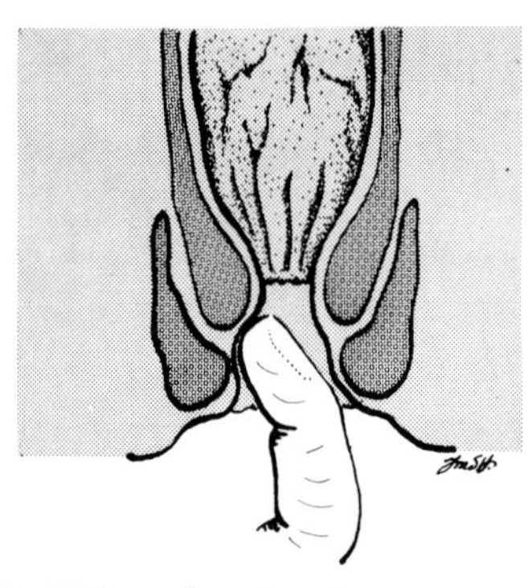

Figure 131–13. Location of the intersphincteric groove by the palpating finger. (Modified from Goligher.[17])

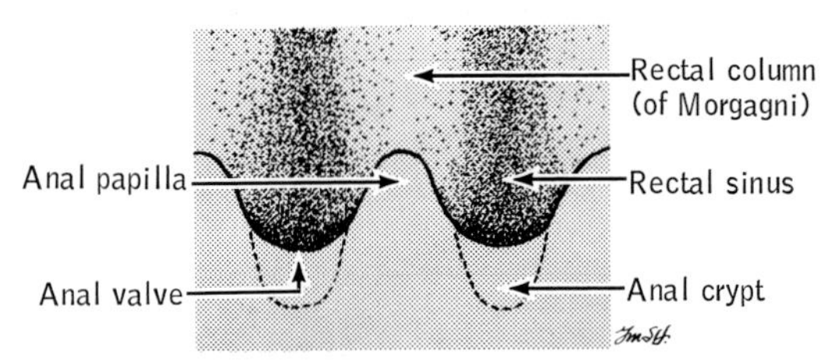

Figure 131–14. The small structures at the pectinate line.

Within the lining of the anal canal is the transition from the columnar epithelium characteristic of the intestine to the stratified squamous epithelium of skin. Contrary to older descriptions, the mucocutaneous junction is neither a sharp nor a constant line[18]; rather, the columnar cells of the rectal mucosa become progressively cuboidal, finally blending into the basal layer of the squamous epithelium, which then becomes more stratified in the true skin at the anal verge.[17] This transition can occur anywhere within the anal canal, most commonly at the anal papillae.

The operator of biopsy forceps does well to distinguish between the columnar and squamous surfaces; the former is insensitive, whereas the latter is equipped with keen pain receptors.

In the submucous space, at the level of the columns of Morgagni and the anal papillae, lies the internal hemorrhoidal venous plexus. In the subcutaneous space, between the intersphincteric groove and the anal verge, lies the external hemorrhoidal plexus.

Perirectal Spaces. Important in the diagnosis and treatment of pelvic infection, often arising from the rectum and anal canal, is an orientation pertaining to the real and potential spaces surrounding the rectum and into which infection may spread. These spaces are delimited by muscle and fascia furnishing support, requiring strength, and yet permitting mobility, which requires elasticity.

In the frontal plane the pararectal spaces are divided by the oblique portion of the levator ani muscle and the heavy fascia in which it is enveloped (Fig. 131–15*A*). Infection penetrating through anal fistulas finds its way into the ischiorectal fossae anterior to the levator partition. Infection or neoplasm originating above the anal canal spreads to the supralevator space.

In the sagittal plane, potential spaces exist behind, beneath, and in front of the rectum

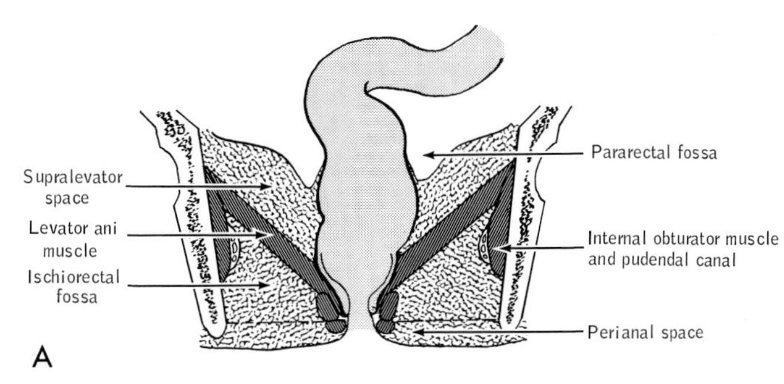

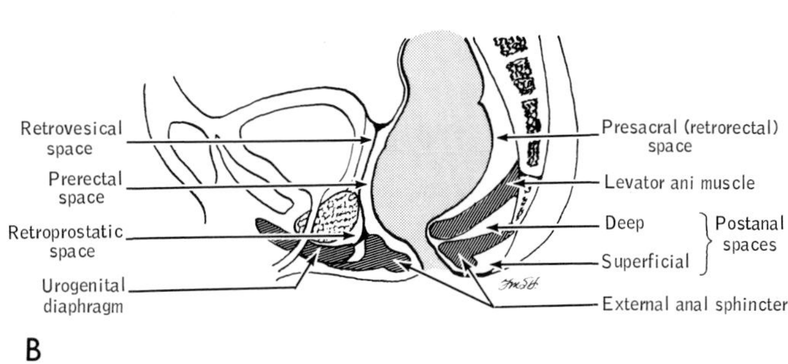

Figure 131–15. The perirectal spaces and the delimiting structures. *A*, Frontal section; *B*, sagittal section (in the male).

(Fig. 131–15*B*). Lateral attachments of the rectum to the pelvic wall by the fascia of the hypogastric sheaths (containing the superior and middle hemorrhoidal vessels, the pelvic nerve plexuses, and lymphatics, on either side) prevent anterior communication from the retrorectal space. Thus, presacral suppurative collections are more likely to drain into the rectum than to spread laterally. The width of the presacral space, as seen in a sagittal projection with the rectum filled by barium, should not exceed 1.5 cm.[19] Below the levator ani muscle, however, there is opportunity for communication anteriorly and posteriorly in the ischiorectal fossae and from one side to the other in the postanal spaces.

Segmental Contractions Simulating Strictures. There are several points of contraction or focal narrowing, inconstantly seen in radiographs of the living colon at barium enema examination, which may simulate organic strictures and may suggest spurious diagnoses of inflammatory or neoplastic defects (Fig. 131–16). Actually, none of these appear in the extirpated dead colon, and it is doubtful that any represent true sphincters. The commonest segment of contraction is *Cannon's ring*, which is observed in the midtransverse colon. This coincides with the junction of the primitive midgut and hindgut, marking a segment in which fibers from the superior and inferior nerve plexuses overlap. The contradiction rings of *Payr-Strauss* and of *Balli* in the descending colon may mark the sites of origin for peristaltic rushes resulting from the defecation reflexes. The contraction of *Rossi* near the rectosigmoid

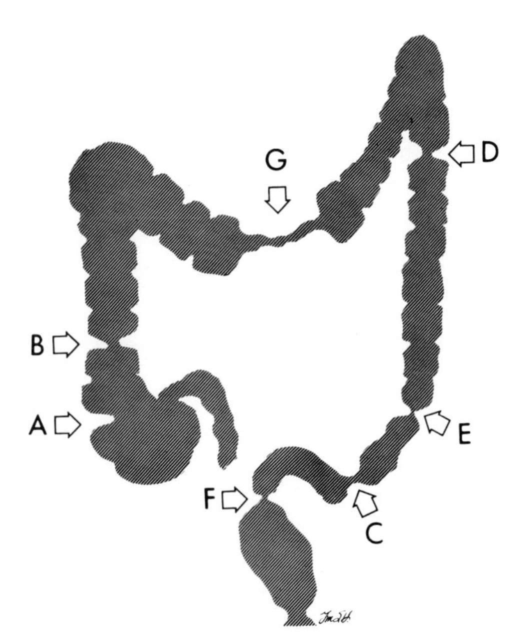

Figure 131–16. The approximate locations of inconstant segmental contractions, which may simulate lesions in the barium-filled colon. They are designated by the names of their describers: A, Busi; B, Hirsch; C, Moultier; D, Payr-Strauss; E, Balli; F, Rossi; G, Cannon's ring. (Modified from Templeton.[20])

junction has been postulated as a reflex barrier to the fecal load normally stored in the sigmoid segment. Shafiroff[21] states that perceptibly thickened circular muscle at the rectosigmoid junction can be identified in 80% of cadavers. The contractions of *Busi* and of *Hirsch* in the ascending colon and of *Moultier* in the sigmoid segment have been described as sites of poorly defined thickening of circular muscle fibers.

Mention of these occasional zones of contraction is not to overemphasize their anatomic or physiologic significance. Any well defined or constant stricture in the barium outline of the colon must first be considered as organic disease. But knowledge of these points of functional contraction may help to explain the appearance of inconstant focal narrowing.

Histology

The wall of the colon consists of 4 layers: the mucosa, the submucosa, the muscular coat, and the serosa. The *mucosa* is covered by a single layer of tall columnar epithelial cells which contain abundant goblet cells, the source of copious mucus (Fig. 131–17). Argentaffin cells are relatively prominent at the depths of the glandular crypts in the rectum.[22] The colon participates in the "gastroenteric pancreatic endocrine system," inasmuch as cells elaborating enteroglucagon and vasoactive intestinal peptide (but not gastrin, secretin, cholecystokinin, or somatostatin) have been demonstrated.[23] The luminal surface of these epithelial cells is a striated border similar to that of the small intestine. Donnellan[24] has provded a comprehensive atlas of the ultrastructure of the colonic epithelium and is underlying tissues. In a similar documentation, the Pittmans[25] have emphasized the filamentous coat overlying the luminal surface of the colon epithelial cells, bearing an intimate, if not integral, relation to the microvillous membrane. Presumably this is a counterpart of the glycocalyx of the small bowel epithelium, although one would guess it has a different function, perhaps as a barrier to colon bacteria. Certain bacteria are capable of dissolving colon mucus.[26] The kinetics of epithelial cell prolifera-

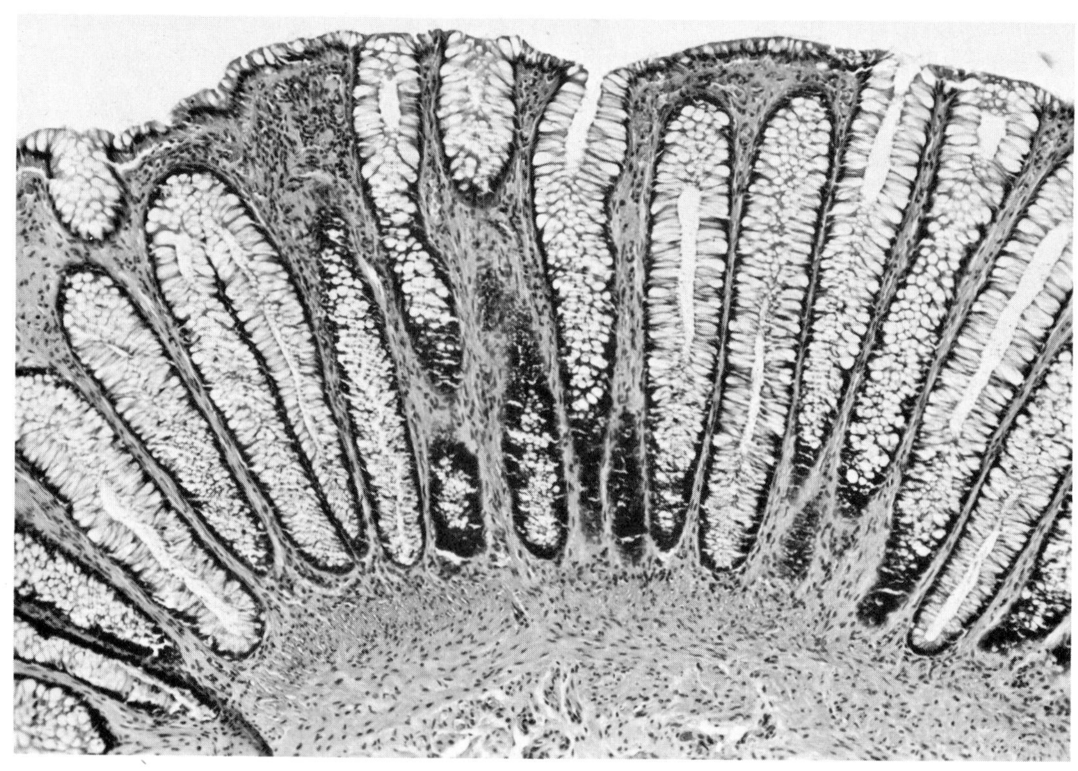

Figure 131–17. Biopsy section of human rectal mucosa showing remarkably uniform glands of Lieberkühn lined by abundant, mucus-laden goblet cells. The mononuclear cell infiltrate in the lamina propria is rather sparse in this specimen. (Obtained by Dr. J. A. Rinaldo, Jr.) (Hematoxylin and eosin, × 115.)

tion in the colon are similar, although somewhat slower, than in the proximal small intestine.[27]

The simple columnar epithelium is supported by the connective tissue of the *lamina propria,* which contains blood vessels, lymphatic channels, and unmyelinated nerve fibers, and which normally is infiltrated by lymphocytes, plasma cells, histiocytes, and other leukocytes. Occasional small clusters of histiocytes reacting with the periodic acid–Schiff (PAS) stain normally occupy the lamina propria[28] and are not indicative of Whipple's disease (Chapter 109). Frequently, the lymphocytes congregate in solitary follicles with germinal centers, and these may extend into the submucosa. Doubtlessly, certain cells populating the lamina propria of the colon are "immunologically competent"; that is, they can participate in various immune responses of which the colon has been found capable (Chapter 243). Immunofluorescent techniques are available whereby these cells can be identified in special preparations.[29] Because of the normal cellular infiltrate, the presence of actual inflammation is sometimes difficult to discern, and biopsies of normal colorectal mucosa are apt to be reported as "chronic colitis" or "chronic proctitis."

In contrast to the fingerlike villi of the small intestine, the mucosa is relatively flat, although its surface is punctuated by closely set, remarkably straight, symmetrical epithelial crypts forming the *glands of Lieberkühn.* These are strikingly evident in scanning electron micrographs of the mucosal surface[30] (Fig. 131–18). Another, and simpler, method of demonstrating the luminal surface of the colorectal mucosa has been described by Poulsen and his Danish colleagues.[31] Alcian green stain applied to a properly mounted biopsy specimen provides a remarkably clear outline of the crypt openings (Fig. 131–19). At sigmoidoscopy, with the sheen of mucus wiped away, the openings of these glands are visible to the naked eye as fine pits *(foveae).* This lends a minutely granular appearance to the healthy mucosa which is not to be confused with the coarser granularity of ulcerative colitis. Sasson[32] has shown that barium can and does enter the epithelial crypts during radiographic examinations and may appear as fine spicules along the profile of the barium-filled colon. These, too, are not to be construed as signs of mucosal disease.

A distinct pericryptal connective tissue sheath has been described by Pascal and his associates,[33, 34] in which the subepithelial fibroblasts originate at the depths of the crypts and migrate upward and mature in concert with the adjacent epithelial cells. This suggests a close and possibly interdependent relationship between entodermal and mesenchymal elements in the colon.

The mucosa is separated from the submucosa by the thin *muscularis mucosae,* which is arrayed in somewhat indistinct circular and longitudinal layers. Within the denser connective tissue of the *submucosa* is a rich network of small arteries, veins, and lymphatic vessels. Here, too, is the submucosal nerve plexus of Meissner.

Peculiar to the colon is that its outer longitudinal *muscle* is represented by 3 separate taeniae rather than by a continuously enveloping coat. This arrangement permits greater distention of the colon wall at the commodious haustra. Interconnections between the taeniae and the circular muscle fibers have been demonstrated, particularly in the proximal segments of the colon.[35] The longitudinal coat again becomes continuous over the rectum. The inner muscle coat is well developed in the colon and forms a series of strictly circular rings.[36–38] Along the external surface of the circular muscle coat are the clusters of ganglion cells and their fine ramifications making up the myenteric plexus of Auerbach. Unmyelinated postganglionic fibers penetrate the muscle to communicate with the submucosal plexus.

The *serosa* is distinctive in containing the fatty *appendices epiploicae,* particularly evident in the sigmoid segment. Where not adherent to the posterior abdominal wall, the colon is enveloped by the mesothelium of the visceral peritoneum. The rectum, of course, has no serosa.

Blood Supply

The ontogeny of the colon is reflected in its blood supply, which derives from 2 sources: the superior mesenteric artery, which serves all of the intestine developing from the embryonic midgut and extending from the descending limb of the duodenum to approximately the midtransverse colon, and the inferior mesenteric artery, which serves that portion of the colon developing from the hindgut and extending from the

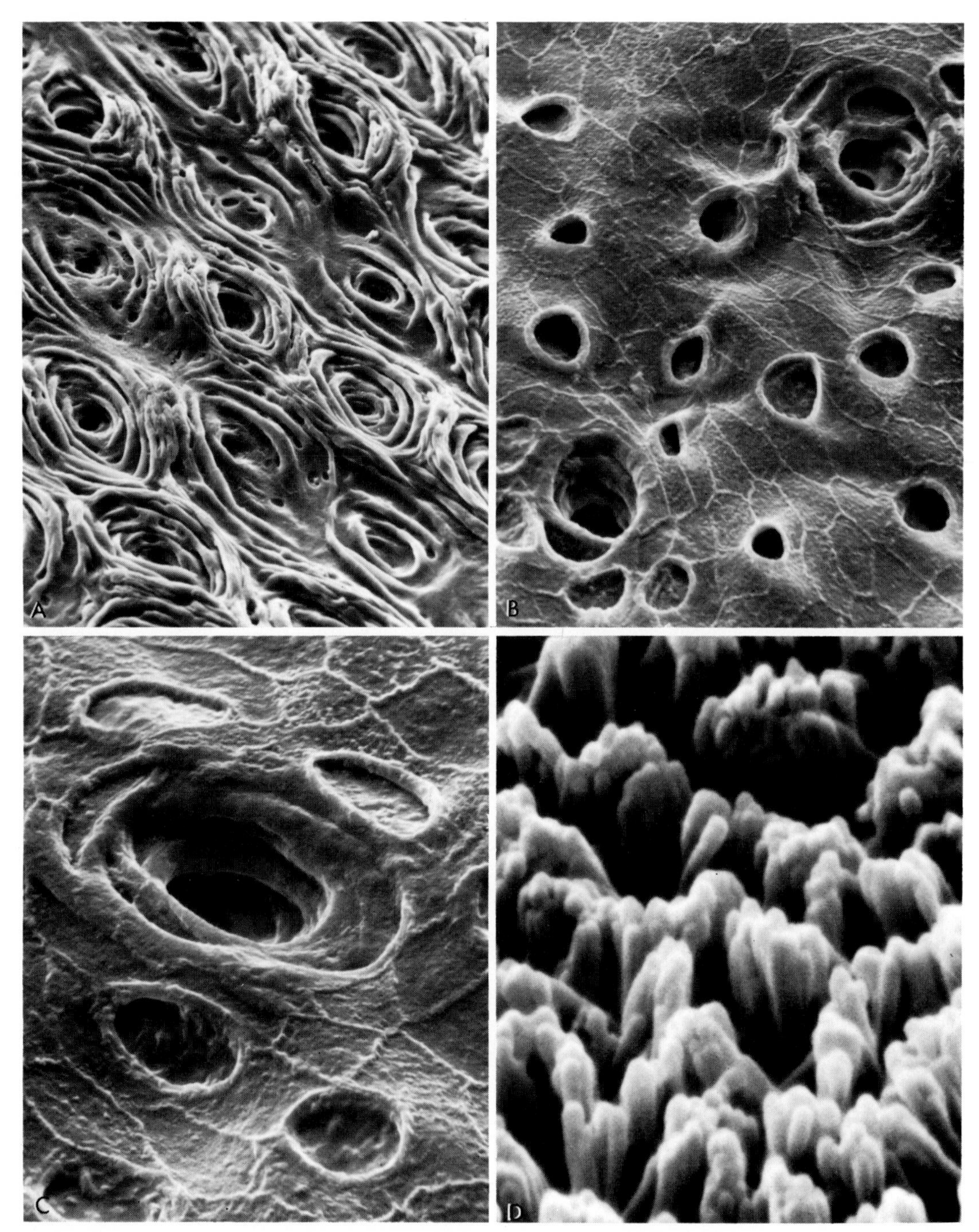

Figure 131–18. In seemingly 3-dimensional photographs obtained by the scanning electron microscope, the surface of the cecum *(A)* is characterized by numerous pits surrounded by raised concentric whorls of mucosa, flecked with randomly scattered goblet cell pores (× 350). In both the colon and rectum *(B)*, however, the mucosal whorls are absent, and the crypts of Lieberkühn are scattered irregularly amid smaller and more numerous goblet cell pores in the undulating epithelial surface; the close-fitting junctions of the polyhedral epithelial cells are distinct (× 1350). At higher magnification of a rectal crypt and its neighboring goblet cell pores *(C)*, the luminal surface of the cells appears rough (× 2300) The ultrastructure of the luminal surface *(D)* becomes apparent at very high magnification (× 25,000); its delicate microvilli resemble the nap of a carpet. (Courtesy of Dr. Joseph A. Burke, University of Kentucky, and reprinted by permission of the publishers of *Hospital Practice.*)

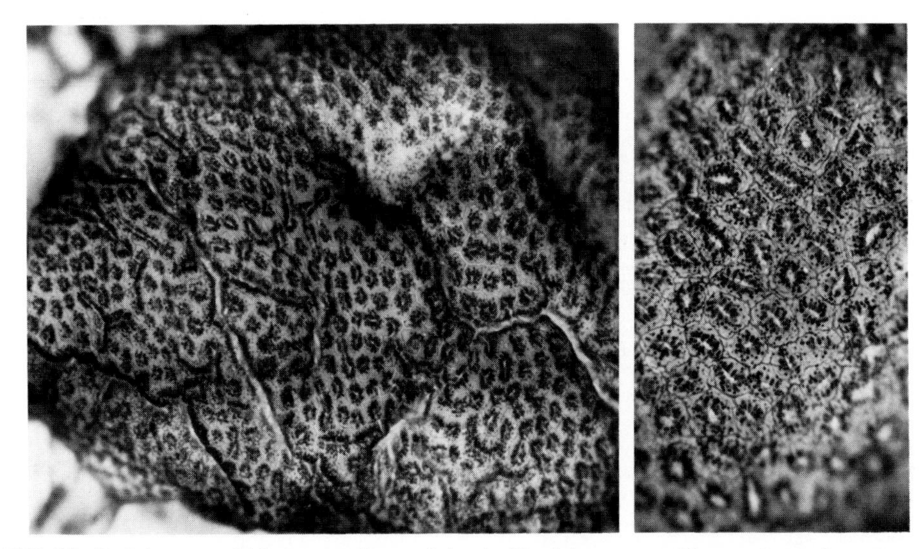

Figure 131–19. Rectal mucosal biopsy specimen stained with alcian green. The crypt openings on the luminal surface, outlined by the punctate staining of goblet cells, form a regular pattern and density (*left,* × 40; *right,* × 65). (From Poulsen SS et al. Scand J Gastroenterol 1978; 13:605. Reproduced with permission.)

midtransverse colon to the rectum (Fig. 131–20). The lowermost rectum and anal canal are served by the paired middle and inferior rectal (hemorrhoidal) arteries, both of which are branches of the internal iliac (hypogastric) artery.

Superior Mesenteric Artery. Generally, the right colon boasts a major arterial branch to each of 3 segments: (1) the cecum and its appendix are served, along with the terminal ileum, by the ileocolic artery; (2) the ascending colon is served by the right colic artery; and (3) the proximal portion of the transverse colon is served by the middle colic artery. These 3 colic branches spring from the right side of the superior mesenteric artery, beginning with the origin of the middle colic branch just beyond the emergence of the parent vessel from beneath the pancreas and over the transverse portion of the duodenum. Curiously, the origins of many of the numerous jejunal and ileal branches, which fan out from the left side, are actually distal to the origins of the colic branches.

Among 600 specimens, Sonneland et al.[39] found 24 varying anatomic patterns in the colic branches of the superior mesenteric artery, but 3 patterns differed only in the points of origin of the 3 colic branches. These authors found the ileocolic branch invariably present, the right colic branch absent in 12.6% and multiple in 9.4%, and the middle colic branch absent in 3.8% and multiple in 8.6%.

The ileocolic artery has 4 chief ramifications. An ileal branch anastomoses in the mesentery with the terminal branch of the superior mesenteric artery to form an arc from which straight branches serve the terminal 15 cm of the ileum. Anterior and posterior cecal branches enhance the cecum. An appendicular branch descends behind the ileum and along the free edge of the mesoappendix to furnish the sole source of blood for the appendix. An ascending branch serves the proximal ascending colon. The distribution of the ileocolic artery explains why surgical resection of the terminal ileum always requires resection of the cecum and proximal ascending colon and vice versa. The ascending branch of the ileocolic artery then proceeds to anastomose with the descending branch of the right colic artery. In turn, the ascending branch of the right colic artery connects with the right branch of the middle colic artery, whose left branch usually communicates with the superior left colic branch of the inferior mesenteric artery. These anastomoses, together with the arcs formed by the several sigmoidal arteries, comprise the *marginal artery of Drummond,* thus forming a chain of collateral circulation for almost the whole length of the colon. As confirmed in the study by Sonneland and his associates,[39]

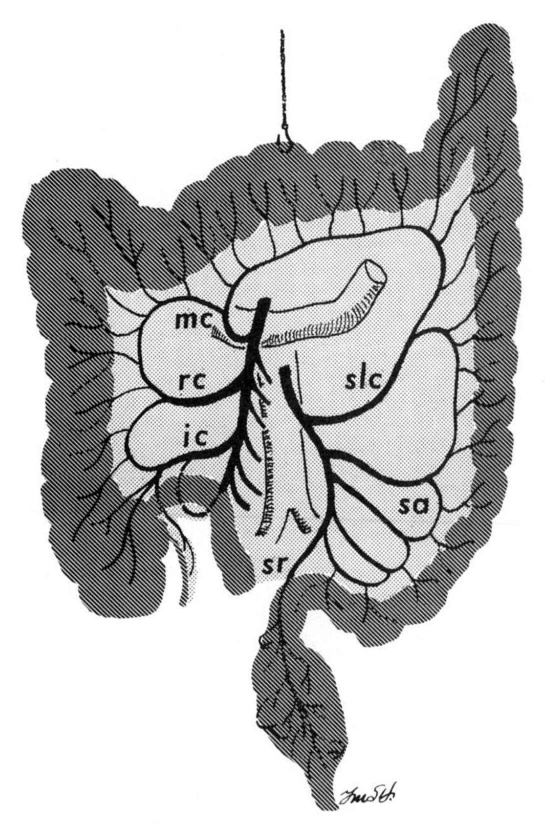

Figure 131–20. In this diagram of the arterial blood supply to the colon the transverse segment is elevated. The major arterial branches of the superior mesenteric artery are: ic, ileocolic; rc, right colic; and mc, middle colic. Those of the inferior mesenteric artery are: slc, superior left colic; sa, sigmoidal arteries; and sr, superior rectal. The connection between the left branch of the middle colic artery and the left colic artery is sometimes called the arc of Riolan.

if there is a weak link in this marginal arterial chain, it will be found most likely between the ileocolic and right colic branches of the superior mesenteric artery or between the middle colic branch and the left colic artery near the splenic flexure. The latter segment is that most vulnerable to ischemic "colitis" (Chapters 115 and 116).

The major branches comprising the marginal artery are situated from 0.5 to 8.0 cm from the wall of the colon; the closest approximation is along the descending and pelvic colon segments. From the marginal artery lead both short and long terminal branches which invest and embrace the colon wall. Their richest ramifications are in the submucosa.

Inferior Mesenteric Artery. Arising from the aorta at the level of the third lumbar vertebra, below the transverse segment of the duodenum, the inferior mesenteric artery descends beneath the peritoneum, directing its branches to the left and inferiorly. The first branch is the superior left colic artery, which bifurcates in the manner of the colic branches of the superior mesenteric artery, contributing an ascending limb and a descending limb to the marginal artery of Drummond. As previously noted, the anastomosis beween the limbs of the middle colic and left colic branches, near the splenic flexure, may be the most precarious communication between segments comprising the marginal artery. Nevertheless, Braithwaite[40] found that ischemic necrosis in the distal colon required not only occlusion of the inferior mesenteric artery but also removal of a large segment of the marginal artery.

The next 2 to 4 branches of the inferior mesenteric artery are known collectively as the inferior colic or sigmoidal arteries. Commonly the uppermost sigmoidal artery arises as a branch of the superior left colic artery. Within the mesentery of the sigmoid colon (pelvic mesocolon), these several branches form anastomosing loops arrayed in one or more tiers to form the distal extent of the marginal artery.

The point of bifurcation between the lowermost sigmoidal branch contributing to the marginal artery and the first independent branch to the rectum has been dubbed "the critical point of Sudeck." The fear has been expressed that extirpation of the inferior mesenteric artery, as in a segmental resection of the descending colon, may imperil the blood supply to the rectum, or, conversely, that removal of the rectum and its uppermost arteries may jeopardize the left colon. However, by injection studies McGowan[41] showed that ligation at the "critical point" still allowed adequate filling of vessels to the sigmoid colon and rectum, presumably because of intramural anastomotic channels. Michels and his associates,[42] based on a study of 400 dissections with a view to the consequence of regional resection, have concluded that the so-called critical point of Sudeck is of no practical significance. In the course of rectal excision in 37 patients, Goligher[43] found that high ligation of the inferior mesenteric artery with sacrifice of the left colic branch gave no sign of impairing the viability of the left colon in 70% of patients, thus permitting the safe use of the left colon for anastomosis or colostomy.

Entering into the pelvis, the inferior mesenteric artery continues as the superior rectal (hemorrhoidal) artery. Its terminal branches encircle the upper rectum, pierce the muscle coat, and ramify in the submucosa, sending twigs as low as the anal columns.

Paired Rectal Branches of the Internal Iliac (Hypogastric) Arteries. The least important contribution to the blood supply of the rectum is by the small and inconstant middle rectal (hemorrhoidal) arteries. Often they are partially obliterated, as is their more prominent neighbor, the erstwhile umbilical artery. The anal canal is supplied by the paired inferior rectal (hemorrhoidal) arteries, which derive from the internal pudendal arteries, themselves major branches of the internal iliac arteries. To varying extents, there are fine communications between the ramifications of all 3 rectal arteries.

Straight Arteries of the Colon. From the marginal artery to the mesenteric border course the "arteriae rectae" or straight arteries. Short branches penetrate the mesocolic taenia, while long branches follow the outer wall of the colon to the antimesenteric taeniae. Rarely do these straight arteries anastomose, and there is little longitudinal spread in their submucosal ramification. For this reason it is important to preserve all the straight arteries at the site of transection.[44] Moreover, the anatomic observation that the straight arteries are strictly terminal arteries helps to explain the susceptibility to segmental ischemic colitis in cases of small artery disease.

Microcirculation. A capillary plexus lies just below the surface epithelium of the colon, the capillary wall being situated as close as 1 μ to the base of the epithelial cells; minute apertures (fenestrae) in the capillary wall are most numerous in the superficial one-third of the mucosa and are oriented toward the basilar portion of the epithelial cells.[45]

Venous Return. In general, the arteries just described are attended by veins bearing the same names. The 3 colic tributaries of the superior mesenteric vein return blood from the right, or proximal, half of the colon. The superior mesenteric vein, coursing to the right of its artery, ascends in front of the vena cava and receives branches from the small intestine. At the level of the second lumbar vertebra and behind the head and neck of the pancreas, the superior mesenteric vein joins the splenic vein to form the portal vein.

The inferior mesenteric vein, beginning with the superior rectal (hemorrhoidal) vein and thence receiving its left colic tributaries, ascends retroperitoneally at the left of its artery and usually empties into the splenic vein, where it lies embedded in the posterior surface of the body of the pancreas. An alternative course carries the inferior mesenteric vein medially across the root of the superior mesenteric artery to join directly the juncture between the superior mesenteric and splenic veins.

Because the mesenteric veins lack valves, portal vein hypertension is reflected in increased venous turgor throughout the intestine,[26] often with edema in the bowel wall.

The lower rectum and anal canal are invested by a rich venous network which comprises the internal hemorrhoidal plexus, in the submucosa at the level of the rectal columns of Morgagni, and the external hemorrhoidal plexus, in the subcutaneous tissue at the anal verge (Fig. 131–21). The internal hemorrhoidal plexus is drained chiefly by the middle rectal (hemorrhoidal) vein, which is much more important than its corresponding artery. The external hemorrhoidal plexus is drained by the inferior rectal (hemorrhoidal) vein. Both the middle and inferior rectal veins are tributaries of the internal iliac (hypogastric) veins, which then lead into the inferior vena cava. Because there are free communications between these plexuses below and ramifications of the superior rectal vein above, portal hypertension is readily transmitted to the hemorrhoidal plexuses, which then distend to form the prominent hemorrhoids so often seen with cirrhosis.

Lymphatics

Endowed with dense networks of lymph capillaries and abundant aggregates of lymphoid follicles, the walls of the colon are drained by lymph channels following 2 main routes marked by the superior and inferior mesenteric vessels. Retrograde flow is retarded by numerous semilunar valves. Fusiform dilatations between valves lend a beaded appearance to the distended lymph channels. The lymph vessels draining those segments of the colon supported by a mesentery are contained within the leaves of the mesentery; from other segments the lymph vessels course beneath the parietal peritoneum.

Astride the gathering lymph channels are

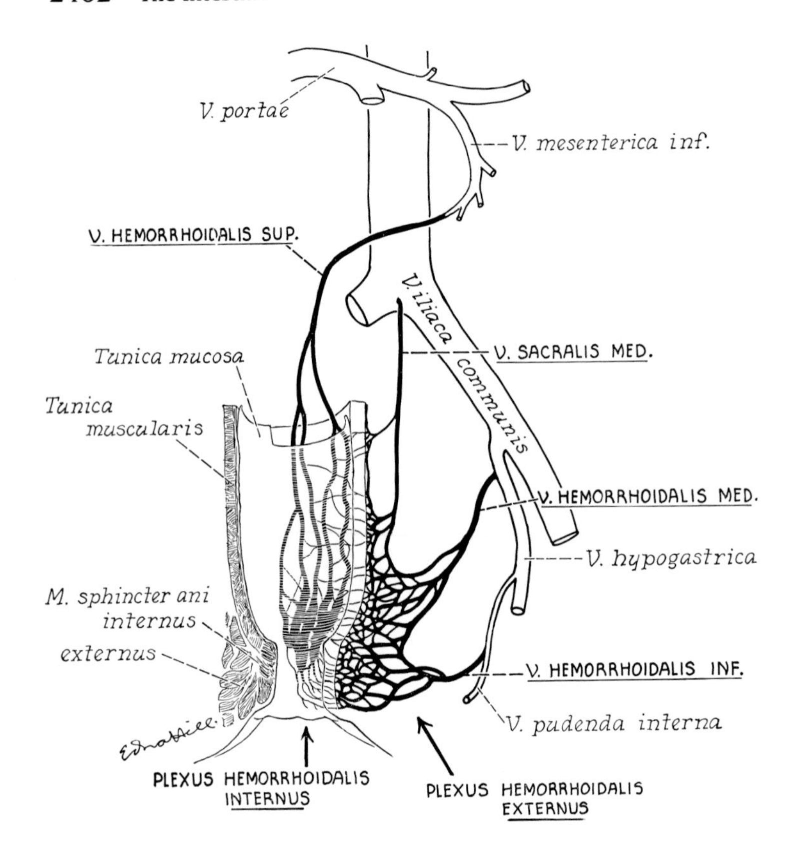

Figure 131–21. Venous drainage from the rectum and anus. Note the dual return to the portal and caval systems, providing for collateral venous circulation through the hemorrhoidal plexuses.

numerous bean-shaped lymph nodes of varying size. In general, the intestinal lymph nodes are disposed in 3 groups which form a sequential chain: the *paracolic nodes* situated along the course of the marginal artery which receive efferent lymph vessels from the colon wall, the *intermediate nodes* grouped along the radiating colic blood vessels, and the *central nodes* congregated at the roots of the vessels near the aorta. Frequent communications between channels permit collateral lymph circulation, which may bypass one or more of these groups. Particularly large clusters of nodes are found in the angle formed by the ileocecal junction, in the transverse mesocolon at the flexures, and in the pararectal spaces.

Efferent lymphatics from the anus join with those of the perineal skin, drain into the superficial inguinal nodes, and thence into the common collecting system from the legs and abdominal wall. Drainage from the anal canal is into the system accompanying the internal iliac (hypogastric) vessels, and that from the rectum is into the inferior mesenteric system.

Between the aorta and the right crus of the diaphragm all the collecting lymph channels from the viscera, the abdominal wall, and the legs converge in an elongate 5-cm sac known as the *cisterna chyli.* The large afferent channel proceeding from the cisterna superiorly through the aortic opening in the diaphragm is the thoracic duct. It is recalled that the thoracic duct eventually collects lymph from all the body except the right side of the head, neck and thorax, the right arm, the right lung, the right side of the heart, and the convex surface of the liver. The thoracic duct empties into the venous system at the left jugulosubclavian angle. This extensive drainage explains why a *Virchow's node* in the left supraclavicular fossa can represent metastatic neoplasm from almost all the viscera both below and above the diaphragm.

Familiarity with the lymphatics of the colon is useful in understanding the growth and spread of cancer and in formulating sound treatment. Knowledge of the rich network of lymph channels, their frequent intercommunications, and their numerous lymph nodes dictates the need for wide excision of potentially cancer-laden tissues in any resection of colon cancer. From a cancer in the rectum, retrograde lymphatic spread is relatively uncommon[46] and probably occurs only if there is a block in proximal channels by already advanced disease[47] (Chapter 139).

Innervation

The neural control of motor and secretory activity in the colon and primary visceral sensation from the colon are mediated exclusively by elements of the autonomic nervous system. Of course, a consideration of sensory impulses traversing somatic fibers of the central nervous system and arising from receptors in the parietal peritoneum is often important in analyzing pain patterns associated with disease in the colon (Chapter 3).

The autonomic innervation comprises both extrinsic and intrinsic components. The former includes the ganglia, plexuses, and fibers that serve the colon but lie outside its wall. The latter consists of the rich network of fibers and ganglion cells that lies within the submucosa and muscular wall of the intestine. Although the extrinsic components are anatomically the more impressive, the intrinsic pathways are probably of greater functional significance. Wood[48] has described the enteric nervous system as "the brain of the gut" that integrates information received and issues an appropriate response. Moreover, Wood maintains the gut is capable of "smart behavior" and gives as an example the response of reverse peristalsis to an advancing bolus that encounters an obstruction.

For the colon, as elsewhere, the autonomic innervation includes both sympathetic and parasympathetic pathways. Neither anatomically nor functionally are these mutually exclusive. In many situations nerve bundles and plexuses are shared by both sympathetic and parasympathetic fibers.[49] Briefly, distinguishing features are: (1) anatomically, preganglionic parasympathetic fibers are remarkably long, extending all the way from the brainstem to the colon before terminating at synapses within the submucosal and myenteric plexuses, whereas the first synapse between sympathetic fibers is situated within ganglia extrinsic to the colon; and (2) functionally, postganglionic discharges by the terminal parasympathetic fibers are effected by the release of acetylcholine (hence, cholinergic fibers), while postganglionic discharges by the terminal sympathetic fibers are effected by adrenaline-like substances (hence, adrenergic fibers).

The traditional, simplistic concept of cholinergic excitation and adrenergic inhibition has been challenged and is rapidly changing.[48–51] Not only are putative neurotransmitters and neuromodulators far more numerous (5-hydroxytryptamine, purine nucleotides, dopamine, somatostatin, vasoactive intestinal peptide, enkephalins, substance P, and bombesin) than the well-known acetylcholine and norepinephrine,[48] but Burnstock[49] has shown that various enteric neurons are capable of elaborating more than one active substance. This tells us that neuropharmacology is vastly more complicated than previously thought and helps to explain why therapeutic response to simple anticholinergic agents often falls far short of expectation. When a clear picture emerges from what is now a bewildering array of information, one can hope that more consistently effective pharmacologic therapy can be recommended.

Sympathetic Innervation. The effector cells of origin for the whole of the sympathetic nervous system are situated in the lateral horns of the spinal cord from the eighth cervical or first thoracic segment to the second or third lumbar segment. The axons of these cells emerge, on either side, as part of the anterior spinal nerve roots corresponding to their levels of origin. They then shortly leave the spinal nerves as myelinated fibers within the white rami communicantes leading to the nearby paired paravertebral chain of ganglia (Fig. 131–22). Within the paravertebral ganglia the sympathetic fibers may synapse with a postganglionic neuron, ascend or descend several segments in the chain, or pass through the ganglion unaltered. The last course is followed by most of the preganglionic fibers serving the abdominal viscera. Beyond the paravertebral ganglia, these fibers are gathered in several bundles as the greater (from the fourth to tenth thoracic segments), the lesser (from the ninth to eleventh thoracic segments), the least (from the eleventh thoracic to the first lumbar segments), and the lumbar (from the second and third lumbar segments) splanchnic nerves. The splanchnic nerves (still preganglionic fibers) pass, in turn, to the prevertebral (pre-aortic) ganglia and plexuses, which are applied to the adventitia of the aorta and the roots of its main branches.

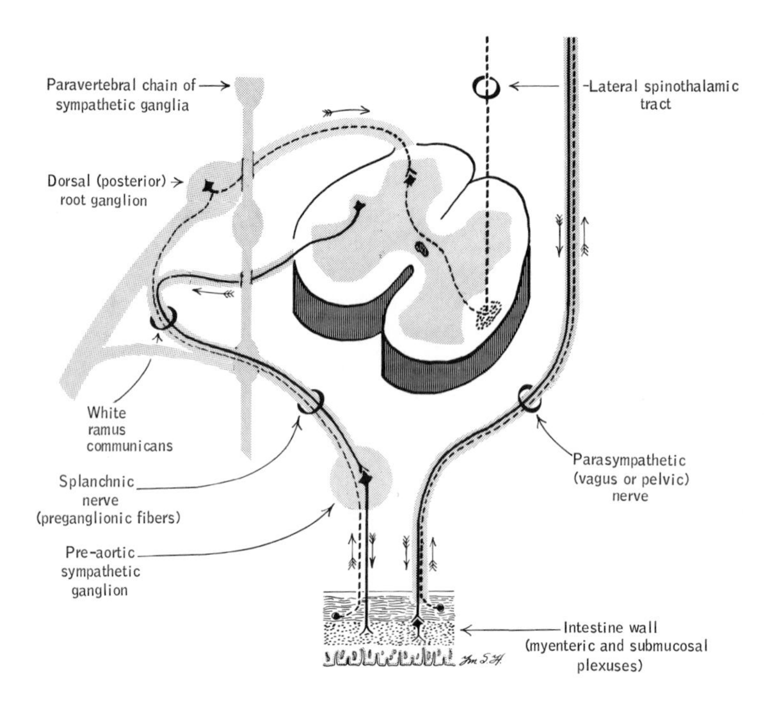

Figure 131–22. Scheme of pathways followed by sympathetic fibers *(left)* and parasympathetic fibers *(right)* serving the intestine. Both efferent *(solid line)* and afferent *(broken line)* pathways are shown.

The several pre-aortic ganglia (Fig. 131–23) take their names from the adjacent arterial trunks. The largest and best defined are the paired celiac ganglia, between which is the celiac (solar) plexus. Just below are the superior mesenteric ganglia and plexus. One would then expect inferior ganglia, but such are rarely identifiable in man. Rather, between the roots of the superior and inferior mesenteric arteries there is a dense intermesenteric (aortic) plexus which doubtlessly contains scattered ganglion cells. Leading from the intermesenteric plexus, receiving the lumbar splanchnics, and situated at the bifurcation of the aorta is the superior hypogastric plexus. Below, and applied to the internal iliac arteries, are the paired inferior hypogastric (pelvic) plexuses and the hypogastric ganglia. Intermingling with these networks are preganglionic parasympathetic fibers from the cranial outflow above and from the sacral outflow below, an anatomic fact that is sometimes forgotten.

The communications between these gan-

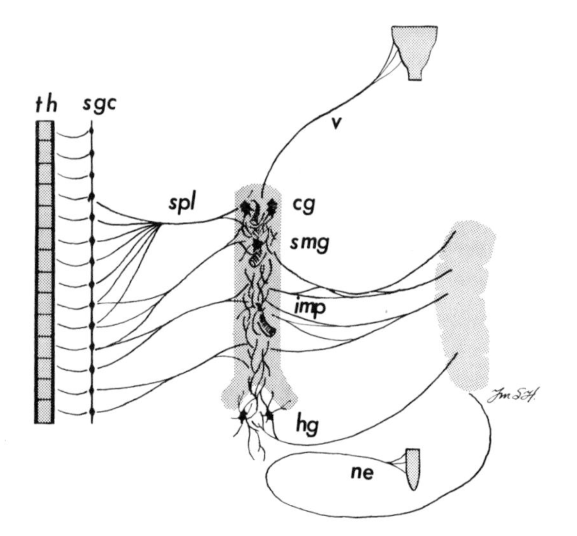

Figure 131–23. Diagram of the autonomic innervation of the colon. Preganglionic sympathetic fibers emanate from the thoracic spinal cord (th), traverse the sympathetic ganglion chain (sgc), emerge as the splanchnic nerve (spl), and synapse in the pre-aortic ganglia (cg, celiac ganglia; smg, superior mesenteric ganglion; imp, intermesenteric plexus; and hg, hypogastric ganglia). Postganglionic fibers then follow the blood vessels to the colon wall. Preganglionic parasympathetic fibers make up the vagus nerve (v) from the medulla oblongata and the nervi erigentes (ne) from the sacral spinal cord.

glia and within these plexuses are so numerous that it is almost impossible to trace the course of a single nerve fiber from its entering splanchnic nerve to its final specific termination. Nevertheless, each preganglionic sympathetic fiber finds a synapse within the pre-aortic ganglia; the fiber emerging is postganglionic and adrenergic. The postganglionic fibers then reach their effector organs by adhering to the adventitia of arteries as they ramify at the wall of the colon.

Parasympathetic Innervation. The preganglionic fibers carrying parasympathetic impulses take their origin at only 2 levels of the central nervous system: from the medulla oblongata as the cranial outflow, and from the anterior horns of the second, third, and fourth sacral segments of the spinal cord as the sacral outflow.

Most of the fibers comprising the cranial outflow are gathered together as the vagus (cranial X) nerves, which descend along the esophagus and profusely ramify at the level of the celiac plexus. As noted, these myelinated preganglionic fibers then intermingle almost indistinguishably with the pre- and postganglionic sympathetic fibers as they pass down through the pre-aortic plexuses. The vagus fibers find their way to the colon both independently in the mesentery and in company with the colic branches of the superior mesenteric artery.

Fibers of the sacral outflow emerge in the anterior roots of the corresponding sacral nerves but soon deviate to be gathered together in bundles as the pelvic nerves *(nervi erigentes)* which, in turn, contribute to the hypogastric plexuses.

The linear extent to which the vagus and the pelvic nerves anatomically permeate and functionally influence the colon has been questioned and disputed. It would seem likely, from the evidence at hand, that the division of innervation is somewhere in the transverse colon, corresponding to the point representing the diverse embryologic derivation of the colon.

The preganglionic parasympathetic fibers entering the colon form synapses (Fig. 131–22) in ganglia clustered in the muscular coats (myenteric plexuses of Auerbach) and within the submucosa (plexuses of Meissner). The myenteric plexuses are larger and are progressively more numerous toward the rectum. Histologic preparations have shown numerous and intricate connections between postganglionic fibers of adjacent myenteric and submucosal ganglia.

These plexuses and their intercommunications constitute the important intrinsic innervation of the intestine, which is capable of functioning independently of the intrinsic components. An isolated segment of gut, kept alive but shorn of its extrinsic nerve connections, can exhibit rhythmic contractions with an appropriate stimulus. Clinicians recognize that patients deprived of extrinsic parasympathetic innervation, as after vagotomy, or of extrinsic sympathetic innervation, as after thoracolumbar sympathectomy, usually maintain essentially normal intestinal function. The bowel appears to have a haughty disregard for the neurosurgeon. Conversely, patients lacking myenteric and submucosal plexuses, congenitally as in Hirschsprung's anomaly or as an acquired aftermath of Chagas' disease, exhibit strikingly impaired intestinal motor activity.

Innervation of Striated Anorectal Muscles. The levator ani, coccygeus, and external anal sphincter muscles are supplied by motor fibers emanating chiefly from the fourth sacral segment of the spinal cord and emerging with the root of the pudendal nerve.

Afferent Pathways from the Colon and Rectum. As elsewhere in the gastrointestinal tract, the intact mucosa of the colon and rectum is insensitive to ordinary stimuli. Biopsy specimens may be taken from the colon and rectal mucosa above the pectinate line with no discomfort to the patient. Sensory receptors within the colon wall react to stretching, as by gaseous distention or at colonoscopy, and to muscular hypertonicity, as in spasm. The mesentery, where present, is sensitive to tugging and stretching. Impulses initiated by these stimuli are mediated by autonomic afferent fibers, chiefly sympathetic. From the peripheral receptors, these fibers pass without interruption through the sympathetic ganglia to their cell bodies situated, along with those of the somatic afferent nerves, in the dorsal root ganglia, from which axons pass to the posterior columns of the spinal cord.

As described in Chapter 3, the pain pattern of disease and disorder in the colon often is augmented by afferent stimuli from sensitive receptors in the parietes and mediated along somatic afferent pathways.

The anal epithelium, being skin and invested by keenly sensitive receptors, is peculiarly susceptible to stimuli producing itch and pain. Even the smallest lesions in the anal canal can be the source of intense distress. These impulses are mediated along somatic afferent pathways.

References

1. Blankenhorn DH, Hirsch J, Ahrens EH Jr. Transintestinal intubation: Technic for measurement of gut length and physiological sampling at known loci. Proc Soc Exp Biol 1955; 88:356.
2. Fleischner FG, Bernstein C. Roentgen-anatomical studies of the normal ileocecal valve. Radiology 1950; 54:43.
3. Buirge RE. Gross variations in the ileocecal valve: A study of factors underlying incompetency. Anat Rec 1943; 86:373.
4. Buirge RE. Experimental observations on human ileocecal valve. Surgery 1944; 16:356.
5. Ulin AW, Shoemaker WC, Deutsch H. The ileocecal valve and papilla. Arch Intern Med 1956; 97:409.
6. Wolfer JA, Beaton LE, Anson BJ. Volvulus of cecum: Anatomical factors in its etiology; Report of a case. Surg Gynecol Obstet 1942; 74:882.
7. Bobroff LM, Messinger NH, Subbarao K, et al. The cecal bascule. Am J Roentgenol 1972; 115:249.
8. Hollinshead WH. Anatomy for Surgeons, 2nd Ed, Vol 2. New York: Harper & Row, 1971: 597.
9. Wakeley CPG. The position of the vermiform appendix as ascertained by an analysis of 10,000 cases. J Anat 1933; 67:277.
10. Maisel H. The position of the human vermiform appendix in fetal and adult age groups. Anat Rec 1960; 136:385.
11. Pace JL. The anatomy of the haustra of the human colon. Proc R Soc Med 1968; 61:934.
12. Whalen JP, Riemenschneider PA. An analysis of the normal anatomic relationships of the colon as applied to roentgenographic observations. Am J Roentgenol 1967; 99:55.
13. Cohen WN. Roentgenographic evaluation of the rectal valves of Houston in the normal and in ulcerative colitis. Am J Roentgenol 1968; 104:580.
14. Shafik A. A new concept of the anatomy of the anal sphincter mechanism and the physiology of defaecation. VIII. Levator hiatus and tunnel: anatomy and function. Dis Colon Rectum 1979; 22:539.
15. Shafik A. A new concept of the anatomy of the anal sphincter mechanism and the physiology of defaecation. IX. Single loop continence. A new theory of the mechanism of anal continence. Dis Colon Rectum 1980; 23:37.
16. Shafik A. A new concept of the anatomy of the anal sphincter mechanism and the physiology of defaecation. X. Anorectal sinus and band: anatomic nature and surgical significance. Dis Colon Rectum 1980; 23:170.
17. Goligher JC. Surgical anatomy of colon, rectum, and anus. *In:* Surgery of the Anus, Rectum and Colon. London: Ballière Tindall, 1975:1.
18. Walls EW. Observations on the microscopic anatomy of the human anal canal. Br J Surg 1958; 45:504.
19. Chrispin AR, Kelsey-Fry I. Presacral space shown by barium enema. Br J Radiol 1963; 36:319.
20. Templeton AW. Colon sphincters simulating organic disease. Radiology 1960; 75:237.
21. Shafiroff BG. Applied anatomy of colon and rectum. Pediatr Clin North Am 1956; 3:3.
22. Funk HU, Weber E, Hedinger C, et al. Number of argentaffin cells in the human gastrointestinal tract under normal and pathological conditions. Virchows Arch Pathol Anat 1966; 340:289.
23. Williams PL, Warwick R. Gray's Anatomy, 36th Ed. Philadelphia: WB Saunders, 1980: 1350–68.
24. Donnellan WL. The structure of the colonic mucosa: The epithelium and subepathelial reticulohistocytic complex. Gastroenterology 1965; 49:496.
25. Pittman FE, Pittman JC. An electron microscopical study of the epithelium of the normal human sigmoid colonic mucosa. Gut 1966; 7:644.
26. Gebbers J-O, Laisme JA, Otto HF. Modern aspects of the functional morphology of the colon. Coloproctology 1981; 3:211.
27. Lipkin M. Newer measurements of cell proliferation in the colon. Gastroenterology 1966; 51:851.
28. Ekuan JH, Hill RB Jr. Colonic histiocytosis: Clinical and pathological evaluation. Gastroenterology 1968; 55:619.
29. Brandtzaeg P, Baklien K. Immunoglobulin-producing cells in the intestine in health and disease. Clin Gastroenterol 1976; 5:251.
30. Crucioli V, Torsoli A, Pallone F, et al. Scanning electron microscopy of the normal human colon. Rendic Gastroenterol 1970; 2:184.
31. Poulsen SS, Christensen KC, Petri M, Jarnum S. Stereomicroscopic examination of stained rectal biopsies. Scand J Gastroenterol 1978; 13:605.
32. Sasson L. Entrance of barium into intestinal glands during barium enema. JAMA 1960; 173:87.
33. Pascal RR, Kaye GI, Lane L. Colon pericryptal fibroblast sheath: Replication, migration, and cytodifferentiation of a mesenchymal cell system in adult tissue. I. Autoradiographic studies of normal rabbit colon. Gastroenterology 1968; 54:835.
34. Kaye GI, Lane N, Pascal RR. Colonic pericryptal fibroblast sheath: Replication, migration, and cytodifferentiation of a mesenchymal cell system in adult tissue. II. Fine structural aspects of normal rabbit and human colon. Gastroenterology 1968; 54:852.
35. Pace JL. The interconnexions of the muscle layers of the human colon. J Anat 1968; 103:289.
36. Elsen J, Arey LB. On spirality in the intestinal wall. Am J Anat 1966; 118:11.
37. McKirdy HC, Macmillan J. Spirality of the muscle layers of the intestine. Experientia 1971; 27:790.
38. Pace JL, Williams I. Organization of the muscular wall of the human colon. Gut 1969; 10:352.
39. Sonneland J, Anson BJ, Beaton LE. Surgical anatomy of arterial supply of colon from superior mesenteric artery based upon study of 600 specimens. Surg Gynecol Obstet 1958; 106:385.
40. Braithwaite JL. The effects of interruption of the inferior mesenteric artery and its branches on the blood supply of the terminal part of the large gut in the experimental animal. Surg Gynecol Obstet 1955; 100:521.
41. McGowan JR. Collateral circulation in the sigmoid colon. Arch Surg 1955; 71:531.
42. Michels NA, Siddharth P, Kornbluth PL, et al. The variant blood supply to descending colon, rectosigmoid, and rectum based on 400 dissections: Its importance in regional resections. Dis Colon Rectum 1965; 8:251.
43. Goligher JC. The adequacy of the marginal blood supply to left colon after high ligation of the inferior mesenteric artery during excision of the rectum. Br J Surg 1954; 41:351.
44. Griffiths JD. Extramural and tramural blood supply of the colon. Br Med J 1961; 1:323.
45. Granger DN, Barrowman JA. Microcirculation of the alimentary tract. I. Physiology of transcapillary fluid and solute exchange. Gastroenterology 1983; 84:846.
46. Cole WH, Packard D, Southwick HW. Carcinoma of the colon with special reference to prevention of recurrence. JAMA 1954; 155:1549.
47. Dockerty MB. Pathologic aspects in control of spread of colonic carcinoma. Proc Staff Meet Mayo Clinic 1958; 33:157.
48. Wood JD. Physiology of the enteric nervous system. *In:* Johnson LR, ed. Physiology of the Gastrointestinal System, Vol I. New York: Raven Press, 1981: 1–37.
49. Burnstock G. Neurotransmitters and trophic factors in the autonomic nervous system. J Physiol 1981; 313:1.
50. Davenport HW. Physiology of the Digestive Tract, 5th Ed. Chicago: Year Book Medical Publishers, 1982.
51. Goyal RK. Neurology of the gut. *In:* Sleisinger MH, Fordtran JS, eds. Gastrointestinal Disease, 3rd Ed. Philadelphia: WB Saunders, 1983. 97–115.

Chapter 132

Pathophysiology of Colonic Motility Disorders

William J. Snape, Jr.

Colonic smooth muscle, like smooth muscle throughout the stomach and small intestine, is controlled by its intrinsic myoelectrical activity, which is composed of slow waves and spike potentials.[1,2] Further control of colonic motility is mediated through neural reflexes or the effects of neurohumoral peptides on the underlying myoelectrical activity.

Myoelectrical Activity of the Colon

Contraction of the colonic smooth muscle is controlled by depolarization of smooth muscle membrane. There are at least 2 basic types of membrane potential activity or myoelectrical activity in humans: slow waves and spike potentials (Fig. 132–1).[3] Oscillation potentials, a third type of phasic myoelectrical activity, occur in animals[4] and also may be present in humans.[5]

Slow Waves. Slow waves are cyclical slow changes in the membrane potential of the colonic smooth muscle. Human colonic slow wave activity appears to be generated from longitudinal smooth muscle,[6–8] whereas in the cat, the source of the activity appears to be the circular smooth muscle.[9] Slow wave activity in the cat colon is dependent upon both sodium and calcium ions,[10, 11] but their importance in the control of human colonic slow wave activity is unknown.

The slow wave pattern is not constant throughout the colon. There is a frequency of 9 to 10 cycles/minute from the ascending colon to the upper sigmoid colon. The frequency decreases from the lower sigmoid colon to the rectum, where it appears to be 6 cycles/minute.[12–14]

It is probable that the pattern of slow wave frequency is important in the control of colonic function. Slow waves relate to the contractile pattern by controlling the interval at which spike potentials occur.[15] In the cat, the propagation of slow wave activity from the transverse colon toward the cecum can impede the forward flow of colonic contents, allowing more complete absorption of salt and water.[16] When this mechanism is disrupted by the administration of an exogenous compound or by illness, diarrhea usually results.[17,18]

Spike Potentials. Spike potentials are rapid changes in membrane potential that occur at the peak of slow wave depolarization.[1] They appear to be dependent upon calcium movement into smooth muscle cells.[11, 19, 20] The major type of spike activity is superimposed on slow wave activity, and its frequency is controlled by the slow wave frequency.[14, 15] This type of spike activity causes a segmental type of contractile response, which most likely has a mixing function within the lumen of the colon.[5, 21] The administration of exogenous neural agonists or gastrointestinal peptides stimulates slow wave–associated colonic spike and contractile activity.[14, 22] The endogenous release of these neurohumoral agents may be important in the physiologic control of colonic motility. Eating stimulates the release of many peptides and initiates many neural reflexes that may alter colonic motor function.

Spike potentials can also exist as migrating spike bursts (Fig. 132–2). In the cat, oscillatory potentials beginning in the ascending colon with a frequency of 35 to 45 cycles/minute initiate migrating action potentials.

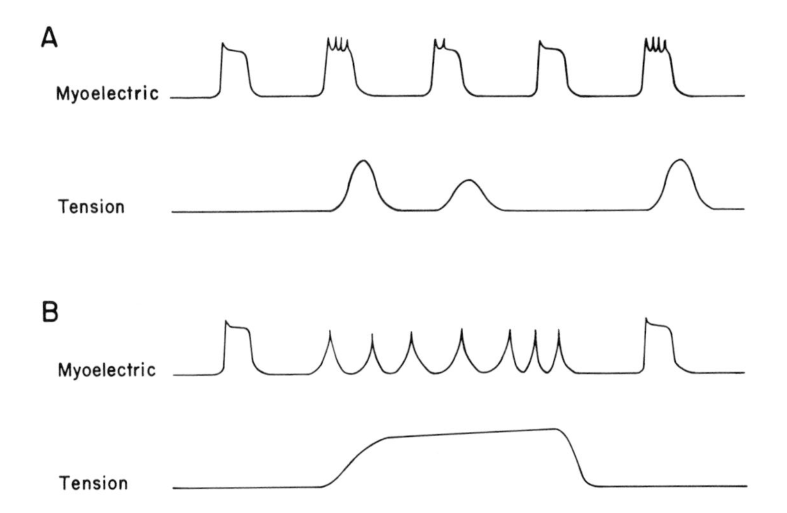

Figure 132–1. Schematic diagram of myoelectric activity. *A*, Slow waves, spike potentials, and contractions are present. Spike potentials must be pressent for phasic contractions to occur. *B*, Tonic contractions associated with oscillatory potentials.

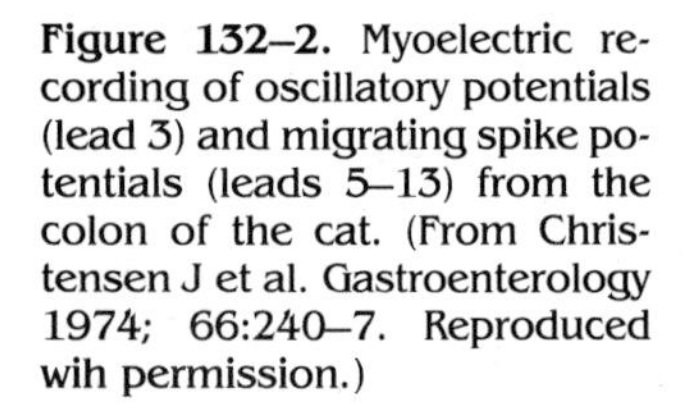

Figure 132–2. Myoelectric recording of oscillatory potentials (lead 3) and migrating spike potentials (leads 5–13) from the colon of the cat. (From Christensen J et al. Gastroenterology 1974; 66:240–7. Reproduced wih permission.)

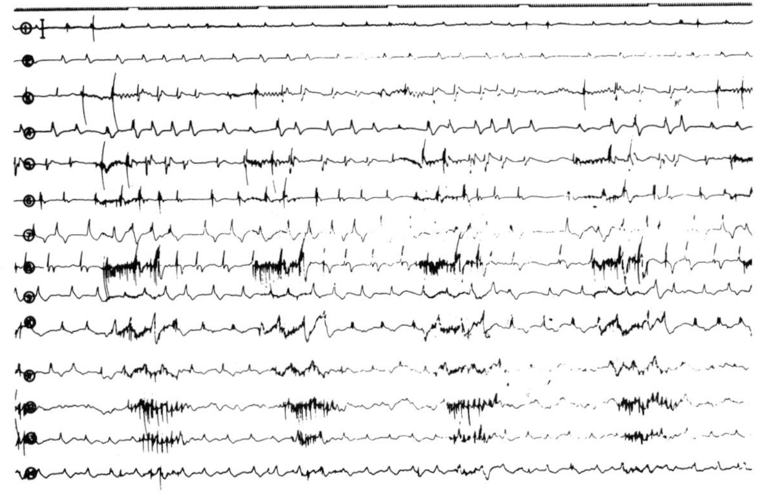

These begin in the transverse colon and migrate aborally.[4] The spike activity is associated with a powerful contraction. This type of spike activity may also occur in humans.[5,23] The duration of the migrating spike burst is controlled by inhibitory neurons within the myenteric plexus.[24] The migrating spike burst may be the electrical correlate for the mass movement described in humans, but this has not been proved.

Gastrocolonic Response

Colonic motility is increased after a meal.[22,25] This increase reflects the net sum of stimulation and inhibition of colonic smooth muscle by neural reflexes and gastrointestinal peptides.[25–27] Called the *gastrocolonic response,* the increase in motility is not related to the pattern of bowel evacuation after eating. In healthy subjects, colonic spike and contractile activity immediately increases after eating a standardized meal.[22,25] The quantity of nutrients in the meal rather than its volume determines the magnitude of stimulation of the gastrocolonic response.

Figure 132–3 shows the effect of dietary components on the gastrocolonic response. Carbohydrate and protein do not stimulate colonic motility. Instead, the fat component of the meal is the major stimulant. Fat stimulates an early increase in colonic motility and also a delayed increase.[25] The mechanism of the bimodal response is unknown. There is some evidence that the early response is mediated through cholinergic nerves and that the late response is mediated humorally.[27] Amino acids inhibit the colonic motor response that occurs after eating fat or a 1000-Kcal mixed meal.[25,26] Thus, *the characteristic change in colonic motility after a mixed meal seems to be a summation of fat stimulation and amino acid inhibition.* Protein eaten with a mixed meal would be digested to amino acids after about 30 minutes, and this action would inhibit the late increase in colonic motility, leaving only the early response.

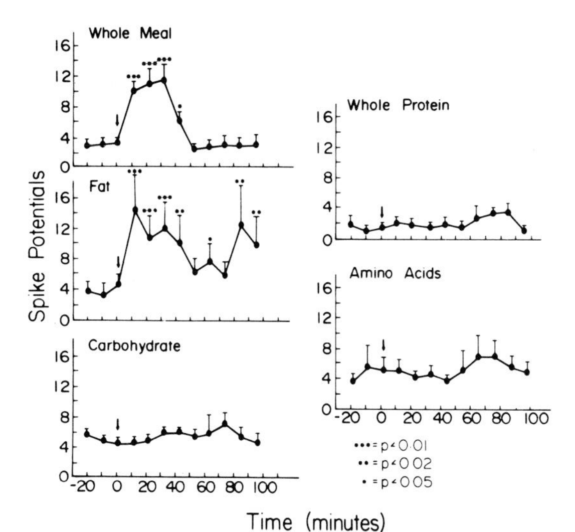

Figure 132–3. Colonic spike response after eating. The number of spike potentials is shown for 10-minute periods before and after ingesting a 1000-Kcal mixed meal or individual dietary components, fat (600 Kcal), carbohydrate (320 Kcal), whole protein or amino acids (200 Kcal). (From Wright SH et al. Am J Physiol 1980; 238:G228–32. Reproduced with permission.)

Studies have begun to clarify the mechanisms that control the gastrocolonic response (Table 132–1). Findings to date include the following:

1. The response is not dependent upon the ingested nutrients' reaching the colon.[28]
2. Anticholinergic drugs inhibit the gastrocolonic response.[27,28] Furthermore, an intact cholinergic muscarinic (afferent) receptor seems to be necessary for stimulation of the gastrocolonic response. This is suggested by the observation that when procaine is added to the stomach prior to eating, the gastrocolonic response is also inhibited.[29]
3. The opioid antagonist naloxone inhibits the gastrocolonic response, whereas morphine stimulates it, so that an intact opioid receptor also is necessary.[29] Indeed, there

Table 132–1. NEUROHUMORAL CONTROL OF THE GASTROCOLONIC RESPONSE

Neural	Peptide
Central Nervous System:	*Neuropeptide:*
Brain:	Opiate (+)
Stress (+)	OP-CCK (+)
Sham meal (n.e.)*	*Humoral:*
Spinal Cord	Gastrin (+)
Transection (n.e.)	
Peripheral Nervous System:	
Mucosal afferent receptors:	
Volume stretch receptors (n.e.)	
Chemical receptors (+)	
Myenteric efferent neurons:	
Cholinergic (+)	
Vagotomy (−)	
Sympathetic ganglia (−)	
Non-adrenergic, non-cholinergic neuron (−)	
5-Hydroxytryptamine (−)	

*n.e. = No effect.

are opioid-containing neurons within the myenteric plexus.

These studies suggest a complex interaction between afferent neural receptors in the gastroduodenal mucosa and cholinergic and opioid neurons in the intrinsic plexuses of the bowel.

The central nervous system (CNS) modifies many functions of the gastrointestinal tract. A modified sham feeding elicits CNS stimulation of acid secretion, but does not stimulate an increase in colonic motility after a meal.[29, 30] In cats, stimulation of the cerebrum, midbrain, and hypothalamus stimulates colonic motility.[31] Emotional stress can stimulate colonic motility in humans.[32] The central nervous system, therefore, can stimulate or mediate an increase in colonic motility under certain circumstances. Lesions of the spinal cord do not seem to affect the increase in colonic motility that occurs after a meal, but there is no gastrocolonic response after vagotomy.[33, 34]

Gastrointestinal peptides may also be involved in the control of colonic motility. Gastrin and cholecystokinin are capable of stimulating colonic smooth muscle and spike activity, both in human subjects and in animals,[35, 36] even though there is some controversy about the potency of gastrin in stimulating colonic smooth muscle.[37] Serum concentrations of these 2 gastrointestinal peptides increase after a meal.[38, 39] However, in healthy subjects the major increase in gastrin occurs later than the increase in postprandial colonic motility.[22] Gastrin, therefore, may not be involved in the gastrocolonic response. Cholecystokinin (CCK) may be the mediator of the late response after eating fat. Further studies are needed to assess accurately the role of CCK in the normal physiologic control of colonic motility. Naloxone also inhibits colonic stimulation by the octapeptide of CCK. The structural similarity between the 2 compounds suggests a similarity in receptors.[40] Further studies are also necessary to evaluate this mechanism.

Luminal bile salts stimulate colonic motility in rabbits and humans.[41,42] Deoxycholic acid stimulates motility in the ascending colon through direct contact with mucosal neuroreceptors.[43] Bile salt stimulation of the colon is mediated by cholinergic and alpha-adrenergic neurons. Placing bile salts in the human ascending colon stimulates distal motility.[42] Inasmuch as bile is excreted into the gastrointestinal tract after eating fat-containing meals, bile salts may be the mediator of the late increase in colonic motility induced by a fatty meal.

Colonic Motility in Disease

Irritable Colon Syndrome (see Chapter 134). A disorder in gastrointestinal motility may be the major cause of symptoms in the irritable colon (irritable bowel) syndrome. In a survey of apparently healthy subjects, about one-third had symptoms suggestive of a functional gut disorder.[44] There were 4 types of symptom patterns in these subjects: (1) spastic (painful) irritable colon syndrome; (2) painless diarrhea; (3) painless constipation; and (4) non-colonic dyspepsia. The question arises: How does motility of the gastrointestinal tract determine symptoms in these patients?

Motor activity is less propulsive throughout the colon than in the more proximal portions of the gastrointestinal tract.[45] Lack of propulsion slows the forward flow of fecal contents and allows more complete absorption of salt and water by the colonic mucosa.[46] Constipated patients were noted to display an increase in segmenting contractions in the descending colon, and patients with diarrhea showed a decrease in colonic contractions.[47] These data suggest that abdominal pain and constipation of the irritable colon syndrome may be secondary to an increased number of segmenting contractions that cause a functional partial obstruction of the colon.[48]

The slow wave pattern is disturbed in patients with abdominal pain and an altered bowel habit.[15, 49, 50] In these subjects, slow waves occur at a frequency of 3 cycles/minute significantly more often than in healthy subjects.[15, 49, 50] The abnormal slow wave rhythm is present only in persons with an irritable bowel, and patients with abdominal pain for other reasons have a normal slow wave rhythm.[5] The abnormal slow wave rhythm is also present during remissions.[51] Thus, there appears to be an underlying abnormality in the colonic smooth muscle that causes an abnormal slow wave pattern in patients with irritable colon syndrome. This abnormality also is present in children with an irritable bowel.[52]

When colonic motility is stimulated by either the IV administration of a gastrointestinal peptide or eating a meal, the pattern of contractile activity is determined by the slow wave frequency.[15] As mentioned, in patients with the irritable colon syndrome the colon contracts at a frequency of 3 cycles/minute. This response appears as localized contractions of circular muscle on cineradiography.[53–55] The abnormal slow wave pattern appears to act as a background, allowing an abnormal contractile pattern during periods of colonic stimulation.

Patients with painless diarrhea have a different motility pattern, similar to that of healthy control subjects.[56] In general, colonic motility is decreased in patients with painless diarrhea.[47] Increased amounts of localized motor activity are occasionally present, but the pattern of the contractility differs from that seen in patients with a spastic colon.[57,58] Apparently, the pattern of the colonic motility disturbance differs between the spastic colon and painless diarrhea variants.

Patients with painless constipation appear to have a pattern of colonic motility similar to spastic colon patients.[56] However, their pain threshold may differ from patients with the irritable bowel syndrome. Patients with the irritable colon syndrome recognize rectal distention just as do healthy subjects, but distention is painful when the rectum is less full.[58,59] Hence, there appears to be hyperalgesia in the patients with the irritable bowel syndrome. Patients with painless constipation appear to have the same underlying motility disorder, but they do not have the colonic hyperalgesia.

Occasionally, abdominal pain is associated with an increase in segmenting contractions in other portions of the intestinal tract.[60] Distention of the esophagus, duodenum, or small intestine may reproduce pain similar to that spontaneously experienced.[61, 62] It is possible, therefore, that an abnormality in motility in other portions of the gastrointestinal tract can lead to symptoms of the irritable colon syndrome. Duodenogastric reflux also occurs in patients with functional bowel disease.[63]

The transit of material through the lumen of the colon is also disturbed in patients with the irritable colon syndrome. Although few studies have been made, it appears that either eating or cholinergic stimulation increases transit through the colon in patients with the irritable colon syndrome[64, 65] and that transit differs in the patient with an irritable colon from that of healthy subjects.

Patients with the irritable colon syndrome frequently have a postprandial exacerbation of their symptoms. Not surprisingly, the postprandial gastrocolonic response is also abnormal.[66] Although the quantity of spike and contractile activity after a meal is similar to that of healthy subjects, the pattern of the response is markedly different. Figure 132–4 shows the gastrocolonic response in healthy subjects and in patients with the irritable colon syndrome. The gastrocolonic response is delayed in patients with the irritable colon syndrome who have abdominal pain and an alteration in their bowel habits, in contrast to healthy subjects.[66] In healthy subjects, the increase in colonic motility occurs immediately after eating, whereas in patients with the irritable bowel syndrome the major in-

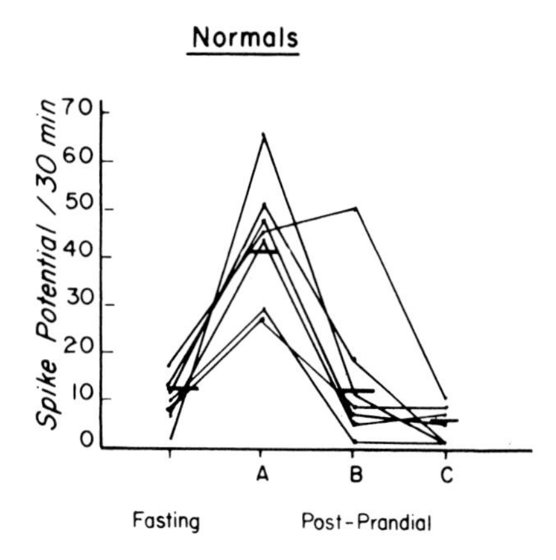

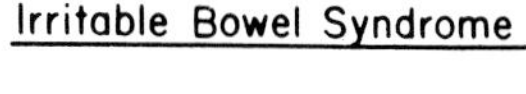

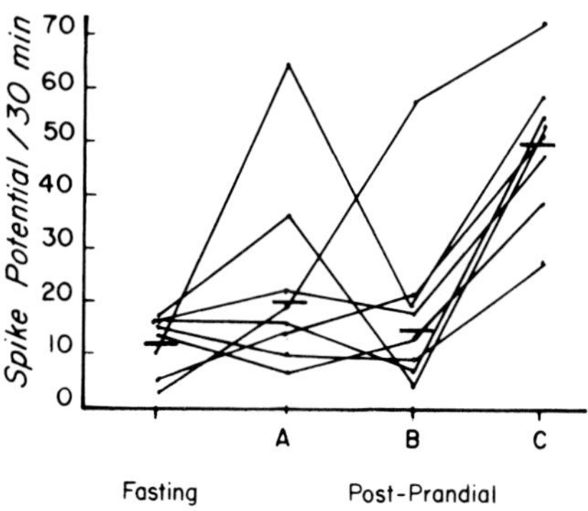

Figure 132–4. The colonic spike response to a standard 1000-Kcal meal in normal subjects and in patients with the irritable bowel syndrome. The individual responses are plotted as SP/30 minutes for the fasting and 3 postprandial periods. Points A, B, and C represent 0 to 30, 30 to 60, and 60 to 90 minutes postprandially. The horizontal line represents the mean responses during the 30-minute period. (From Battle WM et al. Dig Dis Sci 1980; 25:647–52. Reproduced with permission.)

crease in colonic motility occurs 60 to 90 minutes after eating.[23, 66] The delayed increase in colonic motility can be inhibited by anticholinergic agents[66] and by administration of amino acids prior to eating.[67] Thus, as in healthy subjects, the dietary components of a meal may influence the gastrocolonic response in these patients.

The postprandial increase in colonic contractile activity occurs at a frequency of 3 cycles/minute in patients with the irritable colon syndrome.[66] By contrast, the increase in colonic contractile activity occurs at a frequency of 6 cycles/minute in healthy subjects.[22]

The postprandial exacerbation of symptoms in patients with the irritable colon syndrome may be mediated by release of a gastrointestinal peptide or by initiation of autonomic neural reflexes that stimulate the abnormal smooth muscle substrate. The role of the autonomic nervous system or the gastrointestinal peptides in the production of symptoms is still unknown. Cholecystokinin may be involved in symptom production, since CCK stimulates significantly more contractile activity in patients with an irritable colon who have postprandial abdominal pain.[68]

Current accumulated knowledge of the pathophysiology of colonic motor dysfunction in patients with the irritable colon syndrome suggests various modalities of therapy that may be helpful. A low-fat, high-protein diet should decrease the contractile response of the colon. Increased dietary fiber may decrease symptoms if stool frequency is increased,[69, 70] possibly because of the decrease in the segmenting activity that occurs on a high-fiber diet.[71]

Anticholinergic drugs decrease colonic motility and should decrease symptoms.[66] A double-blind study using high doses of an oral anticholinergic did indeed decrease abdominal pain.[72] Simultaneous administration of a mild tranquilizer, dietary fiber, and an anticholinergic drug has the greatest effect.[70] Mild tranquilizers may decrease symptoms, since stress can stimulate colonic motility in healthy subjects and in patients with an irritable colon.[32] Papaverine, a general smooth muscle relaxant, also decreases cholinergic stimulation of colonic motility, but does not decrease cholecystokinin stimulation.[73] Calcium channel blockade inhibits colonic smooth muscle activity,[11] so that drugs with this action may be of some therapeutic value in patients with an irritable colon.

Diverticular Disease (see Chapter 135). Colonic diverticula, i.e., herniations of mucosa through the colonic circular smooth muscle, have a minimal covering of smooth muscle. Patients with the irritable colon syndrome seem to have a proclivity to develop diverticulosis.[74, 75] If the underlying pathogenesis is similar in the 2 conditions, the pathophysiology should also be similar. Unlike the 3 cycles/minute slow wave rhythm observed in patients with the irritable bowel syndrome, however, patients with diverticular disease of the colon have a slow wave frequency of about 18 cycles/minute,[76] which is decreased after administration of bran. Inasmuch as circular and longitudinal smooth muscle of the colon are both thickened,[77–79] diverticular disease of the colon appears to be secondary to dysfunction of colonic smooth muscle.

Although basal colonic intraluminal pressure in these patients is similar to that in healthy control subjects,[78, 80] neostigmine or eating increases the pressure significantly more than in healthy subjects.[81, 82] This encourages the hypothesis that the major disorder in diverticular disease is an excessive amount of segmenting contractions of the colon and suggests that the treatment should be aimed at decreasing contractions.

Anticholinergics inhibit the increase in colonic motility seen in patients with diverticular disease.[81] Increased dietary fiber, which may be useful in the treatment of the irritable colon syndrome,[83] may be helpful as well by decreasing intraluminal pressure and restoring the abnormal myoelectrical pattern toward normal.[76, 84] Glucagon may also alleviate symptoms,[85] perhaps by inhibiting slow wave activity and thus decreasing the abnormal contractile pattern present in those with irritable colon phenomena.[86]

Diabetes Mellitus (see Chapter 252). Gastrointestinal motility disturbances are common among patients with diabetes mellitus.[87] *Constipation* may be the most common gastrointestinal complaint in these patients. Severe constipation has been reported in 20% of patients with significant diabetic neuropathy.[88] A less common gastrointestinal symptom in diabetic patients is unexplained chronic diarrhea.[89] Steatorrhea coincident with diarrhea has generally been attributed to pancreatic insufficiency, celiac disease, or bacterial overgrowth within the small intestine.[87, 89] The colon appears to play a permissive role in patients with diarrhea. In the absence of steatorrhea, colonic dysfunction may be the primary contributor. Atonic dilatation of the colon simulating organic obstruction has been reported with prolonged intractable diarrhea.[90] Indeed, diabetic enteropathy may be a cause of megacolon.

In diabetic patients who require insulin and who have a major complaint of constipation, the colonic slow wave pattern is similar to that present in healthy subjects,[91] but the gastrocolonic response to a meal is disturbed (Fig. 132–5). Diabetic patients who have severe constipation have no increase in postprandial colonic spike activity; in those with a normal bowel habit, the response is similar in amplitude to that of healthy controls but is delayed. These data suggest that the colon in diabetics does not respond normally to the physiologic stimulus of eating, thereby perhaps inducing atonicity and contributing to the development of constipation. The cholinergic neural control of colonic function, which appears to play a vital role in the normal gastrocolonic response, may be disturbed in diabetics with constipation. The smooth muscle appears normal in these patients, insofar as administration of parasympathomimetic drugs or metoclopramide increases colonic spike and contractile activity.[91] The motor defect associated with constipation in patients with diabetes mellitus would seem then to focalize at one or more of several levels of the neuraxis. There may be a defect in the neural receptors of the upper gastrointestinal tract mucosa that inhibits the gastrocolonic response. Previous studies have shown that blockade of these neural receptors with procaine abolishes the gastrocolonic motor response.[29] There may also be a defect in the neural connection between the upper gastrointestinal tract and the colon, or there may be defects in the prevertebral and paravertebral sympathetic ganglia involved with the control of colonic function.[92, 93] There is no correlation between peripheral nerve conduction velocity, gastric emptying, or colonic motility in patients with diabetes mellitus.[91]

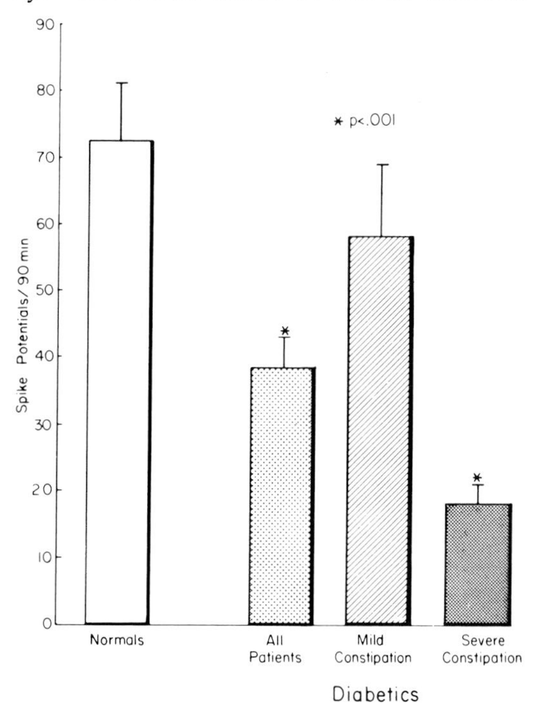

Figure 132–5. Cumulative spike potential response after eating a 1000-Kcal meal in normal subjects and patients with diabetes mellitus who have either severe or mild constipation. (From Battle WM et al. Gastroenterology 1980; 79:1217–21. Reproduced with permission.)

Diarrhea is much less common in patients with diabetes mellitus. Colonic motility has not been reported in diabetic patients with diarrhea, but a smooth muscle dysfunction in the small intestine of patients with diabetic diarrhea has been noted.[92] This consists of decreased tone of the intestinal smooth muscle wall associated with an increased amplitude of phasic small intestinal contractions in the small intestine.[92]

Inasmuch as parasympathomimetic agents or metoclopramide can stimulate the colon, it is reasonable to expect them to alleviate symptoms of constipation. Metoclopramide and neostigmine do indeed improve constipation in diabetic patients.[94] The treatment of diabetic diarrhea, however, has been unsuccessful and no consistently effective therapy is currently available for this condition.

Progressive Systemic Sclerosis (see Chapter 244). When progressive systemic sclerosis (PSS) involves the colon, as it may any portion of the gastrointestinal tract,[95] most of the patients so affected are symptomatic and have severe bowel dysfunction. Colonic myoelectrical activity is abnormal in patients with PSS in that slow waves are present at a frequency similar to healthy subjects, but there is no gastrocolonic response after eating a meal. This was observed in one study[96] in 9 of 10 consecutive patients with PSS; the one patient with a normal response had minimal systemic and gastrointestinal disease.

Exogenous stimulating drugs administered to patients with PSS have been noted to result in a mixed reaction.[96] Four of 10 patients had a normal increase in colonic spike activity after the administration of neostigmine or metoclopramide; the other 6 patients did not respond to either medication. These

2 groups of patients were clinically different. The patients who had no response to the exogenous administration of stimulating agents had a longer duration of disease, were rated clinically as having more severe disease with cardiac, renal, or pulmonary involvement, and also had abnormal radiographic appearances of either the colon or the upper gastrointestinal tract.[96] Four of the 6 patients who had no increase in colonic motility after exogenous stimulation died within a year of the study. Pathologic examination of the gastrointestinal tract of these patients revealed severe fibrosis and muscle atrophy.

Progression of the gastrointestinal involvement parallels progression of the systemic disease, in keeping with previous observations pertaining to the esophagus and small intestine.[97, 98] Early in the disease there is a latent neural defect. However, in patients with longstanding PSS, the response of the smooth muscle is diminished as it atrophies and is replaced by collagen.[97, 98]

Patients early in the course of their disease usually have no clinically evident dysfunction of their bowel habit. Later in the disease, however, they suffer from disturbed motility in both the small intestine and the colon. Unfortunately, the disease at this stage has progressed to a point at which pharmacologic stimulation is unsuccessful.

Idiopathic Pseudo-obstruction (see Chapter 123). The colon is generally involved in patients with idiopathic intestinal pseudo-obstruction.[99] There are at least 2 types of patients with this puzzling derangement: (1) those in whom the gastrointestinal smooth muscle is diseased, and (2) those who have generalized autonomic neuropathy.[99–101] Abnormal colonic motility has been observed only in patients with the neural type of idiopathic pseudo-obstruction. These are patients with abnormal neural control of esophageal and small intestinal motility as well.[102] Slow wave activity is normal in these patients; spike and contractile activity increases after the administration of a parasympathomimetic agent,[102] but after a 1000-Kcal meal was eaten no increase in colonic motility was observed.[103] These data further suggest that the neural connection between the gastroduodenal receptors and the colonic myenteric plexus is disrupted in this condition. They also indicate that the motility pattern of the neural form of the disease is similar to that in patients with early scleroderma or amyloidosis.[96,104]

Neuromuscular Disorders (see Chapter 253). Bowel function is disturbed in patients who have generalized disorders of the neuromuscular system. Patients with myotonic dystrophy have dysphagia or an altered bowel habit in addition to their skeletal muscle dysfunction,[105] and their internal and external anal sphincters show prolonged contraction on rectal distention.

Patients with multiple sclerosis have difficulty with severe constipation[106] associated with an absent gastrocolonic response. There is functional evidence in these patients of a lesion in the somatosensory axis central to the lumbosacral portion of the spinal cord.[106]

Ulcerative Colitis (see Chapter 126). Previous studies have described decreased colonic contractility in patients with ulcerative colitis.[107,108] Myoelectrical activity is also abnormal in these patients. Slow waves have a frequency similar to that of healthy controls. Spike activity before a meal also is similar in both groups.[109] However, patients with ulcerative colitis respond differently after eating a meal than do healthy subjects; the spike response is similar to that seen in healthy subjects, but it is somewhat decreased and shortened, although there is no increase in contractile activity. These data suggest that there is a disturbance in electromechanical coupling in the smooth muscle of patients with ulcerative colitis. This is further confirmed by *in vitro* studies of isolated smooth muscle from patients with ulcerative colitis.

The mechanism of electromechanical uncoupling in patients with ulcerative colitis is presently unknown. Although increased numbers of nerves containing vasoactive inhibitory peptide (VIP) are present in Crohn's disease, this is not true of ulcerative colitis.[110] Other compounds may be involved in this process, since increased levels of tissue kinins and prostaglandins are present in the mucosa of patients with ulcerative colitis.[111–113]

References

1. Bortoff A. Current concepts. Intestinal motility. N Engl J Med 1969; 280:1335–7.
2. Bortoff A. Myogenic control of intestinal motility. Physiol Rev 1976; 56:418–34.
3. Christensen J. Myoelectric control of the colon. Gastroenterology 1975; 68:601–9.
4. Christensen J, Anuras S, Hauser RL. Migrating spike bursts and electrical slow-waves in the cat colon: Effect of sectioning. Gastroenterology 1974; 66:240–7.
5. Sarna SK, Waterfall WE, Bardakjian BL, Lind JF. Types of human colonic electrical activities recorded postoperatively. Gastroenterology 1981; 81:61–70.
6. Vanasin B, Bass DD, Mendeloff AI, Schuster MM. Alteration of electrical and motor activity of human and dog rectum by diphenylhydantoin. Dig Dis 1973; 18:403–10.

7. Duthie HL, Kirk D. Electrical activity of human colonic smooth muscle in vitro. J Physiol 1978; 283:319–30.
8. Chambers MM, Bowes KL, Kingma YJ, Bannister C, Cote KR. *In vitro* electrical activity in human colon. Gastroenterology 1981; 81:502–8.
9. Christensen J, Caprilli R, Lund GF. Electric slow waves in circular muscle of cat colon. Am J Physiol 1969; 217:771–6.
10. Wienbeck M, Christensen J. Cationic requirements of colon slow-waves in the cat. Am J Physiol 1971; 220:513–9.
11. Snape WJ Jr. Effect of calcium on the neurohumoral stimulation of feline colonic smooth muscle. Am J Physiol 1982; 243:G134–40.
12. Sarna SK, Bardakjian BL, Waterfall WE, Lind JF. Human colonic electrical control activity (ECA). Gastroenterology 1980; 78:1526–36.
13. Taylor I, Duthie HL, Smallwood R, Linkens D. Large bowel myoelectrical activity in man. Gut 1975; 16:808–14.
14. Snape WJ Jr, Carlson GM, Cohen S. Human colonic myoelectric activity in response to prostigmine and the gastrointestinal hormones. Am J Dig Dis 1977; 22:881–7.
15. Snape WJ Jr, Carlson GM, Matarazzo SA, Cohen S. Evidence that abnormal myoelectrical activity produces colonic motor dysfunction in the irritable bowel syndrome. Gastroenterology 1977; 72:383–7.
16. Christensen J, Hauser RL. Longitudinal axial coupling of slow waves in proximal cat colon. Am J Physiol 1971; 221:246–50.
17. Christensen J, Weisbrodt NW, Hauser RL. Electrical slow-wave of the proximal colon of the cat in diarrhea. Gastroenterology 1972; 62:1167–73.
18. Barker JD Jr, Christensen J. Some effects of quinidine and quinine on the electromyogram of the colon. Gastroenterology 1973; 65:773–7.
19. Bolton TB. Mechanisms of action of transmitters and other substances on smooth muscle. Physiol Rev 1979; 59:606–718.
20. Johansson B, Somlyo AP. Electro-physiology and excitation-contraction coupling. *In*: Bohr DF, Somlyo AP, Sparks HU Jr, eds. The Handbook of Physiology, Section 2. The Cardiovascular System, Volume II. Bethesda, Md: American Physiological Society, 1980: 301–23.
21. Fioramonti J, Garcia-Villar R, Bueno L, Ruckebusch Y. Colonic myoelectrical activity and propulsion in the dog. Dig Dis Sci 1980; 25:641–6.
22. Snape WJ Jr, Matarazzo SA, Cohen S. Effect of eating and gastrointestinal hormones on human colonic myoelectrical and motor activity. Gastroenterology 1978; 75:373–8.
23. Bueno L, Fioramonti J, Ruckebusch Y, Frexinos J, Coulom P. Evaluation of colonic myoelectrical activity in health and functional disorders. Gut 1980; 21:480–5.
24. Christensen J, Anuras S, Arthur C. Influence of intrinsic nerves on electromyogram of cat colon in vitro. Am J Physiol 1978; 234:E641–7.
25. Wright SH, Snape WJ Jr, Battle W, Cohen S, London RL. Effect of dietary components on gastrocolonic response. Am J Physiol 1980; 238:G228–32.
26. Battle WM, Cohen S, Snape WJ Jr. Inhibition of postprandial colonic motility after ingestion of an amino acid mixture. Dig Dis Sci 1980; 25:647–52.
27. Snape WJ Jr, Wright SH, Battle WM, Cohen S. The gastrocolic response: Evidence for a neural mechanism. Gastroenterology 1979; 77:1235–40.
28. Sillin LF, Schulte SJ, Woods JH, Cowles VE, Condon RE, Bass P. Electromotor feeding responses of primate ileum and colon. Am J Surg 1979; 137:99–105.
29. Sun EA, Snape WJ Jr, Cohen S, Renny A. The role of opiate receptors and cholinergic neurons in the gastrocolonic response. Gastroenterology 1982; 82:689–93.
30. Richardson CT, Walsh JH, Cooper KA, et al. Studies on the role of the cephalic-vagal stimulation in the acid secretory response to eating in normal human subjects. J Clin Invest 1977; 60:435–41.
31. Rostad H. Central and peripheral nervous control of colonic motility in the cat. Acta Physiol Scand 1973; 89:79–181.
32. Narducci F, Snape WJ Jr, Battle WM, London R, Cohen S. Stimluation of colonic myoelectric activity by emotional stress in healthy subjects and the irritable bowel syndrome: Effect of pretreatment with Librium. Gastroenterology 1982; 82:1137.
33. Connell AM, Frankel H, Ittman S. The motility of the pelvic colon following complete lesions of the spinal cord. Paraplegia 1963; 1:98–115.
34. Connell AM, McKelvey STD. Influence of vagotomy on the colon. Proc Roy Soc Med 1970; 63(Suppl):7–9.
35. Logan CHJ, Connell AM. The effect of a synthetic gastrin-like pentapeptide (ICI 50, 123) on intestinal motility in man. Lancet 1966; 1:996–9.
36. Snape WJ Jr, Cohen S. Effect of bethanechol, gastrin I or cholecystokinin on myoelectrical activity in the isolated cat colon. Am J Physiol 1979; 236:E458–63.
37. Misiewicz JJ, Waller SL, Holdstock DJ. Gastrointestinal motility and gastric secretion during intravenous infusions of gastrin II. Gut 1969; 10:732–9.
38. Dockray GJ, Taylor IL. Heptadecapeptide gastrin: Measurement in blood by specific radioimmunoassay. Gastroenterology 1976; 71:971–7.
39. Byrnes DJ, Borody T, Henderson L. Plasma cholecystokinin. Reg Peptides 1980; 1(Suppl):S15.
40. Schiller PW, Lipton A, Horrobin DF, Bodanszky M. Unsulfated C-terminal 7-peptide of cholecystokinin, a new ligand of the opiate receptor. Biochem Biophys Res Comm 1978; 85:1332–8.
41. Snape WJ Jr, Shiff S, Cohen S. Effect of deoxycholic acid on colonic motility in the rabbit. Am J Physiol 1980; 238:G321–5.
42. Kirwan WL, Smith AN, Mitchell WD, Falconer JD, Eastwood MA. Bile acids and colonic motility in the rabbit and the human. Gut 1975; 16:894–902.
43. Shiff SJ, Soloway RD, Snape WJ Jr. Mechanism of deoxycholic acid stimulation of the rabbit colon. J Clin Invest 1982; 69:985–92.
44. Thompson WG, Heaton KW. Functional bowel disorders in apparently healthy people. Gastroenterology 1980; 79:283–8.
45. Adler HF, Atkinson AJ, Ivy AC. A study of the motility of the human colon: An explanation of dysynergia of the colon, or of the "unstable colon." Am J Dig Dis 1941; 8:197–202.
46. Devroede GJ, Phillips SF. Conservation of sodium, chloride and water by the human colon. Gastroenterology 1969; 56:101.
47. Connell AM. The motility of the pelvic colon. Gut 1962; 3:342–8.
48. Connell AM, Jones FA, Rowlands EN. Motility of the pelvic colon. Gut 1965; 6:105–12.
49. Snape WJ Jr, Carlson GM, Cohen S. Colonic myoelectric activity in the irritable bowel syndrome. Gastroenterology 1976; 70:326–30.
50. Taylor I, Darby C, Hammond P, Basu P. Is there a myoelectrical abnormality in the irritable colon syndrome? Gut 1978; 19:391–5.
51. Taylor I, Darby C, Hammond P. Comparison of rectosigmoid myoelectrical activity in the irritable colon syndrome during relapses and remissions. Gut 1978; 19:923–9.
52. Kline J, Hayek M, Hodges V, Barbero G. Myoelectric activity in children with the recurrent abdominal pain syndrome (RAP). Gastroenterology 1982; 82:1101.
53. Ritchie JA, Ardran GM, Truelove SC. Motor activity of the sigmoid colon of humans. Gastroenterology 1962; 43:642–68.
54. Sun EA, Goren R, Snape WJ Jr, Kressel H. Use of a videotaped barium enema for studying colonic motility. Gastroenterology 1981; 80:1297.
55. Lumsden K, Chaudhary NA, Truelove SC. The irritable colon syndrome. Clin Radiol 1963; 14:54.
56. Snape WJ Jr. Unpublished observation.
57. Ritchie JA, Tuckey MS. Intraluminal pressure studies at different distances from the anus in normal subjects and in patients with the irritable colon syndrome. Am J Dig Dis 1969; 14:96–105.
58. Whitehead WE, Engel B, Schuster MM. Irritable bowel syndrome: Physiological and psychological differences between diarrhea-predominant and constipation-predominant patients. Dig Dis Sci 1980; 25:404–13.
59. Ritchie J. Pain from distension of the pelvic colon by inflating a balloon in the irritable colon syndrome. Gut 1973; 14:125–32.
60. Holdstock DJ, Misiewicz JJ, Waller SL. Observations on the mechanism of abdominal pain. Gut 1969; 10:19–31.

61. Moriarty KG, Dawson AM. Functional abdominal pain: Further evidence that whole gut is affected. Br Med J 1982; 284:1670–2.
62. Lasser RB, Bond JH, Levitt MD. The role of intestinal gas in functional abdominal pain. N Engl J Med 1975; 293:524–6.
63. Anderson DL, Boyce HW Jr. Duodenogastric reflux: Association with irritable bowel syndrome. Gastrointest Endosc 1974; 20:112–4.
64. Ritchie JA. The transport of colonic contents in the irritable colon syndrome. Gut 1970; 11:668–72.
65. Manousos OH, Truelove SC, Lumsden K. Transit times of food in patients with diverticulosis or irritable colon syndrome and normal subjects. Br Med J 1967; 3:760–2.
66. Sullivan MA, Cohen S, Snape WJ Jr. Colonic myoelectrical activity in irritable-bowel syndrome. N Engl J Med 1978; 298:878–83.
67. Battle WM, Cohen S, Snape WJ Jr. Inhibition of postprandial colonic motility after ingestion of an amino acid mixture. Dig Dis Sci 1980; 25:647–52.
68. Harvey RF, Read AE. Effect of cholecystokinin on colonic motility and symptoms in patients with the irritable-bowel syndrome. Lancet 1973; 1:1–3.
69. Manning AP, Heaton KW, Harvey RF. Wheat fibre and irritable bowel syndrome. Lancet 1977; 2:417–8.
70. Ritchie JA, Truelove SC. Treatment of irritable bowel syndrome with lorazepam, hyoscine butylbromide and ispaguhla husk. Br Med J 1979; 1:376–8.
71. Fioramonti J, Bueno L. Motor activity in the large intestine of the pig related to dietary fibre and retention time. Br J Nutr 1980; 43:155–62.
72. Snape WJ Jr, Wright SA, Battle WM, London R, Sun EA, Cohen S. Successful treatment of the irritable colon syndrome with high doses of an anticholinergic. Gastroenterology 1981; 80:1289.
73. Snape WJ Jr. Influence of papaverine on bethanechol or OP-CCK stimulation of feline colonic muscle. Gastroenterology 1981; 80:498–503.
74. Havia T, Manner R. The irritable colon syndrome. Acta Chir Scand 1971; 137:569–72.
75. Fleischner FG, Ming S-C, Henken EM. Revised concepts on diverticular disease of the colon. Radiology 1964; 83:859–72.
76. Taylor I, Duthie HL. Bran tablets and diverticular disease. Br Med J 1976; 1:988–90.
77. Morson BC. The muscle abnormality in diverticular disease of the sigmoid colon. Br J Radiol 1963; 36:385–92.
78. Arfwidsson S. Pathogenesis of multiple diverticulae of the sigmoid colon in diverticular disease. Acta Chir Scand 1964; Suppl 342.
79. Hughes LE. Postmortem survey of diverticular disease of the colon. Gut 1969; 10:336–51.
80. Painter NS, Burkitt DP. Diverticular disease of the colon: A deficiency disease of Western civilization. Br Med J 1971; 2:450–4.
81. Painter NS, Truelove SC. The intraluminal pressure patterns in diverticulosis of the colon. Part II. The effect of prostigmine. Gut 1964; 5:365–73.
82. Parks TG, Connell AM. Motility studies in diverticular disease of the colon. Gut 1969; 10:534–42.
83. Painter NS, Almeida AZ, Colebourne KW. Unprocessed bran in treatment of diverticular disease of the colon. Br Med J 1972; 2:137–40.
84. Hodgson J. Effect of methylcellulose on rectal and colonic pressures in treatment of diverticular disease. Br Med J 1972; 3:729–31.
85. Daniel O, Basu PK, Al-Samarar HM. Use of glucagon in the treatment of acute diverticulitis. Br Med J 1974; 3:720–2.
86. Taylor I, Duthie HL, Cumberland DC, Smallwood R. Glucagon and the colon. Gut 1975; 16:973–8.
87. Scarpello JHB, Barber DC, Hague RV, Cullen DR, Sladen GE. Gastric emptying of solid meals in diabetes. Br Med J 1976; 2:671–73.
88. Rundles RW. Diabetic neuropathy. Medicine 1945; 24:111–60.
89. Katz LA, Spiro HM. Gastrointestinal manifestations of diabetes. N Engl J Med 1966; 275:1350–1.
90. Paley RG, Mitchell W, Watkinson G. Terminal colonic dilatation following intractable diarrhea in a diabetic. Gastroenterology 1961; 41:401–7.
91. Battle WM, Snape WJ Jr, Alavi A, Cohen S, Brunstein S. Colonic dysfunction in diabetes mellitus. Gastroenterology 1980; 79:1217–21.
92. Whalen GE, Soergel KH, Geenen JE. Diabetic diarrhea. Gastroenterology 1969; 56:1021–32.
93. Weems WA, Szurszewski JH. Modulation of colonic motility by peripheral neural inputs from neurons of the inferior mesenteric ganglia. Gastroenterology 1977; 73:273–8.
94. Snape WJ Jr, Schwartz SS, Battle WM, Braustein SN, Goldstein HA, Alavi A. Metoclopramide in the treatment of gastroparesis due to diabetes mellitus. Ann Intern Med 1982; 96:444–6.
95. Hodges FJ, Rundles RW, Hanelin J. Roentgenologic study of the small intestine. Dysfunction associated with neurological diseases. Radiology 1947; 49:659–73.
96. Battle WM, Snape WJ Jr, Wright S, Sullivan MA, Cohen S, Meyers A, Tuthill R. Abnormal colonic motility in progressive systemic sclerosis. Ann Intern Med 1981; 94:749–52.
97. Cohen S, Fisher R, Lipshutz N, Turner R, Myers A, Schumacher R. The pathogenesis of esophageal dysfunction in scleroderma and Raynaud's disease. J Clin Invest 1972; 51:2663–8.
98. DiMarino AJ, Carlson G, Myers A, Schumacher HR, Cohen S. Duodenal myoelectrical activity in scleroderma. N Engl J Med 1973; 289:1220–3.
99. Snape WJ Jr. Pseudo-obstruction and other obstructive disorders. Clin Gastroenterol 1982; 11:593–608.
100. Schuffler MD, Lowe MC, Bill AH. Studies of idiopathic intestinal pseudo-obstruction. I. Hereditary hollow visceral myopathy: Clinical and pathological studies. Gastroenterology 1977; 73:327–38.
101. Schuffler MD, Bird TD, Sumi MS, Cook A. A familial neuronal disease presenting as intestinal pseudo-obstruction. Gastroenterology 1978; 75:889–98.
102. Sullivan MA, Snape WJ Jr, Matarazzo SA, Petrokubi RJ, Jeffries G, Cohen S. Gastrointestinal myoelectrical activity in idiopathic intestinal pseudo-obstruction. N Engl J Med 1977; 297:233–8.
103. Snape WJ Jr, Sullivan MA, Cohen S. Abnormal gastrocolic response in patients with intestinal pseudo-obstruction. Arch Intern Med 1980; 140:386–7.
104. Battle SM, Rubin MR, Cohen S, Snape WJ Jr. Gastrointestinal-motility dysfunction in amyloidosis. N Engl J Med 1979; 301:24–5.
105. Harvey JC, Sherbourne DH, Siegel CI. Smooth muscle involvement in myotonic dystrophy. Am J Med 1965; 39:81–90.
106. Glick ME, Meshkinpour H, Halderman S, Bhatia NN, Bradley WE. Colonic dysfunction in multiple sclerosis. Gastroenterology 1982; 88:1002–7.
107. Kern F Jr, Almy TP, Abbot FK, Bogdonoff MD. The motility of the distal colon in non-specific ulcerative colitis. Gastroenterology 1951; 19:492–503.
108. Spriggs EA, Code CF, Bargen JA, Curtiss RK, Hightower NC Jr. Motility of the pelvic colon and rectum of normal persons and patients with ulcerative colitis. Gastroenterology 1951; 19:480–91.
109. Snape WJ Jr, Matarazzo SA, Cohen S. Abnormal gastrocolonic response in patients with ulcerative colitis. Gut 1980; 21:392–6.
110. Bishop AE, Polak JM, Bryant MG, Bloom SR, Hamilton S. Abnormalities of vasoactive intestinal polypeptide–containing nerves in Crohn's disease. Gastroenterology 1980; 79:853–60.
111. Veitlin IJ, Smith AM. Mobilization of tissue kallikrein in inflammatory disease of the colon. Gut 1973; 14:133–8.
112. Ligumsky M, Karmeli F, Sharon P, Zor U, Cohen F, Rachmilewitz D. Enhanced thromboxane A_2 and prostacyclin production by cultured rectal mucosa in ulcerative colitis and its inhibition by steroids and sulfasalazine. Gastroenterology 1981; 81:444–9.
113. Hawkey CJ, Truelove SC. Effect of prednisolone on prostaglandin synthesis by rectal mucosa in ulcerative colitis: Investigation by laminar flow bioassay and radioimmunoassay. Gut 1981; 22:190–3.

Chapter 133

Hirschsprung's Disease

John G. Raffensperger

Hirschsprung's disease is due to the congenital absence of ganglion cells from the myenteric plexus in a segment of intestine that extends proximally from the anus for a variable distance. There were necropsy reports of patients dying with hugely distended colons before Hirschsprung clearly described the disease that is now named for him. His description[1a] of the clinical and gross pathologic findings in 2 boys who died at 8 and 11 months of age with unrelenting constipation, malnutrition, and enterocolitis is a medical classic.

Throughout the early 1900s there were scattered observations of the absence of ganglion cells from the colon in Hirschsprung's disease.[1–3] The significance of this was evidently lost, however, because it seemed more logical to blame the symptoms on the hugely dilated segment of the bowel. Thus, the term "*megacolon*" focused on the wrong end of the disease. Robertson and Kernohan,[4] and later Tiffin and associates,[5] clarified this by stating that Hirschsprung's disease is caused by a lack of peristalsis across a segment of colon that lacked ganglion cells in Auerbach's plexus. At the Boston Children's Hospital, Swenson studied several patients with Hirschsprung's disease who had undergone colostomy. He inserted recording balloons into the dilated colon and distally into the apparently normal segment. His pressure studies demonstrated normal peristalsis proximal to the colostomy, but distally there were only segmental contractions and no propulsive waves. After operations in animals proved that it was possible to remove the rectum and still preserve continence, Swenson resected the aganglionic colon and anastomosed normally innervated bowel to the anus.[6] Swenson published his work exactly 60 years after Hirschsprung's presentation.

Pathophysiology

The intrinsic autonomic nervous system of the bowel consists of 3 distinct plexuses of ganglion cells with their neural connections. Auerbach's plexus lies between the circular and longitudinal muscles; Henle's plexus, or the deep submucosal plexus, is situated along the inner margin of the circular muscularis propria; and Meissner's plexus lies immediately beneath the muscularis mucosa.[7] The myenteric plexus is formed by neuroblasts that arrive at the alimentary tract by craniocaudal migration during the 5th to the 12th week of gestation. The neuroblasts initially appear in the myenteric plexus just outside the circular muscle layers, and then migrate across the muscle to the submucosa.[14] Sympathetic fibers originating from cells in the prevertebral parasympathetic ganglia enter the bowel wall and end in a fibrillar network about the intrinsic ganglion cells. Cholinergic fibers from the vagal and pelvic outflow also terminate in the intrinsic plexus, primarily in the distal rectum and internal sphincter.[8,9] The ganglion cells constitute the intrinsic neuroapparatus of the bowel.

Longitudinal sections through the distal rectum in normal subjects have demonstrated an absence of Auerbach's plexus within 2.5 mm above the pectinate line. The submucosal plexus terminates an average of 2 mm proximal to Auerbach's plexus, and there is an additional 5 mm of distal rectum with a diminished number of ganglion cells.[10, 11] A biopsy to determine the presence or absence of ganglion cells must be taken at least 3 cm above the dentate line, or an erroneous diagnosis of Hirschsprung's disease may be made based upon the absence of ganglion cells from the most distal segment of rectum.

In Hirschsprung's disease, the ganglion

cells are absent from all 3 plexuses. In addition, there are large longitudinally oriented nerve fibers with few branches. These nerve trunks stain intensely for cholinesterase.[12] Further studies have demonstrated an increased tissue concentration of norepinephrine in the aganglionic colon.[13] The adrenergic hyperactivity contributes to muscular spasm. The aganglionic segment extends to the sigmoid colon in about 75% of patients with Hirschsprung's disease. In the remaining patients, the colon is involved to a greater or lesser extent, and in 3% the entire colon and portions of the small bowel are aganglionic. There is no definite relationship of the patient's age to the extent of the aganglionic bowel; some older patients have had aganglionosis to the transverse colon.

Epidemiology

The estimated prevalence of Hirschsprung's disease is 1:5000. A recent survey by the Surgical Section of the American Academy of Pediatrics revealed a male:female ratio of 3.8:1, a similar prevalence of the disease among blacks and whites, and a familial incidence of 7%.[15] The disease appears to be autosomal recessive and sex-linked. In comparison with children who have other birth defects, those with Hirschsprung's disease are remarkably free of associated congenital deformities. The disease has occurred in monozygotic twins and in children with Down's syndrome, as well as in those with a wide variety of other anomalies.[16, 17]

Clinical Features

The presenting signs, symptoms, and age at onset of symptoms are variable. On the one hand, the condition may present in the newborn infant with acute abdominal distention, vomiting, and failure to pass meconium. Although in a few patients constipation may be either ignored or controlled until adulthood, over 90% of patients with Hirschsprung's disease will have failed to pass meconium on the first day of life. This cardinal symptom allows the diagnosis to be made in the neonatal period. If the infant passes stool in response to digital stimulation or an enema, one must consider Hirschsprung's disease, hypothyroidism, cystic fibrosis of the pancreas, and the small left colon syndrome. If the diagnosis of Hirschsprung's disease is overlooked at this time, the infant may move his bowels in response to formula changes, suppositories, or medication for a period of time. Breast feeding ameliorates the symptoms, but when a formula or solid foods are added to the diet, constipation becomes severe.

The usual infant with Hirschsprung's disease will have intermittent, progressive constipation and episodic vomiting. The mother may hear loud borborygmi. Infants with more severe symptoms will exhibit poor weight gain and be fussy and sickly. When constipation is less severe and controllable by diet and simple medication, the child will thrive and appear as healthy as a normal sibling.

Physical examination of the neonate may be totally unrevealing except for an explosive stool as the examining finger is withdrawn from the rectum. There is often an easily visible and palpable loop of bowel extending transversely across the upper abdomen. If peristaltic waves are seen going from right to left, the loop of bowel is likely to be a dilated transverse colon proximal to a aganglionic segment. In the neonatal period, it is clinically difficult to differentiate Hirschsprung's disease from intestinal atresia or stenosis, meconium ileus, and the meconium plug syndrome (Chapter 87). Plain radiographs of the abdomen will usually make the diagnosis of atresia or stenosis. A barium enema examination that reveals multiple plugs of firm stool in the terminal ileum and colon suggests meconium ileus, and a sweat chloride test confirms the presence of cystic fibrosis of the pancreas. If the baby passes a firm plug of meconium after an enema or rectal examination, one must still consider cystic fibrosis of the pancreas and Hirschsprung's disease, as well as hypothyroidism and maternal factors, such as drug ingestion.

A dramatic first symptom of Hirschsprung's disease in infants may be acute, spontaneous perforation of the colon. Usually this is in the cecum or appendix. There is an antecedent history of failure to pass stool and then sudden abdominal distention. Radiographs demonstrate free air in the peritoneal cavity.

An infant also may present with enterocolitis rather than with constipation.[18] This usually occurs in a baby under 3 months of age whose abdomen becomes severely distended and who passes a large amount of watery stool. An upper respiratory tract infection or simple gastrointestinal upset epidemic in the family seems to trigger an acute intestinal decompression. Sepsis and severe dehydration may occur in a few hours and the disease is often fatal.

On physical examination, the abdomen is severely distended and quiet to auscultation. A rectal examination often results in an explosive release of gas and fluid. The passage of a rectal tube into the dilated bowel will release more gas and fluid, with improvement of the patient. This differentiates the enterocolitis of Hirschsprung's disease from a mechanical obstruction.

Plain radiographs reveal generalized bowel distention and, if a barium enema examination is performed, one sees a ragged mucosa signifying ulcerations. Treatment consists of antibiotics, rapid fluid therapy, and continued rectal irrigations with warm normal saline solution until the bowel is completely decompressed.

Some patients tolerate Hirschsprung's disease surprisingly well, and the disease has been found in otherwise healthy adults. Constipation is relieved by dietary changes, and some have learned to control it through the use of suppositories or enemas. However, as these individuals grow older, spontaneous bowel movements become more infrequent and cathartics become progressively less effective. Occasionally there are acute episodes of bowel decompensation, not unlike the enterocolitis seen in babies. Classically, the older child with Hirschsprung's disease is sickly, pale, and undernourished and has a large, protuberant abdomen and skinny legs.

Diagnosis

A barium enema examination is the most important diagnostic test. However, for greatest accuracy it should be performed by an expert pediatric radiologist. The bowel must not be overfilled lest the sigmoid loop overlay and obscure the narrow rectum, which is best demonstrated on a lateral film. A relatively normal-appearing distal aganglionic bowel may be demonstrated, which contrasts sharply with the distended proximal colon, even in the newborn period (Figs. 133–1 and 133–2). However, in our own series, barium enema examination during the newborn period failed to yield a correct diagnosis in 20% of cases because the proximal colon had not yet dilated. Furthermore, the small left colon syndrome, hypothyroidism, and the meconium plug syndrome may all be confused with Hirschsprung's disease.

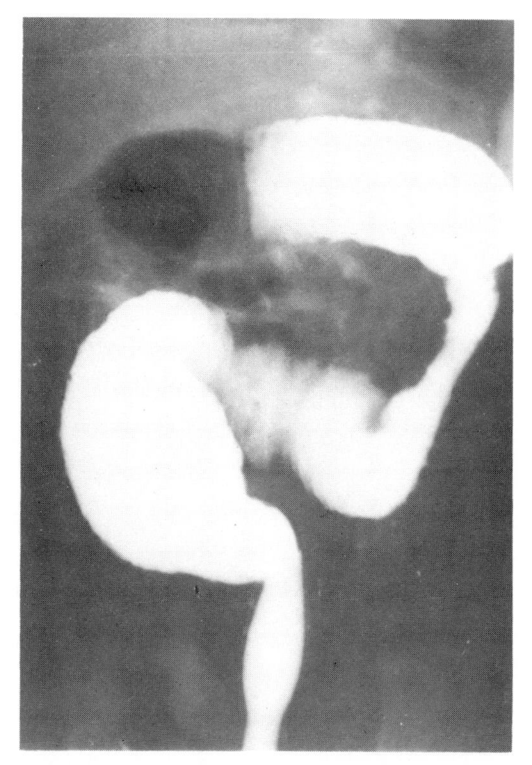

Figure 133–1. Typical "narrow" aganglionic segment in a 3-week-old infant with constipation and abdominal distention.

In the older child or adult, a barium enema study will demonstrate a relatively narrow distal segment of aganglionic bowel. Follow-up radiographs show the barium to be retained in the bowel for many days. When the colon is dilated down to the rectal sphincter, Hirschsprung's disease is an unlikely diagnosis. In the rare case in which the entire colon is aganglionic, the colon is narrow and shortened, while the small bowel is dilated (Fig. 133–3).

A history of constipation going back to the neonatal period and a barium enema examination demonstrating a narrow distal rectum are sufficient to make the diagnosis of Hirschsprung's disease. Nevertheless, many surgeons require further confirmation of the diagnosis before proceeding with surgical treatment. The most reliable diagnostic test is the full-thickness rectal biopsy, in which evidence of Auerbach's plexus is sought by light microscopic examination.[19] Unfortu-

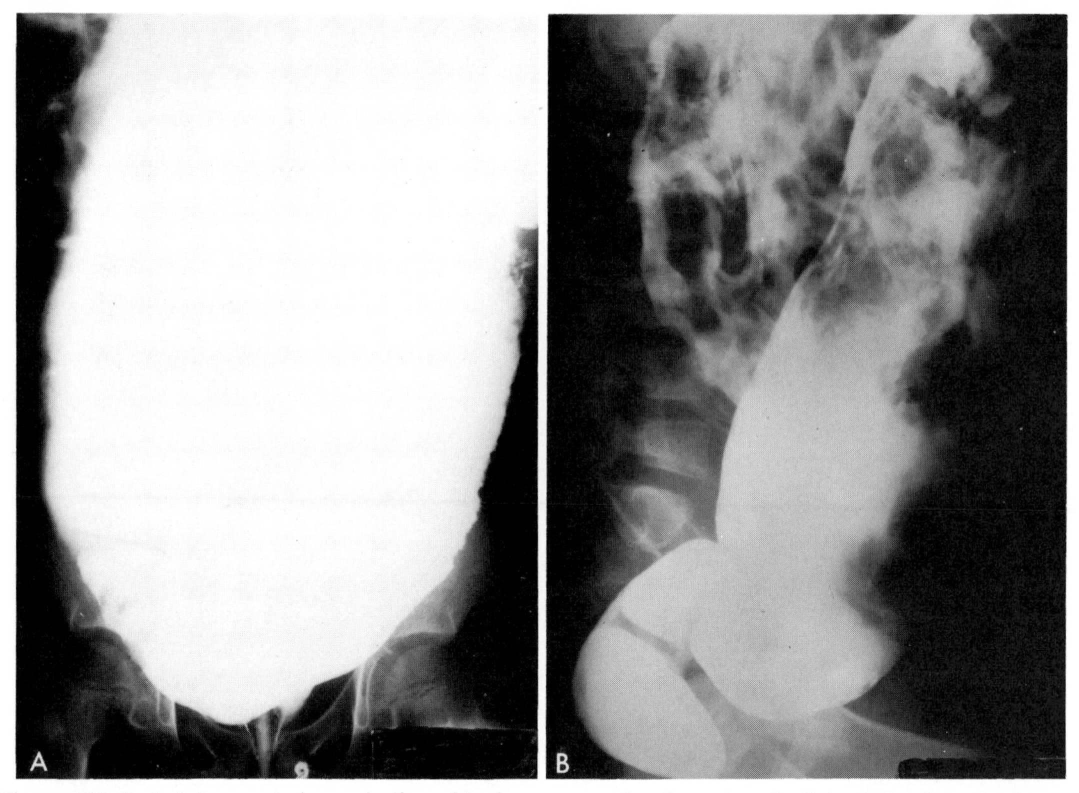

Figure 133–2. *A,* Anteroposterior projection of barium enema showing a hugely distended colon of a 5-year-old child with Hirschsprung's disease. The narrow segment is obscured. *B,* Lateral view demonstrating the narrow, aganglionic rectum.

nately, this requires hospitalization and general anesthesia. The technique of rectal biopsy has been simplified by the use of an intestinal suction biopsy capsule.[20,21] We currently use a 4.7-mm capsule with the following technique: Rectal irrigations are given until the rectum is clean to digital palpation. The capsule is inserted into the anal canal for a distance of 5 to 6 cm with the knife of the capsule closed. The capsule is opened when it is in the proper position, and a negative pressure of at least 20 mm of mercury is applied for several seconds. This allows time for the mucosa and submucosa to be pulled into the capsule. The knife is then pulled shut and the capsule is removed from the rectum. The biopsy specimen is teased from the capsule with a needle and placed on a small square of monofilament Saran net. It is helpful to examine the biopsy with a magnifying lens to make sure that a bit of submucosa is included in the specimen. The specimen is oriented on the cloth with the mucosa down; it must be kept as flat as possible and immediately fixed in Bouin's solution.

In normal subjects, ganglion cells are readily found in a properly obtained submucosal biopsy specimen. As many as 20 to 50 sections may be required to confirm the presence of ganglion cells, however, which are smaller and more difficult to identify than the cells in Auerbach's plexus. No errors of interpretation were found in a series of 42 patients when 2 adequate specimens from each patient were examined.[22]

The rectal suction biopsy procedure has proved to be a most valuable means of excluding Hirschsprung's disease, especially in the newborn infant who has had a delayed passage of meconium. We now perform this test on all infants for whom the diagnosis of meconium plug syndrome has been suggested. Nevertheless, we are not willing at this time to make a definitive diagnosis of Hirschsprung's disease in any patient solely on the basis of an absence of ganglion cells in a suction biopsy.

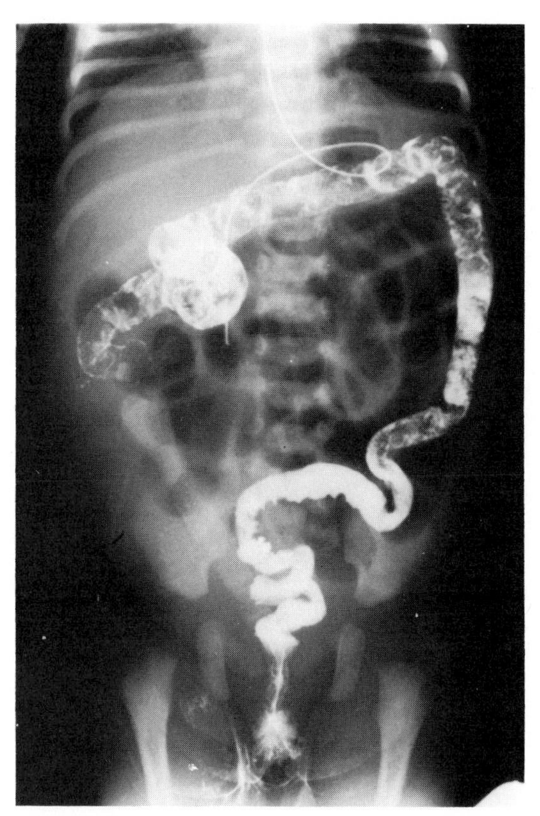

Figure 133–3. Total colonic aganglionosis in a neonate who presented with an almost complete intestinal obstruction.

Rectal suction biopsy is not as helpful in excluding Hirschsprung's disease in older children who may have a short segment lesion. In such cases, the mucosa is thickened and it is more difficult to obtain a specimen sufficiently inclusive of submucosa. In these patients, we continue to prefer full-thickness biopsy. The latter can be extended to an anorectal myotomy if there are no ganglion cells on the frozen section.

Histochemical techniques add to the accuracy of light microscopy.[23,24] Normal persons show barely detectable acetylcholinesterase activity in the intestinal submucosa. When ganglion cells are absent, there is an overabundance of acetylcholine and, consequently, of the corresponding enzyme acetylcholinesterase. When acetylcholinesterase stains are utilized, it is necessary to look at only a single section, rather than multiple sections, to make a definite diagnosis. There is an additional factor, i.e., stains for acetylcholinesterase are positive findings, while the absence of ganglion cells may mean only that one has not looked at enough material.

Measurements of anorectal pressure are helpful. In Hirschsprung's disease, the internal sphincter fails to relax in response to balloon distention of the rectum.[25, 26] Using a triple balloon system and a water manometer (Chapter 28), distention of the rectal balloon with 10 to 15 mm of water results in a gradual fall of internal sphincteric pressure (in contrast to 2 to 4 cm of water in normal children).[27] In our experience, it has been difficult to place the recording balloon or an open catheter system accurately within the internal sphincter. Furthermore, crying and abdominal straining may produce false results. In the newborn period, when one would like to make the diagnosis of Hirschsprung's disease without resort to a biopsy, the anorectal reflex is poorly developed. Holschneider et al.[28] have demonstrated that the normal rectoanal reflex does not develop until 12 days of age. In a highly sophisticated study[29] conducted in a special manometric laboratory, there were 10 false-positive and 8 false-negative results in 229 examinations. There was a 26% error rate in infants under 1 month of age. Although the accuracy of manometry increases with the patient's age, it is never sufficiently accurate to make a definitive diagnosis of Hirschsprung's disease without confirmatory biopsy evidence. The history, physical examination, and barium enema study are just as accurate in determining the need for biopsy in the older child; consequently, manometry is at best only a rough screening test. In our experience, the rectal suction biopsy is simple and fast and provides a greater degree of accuracy in the diagnosis of Hirschsprung's disease than other preliminary tests.

Differential Diagnosis

Anal fissures are a common cause of constipation in infants and children. A hard bowel movement may stretch and tear the mucocutaneous junction. The resultant sphincter spasm results in further pain with each bowel movement, so the baby screams and "holds back his stools." Often there is a history of a few drops of red blood on the stool surface. The diagnosis is made by placing the infant in the knee-chest position, spreading the buttocks, and inspecting the mucocutaneous junction for fissures at the 10 and 6 o'clock locations. Treatment consists of keeping the baby's stools soft with mineral oil and applying zinc oxide ointment to the anus.

Constipation following *repair of an imperforate anus* is a frequent problem. This is probably the result of damaged sensory receptors in the rectum, due either to the corrective surgical procedure or to congenital defects in the pelvic nerve supply. Since the child has no "signals" that his rectum is full and ready to be evacuated, we attempt to train him with suppositories and enemas to empty his bowel according to a daily habit pattern.

Difficulties encountered with the term *"megacolon"* are nowhere better seen than in that group of patients who have psychogenic constipation (Chapter 134). At various times, this has been labeled "idiopathic megacolon," "functional megacolon," or "encopresis." When constipation has its onset later in childhood, after a period of normal bowel habits, it is unlikely that the diagnosis will turn out to be Hirschsprung's disease. Careful probing of the history is essential, because in some cases a mother may claim her child has been constipated all his life, when actually the child was well in infancy. If further history reveals that the child soils his pants, one can be practically certain that he does not have Hirschsprung's disease. Often the mother has forced early toilet training at about the same time a new baby made his appearance or at a time when there was a major family upheaval, such as a divorce.

These children are well nourished and healthy. They may have some abdominal distention and palpable stool in the colon, but not as much as in Hirschsprung's disease. Rectal examination is practically diagnostic. There are feces smeared on the perineum and on the child's underwear. Soft stool fills the rectal ampulla. Barium enema examination reveals no narrow segment, but the colon is dilated down to the anus. If for some reason doubt remains about the diagnosis, a rectal biopsy will settle the matter.

The etiology of psychogenic constipation is unclear, and since it is not as exciting as other diseases, few doctors are willing to spend time with these children. The most complete study has been of 209 children by Bellman in Sweden.[30] The highest incidence was between 3 and 6 years of age. The occurrence rate in 7-year-old schoolchildren was 2.3% in boys and 0.7% in girls. In detailed psychologic studies, common factors in the disease were disturbance in contact with the mother, an early age at toilet training, fear of the toilet, anxiety reaction, inhibited aggression, and a feeling of failure. Of these children, 13% had speech problems and many were depressed. When studied several years after cure of the bowel problem, 158 of the 186 children who were followed seemed to be well adjusted, and few had any but a hazy recollection of their past troubles.

One physician after another is consulted and various cathartics are tried, most of which work for a short while. Many of these patients wind up in a surgeon's office, carrying a stack of radiographs purportedly showing "megacolon." The parents interpret their child's red-faced straining at the stool as an effort to have a bowel movement, rather than holding back. The child has found that more attention is received if there is no bowel movement, and the whole thing becomes an emotionally charged family issue.

Treatment

Treatment for the patient with Hirschsprung's disease must be individualized according to the patient's condition and the surgeon's experience and skill. The extremely ill neonate requires IV fluids, total parenteral nutrition, antibiotics, and rectal irrigations until the bowel has been decompressed and the nutritional condition is optimal. Some children with mild symptoms are treated very well with daily rectal irrigations given by the mother at home until they are a year old and can have a definitive operation. When rectal irrigations fail or if the infant has had enterocolitis, we prefer to place a colostomy just proximal to the aganglionic bowel. A frozen section must be performed on the bowel wall at the time of operation to make certain that the colostomy itself contains ganglion cells. The baby is left with a colostomy until he weighs approximately 9 kg, and then some type of pull-through operation is performed. Older patients with hugely dilated bowels will also require colostomy for several months prior to a pull-through operation in order to allow the bowel to decompress.

There are now several definitive operations that have proved to be successful for the treatment of Hirschsprung's disease. The principle is to bring intestine with normal ganglion cells down to within a centimeter or so from the dentate line. The original operation described by Swenson[6] in 1948 continues to be safe and effective. The patient is prepared with an elemental diet, cathartics, and enemas to ensure perfect mechanical cleansing of the bowel. I give my patients oral neomycin and erythromycin for 24 hours before operation. We continue to utilize Swenson's original technique in which the aganglionic bowel is sharply dissected free from surrounding structures and removed to within a centimeter or so from the dentate line. Bowel with normal ganglion cells is then pulled through and sutured to the distal stump of rectum.

There are a number of other operations described for Hirschsprung's disease. The Duhamel operation leaves the distal rectal stump and brings down bowel with ganglion cells to establish an end-to-side anastomosis posterior to the rectum.[31] The Soave procedure leaves the aganglionic muscle layer intact, but the mucosa is stripped from the rectum; proximal bowel containing ganglion cells is then brought down through this tunnel for anastomosis to mucosa just proximal to the dentate line.[32] Several authors have described a mild or "short segment" form of Hirschsprung's disease that responds to internal sphincterotomy combined with removal of a strip of the distal aganglionic muscle.[33] Very few patients with the short segment form of the disease will respond to an anorectal myomectomy. Also, careful pathologic study is required to differentiate these patients from those with psychologic constipation.

Prognosis

In experienced hands, all of the operations described are followed by satisfactory results. In my own experience, which includes the Duhamel as well as the Soave procedure, the Swenson operation has provided the most satisfactory long-term results.

There have been no operative deaths following the Swenson operation at The Children's Memorial Hospital over the past 11 years. Ten to 15% of children will have one or more episodes of enterocolitis during the first year after operation, but even these patients settle down to an essentially normal existence.

Several long-term studies have shown that following the Swenson operation, patients are continent of feces, cured of their constipation, and enjoy a normal sex life as adults. Many of Swenson's original patients have children of their own, thus laying to rest fears concerning the risks of operative injury to the pelvic nerve plexus.

References

1. Brentano A. Uber einen Fall von Hirschsprungscher Krankheit. Verh Deutsch Ges Chir 1904; 1:365.
1a. Hirschsprung H. Stuhlträgheit Neugeborener in Folge von Dilatation and Hypertrophie des Colons. Jahrb. f. Kinderh. 1888; 27:1.
2. Dalle Valle A. Contributo alla conoscenza della forme famigliare del megacolon congenito. Pediatria 1938; 32:123.
3. Tittel K. Uber eine angeborene Missbildung des Dickdarmes. Wien Klin Wochenschr 1901; 14:903–7.
4. Robertson HE, Kernohan JW. The myenteric plexus in congenital megacolon. Proc Staff Meet Mayo Clin 1938; 13: 123–5.
5. Tiffin ME, Chandler LR, Faber HK. Localized absence of the ganglion cells of the myenteric plexus in congenital megacolon. Am J Dis Child 1940; 59:1071–82.
6. Swenson O, Bill AH. Resection of rectum and rectosigmoid with preservation of the sphincter for benign spastic lesions producing megacolon. Surgery 1948; 24:212–20.
7. Gunn M. Histological and histochemical observations on the myenteric and submucous plexuses of mammals. J Anat 1968; 102:223–39.
8. Jacobowitz D. Histochemical studies of the autonomic innervation of the gut. J Pharmacol Exp Ther 1965; 149:358–64.
9. Garrett JR, Howard ER, Lansdale JM. Myenteric nerves in the hind gut of the cat. J Physiol (London) 1972; 226:103–4.
10. Baumgarten HG, Holstein AF, Stelzner F. Nervous elements in the human colon of Hirschsprung's disease. Virchow's Arch Pathol Anat 1973; 358:113–36.
11. Aldridge RT, Campbell PE. Ganglion cell distribution in the normal rectum and anal canal: A basis for the diagnosis of Hirschsprung's disease by anorectal biopsy. J Pediatr Surg 1968; 3:475–90.
12. Weinberg AG. The anorectal myenteric plexus: Its relation to hypoganglionosis of the colon. Am J Clin Pathol 1970; 54:637–42.
13. Touloukian RJ, Aghajanian G, Roth RH. Adrenergic hyperactivity of the aganglionic colon. J Pediatr Surg 1973; 8: 191–5.
14. Okamoto E, Ueda T. Embryogenesis of intramural ganglia of the gut and its relation to Hirschsprung's disease. J Pediatr Surg 1967; 2:437–43.
15. Kleinhaus S, Boley SJ, Sheran M, Sieber WK. Hirschsprung's disease: A survey of the members of the Surgical Section of the American Academy of Pediatrics. J Pediatr Surg 1979; 14:588–97.
16. Schwarz KB, Keating JP, Holtmann B, Ternberg J. Congenital lip pits and Hirschsprung's disease. J Pediatr Surg 1979; 14:162–4.
17. Shah KN, Dalal SJ, Desai MP, Sheth PN, Joshi NC, Ambani LM. White forelock, pigmentary disorder of irides, and long segment Hirschsprung's disease: Possible variant of Waardenburg syndrome. J Pediatr 1981; 99:432–5.
18. Swenson O, Fisher JH. Hirschsprung's disease during infancy. Surg Clin North Am 1956; 36:1511–5.
19. Swenson O, Fisher JH, MacMahon J. Rectal biopsy as an aid in the diagnosis of Hirschsprung's disease. N Engl J Med 1955; 253:632–5.
20. Dobbins WO, Bill AH. Diagnosis of Hirschsprung's disease excluded by rectal suction biopsy. N Engl J Med 1965; 272:990–3.
21. Aldridge RT, Campbell PE. Ganglion cell distribution in the normal rectum and anal canal: A basis for the diagnosis of Hirschsprung's disease by anorectal biopsy. J Pediatr Surg 1968; 3:475–90.
22. Campbell PE, Noblett HR. Experience with the rectal suction

biopsy in the diagnosis of Hirschsprung's disease. J Pediatr Surg 1969; 4:410–5.
23. Meier-Ruge W, Lutterbeck PM, Herzog B, Morger R, Moser R, Scharli A: Acetylcholinesterase activity in suction biopsies of the rectum in the diagnosis of Hirschsprung's disease. J Pediatr Surg 1972; 7:11–7.
24. Elema JD, deVries JA, Vos LJM. Intensity and proximal extension of acetylcholinesterase activity in the mucosa of the rectosigmoid in Hirschsprung's disease. J Pediatr Surg 1973; 8:361–8.
25. Lawson JON, Nixon HH. Anal canal pressures in the diagnosis of Hirschsprung's disease. J Pediatr Surg 1967; 2:544–52.
26. Schnaufer L, Talbert JL, Haller JA, Reid NCRW, Tobon F, Schuster MM. Differential sphincteric studies in the diagnosis of anorectal disorders of childhood. J Pediatr Surg 1967; 2:538–43.
27. El Shafie M, Suzuki H, Schnaufer L, Haller JA, White JJ. A simplified method of anorectal manometry for wider clinical application. J Pediatr Surg 1972; 7:230–5.
28. Holschneider AM, Kellner E, Streibl P, Sippell WG. The development of anorectal continence and its significance in the diagnosis of Hirschsprung's disease. J Pediatr Surg 1976; 11:151–6.
29. Meunier P, Marechal JM, Mollard P. Accuracy of the manometric diagnosis of Hirschsprung's disease. J Pediatr Surg 1978; 13:411–5.
30. Bellman M. Studies on encopresis. Acta Pediatr Scand 1966; 170(Suppl):1–151.
31. Duhamel B. A new operation for the treatment of Hirschsprung's disease. Arch Dis Child 1960; 35:38–50.
32. Jordan FT, Coran AG, Weintraub WH, Wesley JR. An evaluation of the modified endorectal procedure for Hirschsprung's disease. J Pediatr Surg 1979; 14:681–5.
33. Udassin R, Nissan S, Lernau O, Hod G. The mild form of Hirschsprung's disease (short segment): 14 years experience in diagnosis and treatment. Ann Surg 1981; 194:767–70.

Chapter 134

Irritable Bowel Syndrome

William S. Haubrich

The irritable bowel syndrome defies definition. Everyone knows what it is, yet who can precisely define it? Bergen Evans, an authority on language, has observed, "The obvious is not easy to define; of necessity, the simplest must be defined in terms less simple." Peter Mere Latham, the 19th century medical aphorist, could as well have been talking about the irritable bowel when he remarked, "There are things which will not be defined, and Fever is one of them. Besides, when a word has passed into everyday use, it is too late to lay a logical trap for its meaning and think to apprehend it by a definition."

There are 3 reasons for our difficulty. First, though the irritable bowel can be recognized by certain positive attributes, it usually is described in terms of what it is not, i.e., it is not an anatomic or structural lesion, and it is not an identifiable entity. Second, the irritable bowel is expressed by a nebulous array of protean and nondescript symptoms and signs which are shared by a variety of digestive diseases. Finally, to attempt a definition of a functional disorder is to run the risk of what may be a fallacy of dichotomy. Must disease be either "organic" or "functional"? We are reminded that what is thought "functional" today may be found "organic" tomorrow.

Nevertheless, at our present state of knowledge (or lack thereof), there is an alimentary disturbance that we call "the irritable bowel syndrome" (IBS). It is manifested in various patients by abdominal distress, ranging from mild discomfort to frank pain, and by an erratic bowel action, often with alternating constipation and diarrhea. It is distinguished by an absence of any discernible anatomic or metabolic abnormality. In itself it is invariably benign in the sense that it does not adversely affect the physical well-being or the longevity of the patient. It tends to be chronic. For many, but not all, patients affected by an irritable bowel, it may seem to be provoked or aggravated by emotional disturbances.

The bowel and its function or dysfunction have been a matter of concern to physicians through the ages. Moses ben Maimon, the famed 12th century physician better known as Maimonides, was said to have advised, "Man should always strive to have his intestines relaxed all the days of his life." The first description of spastic bowel in the English language* has been credited by Ryle[1] to John Howslip, who in 1830 wrote a little book entitled "Practical Remarks on the Discrimination and Successful Treatment of Spasmodic Stricture in the Colon Considered as an Occasional Cause of Habitual Confinement of the Bowel." Regrettably, so far as I know, this helpful volume is out of print. Charles Darwin suffered the stigma of chronic hypochondriacal digestive distress, although Sir Peter Medawar has speculated that Darwin's symptoms may have derived from the megagut syndrome acquired as Chagas' disease during his youthful sojourn in South America.[2]

At the turn of the century, European writers considered functional bowel spasm to be rare. At that time, hysterical paralysis of striated muscles seemed a com-

*This was preceded by a description in the Hebrew language, as recorded in the Old Testament: "My bowels, my bowels! I am pained at my very heart; my heart maketh a noise in me, I cannot hold my peace, because thou hast heard, O my soul, the sound of the trumpet, the alarm of war." — Jeremiah 4:19.

mon reaction to stress. Curiously, expressions of emotional disturbance are subject to changing fashions. During the First World War the popular sounding board was the heart, and the common reaction was "neurocirculatory asthenia" or "soldier's heart." Little or nothing was heard of this in the Second World War. According to Palmer,[3] there was a deliberate effort by the military medical authorities to suppress the concept of cardiac neurosis. Not surprisingly, stress found expression in another organ system, the digestive tract. Meanwhile, an understanding of functional gastrointestinal disorders was developed in the writings of Alvarez,[4] Bockus and Willard,[5] Hurst,[6] Jordan and Kieffer,[7] and Spriggs,[8] among others. More recent notable contributors to the subject have included Almy,[9] Chaudhary and Truelove,[10] Drossman et al.,[11,12] Kirsner,[13] Latimer,[14,15] Mendeloff,[16] Snape et al.,[17,18] Taylor et al.,[19,20] Thompson and Heaton,[21] and Lennard-Jones.[21a]

The late Sara Jordan, for many years the esteemed head of gastroenterology at the Lahey Clinic in Boston, wisely noted that oftentimes in medicine the extent of exact knowledge is inversely proportional to the verbosity of designations and the prolixity of pathogenesis. That the present subject of our attention fits this rule is attested by the following terms: spastic colitis, mucous colitis, cathartic colitis, simple colitis, emotional diarrhea, unstable colon, and many others meaning more or less the same thing. The casual use of the term "colitis" is deplored.*

I am resisting the temptation to offer an elaborate classification of functional bowel disorders. Such a classification would be easy enough to concoct, but it might erroneously imply that there are within the category separate entities that can be distinguished on the basis of cause or mechanism, and this has not been my experience. There doubtless are varying expressions of functional bowel disorders, and certainly treatment must be on an almost individual basis.

Pathogenesis

The symptoms of abdominal distress and erratic defecation have their origin largely in muscular tonus changes within the bowel wall. Distention or stretching of the bowel, as by gas, or by harsh muscular contraction, as in spasm, gives rise to disagreeable abdominal sensations. These are transmitted, for the most part, by way of sympathetic afferent fibers and modified along the way by diencephalic relay centers before reaching the sensory cortex of the brain. When the distended or spastic bowel tugs at its supporting mesenteries, painful sensations may be mediated along cerebrospinal afferent pathways and referred to the points of mesenteric attachment. This is an explanation for the complaint of back pain so often attending functional bowel disorders. Ritchie[22] has observed that patients with the IBS have lower than normal pain thresholds.

Normally chyme in the small bowel and feces in the colon are mulled and moved along by orderly, gentle muscular contractions. When these contractions are disorganized, harsh, or spasmodic, the result is abdominal discomfort and erratic propulsion. Sometimes this is reflected in peristaltic rushes resulting in the frequent expulsion of liquid stools (although basal bowel pressures in patients subject to diarrhea are low); sometimes spasm delays normal evacuation with consequent constipation (basal bowel pressures in constipated patients tend to be high). Thus, the same basic fault can account for both constipation and diarrhea, a seemingly paradoxical combination that frequently dismays the patient and confounds the uninformed therapist.

The consistency of expelled stool, watery or desiccated, also may relate to the osmolality of the colon contents.[23, 24] Organic ions (acetate, propionate, butyrate, lactate) constitute the chief solute in the aqueous medium of fecal matter and contribute significantly to its osmotic pressure. Fecal acidorrhea correlates with fecal volume and is increased in malabsorption states, particularly in lactase deficiency, but has not yet been shown to differ qualitatively or quantitatively in patients with functional bowel disorders.

Mucus is regularly secreted by the normal bowel as a lubricant and is not to be construed as a pathologic product. Under conditions of stress the bowel often elaborates excessive mucus, which sometimes is expelled in prodigious quantity (Fig. 134–1). In the early literature concerned with functional intestinal disorders, the discharge of excessive mucus from the rectum in the absence of inflammation was labeled "mucous coli-

*Axel Munthe, in his "Story of San Michele," tells why "colitis" became such a popular term: "It soon became evident that appendicitis was on its last legs, and that a new complaint had to be discovered to meet the demand. The Faculty was up to the mark, a new disease was dumped on the market, a new word was coined, a gold coin indeed, *colitis*!"

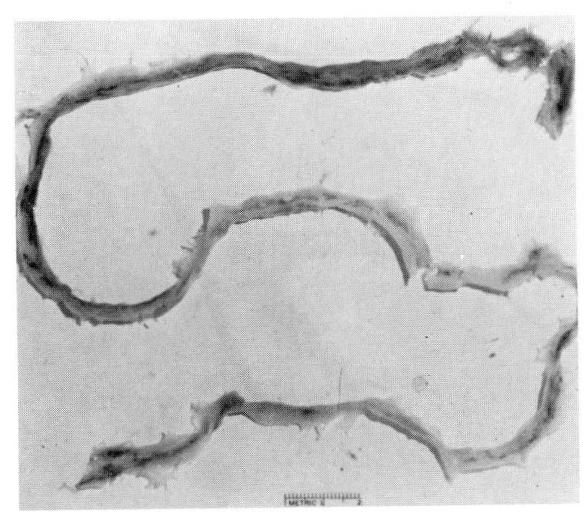

Figure 134–1. A 65-year-old woman afflicted with a markedly irritable colon repeatedly brought to the clinic jars containing "worms" she said she had passed. Invariably these were long strands of coagulated mucus.

tis." This term has been cast into the oblivion it deserves.

Current concepts of the nature of motility disturbances in the irritable colon are thoroughly reviewed by Snape in Chapter 132. In brief, the irritable colon seems to have an inherent and peculiar propensity to "slow-wave activity" that sets the stage for harsh, non-propulsive muscular contractions. Whether further investigation bears this out and, as a consequence, yields a more rational means of treatment remains to be seen.[15,25] What is of tremendous importance is that now we may have a clue to an actual lesion in the so-called irritable colon. This can change our whole perspective of the problem, including our perception of the patient so afflicted. In this light, the patient will be no longer an annoying complainer but will be seen as a sufferer with a definable cause.

Interest has been rekindled in the role of gastrointestinally active hormones[26] (Chapter 241). For example, the gastroenteric reflex, often exaggerated in patients with an irritable bowel, may be triggered by gastrin and cholecystokinin released in response to a meal. The striking effect of glucagon on intestinal tonus is well recognized and put to practical use by radiologists in obtaining hypotonic radiographs of the duodenum and colon (see Chapter 135, Fig. 135–11). Secretin suppresses gastrointestinal motility,[27] whereas the prostaglandins enhance intestinal activity and have been implicated in certain diarrheas[28] (Chapter 242). The adverse effect of various dietary offenders in the IBS has been linked to the stimulation of prostaglandin activity.[29] Some reservation has been expressed as to the significance of the gut hormone responses in the IBS,[30] and the precise role of these substances remains unknown.

There is clear evidence that the pathogenesis of the IBS is not confined to the colon. Aberrant motility in the esophagus has been demonstrated[31] and this, together with reflex pylorospasm, is reflected clinically in the symptoms of proximal alimentary disturbance so often remarked by patients with the IBS. Moreover, functional abdominal distress has been shown to result from tonus changes in the small bowel,[32] where excessively rapid transit often is associated with functional diarrhea.[33] Thus, the whole gut can participate in the IBS.

Etiology

The actual causes of hyperactivity in the irritable bowel often are obscure, though certain stimuli to which the bowel reacts are recognized. These stimuli and their effect on the bowel vary from patient to patient and in the same patient from time to time.

Inherent Sensitivity. So often I have been impressed, in exploring the histories of many patients, that the varying expressions of functional gastrointestinal disorders are longstanding, frequently going back even to childhood. Consequently, I conceive that some of these patients have been endowed by an otherwise beneficent Creator with a keenly sensitive digestive tract and nervous system. This concept is further borne out by the frequent familial occurrence of these disorders.

In addition, the environment of the very young frequently contributes to later bowel disturbances of the adult. Apley and Hale,[34] in their long-term study of children with recurring abdominal pain, have addressed the question: "Do little bellyaches grow up to be big bellyaches?" The answer: many do. Very often the adult patient will recall a mother who was overly solicitous of bowel action in her children. Certainly, attitudes toward diet often have their origin in childhood associations, pleasant and unpleasant. The overly fastidious parent spawns the finicky child.

Diet and Drugs. Unquestionably the bowel

behaves or misbehaves, to some extent, according to the physical and chemical properties of ingested food. The irritable bowel has been shown to exhibit a hypertonic gastroenteric reflex in response to eating.[35, 36] This usually is manifested by increased muscular tone and segmenting contractions but may include heightened peristaltic activity and postprandial urge to stool.

Excessive loads of carbohydrate can exceed the absorptive capacity of the small intestine, and the resulting products of fermentation in the colon can contribute to the symptoms of the IBS. The adverse effect of lactose in persons with diminished lactase activity is now widely appreciated (Chapter 104), and the disagreeable effects of incompletely absorbed wheat flour,[37] fructose,[38] and sorbitol[39] have been recently remarked. Occult lactase deficiency is seldom found to contribute to the IBS in non-Jewish white patients of Northern or Western European descent.[39a]

Aside from the obvious aggravation by cathartic abuse, which is common in patients complaining of alternating constipation and diarrhea, certain drugs may induce hyperirritability, whether ingested inadvertently or taken knowingly for other conditions.[40] Caffeine, sometimes consumed in prodigious quantities by habitual coffee and cola drinkers, is a common offender. A list of medications which can aggravate an irritable bowel would be almost interminable. In practice, among those most often encountered are various antibiotic agents, digitalis, propranolol, quinidine, certain antihypertensive agents (notably guanethidine, hydralazine, and reserpine), and the opiates.

Emotional Factors. The numerous hypotheses that have been advanced to explain presumed psychophysiologic links between emotional disturbances and the IBS have been reviewed by Latimer.[14] He remarks that most of these hypotheses are untested or untestable. Fava and Pavan[41, 42] observed that disturbing interpersonal events were unusually frequent in the experience of patients with the IBS. Whitehead et al.[43] have postulated that somatic complaints are an expression of "learned behavior." What Young and his associates[44] identified as psychiatric illness was found to be unusually prevalent among patients with the IBS.

Yet no correlation could be found by Whitehead and co-workers[45] between psychologic disturbance and specific patterns of colon motility. Moreover, no one has yet defined a peculiar or distinctive pattern of emotional behavior or response in patients exhibiting the IBS.

An important point is that functional bowel disorder is not synonymous with neurosis. All patients with keenly sensitive alimentary tracts are not neurotic; all neurotic persons do not exhibit the IBS. The reaction to stress by the patient with a functional bowel disorder is one of degree rather than of kind. The excitement that is attended by only a brief sense of abdominal uneasiness for one person may induce excruciating and lasting cramps for another.

Often perplexing to the patient is that, even for the susceptible subject, moments of stress are not always and consistently followed by symptoms, or that symptoms can and often do occur during periods of relative tranquility. This is familiar to the military medical officer as the "garrison syndrome," wherein the endangered soldier bears up well when he is on the battle line, only to suffer functional gastrointestinal distress when he is withdrawn to the relative safety of a secure encampment. This has its counterpart in civil life. The harassed person may perform unimpairedly during times of stress, only to suffer the backlash when the crisis has passed. Stewart Wolf[46] explains this by pointing out that emotional conflicts can be shunted out of awareness but lurk in the brain, subject to being recruited on appropriate stimulation.

The physician is seldom rewarded by inquiring of the patient with an irritable bowel whether he or she feels emotionally disturbed. As pointed out in Chapter 14, the patient afflicted by a functional alimentary disorder often is alexithymic, i.e., emotional strain is expressed not verbally but rather by somatic manifestations.

Unproved or Disproved Factors. In my experience, food allergy (Chapter 239) is a minor and infrequent cause of functional bowel disorder. It is true that the reaction to a particular foodstuff by a given patient may be contrary to that in the population at large, but this does not imply an actual antigen-antibody reaction. Diarrhea consequent to eating a lettuce salad does not require an immunologic explanation. True food allergy, when it rarely occurs, usually is abundantly evident in concomitant signs of hypersensitivity in other systems, such as a skin rash.

Infection by microorganisms, either ordinary or exotic, long ago lost its popularity as an explanation for the IBS. There is no evidence that the colon flora of patients afflicted with a keenly sensitive bowel is different in either kind or quantity from that of normal persons. A possible exception might be the egregiously flatulent patient. Therapeutic attempts to eliminate or rearrange the intestinal bacterial population are misguided and futile. Mechanical imperfections in the size, shape, or disposition of the bowel rarely contribute to functional bowel disorders. So-called visceroptosis, sagging colon, and mobile cecum are lame explanations for the irritable bowel, and the folly of surgical adjustment should never be perpetrated. It is true that in an unusual instance a congenitally redundant and capacious colon may contribute to scybalous constipation (see Chapter 131, Fig. 131–1), but this can be adequately managed by means other than partial colectomy.

Clinical Features

The typical patient harboring a sensitive and disordered bowel is a woman in her middle years, usually of a nervous disposition, who has consulted numerous physicians in the past, who often bears one or more surgical scars on her abdomen, and who despairs because her friends say she looks so well yet she feels so miserable. This thumbnail sketch is only typical. There are numerous exceptions.

Prevalence. Functional bowel disorders account for the most frequent digestive complaints heard in the consultation rooms of family physicians, internists, and gastroenterologists alike. They are also commonly heard, though not always recognized, in the offices of surgeons, urologists, and gynecologists. Fully half of all patients seen in any gastroenterology clinic are found to exhibit functional bowel disorders in one form or another. Whoever has entered the practice of clinical medicine and is unprepared or unwilling to deal with this problem has been sadly misled and misplaced.

Women with complaints referable to an irritable bowel outnumber men by almost 3 to 1. However, in those countries, such as India, where traditionally men consult doctors more often than do women, the ratio is reversed.[47] The disorder is manifested in children and adolescents[34, 48] more often than is generally appreciated and accounts for at least some of the "cold" appendices extracted from youngsters. The peak incidence of the IBS is in the fifth and sixth decades when the stresses and frustrations of life are maximal.

In a large clinic catering to a heterogeneous clientele there is little appreciable difference in frequency according to race or nationality. The affluent may be somewhat less tolerant of discomfort resulting from functional bowel disorders; certainly the poor can less easily afford to indulge their complaints, but they are commonly afflicted nonetheless.[49] No occupational group is conspicuous by its absence, though schoolteachers and salespersons seem more affected than farmers and fishermen.

Symptoms. The patients' complaints, in the order of their frequency, are usually directed to (1) abdominal distress, (2) erratic frequency of bowel action, and (3) variation in consistency of stools.* These complaints may occur singly or, more often, in combination. Commonly there are accompanying symptoms otherwise referred to the digestive tract, such as a lump in the throat, nausea, pyrosis, belching, and flatulence, and symptoms referred to other systems, such as giddiness, palpitation, shortness of breath, and frequency of urination. Just as commonly there are protean complaints, such as weakness, fatigue, lassitude, and ennui.

Seldom can a patient with a functional disorder describe her symptoms succinctly. The more compulsive patient brings a long, handwritten narrative (see Fig. 14–2). Often the patient gives an impression of unduly amplifying bodily sensations.[50] The longer the list and duration of symptoms, the more likely is the diagnosis of functional disorder.

Abdominal Distress. The intensity of irritable bowel distress covers a broad spectrum from annoying discomfort to excruciating pain; it varies from patient to patient and from day to day in the same patient. Although distress in the long run may be marked by exacerbations and periods of relative relief, seldom does it occur in clusters, as in peptic ulcer disease, and rarely, if ever, in acute isolated attacks, such as characterize biliary tract pain.

*For a proper perspective, it is instructive that similar symptoms can be elicited in about 1 of 5 persons in the general population who have not felt called upon to seek medical aid.[21, 49a]

Seldom is the distress sharply or consistently localized. Rather, the patient indicates the site of distress by sweeping gestures of the outstretched hand, in contrast to the peptic ulcer patient who typically uses the tip of a single finger to point to one focus. Most often, colon spasm is felt in the area of the left lower abdominal quadrant and hypogastrium. Occasionally it can be referred to the lower back, flanks, and thighs. This is explained by the spastic or distended bowel tugging at its mesentery. Distress arising from a gas-distended colon is usually felt, as expected, in either hypochondrium, more often on the left (Fig. 134–2).

Variations in the characterization of distress are limited only by the patient's vocabulary. Cramping, griping, burning, twisting, and knotting are frequent adjectives. A sense of fullness, heaviness, or pressure is common.

The distress of the irritable bowel fits no fixed diurnal pattern and seldom bears any consistent relation to meals, posture, or exercise. More often than not, the patient feels more comfortable with an empty than with a filled stomach. In some cases, distress is less annoying in the morning and tends to build up toward evening. An exception may be the depressed patient who is discomfited in the morning by the thought of facing still another day. Often the patient admits to being distracted from discomfort when preoccupied with daily tasks and then is miserable when the evening's leisure permits contemplation of the bowel. Contrary to expectation, there often is no consistent relation between abdominal distress and bowel action. Occasionally, a patient asserts that cramping distress is relieved by evacuation, albeit temporarily. Insomnia, particularly the delayed type that is symptomatic of depression, is a frequently concomitant complaint, but when asleep the patient seldom is awakened by an irritable bowel.

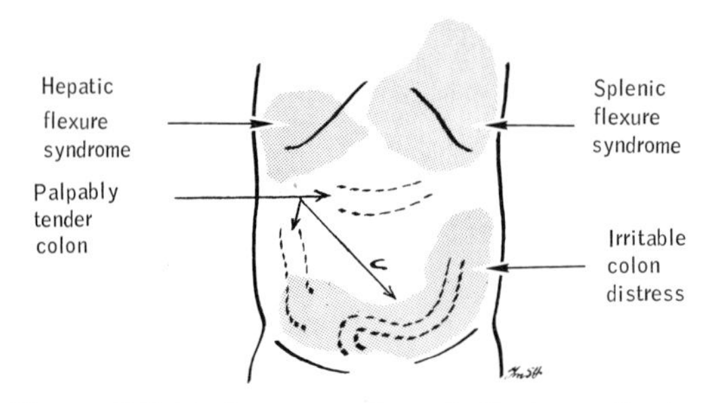

Figure 134–2. Common sites of distress reflecting functional bowel disorder.

Helpful both diagnostically and therapeutically is a searching inquiry for factors provoking or aggravating distress. At the top of the list are circumstances implying emotional stress. Familiar examples are deranged interpersonal relationships, illnesses or deaths among family or friends, loss or change of jobs, and any one or more of a host of trials and tribulations to which human beings are liable.[41] As previously noted, reactive symptoms often appear not coincident with the peak of stress but later when the crisis has passed. In women, functional bowel distress commonly is more troublesome just before or during menstruation. This is not to be construed as significant of intestinal endometriosis. A failure to appreciate the aggravating effect of menstruation on the irritable bowel can cause therapy to be misdirected to the genital system. Many women experience heightened bowel symptoms at the menopause. Fatigue, particularly the asthenia following febrile and infectious illnesses (especially those treated with antibiotic agents), often is marked by disordered bowel function. The relation between diet and drugs has been mentioned and will be discussed further in the section on treatment.

Erratic Bowel Action. Alterations in the frequency of bowel movements from the presumed "normal," either too few or too many, are common. Perplexing to the patient is the frequent and seemingly paradoxical tendency to alternating "constipation" and "diarrhea." By constipation the patient may refer to simple lack of urge or to scybalous dyschezia (difficult passage of hard, dry, or pebbly stools). Diarrhea may be described as merely watery evacuations or the multiple passage of small, fragmented stools.

The consistency of stools varies as often as their frequency. This, together with differences in color and texture, is often alarming to the anxious patient, for whom watery stools connote a loss of nourishment and small, fragmented stools connote an obstructed passage (Fig. 134–3). Visible mucus, sometimes expelled in fantastically long, ropy strands (see Fig. 134–1), is similarly disquieting. Often mucus is mistaken by the patient as "tissue" and the fear is of internal disintegration. Blood in the stools, either fresh or black, can *never* be attributed to functional bowel disorder.

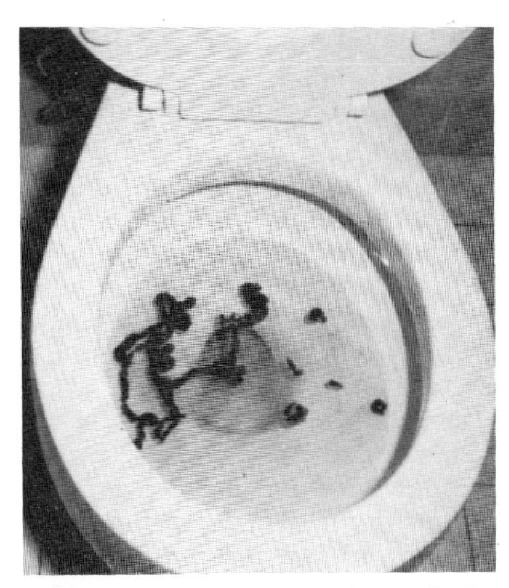

Figure 134–3. A highly introspective, retired gentleman, aged 75, had been so long concerned about his defecation that he felt compelled to submit this photograph he had taken of his home commode. His bowel had been hypertonic for many years.

Gaseousness and flatulence are frequent complaints. The origin and nature of intestinal gas are described in Chapter 9. The hepatic and splenic flexures are natural gas traps. When the descending colon is spastic, entrapped gas can negotiate the hairpin flexures only with difficulty. The ballooned splenic flexure tugs at the phrenocolic ligament (hence, pain extending into the left chest), impinges on the left hemidiaphragm (hence, the feeling of limited inspiration and consequent shortness of breath), and provides reverberation for the beating heart (hence, palpitation). All in all, this comprises the splenic flexure syndrome. To the patient, the fear is that of an impending "heart attack."

A painstaking analysis of symptoms serves not only to rule out evidence of an organic lesion but, just as importantly, serves to marshal positive evidence supporting a diagnosis of a functional disorder.[51]

Physical Clues. There are no physical findings that can be construed as pathognomonic of a functional bowel disorder, but a few are rather suggestive. The patient whose first handshake is cold and clammy is a likely candidate, as is the patient who insists on wearing dark glasses indoors on a cloudy day. Garish make-up and affected dress or mannerisms often betray an insecure personality. Noteworthy observations during examination often include the tremulous voice, the inappropriate laughter, the precipitous weeping, and the wringing of hands.

One of the most striking physical features is the patient's hearty state of nutrition despite many years of digestive complaints. A loss of skin turgor and muscle wasting, characteristic of many truly debilitating diseases, cannot be attributed to functional disorders.

The abdomen, whether flat or protuberant, usually is soft. There may be excessive tympany over the cecum or in either hypochondrium. Tender spasm is often readily palpated along the anatomic course of the lower abdominal quadrant and over the cecum on the right (see Fig. 134–2). During the course of examination when I can palpate a tender colon, I usually call this to the patient's attention. Thus, I have reassured the patient that I recognize a source of symptoms in the abdomen. At the same time, I can briefly describe the mechanism of this palpable soreness. This can be heartening to the patient who has been previously told the problem was "all in the head." Rebound tenderness is never sought; this is a false sign. Any sensitive, distended bowel segment will react painfully when suddenly decompressed. Muscle rigidity in the anterior abdominal wall is the only reliable sign of peritoneal irritation.

Often one or more scars of previous surgical forays will be found to adorn the abdomen of the patient with a long history of functional bowel disorder. Occasionally, closer inquiry substantiates a truly acute suppurative appendicitis to have punctuated the course of irritable colon, but more often the removed appendix yielded no pathologic diagnosis, the removed gallbladder contained only innocent stones, if any, and the uterus was extracted in the vain hope of relieving vague hypogastric discomfort.

Digital examination of the rectum is frequently marked by discomforting spasm and reactivity. In patients with functional bowel disorder, the rectal ampulla often is occupied by feces instead of being empty, as it should be.

Proctosigmoidoscopy is essential to the physical examination of any patient with bowel complaints (Chapter 42). In the irritable bowel, the mucosa is intact, smooth, and glistening throughout. Often intense spasm is encountered as the sigmoidoscope is being advanced, and the rectosigmoid angle is negotiated only with difficulty. With tense contraction of the sigmoid segment in view, the patient may remark that her lower abdominal pain is thus reproduced. This helps substantiate the mechanism of pain for both the examiner and the examinee. Copious mucus may be seen, but this is not a discriminating diagnostic sign, especially if preparatory phosphosoda enemas were employed.

Further Objective Studies. A thorough physical examination and pertinent, comprehensive objective study serve a dual purpose. First, they help to rule out significant organic disease, intrinsic or extrinsic to the bowel, that may explain the patient's symptoms. One is reminded that there is no symptom of the irritable bowel that cannot be exhibited by organic disease. Second, the convincing demonstration that no significant lesion exists permits the physician to reassure the patient with confidence and to advise persuasively a proper regimen.

It is soon learned that the patient with a functional disorder rarely protests the doctor's request for testing procedures. The wise physician, following an exhaustive history and complete physical examination, decides upon and pursues a comprehensive objective survey at the outset. Piecemeal testing betrays an uncertain and desultory attitude in the doctor and engenders doubt and anxiety in the patient. Once done, an initially unequivocal and convincing objective survey should suffice.

Perversely, it seems to be the anxious patient with a patently functional disorder who occasionally comes up with an equivocal or borderline finding among the laboratory reports or in the imaging procedures. Such instances require the most perceptive judgment of whether the study must be repeated in order to confirm or deny the minor aberration at the risk of heightening the patient's anxiety or clouding his doubt. Of paramount importance is to be able to reconcile an objectively demonstrated abnormality with the patient's subjective symptoms. When this is not done, both the doctor and his patient are sadly led astray, sometimes with serious consequences. For example, in the patient with protracted symptoms clearly referable to an irritable bowel, the finding of a small hiatus hernia at a barium meal examination is of no clinical significance. An ill-conceived suggestion that a surgical repair of the esophagogastric defect will remedy the patient's colon distress is fraught with hazard. Or, in a similar patient, if a slight deformity in the duodenal bulb prompts a vagotomy and pyloroplasty, this could have disastrous consequences. These examples may seem outlandish, but they are, unfortunately, not rare.

Laboratory Aids. Regrettably there are no laboratory tests that can yet provide positive evidence of the IBS. The laboratory serves mainly to help the doctor avoid the error of overlooking an unexpected anemia, a latent diabetes, an atypical malabsorption state, or, most importantly, an obscure neoplasm. The inexperienced might conceive of the erythrocyte sedimentation rate or some non-specific enzyme test as an infallible index of the presence or absence of organic disease. Veteran clinicians know this is not so.

An infectious disease in the bowel is not likely to be confused with an irritable bowel. Culture of the feces for "pathogenic" bacteria is almost invariably futile. Depending on the circumstances, it may be worthwhile to examine a stool specimen for trophozoites or cysts of ameba or giardia, inasmuch as these parasitic infections may simulate the IBS (Chapter 232). Testing a series of stool specimens for occult blood can be helpful (Chapter 24); a significantly positive reaction makes mandatory a thorough search for an organic lesion.

Radiographic Examinations. Generally in patients with functional gastrointestinal disorders one expects to find no anatomic or structural defect in the radiographically outlined segments of the digestive tract. Occasionally the fluoroscopist may report or one may see in the films what appears to be unusual spastic contraction in the barium-filled colon (Fig. 134–4). In some cases, distortion in a single film momentarily causes concern which is dispelled by comparing other similar exposures in the series (Fig. 134–4). This may be compatible with an irritable bowel but cannot be construed as pathognomonic. Nevertheless, it can be helpful to point out to the patient a configuration of segmental spasm as a further explanation for the disagreeable symptoms.

A barium meal examination in patients with the IBS may exhibit disturbed motility in the small intestine as well. This can be evident as segmental spasm (Fig. 134–4) and distention (Fig. 134–5) or as excessively rapid small bowel transit, the latter often a feature observed in cases of functional diarrhea.[33] Because of the frequently found evidence of motility disorder in both the small and the large bowel, Bockus preferred the more in-

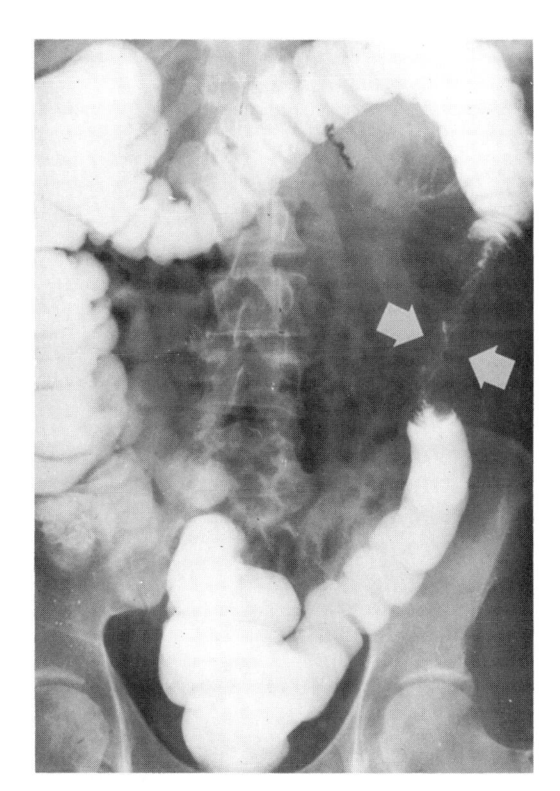

Figure 134–4. Sharp, segmental colon spasm in the barium enema examination of a harried 42-year-old advertising man who often complained of left abdominal pain. Other films, taken later in the same series, showed a relaxed, well-filled, normal descending colon.

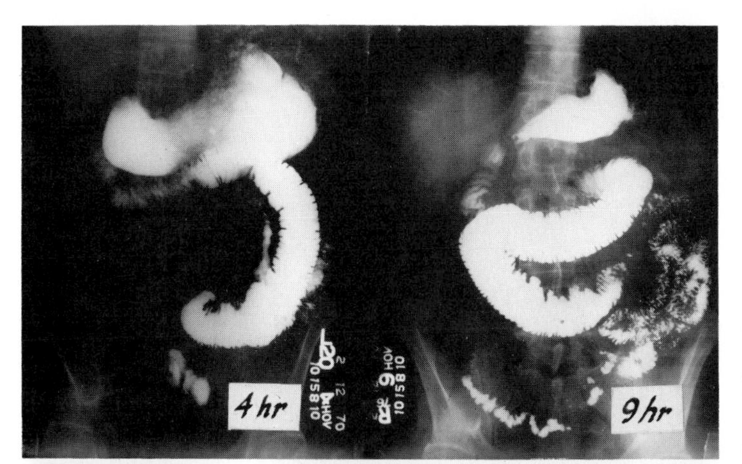

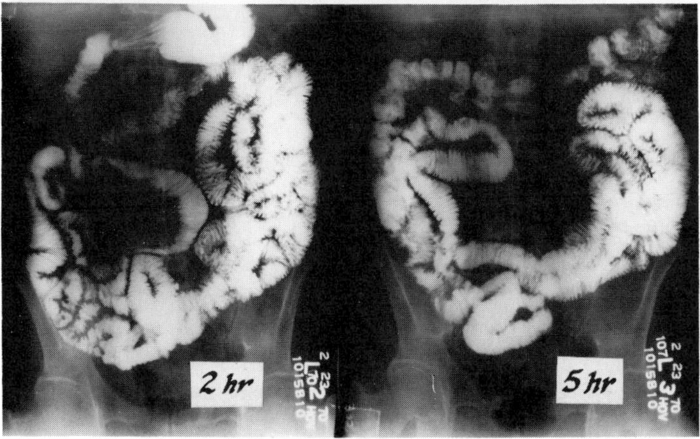

Figure 134–5. A tense 50-year-old executive who had annoying symptoms of functional gastrointestinal disorder received a series of frantic telephone calls from his office while he was undergoing a barium meal examination at the clinic. A startling motor disorder was apparent in the ensuing films (*above*). Eleven days later, under more tranquil circumstances, a repeated examination (*below*) was quite normal.

clusive term "functional enterocolonopathy" when describing these cases.

The habitual use of irritant cathartics can result in a radiographic configuration in the colon sometimes difficult to distinguish from actual inflammatory disease (Fig. 134–6). Reference is made in Chapter 135 to serrations in the sigmoid segment sometimes mistaken for diverticulitis. These are now recognized as the result of circular muscle spasm and hypertrophy and should more properly be considered an expression of altered motility characteristic of functional bowel disorder.

A helpful maneuver in elucidating the actual cause of radiographic distortion in the colon is the hypotonic barium enema examination, more properly designated as a physiologic or pharmacologic study. By observing the response of the colon to various agents administered at the time of barium enema, the physiologically oriented radiologist can deduce the nature of the colon's reactivity. Ferrucci[52] has suggested the use of an IM administered anticholinergic agent such as propantheline (Pro-Banthine, 30 to 45 mg), but many radiologists now prefer the IV administration of glucagon in a dose of 1 mg (see Chapter 135, Fig. 135–11); this is less apt to be attended by undesirable side effects.

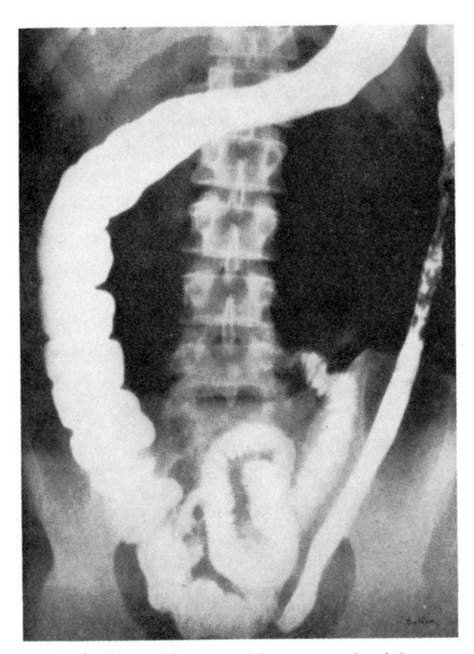

Figure 134–6. A 60-year-old woman had long complained of abdominal discomfort associated with alternating constipation and diarrhea. For many years she had habitually taken irritant cathartics and then wondered why her stools were so often runny. Note the virtual absence of haustra in the tubular transverse and descending segments, a configuration suggesting chronic ulcerative colitis. However, she had never bled, and her colon mucosa was entirely intact, save for melanosis coli.

Saba and his associates[53] rightly assert that the radiologist should be prepared to contribute positively to a diagnosis of the IBS and not merely aim to exclude an organic lesion.

Endoscopy. The essential role of proctosigmoidoscopy in all patients exhibiting bowel symptoms has been noted and deserves reemphasis. Fiberoptic colonoscopy, on the other hand, is seldom required and adds little to the diagnosis of functional bowel disorder except in those instances of equivocal radiographic configuration requiring clarification. Fielding and Doyle[54] performed peroral endoscopy in 100 patients with the IBS and found evidence of "gastritis" in 62; however, they concluded that the gastric mucosal reaction bore no direct relation to the patients' symptoms but rather reflected a propensity for pyloroduodenal dysmotility associated with the IBS, and consequent bile reflux.

Manometry and Measurement of Bioelectric Activity. Mention has been made of the pathogenetic postulate that a "slow wave" bioelectric activity characterizes the IBS and may be responsible for disturbed bowel motility. This, however, is yet to be proved, and the technique involved remains an investigational, not a diagnostic, tool.[55]

Differential Diagnosis

Functional bowel disorders can simulate almost any conceivable disease below the diaphragm and a few above it. Mute testimony to this fact is eloquently given by the multiple scars so often graven on the abdominal wall. The following conditions are those most often confused:

Diverticular Disease of the Colon (see Chapter 135). A truly acute inflammatory complication of diverticula is usually marked by fever and leukocytosis in addition to an exquisitely tender mass most often in the left lower abdominal quadrant. Recurring episodes of acute diverticulitis lasting several days or weeks are often separated by long symptom-free intervals. Sustained hypertonicity of the sigmoid segment in the presence of diverticula has been labeled in the past as "chronic diverticulitis," a term that probably should be cast into limbo. An exception might be the fixed, unyielding distortion of stenosing pericolitis, a complication of diverticular disease. When the presence of obviously uncomplicated diverticula coincides with an irritable colon, attention is properly directed to the latter rather than to the former.

Neoplasm in the Bowel (see Chapters 114, 138, and 139). Here the gravest errors can befall even the experienced clinician. Small, hidden, benign tumors of the small intestine can give symptoms of partial, intermittent bowel obstruction over many years. All the symptoms of colon cancer can, and frequently do, duplicate symptoms characteristic of functional bowel disorder. At particular risk is the patient whose irritable bowel has become so familiar to his physician over the years that his supervening colon carcinoma goes unrecognized. In the elderly patient, the shorter the history, the more likely is the diagnosis of cancer. The patient who claims to have enjoyed a regular bowel habit, free of abdominal discomfort, until a few short weeks or months before seeking medical advice requires the most painstaking, objective study. The appearance of intestinal bleeding, in any form, imposes a similar obligation. It is important to remember that patients with colon cancer seldom lose appreciable weight or show other signs of systemic illness until their disease is far advanced. Further, it is well known that certain villous tumors of the colon can exude copious mucus which might be mistaken for "mucous colitis."

Ulcerative Colitis (see Chapter 126). Seldom, if ever, should this condition be confused with a functional disorder. Rectal bleeding almost invariably occurs with ulcerative colitis (although, strangely, bleeding is sometimes denied by the patient), and in almost all cases the typical mucosal changes of ulcerative colitis are readily identified at proctosigmoidoscopy.

Crohn's Disease (see Chapter 127). Confusion here is more likely. The chief distinguishing features of Crohn's disease are usually the youth of the patient and the signs of systemic illness, notably anemia, fever, and debility. There is no evidence that the IBS is a precursor of inflammatory bowel disease, either ulcerative colitis or Crohn's disease.

Appendicitis (see Chapter 144). Fortunately, in this enlightened era, the concept of chronic appendicitis has fallen into the oblivion it deserves. The large numbers of patients with longstanding functional disorders who bear right lower quadrant scars indicate this day was long in dawning. Acute appendicitis is a disease of only short duration. While unrecognized acute appendicitis may be recurrent, the intervals are relatively symptom-free.

Malabsorption States (see Chapter 101). The course of sprue or adult celiac disease can be prolonged but is marked by progressive inanition. The patient may complain of bloating but only infrequently of painful distress. The diarrhea of sprue seldom is explosive or watery; rather, the stools are mushy and gently expressed. The hallmark of the sprue stool is its extraordinary stench and its fat content.

Peptic Ulcer and Biliary Tract Disease (see Chapters 67 and 189). These are exceedingly common and often coexist with the IBS. They possess characteristic features that should cause little confusion when one or the other accompanies a functional bowel disorder.

Gynecologic Conditions. If the middle-aged woman with an irritable bowel does not bear an appendectomy scar, then very often a scar will be found in the lower midline of her abdomen, marking a previous surgical venture into the pelvis. Typically the reason given was removal of an ovarian cyst or the extirpation of ubiquitous "fibroids." Her functional bowel distress was misinterpreted and wrongly attributed to an innocent ovary or uterus. The only way I know by which this sort of error can be avoided is for the practitioner dealing with gynecologic problems to become fully familiar with the characteristics of functional bowel disorder and to restrain a recommendation for pelvic surgery in cases with marginal indications.

Frequency of urination and dysuria frequently attend an irritable bowel and often are the urinary counterparts of a functional disorder. Unfortunately these urinary symptoms may be attributable to "cystitis" and indiscriminately treated with antibiotics which, in turn, aggravate the irritable bowel.

Cardiopulmonary Disease. It is understandable that a patient with a feeling of painful pressure in the left hypochondrium, a seeming inability to take a deep breath, and palpitation—all symptoms of the splenic flexure syndrome (Chapter 9)—may be fearful of a "heart attack." This patient's anxiety can be dispelled usually by a careful physical examination, the demonstration of a normal electrocardiogram, and a reassuring explanation of the disturbing symptoms. The problem is somewhat more complicated in the patient who actually has developed angina of effort and, as a consequence, becomes aerophagic (Chapter 9). Patients with pulmonary emphysema seem prone to gastrointestinal complaints, particularly postprandial upper abdominal pressure (that often aggravates their dyspnea) and constipation (Chapter 7).

Metabolic Disturbances. Patients with insulin-dependent diabetes mellitus, especially with signs of autonomic neuropathy, have been shown to exhibit colon dysfunction[56] (Chapter 252). The bowel also may share in the neuromuscular disturbance occasioned by excesses or deficiencies in the various electrolytes, notably potassium and calcium. Patients with hyperthyroidism may have abdominal symptoms akin to those of IBS (Chapter 251).

Treatment

Four ingredients are essential to the successful management of functional bowel disorder: (1) A thorough and empathetic understanding of the condition on the part of the physician; (2) a capacity for comprehending the nature of the condition on the part of the patient; (3) a demonstration, convincing both to the physician and to the patient, that no organic disease is contributing to the symptoms; and (4) an abundance of time. Lacking any one of these ingredients, therapeutic efforts are usually doomed to failure. Note that medicaments and psychiatric consultation are *not* included among these essentials, though both are sometimes helpful. At the same time it is important to the physician to examine his own attitudes toward functional disorders and to the patient so afflicted. A slim volume by Steiger and Hansen[57] contains helpful suggestions bearing on this element.

Initial Interview. Proper management of the patient begins with the initial history-taking. The patient is allowed to make a free and full exposition of his or her complaints, even though this can sometimes be rather trying to the listener. Despite frequent protestations of fatigue, the patient seldom seems to tire of telling his or her story. The physician, meanwhile, must try to maintain an attitude of interest without displaying annoyance or alarm and without remonstrance.

The patient seldom will leave much ground to be covered in terms of *what*, but occasionally the physician will find it helpful to ask *why* the patient mentions a certain temporal relationship or *why* the patient tends to associate seemingly unrelated circumstances. Information helpful in formulating later advice is sometimes gained by these questions. Above all, sooner or later, the physician will want to know *why* the patient chose this time for consultation, especially when the symptoms are so longstanding. In some cases, at the conclusion of the interview, I inquire of the patient's own theories regarding the cause of his complaints. Sometimes he will reply, in a huff, that he had hoped *that* is information I might be able to tell him, but at other times he will reveal a suppressed anxiety, a peculiar foreboding, or even a frank psychosis.

Summary Advice. This is the moment of truth for which the physician has been preparing himself since his first interview with the patient and while he has been evaluating the returns from the objective studies. Now he must decide, on the basis of his estimate of the patient and the problem, what he is to say, where he will lay the emphasis, at what level he will try to explain the findings, and, lastly, what he will prescribe. An essay by Tumulty of the Johns Hopkins Hospital is recommended for the sage advice it offers on this score.[58]

If one recognizes in the patient a significant affective disorder, one's approach will be governed by a delineation of the patient's psychic setting (Chapter 245). Pfeifer[59] describes 5 aberrations one might encounter among patients with functional disorders. First, and probably the most common, is the depressed patient. This patient is typically middle-aged and confuses pain as the cause rather than the effect of depression which, in any event, he usually denies. This patient insists that first his symptoms be relieved, then his spirits will lift. Second is the true hypochondriac who sees himself as ill and will not be dissuaded. More often than not he is little interested in either a diagnosis or the prospect of relief by treatment but tends to improve with frequent visits to the doctor. Third is the patient with conversion reaction or hysteria whose visit probably was prompted by a spouse or close friend and whose attitude is "la belle indifference." Fourth is the pain-prone patient with a masochistic personality, typically a woman who is a grave risk to herself and to her doctor. For her, suffering is a way of life, and she sanguinely describes a long history of disagreeable diagnostic studies and trying therapies, often including a number of painful operations. This patient, Pfeifer warns, can "stir rescue fantasies in the most case-hardened doctor—who isn't challenged to succeed where others have failed?" Fifth, and finally, is the patient whose somatic delusions reflect an actual paranoid schizophrenia and who, on recognition, should be referred promptly to expert psychiatric care. Groves[60] cautions of the pitfalls in dealing with intensely dependent patients whom he categorizes as (1) dependent clingers, (2) entitled demanders, (3) manipulative help-rejectors, and (4) self-destructive deniers.

Reassurance. The degree of emphasis to be placed on reassurance that no organic disease exists will depend on an estimate of how much the patient needs or wants this reassurance. How much of a role has anxiety played? This varies remarkably from patient to patient. Some patients have been little discomforted but have been terrified by fancied implications of their discomfort. Others have given little thought to the meaning of their distress but feel entitled to and demand relief. Still others, interestingly, are neither anxious nor entreating but rather ask only for an earnest appreciation of their symptoms to which they hold fast as a bulwark against life's demands. Sapira[61] has outlined an approach to reassurance therapy in a helpful way.

It has been my custom to review, in detail, the results of each and every test and examination with the patient. I show him the radiographs, trying to explain the anatomy in simple terms. I know full well that many of my patients are uncomprehending of what I show them, but they very often express appreciation of the demonstration.

I have learned to avoid using the term "negative" when I discuss the results of examinations. A number of years ago a friendly patient, who was an industrial engineer in charge of a large technical laboratory, pointed out to me that in his business "negative" had the connotation of failure, error, or wrongness. Consequently, I have discarded this word from my vocabulary when talking with patients and in its place I use "satisfactory" or "favorable" or "within a healthy range." I think perhaps this is more than just a matter of Pollyanna semantics.

When reporting the findings, it is worth mentioning specifically that "there is no sign of tumor, growth, or cancer—not that we were worried about cancer in your case, but we always look carefully for it." Even when the patient has not voiced the question, he has tacitly wondered. It is gratifying to observe how often the patient is visibly relieved when these reassuring words are spoken.

If the studies disclose an innocent and unsuspected abnormality, this should be frankly explained to the patient and not ignored. At the same time it is made clear that the minor aberration does not bear on his principal problem nor will it interfere or detract from his course of treatment.

Explaining Normal Bowel Physiology. In venturing to discuss the nature of a functional bowel disorder, the wise physician takes care not to minimize or make light of the patient's distress. The chances are that the patient has consulted numerous physicians who have given the impression, wittingly or not, that the symptoms are imaginary and, hence, fictitious. Such a simplistic dismissal has no therapeutic value. Rather, the somatic aspect of distress should be specifically explained, recalling the tense and tender bowel palpated at physical examination and pointing out the configuration of spasm often evident in the barium enema films. At the same time, it is emphasized that spasm is distressing rather than damaging, intensely annoying rather than injurious.

Two points are worthy of mention to the patient. First, it is explained that spasm or stretching of the bowel does not actually interfere with the normal physiologic process of digestion; that is, the bowel is doing its job, albeit under stress. The patient need fear no impairment of nourishment. Second, and more important to the anxious patient, despite the fact that he has experienced the distress of an irritable bowel for a long time (years in many cases), this condition has not been shown to predispose serious disease. Both of these statements are true, and their mention usually is appreciated. Some writers, notably Burkitt and his associates,[62] might utter a caveat with the second statement. Their contention is that a spastic, constipated bowel is due to depleted dietary fiber; their speculation is that such a diet is associated with an increased prevalence of diverticular disease and cancer of the colon. Although the epidemiologic evidence is suggestive, an actual cause-and-effect relation between bowel spasm and cancer is yet unproved.

Educating patients to tolerate erratic bowel action is a more difficult matter. The belief that it is a vital necessity to have no more or no less than one bowel movement each day is often so deeply ingrained that even the most eloquent dissuasion may be of no avail. Nevertheless, the effort is made. Similarly, it is explained that appreciable variations in the size and consistency of the stool are not signs of disease but are quite compatible with good health. Mucus is mentioned as a normal product of the colon, formed in order to lubricate the smooth passage of the stool.

Generally, I have not found it helpful to advise elaborate rituals as an aid to regular bowel action. Undue ceremony tends to magnify an already excessive bowel consciousness. I do, however, point out that the bowel is a creature of habit, and I suggest to the patient that he take advantage of the well-known gastroenteric reflex and provide at least an opportunity for the bowel to evacuate itself after the breakfast meal. By the same token, if the patient's problem is one of too frequent stools, he should not be disturbed by the expression of a normal gastroenteric reflex following any meal of the day.

More Specific Measures. In the course of his discussion, the alert physician senses the capacity of his patient to absorb and respond to his proffered advice. An intellectual approach will appeal to some but totally unimpress others. Some patients will do better with less explanation and more stern, fatherly advice. This is wholly a matter for the physician's judgment, and his skill in estimating the situation is sharpened by experience. In my opinion, the younger the patient, the more is the need for thorough explanation as the only hope for avoiding a lifelong bowel preoccupation. For the elderly, attempts at re-education often are futile, and the doctor must be content with advising simple, symptomatic measures. Most patients will expect, and are entitled to, a word or two of more specific direction.

DIET. In my view, emphasis should be placed on liberalizing rather than restricting diet selection. Often, in making their rounds of doctors, patients with functional bowel disorders will have been issued a series of printed diet sheets. Collectively, these will have disallowed almost everything edible. The patient comes to feel that any deviation from mush will have dire consequences. It is important to avoid fostering the patient's idea that he is a stomach cripple. I assure the patient with an irritable bowel that no food he ingests will entail any actual injury or produce tissue damage. I hasten to add that I cannot guarantee that every item of food will "sit" comfortably with him. Indeed, I would be surprised if it did. But I would encourage him to feel free to enjoy as nearly a normal, wholesome diet selection as he can within the limits of his own individual taste and tolerance. Jones et al.[29] have revived the idea of an elimination diet to identify intolerance to specific foodstuffs. This, I think, is unnecessary in most cases. There is no justification in arbitrarily proscribing lactose-containing foods in IBS patients of Northern or Western European ancestry.[39a] The sensible patient is best guided by his own good, honest experience. Above all, emphasis is given to what the patient can eat rather than to what he cannot.

A "high fiber" diet has its advocates[63,64] and its doubters.[65] Bran, in various forms, seems to be a popular item nowadays for almost all the ills to which the bowel is heir. Doubtless, bran can sometimes be helpful if one discounts the flatulence it often induces. The rougher forms of bran have been poorly tolerated by many of my patients with the IBS. Patients found to be consuming inordinate amounts of food containing sorbitol[39] or fructose[38] are also well advised to moderate their habits.

On physiologic grounds I feel more justified in emphasizing the *how* rather than the *what* of diet. The patient is told that in contrast to the automatic control characteristic of the other body systems, the digestive tract is almost entirely at his mercy for the work it has to do. All biologic systems work best on a rhythmic basis. Therefore, the patient's stomach and bowel will appreciate his cooperation in affording a fairly even, regular schedule of feeding, which means neither skipping meals nor overloading the stomach at any one sitting.

There are some practitioners who will disagree with this approach, claiming that it is not sufficiently authoritarian. I would grant that some patients require more directive thinking than others. But for most, I am convinced that a more liberal regimen is beneficial.

PHYSICAL AIDS. These are of limited application, but a few deserve mention. Painful spasm in the abdomen often is relieved by local heat. An electric heating pad or a hot-water bottle wrapped in a moist towel is soothing to the patient with bowel spasm. Lying in a tub of warm water is occasionally advised. Simple physical exercise has much to commend it. Many patients with functional bowel disorders lead lives that are unduly sedentary. Much of the energy they expend is in nervous pursuits. Leisurely walking is an almost universally available form of exercise and quite satisfactory. Exercise need not be a highly organized activity.

The proper use of enemas may be considered among physical aids to elimination. The regular use of enemas is not encouraged, but neither is the occasional use disparaged. The patient can be assured that enemas are safe when heed is paid to (1) their content, which should be plain warm water; and (2) their volume, which should not exceed 1 pint. It is explained that the purpose of an enema is not to flush out the entire colon but rather only to distend the rectal ampulla gently so that normal expulsive reflexes may be set in motion.

MEDICATIONS. To read the advertisements of pharmaceutical manufacturers, one would think the millenium has arrived; that the patient need but swallow a pill (long-acting, at that), and his bowel spasm will vanish and his emotional state be one of utter tranquility. Veteran practitioners know this is not so, and patients, in turn, should not be deceived into believing there is a simple quasi-magic remedy for functional bowel disorder. These patients seem to be more than ordinarily susceptible to suggestion. The experienced physician knows that when dealing with a functional bowel disorder, he can expect an early favorable response to any new regimen he invokes. He knows, too, that even the most promising regimen will lose much of its charm sooner or later, and that the patient will return or seek out another practitioner because of much the same complaints for which he was originally treated.

Recognizing the frequent contribution to functional bowel disorder of emotional stress or nervous tension, the physician is tempted to prescribe sedative medication in one form or another. The benzodiazepine compounds such as chlordiazepoxide (Librium), 5 to 10 mg, and diazepam (Valium), 2 to 5 mg, usually prescribed before meals and at bedtime, have been popular with physicians and patients alike. Doubtless there are selected cases wherein such agents have been helpful when given in short courses. Probably more often the IBS is an expression of a reactive or endogenous depression and, if psychotropic drugs are to be used, antidepressant agents are more appropriate than so-called tranquilizers. The concomitant anticholinergic properties of the tricyclic antidepressants, such as imipramine (Tofranil) or amitriptyline (Elavil), may be of added benefit. Again, defined rather than interminable courses are advised.

Although conceptually attractive for the relief of bowel spasm, anticholinergic agents are disappointing in their frequent lack of effectiveness in functional bowel disorders. When incorporated in a combination form with a sedative, the dose is often less than pharmacologically active. Atropine (0.4 to 0.8 mg), tincture of belladonna (10 to 30 drops), propantheline (Pro-Banthine, 15 to 30 mg), or dicyclomine (Bentyl, 10 to 20 mg) can be given before meals or at bedtime. Anticholinergic agents sometimes are helpful in quelling a troublesome gastroenteric reflex. In some cases they may allay painful bowel spasm.[66–67a] In any case, the prudent physician will resolutely resist the use of narcotic drugs.

Again, note is made of the importance of a thorough survey of the patient's previous experience with drugs or medications taken for reasons unrelated to the bowel. Particular attention should be directed to the use of antibiotic, cardiotonic, analgesic, and psychotropic drugs. Perhaps more often than not, subtractions rather than additions are best made to the patient's pharmacy list.

CONTROL OF ERRATIC OR IRREGULAR BOWEL ACTION. Implicit in the management of most cases of functional bowel disorder, at one time or another, is the control of diarrhea and constipation. Essential to appropriate treatment in each case is a precise definition of what the patient means when he complains of "diarrhea" or "constipation." An almost ideal agent to correct erratic bowel action with stools of varying consistency, so typical of functional bowel disorder, is one form or another of Plantago (psyllium) seed derivative, a naturally occurring mucilaginous colloid. It is important to distinguish between such preparations as Hydrocil, Konsyl, and Siblin, which are composed entirely of Plantago mucilloids, and preparations of the nature of Metamucil and L. A. Formula, which are half-and-half mixtures of mucilloids and dextrose. The dose of psyllium mucilloids is 1 heaping teaspoon in ¾ glass of water or juice 1 to 3 times daily as needed. The mucilloids tend to "normalize" stools, i.e., they add consistency to fluid stools and soften hard, pebbly stools. Patients complaining of fragmented stools are particularly pleased with the solidifying effect of mucilloids which can sometimes lessen urgency to stool. In the colon, their bulk may tend to reduce harsh, segmented spasm. Moreover, the mucilaginous colloids exert some adsorptive capacity, thus countering the adverse effects of bile acids and similar substances in the colon. Their long-term use is safe—more dietary additives than drugs. The hemicelluloses, such as agar or the semisynthetic formulations of carboxymethylcellulose, offer no advantage even though preferred by some patients. It is only fair to note that the efficacy of psyllium therapy has been challenged.[68] My patients, however, continue to find it beneficial.

A mild tendency to frequent, loose stools may respond to the measures prescribed above. Aluminum hydroxide gel (Alternagel) can be helpful when there is a concomitant need for an antacid. Preparations containing kaolin and pectin are sometimes useful. More troublesome diarrhea can be controlled with diphenoxylate (Lomotil) or loperamide (Imodium). The usual dose ranges from 2 to 5 mg before meals or at bedtime as needed. The typical pattern of stooling in functional disorders is an early morning "run." This can be often forestalled by the patient's taking the first daily dose on arising.

Suggestions for the assessment and management of constipation, applicable to patients with the IBS, are given in Chapter 7.

BIOFEEDBACK AND OPERANT CONDITIONING. Recent interest has been evident in techniques of conditioned behavior as they may be applied to various disorders, particularly anorectal incontinence.[69–72] The basic idea is that favorable responses can be enhanced and unfavorable responses can be suppressed, the startling concept being that visceral activity, ordinarily thought of as autonomically governed, can be brought under voluntary control. If true, then smooth muscle spasm, such as characterizes the irritable bowel, might be "conditioned" to relax, or a suppressed gastroenteric reflex might be enhanced. Obviously, this is somewhat akin to yoga, devoid of its philosophic trappings and objectified by electronic sensors. The Baltimore City Hospital group led by Schuster, reporting successful correction of aberrant anal sphincter responses,[73, 74] cites 4 conditions requisite to "operant conditioning": (1) the presence of a well-defined and readily measured response, e.g., synchronized sphincteric reflexes; (2) a response that is variable and under neural control; (3) a recognizable clue that signals the patient to initiate control; and (4) a compelling motivation on the part of the patient to bring the desired response under control. The potential rewards of this intriguing approach warrant further investigation.

INDICATIONS FOR PSYCHOTHERAPY. Perhaps it should be restated that functional bowel disorders are *not* to be construed as synonymous with neuroses. A bowel may be keenly sensitive and hyperirritable without its owner being neurotic. True, the conditions often coincide and doubtlessly can contribute to each other. As the patient often explains, "It may be that my nerves upset my bowel, but my bowel gets on my nerves!"

Neurosis, when it attends a functional bowel disorder, may be either of the anxiety or the conversion type. The former is more readily alleviated, albeit temporarily. Experience teaches that, although evidence of neurotic tendencies is common, seldom will the veteran clinician find it necessary to call on the psychiatrist for help in dealing with the patient and with his functional bowel disorder. This is probably fortunate because, in my experience, seldom are psychiatrists particularly interested in seeing this sort of patient.

In most cases it is unwise to probe deeply in a search for grave underlying emotional aberrations. Certainly, inquiry along these lines is inappropriate during the first interview. It has been interesting to me to observe how well the patient himself will introduce the matter at the most propitious time after he has become confident in his doctor's care. Then the patient's problems can be discussed frankly and forthrightly.

Only in comparatively rare cases will there be evident signs of true psychosis, usually a latent schizophrenia. These signs, of course, are ominous, and in such cases expert psychiatric care should be sought without delay.

Prognosis

Functional bowel disorders pose no threat to life or limb. They are compatible with a long and otherwise healthy life. Indeed, a functional disorder may even be a key to longevity if Dr. Oliver Wendell Holmes's formula for a long life is valid: "Have a chronic disease and take care of it." Unfortunately, however, for many persons a life preoccupied by a highly irritable and erratic bowel only seems long.

All of us sometimes feel uneasy about our diagnosis of IBS in a given patient, even when the diagnosis has been seemingly well established. Will the diagnosis hold up over time? We can take heart from the report by Holmes and Salter,[74] a who found their diagnosis of IBS required change in only 4 of 77 patients whose course was followed 6 years or longer.

The question of the patient's being relieved of his symptoms is another matter. The likelihood of remission is inversely related to the duration of symptoms. A majority of patients will have exhibited varying expressions of functional gastrointestinal disturbances for many years, often for as long as they can remember. As a consequence, the physician must content himself with a therapeutic result somewhat short of complete and lasting remission. Among 50 patients followed by Waller and Misiewicz[75] for 1 year, only 6 were symptom-free and the remainder were unchanged or somewhat improved. Chaudhary and Truelove[10] reported a similar experience in 130 cases and pointed out that the prognosis was more favorable in patients with simple diarrhea compared with those having painful spastic colons. Fleischner and Hendrix[76] intimate that treatment of a spastic colon may diminish the likelihood or severity of later diverticular disease. Probably the greatest peril to the patient with functional bowel disorder is that his chronic complaints will mask the later symptoms of a supervening but unrelated malignant disease.[77] To avoid this pitfall, to perceive the glimmer of organic disease beneath the haze of functional complaints, is perhaps the most vexing problem for the physician in whose hands these patients place their care.

In any event, the doctor who has won the confidence of his patient with a functional bowel disorder can expect to be seeing his "familiar face"[78] for a long time to come.

Anorectal Pain Syndromes

These perplexing afflictions may or may not bear a relation to the irritable bowel; surely they can occur in the absence of any other symptoms of the IBS. They are similar only in that no organic lesion has been identified with them, and they are exceedingly vexatious to both patient and doctor alike. Hence, they are considered here along with IBS.

Proctalgia Fugax. This peculiar expression of a presumed functional anorectal disorder is common but seldom appreciated, unless the physician himself has experienced it. The condition has been long recognized.[79,80] Douthwaite[81] described the syndrome in 10 doctor-patients. Occurring most often in adult men, the intense, fleeting rectal pain has the singular propensity of awakening the victim from a sound sleep at night. The boring ache tends to wax and wane, then dissipates after 10 to 30 minutes. Unheralded episodes are isolated by symptom-free intervals of weeks, months, or even years. Rarely does pain occur on successive nights. Usually there are no other manifestations of functional bowel disorder or disturbed bowel action.

The cause and mechanism of proctalgia fugax are unknown. Because it occurs at night and is fleeting, seldom has it been objectively observed. Douthwaite's doctors, who had palpated their rectums during attacks, described a tense band on one or the other side of the rectal canal, suggesting levator muscle spasm. Harvey[82] recorded sigmoid contractions but was unable to substantiate levator or sphincter spasm in 2 patients whose bowel motility was assessed during attacks. The anal sphincters typically are lax. Pain may or may not be attended by an urge to defecate or urinate; in either case, these efforts leave the pain unaltered.

A psychologic profile describing patients so afflicted as perfectionistic and tense has been suggested,[83] but this picture may have been distorted insofar as only complainers were psychometrically tested and the condition is known to affect a substantial fraction of the "normal" population.[84, 85]

Treatment is unsatisfactory and arcane,[85] many patients supposing they have found their own remedies. Hot baths, hot stupes to the perineum, or warm enemas have their advocates; pinching the buttocks or putting pressure on the anus has been tried. Counterirritation is probably the common mechanism of these maneuvers, perhaps by the induction of competing afferent impulses. As the pain is invariably self-limited, efficacy is hard to judge.

The importance of properly identifying proctalgia fugax is, first, to avoid a mistaken diagnosis and misguided treatment (prostatitis is often confused) and, second, to assure the perplexed and anxious victim that his symptom is real and well recognized but not indicative of or related to dire disease.

Familial Rectal Pain. This even more curious and rare condition has been documented[86–88] by pedigrees. Evidently, because of an autosomal dominant genetic determinant, members of families, ranging from infancy to old age, have been afflicted by recurring, intense anorectal pain. The pain sometimes is attended by ocular and jaw pain, often associated with blanching and erythema in the skin near the affected parts. The latter feature implies vascular changes, perhaps mediated by an autonomic neuropathy. No remedy has been described.

Chronic Anorectal or Pelvic Pain. More vexing to the clinician is the problem of persistent, unremitting, distracting anorectal or pelvic pain,[89] which, in my experience, occurs predominantly in postmenopausal women. An explanation for such pain, in most cases, eludes the most extensive and intensive investigation, and the pain often is unallayed despite a variety of medical and surgical attempts at treatment. Many of these poor people appear depressed, but I have found the prescription of antidepressant medications of little avail.

A group of Mayo Clinic physiatrists[90] has described a syndrome they call "tension myalgia of the pelvic floor" which is said to respond to rectal diathermy, massage, and relaxation exercises. Probably this is similar to what has been also called the "levator[91] or Thiele's[92] syndrome." In such cases, pain often extends into the gluteal area and thighs. This is to be distinguished from coccydynia, a sharply localized pain elicited on palpation or manipulation of the coccyx. This condition is a peri-articular reaction, usually consequent to trauma, that tends to be self-limited.

For the sufferer from chronic unexplained and unremitting anorectal pain, the clinician's chief role is to shield the patient from the hazard of opiate addiction and ill-advised surgical forays.

References

1. Ryle JA. Chronic-spasmodic affections of the colon. Lancet 1928; 2:1115.
2. Medawar PB. Darwin's illness. Ann Intern Med 1964; 61: 782–6.
3. Palmer ED. Functional Gastrointestinal Disease. Baltimore: Williams & Wilkins, 1967.
4. Alvarez WC. Nervousness, Indigestion, and Pain. New York: Paul B. Hoeber, 1943: 319–27.
5. Bockus HL, Willard JH. Functional disorders of the colon. Penn Med J 1934; 37:645.
6. Hurst AF. The unhappy colon. Lancet 1935; 1:1483.
7. Jordan SM, Kieffer ED. Irritable colon. JAMA 1929; 93:592.
8. Spriggs EI. Functional disorders of the colon. Q J Med 1931; 24:533.
9. Almy TP. The irritable bowel syndrome; back to square one? (Editorial). Dig Dis Sci 1980; 25:401–3.
10. Chaudhary NS, Truelove SC. The irritable colon syndrome; a study of the clinical features, predisposing causes, and prognosis in 130 cases. Q J Med 1962; 31:307.
11. Drossman DA, Powell DW, Sessions JT Jr. The irritable bowel syndrome. Gastroenterology 1977; 73:811–22.
12. Drossman DA. Diagnosis of the irritable bowel syndrome. (Editorial). Ann Intern Med 1979; 90:431–2.
13. Kirsner JB. The irritable bowel syndrome; a clinical review and ethical considerations. Arch Intern Med 1981; 141: 635–9.
14. Latimer PR. Psychophysiologic disorders; a critical appraisal of concept and theory illustrated with reference to the irritable bowel syndrome. Psychol Med 1979; 9:71–80.
15. Latimer P, Sarna S, Campbell D, Latimer M, Waterfall W, Daniel EE. Colonic motor and myoelectrical activity; a comparative study of normal subjects, psychoneurotic patients, and patients with irritable bowel syndrome. Gastroenterology 1981; 80:893–901.
16. Mendeloff AI. Epidemiology of the irritable bowel syndrome. Practical Gastroenterol 1979; 3:12–8.
17. Snape WJ Jr., Carlson GM, Cohen S. Colonic myoelectric activity in the irritable bowel syndrome. Gastroenterology 1976; 70:326–30.
18. Snape WJ Jr., Carlson GM, Matarazzo SA, Cohen S. Evidence that abnormal myoelectrical activity produces colonic

motor dysfunction in the irritable bowel syndrome. Gastroenterology 1977; 72:383–7.
19. Taylor I, Darby C, Hammond P. Comparison of rectosigmoid myoelectric activity in the irritable colon syndrome during relapses and remissions. Gut 1978; 19:923–9.
20. Taylor I, Darby C, Hammond P, Basu P. Is there a myoelectrical abnormality in the irritable colon syndrome? Gut 1978; 19:391–5.
21. Thompson WG, Heaton KW. Functional bowel disorders in apparently healthy people. Gastroenterology 1980; 79: 283–8.
21a. Lennard-Jones JE. Current concepts: Functional gastrointestinal disorders. N Engl J Med 1983; 308:431–5.
22. Ritchie J. Pain in irritable bowel syndrome. Pract Gastroenterol 1979; 3:16–23.
23. Bustos-Fernandez L, Gonzalez E, Marzi A, Ledesma MI. Fecal acidorrhea. N Engl J Med 1971; 284:295–8.
24. Fordtran JS. Organic ions in fecal contents. (Editorial). N Engl J Med 1971; 284:329–30.
25. Sarna S, Latimer PR, Campbell D, Waterfall WE. Effect of stress, meal, and neostigmine on rectosigmoid electrical control activity (ECA) in normal and in irritable bowel syndrome patients. Dig Dis Sci 1982; 27:582–91.
26. Harvey RF. Effects of hormones in normal subjects and patients with irritable bowel syndrome. Practical Gastroenterol 1979; 3:10–15.
27. Hermon-Taylor J, Code CF. Effect of secretin on small bowel myoelectric activity in conscious healthy dogs. Am J Dig Dis 1970; 15:545–50.
28. Rachmilewitz D. Prostaglandins and diarrhea. (Editorial). Dig Dis Sci 1980; 25:897–9.
29. Jones AV, Shorthouse M, McLaughlan P, Workman E, Hunter JO. Food intolerance: a major factor in pathogenesis of irritable bowel syndrome. Lancet 1982; 2:1115–17.
30. Besterman HS, Sarson DL, Rambaud JC, Stewart JS, Guerin S, Bloom SR. Gut hormone responses in the irritable bowel syndrome. Digestion 1981; 21:219–24.
31. Whorwell PJ, Crouter C, Smith CL. Esophageal motility in the irritable bowel syndrome. Br Med J 1981; 282:1101–2.
32. Moriarity KJ, Dawson AM. Functional abdominal pain; further evidence that whole gut is affected. Br Med J 1982; 284:1670–2.
33. Corbett CL, Read TS, Read NW, Hobson N, Bergman I, Holdsworth CD. Electrochemical detector for breath hydrogen determination; measurement of small bowel transit time in normal subjects and patients with the irritable bowel syndrome. Gut 1981; 22:836–40.
34. Apley J, Hale B. Children with recurrent abdominal pain; how do they grow up? Br Med J 1973; 3:7–9.
35. Connell AM, Jones FA, Rowlands EN. Motility of the pelvic colon. IV. Abdominal pain associated with colonic hypermotility after meals. Gut 1965; 6:105–12.
36. Ritchie JA. The gastrocolic response to food. Digestion 1968; 1:15.
37. Anderson IH, Levine AS, Levitt MD. Incomplete absorption of the carbohydrate in all-purpose flour. N Engl J Med 1981; 304:891–2.
38. Ravich WJ, Bayless TM, Thomas M. Fructose: incomplete intestinal absorption in humans. Gastroenterology 1983; 84:26–9.
39. Hyams JS. Sorbital intolerance: an unappreciated cause of functional gastrointestinal complaints. Gastroenterology 1983; 84:30–3.
39a. Newcomer AD, McGill DB. Irritable bowel syndrome; Role of lactase deficiency. Mayo Clin Proc 1983; 58:339–41.
40. Deren JJ. Iatrogenic diarrhea. Practical Gastroenterol 1980; 4:25–32.
41. Fava GA, Pavan L. Large bowel disorders. I. Illness configuration and life events. Psychother Psychosom 1976/77; 27:93–9.
42. Fava GA, Pavan L. Large bowel disorders. II. Psychopathology and alexithymia. Psychother Psychosom 1976; 27: 100–5.
43. Whitehead WE, Winget C, Fedoravicius AS, Wooley S, Blackwell B. Learned illness behavior in patients with irritable bowel syndrome and peptic ulcer. Dig Dis Sci 1982; 27:202–8.
44. Young SJ, Alpers DH, Norland CC, Woodruff RA Jr. Psychiatric illness and the irritable bowel syndrome; practical implications for the primary physician. Gastroenterology 1976; 70:162–6.
45. Whitehead WE, Engel BT, Schuster MM. Irritable bowel syndrome. Physiologic and psychological differences between diarrhea-predominant and constipation-predominant patients. Dig Dis Sci 1980; 25:404–13.
46. Wolf S. Emotions and the autonomic nervous system. Arch Intern Med 1970; 126:6.
47. Pimparkar BD. Irritable colon syndrome. J Ind Med Assoc 1970; 54:95.
48. Silverberg M, Daum F. Irritable bowel syndrome in children and adolescents. Practical Gastroenterol 1979; 3:25–9.
49. Schwab JJ, Traven VD. Factors related to the incidence of psychosomatic illness. Psychosomatics 1979; 20:307–12.
49a. Drossman DA, Sandler RS, McKee DC, Lovitz AJ. Bowel patterns among subjects not seeking health care: Use of a questionnaire to identify a population with bowel dysfunction. Gastroenterology 1982; 83:529–34.
50. Barsky AG. Patients who amplify body sensations. Ann Intern Med 1979; 91:63–70.
51. Manning AP, Thompson WG, Heaton KW, Morris AF. Towards positive diagnosis of the irritable bowel. Br Med J 1978; 2:653.
52. Ferrucci JT Jr. Hypotonic barium enema examination. AJR 1972; 116:304.
53. Saba GP, Gatewood OMB, Feinstein RS, Gayler BW. Radiological diagnosis of irritable bowel syndrome. Practical Gastroenterol 1979; 3:38–41.
54. Fielding JF, Doyle GD. The prevalence and significance of gastritis in patients with lower intestinal irritable bowel (irritable colon) syndrome. J Clin Gastroenterol 1982; 4:507–10.
55. Greenbaum DS. Can the diagnosis of irritable bowel syndrome be improved by rectosigmoid motility studies? (Editorial). J Clin Gastroenterol 1983; 5:11–3.
56. Battle WM, Snape WJ Jr., Alavi A, Cohen S, Braunstein S. Colonic dysfunction in diabetes mellitus. Gastroenterology 1980; 79:1217–21.
57. Steiger WA, Hansen AV Jr. Patients Who Trouble You. Boston: Little, Brown & Co, 1964.
58. Tumulty PA. The approach to patients with functional disorders. N Engl J Med 1960; 263:123.
59. Pfeifer E. Treating the patient with confirmed functional pain. Hospital Phys, June 1971, pp 68–92.
60. Groves JE. Taking care of the hateful patient. N Engl J Med 1978; 298:883–7.
61. Sapira JD. Reassurance therapy. Ann Intern Med 1972; 77:603–4.
62. Burkitt DP, Walker ARP, Painter NS. Effect of dietary fiber on stools and transit times and its role in the causation of disease. Lancet 1972; 2:1408.
63. Manning AP, Heaton KW, Harvey RF, Uglow P. Wheat fibre and irritable bowel syndrome; a controlled trial. Lancet 1977; 2:417–8.
64. Ritchie JA, Truelove SC. Treatment of the irritable bowel syndrome with lorazepam, hyoscine, butyl bromide, and ispaghula husk. Br Med J 1979; 1:376–8.
65. Søltoft J, Gudmand-Høyer E, Krag B, Kristensen E, Wulff HR. A double-blind trial of the effect of wheat bran on symptoms of irritable bowel syndrome. Lancet 1976; 1: 270–2.
66. Ivey KJ. Are anti-cholinergics of use in the irritable colon syndrome? Gastroenterology 1975; 68:1300–7.
67. Pias G, Mazzacce G. Profinium bromides in the treatment of the irritable colon syndrome. Gastroenterology 1979; 77:500–2.
67a. Ritchie JA, Truelove SC. Comparison of various treatments for irritable bowel syndrome. Br Med J 1980; 281:1317–19.
68. Longstreth GF, Fox DD, Youkeles L, Forsythe AB, Wolo-

chow DA. Psyllium therapy in the irritable bowel syndrome. Ann Intern Med 1981; 95:53–6.
69. Shapiro D, Schwartz GE. Biofeedback and visceral learning; clinical applications. Semin Psychiatry 1972; 4:171.
70. Almy TP, Corson JA. Biofeedback: The light at the end of the tunnel? (Editorial). Gastroenterology 1979; 76:874–6.
71. Schuster MM. Biofeedback treatment of gastrointestinal disorders. Med Clin North Am 1977; 61:907–12.
72. Wald A. Biofeedback therapy for fecal incontinence. Ann Intern Med 1981; 95:146–9.
73. Engel BT, Nikoomanesh P, Schuster MM. Operant conditioning of rectosphincteric responses in treatment of fecal incontinence. N Engl J Med 1974; 290:646–9.
74. Cerulli MA, Nikoomanesh P, Schuster MM. Progress in biofeedback conditioning for fecal incontinence. Gastroenterology 1979; 76:742–6.
74a. Holmes KM, Salter RH. Irritable bowel syndrome—a safe diagnosis? Br Med J 1982; 285:1533–4.
75. Waller SL, Misiewicz JJ. Prognosis in irritable bowel syndrome. Lancet 1969; 2:753.
76. Fleischner FG, Hendrix TR. Diverticular disease of the colon; new observations and revised concepts. Gastroenterology 1971; 60:316–24.
77. Hawkins CF, Cockel R. The prognosis and risk of missing malignant disease in patients with unexplained and functional diarrhea. Gut 1971; 12:208.
78. Kemp R. The familiar face. Lancet 1963; 1:1223.
79. Myrtle AS. Some common afflictions of the anus often neglected by medical men and patients. Br Med J 1883; 1:1061–2.
80. Thaysen T. Proctalgia fugax; a little known form of pain in the rectum. Lancet 1935; 2:243–6.
81. Douthwaite A. Proctalgia fugax. Br Med J 1962; 2:164–5.
82. Harvey RF. Colonic motility in proctalgia fugax. Lancet 1979; 2:713.
83. Pilling LF, Swenson WM, Hill JR. The psychologic aspects of proctalgia fugax. Dis Colon Rectum 1972; 8:372–6.
84. Panitch NM, Schofferman JA. Proctalgia fugax revisited. (Abstract). Gastroenterology 1975; 68:1061.
85. Thompson WG. Proctalgia fugax. Dig Dis Sci 1981; 26: 1121–4.
86. Hayden R, Grossman M. Rectal, ocular, and submaxillary pain; a familial autonomic disorder related to proctalgia fugax; report of a family. Am J Dis Child 1959; 97:479.
87. Mann TP, Cree JE. Familial rectal pain. (Letter). Lancet 1972; 1:1016–7.
88. Dugan RE. Familial rectal pain. (Letter). Lancet 1972; 1:854.
89. Neill ME, Swash M. Chronic perianal pain; an unsolved problem. J Roy Soc Med 1982; 75:96–101.
90. Sinaki M, Merritt JL, Stillwell GK. Tension myalgia of the pelvic floor. Mayo Clin Proc 1977; 52:717–22.
91. Grant SR, Salvati EP, Rubin RJ. Levator syndrome; an analysis of 316 cases. Dis Colon Rectum 1975; 18:161–3.
92. Thiele GH. Tonic spasm of the levator ani, coccygeus, and piriformis muscles; its relationship to coccydynia and pain in the region of the hips and down the leg. Trans Am Proctol Soc 1936; 37:145.

Chapter 135

Diverticula and Diverticular Disease of the Colon

William S. Haubrich

To ponder the problem of diverticula in the colon is to reflect on the distinction between normality, abnormality, and disease. What is normal? Is normality a condition pertaining in a majority of a given population? If so, the presence of colon diverticula is almost "normal" for older adults residing in the United States and other Western countries. If, on the other hand, one looks upon diverticula as representing deviation from normal among colons generally, then is such abnormality a disease? In this chapter, the mere presence of intact diverticula is distinguished from diverticular disease, which then is liable to certain complications. Diverticula in the colon are common; diverticular disease is relatively unusual; complications, fortunately, are even less frequent.

Seasoned clinicians know that one of their daily and often most difficult tasks is to reconcile (a) whatever the patient offers by way of complaints with (b) whatever abnormality may be objectively detected by examination. In all of clinical medicine there is no better example of this dilemma. Almy and Howell[1] estimate that of the millions of people harboring diverticula in their colons, only about 1 in 5 will develop symptoms or illness; only a minority of these will be liable to grave complications; and less than 1 in 10,000 will die because of diverticular disease.

Definition and Historical Background

A colonic diverticulum is an outpouching, protrusion, or herniation of the mucosa through the circular muscular coat of the large intestine, forming a more or less permanent sac composed only of mucosa, connective tissue, and serosa. As such, the outpouching has sometimes been called a "pseudodiverticulum," but no useful purpose is served by this pedantic distinction. The term *diverticulosis,* proposed independently by de Quervain[2] and by Case[3] many years ago, has been taken to mean the mere presence of diverticula in the absence of any morbid change. *Diverticular disease* is properly reserved for the circumstance in which diverticula are associated with inflammation or its sequelae and, hence, productive of symptoms. The acute inflammatory disease is *diverticulitis.* Diverticular disease can sometimes give rise to grave *diverticular complications.* Again, it is emphasized that diverticulosis is common (and often unjustly maligned); diverticular disease, including diverticulitis and its complications, is relatively infrequent.

Until the present century, diverticular disease was looked upon as a rather rare pathologic curiosity of little clinical significance.

The classic account by Telling and Gruner[4] contains an early bibliography. Hurst[5] credits Jean Cruveilhier (1791–1874), the renowned French pathologist, with the earliest description[6] of the disease in 1849, although the first mention may have been by Matthew Baillie in 1793.[7]

There are 2 reasons why early authors paid little heed to the condition. The first is that in years past diverticula were doubtless less common than now; in part, this was because of a predominantly younger population at that time. Moreover, some have contended that the emergence of diverticula followed the introduction of steel rolling mills for pulverizing grain in the late 19th century. The second reason is that before the advent of contrast radiography, at the turn of the century, clinicians had no reliable means of detecting either diverticula or diverticular disease, usually a nonfatal affliction in the living patient.

A common misunderstanding requires a note to be made that "diverticulum" is a Latin term derived from *divertere* "to turn a different way." The *-icul* indicates a diminutive, and *-um* of the noun is the neuter singular ending. A single outpouching is a diverticul*um;* 2 or more are diverticul*a* (*not* diverticuli or diverticulae).

Pathologic Anatomy

Macroscopic Features. The muscular wall of the colon, in common with the alimentary tract generally, is formed by an inner circular layer and outer longitudinal fibers. However, the colon is exceptional in that, while the circular muscle completely surrounds the wall, the longitudinal component consists of 3 distinct bands or *taeniae* extending from the base of the appendix to the rectum (Chapter 131). It is through separations in thickened fascicles of circular muscle and between the *taeniae* that diverticula protrude (Fig. 135–1).

Gross Appearance. Typically, diverticula occur in 2 rows on either side of the colon, frequently clustered in the sigmoid segment, but they can appear anywhere around the circumference and in any segment of the colon; rarely do diverticula protrude from the rectum. Usually globular or fusiform, their average diameter is 0.5 cm to 1 cm, but they can vary in size from a barely perceptible dimple to sacs 2 cm or larger. So-called "giant" diverticula probably in most cases are cyst-like, juxtacolonic spaces representing sites of perforation (these are described in the section on complications). Diverticula are connected to the bowel lumen by necks of varying lengths and calibers.

In many instances, diverticula are enveloped by pericolic fat in such a way that at first glance, at operation or at necropsy, they are concealed. When the colon is opened, it may be difficult to find communication between each diverticulum and the intestinal lumen, particularly if there have been previous attacks of diverticulitis. Fecaliths frequently occupy diverticula in the sigmoid segment; their presence does not indicate diverticular disease. It is possible for a diverticulum to invaginate the lumen (become turned inside out) and assume the appearance of a polyp. Colonoscopists have learned to be wary of this unusual configuration.

Diverticula tend to cluster in the sigmoid colon, mainly in its middle and proximal parts. It is unusual, at least in Western populations, for diverticula to appear in the proximal colon and yet be absent from the sigmoid segment. They may occur singly or be widely and densely disseminated throughout the large intestine but are rarely seen in the rectum. The approximate distribution of diverticula in the colon is shown in Figure 135–2.

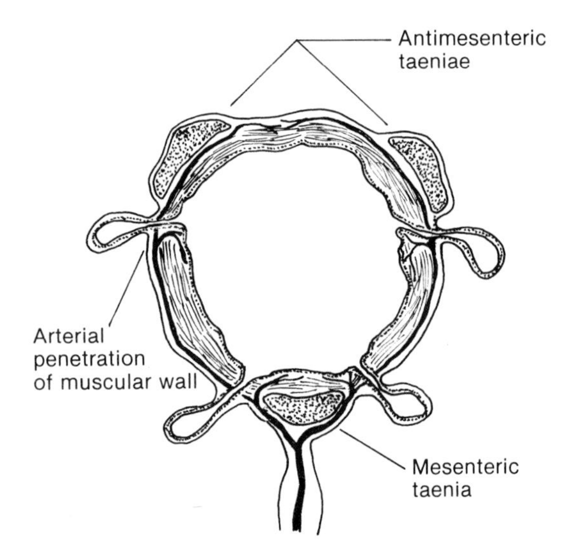

Figure 135–1. Diverticula tend to protrude where nutrient arteries penetrate the circular muscle layer. Most diverticula emerge between the mesenteric and antimesenteric taeniae. The intimate association of diverticula and penetrating arteries explains, in part, the proclivity of diverticula to bleeding (see Fig. 135–15).

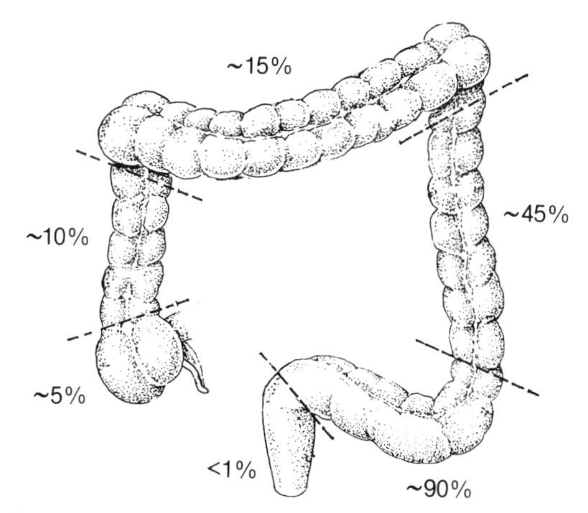

Figure 135–2. Spatial distribution of diverticula in serial segments of the colon, according to previous tabulations of large groups.[8, 9] Comparable up-to-date figures have not been compiled. Probably the distribution has not altered greatly, but with the increasing popularity of high-fiber diets it will be interesting to learn if a change will be effected, particularly a lesser preponderence of diverticula in the sigmoid segment.

In the proximal colon, a diverticulum may be isolated and single. As a general rule, with progression of the condition, the number of diverticula in a given segment increases and the linear extent of involvement lengthens. This is not to say that diverticula naturally or necessarily come to occupy a greater linear extent of the colon. In many instances, diverticula, once established in the sigmoid colon, remain relatively unchanged through the years.

Microscopic Features. A typical uncomplicated diverticulum extends in a flask-like configuration through the muscle layer of the colon. The wall of the diverticulum consists only of mucosa and submucosal connective tissue and, in its base, pericolic connective tissue and serosa. The neck of the "flask" is in continuity with the surface epithelium of the colon lumen and is situated between fascicles of circular smooth muscle. The mucosal protrusion is globular or piriform. The lining mucosa differs from that of the normal colon only in being more frequently underlaid by focal accumulations of lymphocytes, sometimes in follicular configuration. Aside from the diverticulum itself, the most conspicuous feature of the bowel wall is thickening, often marked, of the adjacent muscularis propria. This is an almost invariable feature.[10, 11] No abnormality has been observed in the neural components.[11]

Complicating inflammation may distort or even obliterate the affected diverticulum. Even within a cluster, usually only 1 or at most several diverticula are inflamed at a given time. Inflammation initially consists of a peridiverticular infiltration by neutrophils, which later may be replaced by mononuclear cells. Inflammation spreads into the pericolic fat and connective tissue, often with the formation of small or large abscesses. Occasionally giant cells appear, presumably in response to contamination by feces. A fortuitously selected section of the affected bowel may show the microperforation which has stimulated the inflammatory reaction (Fig. 135–3). When inflammation subsides, the only markers may be the thick muscular coat, focal fibrosis, and a heavier investment by pericolic fat.

It is doubtful, pathologically, that a state of truly chronic inflammation exists with any appreciable frequency. For practical purposes, the inflammatory reaction is either active or has subsided (an exception would be the case of an unresolved pericolic abcess). This is one of the reasons why inflammation has been reported to be absent in as many as one-third of specimens surgically resected because of "diverticulitis."[10] The other reason is that symptoms prompting operation may have been due solely to spasm of the thickened muscle wall.

In segments of colon resected because of diverticular hemorrhage, evidence of concomitant inflammation is conspicuously absent. In sections of such a specimen, one may or may not be able to identify the bleeding vessel.

Prevalence

There are striking differences in prevalence of colon diverticula in various geographic areas of the world. One can argue that the true prevalence of diverticula can never be known until an entire population is subject to meticulous barium enema examination or necropsy. Because these procedures are less often done in certain developing countries, the prevalence of diverticular disease may have been somewhat underestimated. However, this consideration, in itself, cannot account for the clearly evident rarity of the condition in many parts of the world.

The presence of colon diverticula among residents of Western countries bears a

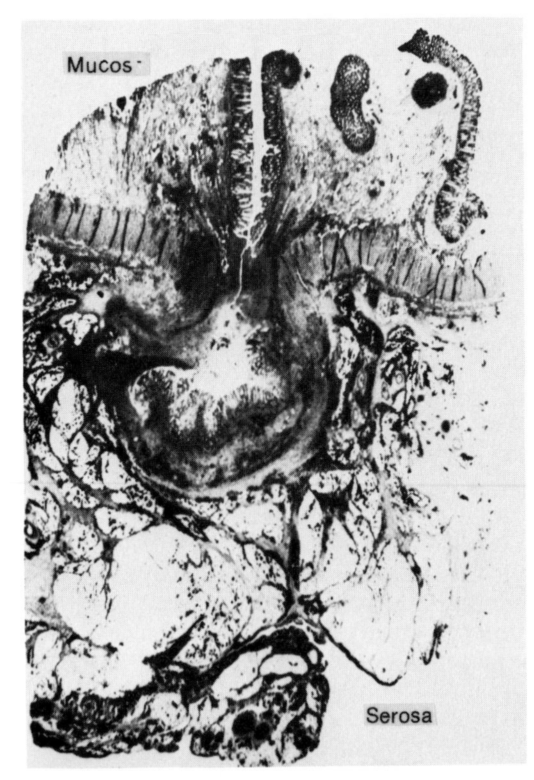

Figure 135–3. A 34-year-old woman was admitted because of symptoms interpreted as almost classic for acute appendicitis. At operation the appendix was normal. Careful search disclosed a single, inflamed diverticulum of the proximal transverse colon, buried in the omentum. Segmental resection and primary anastomosis were accomplished. In a subsequent barium enema examination, no diverticula were apparent in the sigmoid colon. The microscopic features conform with those described in the text. The supposition is that this diverticulum, in this young patient, was congenital rather than acquired. In this instance, the muscular coat through which the diverticulum protrudes is of normal thickness. Perforation appears to have occurred at the side of the diverticulum, just below its neck.

straight-line relation to age, reaching a peak of about 50% among persons in the ninth decade of life[11] (Fig. 135–4). Men and women are nearly equally affected. Diverticular disease, while less frequently encountered in persons under the age of 40 years, nevertheless is relatively more troublesome and more likely to require a surgical remedy in younger patients.[12]

The condition is relatively uncommon, even rare, in Africa, Asia, and many parts of South America. This is true even taking into account a lower average age of populations in these areas. It is interesting to note that there appears to be an increasing prevalence of diverticular disease among urbanized South African blacks.[13] Diverticular disease is seldom encountered in Japan; when it occurs, the site more often is in the proximal rather than the distal segments of the colon.[14]

Burkitt,[15] who served many years as a physician in Africa, gained fame by proclaiming diverse dietary habits as a major reason for demographic differences. The African native subsists on a diet high in vegetable fiber content and low in refined carbohydrates; for the denizens of Western cities the reverse is true. But other genetic and environmental factors would have to be considered, too. Be that as it may, real and significant differences in the prevalence of diverticula and diverticular disease exist.

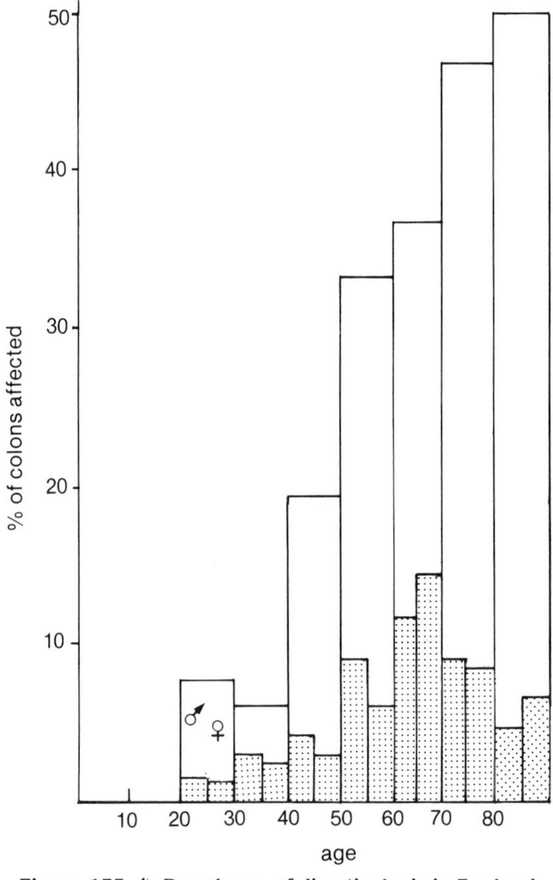

Figure 135–4. Prevalence of diverticulosis in England, according to the age of the population surveyed. The shaded bars indicate the fractions of patients (men on the left, women on the right, in each column) so afflicted who presented with symptoms referable to diverticular disease. (Adapted from data reported by Parks TG. Clin Gastroenterol 1975; 4:53–69.)

This can be observed, too, among diverse populations occupying the same geographic area. For example, de la Vega[16] cited the striking difference in occurrence of diverticula and diverticular disease in Mexico among the mostly native Indian patients treated at the Municipal Hospital Juarez (diverticular disease was nearly nonexistent) and among patients of almost purely Spanish extraction treated at the private Hospital Español (diverticula were noted in 9.2%). These 2 groups of patients differed sharply in dietary custom as well as in racial origin, sharing only a common area of residence.

According to Eusebio and Eisenberg,[12] diverticular disease accounted for 1.3% of hospital admissions in Minneapolis.

Pathogenesis

Man is the only animal known to develop diverticulosis coli in the natural state. Moreover, in addition to man, only the colons of primates, horses, guinea pigs, and rabbits are featured by taeniae coli, a construction conducive to mucosal outpouching. Probably it is significant that all of these species, except for man, are herbivorous. In the laboratory, diverticulosis coli can be produced in rabbits and guinea pigs only by highly contrived means. Because of these facts, the study of diverticular disease in experimental animals has been sharply limited.[17]

Painter[18] joined with Burkitt to be among the first to ascribe diverticula of the colon to modern Western culture and its custom of a highly refined diet. According to this thesis, sustained bowel contraction consequent to a lack of dietary residue increases intraluminal pressure, which then leads to diverticular outpouching. Burkitt[15] extended the onus of a fiber-deficient diet to include appendicitis, colon cancer, hemorrhoids, and varicose veins. In response, Mendeloff[19] urged caution in singling out diet as a sole cause of so many maladies in differing populations.

Those who implicate a fiber-deficient diet in the pathogenesis of diverticula and diverticular disease relate diet to its effect on stooling patterns. Persons consuming a high-fiber diet tend to exhibit faster intestinal transit (hence, more frequent stools and less fecal stasis) and increased collective stool weight. These features are assumed to lessen a tendency to diverticular formation and complications therefrom. The statistical association is impressive. Yet, Eastwood and his associates[20] found in 60 patients with diverticular disease that prolonged intestinal transit, increased luminal pressure, and reduced fecal weight were not significantly different than observed in the general population. These authors suggested that where these features correlated with diverticular disease, they might be the consequence rather than the cause.

The factor of low-volume fecal stasis might explain the development of diverticula such as commonly cluster in the sigmoid and descending segments of the colon. But what of diverticula that not infrequently occur sporadically or in clusters along the transverse or ascending segments or in the cecum? Here the lumen is more capacious, the muscular wall seldom thickened, and luminal pressures are lower. It would seem obvious that yet another factor, that of focal weakness in the bowel wall, probably associated with aging, must pertain. A general debility in connective tissue might help to explain the postulated association of diverticulosis coli with diverticula and hernia elsewhere, as cited by de la Vega.[16] It is interesting to note, moreover, that diverticula occur early and commonly in patients with certain connective tissue disorders, such as Marfan's and Ehlers-Danlos syndromes.[1]

Mention has been made of the consistency with which thickening in the muscular wall accompanies most diverticula in the colon.[10,11] (Fig. 135–5). Whether this is hyperplasia or hypertrophy of muscle has been debated and is unresolved. Again the question of cause or result is raised. Do hypertonicity and thickening of the muscular wall precede the occurrence of diverticula? Or, does the presence of diverticula result in a contraction and foreshortening of the affected segment that gives the appearance of muscular thickening? Either is theoretically possible; neither is supported by hard evidence.

Speculation in this regard prompts the question of what relation, if any, pertains between colon diverticula and the irritable bowel syndrome. In Western countries, both conditions are prevalent, and it is hardly surprising that the 2 conditions would coexist in a substantial portion of the population (Fig. 135–6). Is this coincidence or pathogenesis? To Connell,[21] long a student of both diverticular disease and the irritable bowel (and to most of the rest of us), the

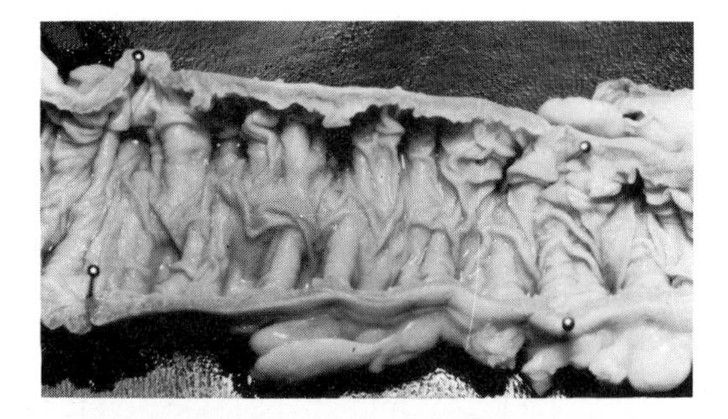

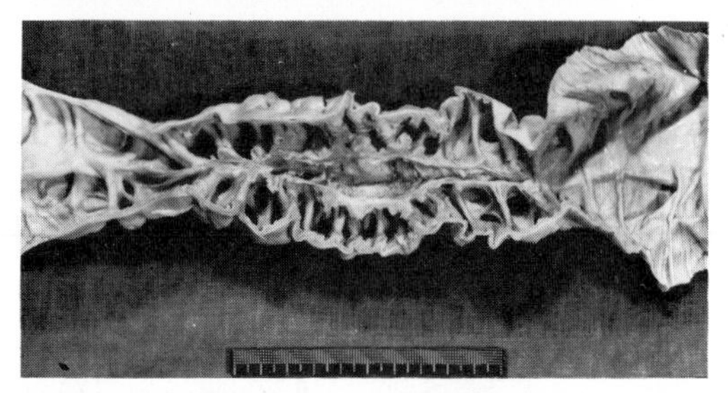

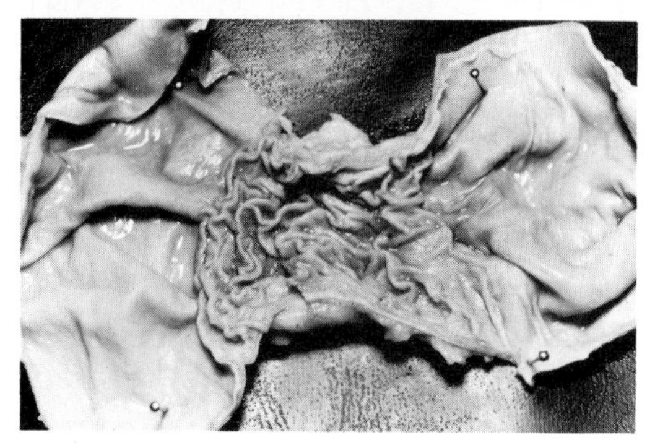

Figure 135–5. Characteristically, bands of circular muscle become thickened and separated (*top*), often constricting the lumen from which an array of diverticular sacs protrude (*middle*). In some cases, contracture involves both circular and longitudinal muscle bands (*bottom*). (Polysiloxane enema technique; photographs of specimens from Hughes LE. Gut 1969; 10:344–351. Reproduced with permission.)

issue remains unsettled. In Parks' series[22] of 521 patients with diverticular disease, nearly half described erratic bowel action that might have been attributable to an irritable bowel, yet over half the patients had bowel symptoms for less than a month before a diagnosis of diverticular disease was made. From another perspective, Holmes and Salter[23] reported that once a diagnosis of irritable bowel syndrome was established, it remained unchanged in all but 4 of 77 patients followed 6 years or longer. In this group at least, diverticular disease was not a sequel to an irritable bowel. Nevertheless, it has been noted by Connell[21] and others that the colon harboring diverticula can exhibit aberrant motility in a manner similar to that of the irritable bowel, particularly an exaggerated tonic response to meals and cholinergic stimuli.

Wynne-Jones[24] has offered a novel postulate for the pathogenesis of diverticular disease. He suggests the condition is related to the unnecessary retention of excessive flatus and the high intraluminal bowel pressure thereby induced. In support of his thesis, Wynne-Jones points out that both retention of flatus and diverticular disease are characteristic of modern urban society. Moreover, the peak prevalence of diverticular disease tends to coincide with that of "adult social consciousness," then declines in later decades of life, possibly, according to Wynne-Jones, "owing to the onset of anal laxity."

Diverticular disease of the colon has been reported to occur with a frequency greater than expected in association with other lesions as well. In years past, reference was made to Saint's Triad, a co-existence of hiatus hernia, cholelithiasis, and diverticulosis coli. The pathogenesis, shared with hiatus hernia, was presumed to be a defect in supporting connective tissue. Many clinicians have thought of Saint's Triad as the mere coincidence of 3 common conditions; however, Capron et al.[25] recently reported that in 2 matched groups, each of 102 patients, one with diverticulosis and one without, the frequency of cholelithiasis was 45% and 22%,

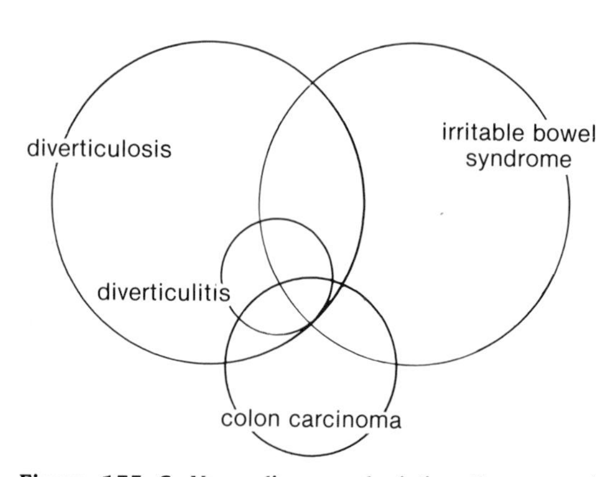

Figure 135–6. Venn diagram depicting the approximate coincident relations between certain conditions frequently affecting the colon. There is substantial overlap between patients harboring diverticula and those exhibiting the irritable bowel syndrome, even though no cause-and-effect relation is known to pertain. In some patients, diverticulitis and carcinoma coexist, again in the absence of any causal association.

respectively. The difference was especially significant in women. A postulated link between diverticula and gallstones might be a high-carbohydrate, low-residue diet; a high-residue diet is said to stimulate endogenous chenodeoxycholic acid and inhibit HMG-CoA reductase that controls synthesis of cholesterol. Thus, it is conceivable that a high-residue diet might, in the long run, protect against both the formation of diverticula and gallstones. Gear et al.[26] observed that in Oxford, England, diverticulosis coli was 3 times more prevalent among omnivorous citizens than among vegetarians.

Diverticula were found in the colons of 10 of 12 patients with renal impairment due to polycystic kidney disease, according to Scheff et al.[27]

Outpouchings of the colon wall, different from those of ordinary diverticulosis, can occur in patients with Crohn's colitis[28] (Chapter 127) and systemic sclerosis (Chapter 244). The wide-mouthed diverticula associated with systemic sclerosis, it may additionally be noted, rarely, if ever, give rise to complications.

A truly inflammatory state of diverticulitis may be explained as follows: constriction of circular muscle in the bowel wall, acting as a collar, is conducive to fecal stasis. Fecal pellets tend to become inspissated within diverticular sacs. Wide-necked sacs empty readily and rarely become inflamed. The lack of a muscular coat in the diverticular pouch impairs ejection of offending fecaliths from narrow-necked sacs. Contrary to former concern, diverticular occlusion rarely, if ever, can be attributed to vegetable seeds or other ingesta. Reactive inflammation in the neck of the sac with associated edema further occludes luminal communication. Under these circumstances, microperforation of the injured diverticular mucosa leads to contamination and infection of the pericolic tissues. This is a process similar to that of obstructive inflammation in the vermiform appendix (Chapter 144).

By virtue of serosal and peritoneal defenses, the inflammatory reaction usually is promptly walled off and thereby contained. Localized suppuration may coalesce as an abscess. A much graver threat is breakdown in local defense and perforation with contamination of the peritoneal cavity.[29] Adjacent structures may adhere to the inflamed colon and the result can be fistulas to the urinary bladder, other intestinal segments, adjacent vascular structures, the vagina, the abdominal wall, and even to the epidural space.[30]

A tendency for the appendices epiploicae to become involved accounts for much of the stiffness and swelling of the affected segment. In some instances the suppurative changes are those of a pericolic phlegmon. Impingement on the lumen and subsequent scarring can lead to partial or complete obstruction and may mimic neoplastic infiltration.

It is important to note that this sequence of events, constituting a true diverticulitis, is an *extra*luminal process. Infection is essentially intramural and periserosal, producing a pericolitis; it is not luminal or mucosal.

Diagnosis

Clinical Symptoms and Signs. The mere presence of innocent, uncomplicated diverticula in a colon gives rise to no characteristic or significant symptoms. This, while long and well known, has been recently confirmed by Thompson and his colleagues in Ottawa.[31] Because of the previously described association of muscular hypertonicity in diverticulosis, such symptoms as might be proffered by patients with uncomplicated diverticula are indistinguishable from those of patients exhibiting the irritable colon syndrome. It is important to remember that the irritable colon syndrome can be marked by peaks of activity which can be easily mistaken for flares of diverticulitis. Conversely, mild attacks of diverticulitis can go unnoticed or might be interpreted as acute exacerbations of the irritable bowel syndrome. In most instances the distinction is of little more than academic interest because the initial management in both conditions would be essentially the same.

The significant problem is to recognize truly inflammatory complications of diverticular disease. In actual diverticulitis, pain becomes more severe and persists, usually in the left lower abdominal quadrant and hypogastrium. Changes of intra-abdominal pressure caused by voluntary contraction of the abdominal musculature may aggravate the pain. Frequently, the pain extends to the low back. Intermittently, severe cramping pain may be attended by nausea and vomiting. Either diarrhea or constipation may usher in the attack. Tenesmus may be severe and mucus is noted in the stools of some patients, but visible hematochezia rarely attends acute diverticulitis. Fever, often spiking and punctuated by chills, is commonplace.

Palpation of the abdomen evokes tenderness over the affected bowel, usually in the left lower quadrant and occasionally across the entire hypogastrium. As in cases of irritable or spastic colon, the outline of the distal colon is often felt as a tender, rope-like mass. When the "colonic rope" is only minimally tender and freely movable, the correct diagnosis is likely to be colonic irritability. If the sausage-like mass is large, markedly tender, and fixed, then an acute suppurative pericolitis is likely. When serosal inflammation occurs, involuntary muscle guarding in the abdominal wall often hampers deep palpation (which is fortunate because brusque massaging would be hazardous) and signals peritoneal irritation. Pertinent physical examination is completed by a gentle digital palpation of the rectum. Often tender induration is felt at the fingertip, and occasionally a firm mass simulating Blumer's shelf is encountered.

The laboratory is of limited help in the assessment of diverticular disease. Leukocytosis bolsters a clinical impression of suppurative complication but is not to be construed as diagnostic, either by its presence or absence.

Sigmoidoscopy and Colonoscopy. With evidence of an acute, fulminating diverticulitis, sigmoidoscopy may not be required. *It should never be performed with air insufflation* (Chapter 42). In less acute circumstances, sigmoidoscopy can help to rule out carcinoma or inflammatory lesions with which diverticulitis may be confused, such as Crohn's disease or ulcerative colitis, irradiation colitis, invasive amebiasis, and bacillary dysentery. The orifices of the diverticula themselves are rarely seen within the range of the ordinary rigid 25-cm sigmoidoscope, and the rectal mucosa in diverticular disease can be expected to appear intact, smooth, and glistening. However, Buie[32] long ago described the following sigmoidoscopic findings as indirectly suggestive of diverticular disease: "(1) limited mobility of the low bowel segment which is normally freely movable, (2) abnormally sharp angulation in the region of the rectosigmoid or above, (3) narrowing of the lumen of the bowel, and (4) sigmoidal sacculations (shallow pouches that extend partially or entirely around the bowel and are separated by ridge-like elevations which are not obliterated by pressure)." Cooper[33] reported the presence of 1 or more of these findings in 58% of 151 cases of diverticulitis of the sigmoid. It should be mentioned, too, that the mucosa at the rectosigmoid junction is often congested and edematous. None of these sigmoidoscopic findings, of course, is pathognomonic.

Sigmoidoscopic examination can be helpful in assessing the condition of the rectosigmoid distal to the lesion with a view to surgical treatment. If the bowel appears normal throughout the extent visible through the 25-cm sigmoidoscope, and an operation is eventually required, the surgeon may confidently count on a distal segment suitable for anastomosis.

The advent of fiberoptic colonoscopy has furnished another useful tool in the differential diagnosis of diverticular disease (Chapter 43). With the extent of the large intestinal lumen visible by flexible colonoscopy, the orifices of diverticula in the affected segment can be plainly evident, the lumen often appearing as the interior of a flute (Fig. 135–7). If the examination is deemed advisable, extreme caution must be exercised. A sigmoid segment sharply angulated or unyieldingly fixed as a result of inflammatory distortion is liable to injury at colonoscopy. Air should be insufflated only with extreme caution, if at all. Colonoscopy probably is of prime value in the detection of bleeding which can emanate from otherwise seemingly uncomplicated diverticula.

Colonoscopy has been shown to resolve uncertainty in the interpretation of barium

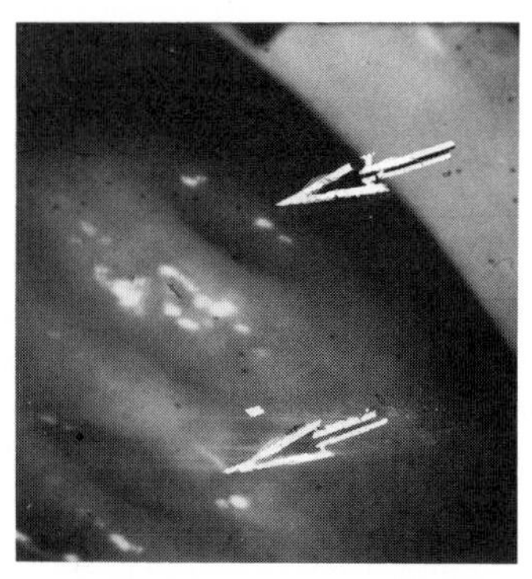

Figure 135–7. The arrows point to 2 of a series of diverticular orifices as seen through the colonoscope.

enema examination when a question of neoplasm has been raised.[34, 35] However, if the issue is a fixed distortion of the sigmoid segment wherein the differential diagnosis is between diverticulitis and carcinoma, colonoscopy probably would be superfluous; the indication for surgical resection pertains in either case.

Radiographic Features. Barium enema examination usually affords the best means of demonstrating the presence of diverticula in the colon. As a general rule, if the purpose of the examination is to seek the presence or extent of diverticular disease, barium enema by the single-contrast, solid-column procedure is preferable to the double-contrast technique with air insufflation. Diverticula and their relation to the bowel wall are more clearly delineated when the colon is filled with barium alone. The double-contrast technique with air insufflation should not be attempted if active diverticulitis is expected, because of the danger of perforation.[36]

Diverticula appear as globular, barium-containing extrusions beyond the normal contour of the colon. Sometimes it is surprising how inconstant these extrusions may appear in various radiographic exposures of the same colon at the same examination. Occasionally, the sacs are not seen when the barium-filled colon is hypertonic but are well demonstrated when the segment is relaxed and distended (Fig. 135–8). The postevacuation film is of decided importance in that some barium-filled diverticular sacs will be noted which were obscured or otherwise inapparent in films taken when the colon was filled. At certain phases in their development, diverticula may be of changeable configuration; they can appear in 1 barium enema series and then fail to appear in a subsequent examination, and vice versa.[37] Frequently, the sacs retain barium for several days or longer after barium enema, even when the main lumen of the colon is clear. Such retention is not to be construed as evidence of complicating disease. Residual clumps of barium along the anatomic course of the colon can be confusing when, as often is the case, a barium meal examination follows a barium enema.

A plain or scout film of the abdomen should precede the barium enema, particularly in the examination of a patient with recent pain (Chapter 32). A scout film can help to exclude other possible causes of an attack simulating diverticular disease, e.g., renal or ureteral calculus, volvulus or other forms of bowel obstruction, ileus resulting from acute vascular compromise, soft tissue masses, or free peritoneal air.

Barium enema examination is not necessarily contraindicated by the suspected presence of diverticulitis, but when undertaken, it should be performed with extraordinary caution to avoid perforation. In most cases of acute diverticulitis, immediate barium enema examination is unnecessary; it is properly deferred a week or longer so as to allow bolstering of the weakened bowel wall. If, as barium is being introduced, a point of obstruction is encountered, the flow of barium should be stopped, even though the remaining proximal colon is left unexamined. Not only is there risk in attempting to force barium above an obstruction, but the barium sequestered proximal to an obstructed segment can seriously complicate a needed surgical procedure.

While the radiologist usually is adept at demonstrating the presence of diverticula in the colon, he is less able to distinguish accurately between diverticulosis, diverticulitis, and carcinoma, particularly when these conditions are conjoined. Schnyder and his San Francisco colleagues[38] reported 92% radiographic accuracy in detecting the presence of diverticula, 82% accuracy in identifying diverticulitis (a remarkable achievement), and only 50% accuracy in clearly distinguishing diverticular disease and carcinoma. The clinician must assume ultimate responsibility for resolving the differential diagnosis.

Supervening inflammation, because it is pericolic, often cannot be discerned in barium enema radiographs. With the possible exception of an isolated diverticulum in the right colon (discussed later), complete absence of diverticula in a well-filled colon means that a diagnosis of diverticulitis is nigh untenable. It is true that an acutely inflamed, edematous diverticulum will not fill with barium and, hence, may be inapparent. But where there is a cluster of diverticula, seldom are all sacs involved, and almost invariably a few will accept barium and thus betray the nature of the disease.

There are only 2 radiographic signs of actual diverticulitis, and neither is pathognomonic. One is the demonstration of extraluminal barium at a segment occupied by diverticula, and the other is a fixed, eccentric,

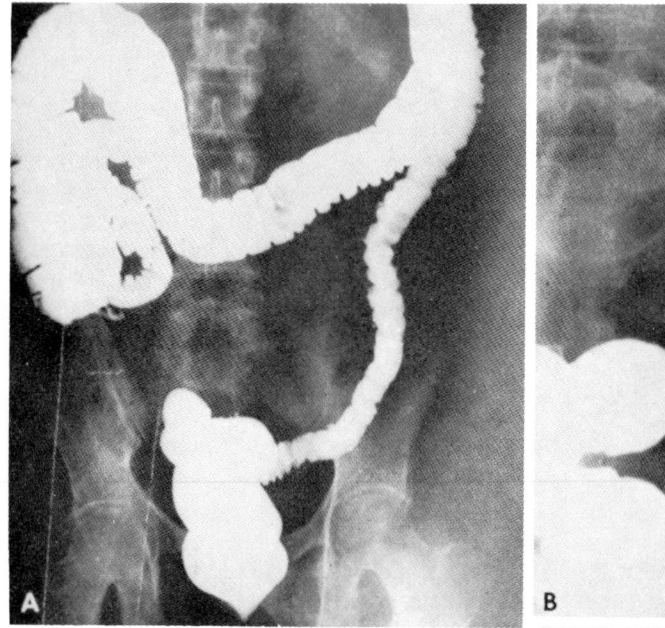

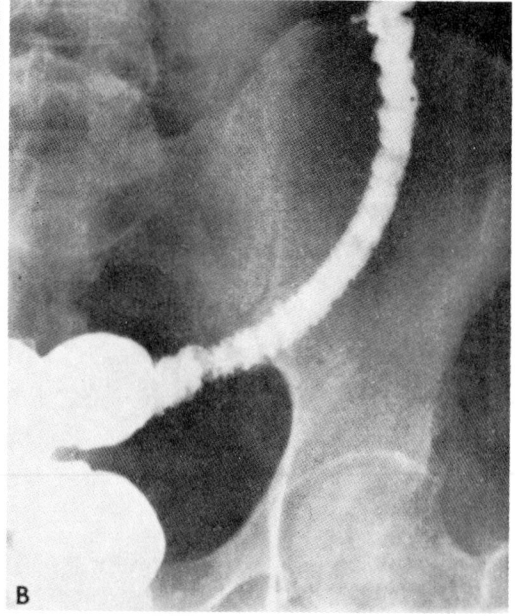

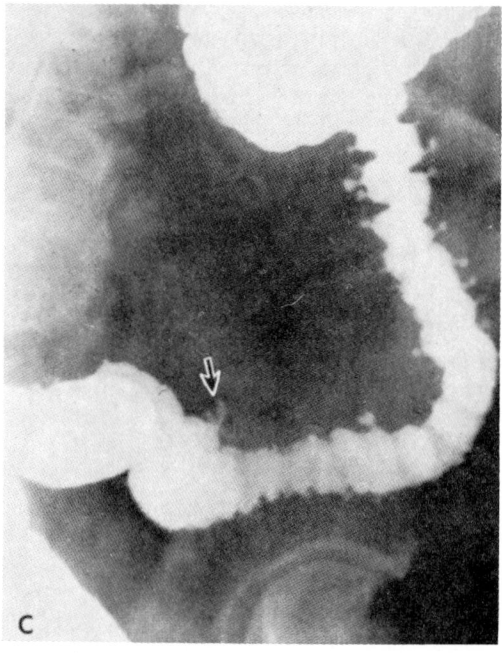

Figure 135–8. These barium enema radiographs, taken of a 40-year-old physician during a single examination, illustrate the inconsistency in appearance of diverticula. *A* and *B* show hypertonicity in the distal colon, but only 1 or 2 diverticula are evident. With further distention and partial relaxation (*C*), numerous small sacs appear; one is partly filled, probably with a fecal fragment (*arrow*).

subtractive defect in the barium column that is produced by an impinging inflammatory mass (Fig. 135–9; also see Figs. 135–12 and 135–14). There is yet another configuration that may, in some cases, signify active or healed diverticulitis. This is the presence of 1 or more fixed, deep, sharply pointed incisuras along 1 side of the barium column (Fig. 135–10) as described many years ago by Willard and Bockus.[39] Often, the incisura points toward diverticula extending from the opposite bowel margin. The focal contraction of the bowel wall is thought to arise in much the same fashion as that of the so-called "opposite incisura" seen on the greater curve of the stomach that points to an ulcer on the lesser curve. The defect probably develops from contraction and spasm of circular muscle bundles opposite the site of an inflamed diverticulum. Fibrotic changes can result in a fixed incisura.

Extended areas of luminal constriction as-

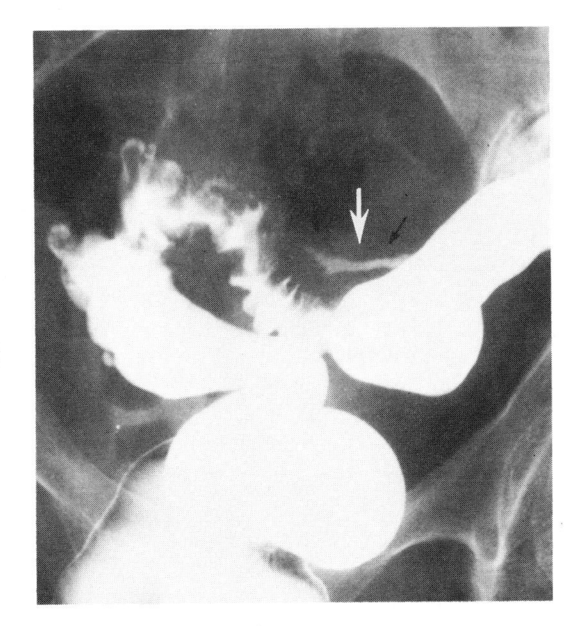

Figure 135–9. Classic signs of diverticulitis are seen in this barium enema radiograph focused on the rectosigmoid segment. The arrow points to a streak of extraluminal barium signifying perforation. Below this is a concave impression on the sigmoid segment, representing impingement by an inflammatory mass.

sociated with irregular, jagged margins and mucosal distortion denote a segment of diffuse inflammation of the bowel wall. Extension of reaction into the appendices epiploicae can also contribute to this appearance. Such configuration may be difficult to distinguish from Crohn's disease. A lengthy segment (>8 cm) so distorted, however, would unlikely be the seat of a neoplasm. Barium extending beyond the contour of the affected segment may signify a sinus tract or fistula. Such a configuration often is more apparent in the postevacuation film than in exposures of the barium-filled colon.

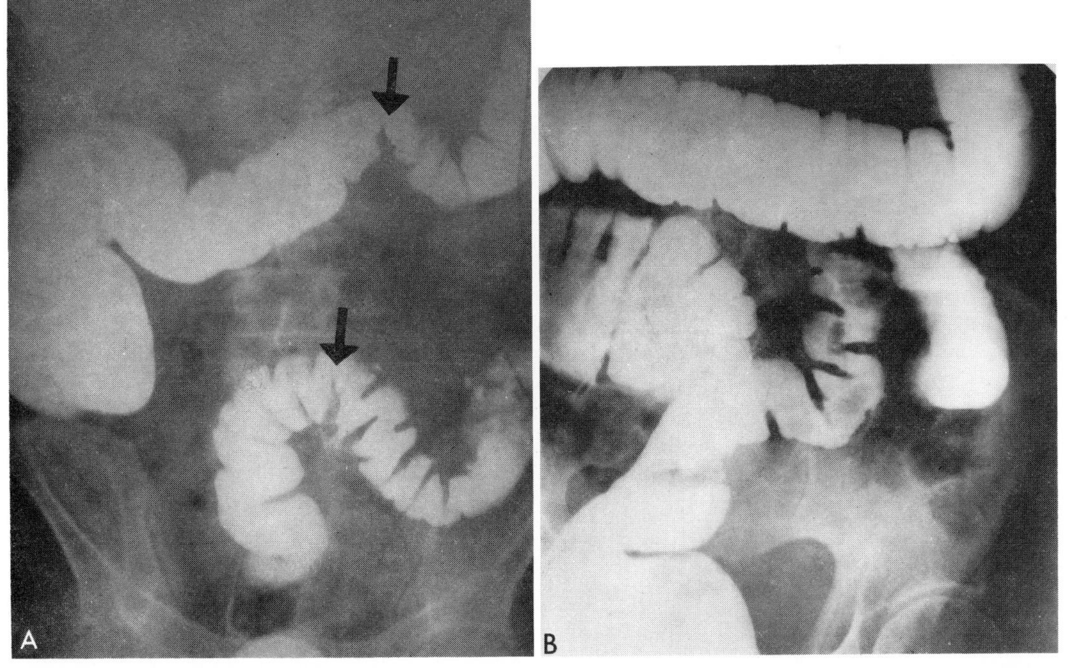

Figure 135–10. *A*, Deep incisural defects in the sigmoid and transverse segments of the colon *(arrows)* in a patient who had recurring attacks of diverticulitis simulating partial bowel obstruction. *B*, Another example of fixed incisurae in the colon of a patient who several weeks earlier had sustained a severe bout of sigmoid diverticulitis.

Segmental constriction or irregularity due to circular muscle spasm may be distinquished from the fixed distortion resulting from inflammation or scarring by the use of glucagon administered IV in a dose of 1 mg at the time of barium enema. Glucagon produces a prompt, dramatic, although transient relaxation of smooth muscle in the wall of the bowel (Fig. 135–11). Its lack of undesirable side-effects makes glucagon far superior to anticholinergic drugs for this purpose.

It should be emphasized that the presence of a few colonic diverticula in a barium enema radiograph ought not blind the examiner to the possibility of a more serious lesion lurking elsewhere in the colon. Never should the mere demonstration of diverticula, in the absence of sound clinical evidence, be construed as necessarily constituting an explanation for a patient's symptoms. Also, as will be explained later, never should the presence of colonic diverticula be assumed as the cause of anemia due to occult intestinal blood loss.

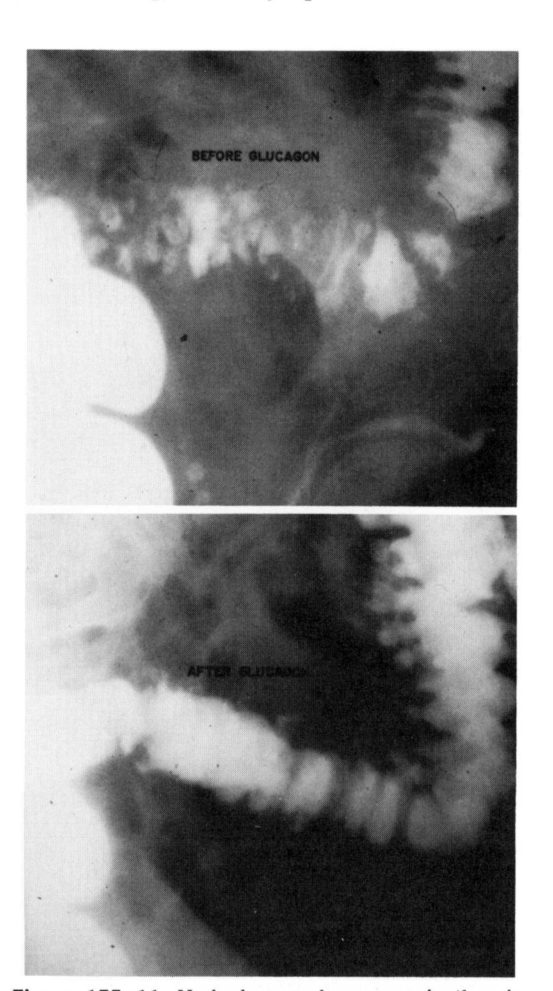

Figure 135–11. Marked muscular spasm in the sigmoid colon *(above)*, which might be confused with the configuration of diverticulitis, disappears within minutes after the IV injection of glucagon *(below)*.

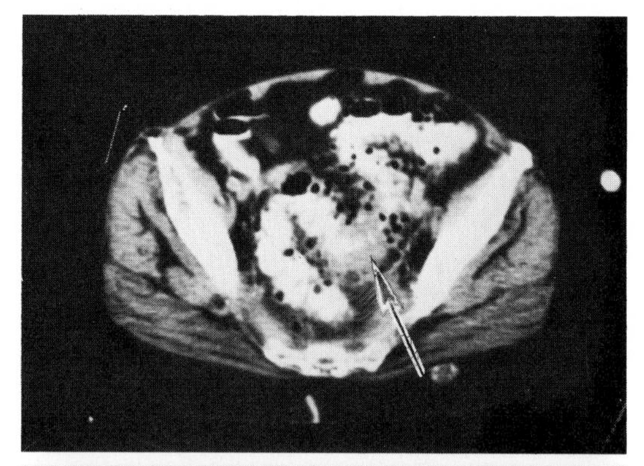

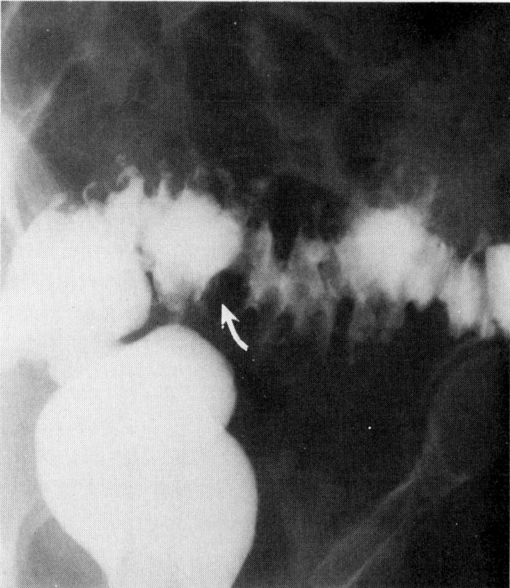

Figure 135–12. Computed tomographic findings in diverticulitis associated with an abdominal mass. *Above*, An 80-year-old woman was admitted because of fever and a tender hypogastric mass; she had recurring isolated episodes of fever and lower abdominal pain for a number of years. The density adjacent to the contrast-filled lumen of the sigmoid colon denotes abscess (*arrow*); numerous focal lucencies represent diverticula. *Below*, Diverticula, together with impingement on the contour of the sigmoid, also are apparent in a barium enema examination performed shortly thereafter.

Because the patient with diverticular disease often will present with an abdominal mass, ultrasonography or computed tomography (CT) may be chosen as a preliminary imaging procedure. Ultrasonography may permit delineation of an abscess cavity; CT scanning may provide a fairly characteristic picture of inflammatory diverticular disease (Fig. 135–12).

Differential Diagnosis

This can be challenging, both in terms of considering diverticular disease as a possible cause of a patient's symptoms and also in properly assessing the role of diverticula when they co-exist with other lesions. In cases warranting surgical intervention, differential diagnosis may be resolved only at the operating table.

Carcinoma. This often poses the most disturbing dilemma because both diverticular disease and carcinoma can co-exist. Morton and Goldman[40] reported neoplasm, benign or malignant, concomitant with diverticulitis in 19% of 141 patients. Conversely, of 180 patients with sigmoid carcinoma, 19% also had diverticulosis or diverticulitis. It is not necessary to assign a cause-and-effect relationship to account for the co-existence of these 2 diseases in the sigmoid colon. Usually, neoplasia does not originate in a diverticulum but in an area of the bowel devoid of a sac. Furthermore, both diseases are relatively common, occur in patients of the same age groups, and frequently involve the same bowel segment, notably the sigmoid.

Barium enema often has the greatest value in differential diagnosis. The following features are described in order of their importance:

1. Annular constriction associated with typical collaring at one or both extremities of a short, deformed segment is almost pathognomonic of carcinoma. This radiographic configuration is rarely simulated by diverticulitis or its complications.

2. The deformities or defects due to diverticulitis are covered by a relatively intact mucosa, whereas in carcinoma there is usually defacement of normal mucosal architecture.

3. The defect in carcinoma usually has sharply defined limits or borders. In diverticulitis the involved segment is often longer, and its limits are less well demarcated. If a sizable subtractive defect is present in complicated diverticulitis, its border is less distinct in outline.

4. In diverticulitis, repeating the examination after a short period of treatment may result in a substantial lessening of the apparent deformity as the irritability, inflammation, and edema subside. The radiographic defect produced by carcinoma is relatively immutable.

While colonoscopy can be helpful in resolving the differential diagnosis in some cases, often the distortion of the affected segment precludes passage of the standard colonoscope or flexible sigmoidoscope. Sometimes this impediment can be overcome by inserting a small-caliber endoscope for inspection and biopsy. In other cases, it may be possible to obtain specimens for cytologic examination by cautiously brushing beyond the point of direct vision (Chapters 47 and 48).

Again the point is made that for cases wherein the radiographic configuration is such as to make a differential diagnosis impossible, there is seldom a need to pursue further invasive procedures. Surgical intervention is justified in any such case.

Acute Appendicitis. Inflammation in a vermiform appendix occupying the left lower abdominal quadrant or pelvis can simulate the clinical picture of acute diverticulitis of the sigmoid. Two complications of diverticular disease may be confused with ordinary acute appendicitis. One is solitary cecal diverticulitis, and the other is an acute diverticulitis in a loop of redundant sigmoid colon which has become adherent in the right lower abdominal quadrant. Statistically, acute appendicitis is more common than either of these conditions, particularly in younger patients; for that reason, appendicitis must take diagnostic precedence. A surgical remedy probably would be chosen in either case (Chapter 144).

We recently observed a case of a young woman found to have isolated, acute diverticulitis in the transverse colon (Fig. 135–3). Whenever acute appendicitis is suspected, but a normal appendix is found at operation, it behooves the surgeon to meticulously search the bowel for another lesion.

Diverticulitis itself has been described in the vermiform appendix. Eight patients with this lesion were reported by Rabinovitch et al.[41] Operation was performed because of a diagnosis of acute appendicitis.

Ulcerative Colitis. There is little reason to confuse ulcerative colitis with diverticular disease. A typical sigmoidoscopic picture and the radiographic signs of ulcerative colitis will serve to establish the diagnosis in most instances. Only rarely do the 2 diseases coexist (Chapter 126).

Crohn's Disease. Segmental enteritis of the colon, with its transmural and hyperplastic inflammatory reaction, may not be so easily distinguished from diverticulitis (Chapter

127). In a report from the St. Mark's Hospital in London, Schmidt et al.[42] described 26 cases in which both diverticular disease and Crohn's disease were present. Twenty-four of the 26 patients had anal lesions or rectovaginal fistulas; 23 showed mucosal involvement at proctosigmoidoscopic examination. In 1 patient the anus and rectum appeared clear, but the rectal biopsy was abnormal. These anorectal features were distinctive when the authors compared the Crohn's group with 50 patients requiring operation for ordinary diverticular disease of the colon.

Marshak,[43] after studying 10 patients in whom there were co-existing diverticula and Crohn's disease, established contrasting radiographic features by which the 2 conditions might be distinguished (Table 135–1).

Ischemic Colitis. Mesenteric vascular disease, both acute and chronic, can lead to a bowel reaction simulating diverticulitis. The chief point of distinction is the affected segment. The splenic flexure is often affected by ischemia, but rarely by diverticulitis. Both conditions can affect the sigmoid segment (Chapter 116).

Other Colon Diseases. Rarer conditions such as actinomycosis, syphilis, amebiasis, tuberculosis, lymphogranuloma venereum, irradiation enteritis, collagen disease, foreign body granuloma, and fecal impaction may give rise to ulcerative, inflammatory, and sometimes granulomatous lesions in the sigmoid or elsewhere in the colon with which diverticulitis might be confused. The reader is referred to the chapters devoted to these conditions for discussion of their distinctive features.

Pelvic Inflammatory Disease. Acute salpingitis, with all its ramifications, usually occurs in women younger than those affected by diverticular disease. A vaginal discharge, together with some irregularity of the menses, may indicate the true nature of the condition. Bowel symptoms are not rare in patients with pelvic inflammatory disease[44] but usually are not typical of those experienced with diverticular disease.

Management

Medical Measures

Diverticulosis. The mere presence of asymptomatic colonic diverticula, in the absence of inflammation or other complications, requires no specific treatment other than such prophylactic measures as may prevent diverticulitis. The obese patient is at a disadvantage and should be encouraged to embark on a weight-reducing program. Erratic bowel action, signifying intestinal motor disorder, is appropriately treated. The use of irritating cathartics and purgatives is forbidden. A sensible bowel regimen should be initiated, such as that advised in Chapter 134 for patients exhibiting functional bowel disorder. A helpful measure in the prophylactic management of diverticulosis is the regular and continuing dietary supplement of a hydrophilic, mucilaginous colloid. This has been borne out by controlled trial.[45] One or 2 teaspoons of a psyllium seed hydrophil daily will tend to prevent harsh constriction and to reduce pressure within the diverticula-laden bowel; this preparation will also pre-

Table 135–1. CONTRASTING RADIOGRAPHIC FEATURES OF DIVERTICULITIS AND CROHN'S COLITIS IN THE DESCENDING AND SIGMOID COLON*

Diverticulitis	Crohn's Colitis
Short process, 3 to 6 cm	Long, usually 10 cm or longer
Diverticula sharply defined; frequently contain fecaliths, but may on occasion simulate abscesses	Abscesses frequently have a triangular configuration but may at times be indistinguishable from the coexistent diverticula
When a diverticulum perforates, the abscess creates an extramural defect or an arcuate configuration of folds that stretch over the abscess	This is an ulcerating mucosal process; folds are straightened, perpendicular (like a picket fence); associated with a thick wall, increased secretions
No transverse fissures; folds may be straightened but more commonly have an arcuate configuration	Transverse fissures with marked edema of mucosa produce a stepladder configuration
A short paracolic tract may be seen occasionally in diverticulitis (usually associated with an extramural defect); on rare occasions a perforation may run parallel to the bowel wall	If a tract is seen, it is long, linear and located in the submucosa or muscular layers

*Based on data from Marshak RH: N Engl J Med 1970; *285*:1080.

vent feces from fragmenting and becoming inspissated in the pouches. Intestinal hypertonicity is so commonly present in diverticula bearers that any and all measures to overcome bowel irritability are well advised.

In years past, patients found to harbor diverticula often were admonished to adhere strictly to bland, low-residue diets. The pendulum of therapeutic fashion has today swung almost to the other extreme. Patients found with diverticula are advised to consume diets high in fiber content (the imprecision of the term "fiber" notwithstanding[46]). As Hall[47] has put it, everyone seems to have jumped on the "bran wagon." While anecdotal testimony abounds, purportedly randomized trials are few.[48–51] Most of these claim some measure of symptomatic benefit. (There can be no such thing as a "doubly-blinded" dietary trial.) Ornstein et al.[51] reported benefit limited to relief of constipation, a conclusion supported by Cann et al.[52] in a study of patients exhibiting the irritable bowel syndrome. Devroede and his Canadian colleagues[49] made the interesting observation that instruction in diet, whether high or low in fiber content, helped more to allay symptoms than no dietary instruction at all, thus confirming Hodgson's contention[53] that simply prescribing a "diet" exerts a favorable placebo effect.

Cummings et al.[54] have pointed out that a doubling of fecal weight is required to induce substantial decreases in intraluminal pressures in the distal colon. To accomplish this by diet alone requires the ingestion of 15 g to 20 g of fiber daily. This is not easily done (Table 135–2). Cello[55] points out that while unprocessed bran is the most efficient fiber supplement, it has "the consistency and palatability of redwood sawdust." Moreover, as many patients testify, bran is good for gas—it produces large volumes.

Table 135–2. AMOUNT OF SELECTED FOODSTUFFS REQUIRED TO PRODUCE 20 g of "FIBER" (AND DOUBLE THE DAILY STOOL WEIGHT)*

		Grams	Ounces
Unprocessed bran		45	1½
All Bran/Bran Buds	cereal brands	68	2¼
Bran Chex	cereal brands	135	4½
Total	cereal brands	270	9
Wholemeal bread		404	13½
Whole carrots		681	22½
Cabbage		775	26
Apples, fresh		1477	49

*Data from Cello.[55]

There is yet no convincing evidence that dietary manipulation alone significantly alters the course of diverticular disease one way or another. Therefore, as stated in the previous edition of this book, our position is that patients whose colons are found to bear diverticula, in the absence of acute inflammatory complication, should be permitted and encouraged to consume wholesome diets, unrestricted except for those items known from the patient's own personal experience to disrupt orderly bowel action or to induce abdominal discomfort.

If and when diverticula become diseased, both medical and surgical measures can be invoked, both contributing to a remedy, according to the individual needs of the patient.

Acute Diverticulitis. The ardor with which therapy is applied will depend on the clinical assessment of the intensity of inflammatory reaction. Two basic principles pertain: "bowel rest" and the combat of infection.

For the patient presenting with an acute onset of pain, fever, abdominal tenderness, and leukocytosis, all in relatively mild degree, hospitalization is not necessarily required. Such a patient can be instructed to rest at home and to subsist on a clear liquid or soft diet. A mild sedative-anticholinergic preparation (e.g., Donnatal or Librax) often is symptomatically meliorating. Warm stupes to the affected area of the abdomen can be soothing. To subdue infection, one is again reminded that diverticulitis is a disease of the bowel wall and its adventitia, not of the bowel lumen or its contents. There is no rational basis for the use of orally administered, nonabsorbable antibiotic agents with the mistaken notion of altering or obliterating intraluminal bowel flora. The choice of antibiotic agents is guided by knowing that infection almost always is by microorganisms indigenous to the colon, viz., *E. coli*, similar coliform bacteria, and *Bacteroides* species. An appropriate agent is ampicillin given orally 2 g daily, usually in 4 divided doses; alternative agents are tetracycline, in similar doses, or deoxycycline, 100 mg every 12 hours.

The patient presenting with more severe, fulminant diverticulitis is best hospitalized for more intensive therapy and vigilant observation. Such a patient is liable to complication that may require prompt surgical intervention. The patient is kept at bed rest, allowing for bathroom privileges when feasible. No food or fluid by mouth is permitted; nutrition is maintained by parenteral means. Even in the absence of frank ileus, nasogastric tube aspiration can be used with gratifying results, particularly in the relief of pain, nausea, or vomiting. Opiates as analgesics should be avoided because of their hypertonic effect on the bowel and because of the danger of masking symptoms of increasing peritoneal irritation.[56, 57] Meperidine (Demerol), when given in moderate doses, and perhaps together with atropine, is permissible.

When fulminant infection threatens and intestinal absorption is uncertain, parenteral antibiotic agents are administered. Blood cultures in appropriate sequence (Chapter 21) are obtained before antibiotics are given. This done, empiric antibiotic therapy is begun without delay; the results of culture can guide later adjustment of treatment. Combination IV therapy usually is indicated, employing an aminoglycoside (e.g., gentamicin or tobramycin, 5mg/kg/day) and clindamycin, 1.2 g to 2.7 g daily, or chloramphenicol, 50 mg to 100 mg/kg/day, or cefoxitin, 4 g to 6 g daily, all in divided doses, usually every 6 hours. Antibiotic therapy, even with a prompt and favorable response, should be continued for 7 to 10 days.

Obstipation may require attention as the more acute symptoms subside. Small oil retention enemas (90 ml to 180 ml) may be given initially. Gently administered saline enemas may then be given safely in most instances.

If signs of a complication have not become manifest and as the symptoms of inflammation subside, liquids are permitted by mouth and the diet is gradually liberalized, ambulation is resumed, and the patient is discharged on a follow-up regimen as described next.

Follow-up Care and Prevention. Too little attention has been given to the follow-up care of the patient who has experienced an acute attack of diverticulitis. Assisting the patient to surmount a bout of acute illness is gratifying, but this represents only the initial phase of treatment for diverticular disease. While it may not be possible to wholly prevent further attacks and to eliminate liability to complications, measures can be taken that will be helpful in many cases. An explanation of possibly aggravating factors and instruction in bowel hygiene are in order. A determined effort should be made to enable the patient to manage a regular, comfortable evacuation of the bowel. Physical stresses which increase intra-abdominal and, hence, intracolonic pressure, such as heavy lifting and prolonged stooping, should be avoided. Wracking cough or violent sneezing is to be suppressed.

As advised for the patient whose diverticula are unsullied, the diet need not be rigidly or arbitrarily restricted. The patient's own individual tastes and tolerances are to be respected as the foremost guide in the selection of diet. If milk is poorly tolerated, then lactose-containing dairy foods should be avoided (Chapter 104). Gassy foods and excesses in caffeine-containing or alcoholic beverages are to be shunned. Emphasis is given to the need for an orderly schedule of moderate meals. The stout patient with a history of diverticulitis is well advised to reduce excessive weight. The risk of operation, if later required, will thereby be lessened, and the result of surgery is likely to be more satisfactory. Above all, the sensible physician is perceptive of his patient's dietary idiosyncrasies and advises the patient accordingly.

Most importantly, erratic bowel action, either diarrhea or constipation, must be corrected. Harsh cathartics and irritating enemas are to be avoided, as are costive opiates. Both constipation and diarrhea can reflect bowel spasm. We are convinced that the most effective way to promote gentle bowel action is the daily dietary supplement of one of the psyllium seed derivatives. The patient can also be assured that such a supplement will provide an adequate "fiber" content. For the proper use of these agents, see Chapter 134. Our favorable experience has been borne out by others.[45, 48, 49, 53] It is conceived that the fecal mass constituted with hydrophilic colloids tends not to fragment and impact diverticular sacs. Bulky stools inhibit segmentation and constriction of the bowel, thereby lessening intraluminal pressure. The occasional use of anticholinergic agents, when needed, may be helpful, but their ritualistic or indefinite use is discouraged. So-called prophylactic administration of antibiotic agents is to be deplored.

Surgical Treatment

Segmental Resection. In cases of diverticulitis, surgical intervention is warranted in 4 settings:

1. In an emergency, as when the patient presents with a life-threatening complication, such as acute free perforation

2. In an urgent situation, when medical measures fail to halt a grave progression of disease or when a jeopardizing complication supervenes during medical treatment, as in the case of persistent or enlarging abscess

3. As an elective undertaking, during remission of repeated attacks of acute diverticulitis

4. In cases of uncertain differential diagnosis, when the presence of carcinoma can be determined only by resection of the deformed segment.

The frequencies of various indications for operation in actual practice are given in Table 135–3. Among patients with diverticular disease of the right colon, Peck et al.,[59] reporting their experience in Hawaii with a largely Oriental population, noted that surgery was invoked because of acute or recurrent diverticulitis in 101 of 108 patients, because of hemorrhage in 6, and because of obstruction in only 1.

The need for surgery under emergent or urgent circumstances is described in subsequent sections dealing with the various complications of diverticular disease. A requisite to operation in such cases, of course, is restoration of fluid and electrolyte balance and full antibiotic coverage.

The role of operative intervention to resolve a differential diagnosis has been cited in the foregoing section given to that concern. Again, it is emphasized that if deformity in the sigmoid segment is so great as to preclude distinction between inflammatory disease and carcinoma, surgery is indicated in either case. An unusual but important exception is the instance wherein amebic colitis might be suspected. This condition is amenable to medical treatment and may be identified by examination of the fecal flux and by amebic serology (Chapter 232).

Table 135–3. INDICATIONS FOR SURGICAL INTERVENTION IN 144 CASES OF DIVERTICULAR DISEASE*

Indication	No.	%
Recurrent diverticulitis	51	35
Hemorrhage	36	25
Perforation	31	22
Suspected carcinoma	24	17
Obstruction	23	16
Fistula	15	10
>1 major indication	36	25

*As reported by Orebaugh et al.[58]

The election of a surgical remedy should always be considered in the minority of patients who suffer repeated attacks of diverticulitis. Only about one-fourth to one-third of patients whose initial attack of diverticulitis is identified will be in this category; at least 2 of every 3 patients who recover from an initial attack will require no further hospitalization for treatment of their disease.[60, 61] Nevertheless, it is well to call in the surgeon to observe any episode of acute diverticulitis, even the first. In this way the surgeon can not only assist in assessment of possible complication, but also will be better able to judge the need for later elective intervention.

Elective operation is favored over emergency intervention, whenever possible, because of appreciably lower morbidity and mortality. For example, in a series of 144 patients treated surgically by Orebaugh et al.,[58] the operative mortality was 17.8% (8/45) in cases requiring emergency intervention, 5.8% (1/17) when operation was undertaken in urgent circumstances, but zero (0/82) when conditions permitted elective operation. No deaths ensued among 103 patients who underwent elective operation at Saint Mark's Hospital in London.[62]

In the immediately previous edition of this work, Parks[63] listed 10 indications for elective resection in diverticular disease. These still pertain and, slightly paraphrased, are repeated here: (1) recurrent attacks of localized inflammation; (2) a persistently palpable mass on abdominal, rectal, or vaginal examination; (3) radiographic evidence of persistent, marked deformity or pericolic abscess; (4) associated urinary symptoms, such as may warn of impending fistula; (5) other evidence of internal or external fistulas; (6) clinical or radiographic signs of bowel obstruction; (7) recurring hemorrhage; (8) an unresolved suspicion of carcinoma; (9) severe diverticulitis in a patient under 55 years of age; and (10) rapid progression of diverticular disease. As Parks pointed out, some indications are absolute, while others are relative. He noted, and most seasoned clinicians will agree, that in the absence of a compelling complication, surgical intervention is best withheld at the initial presentation of diverticular disease. Most such patients, on full recovery, will not be again so afflicted.

Elective operation requires thorough and

methodical cleansing and preparation of the bowel. This is a *sine qua non* for safe resection and primary anastomosis.

Whereas in former years a series of staged procedures (first a diverting colostomy, then resection of the affected segment, and finally closure of the colostomy) was considered *de rigueur*, surgeons are now more often opting for a single operation (Fig. 135–13). Obviously the choice of a 1-, 2-, or 3-stage procedure can be judged only according to the circumstances pertaining in an individual case, and often only at the time of laparotomy. Nonetheless, the safety and efficacy of the single operation are evident in reported data. For example, in the experience of Graves and his Vanderbilt associates,[64] among 74 patients in whom the extent of inflammatory reaction precluded initial resection of a perforated colon, operative morbidity was 35% and mortality was 12%, compared with 7% and 4%, respectively, among 43 patients in the same series whose lesions could be removed at the first operation. Howe et al.[65] reported reduced postoperative morbidity, shortened hospital stay, and diminished need for additional drainage procedures when the results of the Hartmann procedure (resection of the perforated segment, oversewn rectal stump, and proximal colostomy) were compared with those of the 3-stage series.

Resection, when it is accomplished, should be of sufficient extent to include all of the affected segment (Fig. 135–14). In cases of sigmoid diverticulitis, which make up the vast majority, the distal line of resection should be close to the peritoneal reflection, i.e., near the rectosigmoid junction. The reason is that the thickened, hypertonic, muscular wall of the whole sigmoid segment is thereby extirpated. The line of proximal transection need be above the lesion only insofar as to provide intact, healthy bowel suitable

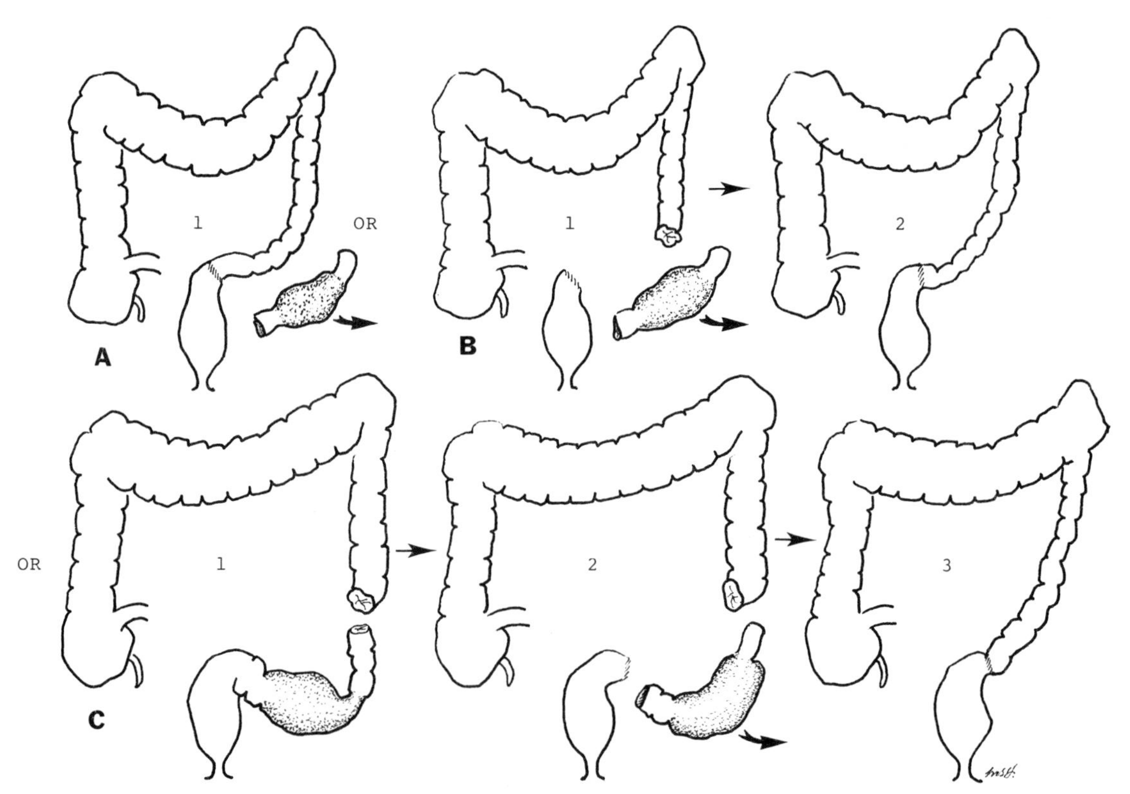

Figure 135–13. Schematic depiction of 1-, 2-, and 3-stage operative procedures for diverticular disease. In the 1-stage operation *(A)*, the affected segment is resected and continuity restored therewith as a primary anastomosis. In the 2-stage procedure *(B)*, the affected segment is resected, a diverting colostomy is constructed, and the rectal remnant is closed as a Hartmann procedure, or its proximal end is brought out as a mucous fistula; later, continuity is restored. In the 3-stage operation *(C)*, the colon is transected above the affected segment and only a diverting colostomy and mucous fistula are effected; later the diseased segment is resected; still later, continuity is restored.

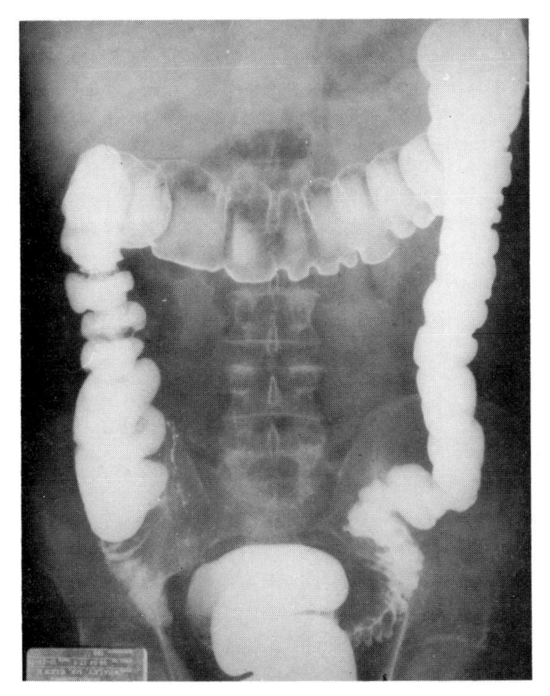

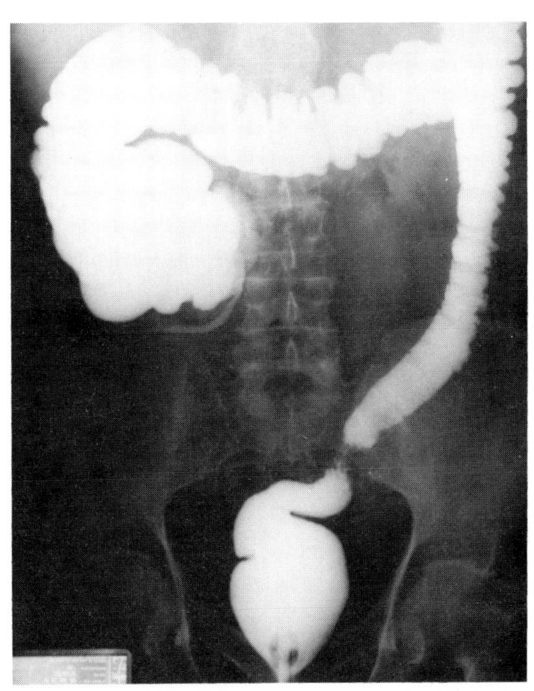

Figure 135–14. A 55-year-old engineer presented because of semiannual attacks of left lower quadrant pain with fever and chills over the preceding 9 years. Barium enema *(left)* showed impingement at the site of diverticular disease in the sigmoid segment. At elective operation, segmental sigmoid resection with primary anastomosis was accomplished. The resected segment contained numerous small intramural and pericolic abscesses. Postoperative barium enema *(right)* showed a foreshortened distal colon with transient spasm at the point of anastomosis. The patient has remained free of his previous symptoms.

for primary anastomosis or temporary diverting colostomy. Even when uninvolved diverticula are known to be present proximal to the inflamed segment, these are properly left undisturbed; the likelihood of recurrent diverticulitis elsewhere in the colon is slight.

Having recovered from segmental resection, the patient is well advised in a follow-up program, such as that described in the foregoing section on medical management.

Sigmoid Myotomy. Because of the recognized role of muscular hypertonicity and thickening,[10, 11] previously mentioned as a pathogenetic factor, and from a desire to spare patients the presumably more formidable operation of segmental resection, the idea of sigmoid myotomy has surfaced from time to time. Longitudinal myotomy was first advanced by Reilly in 1964.[66] Depending on the apparent extent of thickened muscle, a cut 20 cm to 50 cm long is made along the antimesenteric border of the sigmoid colon, severing all circular muscle fibers but sparing the submucosa. The latter is carefully preserved intact. Reilly preferred to leave an open cut, but Daniel[67] recommended an overlying peritoneal graft to reduce the risk of mucosal perforation. While early favorable reports were issued, myotomy never has gained favor with most surgeons, including those with long experience with diverticular disease.[63] Prasad and Daniel[68] observed that reduction in intraluminal pressure, even when achieved early, is not maintained, and motility returns to its preoperative state within 3 years.

More recently, Hodgson and his colleagues[69] at the Bronx (N.Y.) Veterans Administration Hospital have proposed taeniamyotomy (i.e., transverse severance of the longitudinal muscle bands at the affected site) in preference to Reilly's operation. The notion is that plication of the bowel, and hence intraluminal pressure, will be thereby reduced.

It is difficult to conceive that sigmoid myotomy, in any form, is likely to alter diverticular disease favorably, except possibly in supposed cases in which actual diverticula are nonexistent.

Complications

Hemorrhage. Bleeding from colon diverticula is typically abrupt, brisk, and brief. It can be massive, but rarely is it exsanguinating; in the great majority of cases, hemorrhage from diverticula is self-limiting. Bleeding is seldom coincident with diverticulitis.[70] Diverticula are rarely, if ever, a source of occult bleeding such as might be postulated to account for iron-deficiency anemia; this type of blood loss almost always is from another source.

The actual frequency of bleeding from colon diverticula is not known. Early writers gave the impression that hemorrhage was a rare expression of diverticula, but then a spate of reports suggested a greater frequency and severity of bleeding associated with diverticula of the colon.[16] Parks[71] noted hemorrhage as a complication in 119 of 521 patients presenting with diverticula. This, of course, does not mean that one-fifth of all patients who harbor diverticula will bleed; this figure will be much smaller, probably less than 5%.

Vascular injection studies have shown a close relation between blood vessels and diverticula, as well as increased vascularity adjacent to diverticula.[72] Histologic sections in some instances have disclosed replacement of mucosa in diverticular sacs by vascular dysplasia. Probably this is the result of stercoral trauma which further provokes vascular rupture and hemorrhage[73] (Fig. 135–15). It has been postulated, too, that vascular dysplasia in diverticular sacs may be similar in pathogenesis to that affecting the fine vasculature elsewhere in the aging colon.[74]

Because most bleeding diverticula are in the distal colon, the expelled blood usually is red, often accompanied by liver-like clots. Bleeding from the proximal colon can produce dark stools, erroneously suggesting upper gastrointestinal hemorrhage. Typically, however, the color resembles more that of Bordeaux wine rather than being black. The stools also are devoid of the shiny, sticky characteristics of pitch or tar, as are found with melena (Chapter 6).

Ordinary sigmoidoscopy cannot be expected to disclose the bleeding site but does provide the helpful information that fresh blood is coming from a proximal source. Flexible sigmoidoscopy or colonoscopy can be tried, but with copious hemorrhage the visual field often is hopelessly obscured. In cases of lesser bleeding, colonoscopy can be definitive when cleansing is possible. Using colonoscopy, Tedesco et al.[75] found that diverticula were the source in 20% of patients with distal intestinal bleeding. More important was their observation that in 85 patients with diverticulosis who bled, 40% were dis-

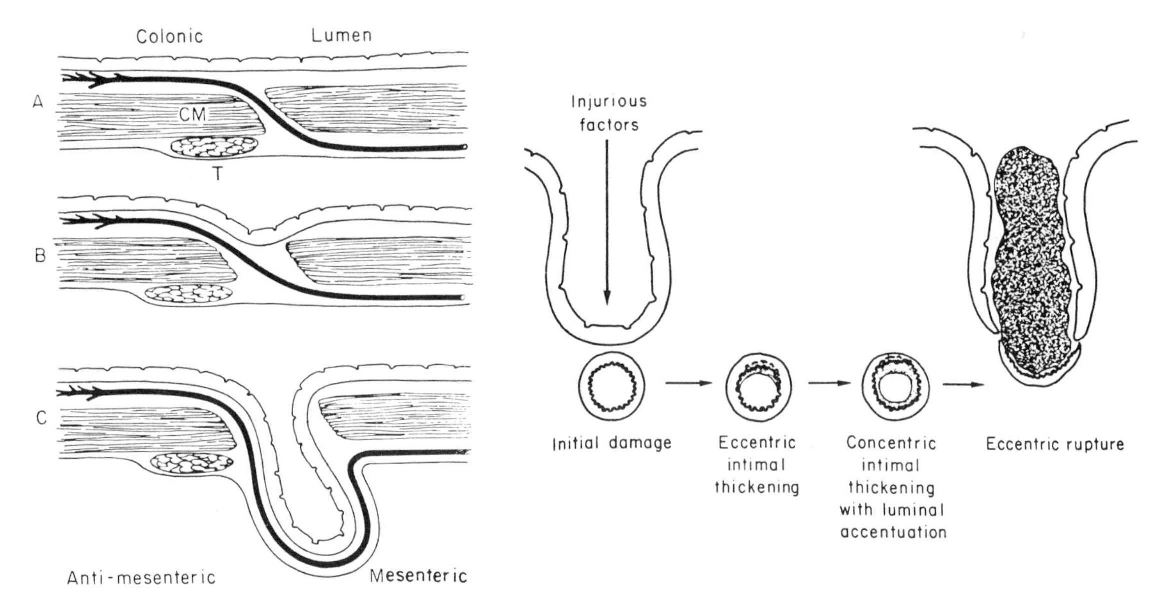

Figure 135–15. *Left,* Formation of a diverticulum in relation to a straight artery as it penetrates the muscular wall of the colon. *Right,* Proposed pathogenesis of injury in the adjacent arterial wall leading to diverticular hemorrhage. (From Meyers MA et al. Gastroenterology 1976; 71:577–830. Reproduced with permission.)

covered to harbor lesions other than diverticula that were likely sources of bleeding.

Adequate barium enema examination of an actively bleeding colon is frequently impossible or unrevealing. While it has been claimed that the introduction of barium into a bleeding colon may stop hemorrhage,[76] presumably by its astringent effect, the cessation of bleeding in such circumstances also may be coincidental.

If emergency operation is too hastily undertaken, the large bowel may be found filled with blood from cecum to rectum, making difficult the decision where to resect. Lacking a precise diagnosis, zealous and desperate surgeons have been known to resort to subtotal or even total colectomy. This is unfortunate because massive arterial hemorrhage often derives from a single diverticulum and can be controlled by properly selective resection. Moreover, examination of a blindly extirpated colon often fails to reveal the actual site of hemorrhage.[77] The wiser course is to provide the bleeding patient with all necessary resuscitative support that will allow definition of the bleeding site.

The need for precise localization of diverticular bleeding can be met, in many cases, by selective arteriography (Chapter 35) or radionuclide scintigraphy (Chapter 36). Either of these procedures must precede, not follow, the introduction of contrast medium into the alimentary tract. Extravasation at a rate of not less than 0.5 ml/minute at the time of examination probably is necessary for identification of an actively bleeding vessel.

Selective arteriography offers not only a chance to pinpoint the site of bleeding (Fig. 135–16) but also provides a means of stopping hemorrhage.[78] A bleeding point was identified in all 15 patients with massive diverticular hemorrhage examined by Baum et al.[79]; hemorrhage was controlled by vasopressin infusion in 7, while the remaining 8 patients required urgent or elective resection. Goldberger and Bookstein[80] have shown the efficacy of arteriographically guided embolization in the abatement of diverticular hemorrhage. Moreover, microangiographic techniques may disclose vascular abnormalities that predispose to hemorrhage, even in the absence of active bleeding. As described by Meyers and his associates,[73] these include asymmetric or eccentric intimal thickening of the straight arteries (vasa recta) in the colon wall, often with medial thickening of the internal elastic lamina. If operation is required, arteriography can guide the surgeon to a highly selective resection[81] or arterial ligation.[82]

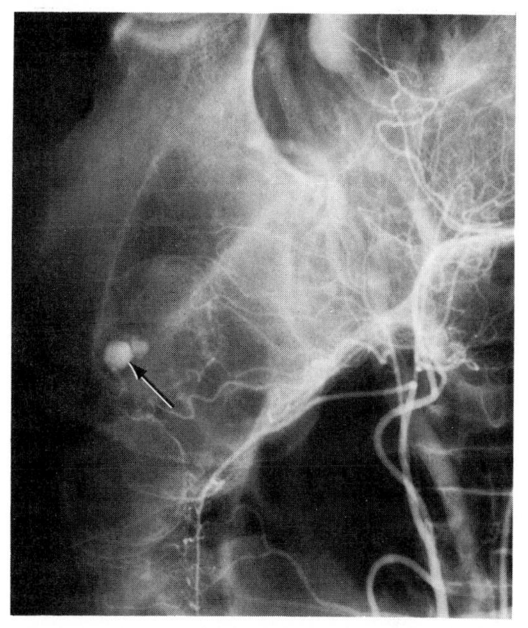

Figure 135–16. In this inferior mesenteric arteriogram, a dense accumulation of contrast medium *(arrow)* delineates a bleeding diverticulum in the proximal sigmoid colon. Also seen is an artery leading to this diverticulum. (From Hill GJ II, Taubman O. Dig Dis 1973; 18:808. Reproduced with permission.)

An even simpler means of localizing active bleeding in the colon, though not defining vascular architecture, is by injecting an aliquot of the patient's own erythrocytes labeled with ^{99m}technetium. Positive findings usually are obtained in patients requiring transfusion of more than 1 unit of blood or packed red blood cells during 24 hours. Both the sensitivity and specificity of this test for intestinal bleeding are promising.[83]

Intestinal Obstruction. Varying degrees of impingement on the bowel lumen have been noted in approximately 5% to 10% of patients with diverticular disease.[58, 71] For reasons readily apparent, obstruction usually involves the sigmoid segment. Only rarely does obstruction complicate diverticular disease in the proximal colon.[59] However, a knuckle of small intestine occasionally is entrapped in the inflammatory process with ensuing small bowel obstruction.[84] A cautious preliminary barium enema examination can clarify the picture.

With acute diverticulitis, symptoms of obstruction can be abrupt, consequent to rapidly developing edema and inflammatory swelling. In the absence of acute peritonitis, shock, or vascular compromise, obstruction may subside with conservative management. Repeated episodes of acute diverticulitis and pericolitis predispose to increasing bowel obstruction as a result of fibrotic constriction. It will be recalled that the development of diverticula is attended by shortening, distortion, and fixation of the colon. This renders the diverticula-laden segment especially liable to compromise of the narrowed lumen. Silberman and Thorner[85] described an instance of volvulus of a giant sigmoid diverticulum.

Complete obstruction produced by diverticular disease in the sigmoid segment requires urgent surgical decompression when marked by progressive distention of the proximal colon, especially when accumulating gas and fluid are confined by a competent ileocecal valve. This can usually be accomplished by a loop-colostomy in the transverse segment; the obstructed segment is then resected after a few weeks of restorative care. When obstruction is only partial and intermittent, opportunity is provided for adequate bowel preparation and then elective operation with a view to segmental resection and primary anastomosis. In any case wherein exploration is undertaken because of obstructive signs, a thorough assessment of the small intestine is in order, even when a focus of diverticular disease in the colon is clearly evident.

Abscess. A substantial suppurative collection occurs in about 10% of cases.[71] Abscess is suspected as an aftermath of acute diverticulitis when clinical improvement does not progress and there are symptoms and signs of sepsis, including spiking fever and rising leukocytosis. A defined mass may be detected near the site of the original pain, which tends to become continuous. Tenderness often is associated with muscle guarding and localized abdominal rigidity. A tender mass may be palpated in the cul-de-sac on rectal examination. In some cases, a suppurative mass becomes apparent only after acute symptoms have subsided.

A palpable mass may represent a "gas cyst" as a complication of diverticular disease.[86] Typically these are unlined by epithelium and are the consequence of confined perforation. They may be mistaken for what have been described as "giant" diverticula.

A localized perforation with abscess may be confined entirely within the mesocolon. When limited to the female pelvis, the abscess may involve the uterus, fallopian tube, or ovary. Adjacent loops of small intestine may be affected. Metastatic suppuration, fortunately, is rare.

It is important to remember that an inflammatory diverticular mass can compress neighboring structures, giving rise to extracolonic symptoms. Hersch and Schwabe[87] reported 2 cases of left hydronephrosis caused by diverticular abscess impinging on the distal ureter.

Fistula. A fistula may form as a result of perforation into (1) the bowel, as an enterocolic or colocolic fistula; (2) the urinary bladder, as a vesicocolic fistula; (3) the adjacent integument, as a colocutaneous fistula; (4) the pelvic floor, resulting in ischiorectal abscess or perianal fistula; or (5) the vagina, as a rectovaginal fistula. Fistulization may be a direct complication of diverticular disease. It may also be a sequel to operation for diverticular disease wherein a precarious suture line becomes disrupted.[88]

The urinary bladder, because of its fixed proximity to the sigmoid colon, is the most common site of fistula formation. Most vesicocolic fistulas are in the lower posterior wall of the bladder. Although diverticulitis occurs without predilection for sex, vesicocolic fistulas are much more frequent in men. The relative rarity of vesicocolic fistulas in women is attributed to the protection afforded the female bladder by the uterus and fallopian tubes.

Vesicocolic fistulas have been reported in about 10% of patients undergoing surgery for complicated diverticulitis.[58] Hafner et al.,[89] in a review of 500 consecutive cases of diverticular disease, found symptoms referable to the genitourinary system in 178 (35.6%). Vesicocolic fistulas were identified in one-tenth of these patients (3.6% of the total group). Colovaginal fistulas were found in 7 cases.

Urinary frequency and urgency, sometimes attended by dysuria, are common in otherwise uncomplicated sigmoid diverticulitis. These symptoms are accentuated with fistulization. The classic (and startling!) symptom that is pathognomonic of enterovesical fistula is the passage of flatus (pneumaturia) and feces through the urethra. Pyuria and hematuria also may be noted.

The introduction of barium or other radio-

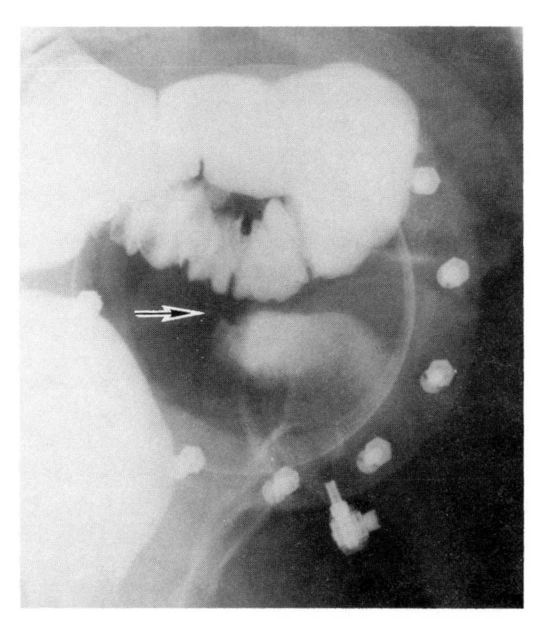

Figure 135–17. A 70-year-old man complained of recurring dysuria and pneumaturia. At cystoscopy the urologist discovered 2 fistulas in the urinary bladder wall. Barium enema disclosed a fistulous tract *(arrow)* extending from a deformed sigmoid segment to the bladder. At operation there was dense adhesion between the bladder wall and a segment of suppurative diverticulitis in the sigmoid colon. Somewhat surprisingly, the patient denied any previous bowel symptoms. Resection of the sigmoid segment with primary anastomosis and repair of the bladder wall relieved the urinary complaint.

paque media into the colon will sometimes, but not always, show the fistulous tract (Fig. 135–17). Cystoscopy should establish the diagnosis, but the fistulous opening is not always seen owing to the marked inflammatory reaction in the adjacent bladder mucosa.

Enteroenteric fistulas are relatively unusual.[90] Among 202 complicated cases of diverticulitis, Mayo and Blunt[91] encountered a fistulous communication with the small intestine in 5 and with the colon in 3.

Bizarre fistulization has been reported,[30] as, for example, to the hip joint, to the mesenteric and portal veins, and to the epidural space. Extension to the abdominal wall can result in subcutaneous emphysema.[92]

Minor cutaneous fistulas, such as can follow slight leakage at suture lines, when unattended by signs of intra-abdominal suppuration, may be treated by expectant measures; sometimes they heal spontaneously. A fistula of any magnitude, however will require prompt surgical attention. Colovesical fistulas, even when initial symptoms seem minor, almost always warrant surgical correction; the risk of serious urinary tract infection and spreading sepsis is too great to permit procrastination. Moreover, when such a fistula is small, often the bladder wall can be repaired, the affected sigmoid segment resected, and a primary anastomosis effected. Minor colovaginal fistulas may be similarly treated. Larger fistulas, including most enteric fistulas, will require staged surgical procedures.

Perforation and Peritonitis. It can be argued, justifiably, that all diverticulitis is the result of perforation, which is to say that there must be at least microperforation of the diverticular mucosa to set up an intramural or pericolic inflammatory reaction. However, more flagrant penetration of the bowel wall may occur, resulting either in a confined suppurative collection (single or multiple abscesses, as previously described) or more or less generalized peritonitis. In the experience of Graves and his Vanderbilt associates,[64] perforation was confined in two-thirds of 117 cases. Rupture of an inflamed diverticulum into the peritoneal cavity with ensuing generalized peritonitis is a relatively rare complication.

The clinical configuration of *acute free perforation* is almost identical with that of a ruptured appendix. Symptoms and signs of acute, simple diverticulitis are likely to precede perforation by a few days, but rupture can occur with little warning. Severe pain occurs at the site of primary peritoneal insult, often accompanied by nausea and vomiting. Rigidity of the abdominal wall may be confined to the left lower abdominal quadrant in sigmoid perforation. Peristaltic sounds disappear. Exquisite tenderness is elicited on rectal examination as the probing finger contacts the cul-de-sac anterior to the rectum. Fever, leukocytosis, and neutrophilia are evident in most cases.

A *forme fruste* type of perforation is much more common than free perforation in sigmoid diverticulitis. The site of rupture, especially when it occurs at the tip of a diverticulum (which, as Fleischner[93] has pointed out, is the most common site), becomes walled off by contiguous structures. When this occurs, signs of free perforation as may have presented, quickly disappear. The pain lessens, local signs become less striking, and peristaltic activity is resumed. The inflammation may only slowly resolve, and residual abscess or bowel obstruction may be a later complication.

It is possible for localized peritonitis to accompany acute diverticulitis in the absence of evident rupture. For example, an inflamed sac embedded in an epiploic appendix can induce a pericolic serosal reaction. Serosal inflammation may resolve slowly, leaving no significant aftermath. Adhesions to adjacent structures can develop and may result in eventual bowel obstruction. Continued inflammation may lead to fistulization.

Acute free perforation with unconstrained *peritonitis* is the most grave complication that can befall the patient with diverticular disease. While the picture of catastrophe often is clear, a correct preoperative diagnosis of a perforated diverticulum can be expected in less than half the cases.[94] The attendant gram-negative sepsis and shock combine with intense peritoneal reaction to constitute a potentially lethal combination. In former years, mortality rates as high as 40% were not unusual; today the prospect is more favorable, but the threat remains formidable. Prompt attention to the need for surgical intervention is often the deciding factor.

For flagrant peritonitis in a desperately ill patient, a 2- or 3-stage procedure is mandatory. The 2 principal aims are thorough drainage of the infected peritoneal cavity and construction of a diverting proximal colostomy. If at all possible, the perforated segment of colon should be removed. The rectal stump is dealt with by the Hartmann procedure. To attempt any sort of anastomosis is fraught with hazard. During the recovery period, the clinician must be vigilant for signs of undrained suppurative collections. Only when the patient is deemed secure can plans be made for restoring bowel continuity.

Even in cases of lesser gravity, wherein perforation has been spontaneously sealed off and infection contained within natural confines, deciding on a 2-stage procedure often is preferable to taking the risk of primary anastomosis.

Taking into account the advantage of operation by the most experienced and deft surgeon and the protection afforded by the newest antibiotic agents, the patient's recovery is due largely to assiduous nursing care and supportive medical measures.

Diverticula of the Cecum and Proximal Colon

Relatively uncommon in the United States and other Western countries, diverticulitis in this location is of interest because it can resemble other diseases more frequently found in the area, viz., appendicitis, carcinoma, and certain granulomatous lesions. Doubtless some of the cases referred to in years past as "acute typhlitis" were actually instances of cecal diverticulitis. As previously mentioned, right-sided diverticular disease tends to predominate even today in other areas of the world where diverticulosis is less prevalent, especially among Oriental patients.[14, 59]

Pathogenesis. In contrast to the typically clustered, acquired diverticula in the distal colon, most of the solitary or scattered sacs characteristic of the proximal colon have been thought to be congenital or "true" diverticula.[95, 96] Lauridsen and Ross[97] found that 70% were true diverticula in the sense of being composed of all layers of the bowel wall. Solitary congenital sacs have been attributed to the persistence of the embryonic "transient appendix," i.e., an appendix which appears early in embryonic life before the true vermiform appendix develops. Solitary diverticula of the cecum usually occur in close proximity to the ileocecal junction. Others are occasionally found in the ascending and transverse segments of the colon.

Multiple or clustered diverticula in the proximal colon are considered to be acquired, almost invariably being associated with similar clusters of diverticula in the distal colon.[98] Such diverticula probably develop in a manner similar to that previously described for acquired diverticula elsewhere in the colon. A recent study from Japan[98a] showed that in patients with right-sided diverticular disease, intraluminal pressures, both in rising and stimulated states, were greater in the affected segments when compared with those of control subjects.

Frequency. Potier[99] is credited with reporting the first case of diverticulum of the cecum in 1912. Subsequent case reports and reviews have been numerous.[97, 98, 100] Nevertheless, diverticula limited to the cecum and ascending colon probably account for less than 1% of all cases of diverticulosis in the Western world. Leichtling[101] stated that cecal diverticulitis occurred in only about 0.1% of all cases of diverticular disease. According to Greaney and Snyder,[102] acute cecal diverticulitis is found in 1 of every 1100 emergency laparotomies.

Patients with acute diverticulitis of the right colon tend to be about 10 years younger than patients with diverticulitis of the left colon.[98, 103] This has been attributed to the presumably congenital sacs occurring in the cecal region.[98] Both sexes are equally susceptible.[98, 101]

Clinical Manifestations and Diagnosis. Pain is the most common symptom, being almost universally present.[101, 104, 105] The character and location of the pain are highly suggestive of acute appendicitis but can also simulate hepatobiliary disease (Fig. 135–18). With confinement and walling off of the inflamed area, pain may be of more gradual onset and less intense. A preoperative diagnosis of acute appendicitis is made in at least half the cases that are found at the operating table to have cecal diverticulitis. Marked tenderness in the area of the cecum is encountered in most patients, sometimes attended by a palpable mass. The presenting complaint was bleeding in the absence of pain in 4 of 25 patients reported by Nicholas et al.[104]

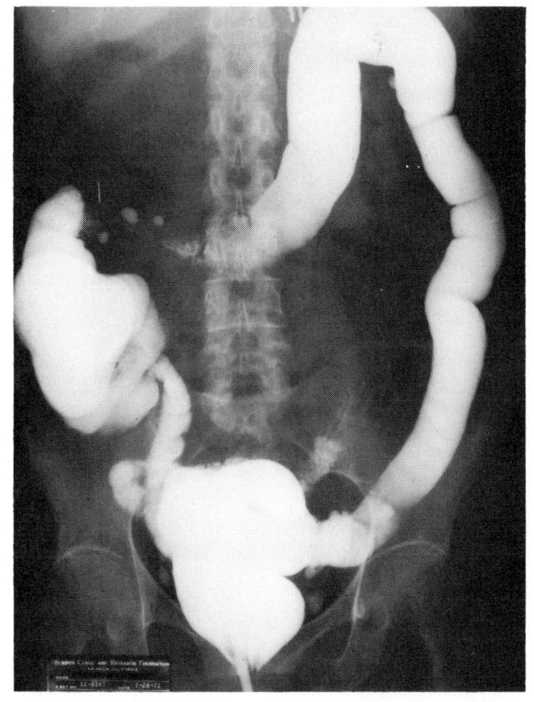

Figure 135–18. A 65-year-old physician's wife was referred because of "recurrent hepatitis." In the preceding year she had 2 episodes of fever, chills, and cramping pain in the right upper abdomen attended by obstructive jaundice. There was persistent elevation in serum alkaline phosphatase activity. Cholecystograms were normal. Barium enema *(above)* revealed diverticular disease at the hepatic flexure. Operation disclosed partially resolved inflammation at this site; the liver was grossly and microscopically normal. The hepatic flexure of the colon was resected, primary anastomosis was accomplished, and the patient has remained free of symptoms.

Free perforation or obstruction is rare. Fecaliths have been found in 55% of 104 patients in whom pathologic study was carried out.[97]

Barium enema affords the best opportunity for preoperative diagnosis, except in those instances wherein such examination is contraindicated because of need for urgent operation.[105] Any of the radiographic signs previously described for diverticulitis may be present. Wolf[106] has emphasized the discrete, localized, eccentric, intramural indentation of the barium-distended colon, with an intact mucosa and often a crowding of the transverse folds. If adjacent diverticula are apparent, the correct diagnosis is suggested. The offending diverticulum usually does not fill with barium but at times may appear as a ring shadow.[106]

Treatment. If acute appendicitis or other compelling surgical indication is not evident and the inflammatory process appears to be contained, conservative medical treatment may be cautiously undertaken. Bed rest, nothing by mouth, nasogastric aspiration, parenteral fluids, and antibiotic coverage constitute the essentials of conservative therapy. A failure of response or signs of spreading infection call for prompt surgical intervention.

A majority of patients will require an urgent abdominal laparotomy because of uncertainty of the diagnosis or because of the threat of unconstrained suppuration. The most conservative surgical procedure is advised. It is noteworthy that recurrence is unusual after any type of treatment for cecal diverticulitis.[101, 105] Diverticulectomy is attempted only if the infected sac can be isolated and readily mobilized. Ligation and eversion occasionally may be possible. When a large inflammatory mass is encountered, the problem is more difficult. Simple drainage will seldom suffice. Resection and exteriorization or ileocolostomy are preferable when feasible.[105] When carcinoma is simulated, palpation of the mucosal portion of the apparent tumor by cecotomy, or with a finger invaginating a healthy, pliable portion of the adjacent cecum, may be helpful in deciding whether cancer is present.[101] If carcinoma cannot be excluded, resection should be carried out to the extent permitted by the inflammatory mass. An inability to exclude the presence of carcinoma in the inflammatory mass was reflected in the need to carry out a hemicolectomy in 26 of 132 cases reported by Leichtling.[101] Supplementary appendectomy should be performed at the time of laparotomy if the appendix is accessible and not involved in the inflammatory mass.

Prognosis

For the patient found to harbor colon diverticula, the outlook is favorable. This statement is not to be construed, however, as an excuse for complacency on the part of either the patient or his medical advisor. A number of years ago, Boles and Jordan[107] reported a 15-year follow-up of 294 persons with initially asymptomatic diverticulosis. The majority remained well, but diverticulitis supervened in 25%, and hemorrhage, perforation, and obstruction were complications, each in about 5%. While no recent similar survey has been conducted, there is little reason to expect a major change in the figures.

Horner[108] compared serial barium enema radiographs taken at an average interval of 4.4 years in 183 patients; in 129 (70%) there was no progression of the condition. In the same report, Horner observed that among 503 persons who harbored diverticula, diverticulitis occurred in 9.7% within 5 years, in 25% observed for 6 to 10 years, and in 36.7% followed as long as 18 years. From these data one can estimate an incidence risk of diverticulitis of about 2% annually among patients harboring diverticula.

Larson et al.[61] followed the courses of 132 patients admitted to the Yale–New Haven Hospital, having had their first bout of severe diverticulitis. What happened to these patients in ensuing years is depicted in Figure 135–19. This study bears out the generally accepted dictum that a considerable majority of patients recover and have little or no difficulty consequent to an initial attack of diverticular disease. There is, therefore, no justifiable warrant for so-called prophylactic elective colon resection in this group of patients.

Recurrence of diverticular disease, if and when it befalls the patient, usually is evident within the first year or so following the initial attack. This means that (1) patients requiring a more definitive remedy will in most cases be readily identified, and (2) those whose long-term course is satisfactory are not likely to be threatened.

The linear extent of diverticulosis in the colon is not a prognostic factor. The course of patients with diverticula throughout the colon is similar to that of patients with only limited involvement.[22]

For the patient whose colon is known to bear diverticula, advancing age brings a mixed prospect. The chance of encountering complication is relatively greater during the middle years of life, but the morbidity and

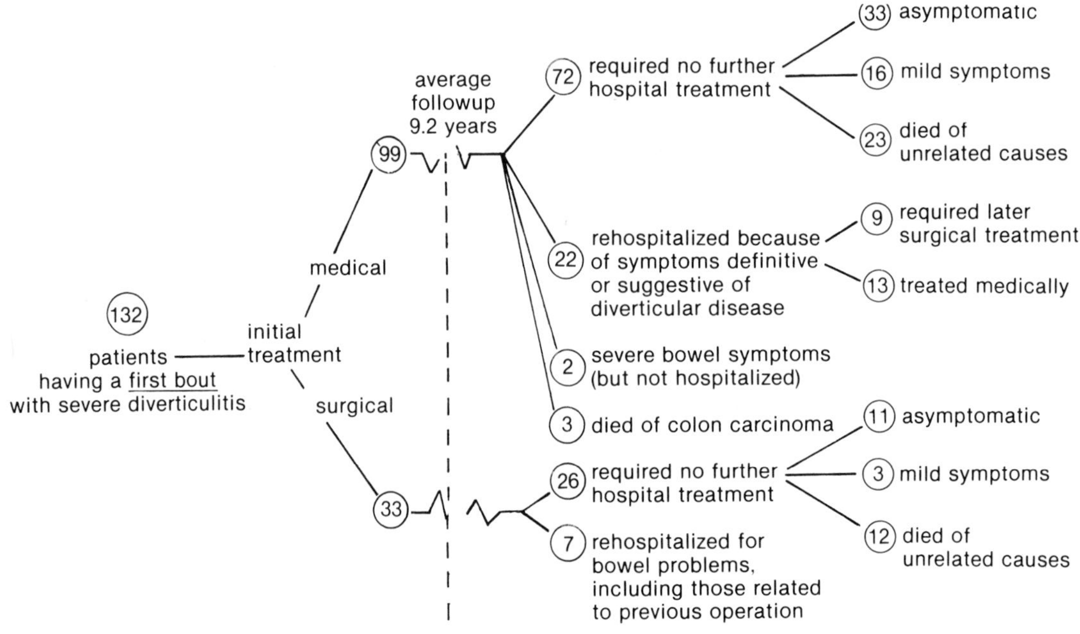

Figure 135–19. Schematic depiction of the courses of 132 patients followed an average of 9.2 years after initial hospitalization prompted by a first bout with diverticulitis. The majority (74%) required no further hospital admission because of diverticular disease. (From data reported by Larson et al.[61])

mortality of diverticular disease, are greater among the elderly.

Patients recovering from an elective surgical correction can be assured of a favorable prognosis. Recurrence of diverticular disease, once the affected segment has been properly removed and once healing is secure, is almost nil.

An occurrence rate of colon carcinoma somewhat greater than that predicted in the general population can be expected in the follow-up of any large group of patients whose diverticular disease has been treated medically. The reason is not that diverticular disease predisposes to carcinoma. It would seem rather that carcinoma can be present when diverticulitis is apparent or that a perforating carcinoma can simulate diverticulitis and only later be discovered. Uncertainty that carcinoma may exist at the site of what appears to be diverticulitis is a justifiable warrant for elective resection; the fear that carcinoma might be engrafted at a site of previous diverticulitis is not.

Can diverticulosis or diverticulitis be prevented? There is no proven answer. Circumstantial evidence suggests that persons whose diet is conducive to frequent, bulky stools may be less liable to the development of diverticula in their colons. There is no evidence, and it would be surprising if evidence were forthcoming, that a change in dietary custom will cause regression in diverticula once formed. There is a suggestion that dietary modification, i.e., institution of a high-fiber diet, may reduce the frequency of diverticulitis and its complications. Hyland and Taylor[109] so treated, then followed for 5 years or longer, 75 patients who had been hospitalized because of diverticular disease; 91% remained symptom-free. If this benefit can be confirmed by repeated and more extensive investigation, then the prospect for the patient whose colon bears diverticula will be even more favorable than at present.

References

1. Almy TP, Howell DA. Diverticular disease of the colon. N Engl J Med 1980; 302:324–31.
2. de Quervain F. Zur Diagnose der erworbenen Dickdarmdivertikel und der Sigmoiditis diverticularis. Dtsch Z Chir 1914; 128:67.
3. Case JI. The roentgen demonstration of multiple diverticula of the colon. AJR 1915; 2:645.
4. Telling WHM, Gruner OC. Acquired diverticula, diverticulitis and peridiverticulitis of the large intestine. Br J Surg 1917; 4:468.
5. Hurst AF, Rowlands RP. Diverticula of the colon. Guy's Hosp Rep 1925; 75:462.
6. Cruveilhier J. Traite de'Anatomie Pathologique. Paris: Bailliere et Cie, 1849: 1:595.
7. Baillie M. Quoted by Bacon HE, Sherman LE. Am J Surg 1950; 80:3.
8. Horner JL. A study of diverticulitis of the colon in office practice. Gastroenterology 1952; 21:223–9.
9. Goodwin FH, Collins EN. Diverticulosis of the colon. Cleveland Clin Quart 1948; 15:194–201.
10. Morson BC. The muscle abnormality in diverticular disease of the sigmoid colon. Br J Radiol 1963; 36:385.
11. Morson BC. Pathology of diverticular disease of the colon. Clin Gastroenterol 1975; 4:37–52.
12. Eusebio EB, Eisenberg MM. Natural history of diverticular disease of colon in young patients. Am J Surg 1973; 125:308.
13. Segal I, Solomon A, Hunt JA. Emergence of diverticular disease in the urban South African black. Gastroenterology 1977; 72:215–9.
14. Kurosu Y, Suzuki T, Koga T. Cecal diverticulitis in the Japanese. Henry Ford Hosp Med J 1971; 19:251–6.
15. Burkitt DP. A deficiency of dietary fiber may be one cause of certain colonic and venous disorders. Am J Dig Dis 1976; 21:104–8.
16. de la Vega JM. Diverticular disease of the colon. In: Bockus HL, ed. Gastroenterology. 3rd Ed. Vol. II. Philadelphia: WB Saunders, 1976.
17. Hodgson J. Animal models in the study of diverticular disease. Clin Gastroenterol 1975; 4:201–19.
18. Painter NS, Burkitt DP. Diverticular disease of the colon: A deficiency of western civilization. Br Med J 1971; 2:450.
19. Mendeloff AI. A critique of "fiber deficiency." Am J Dig Dis 1976; 21:109–12.
20. Eastwood MA, Brydon WG, Smith AN, Pritchard J. Colonic function in patients with diverticular disease. Lancet 1978; 1:1181–2.
21. Connell AM. Applied physiology of the colon: factors relevant to diverticular disease. Clin Gastroenterol 1975; 4:23–36.
22. Parks TG. Natural history of diverticular disease of the colon; review of 521 cases. Br Med J 1969; 4:639–42.
23. Holmes KM, Salter RH. Irritable bowel syndrome—a safe diagnosis? Br Med J 1982; 285:1533–4.
24. Wynne-Jones G. Flatus retention is the major factor in diverticular disease. Lancet 1975; 2:211–2.
25. Capron JP, Piperaud R, Dupas J-L, Delamarre J, Lorriaux A. Evidence for an association between cholelithiasis and diverticular disease of the colon. Dig Dis Sci 1981; 26:523–7.
26. Gear JSS, Ware A, Fursdon P, Mann JI, Nolan DJ, Brodribb AJM, Vessey MP. Symptomless diverticular disease and intake of dietary fibre. Lancet 1979; 1:511–4.
27. Scheff RT, Zuckerman G, Harter H, Delmez J, Kochler R. Diverticular disease in patients with chronic renal failure due to polycystic kidney disease. Ann Intern Med 1980; 92:202–4.
28. Meyers MA, Alonso DR, Morson BC, Bartram C. Pathogenesis of diverticulitis complicating granulomatous colitis. Gastroenterology 1978; 74:24–31.
29. Nahrwold DL, Demuth WE. Diverticulitis with perforation into the peritoneal cavity. Ann Surg 1977; 185:80–3.
30. Smith HJ, Berk RN, Janes JO, Clayton RS, Williams JL. Unusual fistulae due to colonic diverticulitis. Gastrointest Radiol 1978; 2:387–92.
31. Thompson WG, Patel DG, Tao H, Nair RC. Does uncomplicated diverticular disease produce symptoms? Dig Dis Sci 1982; 27:605–8.
32. Buie LA. Diverticula of the colon. N Engl J Med 1939; 221:593.
33. Cooper WL. Sigmoidoscopic findings that suggest diverticulitis. Dis Colon Rectum 1958; 1:120.
34. Forde KA. Colonoscopy in complicated diverticular disease. Gastrointest Endosc 1977: 23:192–3.
35. Max MH, Knutson CO. Colonoscopy in patients with inflammatory colonic strictures. Surgery 1978; 84:551–6.
36. Yudis N, Cohen A, Pearce AE. Perforation of the transverse colon during barium enema and air contrast studies. Am Surg 1968; 97:418.
37. Herbert WW. Dynamic or disappearing diverticula of the colon. Radiology 1968; 91:508.

38. Schnyder P, Moss AA, Thoeni RF, Margulis AR. A double-blind study of radiologic accuracy in diverticulosis, diverticulitis, and carcinoma of the sigmoid colon. J Clin Gastroent 1979; 1:55–66.
39. Willard JH, Bockus HL. Clinical and therapeutic status of cases of colonic diverticulosis seen in office practice. Am J Dig Dis 1936; 3:580.
40. Morton DL, Goldman L. Differential diagnosis of diverticulitis and carcinoma of the sigmoid colon. Am J Surg 1962; 103:55.
41. Rabinovitch J, Arlen M, Barnett T, et al.: Diverticulitis of vermiform appendix. Ann Surg 1962; 155:434.
42. Schmidt GT, Lennard-Jones JE, Morson BC, et al.: Crohn's disease of the colon and its distinction from diverticulitis. Gut 1968; 9:7.
43. Marshak RH. Granulomatous colitis in association with diverticula. N Engl J Med 1970; 285:1080.
44. Balz FF. Diverticulitis as a diagnostic problem in gynecology. Am J Obstet Gynecol 1968; 101:372.
45. Ewerth S, Ahlberg J, Holmström B, Perrson U, Uden R. Influence on symptoms and transit-time of Vi-Siblin in diverticular disease. Acta Chir Scand 1980; 500(Suppl):49–50.
46. Connell AM. Dietary fiber and diverticular disease. Hosp Practice 1976; March, 119–24.
47. Hall RC. The bran-waggon. Br Med J 1976; 1:1076.
48. Brodribb AJ. Treatment of symptomatic diverticular disease with a high-fibre diet. Lancet 1977; 1:664–6.
49. Devroede G, Vobecky JS, Vobecky JM, Beaudry R, Haddad H, Navert H, Pçrey B, Poisson J. Medical management of diverticular disease; a random trait. Gastroenterology 1977; 72:A134/1157 (Abstract).
50. Eastwood MA, Smith AN, Brydon WG, Pritchard J. Comparison of bran, ispaghula, and lactulose in colon function in diverticular disease. Gut 1978; 19:1144–7.
51. Ornstein MH, Littlewood ER, Baird IM, Fowler J, North WRS, Cox AG. Are fibre supplements really necessary in diverticular disease of the colon? A controlled clinical trial. Br Med J 1981; 282:1353–6.
52. Cann PA, Read NW, Holdworth CD. What is the benefit of coarse wheat bran in patients with the irritable bowel syndrome? Gut 1984; 25:168–73.
53. Hodgson WJB. The placebo effect; is it important in diverticular disease? Am J Gastroenterol 1977; 67:157–62.
54. Cummings JH, Branch W, Jenkins DJA, Southgate DAT, Houston H, James WPT. Colonic response to dietary fibre from carrot, cabbage, apple, bran, and guar gum. Lancet 1978; 1:5–8.
55. Cello JP. Diverticular disease of the colon. West J Med 1981; 134:515–23.
56. Painter NS, Truelove SC. Potential dangers of morphine in acute diverticulitis of the colon. Br Med J 1963; 2:33.
57. Painter NS, Truelove SC, Ardran GM, Tuckey M. Effect of morphine, Prostigmin, pethidine, and Pro-Banthine on the human colon, and diverticulosis studied by intraluminal pressure recording and cineradiography. Gut 1965; 6:57.
58. Orebaugh JE, Macris JA, Lee JF. Surgical treatment of diverticular disease of the colon. Am Surg 1978; 44:712–5.
59. Peck DA, Labat R, Waite VC. Diverticular disease of the right colon. Dis Colon Rectum 1968; 11:49–54.
60. Parks TG, Connell AM. The outcome in 455 patients admitted for treatment of diverticular disease of the colon. Br J Surg 1970; 57:775.
61. Larson DM, Masters SS, Spiro HM. Medical and surgical therapy in diverticular disease. Gastroenterology 1976; 71:734–7.
62. Penfold JCB. Management of uncomplicated diverticular disease by colonic resection in patients at St. Marks Hospital, 1964–9. Br. J Surg 1973; 60:695–8.
63. Parks TG. Surgery of diverticular disease of the colon. *In:* Bockus HB, ed. Gastroenterology. 3rd Ed. Vol II. Philadelphia: WB Saunders, 1976: 1001–8.
64. Graves HA Jr, Franklin RM, Robbins LB II, Sawyers JL. Surgical management of perforated diverticulitis of the colon. Am Surg 1973; 39:142–7.
65. Howe HJ, Casali RE, Westbrook KC, Thomson BW, Read RC. Acute perforations of the sigmoid colon secondary to diverticulitis. Am J Surg 1979; 137:184–7.
66. Reilly M. Sigmoid myotomy. Proc R Soc Med 1964; 57:576.
67. Daniel O. Sigmoid myotomy with peritoneal graft. Proc R Soc Med 1969; 62:811.
68. Prasad JK, Daniel O. Recurrence of high intracolonic pressure following sigmoid myotomy. Br J Surg 1971; 58:304.
69. Hodgson WJB, Schanzer H, Babare S, McElhinney AJ. Transverse taeniamyotomy in localized acute diverticulitis. Am J Gastroenterol 1979; 71:61–7.
70. Heald RJ, Ray J. Bleeding from diverticula of the colon. Dis Colon Rectum 1973; 14:420.
71. Parks TG. Reappraisal of clinical features of diverticular disease of the colon. Br Med J 1969; 4:642–5.
72. Slack WW. Diverticula of the colon and their relation to the muscle layers and blood vessels. Gastroenterology 1960; 39:708.
73. Meyers MA, Alonso DR, Gray GF, Baer JW. Pathogenesis of bleeding colonic diverticulosis. Gastroenterology 1976; 71:577–83.
74. Boley SJ, Sammartano R, Adams A, DiBiase A, Kleinhaus S, Sprayregen S. Nature and etiology of vascular ectasias of the colon: degenerative lesions of aging. Gastroenterology 1977; 72:650–60.
75. Tedesco FJ, Waye JD, Raskin JB, Morris SJ, Greenwald RA. Colonoscopic evaluation of rectal bleeding; a study of 304 patients. Ann Intern Med 1978; 89:907–9.
76. Adams JT. Therapeutic barium enema for massive diverticular bleeding. Arch Surg 1970; 101:457–60.
77. Rigg BM, Weing MR. Current attitudes with particular reference to colonic bleeding. Arch Surg 1966; 92:321.
78. Freedman AR, Kerr JC, Swan KG, Hobson RW II. Primate mesenteric blood flow; effects of vasopressin and its route of delivery. Gastroenterology 1978; 74:875–8.
79. Baum S, Rosch J, Otter CT, et al. Selective mesenteric arterial infusions in the management of massive diverticular hemorrhage. N Engl J Med 1973; 288:1269.
80. Golberger LE, Bookstein JJ. Transcatheter embolization for treatment of diverticular hemorrhage. Radiology 1977; 122:613–7.
81. Hill GJ II, Taubman O. Localised microscopic diverticulitis revealed by arteriography at the site of haemorrhage in diverticulosis of the colon. Dig Dis 1973; 18:808.
82. Gieske JC, Kahn PC, Moran JM. Arterial ligation for control of colonic diverticular hemorrhage. JAMA 1971; 217:1100.
83. Winzelberg GG, Froelich JW, McKusick KA, Waltman AC, Greenfield AJ, Athanasoulis CA, Strauss HW. Radionuclide localization of lower gastrointestinal hemorrhage. Radiology 1981; 139:465–9.
84. Welch JP, Warshaw AL. Isolated small bowel obstruction as the presenting feature of colonic disease. Arch Surg 1977; 112:809–12.
85. Silberman EL, Thorner MC. Volvulus of giant sigmoid diverticulum. JAMA 1961; 177:782.
86. Gallagher DM, Russell TR. Surgical management of diverticular disease. Surg Clin North Am 1978; 58:563–72.
87. Hersch RA, Schwabe AD. Left hydronephrosis as a complication of acute sigmoid diverticulitis. Gastroenterology 1963; 45:269.
88. Colcock BP, Stahmann FD. Fistulae complicating diverticular disease of the sigmoid colon. Ann Surg 1972; 175:838.
89. Hafner CD, Ponka LJ, Brush BE. Genitourinary manifestations of diverticulitis of the colon: a study of 500 cases. JAMA 1962; 179:76.
90. Kroening PM. Sigmoid ileal fistulas; a complication of diverticulitis. AJR 1966; 96:323.
91. Mayo CW, Blunt CP. The surgical management of the complications of diverticulitis of the large intestine: Analysis of 202 cases. Surg Clin North Am 1950; 30:1005.
92. Lipsit ER, Lewicki AM. Subcutaneous emphysema of the abdominal wall from diverticulitis with necrotizing fasciitis. Gastrointest Radiol 1979; 4:89–92.
93. Fleischner FG. Diverticular disease of the colon; new observations and revised concepts. Gastroenterology 1971; 60:316.
94. Sweatman CA Jr, Aldrete JS. The surgical management of diverticular disease of the colon complicated by perforation. Surg Gynecol Obstet 1977; 144:47–50.
95. Case TC, Shea CE Jr. Acute diverticulitis of the cecum. Am J Surg 1953; 85:134.

96. Riesenfend G. Acute solitary diverticulitis of the cecum. Int Surg 1968; 49:50.
97. Lauridsen J, Ross FP. Acute diverticulitis of the cecum: report of our cases and review of 153 surgical cases. Arch Surg 1952; 64:320.
98. Daniels VC, Wood EH. Diverticulitis of the cecum and ascending colon. JAMA 1960; 172:519.
98a. Sugihara K, Muto T, Morioka Y. Motility study in right-sided diverticular disease of the colon. Gut 1983; 24:1130–4.
99. Potier F. Diverticulite et appendicite. Bull Mem Soc Anat Paris 1912; 87:29.
100. Paulino F, Roselli A, Martins U. Pathology of diverticular disease of the colon. Surgery 1971; 69:63.
101. Leichtling JJ. Acute cecal diverticulitis. Gastroenterology 1955; 29:453.
102. Greaney EM, Snyder WH. Acute diverticulitis of cecum encountered at emergency surgery. Am J Surg 1957; 94:270.
103. Inglis FG, Hampson LG. Solitary diverticulitis of cecum and ascending colon. Can J Surg 1959; 2:166.
104. Nicholas EE, Frimark WB, Raffensperger JR. Acute cecal diverticulitis. Report of 25 cases. JAMA 1962; 182:157.
105. Schapiro A, Leichtling JJ, Wolf BS, et al. Diverticulitis of the cecum and right colon: clinical and radiographic features. Am J Dig Dis 1958; 3:351.
106. Wolf BS. Roentgen finding in diverticulitis of right side of colon. J Mt Sinai Hosp New York 1956; 23:697.
107. Boles RS, Jordan SM. The clinical significance of diverticulosis. Gastroenterology 1958; 35:579–82.
108. Horner JL. Natural history of diverticulosis of colon. Am J Dig Dis 1958; 3:343.
109. Hyland JMP, Taylor I. Does a high fibre diet prevent the complications of diverticular disease? Br J Surg 1980; 67:77–9.

136

Pneumatosis Cystoides Intestinalis

Robert J. Priest • Franz Goldstein

Pneumatosis cystoides intestinalis is a relatively rare condition characterized by multiple intramural pockets of gas involving any portion of the gastrointestinal tract and occasionally the mesenteric attachments. Pneumatosis in adults frequently has a benign course and prognosis, depending upon associated diseases of the gastrointestinal or pulmonary organs. Infantile pneumatosis intestinalis associated with necrotizing enteritis, however, is a more serious condition and has a high mortality rate.

The many theories regarding the origins of pneumatosis are reflected in its numerous synonyms. It has been called gas cysts of the intestine, peritoneal pneumatosis, intestinal emphysema, cystic lymphopneumatosis, bullous emphysema of the intestine, interstitial abdominal emphysema, intestinal intramural gas, and, most often, pneumatosis cystoides intestinalis. The gas-filled areas of pneumatosis intestinalis of infants may be linear rather than cystic, and the "cystoides" term is less descriptive.

In 1952, Koss[1] made an extensive review of the earliest records of the disease, noting that it was described in the 18th century by Duvernoy, John Hunter, and Jenner. Bernhard Bang, the Danish physician whose name also is associated with undulant fever, described the first well-documented human disease in 1876 and commented that a similar condition occurring in hogs had been known to butchers. Thirteen years after Bang's report, Hahn made the first observation of the disease in a living patient. Finney[2] described the first case in the United States literature in 1908.

Etiology and Pathogenesis

The etiology of pneumatosis cystoides intestinalis is not fully established, nor is the natural history of the disease well understood. It is probable that more than one mechanism is responsible for the formation of these gas cysts. The various theories of etiology have been grouped as either mechanical or bacterial.

Mechanical Theory. This holds that a break in continuity of the mucosa permits air to pass from the intestinal lumen to the submucosal spaces. Table 136–1 lists many of the conditions that have been associated with pneumatosis. Intestinal obstruction is theorized to increase the pressure of intraluminal gas, which then penetrates the wall and forms cysts. Enteritis, ulcerations, tumors, scleroderma, and procedures such as proctosigmoidoscopy, colonoscopy, or polypectomy may give rise to mucosal perforation. Actual proof for this theory is speculative, and breaks in the mucosa are difficult to find except in patients with ulcerative lesions of the intestinal tract. Kay-Butler[3] forced air through mucosal incisions of the cecum in fresh postmortem specimens. He concluded that gas in a continuous line developed from a break in the mucosa. This was different in appearance from the gas-filled cysts of varying size in pneumatosis coli.

A variation of the mechanical theory appears more logical. It is postulated that straining, as by coughing, causes painless alveolar rupture; alveolar air seeps into the perialveolar tissue, ultimately collecting to form a pneumomediastinum; the tension pneumo-

Table 136–1. CONDITIONS REPORTED IN ASSOCIATION WITH PNEUMATOSIS CYSTOIDES INTESTINALIS

Condition
Intestinal Obstruction:
Esophageal stricture[47]
Pyloric[48, 49]
Jejunal[50]
Peptic ulceration:
Stomach[1]
Duodenum[1]
Diverticula:
Jejunal[51]
Small intestine[52]
Sigmoid[53]
Ascites[54, 55]
Intestinal scleroderma[56–64]
Dermatomyositis[65, 66]
Cystic fibrosis of the pancreas[67, 68]
Crohn's disease[69, 70]
Acute appendicitis[71]
Lupus erythematosus[72, 73]
Ischemia of the bowel[74]
Jejunoileal bypass operations for obesity[14–18, 43, 44, 75–78]
Volvulus:
Stomach[79]
Sigmoid[80, 81]
Proctosigmoidoscopy and colonoscopy[82]
Acute and chronic leukemia, Hodgkin's disease and immunologic compromised patients[83–89]
Needle catheter jejunostomy[90]
Necrotizing enterocolitis of children[8, 91]

mediastinum decompresses itself by spread of the air retroperitoneally, advancing along vascular routes of the submucosal and subserosal areas of the bowel wall. Thus, Doub and Shea[4] described 16 cases of pneumatosis coli, of which 15 were associated with asthma and one with pulmonary fibrosis.

Keyting et al.,[5] explained all cases on a mechanical basis: obstruction (duodenal ulcer), trauma (proctosigmoidoscopy), or pulmonary disease with severe cough. By experimentally injecting air into the dog, pig, and unembalmed human cadaver, they demonstrated dissection of the air along the vascular channels of the mesocolon. Non-bacterial gastric emphysema has been described as being the result of rupture of adherent pulmonary bullae into the esophagus and downward extension of the air into the submucosa of the stomach. The vomiting that accompanies ulcerative or obstructive diseases of the stomach and duodenum may result in increased intrapulmonary pressure and the production of alveolar rupture. Chronic coughing may also be associated with this mechanism of alveolar rupture, mediastinal emphysema, and air tracking downward.

Formation of air cysts in the gut by this postulated modification of the mechanical theory would explain the absence of clinical, pathologic, and laboratory evidence of infection in cases of pneumatosis. The gaseous composition of the pneumatosis cyst is usually similar to air; nitrogen and carbon dioxide gases are relatively increased in concentration, while the oxygen content is lowered, owing to absorption.[6]

Keyting et al.[5] also implicated adrenocorticosteroids in the causation of pneumatosis, but there does not appear to have been any increase in frequency of this condition since the introduction of these hormones. Indeed, it is probable that a single mechanism cannot account for all cases of pneumatosis cyst formation. Moreover, even though a coexistent lesion or condition may not be apparent, it is quite likely that pneumatosis is nearly always a secondary development.[5]

Bacterial Theory. There is some clinical as well as experimental evidence that the gas produced in pneumatosis is of bacterial origin. While pneumatosis intestinalis has been reported in newborns following pneumomediastinum in the absence of enterocolitis or gastrointestinal obstruction,[7] the disorder is most often associated with severe enterocolitis in newborns, particularly premature infants. Thus, for example, a review of 100 cases of neonatal necrotizing enterocolitis by Stevenson and associates[8] disclosed radiographic manifestations of pneumatosis intestinalis in 98. Bacteria are thought to be responsible for the gas cysts in these infants, with increased permeability of the intestinal mucosa to gas-forming bacteria perhaps being related to prematurity, malnutrition, extracellular fluid depletion, and severe enteritis.

Lactulose, which depends on bacterial fermentation for its action, may aggravate the symptoms.[9] Yale et al.[10] produced pneumatosis cystoides intestinalis by injecting *Clostridium perfringens* into an isolated segment of strangulated intestine in germ-free rats. Similarly, Stone and his associates[11] tested the bacterial theory of infantile pneumatosis by injecting suspensions of gram-negative gas-forming bacteria and *Clostridium welchii* into the submucosal area of guinea pig colons. A pathologic condition was produced that was identical to the pneumatosis intestinalis of human infants.

The hypothesis that gas production by bacteria may be an etiologic factor in pneumatosis is supported by the finding that unusually high levels of breath hydrogen may be present,[12, 13] although hydrogen is not produced by human cells. Treatment by feeding an elemental diet, which is largely absorbed before reaching the colon, decreased the expiratory hydrogen and resulted in regression of pneumatosis cysts.[13]

Pneumatosis as a sequel of jejunoileal bypass operations has been explained as the fermentation of undigested lactose in the colon and reflux of the excessive gas into the excluded segment of small intestine.[14] Pneumatosis has been seen in the defunctionalized intestine and its mesentery,[15] as well as in the right colon.[16] Shortening the small intestine creates a long blind loop with stasis, relative lack of peristalsis, and diversion of bile acids, thereby creating an environment for bacterial overgrowth and gas formation.[17] Although *Clostridium perfringens* has been cultured from the contents of bypassed jejunoileal segments, it is possible that the pathogenetic mechanism is gas dissecting through the surgical anastomosis.[18]

Pathology

The gross appearance of pneumatosis cystoides intestinalis resembles bubbles under the serosa of the involved segment of intestinal wall (Fig. 136–1). The bowel wall feels spongy in the affected area. The gas cysts vary in size from a few millimeters in diameter to several centimeters. The cysts occur singly, in clusters, or are confluent. If the air cysts are located within the submucosa and not subserosally, diagnosis is not apparent from examination of the exterior of the bowel. However, the involved area may have a resilient consistency. When the intestine is cut transversely, the cystic portion of bowel is seen to be honeycombed with air cysts (Fig. 136–2).

The cysts are thin-walled and break easily. Pneumoperitoneum may result from spontaneous rupture of their serosal surface. Gas does not usually travel from one cyst to another, and there is no apparent connection between the cysts and the lumen of the bowel. The muscular coats of the bowel are usually involved to a lesser degree than the submucosa and subserosa.

Cysts may occur in the stomach, duodenum, small intestine, colon, gastrohepatic ligament, and any mesenteric attachment of the intestine, including the mesocolon, omentum, and parietal and diaphragmatic peritoneum.

Cysts predominate in the subserosa, and submucosal involvement is usually associated with subserosal cysts. A well-defined lining is lacking (Fig. 136–3A), but a layer of endothelial cells may be present. It has been suggested that the cysts represent distended lymphatics. Koss[1] has suggested that the endothelial lining cells have a tendency to coalesce. It is characteristic of the microscopic picture that the lining of the cysts may include large, multinucleated giant cells (Fig.

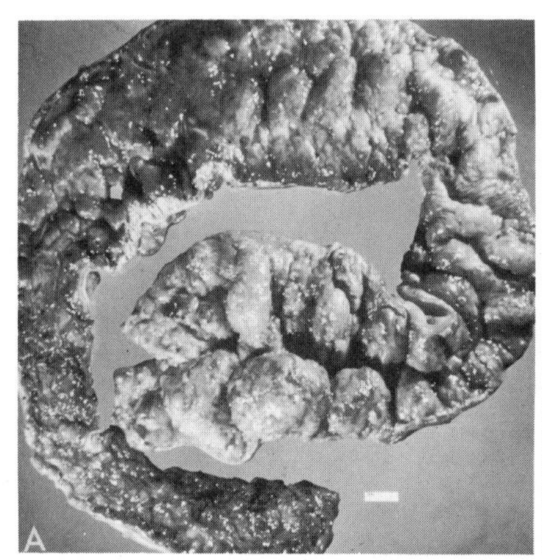

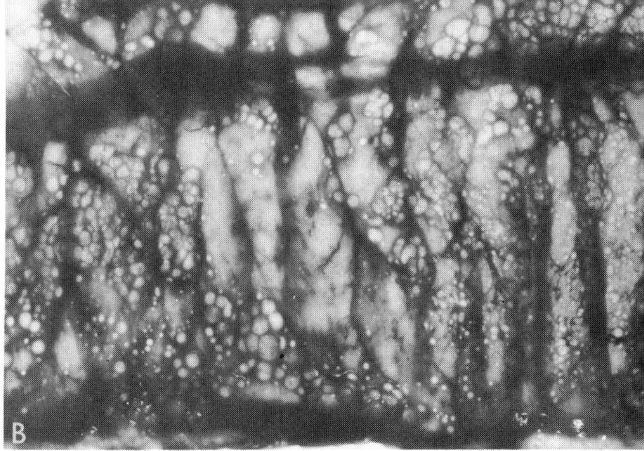

Figure 136–1. *A,* Large and small gas-filled blebs abound in the wall of this necropsy specimen of a colon; the patient had died of pulmonary emphysema. *B,* Bubbles of gas are seen by transillumination throughout the mucosa of the small intestine. The massed cysts have the appearance of soap bubbles in a basin of suds. Some are distorted by the pressure of adjacent gas cysts.

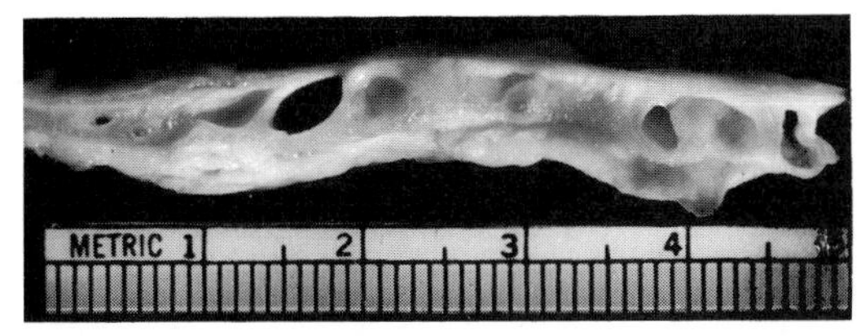

Figure 136–2. The wall of this ascending colon is honeycombed by gas-filled cysts.

136–3*B*). When the giant cells slough, the cyst is bare of any lining. An inflammatory reaction develops in the connective tissue surrounding the cysts, and granulomas with epithelioid cells may form in chronic cases. Finally, fibrosis of the stroma occurs around cyst spaces and scarring of the area progresses, with decrease in size and ultimate disappearance of the cysts.

Pneumatosis of the intestine may occur concomitantly with other lesions of the gastrointestinal tract and lungs. It is this relation to associated diseases that has led to the various theories of pathogenesis. Obstructive pulmonary disease, asthma, bullous lesions of the lungs, and pneumomediastinum have been reported increasingly with concomitant pneumatosis. Pneumatosis has been reported in association with collagen disorders of the intestines, with cystic fibrosis of the pancreas, and with acute and chronic leukemias. As noted, pneumatosis intestinalis of infants is commonly found in association with necrotizing enterocolitis that often spares the sigmoid colon and rectum.

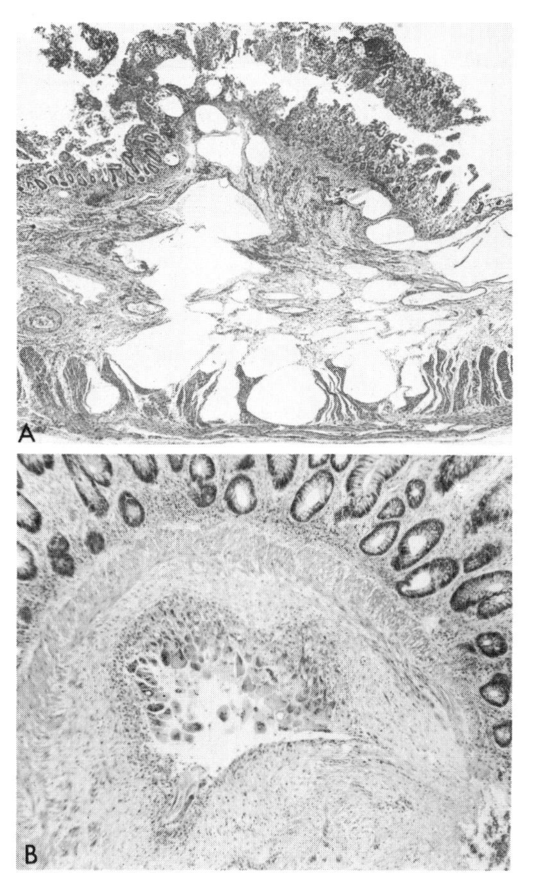

Figure 136–3. *A,* These cystic spaces in the subserosa of the colon have no epithelial or endothelial lining. (Hematoxylin and eosin, × 26.) *B,* Biopsy section of colonic mucosa obtained at sigmoidoscopy. The submucosa is somewhat congested, and abundant giant cells cluster in a cyst-like fashion. The pneumatosis coli in this patient was associated with an 8-year history of asthma.

Classification

Patients with pneumatosis have been divided into 2 general clinical groups, depending upon the coexistence of associated lesions of the gastrointestinal tract.[19] If no other *gastrointestinal* abnormalities are present, the disease is considered *primary* or *idiopathic.* The *secondary* group exhibits intramural gas collections associated with a broad variety of lesions of the gastrointestinal tract. Approximately 15% of the reported cases have been estimated to fall into the primary group and 85% into the secondary group. The primary group occurs mostly in adults, and the colon is usually involved; involvement of the left colon has been described more frequently in recent years.[20,21] The small intestine is involved most commonly in the secondary group.

Classification by clinical groups has also been suggested.[21] *Group I* is composed of patients with severe chronic pulmonary disease, *Group II* includes those patients with no known chronic pulmonary disease but with severe acute pulmonary conditions requiring mechanical ventilation, and *Group III* is composed of patients with severe clinical illness overshadowing the pneumatosis, such as myasthenia gravis and traumatic injuries for which vigorous therapy is required to ensure survival.

Prevalence

Although pneumatosis cystoides intestinalis is a relatively uncommon disease, it is being recognized more frequently. Koss,[1] in a review of 213 patients, found that the disease occurs more frequently in adult men, the sex ratio being approximately 3.5 men to 1 woman. In a review of 919 cases, Jamart[22] also found pneumatosis more often in men, the ratio being 1.9 men to 1 woman. It has been diagnosed most commonly in men aged 30 to 50 and among women in the sixth decade. Smith and Welter[23] found a mean age of 56.6 years (median, 46 years) in a group of adults. One report of pneumatosis in a woman, age 61, and her son, age 34 represents a unique familial cluster.[24]

Clinical Aspects

In Adults. The symptoms of pneumatosis cystoides intestinalis in adults are in no sense specific and may be expressions of one of the concomitant diseases with which pneumatosis is often associated. During some phase of the illness the majority of patients have gastrointestinal complaints. Diarrhea, with as many as 8 to 10 passages daily, may occur episodically for days or weeks. Abdominal cramps are associated with constipation and diminished stool caliber, possibly related to varying degrees of obstruction by the cysts that encroach on the lumen of the bowel and interfere with normal motility. Stools may be loose, float on water, and contain much mucus. Hematochezia is not uncommon, and occasionally rectal bleeding may be profuse. The fecal discharge may be frothy pink and mucoid or, if solid, may be mixed with streaks of blood.

Many patients with pneumatosis suffer symptoms of chronic obstructive pulmonary diseases, including emphysema, chronic asthma, chronic bronchitis, and atelectasis. The use of a nebulizer has been associated with aggravation of abdominal tenderness, flatulence, constipation, and hematochezia. To explain this, it has been conjectured that the nebulizer provoked pneumomediastinum with air dissecting retroperitoneally.

Abdominal signs may be absent, although mild abdominal tenderness may be detected. Pneumatosis of the left colon is palpated occasionally as a spongy resistance in the lower left quadrant of the abdomen. Tender, hard, cystic masses rarely are felt through the abdominal wall or in an abdominal hernia. Pneumatosis affecting the small intestine is generally without physical signs. Abdominal or pulmonary diseases associated with pneumatosis may be recognized by physical examination and can contribute to the diagnosis.

In Infants. Pneumatosis intestinalis in infants is frequently associated with septicemia and shock because of its common concurrence with necrotizing enterocolitis in this age group. Bowel perforation and peritonitis are also encountered fairly often in infants, in contrast to adults in whom cyst rupture and pneumoperitoneum are rarely associated with peritonitis.

Diagnosis

Diagnosis in former years was often made at the time of operation or at necropsy. It is difficult to make the diagnosis of pneumatosis by clinical features, although the diagnosis of coexisting disease is usually evident. However, a clinical diagnosis may be established from typical radiographic findings and, in those patients with disease involving the left colon or sigmoid, by proctosigmoidoscopy or fiberoptic colonoscopy. Often the patient does not appear as ill as might be suggested by the radiographic or endoscopic appearance of the affected bowel.

Radiography. Pneumatosis is suspected when radiolucent clusters are seen along the contours of the bowel[25] (Fig. 136–4). This sign may be seen in a plain film of the abdomen, an IV pyelogram, a barium enema, or even a gas-cystic pattern noted below the diaphragm on a chest film. Computed tomography has detected intramural gas prior to confirmation by other radiologic techniques.[26]

The translucent areas of gas seen in the roentgenogram may lie within the contour of the bowel wall (Fig. 136–5). The lumen of the bowel may not completely fill out with contrast barium and filling defects are evident. These radiolucencies are often misinterpreted as colonic polyps. However, the gas within the cysts is compressible and, unlike solid tumors, the defects change shape. Also, there is relatively more radiolucency than would be expected from solid tissue, and the radiolucent base is broader, especially in the area of overhanging edges near an obstruction.

In adults, the gas accumulates more frequently under the serosa than in the submucosa. Pneumatosis cysts may force the bowel wall inward and produce filling defects of variable size that change position in barium meal progress examinations. The lumen may be compressed concentrically, with air shadows extending on either side of the

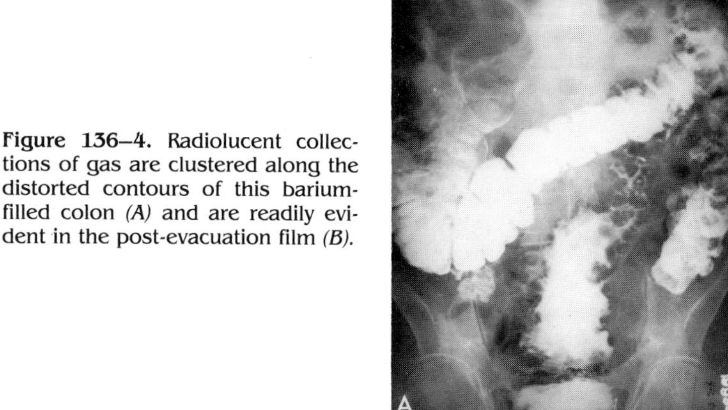

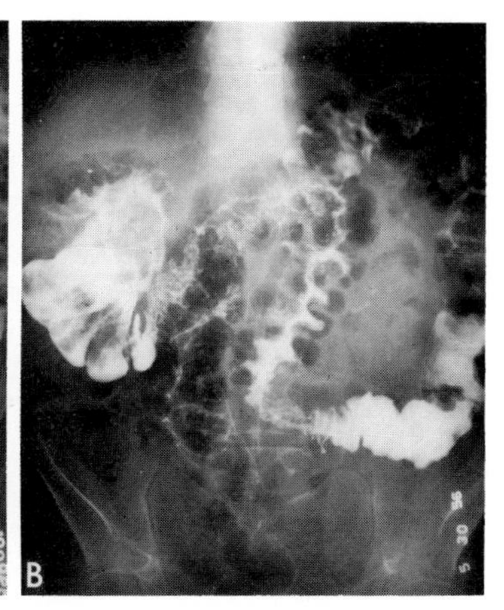

Figure 136–4. Radiolucent collections of gas are clustered along the distorted contours of this barium-filled colon *(A)* and are readily evident in the post-evacuation film *(B)*.

bowel contour and the barium appearing as a thin, irregular stream in the midline of the colon silhouette (Fig. 136–6).

Gas present between the layers of mesentery may simulate free air in the abdomen. Lateral decubitus films will distinguish the 2 findings and indicate that the radiolucency is not free air in the peritoneal cavity. The finding of pneumoperitoneum may suggest pneumatosis when, despite what appears to be free air, there is an absence of the clinical signs of peritonitis or ruptured viscus. Pneumatosis of the small intestine is more difficult to diagnose radiologically than is involvement of the colon. In pneumatosis of the small intestine, a loop of bowel may be interposed between the liver and the diaphragm (the so-called Chilaiditi sign). Radiographic signs of advanced pulmonary disease are common in elderly patients with pneumatosis intestinalis (Fig. 136–7).

Radiographic signs have been described following decompression of a silent pneumomediastinum that in turn resulted from painless pulmonary alveolar rupture.[27] These include paravertebral air in the mediastinum; double ring contour outline of the stomach; translucent bubbles mixed with the shadows of small intestinal gas; translucent defects along the contours of the colon; air in the lateral abdominal walls, inguinal canals, or the retroperitoneal space around kidneys; and air tracking along iliofemoral arterial fascial sheaths. However, gas was not seen to extend along the vessels of 2 patients with pneumatosis who were studied by angiography of the superior and inferior mesenteric arteries.[28] Gas in the portal venous system has been reported in an elderly patient with pneumatosis involving several jejunal loops.[19] Portal venous gas in infants with pneumatosis usually is associated with necrotizing enterocolitis. Intramural gas collections are usually linear or parallel to the long axis of the lumen of the intestine in such infants.[29,30]

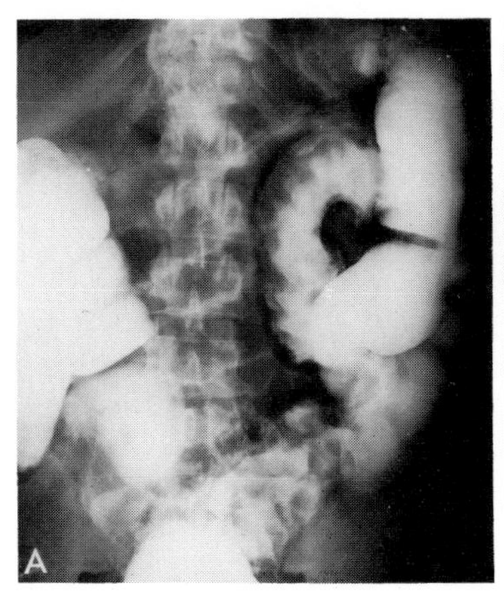

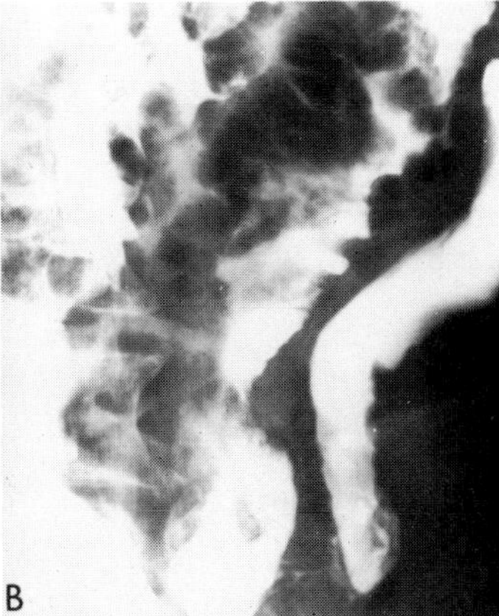

Figure 136–5. *A*, Note the subserosal gas lucencies and scalloping of the barium silhouette in the descending and sigmoid segments of this colon. *B*, These multiple filling defects in a large redundant sigmoid colon should not be confused with polyposis.

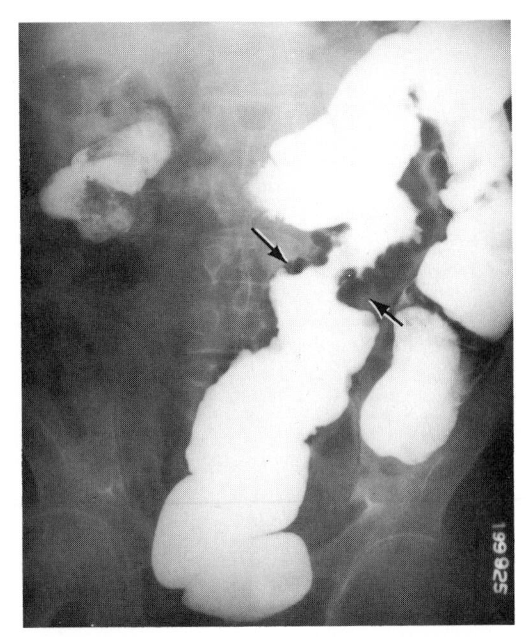

Figure 136–6. Gas-filled cysts, clearly evident by their lucency, concentrically constrict the lumen of this sigmoid colon and help distinguish the defect from neoplasm.

Differential radiographic diagnosis includes enterogenous cysts, which are usually single, although they are occasionally multiloculated. Emphysematous gastritis, the result of intramural infection, may give rise to gas in the stomach wall. The radiographic appearance of pneumatosis must be distinguished from polyposis and carcinoma. This can be done but requires careful observation of the filling defects with attention to the distinguishing features of pneumatosis that have been noted.

Endoscopy. The diagnosis of pneumatosis is often made by proctosigmoidoscopic or fiberoptic colonoscopic examinations[31–33] (Fig. 136–8). Involvement of the left colon and sigmoid areas, being typical, lends itself to detection by this means. The appearance of pneumatosis on endoscopic examination is that of submucosal cyst-like lesions resembling tapioca particles or large globular masses protruding into the lumen, often interfering with deeper passage of the diagnostic instrument. The mucosa overlying the gas cysts is usually intact and appears pale, transparent, or slightly bluish. An initial diagnosis may have been made of polyposis, submucosal lymphoid hyperplasia, granulomatous disease, or malignancy; however, the air-filled space is seen to collapse when biopsy is taken. Spontaneous deflation of a cyst has been observed[20] and, when seen, will of course indicate the correct diagnosis.

Rounded soft mucosal masses may be felt by the examining finger preceding proctosigmoidoscopic examination. When proctosigmoidoscopy has been performed previous to the onset of pneumatosis, it has been suggested as a traumatic etiologic agent. Endoscopy may be diagnostic in cases of asymptomatic pneumoperitoneum. Fiberoptic colonoscopy will establish the extent of colonic involvement by pneumatosis.[31]

Complications

Pneumatosis cystoides intestinalis may be associated with free air in the peritoneal cavity, presumably from rupture of gas cysts. As discussed earlier, pneumoperitoneum has been described as the sequel of air dissecting retroperitoneally from a ruptured alveolus of

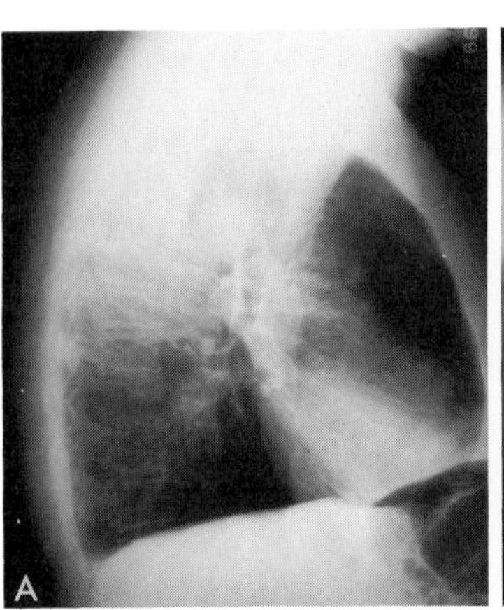

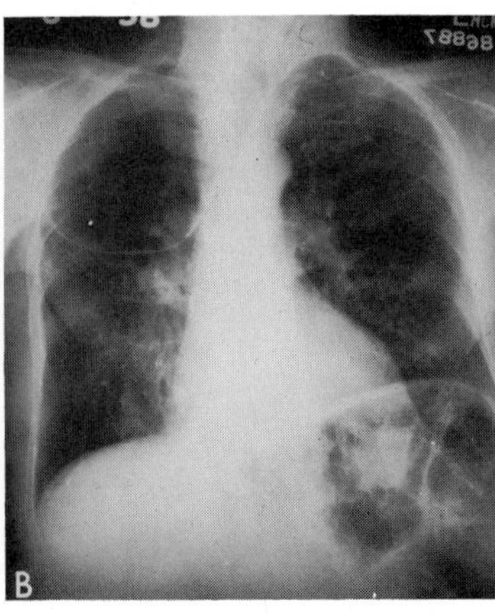

Figure 136–7. Classic chest radiographs in elderly patients with pneumatosis cystoides intestinalis. *A,* Lateral view showing marked emphysema in the patient whose bowel lesions are illustrated in Figure 136–3. *B,* Frontal view of another patient with pulmonary fibrosis and a large bleb in the right upper lung field. In both instances the appearance of the subdiaphragmatic gaseous lucencies might suggest the attending pneumatosis cystoides intestinalis.

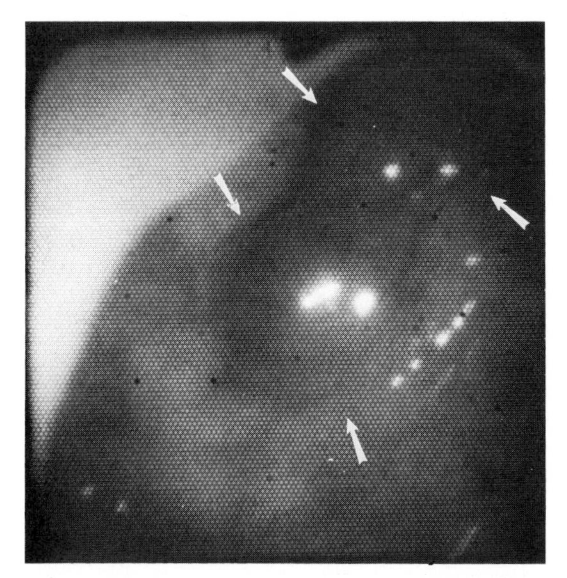

Figure 136–8. The arrows point to submucosal gas cysts as seen through the colonoscope. (From Gruenberg JC et al. Arch Surg 1977; 112:62–4. Copyright 1977, American Medical Association. Reproduced with permission.)

the lung. Pneumoperitoneum in such cases is usually not associated with peritonitis.

Pneumatosis of the small intestine may be complicated by ileus, intussusception, volvulus, and partial or complete obstruction. The last may occur from the encroachment of submucosal cysts into the lumen of the bowel, from compression of large, extrinsic masses of cysts, or from adhesions forming in relation to the cysts of adjacent organs. Extensive cyst pressure may cause bowel obstruction, fecal impaction, and bowel perforation secondary to stercoral ulceration.[34] Extensive intestinal hemorrhage may also occur.

Pneumatosis cystoides intestinalis has been reported to be associated with severe ascites, acute leukemia, and chronic lymphatic leukemia. Cases of malabsorption celiac (sprue) have also been described with pneumatosis.[35, 36] It is not clear whether intestinal malabsorption and pneumatosis are causally related in such cases. It is doubtful that pneumatosis contributes to malabsorption in the many cases reported with intestinal scleroderma or collagen disorders.

Treatment

The cystic areas of pneumatosis may regress spontaneously. In many cases no treatment is indicated, except for management of associated diseases of the intestinal tract or obstructive pulmonary diseases. Although the disease often follows a benign course, the symptoms of abdominal cramping, diarrhea, or constipation may require symptomatic relief.

Oxygen breathing is used to alter the balance in favor of absorption in the process of diffusion of gases into and out of cysts.[37] An oxygen-nitrogen gas mixture (about 75:25, the reverse of the composition of gas within the cysts) is used. Pure oxygen cannot be used safely because of the risk of oxygen toxicity and carbon dioxide narcosis. Breathing high concentrations of oxygen washes nitrogen out of the tissues, altering the cyst-capillary diffusion gradient and thus promoting absorption of gas.

Oxygen has been administered by head tent,[37] by non-rebreathing face mask, or by nasal catheter.[33,38] Lee and co-workers[39] found that continuous oxygen administration was not necessary, allowing a half-hour break for meals. Oxygen in a concentration of 40% has been used successfully through a non-rebreathing face mask with less risk of oxygen toxicity.[40] The potential hazard of toxic effects from oxygen can be detected by the frequent measurement of vital capacity, daily blood gases, and chest radiography.[33,41] Recurrence of gas cysts has been reported as long as a year after oxygen therapy.[41] Hyperbaric oxygen has been used successfully at 2.5 atmospheres (ATA) for 2 hours on successive days.[42]

Metronidazole has been used with success when oxygen treatment failed to relieve symptoms permanently.[9] Metronidazole may be given in pulsed doses for 5 days every 2 to 3 weeks. The successful use of this drug as an antimicrobial agent suppressing anerobic bacteria may support the thesis that gas-forming bacteria contribute to pneumatosis. Metronidazole has also been used in bypass enteropathy to suppress anerobic organisms in the excluded segment of intestine.[43,44] However, it has been reported that the drug may have to be abandoned because of rapid worsening of symptoms.[45]

Pneumatosis has been reported to disappear coincident with reduction of endotracheal suctioning, which had stimulated forceful coughing.[46] The same phenomenon has been observed after discontinuance of nebulizer treatment for asthma.[46a]

Surgical treatment of pneumatosis is usually indicated for complications rather than for the disease itself. Occasionally, cystic lesions of the small intestine disappear and do not recur after operation for coexistent peptic ulcer or intestinal obstruction. Resection may be done if pneumatosis is localized to a short segment of grossly obstructed bowel. Pneumatosis coli involving the left colon, however, does not usually require resection, but surgery may be needed on occasion when pneumatosis of the left more proximal segments of the colon are resected; rectal involvement usually regresses after proximal resection.

Prognosis

The course of pneumatosis cystoides intestinalis in the adult is usually benign. More often it is dependent on the underlying disease associated with its pathogenesis. Following jejunoileal bypass, pneumatosis is usually self-limited and responds to conservative treatment.[16] Occasionally, clinical symptoms continue after jejunoileal bypass and further surgical intervention is required.[17] Gas cysts may disappear spontaneously or may persist for many years, and the disease may recur after segmental resection of the intestine.

Pneumatosis intestinalis in infants is a more hazardous condition, being associated with an underlying necrotizing enterocolitis from which survival is limited.

References

1. Koss LG. Abdominal gas cysts (pneumatosis cystoides intestinorum hominis). An analysis with a report of a case and a critical review of the literature. Arch Pathol 1952; 53:523–49.
2. Finney JMT. Gas cysts of the intestine. JAMA 1908; 51:1291–7.
3. Kay-Butler JJ. Interstitial emphysema of the caecum. Gut 1962; 3:267–8.
4. Doub HP, Shea JJ. Pneumatosis cystoides intestinalis. JAMA 1960; 172:1238–42.
5. Keyting WS, McCarver RR, Kovarik JL, Daywitt AL. Pneumatosis intestinalis: A new concept. Radiology 1961; 76:733–41.
6. Mujahed Z, Evans JA. Gas cysts of the intestine (pneumatosis intestinalis). Surg Gynecol Obstet 1958; 107:151–9.
7. Lee SB, Kuhn JP. Pneumatosis intestinalis following pneumomediastinum in a newborn infant. J Pediatr 1971; 79:813–5.
8. Stevenson DK, Graham CB, Stevenson JK. Neonatal necrotizing enterocolitis: 100 new cases. Adv Pediatr 1980; 27:319–40.
9. Ellis BW. Symptomatic treatment of primary penumatosis coli with metronidazole. Br Med J 1980; 1:763–4.
10. Yale CE, Balish E, Wu JP. The bacterial etiology of pneumatosis cystoides intestinalis. Arch Surg 1974; 109:89–94.
11. Stone HH, Allen WB, Smith RB III, Haynes CD. Infantile pneumatosis intestinalis. J Surg Res 1968; 8:301–7.
12. Gillon J, Tadesse K, Logan RFA, Holt S, Sircus W. Breath hydrogen in pneumatosis cystoides intestinalis. Gut 1979; 20:1008–11.
13. Van Der Linden W, Marsell R. Pneumatosis cystoides coli associated with high H_2 excretion. Treatment with an elemental diet. Scand J Gastroenterol 1979; 14:173–4.
14. Sicard GA, Vaughan R, Wise L. Pneumatosis cystoides intestinalis: An unusual complication of jejunoileal bypass. Surgery 1976; 79:480–4.
15. Ikard RW. Pneumatosis cystoides intestinalis following intestinal bypass. Am Surg 1977; 43:467–70.
16. Doolas A, Breyer RH, Franklin JL. Pneumatosis cystoides intestinalis following jejunoileal by-pass. Am J Gastroenterol 1979; 72:271–5.
17. Ganel A, Haspel Y, Ben-Ari G, David R. Surgical treatment for pneumatosis cystoides intestinalis complicating jejunoileal by-pass. Am J Gastroenterol 1979; 71:306–10.
18. Martyak SN, Curtis LE. Pneumatosis intestinalis. A complication of jejunoileal bypass. JAMA 1976; 235:1038–9.
19. Seaman WB, Fleming RJ, Baker DH. Pneumatosis intestinalis of the small bowel. Semin Roentgenol 1966; 1:234–42.
20. Smith WG, Anderson MJ Jr, Pemberton HW. Pneumatosis cystoides intestinalis involving left portion of colon. Report of four cases diagnosed at sigmoidoscopy. Gastroenterology 1958; 35:528–33.
21. Gruenberg JC, Grodsinsky C, Ponka JL. Pneumatosis intestinalis: A clinical classification. Dis Colon Rectum 1979; 22: 5–9.
22. Jamart J. Pneumatosis cystoides intestinalis. A statistical study of 919 cases. Acta Hepato-Gastroenterol 1979; 26:419–22.
23. Smith BH, Welter LH. Pneumatosis intestinalis. Am J Clin Pathol 1967; 48:455–65.
24. Underwood JW, Finnis D, Scott W. Pneumatosis coli: a familial association. Br J Surg 1978; 65:64–5.
25. Marshak RH, Lindner AE, Milano AM. Pneumatosis coli. Am J Gastroenterol 1971; 56:68–73.
26. Hutchins WW, Gore RM, Foley MJ. CT demonstration of pneumatosis intestinalis from bowel infarction. Comput Radiol 1983; 7:283–5.
27. Elliott GB, Elliott KA. The roentgenologic pathology of so-called pneumatosis cystoides intestinalis. AJR 1963; 89: 720–9.
28. Lunderquist A, Svendler CA, Kornhall S. Angiography findings in pneumatosis cystoides intestinalis. AJR 1973; 117:314–6.
29. Rigler LG, Pogue WL. Roentgen signs of intestinal necrosis. AJR 1965; 94:402–9.
30. Nelson SW. Extraluminal gas collections due to diseases of the gastrointestinal tract. AJR 1972; 115:225–48.
31. Varano VJ, Bonanno CA. Colonoscopic findings in pneumatosis cystoides intestinalis. Am J Gastroenterol 1973; 59:353–60.
32. Forde KA, Whitlock RT, Seaman WB. Pneumatosis and cystoides intestinalis. Report of a case with colonoscopic finding of inflammatory bowel disease. Am J Gastroenterol 1977; 68:188–90.
33. Gruenberg JC, Batra SK, Priest RJ. Treatment of pneumatosis cystoides intestinalis with oxygen. Arch Surg 1977; 112: 62–4.
34. Meikle G. A case of pneumatosis coli. Pneumatosis cystoides intestinalis of the sigmoid colon causing intestinal obstruction, stercoral ulcer and perforation. J R Coll Surg Edinb 1965; 11:65–7.
35. Yunich AM, Fradkin NF. Fatal sprue (malabsorption) syndrome secondary to extensive pneumatosis cystoides intestinalis. Gastroenterology 1958; 35:212–7.
36. Breiter J, Levine JB, Forouhar FA. Pneumatosis cystoides intestinalis associated with refractory sprue. Am J Gastroenterol 1982; 77:322–5.
37. Forgacs P, Wright PH, Wyatt AP. Treatment of intestinal gas cysts by oxygen breathing. Lancet 1973; 1:579–82.
38. Simon NM, Nyman KE, Divertie MB, Rovelstad RA, King JE. Pneumatosis cystoides intestinalis. Treatment with oxygen via close-fitting mask. JAMA 1975; 231:1354–6.

39. Lee SP, Coverdale HA, Nicholson GI. Oxygen therapy for pneumatosis coli: A report of two cases and a review. Aust NZ J Med 1977; 7:44–6.
40. Miralbés M, Hinojosa J, Alonso J. Berenguer J. Oxygen therapy in pneumatosis coli. What is the minimum oxygen requirement? Dis Colon Rectum 1983; 26:458–60.
41. Holt S, Gilmour HM, Buist TAS, Marwick K, Heading RC. High flow oxygen therapy for pneumatosis coli. Gut 1979; 20:493–8.
42. Masterson JST, Fratkin LB, Osler TR, Trapp WG. Treatment of pneumatosis cystoides intestinalis with hyperbaric oxygen. Ann Surg 1978; 187:245–7.
43. Drenick EJ, Ament ME, Finegold SM, Passaro E Jr. Bypass enteropathy: an inflammatory process in the excluded segment with systemic complications. Am J Clin Nutr 1977; 30:76–89.
44. Leung FW, Drenick EJ, Stanley TM. Intestinal bypass complications involving the excluded small bowel segment. Am J Gastroenterol 1982; 77:67–72.
45. Gillon J, Logan RFA, Sircus W, Heading RC. Symptomatic treatment of primary pneumatosis coli with metronidazole. Br Med J 1980; 1:1087.
46. Reyna R, Soper RT, Condon RE. Pneumatosis intestinalis. Report of 12 cases. Am J Surg 1973; 125:667–71.
47. Vanasin B, Wright JR, Schuster MM. Pneumatosis cystoides esophagi. Case report supporting theory of submucosal spread. JAMA 1971; 217:76–7.
48. Dhall DP, Mahaffy RG, Matheson NA. Intestinal pneumatosis treated by pyloroplasty. J R Coll Surg Edinb 1968; 13:226–9.
49. Hoffman RV Jr, Gyorgy TRM, Bradley RL. Pneumatosis intestinalis. Report of a case associated with pyloric obstruction. Am Surg 1968; 34:300–2.
50. Kleinman PL, King DR. Ischemic jejunitis and pneumatosis intestinalis secondary to anastomotic obstruction following jejunal atresia repair. Gastrointest Radiol 1977; 2:113–5.
51. Scott PM. Case report of pneumatosis cystoides intestinalis and syringocystadenomata associated with asymptomatic pneumoperitoneum and jejunal diverticulosis. Neb State Med J 1970; 55:217–9.
52. Dammert K, Stenbäck F, Räsänen O. Pneumatosis intestinalis. A pathogenetic study. Acta Pathol Microbiol Scand 1967; 71:25–34.
53. Jørgensen A, Wille-Jørgensen P. Pneumatosis intestinalis and pneumoperitoneum due to a solitary sigmoid diverticulum. Acta Chir Scand 1982; 148:625–6.
54. Tsega E. Pneumatosis cystoides intestinalis with unexplained ascites in Ethiopian patients. Br J Surg 1975; 62:379–82.
55. Cloete GNP, van Rooyen RJ. Pneumatosis cystoides intestinalis. S Afr Med J 1967; 41:795–800.
56. Meuwissen SGM, Hausman R, Dingemans KP, Reiss M, Hovius SER. A patient with scleroderma of the small intestine complicated by chronic intestinal obstruction, volvulus and intestinal pneumatosis. Neth J Med 1982; 25:354–9.
57. Fallon RH. Pneumatosis cystoides intestinalis, associated with scleroderma and presenting with pneumoperitoneum. Mo Med 1967; 64:117–8.
58. Gompels BM. Pneumatosis cystoides intestinalis associated with progressive systemic sclerosis. Br J Radiol 1969; 42: 701–3.
59. Hughes DTD, Gordon KCD, Swann JC, Bolt GL. Pneumatosis cystoides intestinalis. Gut 1966; 7:553–7.
60. Meihoff WE, Hirschfield JS, Kern F Jr. Small intestinal scleroderma with malabsorption and pneumatosis cystoides intestinalis. Report of three cases. JAMA 1968; 204:854–8.
61. Miercort RD, Merrill FG. Pneumatosis and pseudo-obstruction in scleroderma. Radiology 1969; 92:359–62.
62. Speed T. Cystic pneumatosis intestinalis with pseudosurgical manifestations. Surg Clin North Am 1972; 52:453–7.
63. White WD, Treece TR, Juniper K Jr. Pneumatosis in scleroderma of the small bowel. JAMA 1970; 212:1068.
64. Morrison WJ, Siegelman SS. Pneumatosis intestinalis in association with connective tissue disease. South Med J 1976; 69:1536–9.
65. Braunstein EM, White SJ. Pneumatosis intestinalis in dermatomyositis. Br J Radiol 1980; 53:1011–2.
66. Mueller CF, Morehead R, Alter AJ, Michener W. Pneumatosis intestinalis in collagen disorders. AJR 1972; 115:300–5.
67. Wood RE, Herman CJ, Johnson KW, di Sant'Angnese PA. Pneumatosis coli in cystic fibrosis. Clinical, radiological and pathological features. Am J Dis Child 1975; 129:246–8.
68. Berk RN, Lee FA. The late gastrointestinal manifestations of cystic fibrosis of the pancreas. Radiology 1973; 106:377–81.
69. Ghahremani GG, Port RB, Beachley MC. Pneumatosis coli in Crohn's disease. Dig Dis Sci 1974; 19:315–23.
70. Rienhoff WF III, Collins NP. Pneumatosis cystoides intestinalis and regional enteritis. Ann Surg 1959; 149:593–9.
71. DiDonato LR. Pneumatosis coli secondary to acute appendicitis Case report. Radiology 1976; 120:90.
72. Freiman D, Chon H, Bilaniuk L. Pneumatosis intestinalis in systemic lupus erythematosus. Radiology 1975; 116:563–4.
73. Kleinman P, Meyers MA, Abbott G, Kazam E. Necrotizing enterocolitis with pneumatosis intestinalis in systemic lupus erythematosus and polyarteritis. Radiology 1976; 121:595–8.
74. Roscher AA, Endlich HL. Pneumatosis cystoides intestinalis. Clinical-pathological correlation. Int Surg 1972; 57:623–9.
75. Passaro E Jr, Drenick E, Wilson SE. Bypass enteritis. A new complication of jejunoileal bypass for obesity. Am J Surg 1976; 131:169–74.
76. Feinberg SB, Schwartz MZ, Clifford S, Buchwald H, Varco RL. Significance of pneumatosis cystoides intestinalis after jejunoileal bypass. Am J Surg 1977; 133:149–52.
77. Clements JL Jr. Intestinal pneumatosis—A complication of the jejunoileal bypass procedure. Gastrointest Radiol 1977; 2:267–71.
78. Wandtke J, Skucas J, Spataro R, Bruneau RJ. Pneumatosis intestinalis as a complication of jejunoileal bypass. AJR 1977; 129:601–4.
79. Elidan J, Gimmon Z, Schwartz A. Pneumoperitoneum induced by pneumatosis cystoides intestinalis associated with volvulus of the stomach. Am J Gastroenterol 1980; 74:189–95.
80. Wertkin MG, Wetchler BB, Waye JD, Brown LK. Pneumatosis coli associated with sigmoid volvulus and colonoscopy. Am J Gastroenterol 1976: 65:209–14.
81. Gillon J, Holt S, Sircus W. Pneumatosis coli and sigmoid volvulus: a report of 4 cases. Br J Surg 1979; 66:802–5.
82. Heer M, Altorfer J, Pirovino M, Schmid M. Pneumatosis cystoides coli: A rare complication of colonoscopy. Endoscopy 1983; 15:119–20.
83. Shindelman LE, Geller SA, Wisch N, Bauer JJ. Pneumatosis cystoides intestinalis. A complication of systemic chemotherapy. Am J Gastroenterol 1981; 75:270–4.
84. Crider RJ Jr, Bentlif P. Pneumatosis cystoides intestinalis: The report of a case associated with severe pulmonary disease and chronic lymphocytic leukemia. Henry Ford Hosp Med J 1969; 17:285–94.
85. Jaffe N, Carlson DH, Vawter GF. Pneumatosis cystoides intestinalis in acute leukemia. Cancer 1972; 30:239–43.
86. Navari RM, Sharma P, Deeg HJ, McDonald GB, Thomas ED. Pneumatosis cystoides intestinalis following allogeneic marrow transplantation. Transplantat Proc 1983; 15:1720–4.
87. Kleinman PK, Brill PW, Winchester P. Pneumatosis intestinalis. Its occurrence in the immunologically compromised child. Am J Dis Child 1980; 134:1149–51.
88. McCarthy D, Holland I, Lavender JP, Catovsky D. Pneumatosis coli in adult acute myeloid leukaemia. Clin Radiol 1979; 30:175–8.
89. O'Connell DJ, Thompson AJ. Pneumatosis coli in non-Hodgkin's lymphoma. Br J Radiol 1978; 51:203–5.
90. Cogbill TH, Wolfson RH, Moore EE, VanWay CW, Jones TN, Strain JD, Rudikoff JC. Massive pneumatosis intestinalis and subcutaneous emphysema: complication of needle catheter jejunostomy. J Parenteral Enteral Nutr 1983; 7:171–5.
91. Gupta A. Pneumatosis intestinalis in children. Br J Radiol 1978; 51:589–95.
92. Priest RJ, Chun R. Pneumatosis coli masquerading as tumor. Proceedings of the VIII Congress Bockus International Society of Gastroenterology, Honolulu, 1966, 117–21.

Chapter 137

Enteric Endometriosis

William S. Haubrich

The finding of endometrial glands deep in the muscular wall of the uterus is called *adenomyosis*. The term *endometriosis* generally refers to the presence of heterotopic foci of elements characteristic of endometrium in tissues apart from the uterus. Although not in contiguity with the uterine lining, these foci are usually, but not always, in the vicinity of the uterus. Enteric involvement, then, typically is of those bowel segments within or near the female pelvis. Meyers et al.[1] have estimated that 8% to 15% of menstruating women harbor endometriosis. Among these patients in whom endometriosis is found, the bowel has been reported to be involved in about 12%[2] to 37%.[3]

Among the earliest descriptions of endometriosis is that of Rokitansky[4] in 1860. Sporadic reports followed. It was not until 1921, however, that endometriosis was classically described by Sampson[5] as a clinical and pathologic entity. Sampson included in this description reference to involvement of the sigmoid colon.

Pathology

The enteric lesions of endometriosis are generally serosal, sometimes intramural, and only rarely mucosal. They usually are eccentric but occasionally envelop the circumference of the bowel. They are typically multiple and vary in size from minute, hardly visible nodules to extensive areas of cystic hemorrhagic necrosis and fibrosis. Among 63 cases described by LiVolsi and Perzin,[6] the appendix was involved in 21, the sigmoid colon in 20, the rectum and perirectal tissues in 9, the ileum in 8, the cecum in 2, and the mesocolon, anal canal, and a colostomy in 1 each. This distribution is similar to that described by others.[7–9] Extension to the pleural cavity through diaphragmatic channels has been reported.[10]

As encountered at operation, serosal endometriosis grossly appears as a focal puckering associated with red-brown mottled nodules in a setting of gray fibrosis (Fig. 137–1). Typically there is induration and thickening of the bowel wall, occasionally circumferential and stenotic. When the bowel is severely constricted, kinked, or intussuscepted, obstruction may be evident by proximal dilatation. Less common is circumscribed, cystic tumefaction resembling intramural neoplasia. Affected bowel segments often are adherent or fixed to the adjacent parietes, internal genitalia, or urinary bladder. Enteric lesions usually, but not always, are accompanied by endometrial implants elsewhere in the internal genitalia and their adnexa; nodules in the uterosacral ligaments or a "chocolate cyst" in an ovary is often a clue to the nature of concomitant bowel lesions.[11] It has been estimated that endometriosis can be found in about 0.8% of resected specimens of the appendix.[12]

The histologic appearance is that of multiple, irregular acinar spaces lined by pleomorphic columnar epithelium and interspersed with areas of hemorrhagic necrosis, chronic inflammatory reaction, and fibrosis. Within the wall of the bowel, the aberrant endometrial tissue is attended by hyperplasia of muscular and connective components. The overlying bowel mucosa may be puckered or edematous but tends to remain intact, only rarely being penetrated or ulcerated.

Pathogenesis

Traditionally, there are 3 postulated explanations for the heterotopic endometrial growths, none of them proved or wholly satisfactory:

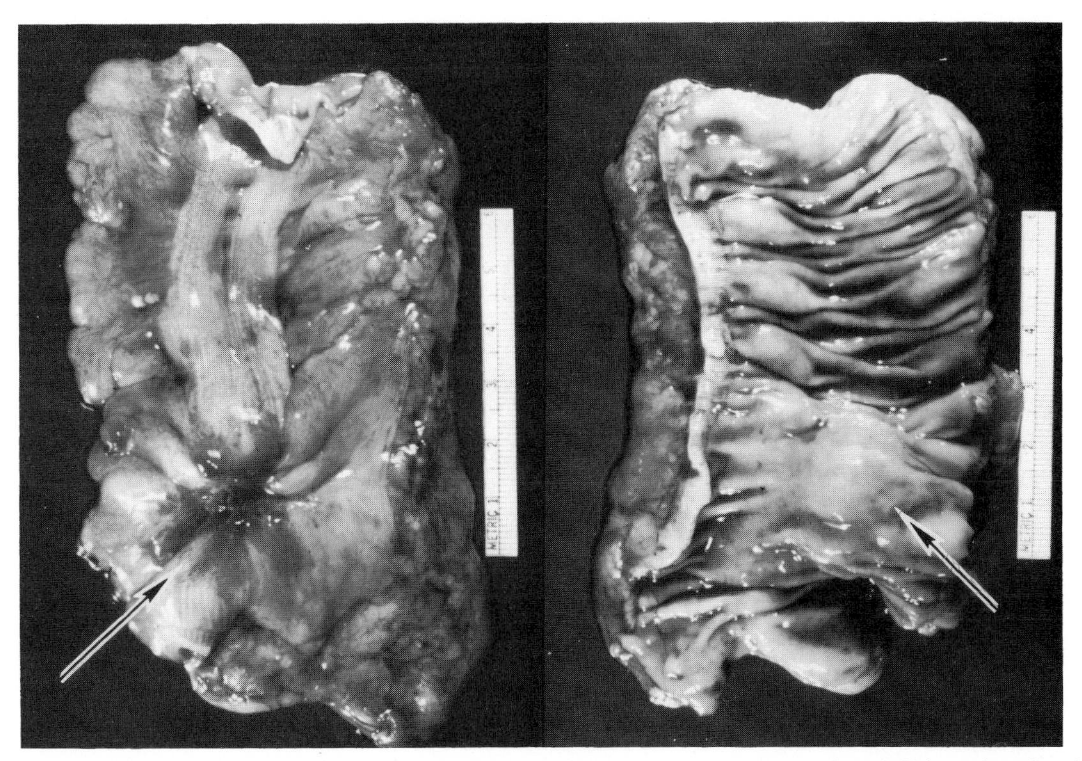

Figure 137–1. A focus of endometriosis embedded in the colon wall. The serosal surface *(left)* is puckered and mottled, while in the opened specimen *(right)* intact mucosa covers a bulging intramural implant. (Photographs kindly furnished by Dr. Joseph L. Ponka, from Dis Colon Rectum 1973; 16:490. Reproduced with permission.)

1. Sampson[5] suggested that endometrium might be spilled into the peritoneal cavity by reflux through the fallopian tubes during menstruation, then implanted on serosal surfaces. This would imply an associated impediment to the normal egress of menstrual fluid, and such impediment has been found as cervical stenosis in some cases of endometriosis. Further, it has been demonstrated that menstrual fluid contains viable cells capable of growth on the receptive peritoneum. The reflux theory alone, however, can hardly account for the curiously selective implantation observed in many cases.

2. Ivanoff[13] and Meyer[14] were among those who recognized a common embryonic derivation of endometrium and serosa from the coelomic membrane and theorized that endometriosis might arise in metaplasia of serosal epithelial cells. This could explain multiple foci at distant sites but leaves the question of cause unanswered.

3. Vascular dissemination of endometrial tissues, especially through lymphatic channels, was suggested by Halban.[15] This would be tantamount to lymphatic metastasis and is discounted by the rarity of finding endometriosis in lymph nodes.

All these postulates require a peculiar viability of endometrial epithelial cells at distant and alien sites, a property shared only by neoplastic cells of other tissues. Furthermore, endometrium at heterotopic sites appears to remain under hormonal control, proliferating and degenerating in a cyclic fashion during the reproductive span. Proliferating endometrium at ectopic sites also has a peculiarly invasive propensity. Cyclic hemorrhage, being confined, tends to cause cystic distortion and consequent necrosis and fibrosis, all of which are destructive to the host tissue.

Just as malignant neoplasia can occur in normal endometrium, so adenocarcinoma has been reported in endometrial implants.[16, 17] Cancer is found in less than 1% of ovarian lesions and is even rarer at other ectopic sites.

With the menopause, hormonal stimulation ceases and the aberrant endometrial tissue becomes inactive. By then, however, much of the damage has been done and the scar remains.

Clinical Features

Endometriosis flourishes only when ovarian function is active; hence, the disease is usually evident in women between the ages of 20 and 45 years. However, symptoms have been reported in teenagers,[18] and the ravages of enteric lesions have become manifest after the menopause.[19] The condition is said to be more frequent in women of the upper socioeconomic classes, presumably because they tend to be older at the time of initial pregnancy and they tend to have fewer pregnancies. Nulliparity, whether it is the cause or effect of the disease, is relatively common among patients with endometriosis.

There are 3 settings in which patients may present: (1) with chronically recurring abdominal or pelvic pain wherein endometriosis may or may not directly involve the bowel; (2) with symptoms of bowel obstruction consequent to enteric endometriosis; and (3) with acute, intense abdominal pain due to hemoperitoneum arising from rupture of an endometrial cyst.

The commonest symptom is *pain,* typically cramping and usually referred to the hypogastrium and pelvic area. Menstrual irregularities, dysmenorrhea, and dyspareunia are frequent concomitants. However, the orthodoxy that symptoms of endometriosis necessarily attend the menses or that abdominal distress accentuated during menstruation is indicative of endometriosis can be misleading. This is particularly true of intestinal involvement.[1, 7, 9] Consider, for example, that many women without endometriosis find the discomfort of an irritable bowel more troublesome just before or during the menstrual flow. Disturbed bowel action, either constipation or diarrhea, often is attended by tenesmus or dyschezia. Intestinal bleeding is unusual.[1, 9] When it occurs, it probably is more often due to ischemic mucosal injury than actual penetration by endometrial tissue.[20]

The most significant symptom of intestinal involvement is *obstruction* (Fig. 137–2).[21, 22] In the rectosigmoid segment, obstruction usually is caused by tumefaction or circumferential stenosis, whereas in the mesenteric small intestine, kinking at the site of endometrial implants is more likely. Other mechanisms of obstruction are intussusception and volvulus. Intermittent colicky or crampy pain, often with abdominal distention, typical of bowel obstruction due to any cause, is the usual expression.

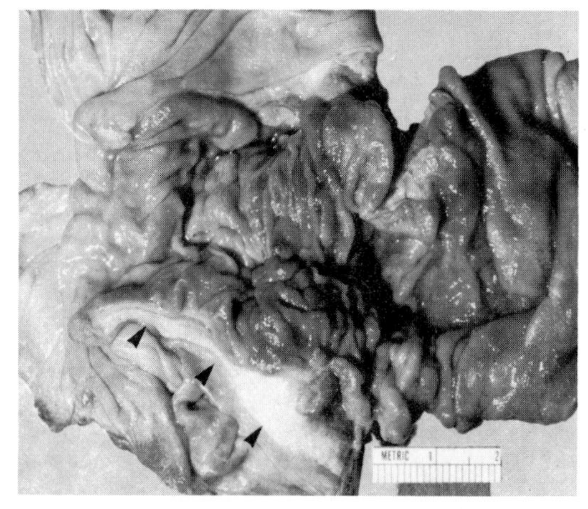

Figure 137–2. A young woman complained of recurring periumbilical pain for 3 weeks, attended by distention and relieved by vomiting. Small bowel radiographs revealed coarse mucosal folds with luminal narrowing in the terminal 12 cm of ileum, suggesting Crohn's disease. At operation a thickened and stenotic ileocecal segment was adherent to the right fallopian tube. Microscopic examination of the resected specimen disclosed endometriosis with constrictive scarring of the serosa and muscular wall. (Photograph kindly furnished by Dr. Bernard M. Schuman.)

A rare but dramatic complication of endometriosis is *hemoperitoneum* arising from eroded or ruptured implants.[23, 24] Such a condition should be included in the differential diagnosis of acute abdominal pain in barren women who have had severe dysmenorrhea. Bleeding from endometrial implants may be triggered by nonpenetrating trauma to the abdomen. Ascitic effusion has been attributed to endometriosis.[25] Disseminated endometriosis can also simulate abdominal and pelvic carcinomatosis.[26]

Endometriosis in the appendix is frequent but only rarely symptomatic,[27] even though the involved appendix can intussuscept and produce a cecal tumor.[28] A syndrome simulating acute appendicitis has been reported.[29] In only about half the cases of appendiceal involvement is the adjacent right ovary affected.[27] Endometriosis has been found in a Meckel's diverticulum.[30]

Physical Findings. In the absence of intestinal obstruction or hemoperitoneum, the disorder is seldom betrayed by abdominal examination. Rarely, endometrial tissue can embed and proliferate in an abdominal scar, particularly after a previous operation for endometriosis or after cesarean section.[31] Endometrioma may be evident at the umbilicus.[32] Occasionally, a poorly defined induration or even a mass may be encountered.[33] Tenderness is more likely to be elicited when the ectopic endometrium is in the late proliferative and decidual phases of the menstrual cycle, just before or during the menses. Bimanual examination of the rectovaginal septum for submucosal nodules can be helpful when endometriosis is suspected. Extraordinary pain on manipulation of the uterine cervix is suggestive. The appearance of blue or purple nodules in the posterior vaginal wall at speculum examination is almost pathognomonic.

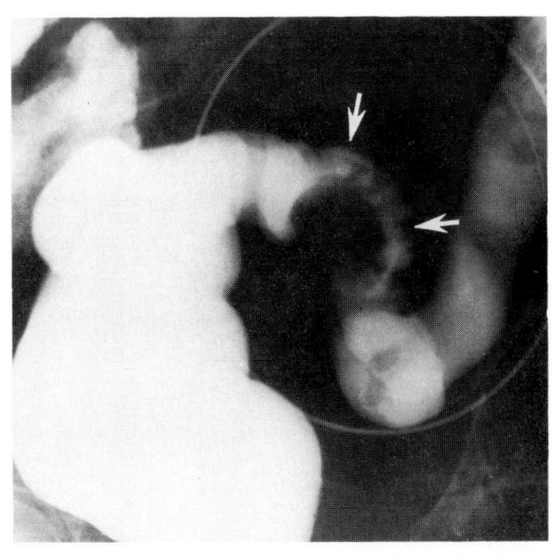

Figure 137–3. Intermittent lower abdominal pain was the complaint of this woman in whom an endometrioma appeared as an intramural tumor of the sigmoid colon at barium enema examination. The overlying mucosa is preserved. (Radiograph kindly furnished by Dr. Joseph P. Whalen, The New York Hospital, and reproduced with permission of *Resident and Staff Physician.*)

Diagnostic Studies

Although narrowing or fixation of the rectosigmoid lumen may be encountered at *sigmoidoscopy*, seldom are underlying endometrial implants apparent through the bowel mucosa.[9, 34]

There are no distinctive *radiographic features* of endometriosis. In the absence of impingement on the bowel or of peritoneal effusion, radiographs are unrevealing. Impingement on the bowel may be evident as (1) a tapered, often eccentric, poorly defined, constricting deformity—the result of endometrial infiltration and scarring in the wall; or (2) a submucosal, polypoid, subtractive defect produced by a cystic endometrioma (Fig. 137–3). In either case, the mucosal pattern usually remains intact, indicating an intramural lesion. According to Gordon et al.,[35] mucosal crenulation in double-contrast radiographs is highly suggestive, though not pathognomonic, of endometrial involvement of the bowel wall. With peritoneal effusion there may be a hazy cast in plain radiographs.

Endometriosis can be diagnosed with certainty only by actually seeing the lesions and confirming their structure in histopathologic sections. Usually the diagnosis is made at *laparotomy* and, in the majority of cases, the finding of endometriosis is incidental.[3, 21] The mere discovery of ectopic endometrial implants, even those involving the bowel wall, cannot be supposed as an explanation for vague abdominal discomfort or erratic bowel action. For example, only 2 of 31 patients in Panganiban and Cornog's series[7] were symptomatic on that account, the exception being a single instance of appendiceal intussusception.

Attempts at *proctoscopic* or *colonoscopic* biopsy, even at sites of apparent impingement or fixation, are almost invariably futile.

Laparoscopy in the hands of qualified gynecologists has become the principal means of establishing a diagnosis of pelvic endometriosis. Moreover, the procedure can lend itself to therapeutic maneuvers, such as fulguration of small implants and lysis of filmy adhesions.[36]

Treatment

Because a variety of therapeutic modalities are available and because none of them is universally applicable, each case of endometriosis requires an individual approach. Gynecologic consultation is well advised.

It has been noted that many instances of endometriosis are discovered incidentally at laparotomy undertaken because of unrelated indications. For asymptomatic lesions, even those involving but not injuring the bowel wall, leaving them undisturbed probably is the judicious course.[2]

Insofar as the course of endometriosis is hormonally dependent, suppression by various endocrine agents has been suggested (Chapter 251). Androgen therapy had been recommended in the past, but its unpredictability and masculinizing side-effect led to its abandonment.

Based on the observation that pregnancy tends to ameliorate endometriosis, progestin therapy has been advocated. The induction of an anovulatory pseudopregnancy state by the use of birth control pills has been a frequently used approach; however, breakthrough bleeding, fluid retention, and depression have been detracting effects. Castration can be beneficial but is undesirable in the premenopausal patient and probably superfluous after a natural menopause. Oophorectomy alone in the presence of enteric lesions is not recommended.[37] The administration of estrogens following induced or spontaneous menopause may aggravate residual or otherwise indolent endometriosis.[2, 22]

Currently, when a trial of medical therapy is invoked, the use of danazol (Danocrine) is recommended.[38–40] This is a synthetic androgen that suppresses pituitary gonadotropin activity and inhibits estrogenic stimulus to endometrial cells; it exhibits only a weak masculinizing effect. Favorable responses have been reported in 60%[38] to 80%[39] of cases. However, it is emphasized that when enteric involvement is symptomatic, hormonal therapy alone cannot be relied upon to lastingly resolve the endometrial lesion or to relieve the symptoms of intestinal obstruction.

When a significant enteric or peritoneal lesion has been determined, surgical intervention is the preferred approach. Often it is only at operation that a differential diagnosis can be resolved and that neoplasia or inflammatory bowel disease can be convincingly ruled out. Examinations of frozen sections may be necessary to avoid either unduly extensive or insufficient resections. The surgical treatment of choice is complete excision of the endometrial implant.[2] In many cases this can be accomplished without entering the bowel lumen. For deeper or more extensive lesions, segmental resection with primary anastomosis is advised. Low lying rectosigmoid lesions, especially those complicated by obstruction, may require a temporary diverting colostomy; abdominoperineal resection is rarely required.

Among 179 cases of bowel involvement encountered in approximately 1500 operations for endometriosis, Gray[2] accomplished total superficial excision of the lesions in 81, partial excision in 61, and segmental resection in 37; he reported subsequent clinically evident recurrences in 16, 10, and 9 cases, respectively.

With prudent management undertaken by a consortium of internist, surgeon, and gynecologist, the long-term prognosis of endometriosis is favorable in the vast majority of patients.

References

1. Meyers WC, Kelvin FM, Jones RS. Diagnosis and treatment of colonic endometriosis. Arch Surg 1979; 114:169–75.
2. Gray LA. Endometriosis of the bowel: Role of bowel resection, superficial excision and oophorectomy in treatment. Ann Surg 1973; 177:580.
3. Williams TJ, Pratt JH. Endometriosis in 1000 consecutive celiotomies. Am J Obstet Gynecol 1977; 129:245–50.
4. Rokitansky C. Über Uterus-Neubildung in uterus-und ovarial-sarcomen. ZKK Gesell d'Ärzte Wien 1860; 16:576.
5. Sampson JA. Perforating hemorrhagic (chocolate) cysts of ovary; Their importance and especially their relation to pelvic adenomas of the endometrial type. Arch Surg 1921; 3:245.
6. LiVolsi VA, Perzin KH. Endometriosis of small intestine producing intestinal obstruction or simulating neoplasm. Am J Dig Dis 1974; 19:100.
7. Panganiban W, Cornog JL. Endometriosis of the intestines and vermiform appendix. Dis Colon Rectum 1972; 15:253.
8. Tedeschi LG, Masand GP. Endometriosis of the intestines: a report of 7 cases. Dis Colon Rectum 1971; 14:360.
9. Teunen A, Ooms ECM, Tytgat GNJ. Endometriosis of the small and large bowel; study of 18 patients and survey of the literature. Neth J Med 1982; 25:142–150.
10. Slasky BS, Kiewers RD, Lecky JW, Zajko A, Burkholder JA. Pleural catamenial pneumothorax: the roles of diaphragmatic defects and endometriosis. AJR 1982; 138:639–43.
11. Ponka JL, Brush BE, Hodgkinson CP. Colorectal endometriosis. Dis Colon Rectum 1973; 16:490.
12. Martin LF, Tidman MK, Jamieson MA. Appendiceal intussusception and endometriosis. J Can Assoc Radiol 1980; 31:276–7.
13. Ivanoff NS. Adenofibromyoma cysticum sarcomatodes carcinomatosum. Monotrehr Geburtsh Gynäk 1898; 7:295.
14. Meyer R. Über den Stand der Frage der Adenomyositis und Adenomyoma im Allgemeinen und im besonders über Adenomyositis seroepithelialis. Zbl Gynäk 1919; 43:745.
15. Halban J. Hysteroadenosis nutastica (die lymphogene Genese der sog. Adenofibromatosis Heterotopica). Wien Klin Wochenschr 1924; 37:1205.
16. Beyoung EE, Gambler CN. Primary adenocarcinoma of the rectovaginal septum arising from endometriosis; report of a case. Cancer 1969; 24:597.
17. Scully RE, Richardson GS, Barlow JF. The development of malignancy in endometriosis. Clin Obstet Gynecol 1966; 9:384.
18. Schifrin BS, Erez S, Moore JG. Teen-age endometriosis. Am J Obstet Gynecol 1973; 116:973.
19. Williams C. Endometriosis of colon in elderly women. Ann Surg 1963; 157:974.
20. Aronchick CA, Brooks FP, Dyson WL, Baron R, Thompson JJ. Ileocecal endometriosis presenting with abdominal pain and gastrointestinal bleeding. Dig Dis Sci 1983; 28:566–72.
21. Martinbeau PW, Pratt JH, Gaffey TA. Small bowel obstruction secondary to endometriosis. Mayo Clin Proc 1975; 50:237–43.
22. Venable JH. Endometriosis of the ileum; 4 cases with obstruction. Am J Obstet Gynecol 1972; 113:1054–5.

23. Carmichael JL, Williams DB. Hemoperitoneum from erosion of ectopic endometrial tissue. South Med J 1972; 65:371.
24. Pratt JH, Shamblin WR. Spontaneous rupture of endometrial cysts of the ovary presenting as an acute abdominal emergency. Am J Obstet Gynecol 1970; 108:56.
25. Chervenak FA, Greenlee RM, Luvenstein L, Tovell HMM. Massive ascites associated with endometriosis. Am J Obstet Gynecol 1981; 57:379–81.
26. Bergen S, Snider WR, Lim YC. Disseminated adenomyosis of abdominal and pelvic cavities. Am Surg 1981; 47:232–5.
27. Langman J, Rowland R, Vernon-Roberts B. Endometriosis of the appendix. Br J Surg 1981; 68:121–4.
28. Schmidt FR, McCarthy JD. Intussusception of the appendix with endometriosis presenting as a cecal tumor. Arch Surg 1971; 103:515.
29. Heupel HW, Reece RL, Pincus M. Stromal endometrioma mimicking acute appendicitis. Minn Med 1970; 53:153.
30. Honore LH. Endometriosis of Mechel's diverticulum associated with intestinal obstruction; a case report. Am J Proctol 1980; 31:11–2.
31. Steck WD, Helwig EB. Cutaneous endometriosis. Clin Obstet Gynecol 1966; 9:373–83.
32. Williams HE, Barsby S, Storing W. Umbilical endometrioma (silent type). Arch Dermatol 1976; 112:1435–6.
33. Miller WB Jr, Melson GL. Abdominal wall endometrioma. AJR 1979; 132:467–8.
34. Farinon AM, Vadora E. Endometriosis of the colon and rectum; an indication for peroperative coloscopy. Endoscopy 1980; 12:136–9.
35. Gordon RL, Evers K, Kressel HY, Laufer I, Herlinger H, Thompson JJ. Double contrast enema in pelvic endometriosis. AJR 1982; 138:549–52.
36. Sulewski JM, Curcio FD, Brontisky C, Stenger VG. The treatment of endometriosis at laparoscopy for infertility. Am J Obstet Gynecol 1980; 138:128–32.
37. McSwain B, Linn RJ, Haley RL Jr, et al. Endometriosis of the colon. South Med 1974; 67:651.
38. Chalmers JA. Danazol in the treatment of endometriosis. Drugs 1980; 19:331–41.
39. Saleh N, Daw E. Endometriosis in non-gynaecological sites. Practitioner 1980; 224:1189-1195.
40. Riddick DH. Drug therapy of endometriosis. Drug Therapy 1982; May:49–53.

Chapter 138

Benign Tumors of the Colon

Arthur D. Schwabe • Klaus J. Lewin

Polyps (Isolated, Sporadic)

Klaus J. Lewin • Arthur D. Schwabe

The tendency of most benign tumors of the large intestine to project into the lumen has led to their common designation as "polyps." The term polyp is not synonymous with adenoma, since polyp is also applied to other neoplastic as well as to hyperplastic, hamartomatous, and inflammatory mucosal excrescences. Adenomas, of course, have assumed considerable clinical significance because of their suspected role as precursors of large bowel cancer, now the second most common malignancy in man. However, some histologic types of polyps are of little clinical consequence, while others may give rise to a variety of symptoms but present little or no risk of undergoing malignant change. This portion of this chapter defines and characterizes the various types of discrete polyps of the colon and their associations. In the portion that follows, the polyposis syndromes are described.

Definitions and Classifications

Polyps are defined as any visible masses of tissue protruding into the lumen of the gastrointestinal tract regardless of size, shape, or histologic type. This descriptive term should be qualified with a more precise designation by histologic appearance; e.g., tubular adenomatous or hyperplastic polyp. In addition, the manner of attachment to the bowel wall, the dimensions, configuration, and color should be indicated. For example, a polyp may be described as a sessile, 2 × 5 cm, soft, cauliflower-like, pink, villous adenoma.

A classification of discrete polypoid tumors of the colon that emphasizes the component nature of the lesions and indicates the syndromes with which they may be associated is given in Table 138–1.

Hyperplastic (metaplastic) polyps are common mucosal excrescences representing foci of epithelial hyperplasia. They are characterized by non-neoplastic proliferation of mucosal glands that is thought to result from excessive glandular maturation. The stimulus to their growth is unknown. They tend to remain unchanged for long periods and have not been shown to be precancerous.

Adenoma is the generic term for 3 types of

Table 138–1. CLASSIFICATION OF POLYPOID TUMORS OF THE COLON

I. Epithelial Tumors
  A. Hyperplastic (metaplastic polyps)
  B. Adenomas
    1. Tubular (adenomatous polyps)
    2. Villous
    3. Tubulovillous (papillary)
  C. Adenomatosis
    1. Familial polyposis coli
    2. Gardner's syndrome
    3. Turcot's syndrome
II. Non-epithelial Tumors
  A. Smooth muscle tumors (leiomyomas)
  B. Vascular tumors
    1. Hemangiomas
    2. Lymphangiomas
  C. Lipomas
III. Hamartomas
  A. Peutz-Jeghers polyps and polyposis
  B. Juvenile polyps and polyposis
    1. Juvenile polyps in childhood
    2. Juvenile polyposis syndromes
    3. Cronkhite-Canada syndrome
  C. Neurofibromas and ganglioneuromas
IV. Inflammatory or Reactive Tumors
  A. Inflammatory pseudopolyps
  B. Lymphoid polyps
  C. Lipoid granulomas and barium granulomas
V. Miscellaneous Tumors

benign epithelial neoplasms: *tubular* adenoma, *villous* adenoma, and *tubulovillous* adenoma. Histologically, adenomas show cellular changes commonly found in malignant neoplasms. Thus, there is nuclear atypia consisting of loss of basal polarity, variation in size and shape, nuclear hyperchromasia, increase in number of mitoses, and a change in the nuclear-cytoplasmic ratio. In addition, there is frequently a qualitative and quantitative change in the cytoplasmic mucin.

Hamartomatous polyps are non-neoplastic tumor-like proliferations characterized by a haphazard mixture of tissues native to the segment of involved gut. They may be composed predominantly of epithelial elements or connective tissue or both. Although frequently present at birth, they tend to grow in size and increase in number with age.

Inflammatory polyps (pseudopolyps) are not neoplasms but rather inflammatory lesions, often showing regenerative changes.

Frequency and Distribution

Polyps of the colon and rectum are uncommon before the age of 30. Thereafter, they become increasingly more prevalent so that by the age of 60 to 80, up to 60% of the population will have one or more polyps.[1] The lesions are found more often in men, with a male to female ratio of about 1.4:1.

The majority of polyps are found on the left side of the colon and rectum. However, the precise number of polyps in the different parts of the large bowel varies, often depending on the method of visualization employed in the study. Thus, in a recent surgical study,[2] 70% of all polyps were located in the rectum, 20% in the sigmoid, and only 10% in the remaining colon. In contrast, the distribution of polyps reported from a large endoscopic study[3] showed 3% of polyps in the rectum, 47% in the sigmoid, 29% in the descending colon, 10% in the transverse colon, and 10% on the right side of the colon. Finally, careful necropsy studies place approximately 20% of large bowel polyps in the rectum, 30% in the sigmoid and descending colon, 20% in the transverse colon, and 30% in the cecum and ascending colon.[1, 4, 5] The distribution of polyps also appears to vary with age. After the age of 60 years, there is an apparent increase in the number of polyps on the right side.[1]

Adenomatous and hyperplastic polyps make up the vast majority of large bowel polyps (98% or more).[6] Approximately 75% are adenomatous, but, of the small lesions (<5 mm), 90% consist of hyperplastic polyps.[7–10] A substantial number of patients have synchronous polyps at the time of diagnosis. Approximately 19% of patients have between 2 and 10 polyps, while 2% have more than 10.[11, 12]

Etiology

The etiology of benign polyps of the colon and rectum varies and depends on the specific type of polyp. In inflammatory pseudopolyps, for example, the lesions result from inflammatory injury and regenerative changes. In the polyposis syndromes (discussed in the latter portion of this chapter), there is clearly a hereditary predisposition. Even though the etiology of neoplastic and hyperplastic tumors remains unclear, several factors merit consideration.

Heredity. Sporadically occurring polyps are neither inherited nor encountered in kindreds with the frequency or regularity seen in the familial polyposis syndromes (see later). However, there appears to be some evidence to suggest that a recessive gene renders patients susceptible to environmental factors.[13–15]

Embryonal Anomaly. The rarity of common polyps in infants or children and the sharply ascending occurrence rate in older age groups are evidence that these lesions are acquired in later life. This does not deny an embryonal origin of certain hamartomatous polypoid lesions, notably "juvenile polyps."

Age. The observation that adenomas occur chiefly in the middle and later years of life suggests either that oncogenic agents require a prolonged time for their influence to become manifest or that restraint to aberrant epithelial growth is reduced in later life, or both. These are merely speculations, but the fact remains that adenomas tend to appear most commonly in aging colons.

Endocrine Influence. The simple observation that common polyps occur more often in men than in women suggests the possibility of a sex-linked or hormonal factor. However, the lack of unusual frequency of these tumors in any known endocrinopathy suggests that the endocrine system has no substantial role in the development of polyps.

Infection. A distinction should be made between polypoid granulomas and adenomatous polyps. Infectious diseases characterized by granulomatous inflammation to which the intestinal mucosa is susceptible may give rise to polypoid lesions in the colon. These include not only specific diseases in which the infecting agent is known, but also chronic inflammatory conditions of uncertain cause. While polypoid granulomas may superficially resemble adenomas, they are not actually new growths. As previously indicated, the so-called pseudopolyp occurring in chronic inflammatory bowel disease really represents epithelial regeneration, mucosal granulomas, or a remaining islet of normal mucosa on a partially denuded luminal surface.

Viral infection has yet to be proved to be a cause of polypoid tumors of the colon. Of current concern is the possibility of a causal relationship between bacteria normally present or infecting the colon and oncogenesis.

Diet. The majority of nutrition-related studies on the etiology of large bowel tumors have been done on carcinomas. However, there is now strong evidence to support the view that discrete adenomatous polyps predispose to the development of cancer of the colon and rectum and that both adenoma and carcinoma share many of the same etiologic factors.[16] This is further discussed in the following paragraphs and in Chapter 139.

Geographic and Environmental Factors. Adenomas of the large bowel show a marked variation in geographic distribution.[16] For example, they are among the most common tumors in North America, Western Europe, and Australia; are uncommon in South America, Africa, and Asia; and are exceedingly rare among blacks in South Africa.[13, 17–19] Epidemiologic studies indicate that these geographic variations are due not to racial or climatic factors, but rather to dietary factors.[17] Protein, fats, and unrefined carbohydrates have all been implicated as causative agents in the etiology of these tumors. Studies point to an important role for dietary fat, bile acids, and the fecal microflora.[16, 17, 19] Thus, it has been shown that: (1) people living in areas with a high prevalence of colon cancer have a higher fecal concentration of bile acids than do people living in areas of low prevalence; (2) feces from persons in the high risk populations have higher counts of anaerobes, such as bacteroides, and lower counts of aerobic bacteria than in populations where cancer of the colon and rectum is rare; and (3) there is a strong association between the number of anaerobic bacteria, metabolized bile acids, and degraded cholesterol on the one hand and the risk of colon cancer among different populations on the other.[19–21] Finally, it is known that the fecal concentration of bile acids is dependent on the amount of dietary fat.[19]

How do all these facts relate to the etiology and pathogenesis of large bowel tumors? The current concept in chemical carcinogenesis is that agents that cause cancer are usually transformed by biochemical means, in this case by the intestinal microflora, into the ultimate carcinogen.[17] Thus, it has been postulated that excess dietary intake of fat produces an increased concentration of fecal bile acids that are metabolized by anaerobic bacteria into carcinogenic agents. Another factor that may contribute to the carcinogenic effects of metabolized bile acids is constipation or irregular bowel action, allowing carcinogens to act on the mucosa for longer than normal periods before being expelled. In support of this, it has been found that persons consuming diets high in fiber content have frequent, bulky stools and seem to be protected from carcinoma. Conversely, persons who consume low-residue diets tend to have scybalous stools and seem more prone to polyps and carcinoma.[22]

Pathogenesis

The normal healthy colon mucosa is an ever changing and dynamic structure. Epithelial cells are born, proliferate, and die at an astonishing rate. It has been estimated that rectal epithelial cells are renewed every 6 to 8 days.[23, 24] Obviously, there are real and potent, albeit undefined, factors that govern a steady state wherein exactly as many cells proliferate as die, thus maintaining the integrity of the colon epithelium.

Colon epithelial cells normally proliferate in the basal third of the glandular crypts and migrate upward into the middle third, which is a transitional zone. Here the intracellular synthesis of DNA and RNA, characteristic of proliferating and growing cells, diminishes and finally stops. As the cells move into the upper third of the crypt toward the surface, they are fully mature. In short order they become senescent, die, and are extruded into the lumen of the colon. There is evidence that the pericryptal fibroblast sheath runs a course in concert with its neighboring epithelium.[25] In light of the precise control exerted on normal epithelial cell growth and renewal, it seems small wonder that occasionally an error may result in a focal expression of abnormal growth recognized as a polyp.

The cells of polypoid growths differ from those of the normal epithelium in that the process of proliferation and maturation is altered. Adenomatous epithelial cells retain their immature characteristics of DNA and RNA synthesis after they move into the upper portions of the crypts toward the surface, where extrusion is retarded and replication persists.[26–31] A similar disorganization is said to occur in apparently normal mucous membranes adjacent to polyps.[24, 29, 30] The cryptal connective tissue sheath is concomitantly immature.[32,33] This abnormally retarded sequence has been confirmed also for the lesions of familial polyposis.[24, 34]

Such kinetic cellular studies may help explain the histogenesis of adenomatous polyps. Originally, adenomatous polyps were thought to result from the proliferation of glands within the mucosa.[35] Once it was realized that cellular replication in adenomatous polyps persists in the upper portions of the glands and in the surface of the mucosa,[27–30] it was proposed that these lesions result from the outward projection of proliferating cells as well as their extension into adjacent normal glands.[28, 36] This explanation, however, does not adequately account for the increased number of glands often seen within adenomatous polyps.

In a study on the histogenesis of minute adenomatous polyps, Maskens[31] showed that new glands result from an infolding of the surface epithelium between normal pre-existing glands. In addition, branching of adjacent glands may contribute to the new gland formation. Can the morphologic differences of tubular and villous adenomas be explained histogenetically? According to Maskens,[31] the differences depend upon whether there is proliferation of the underlying mesenchymal tissues. If there is no accompanying mesenchymal proliferation, the replicating epithelial cells will encounter resistance to upward and outward growth, and infolding is likely to occur because of simple mechanical reasons. The resulting lesion will be a tubular adenoma. The mesenchymal resistance to epithelial growth may also explain why these polyps are usually small. Conversely, if proliferation of the lamina propria accompanies the epithelial growth, there will be outward folding of the neoplastic tissue, resulting in a villous adenoma.

Hyperplastic polyps represent a different aberration. These lesions are characterized by an expansion of the zone of cell division and a minor imbalance in the cycle of cell renewal. As a result, there is increased cell production leading to crowding of cells with papillary infolding. However, in contrast to the adenomas, cell division remains restricted to the lower portion of the crypt, and the epithelial cells of the glands undergo full maturation to goblet and absorptive cells.[9] This, then, suggests a divergent pathogenesis for hyperplastic and adenomatous polyps and argues against a progression from hyperplasia to neoplasia.

The single adenomatous polyp itself is evidence that a control or "brake" on its growth exists. If a polyp begins as an abnormal proliferation of either epithelial or subepithelial cells, why does it so often remain so small and why does it not invariably and infinitely increase in size? Obviously, there is a degree of restraint imposed, even on mucosal neoplasia. Indeed, the restraint of growth in the benign neoplasm appears greater than that imposed on the normal mucosa.

What provokes the aberrant growth pattern? For the naturally occurring polyp, no one yet knows. In nature, polypoid tumors of the colon rarely occur in animals other than man. In the laboratory, however, a full spectrum of lesions, including hyperplasia, adenoma, and carcinoma, can regularly be induced in the colon of the rat by administration of various oncogenic chemicals.[37] Among these are 3:2-dimethyl-4-aminobiphenyl (DMAB)[38] and *N*-methyl-*N*-nitronitrosoguanidine.[39] The oncogenic effect has been elicited when these substances are administered parenterally, encouraging the postulation that the actual tumor-inducing agent is a metabolite produced in the liver or within the fecal milieu of the intestine. The oncogenic effect of cycasin,[40] on the other hand, is observed only when the agent is introduced directly into the alimentary tract and is not evident when it is administered parenterally. This substance seems to require intra-intestinal transformation. Worthy of note is that these or related substances have not thus far been incriminated as causes of intestinal neoplasia in man.

Significantly, the growth and microscopic features of these experimentally induced lesions are similar to those of the naturally occurring tumors in man. The types of lesions, i.e., whether adenomas or carcinomas, are distinct, and transitional forms have not been observed. Unfortunately, no agent has yet been found that induces only adenomas and not carcinomas in laboratory animals. Such an agent would permit interesting experiments on the long-term growth characteristic of benign colon tumors.

Polyp-Cancer Relationships

With the exception of adenomas, all other benign epithelial polyps of the large intestine are without malignant propensity. Villous adenomas have a marked malignant predisposition, up to 50% of excised villous lesions showing evidence of carcinoma.[41, 60] By contrast, a lesser number of tubular adenomas, no more than 5%, show malignant change. Hence, it has been proposed that the relationship between tubular adenomas and carcinoma of the colon is more casual than causal, but this remains a controversial issue. Studies point more and more to a "polyp-cancer" sequence. Enterline[41] has categorized the evidence for a polyp-cancer sequence into 3 major lines: (1) age, site, and incidence comparisons of adenomas and cancers that weigh against random association; (2) the underlying mucosal milieu in which adenomas and carcinomas occur; and (3) the influence of prophylactic treatment of adenomas on the subsequent development of carcinoma.

Age. If adenomas are precursors of carcinoma, adenomas would be expected to occur in a younger age group than carcinoma. Earlier studies showed no such age difference.[41,42] However, these were based on surgical studies, and it is known that many adenomas are clinically silent and go unrecognized for many years. More recent studies by Morson[43] based on findings from a cancer detection clinic have shown a 7-year age differential for adenoma and carcinoma. Furthermore, Morson points out that in familial polyposis coli there is a 15-year lag between the appearance of adenomas in the colon and the subsequent development of carcinoma.

Distribution. For a long time it was accepted that the distribution of adenomas and carcinomas was not the same and that the 2 lesions were therefore unrelated.[44] However, as previously discussed, the recognition of polyps in the different sites of the bowel depends on the method of visualization and may not always reflect the true occurrence. In fact, more recent careful studies have shown a rough relationship in the distribution of adenomas and cancer.[45] Additional evidence for the association of adenoma and carcinoma comes from studies on the prevalence of these lesions. Thus, in those countries in which there is a high prevalence of cancer, there is a similarly high rate of adenoma; the converse is also true.[46] Patients with adenoma are at an increased risk of developing cancer, and, furthermore, adenomas and carcinomas are frequently found in the same colon.[45, 47]

Morphologic Relationships. Early carcinomas appear to be invariably associated with adenomas, and pure, minute carcinomas are exceedingly rare. The factors determining malignant change are unknown, but we do know that (1) the larger the lesion, the more atypical the cytology; and (2) the greater the villous component of the adenoma, the more likely the malignant change in it. Adenomas with severe atypia and carcinomas also show similar abnormal chromosomal and histochemical patterns.[48, 49]

Influence of Prophylactic Treatment. These studies are complicated by the fact that most patients with adenomas are asymptomatic. Thus, population studies must include all patients over a given age to obtain statistically reliable results. One such study[50] indicates that removal of adenomas results in a marked reduction in later occurrence of carcinoma. Furthermore, in a study done at St. Mark's Hospital in London on patients with familial polyposis coli who had colectomies and ileorectal anastomoses, it was shown that fulguration of polyps prevented the subsequent development of carcinoma.[16]

It would seem that it is not so much a question of whether polyps undergo malignant change as why only a small percentage do so, which polyps will become malignant, and how they can be detected. As noted, only about 5% of all adenomatous polyps undergo malignant change. However, there is a distinct cancer risk in large polyps, those showing marked epithelial atypia, and those with villous features. Thus, polyps smaller than 1 cm in diameter rarely show malignant change, whereas polyps 1.5 cm in diameter show a 10% frequency of malignancy, and adenomas greater than 2 cm in diameter show a 30% to 50% malignant propensity. The time interval for the development of cancer has been estimated as between 5 and 15 years.

Pathologic Features

Hyperplastic Polyps (Metaplastic Polyps, Focal Polypoid Hyperplasia)

In past years it was necessary to distinguish between tubular and villous adenomas to clarify the problem of "polyps" in the colon and rectum. Now it is essential to distinguish hyperplastic polyps. Hyperplastic polypoid lesions were usually labeled "adenomas" before their identity was established by Morson[51] in 1962 and Lane and Lev[52] in 1963. They are neither neoplastic nor precancerous, and they have a distinctive pathogenesis. When indiscriminately grouped with polyps generally, they skew statistics and distort the overall picture. The lesions occur primarily in the colon and rectum, although they have also been described in the appendix.[53]

Typically, minute hyperplastic polyps are easily overlooked. Arthur[7] reported "metaplastic nodules" in 95% of 45 specimens obtained at resection for anorectal carcinoma, in 75% of 51 "normal" rectums at necropsy in persons older than 40 years, and in 40% of 25 specimens at necropsy in younger persons. Of 2136 polyps of the rectum studied by Lane et al.,[8] 90% of those 3 mm or less in diameter were found to be hyperplastic.

Pathology. Hyperplastic polyps cannot always be readily distinguished grossly from adenomas. When viewed endoscopically or in surgical or necropsy specimens, hyperplastic foci almost invariably are minute (3 mm or smaller), sessile, well-circumscribed excrescences. Their surfaces are similar in color and texture to the adjacent mucosa, although sometimes they appear pearly gray and translucent. They tend to be distinctly paler than adenomas, less friable, and only rarely pedunculated.

Microscopically, hyperplastic polyps are composed of elongated, somewhat tortuous, often dilated glandular crypts (Figs. 138–1 and 138–2). The epithelial cells are orderly

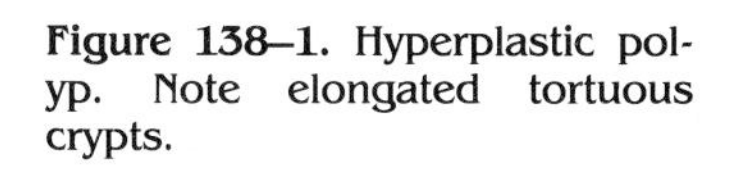

Figure 138–1. Hyperplastic polyp. Note elongated tortuous crypts.

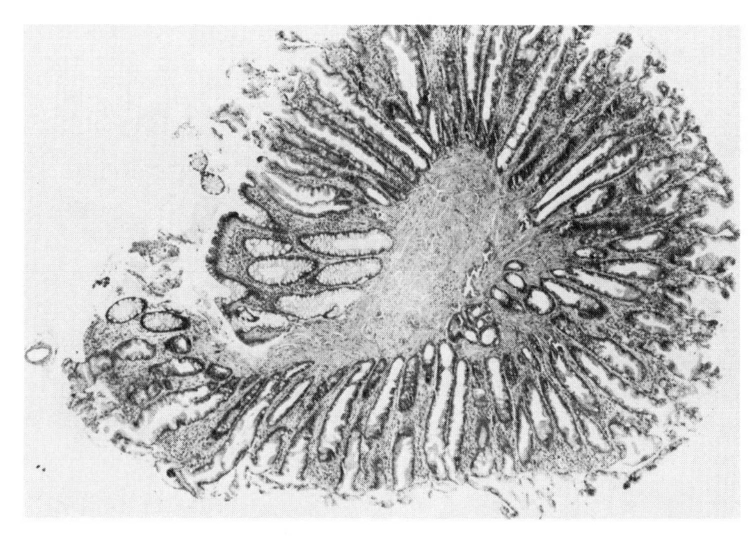

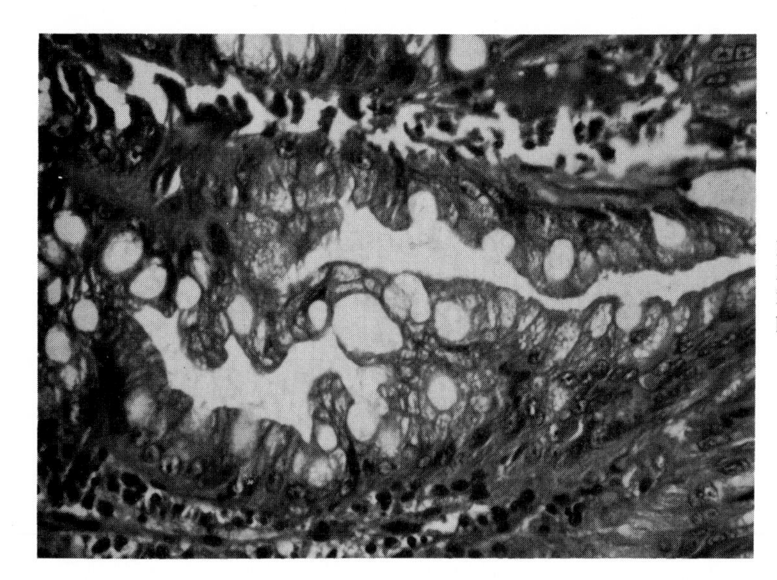

Figure 138–2. Hyperplastic polyp. High power view to show papillary infoldings producing a sawtooth pattern and lack of cytologic atypia.

and, in the basilar portions of the crypts, hardly distinguishable from cells of normal epithelium. Toward the luminal surface, the epithelial cells become irregular in height and develop papillary infoldings, resulting in a serrated, saw-toothed pattern on longitudinal section and a stellate appearance on cross section. The nuclei remain basal and lightly stained, but lack the crowding and atypia characteristic of adenomas. The cytoplasm becomes eosinophilic and contains less mucin than normal. There is thickening of the basement membrane underlying the glands.

The relationship, if any, between hyperplastic polyps and adenomas is uncertain. Hyperplastic polyps, adenomas, and cancers often co-exist in the same colon, and hyperplastic glands may be found at times in adenomas. This has led some to postulate that the lesions share a common histogenesis[39, 54] and that there may be a pathogenetic sequence of transition from epithelial proliferation to hyperplasia, to adenomatous hyperplasia, and even to carcinoma. However, most of the evidence points to divergent pathways of cellular proliferation in hyperplastic and adenomatous polyps.[8, 25, 31–33] Thus, although hyperplastic glands are found in adenomatous polyps, they are also found in juvenile and inflammatory polyps and in the proximity of carcinomas, suggesting that this finding may be non-specific.[55–57] Furthermore, tiny adenomas do not contain hyperplastic areas.[8] The 2 types of polyps also show differences in the distribution of the proliferative zones. Lastly, there is an absence of new gland formation in hyperplastic polyps compared with adenomas.[24, 37]

Adenomatous Polyps

Adenomas are the benign epithelial neoplasms of the large bowel. They can be divided into 3 types, according to their growth pattern: (1) *tubular* adenomas, characterized by proliferating tubules; (2) *villous* adenomas, characterized by finger-like proliferation of the mucosal epithelium; and (3) *tubulovillous* adenomas, characterized by a mixture of both tubular and villous elements. It should be noted that the names of the polyps reflect the architectural differences and that the cytologic features are the same in all adenomas.[16]

The percentage of the different types of adenomatous polyps found in the large bowel depends on individual definitions. There are very few pure histologic types, and most adenomatous polyps contain a mixture of both tubular and villous elements. Shinya and Wolff[11] have defined tubular and villous adenomas as those lesions containing more than 75% of tubular or villous elements, respectively. If more than 25% of the epithelial elements differ from the major epithelial component, the lesion is designated as intermediate or mixed, i.e., tubulovillous. Using these definitions, approximately 64% of benign large bowel polyps consist of tubular adenomas, 9% are villous adenomas, and 27% are tubulovillous adenomas.[10,11] In contrast, Appel et al.[58] found that 37% of adenomatous polyps were tubular, 18% villous, and 45% tubulovillous. However, their criteria for adenomatous polyps were different; tubular adenomas were defined as having less than 5% of a villous component, tubulovillous as having between 5% and 50% of a villous component, and villous adenomas as having more than 50% of a villous component. The relative frequency of the different types of adenoma does not vary in different regions of the colon and rectum.

There is a very significant difference in cancer risk between the different polyps, the risk being related to the extent of villous elements. Thus, the cancer risk is smallest in tubular adenomas, maximal in the pure villous adenomas, and intermediate in the tubulorvillous adenomas.[58]

Tubular Adenomas

Frequency and Distribution. Tubular adenomas are found in the colon and rectum with widely ranging frequencies, depending on the make-up of the population surveyed, the manner and extent of examination, the intensity of scrutiny, and the examiner's definition of a polyp. For example, there is a great difference in the frequency of polyps encountered at proctoscopy in children (<1%) compared with the frequency of polypoid lesions found in adults at necropsy (as high as 75% in whole colons examined with a hand lens).[1, 59, 75] The clinician, who relies largely on proctosigmoidoscopy and barium enema examination, encounters a majority of polypoid tumors in the rectum and lower sigmoid segment. The pathologist, who scrutinizes whole colons at necropsy, finds a more uniform distribution. The oft-quoted statement that up to 75% of polyps occur within the range of the 25-cm sigmoidoscope is valid only in terms of clinically recognized polyps. From their necropsy material, Arminski and McLean[4] estimated that not more than 40% of polyps would have been detected at proctosigmoidoscopy; only 15% of their whole specimens showed polyps limited to the rectum.

Proctosigmoidoscopic examinations of a random adult population in the United States would be expected to disclose polyps in about 7% to 10% of subjects.[60] Polypoid lesions can be discerned at barium enema examinations with comparable frequency (although it should be noted these may not be the same polyps found at proctosigmoidoscopy). Using the double-contrast, air-barium technique and the utmost scrutiny, Welin[61] found polypoid lesions in 3101 (12.5%) of 240,783 colons examined radiographically. This corresponds remarkably well with Ekelund's report[62] of what he took to be significant polypoid lesions in 12.5% of 3398 colons examined at necropsy.

The prevalence of polyps increases with age, reaching a peak in the seventh decade.[1] They are half again as frequent in men as in women,[1] in contrast to the approximately equal distribution of colon cancers. White persons harbor polyps more often than do non-whites. In South Africa, Bremmer and Ackerman,[63] working in a 2000-bed hospital with a largely Bantu population, found only 6 adenomatous polyps during a 12-year period. Polyps occur in black Americans with a frequency intermediate between that of indigenous Africans and whites. Native Japanese have a low frequency of colon polyps, whereas the frequency in Japanese living in Hawaii is higher, generally approaching that of the island population.[64] Colon polyps are relatively uncommon in South Americans.[65]

More than a single polyp is found in one-fourth to one-third of patients. Usually the number is 2 to 5, seldom more than 10.[11,12] The anatomic features of multiple polyps occurring synchronously do not differ from those occurring singly. At the same time, the presence of multiple polyps in the rectosigmoid segment signals the need for a diligent search of the proximal colon for other lesions, including occult carcinoma.[66]

Gross Appearance. Tubular adenomas of the colon may be sessile or pedunculated. They vary in size from minute, barely visible mucosal excrescences to large pedunculated growths (Fig. 138–3). However, as has been previously noted, most tubular adenomas tend to reach a given size and then remain static. In fact, most adenomas remain small, measuring less than 1 cm in diameter. Lesions larger than 2 cm are relatively unusual. The small adenomas are typically dome-shaped and purplish in color. Larger lesions are pedunculated and have irregularly fissured and lobulated surfaces. The stalk (which is composed of normal mucosa and is formed by peristaltic action on the mucosal excrescence) may be thin or thick, short or long, and almost always is smooth and pale. The presence of a stalk is not always apparent on gross examination, and some hemispheric tumors called "sessile" actually overhang a

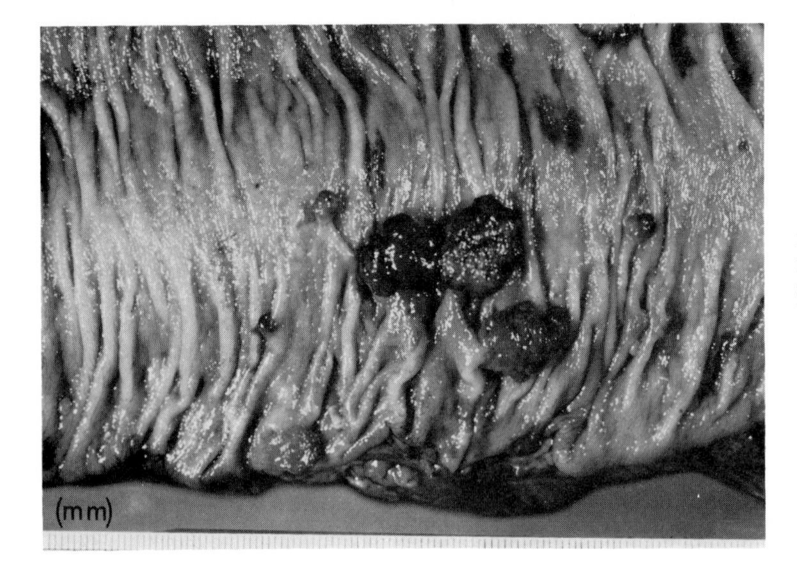

Figure 138–3. Tubular adenomas. Note the 3 pedunculated lesions, each of which has a lobulated surface.

short central pedicle. It has been suggested that the presence of a stalk can be reliably demonstrated by moving a polyp in any direction through a 90° arc without exerting traction on the bowel wall.[67] The clinical importance of a pedicle rests on the observation that lesions with long, thin stalks are almost always benign.[68] However, the absence of a demonstrable pedicle does not necessarily denote malignancy.

Endoscopically, the smallest tubular adenomas appear as minute, sessile, well-circumscribed hemispheric elevations, often barely discernible from undulations in the normal colon mucosa. A distinction between hyperplastic polyps and adenoma is difficult from the gross appearance of lesions this small. Their color is often the clue. Excrescences paler than the surrounding mucosa usually represent hyperplastic polyps; those a shade redder than the normal mucosa tend to be adenomas. Larger benign adenomas, often pedunculated, tend to have more granular, lobulated surfaces that are darker red than the adjacent mucosa and sometimes mottled, resembling a mulberry. The surface may be eroded, although adenomas are generally less friable than small carcinomas.[10, 69]

Microscopic Appearance. Adenomas are composed of tubular glands embedded in the lamina propria. They differ from normal mucosa because of the architectural complexity of the glands and the cytologic atypia of the epithelial cells (Fig. 138–4).

The earliest lesions are confined to the superficial portion of the glands and show only cytologic changes.[31] Later, with continued epithelial proliferation, adenomas are composed of crowded, closely packed, often branched glands set in a sparse lamina propria. As previously mentioned, the glandular crowding probably results from new gland formation produced by infolding of the proliferating surface epithelium and branching of existing glands.[31] Cytologically, the epithelial cells show neoplastic changes character-

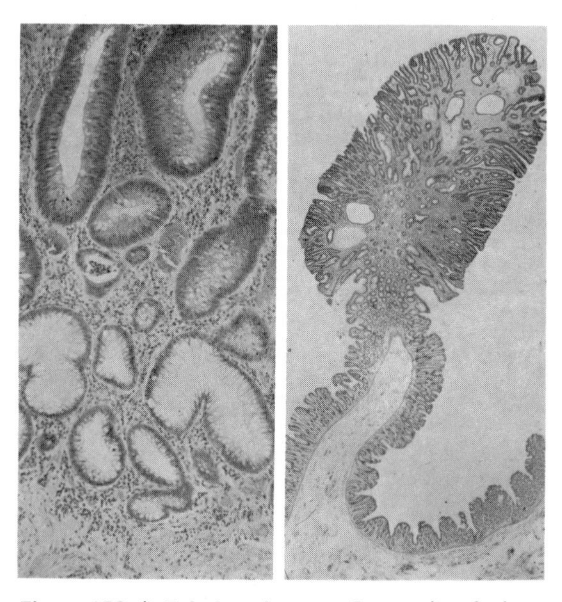

Figure 138–4. Tubular adenoma. Composite of microscopic appearance. The low power view *(right)* shows tubular glands embedded in lamina propria. Higher magnification *(left)* shows adenomatous change in superficial half of gland crypt.

ized by enlarged hyperchromatic nuclei, an increased nuclear-cytoplasmic ratio, and cytoplasmic basophilia with decreased mucin production. In addition, there is increased mitotic activity. Paneth cells and enterochromaffin cells may be found dispersed between the neoplastic cells. Focal villous change is not uncommon, the frequency and extent of which are related to the size of the polyp, as already discussed.[58] The transition from normal to adenomatous epithelium at the base of the polyp is abrupt.

Most tubular adenomas show only minimal epithelial atypia. However, in up to 20% of lesions,[10, 11] especially the larger ones, there may be a spectrum of atypia, ranging from mild to severe to in situ or invasive carcinoma. The epithelial atypia is characterized by a combination of architectural irregularities of the glands and cytologic changes. The former consist of both complex glandular budding culminating in a back-to-back arrangement of the tubules and intraglandular bridging resulting in a cribriform pattern. Necrosis sometimes accompanies these changes. The severity of the cytologic alterations is usually related to the degree of the glandular changes. There is loss of basal orientation of nuclei with nuclear crowding and pseudo-stratification. Nuclei become progressively larger and pleomorphic, with multiple prominent irregular nucleoli. A cardinal criterion of the benign adenoma is that the glandular tubules, no matter how distorted, must remain superficial to the muscularis mucosae. Glandular invasion of the stalk of the polyp or the bowel wall is a sign of malignancy. This is because the lymphatic plexus of the large bowel reaches only to the muscularis mucosae and the base of the gland crypts. Hence, lymphatic metastases cannot occur until the muscularis mucosae has been breached by the proliferating glands.[9] It is important to note that a spectrum of cellular differentiation and complexity in the glandular array is often seen within a single lesion. For this reason a fragmentary biopsy specimen may not be truly representative.

Significance of Dysplasia, Carcinoma-in-Situ, and Early Invasive Carcinoma. *Carcinoma-in-situ* (Fig. 138–5) is the designation used by some pathologists for lesions showing severe atypia, and *intramucosal carcinoma* is the designation for lesions in which there is invasion of single cells or clusters of cells within the mucosa. The natural history of these lesions is unknown; it is unclear whether they will invariably give rise to invasive carcinoma and, if so, over what period of time. What is known is that if the polyp bearing such foci is totally removed and if there is no neoplastic invasion of the stalk, the "cancer" is cured. Hence, many clinicians and pathologists are reluctant to designate these lesions as carcinoma. Lymph node metastases in adenomatous polyps with foci of superficially invasive cancer are exceedingly rare. For example, although the frequency of early invasive carcinoma in tubular adenomas is between 4% and 5%,[10, 11, 53, 70, 71] no regional lymph node metastases were re-

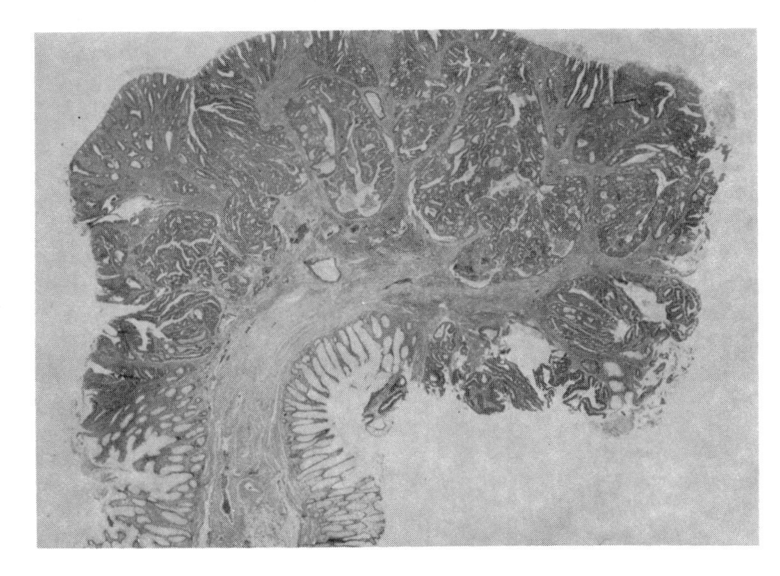

Figure 138–5. Early invasive carcinoma in a tubular adenoma. Note the marked cytologic atypia and architectural irregularity of the glands.

ported in one careful study of 1619 adenomatous polyps in which gastrointestinal adenomas with focal carcinoma were found.[70]

Pseudo-invasion (Epithelial Misplacement). This is a benign condition marked by the presence of "misplaced" adenomatous tissue in the submucosa of an adenomatous polyp that may be confused with an early invasive carcinoma.[51–53] The "misplaced" glands are frequently cystic and may sometimes rupture, resulting in the extravasation of pools of mucin into the submucosa. Inflammation, hemorrhage, and hemosiderin deposit often accompany the glandular changes. Pseudo-invasion differs from adenomas with early invasive carcinoma in the following respects: In the former (1) the "misplaced" epithelium is morphologically similar to that of the overlying adenoma; (2) the "misplaced" glands are surrounded by lamina propria instead of a desmoplastic reaction, as is usually seen in invasive carcinoma; and (3) the presence of extravasated blood and hemosiderin is indicative of ischemic injury. This lesion has been reported in up to 6% of adenomatous polyps, especially in those with long stalks. It is thought to result from ischemic injury following repeated torsion and hemorrhage; there is subsequent downgrowth of the epithelium into the submucosa during the healing phase in a manner similar to colitis cystica profunda.[74]

Villous Adenomas. The villous adenoma is distinct from the tubular adenoma in its occurrence, morphology, and behavior. In contrast to tubular adenomas, villous adenomas are frequently associated with carcinoma of the colon and rectum so that distinction between the 2 types is important in management and prognosis. Compared with tubular adenomas, villous adenomas are uncommon. Thus, in large studies of adenomatous polyps in the colon and rectum, villous adenomas constituted only about 4% to 10% of these lesions. They develop more often in men than in women (in a ratio of about 3:2) and their peak occurrence rate is in the sixth and seventh decades of life; they rarely, if ever, occur in children or adolescents.[75–77]

While tubular adenomas are more evenly distributed throughout the large intestine, villous adenomas occur predominantly in the rectum.[78, 79] For example, of 219 villous adenomas found in 215 patients, Quan and Castro[78] reported 144 in the rectum and 54 in the sigmoid.

Pathology. Villous adenomas are typically sessile and only occasionally pedunculated. They arise from the mucosa over a broad and spreading base, sometimes involving the entire circumference of the bowel, varying in size from 0.5 to 12.0 cm. The surface of the lesion has a cauliflower-like appearance (Fig. 138–6) and is soft and velvety. The lesion is so soft it may be easily missed by digital examination, even when situated in the lower rectum. Areas of firmness should raise suspicion of malignancy.[78] They are often so friable as to be shaved off by the tip of the proctosigmoidoscope. Villous adenomas may attain a bulk sufficient to disturb bowel habits, but because they are soft, they seldom completely obstruct the bowel. When in the rectum, they may prolapse at the anus, and patients have been known to recognize fragments of tumor tissue expelled with the stool.

Villous adenomas are distinguished morphologically by their thin, delicate epithelial fronds that resemble the villi of the small intestinal mucosa (Fig. 138–6). Individual fronds may be single or branched and are lined by atypical neoplastic epithelium, which may contain abundant goblet cells and extend down to the muscularis mucosae. The supporting connective tissue is scant, and there is hardly any central stalk. As in tubular adenomas, foci of pseudo-invasion may occur.

Although the frequency of carcinoma complicating tubular adenomas is still the subject of much debate, there is universal agreement that carcinoma is often found in villous adenomas. The reported frequency varies from 30% to 70% of villous adenomas,[78, 80–86] the likelihood of malignancy increasing with the size of the lesion.[85] Synchronous and metachronous carcinomas are also common.[70, 78] Quan and Castro[78] reported that 49% of their patients had more than one adenoma, 16% had associated bowel malignancies, and, remarkably, 12% had extracolonic cancer. Although the gross appearance of many villous adenomas is sufficiently characteristic to permit a presumptive diagnosis, fragmentary biopsy specimens may be misleading. In Quan and Castro's series[78] of 219 villous adenomas, over half the initial biopsies called "benign" were from tumors later found, when examined whole, to have malignant changes. Biopsy is notoriously unreliable as a means of ruling out the presence of carcinoma. It is important, therefore, to totally

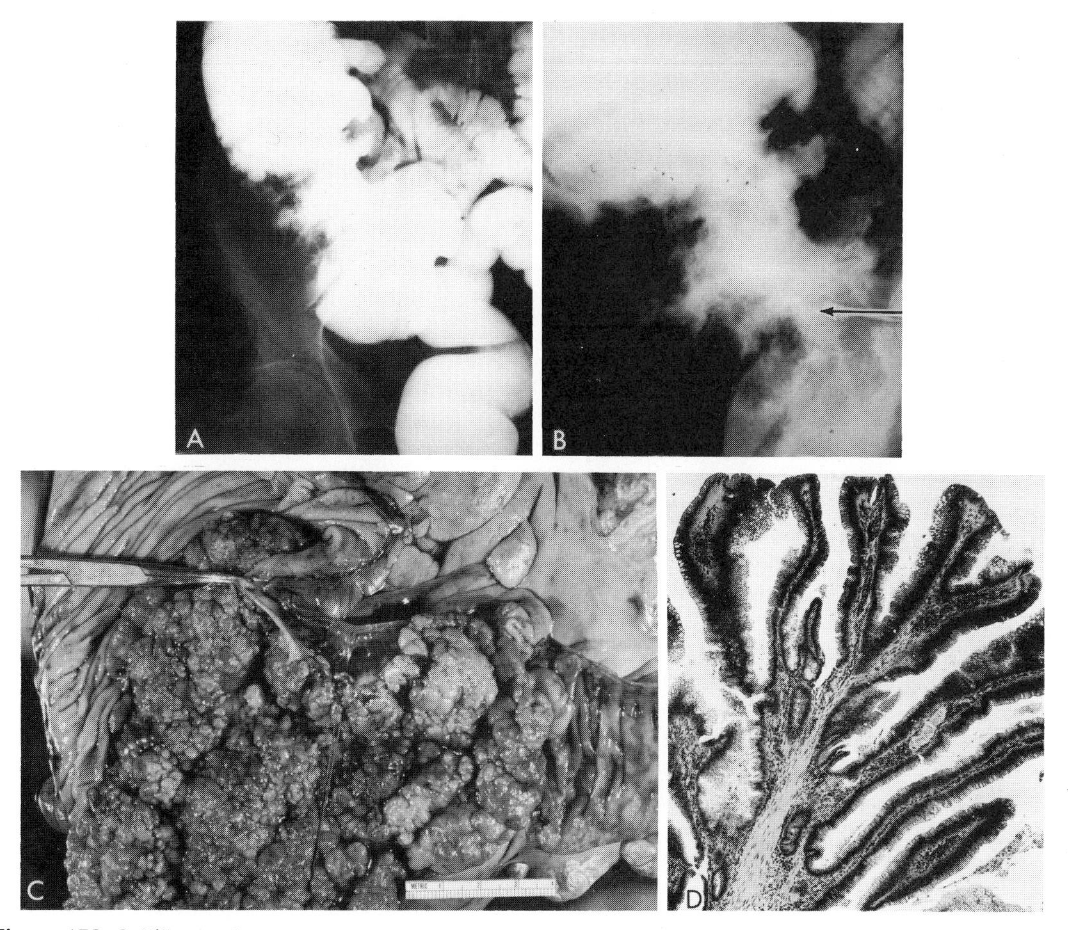

Figure 138–6. Villous adenoma. *A*, Irregular filling defect in the barium column at the junction of the cecum and ascending colon. *B*, The nebulous outline of the lesion is well seen in this spot compression film. *C*, The cauliflower-like tumor as it appeared in the freshly resected specimen. *D*, Fine, delicate, branching epithelial fronds are seen in this typical microscopic view.

excise and carefully section the whole lesion.

Tubulovillous Adenomas (Villoglandular Adenoma, Papillary Adenoma, Mixed Villous and Adenomatous Polyp). These adenomatous polyps are characterized by an admixture of tubular and villous components (Fig. 138–7). As previously noted, there are very few pure histologic types; consequently, the designation of tubulovillous adenomas depends on the definition employed. Adenomas principally of the tubular type but containing from 5% to 25% of the epithelial elements of the villous type have been called tubulovillous. In practice, however, the term is more loosely applied to tubular adenomas that have a villous component. More important than the terminology is the realization that the greater the villous component, the greater the likelihood of carcinoma developing in the polyp.[58] Thus, it is important to specify the percentage of the villous component.

Non-epithelial Tumors

Leiomyomas. Tumors composed of smooth muscle cells are very uncommon in the large intestine. When found, they are usually in the rectum.[91] MacKenzie et al.[87] collected 37 cases of smooth muscle tumors of the colon, of which 24 were reported as benign. In more recent reports, leiomyosarcomas are at least as common, if not more so, than leiomyomas.[89–91] Morphologically, the distinction between benign and malignant smooth muscle tumors may be difficult and not all lesions can be accurately categorized. Their clinical course is often unpre-

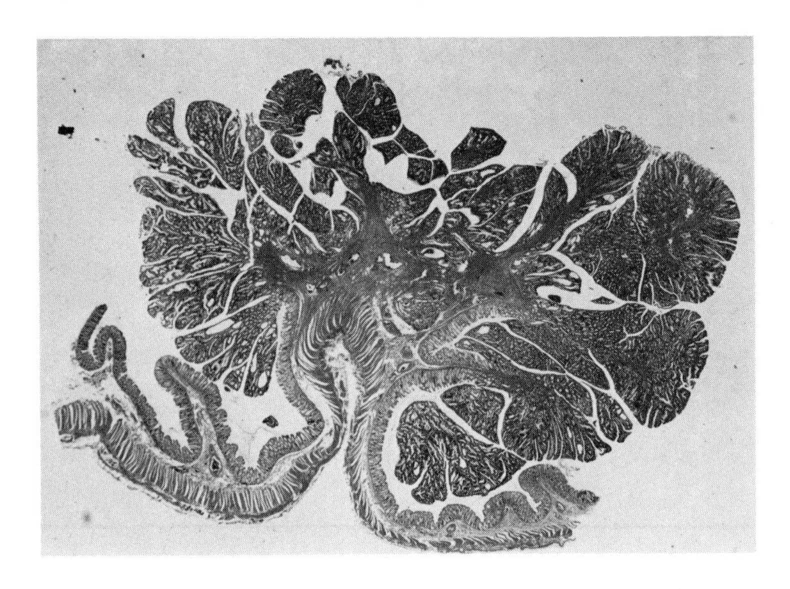

Figure 138–7. Tubulovillous adenoma showing admixture of tubular and villous components.

dictable, making diagnosis and treatment of the individual patient a dilemma. If lesions are larger than 5 cm in diameter and show necrosis and more than the occasional mitosis, they should be treated as malignant and excised with a margin of normal tissue.[89, 90]

Hemangiomas. Vascular tumors of the gastrointestinal tract may assume a polypoid configuration but are rare. Of 290 benign vascular tumors of the gastrointestinal tract collected by Gentry et al.,[92] 107 involved the large intestine. The lesions may be solitary, multiple, or part of a more widespread vascular malformation, such as in the Rendu-Osler-Weber syndrome. Histologically, hemangiomas are generally divided into capillary and cavernous types, with admixtures of both being encountered. The *capillary hemangiomas* usually occur singly and are found in the perianal skin. *Cavernous hemangiomas,* which are composed of large, blood-filled, endothelium-lined channels loosely supported by scanty connective tissue, are often multiple and range from small polypoid lesions to large expansive tumors. Endoscopically, they appear as plum-colored masses with sessile, irregular, but well-circumscribed borders. A characteristic radiographic clue to the presence of a hemangioma is sometimes provided by focal calcific densities representing phleboliths (Fig. 138–8).

The common mode of presentation is bleeding that may be massive. Polypoid lesions may present with intussusception.[93,94] Segmental resection is the treatment of choice for uncontrolled bleeding. Endoscopic biopsy and fulguration can cause massive hemorrhage and perforation.[95]

Lipomas. These tumors are composed of mature adipose tissues supported by fibrous stroma. They can protrude from the mucosal or serosal surface of any segment of the gastrointestinal tract (Fig. 138–9). Mayo et al.[96] reported that lipomas accounted for 4% of benign neoplasms of the gut. Fully two-thirds to three-fourths of alimentary tract lipomas are found in the large intestine,[97, 98] a great majority around the ileocecal valve. Lipomas usually occur singly, although diffuse lipomatosis of the colon has been reported.[99, 100] The lesions are ordinarily submucosal and range in size from 0.5 to 15.0 cm.

Many lipomas are quite unobtrusive, but of those discovered during life, a majority have been symptomatic. As might be expected, lesions larger than 2 cm are those that most often give rise to symptoms, such as intussusception.[101] Of 35 symptomatic lipomas described by Horwitz et al.,[97] 21 caused pain or partial intestinal obstruction, 13 bled, and 1 presented as an abdominal mass. Of 67 patients found with submucous lipomas of the colon and rectum, Wychulis et al.[102] reported that operation was undertaken in 38, primarily because of abdominal pain or bleeding. Because lipomas seem to have a predilection for the region of the ileocecal valve and cecum, recurring right lower abdominal pain is a frequent presenting complaint.

Lipomas are pliant and rubbery as palpated

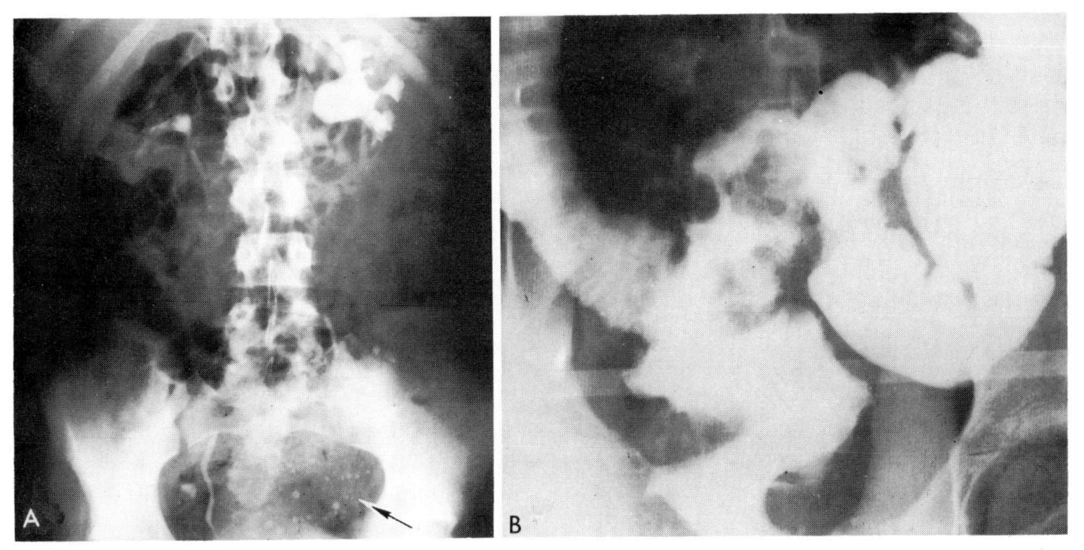

Figure 138–8. The diagnosis of hemangioma is confirmed in the pyelogram *(A)*, in which an extensive cluster of calcific phleboliths occupies the left lower abdomen. It is in this same area that a large, irregular filling defect distorts the barium enema column at the rectosigmoid junction *(B)*. (Courtesy of Dr. Henry Goldberg, Department of Radiology, University of California, San Francisco.)

in the rectum. When examined endoscopically, they appear yellowish and covered by smooth, intact, glistening, normal mucosa. Two almost pathognomonic characteristics of lipomas are their radiolucency and their apparent change in size and shape when compressed.[97] Welin et al.[103] observed no growth in polypoid lipomas in serial radiographic examinations over extended periods. When local excision of lipomatous polypoid lesions is complete, there is no recurrence. Removal through the colonoscope has been shown to be feasible in selected cases.[104]

Hamartomas

Juvenile (Retention) Polyps. Most polyps occurring sporadically in the colons of children are of a unique structure that distinguishes them from common adenomas or familial polyposis and suggests that they represent hamartomatous developmental defects in the colorectal mucosa. Their designation as "juvenile polyps" derives from the fact that a majority are found in children under the age of 10 years. Actually, there is a bimodal occurrence curve; about one-

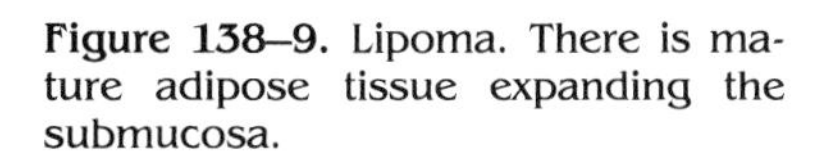

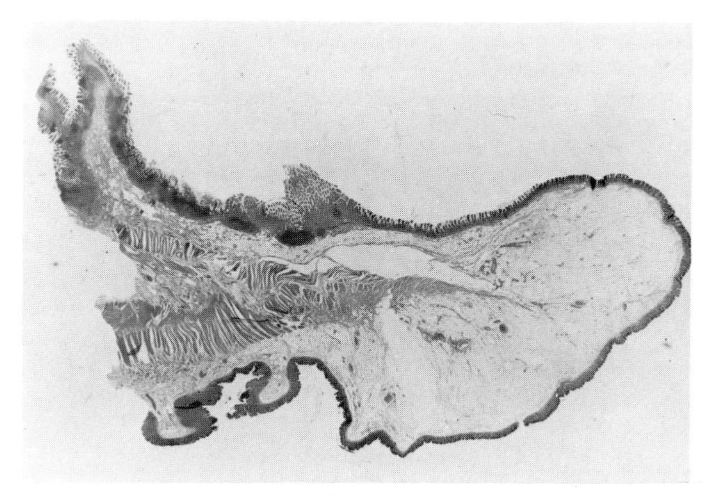

Figure 138–9. Lipoma. There is mature adipose tissue expanding the submucosa.

third are encountered in adults. Roth and Helwig[105] pointed out that juvenile polyps have been found only rarely in the second decade of life. The tumefactions are also sometimes referred to as "retention polyps" because of their cystic structure.

The cause of these polyps has been variously ascribed to an allergic diathesis, an inflammation, and a hamartomatous malformation.[105–107] The age of presentation of the majority of patients with these polyps, coupled with the rarity of morphologically similar lesions in inflammatory bowel disease, argues against an inflammatory cause and more in favor of a hamartomatous malformation. It has been suggested that there is an interrelationship between juvenile polyps, hyperplastic polyps, and adenomatous polyps. However, evidence for this is sparse, and a correlation remains to be proved.[108]

The true prevalence of colorectal polyps during the first or second decade of life is unknown because children seldom are the subject of screening surveys or necropsies. Among 105 asymptomatic boys and girls ranging in age from 6 to 16 years, Turrell and Maynard[109] discovered 2 polyps. Kerr[110] examined 349 children because of rectal bleeding, anal protrusion, or lower abdominal pain and found 68 with solitary polyps and 32 with multiple polyps. In 304 cases of childhood polyps collected by Horrilleno and his associates,[111] the peak frequency was from 2 to 4 years of age; 59.2% occurred in males. In a majority of cases, juvenile polyps are found in the rectosigmoid segment and occur singly. Only 14 of 55 youngsters observed by Holgersen et al.[112] harbored more than one lesion.

Pathology. Juvenile polyps have a characteristic gross appearance (Fig. 138–10). They are cherry-red, pedunculated, round polyps

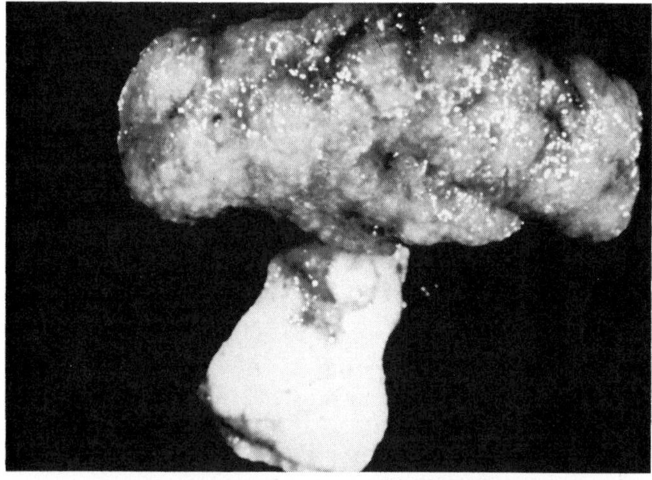

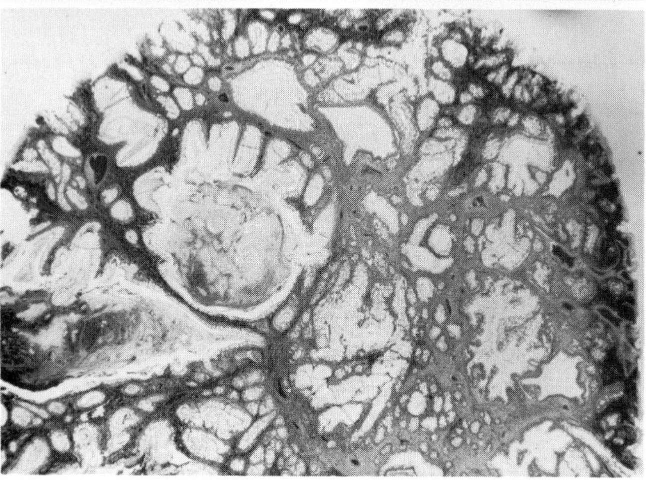

Figure 138–10. Juvenile polyp. In the microscopic view *(below),* note the smooth, round contour and the numerous mucus-filled cysts.

that have a smooth contour and are found on sectioning to contain many mucus-filled cysts. Microscopically, they consist of tubular glands, morphologically resembling those of the adjacent mucosa, embedded in abundant lamina propria. The glands may be elongated and tortuous or cystically dilated and are lined by goblet cells and mucus-containing columnar cells, some of which have a rather eosinophilic cytoplasm. There is usually no cytologic atypia unless severe inflammation is present, in which case some reactive atypia may develop. The stroma is edematous and contains an unusually abundant vascular tissue. It may also contain lymphoid follicles and rarely shows foci of metaplastic bone. The polyps frequently show a focally severe acute and chronic inflammation. This may result in ulceration of glands with spillage of mucus into the surrounding stroma. The polyps are also subject to volvulus with resultant ulceration, hemorrhage, and auto-infarction.

Blood appearing at the anus or streaking the stool is the most common presenting symptom, owing to the friable and highly vascular nature of juvenile polyps. Prolapse of the tumor is common. Classically, an anxious mother brings her child because a "cherry" is lodged at the anus. Among several series compiled by Horrilleno et al.,[111] hemorrhage was noted in 88% to 100%, a visible mass protruded from the anus in 17% to 62%, and diarrhea occurred in 5% to 19%, with constipation in 2% to 13%. Of all juvenile polyps that are recognized, 85% are found within the range of the 25-cm sigmoidoscope. MacEwan and Dunbar[113] have described the radiographic configuration of colon polyps in children, and the arteriographic diagnosis of a juvenile polyp has been illustrated by Korobkin et al.[114]

Treatment of juvenile polyps in the child is the same as that of common polyps in the adult. Complete local excision is indicated for the relief or prevention of symptoms rather than for cancer prophylaxis. Endoscopic excision of juvenile polyps is facilitated by the proportionately capacious rectum and colon of the child that usually accommodates standard instruments.

Prognosis following excision of juvenile polyps is excellent. After observing 68 patients for 3 years, Turrell and Maynard[109] found only 2 newly discovered polyps. No relationship between the juvenile polyps and the later occurrence of ordinary adenomas or carcinomas has been established.

Neurofibromas and Ganglioneuromas. These tumors are very rare in the colon. They may be single or multiple and may appear either as a diffuse thickening of the affected bowel or as polypoid tumors (Fig. 138–11). The majority are associated with von Recklinghausen's disease[115–117] or multiple endocrine neoplasia of the MEN-II type.[118–120] However, isolated cases without systemic involvement have been described.[121, 122] Histologically, neurofibromas can involve any or all layers of the bowel, including the mucosa, and are composed of spindle-shaped nerve fibers and Schwannian elements set in a rather edematous stroma. They may be confused with smooth muscle tumors. Ganglioneuromas are similar to neurofibromas but additionally contain admixed ganglion cells. The latter may bear a superficial resemblance to epithelioid cells and be confused with granulomas.

Inflammatory or Reactive Tumors

Inflammatory Polyps (Pseudopolyps). These are not neoplasms but rather inflammatory lesions, which often show regenerative changes resulting from ulcerative inflammatory injury. Pseudopolyps may be of 2 types: (1) residual islands of intact mucosa projecting from a denuded luminal surface, or (2) redundant tags of regenerated mucosa that was previously ulcerated and undermined. Heavily inflamed granulation tissue is often present. These polyps are most commonly seen in ulcerative colitis but can also occur in other inflammatory diseases, such as Crohn's disease, bacillary dysentery, and amebiasis. Although the pseudopolyps in themselves have no malignant potential, the diseased mucosa in which they form may be susceptible to malignant change after long periods.

Lymphoid Hyperplasia. Lymphoid tissue is normally present throughout the mucosa of the colon and rectum both as a diffuse infiltrate of lymphocytes and plasma cells in the lamina propria and as solitary lymphoid follicles, which are most frequent in the distal colon. Lymphoid hyperplasia can involve both components of lymphoid tissue and result in 2 distinct polypoid lesions: (1) the benign lymphoid polyp (focal lymphoid hyperplasia), and (2) nodular lymphoid hyperplasia.[123] Familiarity with these lesions is especially important in the differential diagnosis of malignant lymphoma and the polyposis syndromes of the gastrointestinal tract.

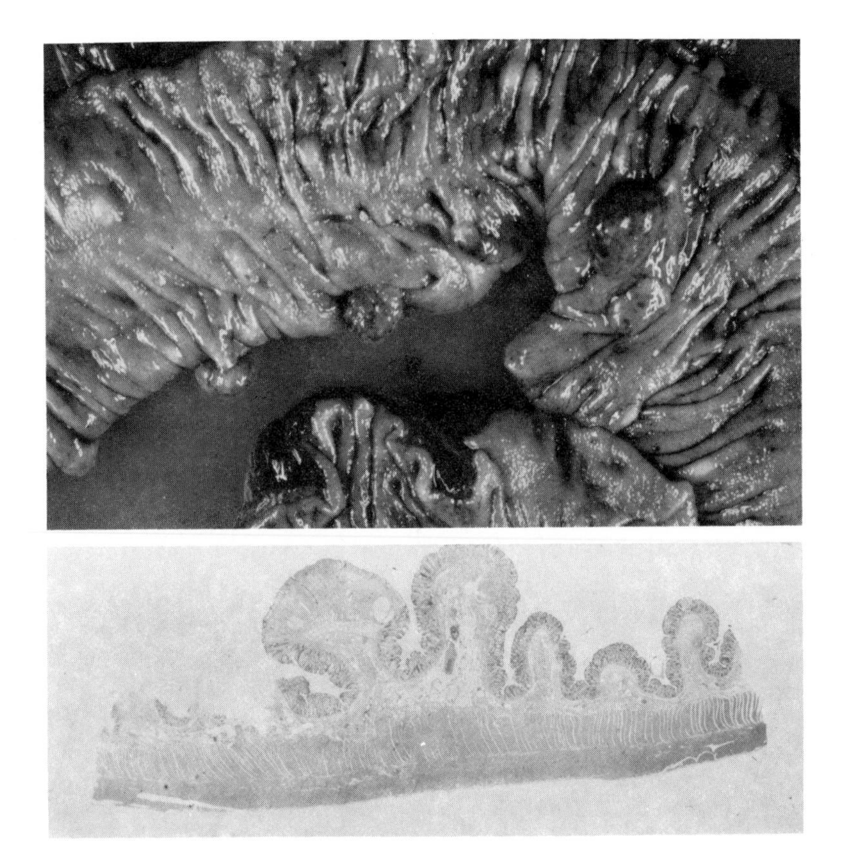

Figure 138–11. Neurofibroma. Composite picture showing gross appearance and submucosal proliferation of neural tissue seen microscopically.

Lymphoid Polyps (Benign Lymphoid Polyp, Rectal Tonsil, Focal Lymphoid Hyperplasia of the Rectum). Lymphoid polyps of the large intestine appear to be located almost exclusively in the rectum.[124–126] They occur in all age groups, including children, but are most common in the second to fifth decades and show a female predominance.[127–130] Patients are usually asymptomatic but may present with a variety of symptoms such as rectal bleeding, constipation, anal discomfort, prolapse of a rectal mass, and diarrhea.[125] These symptoms, of course, are more likely due to hemorrhoids, anal fissures, and colonic carcinoma.

Lymphoid polyps (Fig. 138–12) are usually found in the lower 10 to 15 cm of the rectum and are usually single.[131] When multiple, they generally number less than 6 lesions, although on rare occasions they may be numerous and impart a cobblestone appearance to the rectal mucosa.[132,133] They are most commonly sessile, have a smooth surface that appears pale yellow or white as viewed through an endoscope, and range in size from a few mm to 5 cm in diameter.[123,124,128,134]

Microscopically, the majority of polyps are covered by intact, although at times attenuated, colonic epithelium. They are composed of a heavy lymphoid infiltrate admixed with numerous lymphoid follicles containing large germinal centers. The lymphoid follicles are heaped on one another and straddle the mucosa and submucosa in a manner similar to that of solitary lymphoid nodules found in the normal colon.

Lymphoid polyps of the rectum should be treated by excisional biopsy for diagnostic purposes. If the lesions are multiple and the patient is asymptomatic, excision of all the polyps is probably not necessary since they may regress spontaneously. Moreover, the likelihood of local recurrence is low even after incomplete excision.[127]

Nodular Lymphoid Hyperplasia. Nodular lymphoid hyperplasia (NLH) of the gastrointestinal tract produces multiple discrete mucosal nodules in a variable segment of the small intestine, large intestine, or both. It is most commonly encountered incidentally

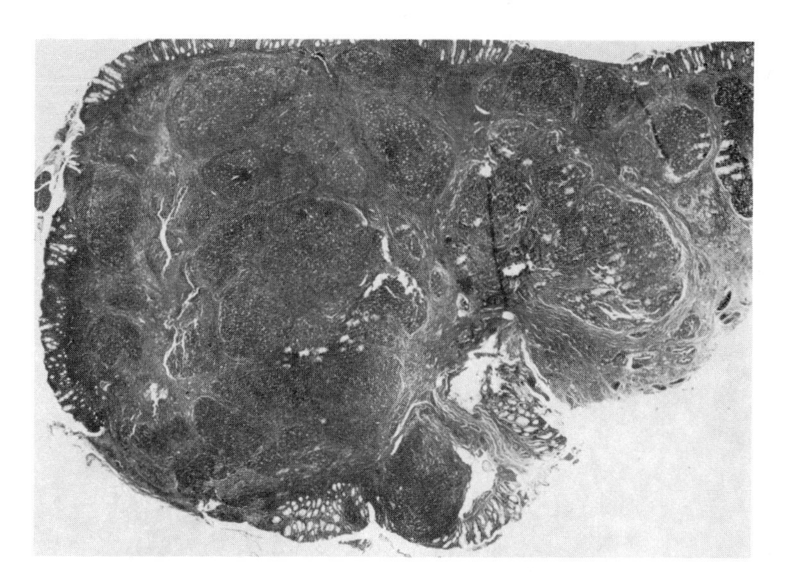

Figure 138–12. Lymphoid polyp. Note the hyperplastic lymphoid tissue covered by attenuated but intact epithelium.

during radiographic examination or at necropsy.[135, 136] NLH may be found in association with hypogammaglobulinemia, especially the late-onset, acquired type.[137, 138] Robinson et al.,[139] in a study of 1000 consecutive necropsies, found 30 cases of NLH distributed as follows: small intestine alone, 13%; large intestine alone, 40%; small and large intestine together, 47%. The patients died of a variety of causes, and none had gastrointestinal symptoms, giardiasis, or hypogammaglobulinemia. Robinson and associates used the term "enterocolitis lymphofollicularis" for the lesion in their patients. We prefer the term "nodular lymphoid hyperplasia" because "enterocolitis" seems inappropriate for a process characterized by the absence of classic inflammation and mucosal destruction.

NLH of the colon has been observed in children who have had barium enema examinations for a variety of gastrointestinal complaints. Indeed, so frequently is the change encountered that it is regarded as a common incidental finding in children and unrelated to their symptoms.[135, 136] The lymphoid nodules are usually small, measuring a few mm in diameter. However, one of the cases described by Louw[129] is exceptional in that the colon contained nodules that measured up to 2 cm in diameter and were easily detected on proctosigmoidoscopic examination.

On gross examination the mucosa is studded with sessile or polypoid nodules measuring up to 5 mm in diameter (Fig. 138–13).[123, 138, 140] Microscopically, the nodules are composed of one or a cluster of hyperplastic lymphoid follicles with prominent germinal centers. When large, these nodules may produce distortion of the overlying glands, but mucosal ulceration is absent. The lymphoid nodules are confined to the lamina propria and superficial submucosa. A decrease or absence of plasma cells is usually noted in the lamina propria of those patients who have accompanying hypogammaglobulinemia.

It is probable that the nodules in NLH without hypogammaglobulinemia represent hyperplasia of the solitary lymphoid follicles normally present in the gastrointestinal tract. Solitary lymphoid follicles are certainly present in sufficient numbers in the normal intestine (approximately 7000 to 21,000 in the colon[123]) to give rise to the characteristic radiologic and gross findings of NLH.[135, 136] Further evidence that NLH represents hyperplasia of pre-existing solitary follicles is provided by the finding of umbilication of the colonic nodules, a feature of normal lymphoid follicles and one that Franken[136] and Capitano and Kirkpatrick[135] consider helpful in making the diagnosis radiographically.

An awareness that NLH may give rise to multiple filling defects in the colon is important in the differential diagnosis of multiple colonic polypoidal lesions. NLH is especially to be kept in mind in patients being evaluated for familial polyposis. In some of these individuals, unnecessary colonic resections have been performed on occasion.[141, 142] NLH must also be distinguished histologically from lym-

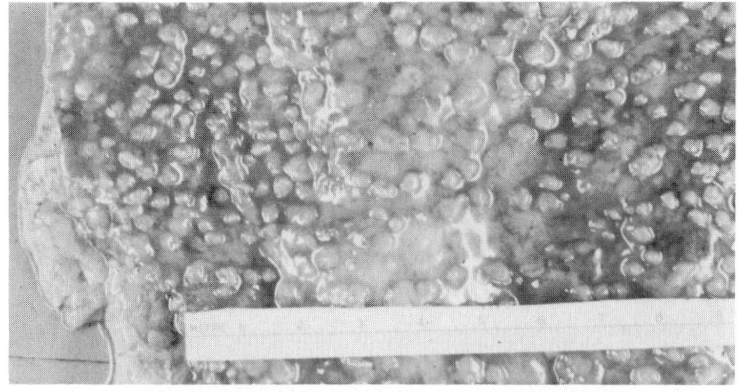

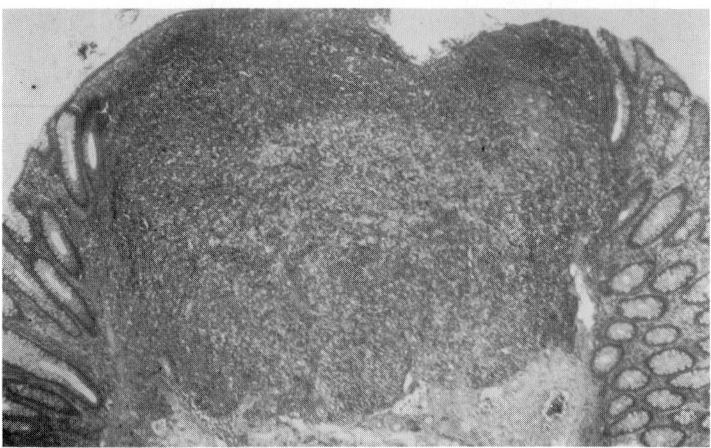

Figure 138–13. Nodular lymphoid hyperplasia. Composite picture showing mucosa studded with numerous small sessile nodules and low power microscopic view of a hyperplastic lymphoid follicle.

phomatous polyposis of the intestine, especially the follicular type.[143] The distinction is easily made insofar as the nodules in NLH are largely confined to the lamina propria and contain prominent germinal centers. In a few instances, NLH has been complicated by the development of lymphoma.[144, 145]

Miscellaneous Polypoid Lesions

A number of rare lesions occasionally produce polypoid tumors of the colon and rectum, with or without symptoms of obstruction, and must be considered in the differential diagnosis of benign polyps.

Lipoid granulomas, sometimes called "oleomas," can result from the inflammatory reaction induced by sclerosing agents with an oil base (usually mineral or cottonseed oils) employed in the injection treatment of hemorrhoids.[146] Their polypoid appearance in the lower rectum can simulate adenomas or even carcinomas. Oleomas are composed of fibrous tissue and a mononuclear cell infiltrate characteristic of chronic inflammation. They may be further identified by the presence of foreign-body giant cells or macrophages containing oil.

Similarly, *barium granulomas* can result from impregnation of the rectum or colon mucosa as a rare complication of barium enema examinations.[147] The lesions are grossly evident as minute, circumscribed, yellow plaques, and are characterized microscopically by a chronic granulomatous inflammatory reaction surrounding crystals of barium sulfate.

Colitis cystica profunda,[74] distinguished by epithelial-lined mucous cysts deep to the muscularis mucosae in the wall of the colon and rectum, may appear as projections into the lumen (Fig. 138–14). The condition may be localized to the rectum or diffuse throughout the colon. An important differentiation is from invasive carcinoma.

Endometriosis may on occasion produce nodular masses with obstruction. The endometrial tissue elicits secondary smooth muscle hypertrophy in the bowel wall (Chapter 137).[148, 149]

Inflammatory fibroid polyps occur at times in the cecum, although they are most commonly found in the stomach.[150–154] They have

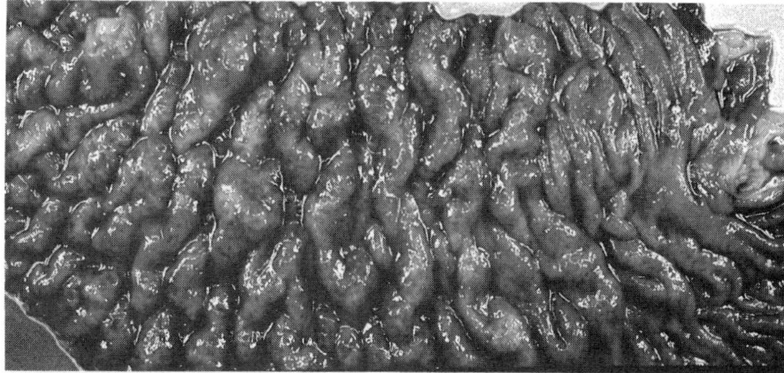
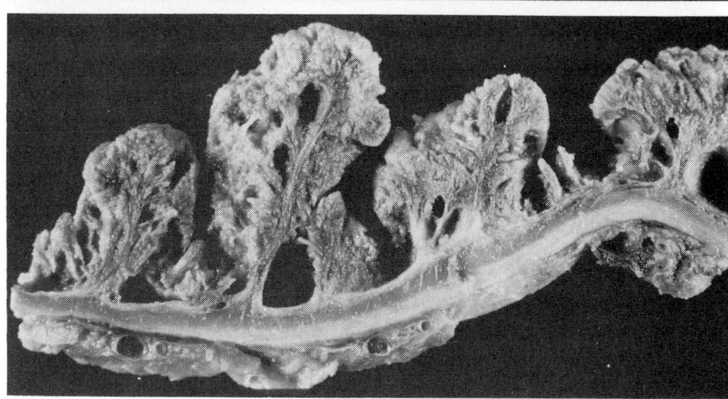

Figure 138–14. Colitis cystica profunda.

a distinct histologic appearance: loose fibrous tissue with a prominent vasculature, surrounded by concentrically laminated fibrous tissue with an accompanying inflammatory infiltrate that frequently contains numerous eosinophils.[150,151] Whether this lesion represents an allergic inflammatory response or a neoplastic process remains to be determined.[151, 152, 155]

Other lesions such as *pneumatosis intestinalis* (Fig. 138–15), lymphangiomas, granular cell myoblastomas, and Kaposi's sarcoma have also been reported to produce polypoid lesions in the large bowel. *Metastatic carcinoma,* most commonly malignant melanoma and lymphoma, may produce polypoid lesions of the colon and rectum and mimic benign tumors. *Carcinoid tumors* are rare low-grade malignant tumors that may occasionally present as polypoid masses (Chapter 113). Lastly, *anal lesions,* such as enlarged anal papillae, hemorrhoids, and condylomata, may be polypoid in appearance and must be distinguished from polypoid tumors (Chapter 143).

Clinical Manifestations

Most patients with discrete colonic polyps are asymptomatic. The lesions are usually detected incidentally during routine physical examinations or during endoscopic or radiographic studies performed to explain symptoms emanating from other usually unrelated disorders. When symptoms do occur, they are more apt to be associated with large polyps, i.e., greater than 1 cm in diameter,[156] and with their complications, such as ulceration, intussusception, and prolapse. Statistics on the frequency of symptoms in hospitalized patients tend to pertain to a selected group with these complications. Thus, in a series of 809 patients with simple adenomas seen at the Massachusetts General Hospital, only 32% were reported to be asymptomatic.[12]

The most common symptom attributable to adenomatous polyps is *rectal bleeding.* In the series just cited, bleeding was present in 44% of the patients. The blood is bright red, rarely profuse, and in the beginning may only coat the stool. Once it has started, it tends to appear with every bowel movement and may eventually be mixed with the feces. In some cases, particularly in tumors situated on the right side of the colon, bleeding may be detected only by testing the stool for occult blood. Juvenile polyps also frequently present with bleeding due to ulceration and auto-amputation. *Changes in bowel habit* may

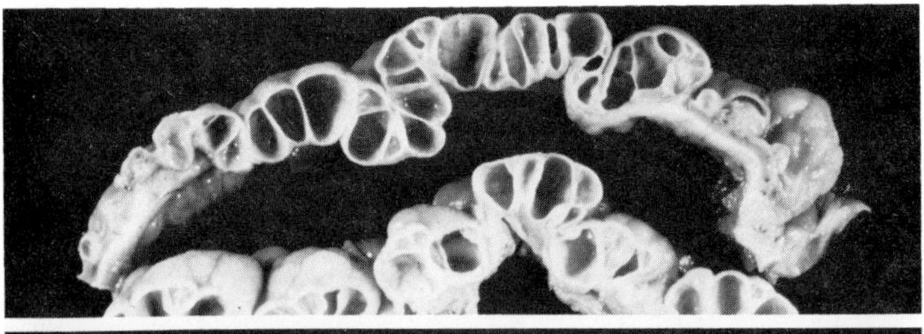

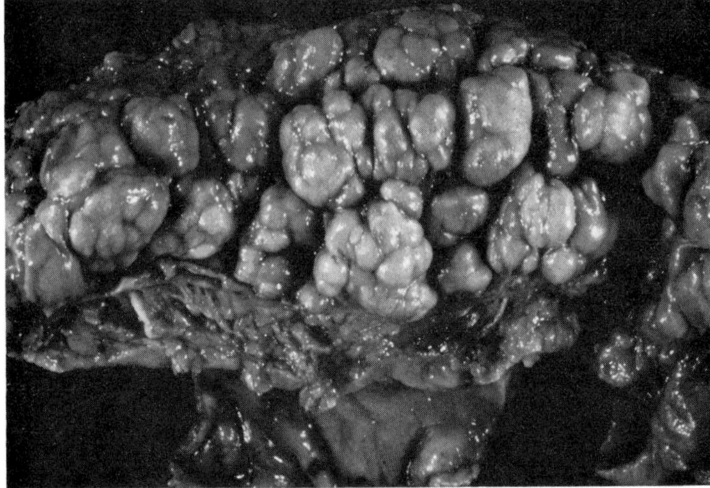

Figure 138–15. Pneumatosis intestinalis. The gas-filled spaces are best visualized in the section of colon cut "end-on" *(above)*. (See Chapter 136.) (Courtesy of Dr. Mahendra Ranchod, Good Samaritan Hospital, San Jose, California.)

be associated with large polyps in a small percentage of cases. Constipation is more apt to occur with lesions in the distal sigmoid colon and rectum, while diarrhea may be the presenting symptom of large villous adenomas. *Abdominal pain,* usually of a cramping character, may be induced by large polyps, which are subjected to varying degrees of intussusception. Other less commonly encountered symptoms are flatulence, excessive discharge of mucus, and distention.

An interesting syndrome sometimes associated with large villous adenomas consists of profuse diarrhea with massive fluid and electrolyte depletion. Patients complain of dehydration, confusion, weakness, weight loss, nausea, depression, and incontinence and may present with severe hypotension and circulatory collapse. Hypovolemia, prerenal azotemia, severe hypokalemia, hyponatremia, and hypochloremia are often found. Unless prompt replacement therapy is provided, death from circulatory collapse may ensue. Babior[157] has summarized the clinical features of all cases reported in the literature up to 1966 and emphasized the presence of large stool volumes, sometimes up to 4 liters in 24 hours, and the high incidence of hypokalemia. Approximately 36 cases had been reported by 1975.[12] The definitive treatment is resection of the tumor.

Benign tumors are seldom detected during physical examination. Rectal polyps tend to be small, pliable, and movable and therefore often escape detection by the palpating finger.

Diagnostic Procedures

Polypoid lesions of the large bowel are best demonstrated by endoscopic or roentgenologic techniques. Proctosigmoidoscopy, colonoscopy, and barium enema examinations are commonly employed for optimum detection. The techniques and other fundamental aspects of these procedures are given in Chapters 33, 42, and 43. Their relative merits and indications as regards benign tumors of the colon are reviewed here.

Proctosigmoidoscopy. In a study of 342 patients reported by Winnan et al.,[158] the average length of large bowel visualized with the conventional 25-cm rigid sigmoidoscope was only 20 cm. Nevertheless, this instrument does detect a substantial number of benign and malignant lesions. The flexible fiberoptic instrument was found by Winnan and associates to be capable of being advanced to 35 cm in 88 and to 50 cm in 52 of their patients. Of 51 polypoid lesions found with the flexible sigmoidoscope, 42 (82%) were beyond the average length of colon visualized by the rigid instrument. The authors also reported no complications in more than 1000 examinations with the flexible sigmoidoscope. It seems clear, therefore, that the flexible sigmoidoscope is superior to the conventional rigid instrument in the detection of polypoid lesions.

Colonoscopy. In 1600 diagnostic colonoscopic examinations, Wolff and Shinya[159, 160] encountered no complications from the procedure, although bleeding and perforations have been reported to occur occasionally. In several large series, complications of colonoscopy alone have ranged from 0.2% to 0.4%; when combined with polypectomy, the complication rate has ranged from 1% to 2.3%.[160–162] The ability to examine the entire colon with the fiberoptic colonoscope has provided new data on the distribution and histologic features of polypoid lesions in various parts of the colon. Thus, of 5786 adenomas found by Wolff and Shinya, 52% were in the rectosigmoid, 25% in the descending colon, 10% in the transverse colon, and 13% in the right colon.[11]

Radiography. High quality double-contrast barium enema, the preferred method of examining the colon today, may detect polyps missed by other radiographic techniques and even during colonoscopy.[162, 163] Some advocate it as the initial screening procedure for polyp detection,[164] but whether it is as accurate in identifying polypoid lesions as colonoscopy remains to be settled. What does seem clear from comparison studies is that the accuracy of either procedure depends on the expertise of the examiner and thorough cleansing of the colon. The emerging consensus among unbiased physicians is that the colonoscopic and radiographic examinations are complementary rather than competitive in the detection of large bowel polyps.

Screening Procedures. The rarity of symptoms in patients with colorectal polyps poses a number of difficult questions for the physician. Who should be screened? At what age should screening begin? What modality should be employed and how frequently should it be repeated? No answers applicable to all patients are available, but a logical approach has been formulated over the past decade.[165, 166]

Asymptomatic patients over the age of 40 should have basic screening procedures, consisting of complete blood counts, stool examinations for occult blood, and proctosigmoidoscopy, as part of their periodic physical examination. If evidence of blood loss is found and upper gastrointestinal causes for bleeding have been ruled out, a double-contrast barium enema study should be obtained. If this is negative, the colon is examined colonoscopically. On the other hand, if polyps are found on proctosigmoidoscopic examination, a complete colonoscopy with biopsy or removal of polyps is undertaken. Once benign polyps have been discovered and removed, patients should be followed with annual colonoscopic examinations for 3 years. If no new lesions are discovered during this period, the routine periodic basic screening procedures are reinstituted. Gilbertson et al.[167] have an ongoing screening study of more than 48,000 patients, aged 50 to 80 years, who have no gastrointestinal symptoms. Thus far, 873 patients with positive Hemoccult slide tests have had further evaluations with endoscopic and radiographic studies, whereby 690 polyps and carcinomas were found. This study indicates that colon neoplasms develop appreciably often in asymptomatic patients over age 50 with occult blood in the stool.

Relatives of patients with one of the gastrointestinal polyposis syndromes should also be screened. The criteria governing such screening are detailed in the following section of this chapter.

Complications

The major complication associated with adenomatous polyps is *malignant change.* Less common are *intussusception* and *prolapse.* Intussusception occurs occasionally with large polyps of the colon, particularly submucous lipomas, adenomas, and polypoid carcinomas.[12] However, intussusception is less common with tumors of the colon than with tumors of the small intestine because the colon for the most part is firmly fixed to the posterior parietes and has a wide lumen.

Prolapse of rectal polyps through the anus occurs occasionally. It has been reported most commonly with juvenile polyps, which may also be complicated by bleeding, infarction, and auto-amputation.

Management

The availability now of colonoscopy and colonoscopic polypectomy has made many of the rules previously applied to polypoid lesions of the colon obsolete and has significantly simplified and facilitated management. No longer is it necessary for the physician to agonize over the possible malignant potential of a polyp beyond the reach of the sigmoidoscope. No longer must he apply specific criteria of size, configuration, and rate of growth before deciding whether a patient's polyp can be watched or requires surgical removal. Endoscopic polypectomy is now accepted as the treatment of choice for discrete, pedunculated polypoid lesions of all types, provided the patient is able to tolerate the colonoscopy and the preceding cleansing process. The techniques of colonoscopy and polypectomy, as well as the contraindications, hazards, and complications, are described in Chapter 43. Polypectomy should not be done when submucous lipomas or large, flat villous adenomas or obvious carcinomas are encountered. Some guidelines for the management of polyps of various sizes, number, configuration, and histologic type are detailed below.

Size of Polyps. The previously set limits applied to the size of polyps that require removal have largely been discarded as new techniques have been introduced. Since it has been shown that carcinoma may exist even in polyps 0.5 to 1 cm in diameter, all polyps should be removed whenever possible.[11] Those 4 cm or greater in largest dimension should first be biopsied, inasmuch as a high percentage of them harbor malignancy. If the histologic examination of the biopsy specimen confirms the presence of malignant change, prompt surgical resection is indicated. If no such change is seen, endoscopic removal, either *in toto* at one visit or in stages, may be undertaken, provided the endoscopist has the experience and training necessary and a stalk can be identified. Isolated minute polyps (i.e., those less than 0.5 cm in diameter) encountered on contrast barium enema examinations are almost always benign lesions and do not by themselves justify the risk of colonoscopy and polypectomy. However, if such small lesions are found during colonoscopy performed for other reasons, they should be removed.

Number of Polyps. Patients found to have a large number of polyps, i.e., 50 or more, should be evaluated for the existence of one of the polyposis syndromes. Several biopsy specimens will usually suffice to establish the predominant histologic type, which, in turn, will dictate subsequent management. In patients with a few isolated, benign-appearing lesions, the most proximal one is removed first. The distance of each from the anus should be noted and indicated on the specimen bottle. In the event that malignant changes are subsequently found on histologic examination, this localization will greatly facilitate further therapy. The maximum number of polyps removed at one procedure should usually be restricted to 5. The major reasons for this limit are the comfort of the patient and the tolerance of the endoscopist.

Configuration of Polyps. Pedunculated lesions are most amenable to easy and safe endoscopic removal. Flat, diffuse, or infiltrating lesions and large sessile polyps present technical problems and should therefore be biopsied from multiple areas so as to obtain representative samples. Most of these will prove to be villous adenomas or carcinomas, which require surgical removal. Smaller sessile polyps may be amputated if a false pedicle of mucosa can be created around their bases. The judgment and experience of the endoscopist are crucial in the selection of sessile lesions amenable to this technique.

Histologic Type. Hyperplastic, hamartomatous, and lymphoid polyps are usually multiple, but carry little or no risk of undergoing malignant transformation. Their gross appearances, as described earlier in this chapter, may enable the endoscopist to suspect their histologic type. It is nevertheless prudent to biopsy several of the largest lesions and subject them to histologic examination.

How does the physician proceed when the pathologic analysis of a successfully removed adenomatous polyp reveals the presence of cancer? If the adenoma contains a focus of carcinoma-in-situ on histologic examination, no further therapy is necessary.[168–170] The patient should merely have the same periodic follow-up outlined for other patients with benign polyps. Patients with polyps containing invasive carcinoma extending into the stalk and/or adjacent mucosa require surgical resection.

Some controversy exists in the management of pedunculated tubular adenomas containing foci of invasive carcinoma confined to the head of the polyp. Shatney et al.[168] recommend only local removal unless there are tumor cells in the lymphatic vessels within the head of the polyp, or the carcinoma is highly undifferentiated, or the pedicle is extremely short and malignant changes extend to the neck of the adenoma. These authors treated 8 patients with only superficially invasive carcinoma by local excision of the polyps and found no evidence of tumor during a prolonged follow-up averaging 87 months. Witt and Winawer[169] also found support for local excision of polyps with invasive carcinoma confined to the head after analyzing the available data. However, Colacchio et al.[170] reviewed their experience with 39 patients with invasive carcinoma in pedunculated adenomas and found that 6 (25%) had lymph node metastases. After analyzing the parameters of size, depth of invasion into the stalk, degree of differentiation, and involvement of lymphatics within the polyp, they determined that it was not possible to predict which lesions would have lymph node metastases at the time of resection. They concluded, therefore, that all patients with polyps containing invasive carcinoma should undergo transabdominal sleeve resection of the colon. Our own experience with pedunculated tubular adenomas containing foci of invasive carcinoma confined to the head of the polyp is similar to that of Shatney and co-workers, and we concur with their recommendations.

References

1. Chapman I. Adenomatous polypi of large intestine: Incidence and distribution. Ann Surg 1963; 157:223–6.
2. Leffall LD. Colorectal cancer prevention and detection. Cancer 1981; 47:1170–2.
3. Wolff WI, Shinya H. Endoscopic polypectomy therapeutic and clinical pathologic aspects. Cancer 1975; 36:683–90.
4. Arminski TC, McLean DW. Incidence and distribution of polyps of colon and rectum based on 1000 autopsy examinations. Dis Colon Rectum 1964; 7:249–61.
5. Feyrter F. Zur Geschwulstlehre (Nach Untersuchungen am Menschlichen Darm) Polypen und Krebs. Beitr Pathol Anat Allgemeinen Pathol 1936; 86:663–760.
6. Behringer GE. Changing concepts in the histopathologic diagnosis of polypoid lesions of the colon. Dis Colon Rectum 1970; 13:116–8.
7. Arthur JF. Structure and significance of metaplastic nodules in the rectal mucosa. J Clin Pathol 1968; 21:735–43.
8. Lane N, Kaplan H, Pascal RR. Minute adenomatous and hyperplastic polyps of the colon: Divergent patterns of epithelial growth with specific associated mesenchymal changes. Gastroenterology 1971; 60:537–51.
9. Fenoglio CM, Lane N. The anatomical precursor of colorectal carcinoma. Cancer 1974; 34:819–23.
10. Shinya H. Colonoscopy: diagnosis and treatment of colonic diseases. New York, Tokyo: Igaku-Shoin, 1982.
11. Shinya H, Wolff WI. Morphology, anatomic distribution and cancer potential of colonic polyps. An analysis of 7,000 polyps endoscopically removed. Ann Surg 1979; 190:679–83.
12. Welch CE, Hedberg SE. Polypoid Lesions of the Gastrointestinal Tract. 2nd Ed. Philadelphia: WB Saunders, 1975.
13. Haenszel W, Correa P. Cancer of the colon and rectum and adenomatous polyps. Cancer 1971; 28:14–24.
14. Hill MJ, Morson BC, Bussey HJR. Aetiology of adenoma-carcinoma sequence in large bowel. Lancet 1978; 1:245–7.
15. Bussey HJR. Familial polyposis coli. *In*: Pathology Annual. New York: Appleton-Century-Crofts, 1979; 61–81.
16. Muto T, Bussey HJR, Morson BC. The evolution of cancer of the colon and rectum. Cancer 1975; 36:2251–70.
17. Wynder LE, Reddy BS. Metabolic epidemiology of colorectal cancer. Cancer 1974; 34:801–6.
18. Berg JW, Howel MA. The geographic pathology of bowel cancer. Cancer 1974; 34:807–14.
19. Hill MJ. Bacteria and the etiology of colonic cancer. Cancer 1974; 34:815–8.
20. Aries V, Crowther JS, Drasar BS, et al. Bacteria and the etiology of cancer of the large bowel. Gut 1969; 10:334–5.
21. Drasar BS, Hill MJ. Intestinal bacteria and cancer. Am J Clin Nutr 1972; 25:1399–1404.
22. Burkitt DP. Epidemiology of cancer of the colon and rectum. Cancer 1971; 28:3–13.
23. Lipkin M. Proliferation and differentiation of normal and neoplastic cells in the colon of man. Cancer 1971; 28:38–40.
24. Lipkin M. Phase 1 and phase 2 proliferative lesions of colonic epithelial cells in diseases leading to colonic cancer. Cancer 1974; 34:878–88.
25. Kaye GI, Fenoglio CM, Pascal RR, et al. Comparative electron microscopic features of normal, hyperplastic and adenomatous human colonic epithelium. Gastroenterology 1973; 64:926–45.
26. Lipkin M, Bell B. Cell proliferation. *In*: Code CF (ed.): Handbook of Physiology. Section 6. Washington, DC: American Physiological Society, 1968: 2861–79.
27. Deschner E, Lewis CM, Lipkin M. In vitro study of human rectal epithelial cells. Atypical zone of H3-thymidine incorporation in mucosa of multiple polyposis. J Clin Invest 1963; 42:1922–8.
28. Cole JW, McKalen A. Studies on the morphogenesis of adenomatous polyps in the human colon. Cancer 1963; 16:998–1002.
29. Deschner E, Lipkin M, Solomon C. Study of human epithelium cells in vitro. J Natl Cancer Inst 1966; 36:849–57.
30. Deschner E, Lipkin M. Study of human rectal epithelial cells in vitro. III. RNA, protein, and DNA synthesis in polyps and adjacent mucosa. J Natl Cancer Inst 1970; 44:175–85.
31. Maskens AP. Histogenesis of adenomatous polyps in the human large intestine. Gastroenterology 1979; 77:1245–51.
32. Kaye GI, Lane N, Pascal RR. Colonic pericryptal fibroblast sheath: Replication, migration, and cytodifferentiation of a mesenchymal cell system in adult tissue. II. Fine structural aspects of normal rabbit and human colon. Gastroenterology 1968; 54:852–65.
33. Kaye GI, Pascal RR, Lane N. The colonic pericryptal fibroblast sheath: Replication, migration and cytodifferentiation of a mesenchymal cell system in adult tissue. III. Replication and differentiation in human hyperplastic and adenomatous polyps. Gastroenterology 1971; 60:515–36.
34. Bleiberg H, Mainguet P, Galand P. Cell renewal in familial polyposis: Comparison between polyps and adjacent healthy mucosa. Gastroenterology 1972; 63:240–5.
35. Dukes CE. An explanation of the difference between a papilloma and an adenoma of the rectum. Proc Roy Soc Med 1947; 40:829–30.
36. Lane N, Lev R. Observations on the origin of adenomatous epithelial polyps of the colon. Cancer 1963; 16:751–64.

37. Maskens AP, Dujardin-Loits RM. Experimental adenomas and carcinomas of the large intestine behave as distinct entities. Cancer 1981; 47:81–9.
38. Spjut HJ, Spratt JS Jr. Endemic and morphologic similarities existing between spontaneous colonic neoplasms in man and 3:2-dimethyl-4-aminobiphenyl induced colonic neoplasms in rats. Ann Surg 1965; 161:309–24.
39. Kikkawa N, Yasutomi M, Hirose S, et al. Studies on the morphogenesis of polyp and cancer in the colon and rectum. Stomach Intest (Japan) 1973; 8:1519.
40. Laqueur GL. Symposium on carcinogenic action of cycads. Fed Proc 1972; 31:1481–99.
41. Enterline HT. Polyps and cancer of the large bowel. *In:* Morson BC (ed). Current Topics in Pathology, Pathology of the Gastrointestinal Tract. New York: Springer Verlag 1976; 97–137.
42. Grinell RS, Lane N. Benign and malignant adenomatous polyps and papillary adenomas of the colon and rectum. Surg Gynecol Obstet 1958; 106:519–38.
43. Morson BC. The polyp-cancer sequence in the large bowel. Proc Roy Soc Med 1974; 67:451–7.
44. Spratt JS, Ackerman LV, Moyer CA. Relationship of polyps of colon to colonic cancer. Ann Surg 1958; 148:682–96.
45. Ekelund G, Lindstrom C. Histopathological analysis of benign polyps in patients with carcinoma of the colon and rectum. Gut 1976; 15:654–63.
46. Correa P, Strong JP, Reif A. The epidemiology of colorectal polyps. Prevalence in New Orleans and international comparisons. Cancer 1977; 39:2258–64.
47. Rider JA, Kirsner JB, Moeller HC, et al. Polyps of the colon and rectum. JAMA 1959; 170:633–8.
48. Enterline HT, Arvan PA. Chromosome constitution of adenomas and adenocarcinoma of the colon. Cancer 1967; 20:1746–59.
49. Filipe M, Branford AC. Mucin histochemistry of the colon. *In*: Morson BC (ed). Current Topics in Pathology. Pathology of the Gastrointestinal Tract. New York: Springer Verlag 1976; 143–70.
50. Gilbertsen VA. Proctosigmoidoscopy and polypectomy in reducing the incidence of rectal cancer. Cancer 1974; 34: 936–9.
51. Morson BC. Some peculiarities in the histology of intestinal polyps. Dis Colon Rectum 1962; 5:337–44.
52. Lane N, Lev R. Observations on the origin of adenomatous epithelium of the colon. Serial section of minute polyps in familial polyposis. Lancet 1963; 16:751–4.
53. Qizilbash AH. Hyperplastic (metaplastic) polyps of the appendix. Report of 19 cases. Arch Pathol 1974; 97:385–8.
54. Oohara T, Ogino A, Tohma H. Histogenesis of microscopic adenoma and hyperplastic (metaplastic) gland in nonpolyposis coli. Dis Colon Rectum 1981; 24:375–84.
55. Goldman H, Ming S, Hickock DP. Nature and significance of hyperplastic polyps of the human colon. Arch Pathol 1974; 89:349–56.
56. Estrada RG, Spjut HJ. Hyperplastic polyps of the large bowel. Am J Surg Pathol 1980; 4:127–33.
57. Lev R, Grover R. Precursors of human colon carcinoma. A serial section study of colectomy specimens. Cancer 1981; 47:2007–15.
58. Appel MF, Spjut HJ, Estrada RG. The significance of villous component in colonic polyps. Am J Surg 1977; 134:770–1.
59. Atwater JS, Bargen JA. The pathogenesis of intestinal polyposis. Gastroenterology 1945; 4:395–408.
60. Moertel CG, Hill JR, Dockerty MB. Routine proctoscopic examination. Second look. Mayo Clin Proc 1966; 41:368–74.
61. Welin S. Results of the Malmö technique of colon examination. JAMA 1967; 199:369–71.
62. Ekelund G. On cancer and polyps of the colon and rectum. Acta Pathol Microbiol Scand 1963; 59:165–70.
63. Bremmer CG, Ackerman LV. Polyps and carcinoma of the large bowel in the South African Bantu. Cancer 1970; 26: 991–9.
64. Stemmermann GN, Yatani R. Diverticulosis and polyps of the large intestine. A necropsy study of Hawaii Japanese. Cancer 1973; 31:1260–70.
65. Correa P, Duques E, Cuello C, et al. Polyps of the colon and rectum in Cali, Columbia. Int J Cancer 1972; 9:86–96.
66. Bockus HL, Tachjian V, Ferguson LK, et al. Adenomatous polyp of the colon and rectum. Its relation to carcinoma. Gastroenterology 1961; 41:225–32.
67. Castelman B, Krickstein HI. Do adenomatous polyps of the colon become malignant? N Engl J Med 1962; 267:469–75.
68. Marshak RH. The pedunculated adenomatous polyp. Am J Dig Dis 1965; 10:958–67.
69. Sato E. Adenomatous polyps of large intestine in autopsy and surgical material. Gann 1974; 65:295–306.
70. Enterline HT, Evans GW, Mercado-Lugo R, et al. Malignant potential of adenomas of colon and rectum. JAMA 1962; 179:322–30.
71. Fechner RE. Adenomatous polyps with submucosal cysts. Am J Clin Pathol 1973; 59:498–502.
72. Muto T, Bussey HJR, Morson BC. Pseudo-carcinomatous invasion in adenomatous polyps of the colon and rectum. J Clin Pathol 1973; 26:25–31.
73. Greene FL. Epithelial misplacement in adenomatous polyps of the colon and rectum. Cancer 1974; 33:206–17.
74. Magidson JG, Lewin KJ. Diffuse colitis cystica profunda. Am J Surg Pathol 1981; 5:393–9.
75. Begelow B, Winkelman J. Polyps of the colon and rectum. A review of 12 years' experience and report of unusual case. Cancer 1964; 17:1177–86.
76. Behringer GE. On pedunculated adenomatous polyps of the colon and rectum with particular reference to their malignant potential. Dis Colon Rectum 1970; 13:116–8.
77. Horn RC Jr. Malignant potential of polypoid lesions of the colon and rectum. Cancer 1971; 28:146–52.
78. Quan SHQ, Castro EB. Papillary adenomas (villous tumors). A review of 215 cases. Dis Colon Rectum 1971; 14:267–80.
79. Hanley PH, Hines MO, Ray JE. Villous tumors. Experience with 217 patients. Am Surg 1971; 37:190–7.
80. Bacon HE, Eisenberg SW. Papillary adenoma or villous tumor of the rectum and colon. Ann Surg 1971; 174:1002–8.
81. Welch JP, Welch CE. Villous adenomas of the colo-rectum. Am J Surg 1976; 131:185–91.
82. Wheat MW, Ackerman LV. Villous adenomas of the large intestine. Clinicopathologic evaluation of 50 cases of villous adenomas with emphasis on treatment. Ann Surg 1958; 147:476–87.
83. Ramirez RF, Culp CE, Jackman RJ, et al. Villous tumors of the lower part of the large bowel. JAMA 1965; 194:863–7.
84. Porter SD, Liechty RD. Villous adenoma in 108 patients. Am J Surg 1968; 116:13–6.
85. Olson RO Sr, Clayton DW. Villous adenomas of the colon, benign and malignant. Arch Surg 1969; 98:487–92.
86. Orringer MB, Eggleston JC. Papillary (villous) adenomas of the colon and rectum. Surgery 1972; 72:378–81.
87. MacKenzie DA, McDonald JR, Waugh JM. Leiomyoma and leiomyosarcoma of the colon. Ann Surg 1954; 139:67–75.
88. Quan SHQ, Berg JW. Leiomyoma and leiomyosarcoma of the rectum. Dis Colon Rectum 1962; 5:418–25.
89. Ranchod M, Kempson RL. Smooth muscle tumors of the gastrointestinal tract and retroperitoneum. A pathologic analysis of 100 cases. Cancer 1977; 39:255–62.
90. Nemer FD, Stoeckinger JM, Evans T. Smooth muscle rectal tumors. Dis Colon Rectum 1977; 20:405–13.
91. Akwari OE, Dozois RE, Weiland LH, et al. Leiomyosarcoma of the small and large bowel. Cancer 1978; 42:1375–84.
92. Gentry RW, Dockerty MB, Clagett OT. Collective review: Vascular malformations and vascular tumors of the gastrointestinal tract. Int Abstr Surg 1949; 88:281–323.
93. Allred HW Jr, Spencer RJ. Hemangiomas of the colon, rectum and anus. Mayo Clin Proc 1974; 49:739–41.
94. Head HD, Baker JQ, Muir RW. Hemangioma of the colon. Am J Surg 1973; 126:691.
95. Bell GA, McKenzie AD, Emmons H. Diffuse cavernous hemangioma of rectum; report of case and review of literature. Dis Colon Rectum 1972; 15:282–377.
96. Mayo CW, Pagtalunan RJG, Brown DJ. Lipoma of the alimentary tract. Surgery 1963; 53:598–603.
97. Horwitz MM, Redleaf PD, Williams HJ, et al. Lipomas of the gastrointestinal tract: An analysis of 72 tumors. AJR 1967; 99:84–9.

98. Weinberg T, Feldman M. Lipomas of the gastrointestinal tract. Am J Clin Pathol 1955; 25:272–81.
99. Ling CS, Leagus C, Stahlgren LH. Intestinal lipomatosis. Surgery 1959; 46:1054–9.
100. Swain VAJ, Young WF, Pringle EM. Hypertrophy of the appendices epiploicae and lipomatous polyposis of the colon. Gut 1969; 10:587–9.
101. Haller JD, Roberts TW. Lipomas of the colon. Clinical pathologic study of 20 cases. Surgery 1964; 55:773–81.
102. Wychulis AR, Jackman RJ, Mayo CW. Submucous lipomas of colon and rectum. Surg Gynecol Obstet 1964; 118:337–340.
103. Welin S, Youker J, Spratt JS Jr. The rates and patterns of growth of 375 tumors of the large intestine and rectum observed serially by double contrast enema study (Malmö technique). AJR 1963; 90:673–81.
104. Papp JP, Haubrich WS. Endoscopic removal of colon lipomas. Gastrointest Endosc 1973; 20:66–7.
105. Roth SI, Helwig EG. Juvenile polyps of the colon and rectum. Cancer 1973; 16:468–79.
106. Alexander RH, Beckwith JB, Morgan A, et al. Juvenile polyps of the colon and their relationship to allergy. Am J Surg 1970; 120:222–5.
107. Silverberg SG. "Juvenile" retention polyps of the colon and rectum. Am J Dig Dis 1970; 15:617–25.
108. Goodman ZD, Yardley JH, Milligan FD. Pathogenesis of colonic polyps in multiple juvenile polyposis. Cancer 1979; 43:1906–13.
109. Turrell R, Maynard A de L. Adenomas of rectum and colon in juvenile patients. JAMA 1956; 161:57–60.
110. Kerr JG. Polyposis of colon in children. Am J Surg 1948; 76:667–71.
111. Horrilleno EG, Eckert C, Ackerman LV. Polyps of rectum and colon in children. Cancer 1957; 10:1210–20.
112. Holgersen LO, Miller RE, Zintel HA. Juvenile polyps of the colon. Surgery 1971; 69:288–93.
113. MacEwan DW, Dunbar JS. Radiologic diagnosis of polyps of the colon in children. Radiology 1961; 77:196–206.
114. Korobkin M, Shapiro H, Lawson D, et al. Arteriographic diagnosis of a juvenile cecal polyp. Gastroenterology 1972; 63:1059–61.
115. Lukash WM, Morgan RI, Sennett CO, et al. Gastrointestinal neoplasm in von Recklinghausen's disease. Arch Surg 1966; 92:905–8.
116. Raszkowski HJ, Hufner RF. Neurofibromatosis of the colon: A unique manifestation of von Recklinghausen's disease. Cancer 1971; 27:134–42.
117. Hochberg FH, DaSilva AB, Galdabini J, et al. Gastrointestinal involvement in von Recklinghausen's neurofibromatosis. Neurology (Minneapolis) 1974; 24:1144–51.
118. Carney JA, Go VLW, Sizemore GW, et al. Alimentary tract ganglioneuromatosis: A major component of the syndrome of multiple endocrine neoplasia, type 2b. N Engl J Med 1976; 295:1287–91.
119. Whittle TS Jr, Goodwin MN Jr. Intestinal ganglioneuromatosis with the mucosal neuroma-medullary thyroid carcinoma pheochromocytoma syndrome: A case report and review of the literature. Am J Gastroenterol 1976; 65:249–57.
120. Snover DC, Weigent CE, Sumner HW. Diffuse mucosal ganglioneuromatosis of the colon associated with adenocarcinoma. Am J Clin Pathol 1981; 75:225–9.
121. Donnelly WH, Sieber WK, Yunis E. Polypoid ganglioneurofibromatosis of the large bowel. Arch Pathol 1969; 87:537–41.
122. Haff RC, San Diego AG. Ganglioneuroma of the ileocecal valve: Review of the literature. Arch Pathol 1972; 93:549–51.
123. Ranchod M, Lewin KJ, Dorfman RF. Lymphoid hyperplasia of the gastrointestinal tract: A study of 26 cases and review of the literature. Am J Surg Pathol 1978; 2:383–400.
124. Helwig EB, Hansen J. Lymphoid polyps (benign lymphoma) and malignant lymphoma of the rectum and anus. Surg Gynecol Obstet 1951; 92:233–43.
125. Holtz F, Schmidt LA. Lymphoid polyps (benign lymphoma) of the rectum and anus. Surg Gynecol Obstet 1958; 106:639–42.
126. Keeling WM, Beatty GL. Lymphoid polyps of the rectum. Arch Surg 1956; 73:753–6.
127. Swartzlander FC, Jackman RJ, Dockerty MB. Submucosal rectal nodules. Am J Surg 1956; 92:657–65.
128. Cornes JS, Wallace H, Morson BC. Benign lymphomas of the rectum and anal canal: A study of 100 cases. J Pathol Bacteriol 1961; 83:371–82.
129. Louw JW. Polypoid lesions of the large bowel in children with particular reference to benign lymphoid polyposis. J Pediatr Surg 1968; 3:195–209.
130. Shattock SG. Polypi of lymphatic tissue from a child's rectum. Trans Pathol Soc Lond 1890; 40:137–9.
131. Granet E, Kagan MB, Solomon C. Lymphomas of the anorectum. Am J Surg 1950; 80:311–5.
132. Meissner WW. Benign lymphoma of the rectum. J Int Coll Surg 1956; 26:739–49.
133. Sheehan DG, Martin F, Baginsky S, Mallory GK, Zamcheck N. Multiple lymphomatous polyposis of the gastrointestinal tract. Cancer 1971; 28:408–25.
134. Heller EL, Lewis HH. Benign lymphoma of the rectum. Am J Pathol 1950; 26:463–71.
135. Capitano MA, Kirkpatrick JA. Lymphoid hyperplasia of the colon in children. Radiology 1970; 94:323–7.
136. Franken EA. Lymphoid hyperplasia of the colon. Radiology 1970; 94:329–34.
137. Hermans PE, Huizenga KA, Hoffman HN, et al. Dysgammaglobulinemia associated with nodular lymphoid hyperplasia of the small intestine. Am J Med 1966; 40:78–89.
138. Hermans PE, Dias-Buxo JA, Stobo JD. Idiopathic late-onset immunoglobulin deficiency: Clinical observations in 50 patients. Am J Med 1976; 61:221–37.
139. Robinson MJ, Padron S, Rywlin AM. Enterocolitis lymphofollicularis. Arch Pathol 1973; 96:311–15.
140. Milano AM, Lawrence LR, Horowitz L. Nodular lymphoid hyperplasia of the small intestine and colon with giardiasis. Am J Dig Dis 1971; 16:745–7.
141. Collins JO, Falk M, Guibone R. Benign lymphoid polyposis of the colon: A case report. Pediatrics 1966; 38:897–9.
142. Gruenberg J, Mackman S. Multiple lymphoid polyps in familial polyposis. Ann Surg 1972; 175:552–4.
143. Cornes JS. Multiple lymphomatous polyposis of the gastrointestinal tract. Cancer 1961; 14:249–57.
144. Matuchansky C, Morchau-Beauchant M, Touchard G, et al. Nodular lymphoid hyperplasia of the small bowel associated with primary jejunal malignant lymphoma. Gastroenterology 1982; 78:1587–92.
145. Kahn LB, Novis BH. Nodular lymphoid hyperplasia of the small bowel associated with primary small bowel reticulum cell lymphoma. Cancer 1974; 33:837–44.
146. Wittoesch JH, Jackman RJ, McDonald JR. Lipoid granulomas of rectum. Proc Staff Meet Mayo Clin 1956; 31:265–71.
147. Gordon BS, Clyman D. Barium granuloma of rectum. Gastroenterology 1957; 32:943–51.
148. Jenkinson EL, Brown WH. Endometriosis. A study of 117 cases with special reference to constricting lesions of the rectum and sigmoid colon. JAMA 1943; 122:249–53.
149. McSwain B, Kinn RJ, Haley RL, et al. Endometriosis of the colon. Report of 14 patients requiring partial colectomy. Medicine 1974; 67:651–8.
150. McGee HJ. Inflammatory fibroid polyps of the ileum and cecum. Arch Pathol 1960; 70:203–7.
151. Samter TG, Alstott DF, Kurlander GJ. Inflammatory fibroid polyps of the gastrointestinal tract. Am J Clin Pathol 1966; 45:420–36.
152. Goldman RL, Friedman NB. Neurogenic nature of so-called inflammatory fibroid polyps of the stomach. Cancer 1967; 20:134–47.
153. Benjamin SP, Hawk WA, Turnbull RB. Fibrous inflammatory polyps of the ileum and cecum. Cancer 1977; 39: 1301–5.
154. Johnstone J, Morson BC. Inflammatory fibrous polyps of the gastrointestinal tract. Histopathology 1978; 2:349–61.
155. Williams RM. An ultrastructural study of a jejunal inflammatory fibroid polyp. Histopathology 1981; 5:193–203.
156. Welch CE. Polyps and cancer of the colon. Am J Surg 1979; 138:625–6.

157. Babior BM. Villous adenoma of the colon. Study of a patient with severe fluid and electrolyte disturbances. Am J Med 1966; 41:615–21.
158. Winnan G, Berci G, Panish J, Talbot TM, Overholt BF, McCallum RW. Superiority of the flexible to the rigid sigmoidoscope in routine proctosigmoidoscopy. N Engl J Med 1980; 302:1011–2.
159. Wolff WI, Shinya H. Colonofiberoscopy. JAMA 1971; 217:1509–12.
160. Wolff WI, Shinya H. Polypectomy via the fiberoptic colonoscope. N Engl J Med 1973; 288:329–32.
161. Silvis SE, Nebel O, Rogers G, Sugawa C, Mandelstam P. Endoscopic complications. Results of the 1974 American Society of Gastrointestinal Endoscopy Survey. JAMA 1976; 235:928–30.
162. Dodds WJ, Stewart ET, Hogan WJ. Role of colonoscopy and roentgenology in the detection of polypoid colonic lesions. Dig Dis 1977; 22:646–9.
163. Laufer I, Smith NCW, Mullens JE. The radiological demonstration of colorectal polyps undetected by endoscopy. Gastroenterology 1976; 70:167–70.
164. Fork FT. Double contrast enema and colonoscopy in polyp detection. Gut 1981; 22:971–7.
165. Eddy D. Guidelines for the cancer-related checkup. Recommendations and rationale. Cancer of the colon and rectum. CA 1980; 30:208–15.
166. Tedesco FJ, Waye JD, Raskin JB, Morris SJ, Greenwald RA. Colonoscopic evaluation of rectal bleeding. A study of 304 patients. Ann Intern Med 1978; 89:907–9.
167. Gilbertson VA, McHugh R, Schuman L, Williams SE. The earlier detection of colorectal cancers. A preliminary report of the results of the occult blood study. Cancer 1980; 45:2899–901.
168. Shatney CH, Lorber PH, Gilbertsen VA, Sosin H. The treatment of pedunculated adenomatous colorectal polyps with focal cancer. Surg Gynecol Obstet 1974; 139:845–50.
169. Witt TR, Winawer SJ. Cancer in a colonic polyp, or malignant colonic adenomas—is polypectomy sufficient? Comment. Gastroenterology 1981; 81:625–6.
170. Colacchio TA, Forde KA, Scantlebury VP. Endoscopic polypectomy. Inadequate treatment for invasive colorectal carcinoma. Ann Surg 1981; 194:704–7.

Polyposis Syndromes

Arthur D. Schwabe • Klaus J. Lewin

The occurrence of multiple benign tumors, predominantly in the colon, is the cardinal feature of a group of disorders collectively known as the gastrointestinal polyposis syndromes.[1,2] They are differentiated by the extent of their gastrointestinal involvement, their associated extraintestinal manifestations, their patterns of inheritance, and the gross and histologic features of the polyps themselves. Although most of these syndromes are relatively rare, afflicted persons are commonly referred to gastroenterologists and colorectal surgeons for diagnosis, genetic counseling, and therapy.

The principal locations of polyps in the various polyposis syndromes are given in Table 138–2. Because the lesions are not confined to the colon (except perhaps for juvenile polyposis coli and Turcot's syndrome), the polyposis syndromes require consideration as well in discussions concerned with tumors of the stomach (Chapters 74 and 76) and tumors of the small bowel (Chapter 114). This overlap in interest, therefore, makes some modicum of duplication of discussion unavoidable.

The polyps found in these syndromes demonstrate great variation in size, density, and manner of attachment to the bowel wall. Histologically, they may be predominantly neoplastic (adenomas) or non-neoplastic (hamartomas). In spite of obvious clinical and pathologic differences, relationships among several syndromes have been observed.

Adenomatous Polyposis Syndromes

Three hereditary syndromes, familial polyposis coli, Gardner's syndrome, and Turcot's syndrome, are characterized by the presence of multiple adenomatous polyps and a high occurrence rate of associated cancer in the colon and rectum.

Familial Polyposis Coli (FPC)

FPC, the most common of the polyposis syndromes attributable to a genetic defect,

Table 138–2. LOCATION OF POLYPS IN THE POLYPOSIS SYNDROMES

Syndrome	Esophagus	Stomach	Small Intestine	Large Intestine
Familial polyposis coli	−	+	+	+ + +
Gardner's syndrome	−	+	+	+ + +
Turcot's syndrome	−	−	−	+ + +
Peutz-Jeghers syndrome	−	+ +	+ + +	+ +
Juvenile polyposis coli	−	−	−	+ + +
Familial generalized juvenile polyposis	−	+ +	+ +	+ + +
Cronkhite-Canada syndrome	+ (?)	+ + +	+ +	+ + +
Neurofibromatosis	+	+ + +	+ + +	+ +
Multiple hamartoma syndrome	+ +	+ +	+ + +	+ +

Key: − None; + Rare; + + Common; + + + Predominant.

has been recognized for more than 100 years. Tonneson,[3] Shiffman,[4] and Bussey[1] have chronicled the historical background of this disorder. Diagnosis depends on the demonstration of at least 100 adenomatous polyps in the large intestine. In the cases studied by the St. Mark's Hospital group in London, the total number of polyps in each specimen varied from 104 to 5000 and the average was just over 1000.[1]

Prevalence. Estimates of the proportion of FPC patients in the general population range from 1 in 6850 to 1 in 24,000.[1,5] Accurate statistics are difficult to obtain in most parts of the world. In Sweden, where excellent population records are available, the prevalence of FPC was calculated to be 1 in 7646. FPC has been detected in Orientals, African and American blacks, Indians, and Arabs. Bussey[1] states that it seems likely that the prevalence of FPC is fairly constant throughout the world.

Inheritance. FPC is inherited as an autosomal dominant trait. It is not sex-linked and therefore can be inherited from either parent by offspring of either sex in equal ratio. Each child of an afflicted parent has a 50:50 chance of developing the disease.[5, 6] In addition to the cases encountered in the setting of an obvious family history, FPC is occasionally detected in persons who have no known afflicted relatives. It has been estimated that polyposis represents the phenotypic expression of a spontaneous mutation in 30% of patients. Uncertain parentage or inaccurate medical information about close relatives may also be responsible for apparently isolated cases. Offspring of such individuals are exposed to the same risk of inheriting polyposis as are those with a strong family history of the disorder.[1, 6] Young adults with FPC should be acquainted with the potential risks to their children and advised to seek genetic counseling.

Clinical Features. Patients with FPC may seek medical attention because of a family history of polyposis or cancer or because of gastrointestinal symptoms. Some cases are detected during routine proctoscopic or incidental radiographic examinations. The diagnosis of FPC is most commonly established between the ages of 20 and 40 years. The mean age of patients at diagnosis at St. Mark's Hospital was 36 years, with a range of 4 to 73 years.[1, 6] However, when relatives of probands were called in for examination, the mean age of patients with polyposis was 24 years. Polyps appear in most patients after the age of 10 years and then rapidly increase in size and number. There is no evidence that adenomatous polyps have ever been present at birth.[1]

Many patients with FPC are asymptomatic even when the colon is studded with polyps. The average interval before symptoms occur after the appearance of polyps is 10 years.[7] The earliest symptom is mild to moderate diarrhea.[2] Cramping abdominal pain, bleeding, weakness, and weight loss may occur, but such symptoms should also alert the clinician to the possible presence of carcinoma. The physical examination is usually unrevealing, unless bowel obstruction from a supervening carcinoma has occurred.

Laboratory Abnormalities. Patients with FPC may have an iron deficiency anemia secondary to prolonged bleeding and, less commonly, electrolyte disturbances associated with chronic diarrhea.[2] The polyps are demonstrated by proctosigmoidoscopy, colonoscopy, and air-contrast barium enema examination (Fig. 138–16). In several series,

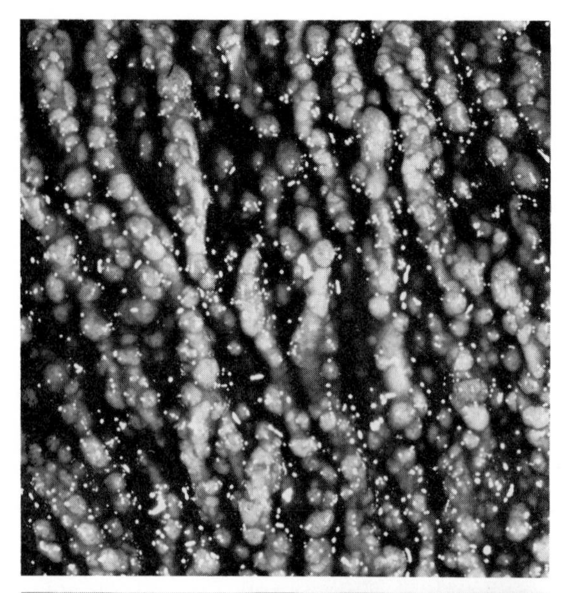

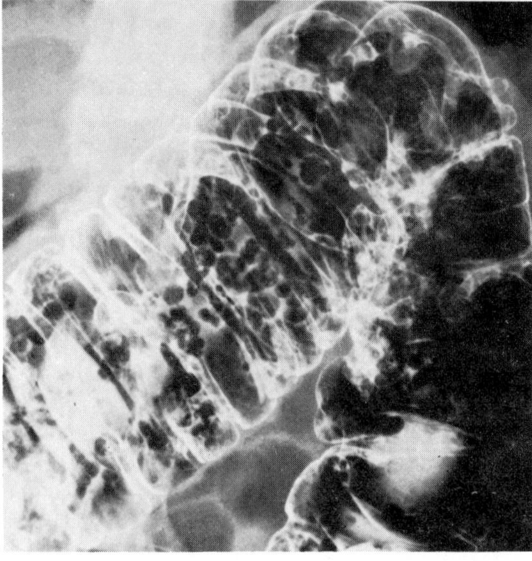

Figure 138–16. Gross appearance of the colon *(above)* in familial polyposis coli, demonstrating myriads of small sessile polyps carpeting the mucosa. Air contrast barium enema *(below)* demonstrating numerous polyps. (Courtesy of Dr. J. A. Hamlin, Department of Radiology, Cedars-Sinai Medical Center, Los Angeles.)

radiographs have revealed osteomas of the mandible and maxilla in FPC patients without any other extracolonic manifestations, suggesting a relationship to Gardner's syndrome.[8,9]

Distribution of Polyps. The polyps in FPC are confined to the colon and rectum in the vast majority of cases. Earlier reports stressed that the adenomas never occurred in the stomach or small intestine, and many authorities still hold to this viewpoint. In the last decade, however, evidence has accumulated in many parts of the world that a few patients, who seem to satisfy all other diagnostic criteria for FPC, have had gastric and small bowel involvement as well. Ushio et al.[9] examined the entire gastrointestinal tract radiographically and endoscopically in a series of patients with FPC. They found polyps in the stomach in 15 of 22 patients and in the duodenum in 9 of 10 patients. The simultaneous discovery of skeletal abnormalities (50%), osteosclerotic lesions in the mandible (81%), and soft tissue tumors (13%) in this series prompted the authors to postulate that "FPC and Gardner's syndrome are substantially the same entity" and should be considered as one systemic disorder with predisposition to multiple tumor formation. Others would classify many of these cases as clear examples of Gardner's syndrome. Yao et al.[10] found duodenal polyps in 13 of 14 patients with adenomatous polyposis of the colon and cited another 29 cases from the literature. At least half of these patients had extracolonic lesions. Bussey[7] cites 4 patients with adenomas in the colon, duodenum, and jejunum; 2 of these also had carcinomas of the duodenum. Sivak and Jagelman[10a] performed esophagoduodenoscopy in a group of 49 patients with familial polyposis coli and Gardner's syndrome. Of the patients in this group who had familial polyposis coli, half had polyps in the upper gastrointestinal tract. On biopsy, many of these, particularly in the stomach, were hyperplastic polyps rather than adenomas. Lymphoid polyps in the terminal ileum have also been noted in patients with FPC.[11]

Pathology. The density of polyps may vary from 100 to many thousands. They may be discrete or situated in groups separated by apparently normal mucosa, or, in their most florid form, they may carpet the entire large bowel as myriads of tiny, sessile mamillations (Fig. 138–16A). The number of polyps is greatest in the left side of the colon in the majority of cases.[1,7] According to Bussey,[1] 98% of the polyps are less than 0.5 cm in diameter and only 1% exceed 1 cm. On rare occasions, benign adenomas greater than 4 cm in diameter may be found.

Grossly, the polyps are either sessile or pedunculated and may have a smooth, lobulated, or shaggy surface. Histologically, they are predominantly tubular adenomas, but on rare occasion a few may demonstrate hyperplastic, villous, tubulovillous, or juvenile features. The earliest changes, seen in the columnar cells of single or groups of glandular crypts of Lieberkühn, are characterized by an increased nuclear-cytoplasmic ratio and loss of cytoplasmic mucin.[7,12] The typical histologic appearances of the fully formed adenomatous polyps were detailed at the beginning of the preceding section of this chapter.

Development of Carcinoma. Accurate information about the exact interval between the first appearance of polyps and the development of cancer in FPC is not available. Muto et al.[13] indicated that available data on the polyp-cancer sequence under these circumstances are likely to underestimate the actual interval. They also cited 59 patients at St. Mark's Hospital who, for various reasons, had no treatment for their disease. During the first 5 years after diagnosis, 12% developed cancer; at 15 to 20 years, cancer had occurred in more than 50% of the patients. The average age of detection of carcinoma has been determined to be approximately 39 years. This is 20 to 25 years earlier in life than the detection of colon carcinoma in patients without polyposis.

The available evidence supports the widely held concept that cancers in FPC arise from adenomatous polyps. In the St. Mark's Hospital series, 36% of the patients had adenomas in continuity with invasive cancer.[1] The simultaneous presence of multiple carcinomas in FPC may also support this concept but could merely be a reflection of the high proliferating potential of the colonic mucosa in this disease. At operation, more than 40% of the FPC patients cited by Bussey[1] had multiple carcinomas.

Treatment. All authorities agree that patients with FPC require surgical resection of the diseased colon. Controversy exists only regarding the timing of the operation and the extent of the resection. Surgery should be advised at the time of diagnosis in almost all cases. From the data accumulated from several large series of FPC patients, it is apparent that the duration of the disease cannot be accurately determined in the vast majority of cases and that cancer may be present in the absence of symptoms. In most patients, polyps are present by the age of 15 years.[2,14] Cancer has been observed in a patient only 8 years of age,[14] but most often cancer supervenes about 15 years after the appearance of polyps.[1,2] Surgery therefore may be delayed in asymptomatic children until they have reached physical and psychologic maturation, provided they can be followed closely with biennial colonoscopic and cytologic examinations.

Initially, total proctocolectomy and ileostomy was advocated for all patients with FPC and is still the procedure of choice of many surgeons familiar with this disease. An alternative procedure, preferred by others and the standard treatment of the St. Mark's Hospital group, is total colectomy with ileorectal anastomosis. Muto et al.[13] recommend that if this procedure is selected, any polyps in the rectum should be treated by fulguration before or after colectomy. Patients so treated should have proctoscopic examinations every 6 months, and any new tumors must again be removed by fulguration.

The risk of cancer of the rectal stump was analyzed in 86 patients followed for up to 25 years.[13] Cancer developed in only 2 patients, at 2 and 7 years after colectomy. This low cancer rate in the rectal stump is at variance with that reported by the Mayo Clinic.[15] Muto et al.[13] feel that the periodic and complete removal of all new polyps in the rectum may be a significant reason for their better results. Another possible explanation is the observation by several groups that polyps in the rectal stump may regress after colectomy, presumably by an inhibition of neoplastic activity from the altered environment.[2,14]

It may be concluded that ileoproctostomy should be reserved for selected patients whose rectums are not carpeted with adenomas, who have no rectal cancer, and who agree to have regularly scheduled examinations and removal of any new tumors.[16]

For more than 30 years, surgeons have attempted to develop other procedures for generalized colorectal disease, designed to remove all of the large bowel mucosa and yet to maintain rectal continence by preserving the anorectal sphincter mechanism. The technique of total colectomy with endorectal pull-through seemed to accomplish these goals. However, it resulted in fecal urgency and frequency or, not infrequently, only partial continence. The procedure basically consists of resection of the colon down to the rectosigmoid junction, dissection and excision of the mucosa below this level to within 1 to 4 cm of the dentate line, and anastomosis of the ileum to the remaining cuff of rectal mucosa. Various modifications for the prevention of dehiscence of the ileorectal anastomosis and the creation of an ileal reservoir have been introduced. Fonkalsrud[17] has reviewed the various modifications and reported on his 10-year experience with 29 patients. He advocates the addition of a lateral internal ileal reservoir because it reduced fecal urgency and frequency in most of his patients. This procedure has not yet achieved wide acceptance among surgeons but may be an attractive alternative to the other customary operations. Long-term follow-up may establish whether this procedure deserves a more prominent place in the management of patients with FPC.

Another approach, the Kock "continent ileostomy," consists of the construction of an ileal pouch subsequent to proctocolectomy. This procedure is described in detail in Chapter 126. It may be employed when preservation of the rectum is not possible or because of rectal cancer or extensive involvement of the rectum with myriads of polyps.

Gardner's Syndrome (GS)

The association of cutaneous abnormalities, bone tumors, colonic polyposis, and cancer was first described in a 36-year-old woman by Devic and Bussey in 1912.[18] In the early 1950s Gardner and his co-workers[19, 20] examined 51 members of a large family and found a combination of osteomas of the skull, mandible, and long bones; soft tissue tumors of the skin; colonic polyposis; and a high incidence of colon cancer. They subsequently defined the manner of inheritance. Extensive analysis conducted over the next 30 years identified 224 members in 6 generations of this family, 28 of whom had the typical clinical manifestations of the syndrome.[21] Over the past 3 decades, numerous reports of similar families, as well as isolated cases from all parts of the world, have appeared in the literature. A variety of other intestinal and extraintestinal lesions have been detected in this disorder, now known as *Gardner's syndrome* (GS).

Frequency. GS has been determined to affect both sexes equally.[22, 23] The gene frequency at birth has been calculated to be 1 in 14,025, or slightly less than that estimated for FPC.

Inheritance. An autosomal dominant pattern of inheritance for GS was first indicated by the early studies of Gardner.[19, 20] He postulated that either a single pleiotropic gene gave rise to the 3 major clinical manifestations or that 3 closely linked genes were responsible. The single gene concept has been favored by several other investigators. Analysis of 161 sibships indicates that the gene has a penetrance of nearly 100%, but there is considerable variation in expressivity.[23]

Clinical Features. Although intestinal polyps in GS have been observed in children as young as 5 years of age, they usually appear between the ages of 15 and 25 years.[23] The diagnosis may be made in early childhood by the presence of epidermoid cysts followed by osteomas, dental abnormalities, and fibromas.

Initially, very few small polyps are present on endoscopic examination, but they increase in size and number as the patients grow older. Most of the patients reported by Gardner et al.[24] have had less than 100 adenomatous polyps in the colon and rectum, and none has had more than 200 polyps. McKusick[25] also has indicated that the polyps in GS are fewer, larger, and more widely scattered than in FPC. Others have not been impressed with any significant differences in the number and size of polyps in the 2 entities.[9, 14] The polyps are confined to the colon and rectum in the vast majority of patients. However, a number of cases have been reported in recent years of adenomatous or hyperplastic polyps in the stomach, duodenum, and small intestine as well.[7, 9, 10a, 26] Hamartomas of the stomach and lymphoid polyps of the ileum have also been detected in a few isolated patients with GS.[23, 26]

The bony abnormalities in GS consist of osteomas, exostoses, and cortical thickening. Osteomas, the most frequently reported osseous lesions, have been found in the mandible, maxilla, the sinuses of the cranium, the frontal and parietal bones, the zygomas, and the long bones of the extremities.[27] The exostoses have been observed on the skull, digits, and long bones. Localized cortical thickening occurs primarily in the long bones and less commonly in ribs, metacarpals, and phalanges. Japanese reports indicate a high occurrence rate of osteomas and small sclerotic areas in the mandible in patients with colonic polyposis but without any other extracolonic manifestations.[8–10] While this finding may indicate a variation in expressivity of the GS gene, it may also suggest a relationship to FPC.

The cutaneous and subcutaneous lesions of GS are epidermoid cysts, fibromas, desmoids, and lipomas.[14, 20, 21] The epidermoid cysts, previously often designated as sebaceous cysts, are frequently found on the face, neck, and trunk. Subcutaneous fibromas have been reported on the scalp, shoulders, arms, and back. Desmoid tumors, appearing as benign though locally invasive fibrous tissue masses, develop most often in surgical scars or after trauma to the skin, but have also appeared spontaneously without known prior injury. Both fibromas and desmoids have been shown to occur in the abdominal cavity, particularly after surgery. They have been found in the mesentery, the retroperitoneal area, and the ligamentous attachments. The development of these desmoid reactions is a dire complication of colectomy in GS and has been responsible for several deaths from inoperable small bowel and ureteral obstruction.

Dental abnormalities in GS patients consist of odontomas, dentigerous cysts, and supernumerary and unerupted teeth. There are also reports in several families of early dental caries and premature loss of teeth, but these may be coincidental findings.

Other abnormalities and tumors described in association with GS are listed in Table 138–3. Carcinoma of the thyroid has been reported in association with FPC and Turcot's syndrome, as well as GS.[1,14] Camiel et al.[28] found papillary carcinomas of the thyroid in 2 sisters with GS. Periampullary carcinomas have been found in 12% of patients with colorectal polyposis as compared with 0.4% in the general population.[23] Carcinomas of the ampulla of Vater, duodenum, and pancreas have been described; such lesions occurred in 14 of 19 patients with GS, whose cases were summarized by Jones and Nance.[29] These authors concluded that periampullary malignancy develops approximately 15 years after the onset of colorectal polyps. The first patient reported with the array of findings that typify GS was also found by Devic and Bussey[18] to have an adrenal adenoma. Subsequently 3 adenomas and 1 carcinoma of the adrenal gland have been reported in GS patients. Whether these tumors constitute an integral component of this syndrome must await more detailed analysis of afflicted kindreds.

Table 138–3. EXTRACOLONIC MANIFESTATIONS OF GARDNER'S SYNDROME

Cutaneous Lesions
Desmoids
Epidermoid cysts
Fibromas
Lipomas
Dental Abnormalities
Dentigerous cysts
Odontomas
Supernumerary teeth
Unerupted teeth
Skeletal Changes
Cortical thickening
Exostoses
Osteomas
Miscellaneous Tumors
Adrenal tumors
Leiomyomas
Mesenteric desmoids
Mesenteric fibromas
Mesenteric fibrosarcomas
Periampullary carcinomas
Ampullary carcinomas
Duodenal carcinomas
Pancreatic carcinomas
Thyroid carcinomas

Pathology. The gross and histologic appearances of the gastrointestinal tumors in GS are identical with other adenomatous polyps and span the histologic spectrum observed in FPC. The intra-abdominal desmoid tumors occur most commonly at the base of the mesentery. They are grossly distinguished as fibrous tissue masses with ill-defined margins extending into adjacent tissues. Microscopically, they are composed of mature fibroblasts with few nuclei, prominent intercellular matrices of collagen, and multinucleated giant cells.[21]

Treatment. The management of the colorectal polyposis in GS follows the same principles and recommendations as those described for FPC because of the high risk of carcinoma developing in the diseased large intestine in both disorders. A more difficult problem arises when polyps are also present in the stomach. The first steps in such cases are biopsy and histologic delineation of the polyps. If they are found to be hamartomas, microcarcinoids, hyperplastic, regenerative, or lymphoid polyps, no treatment is necessary. If adenomatous gastric polyps are discovered, close surveillance with frequent cytologic examinations and biopsy of larger tumors is recommended by some; subtotal gastrectomy is recommended by others. However, because accurate statistics of the malignant potential of these gastric adenomas are not available and because their regression following colectomy has been observed, the more conservative approach seems preferable at this time.[23]

Periampullary carcinomas are treated aggressively with pancreaticoduodenectomy, provided no hepatic or distant metastases are present. Desmoid tumors producing bowel obstruction are resected when technically feasible. When vital structures are encased by the tumor or the involvement of the mesentery or retroperitoneal area is too extensive to permit resection, chemotherapy with theophylline and chlorothiazide has been reported to reduce tumor size in some patients.[23]

Relationship of Gardner's Syndrome to Familial Polyposis Coli. The designation of GS as an entity distinct from FPC has been the subject of considerable debate in the literature for almost 3 decades. Based on certain phenotypic differences and the distribution, number, and size of polyps, McKusick[25] suggested that the gene in GS is different from that of FPC. The separate entity hypothesis has also gained support from the demonstration of increased tetraploidy in skin cultures from patients with GS, but not from those with FPC.[23] Naylor and Lebenthal[23] emphasize that if members of different kindreds are fully evaluated, it will invariably be found that patients with GS have offspring who will eventually develop the full-blown syndrome, while children of those with established FPC will be devoid of extracolonic manifestations. Most authorities, however, favor the concept that GS represents merely a more complete phenotypic expression of the same genotype than does FPC. This view is based on the occurrence of osteomas, desmoids, and gastric and small intestinal polyps and the risk of carcinoma in both entities.[8–10] In addition, more detailed analyses of patients have shown the same variation in age of onset as well as in the number, size, location, and the histologic features of the polyps in both disorders. It may be concluded that the weight of evidence at this time favors the concept that GS and FPC represent a single disorder produced by a simple pleiotropic gene.

Turcot's Syndrome (TS)

In 1959, Turcot, Després, and St. Pierre[30] reported a brother and sister with polyposis of the colon and malignant tumors of the central nervous system. The brother, who died of a medulloblastoma of the spinal cord, also had carcinoma of the colon and rectum. The sister had a subtotal colectomy and later died of a glioblastoma of the left frontal lobe; an incidental chromophobe adenoma of the pituitary was also found at necropsy. A survey of the 2 preceding generations in this family failed to reveal any other relative with polyposis or central nervous system tumors. In the subsequent 2 decades, 7 siblings in 2 additional families[31,32] and a number of other isolated cases have been described. The disorder is now known as the *Turcot* or *glioma-polyposis syndrome.*

Nearly all cases have been detected between the ages of 10 and 25 years. The colonic polyps have been adenomas of the tubular type and occasionally of the villous or adenovillous types. In 4 cases, carcinomas of the large intestine were also found. The central nervous system tumors were identified as glioblastomas in 8 cases and medulloblastomas in 3. Co-existent papillary carcinomas of the thyroid were observed in 3 cases.[33] The manner of inheritance has not been conclusively established. The family history of the 3 siblings reported by Todd et al.[32] was also unrevealing of additional cases. Baughman et al.[31] reviewed 76 family members in 5 generations and found only one distant relative with a posterior fossa ependymoma. Although these observations suggest that this syndrome is transmitted as an autosomal recessive trait, a dominant trait with incomplete penetrance cannot be excluded.[30–33]

Some evidence suggests a relationship between Turcot's and Gardner's syndromes. Binder et al.[34] described the association of polyps of the colon and sebaceous cysts in a large family. One of 4 affected siblings also had a medulloblastoma of the cerebellum; another also had gastric polyps. Parks et al.[35] reported the occurrence of polyposis coli and multiple extraintestinal abnormalities in 15 of 46 family members in 3 generations; one of whom died of a brain tumor. These and other sporadic cases have led some authors to postulate that any form of familial adenomatous intestinal polyposis may be associated with mesodermal, endodermal, or ectodermal abnormalities in varying combinations.

Hamartomatous Polyposis Syndromes

The hamartomatous polyposis syndromes comprise a group of disorders characterized by non-neoplastic, tumor-like proliferations of haphazard mixtures of tissues native to the segment of gut involved. Most of them may be recognized by distinctive extraintestinal manifestations. The mode of inheritance has been established for the Peutz-Jeghers syndrome, some forms of juvenile polyposis, and neurofibromatosis, but is not conclusively settled for the multiple hamartoma syndrome. No evidence for transmissibility has been found in the Cronkhite-Canada syndrome.

Peutz-Jeghers Syndrome (PJS)

The hallmarks of PJS are mucocutaneous pigmentation (melanin spots) and gastrointestinal polyposis.[36, 37] The polyps occur in the stomach and throughout the small and large intestine, but are most common and numerous in the jejunum and ileum. Associated carcinomas of the gastrointestinal tract in PJS are estimated to occur in only about 2% of cases. Typical hamartomatous polyps were present in the large intestine in 19 of 31 patients and carcinoma in 1 patient in 2 series.[36,37] The most frequent complications of PJS are intussusception and bleeding due to ulceration or infarction of the polyps. Treatment of this syndrome is conservative and directed only at the complications.

Juvenile Polyposis Syndromes

Familial and non-familial forms of juvenile polyposis have been described in both children and adults.[38–43] These polyps most commonly occur in the rectum, but may be present throughout the entire colon and occasionally in the stomach and small intestine as well. Clinical and genetic studies along with examinations of pathologic material of patients from many countries have raised the possibility that at least 4 syndromes of juvenile polyposis may exist: (1) juvenile polyposis coli (JPC), (2) familial juvenile polyposis coli (FJPC), (3) familial generalized juvenile polyposis (FGJP), and (4) the Cronkhite-Canada syndrome (CCS). Relationships between 2 or more of these entities, as well as with the adenomatous polyposis syndromes, have been suggested.[39, 40]

Juvenile Polyposis Coli (JPC). JPC was established as an entity clinically and pathologically distinct from other forms of polyposis of the large intestine by a group of investigators from St. Mark's Hospital in London.[38, 39] They indicated that JPC should be classified among the hamartomatous syndromes. Following their initial reports, Bussey[1] cited 37 cases, most of which were solitary and not familial.

The average age of onset of JPC is 6 years.[1] The primary clinical symptom is bleeding, associated often with anemia, hypoproteinemia, malnutrition, and retarded development. Non-familial cases appear to be associated with a high frequency of congenital malformations,[39] such as malrotation of the gut, umbilical fistula, hydrocephalus, and hypertelorism. Co-existent adenomatous and villoglandular polyps in solitary cases have been described.[39,40]

Familial Juvenile Polyposis Coli (FJPC). This entity was clearly documented in 7 cases in 4 families by Veale et al. in 1966.[39] In 2 families there were 2 or more patients with juvenile polyps; in the other 2 pedigrees some relatives had adenomatous polyps.[1,39] A total of 14 cases of cancer of the colon and rectum were found in the relatives of these families. Smilov et al.[41] subsequently identified juvenile polyposis in the large intestine of a boy, his mother, and his maternal grandfather; at age 60 the grandfather also had adenomatous polyps and a carcinoma of the colon. Extensive surveys for polyps in the upper gastrointestinal tract and small bowel were not performed in these cases. Haggitt and Pitcock[42] added 2 cases in 2 generations of a sixth family. Some of the polyps were described as having both juvenile and adenomatous features. A typical adenomatous polyp was found in the jejunum in one of these patients and carcinomas of the large bowel had occurred in 2 close relatives. Recently, Grotsky et al.[43] reported 19 patients with definite polyposis in one family of 92 individuals in 5 generations; 7 patients had symptoms of polyposis and 2 had carcinomas of the large bowel. The polyps in most of the patients examined had typical juvenile characteristics, but a few had features of both juvenile and adenomatous types.

From these observations it is apparent that FJPC, like familial adult polyposis coli, is inherited as an autosomal dominant trait but appears to differ in the age of onset, clinical manifestations, and pathologic features. In FJPC, symptoms tend to occur approximately 15 years earlier. Rectal bleeding, rectal prolapse, and failure to thrive are much more common. The histologic appearance of juvenile polyps is usually quite distinct, although some may exhibit mixed features or may coexist with other polyps.[43, 44] Goodman et al.[44] propose a possible sequence of events in the pathogenesis of juvenile polyps, beginning with focal mucosal hyperplasia and progressing in some instances to adenomas, which in turn may undergo malignant transformation. Others suggest that the possible increased cancer risk in FJPC may be independent of the polyps.[43] There is no question that chronic bleeding, rectal prolapse, intussusception, failure to thrive, and obvious malignancy require appropriate and prompt therapy. Prophylactic colectomy, however, cannot be advocated until a more precise relationship between these polyps and cancer can be documented and quantified.

Familial Generalized Juvenile Polyposis (FGJP). This form of hereditary polyposis was identified in 3 generations of one family by Sachatello et al. in 1970.[45] Typical juvenile polyps were found in both the stomach and colon in 2 patients, in the small bowel and colon in a third, and in the colon alone in a fourth. The authors concluded that FGJP was quite distinct from other forms of hereditary polyposis, including FJPC. Subsequently, Stemper et al.[46] reported juvenile polyposis in 4 generations of a large kindred. In 11 subjects the polyps were confined to the large intestine; in 4 patients the stomach or jejunum was involved either alone or in combination with the large bowel. Eleven members of the kindred had carcinomas of the stomach, duodenum, pancreas, or colon. The occurrence of both generalized and isolated colonic polyposis in the same kindred raised the possibility that FJPC and FGJP were expressions of a single disorder, rather than distinct syndromes. More recently, Cox et al.[47] described a mother and daughter with FGJP, arteriovenous malformations of the lung, and digital clubbing. On the basis of these features, they proposed another new hereditary syndrome. A second family with generalized juvenile polyposis, arteriovenous malformations, and colon carcinoma has been reported by Conte et al.[48]

These and other cases of extensive juvenile polyposis indicate that all forms have an autosomal dominant pattern of inheritance and are associated with an appreciable frequency of gastrointestinal malignancies. The existence of one or more discrete juvenile polyposis syndromes and the possible relationships to other hereditary forms of polyposis have not been settled.

Cronkhite-Canada Syndrome (CCS)

The cardinal features of the Cronkhite-Canada syndrome (CCS) are: (1) the presence of hamartomatous polyps of the juvenile (retention) type throughout the stomach and intestines; (2) ectodermal changes consisting of alopecia, onychodystrophy, and hyperpigmentation; (3) the absence of a family history of polyposis; (4) adult onset; and (5) the eventual development of profuse diarrhea and weight loss. In 1955, a report of 2 patients by Cronkhite and Canada[49] established this entity as clinically distinct from any of the other known forms of gastrointestinal polyposis. Since that time, at least 53 similar cases have been described in the world literature.[50] Most of the patients reported have been whites from Western Europe and North America and Orientals from Japan.[50–52]

Sex and Age. The existing 55 well-documented cases comprise 31 men and 24 women. The average age of onset of symptomatic disease in this group was 59 years, with a range of 31 to 86 years. At the time of presentation, 80% of the patients were over 50 years of age.

Etiology. The cause of CCS is unknown. Malabsorption, malnutrition, deficiencies of one or more vitamins, infection, and impaired immune mechanisms have been suggested as etiologic factors. None of these are supported by any consistent laboratory evidence. However, a report by Russell et al.[52a] of complete remission of the syndrome in a 72-year-old man after 10 weeks of enteral feeding would lend some support to nutritional deficiency as a cause. Inheritance has also been eliminated as a cause of CCS, insofar as this disorder has not occurred in any blood relative of the 55 patients.

Clinical Features. Diarrhea is the most common symptom of CCS and has been observed in more than 80% of all cases.[50] The stools may be of large volume and may contain fat or gross blood. Significant weight loss, ranging from 12 to 81 pounds (5.5 to 36.8 kg), has been documented in 78% of patients. Other frequently reported symptoms are abdominal pain, anorexia, weakness, vomiting, and diminished acuity of taste. Changes in the fingernails and toenails, hair loss, and pigmentary disturbances are almost always present (Fig. 138–17). The nails

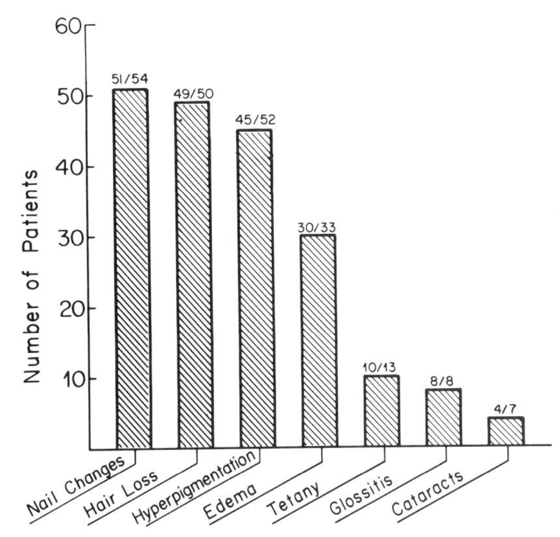

Figure 138–17. Physical findings in patients with Cronkhite-Canada syndrome. (From Daniel ES et al. Medicine 1982; 61:293–309. Reproduced with permission.)

exhibit varying degrees of dystrophy and partial separation of the nail beds and occasionally are shed completely (Fig. 138–18). Hair loss occurs rapidly and involves not only the scalp, but frequently also the face, axillae, extremities, and pubic area. Brownish macules, particularly on the extremities and face, are the most commonly observed pigmentary changes. These changes appear to be due to an increase of melanin in the skin. Generalized hyperpigmentation or patchy vitiligo has also been noted in a few patients. Regrowth of nails and hair and reversal of the hyperpigmentation may take place during spontaneous symptomatic remissions or after treatment, or in spite of continued active

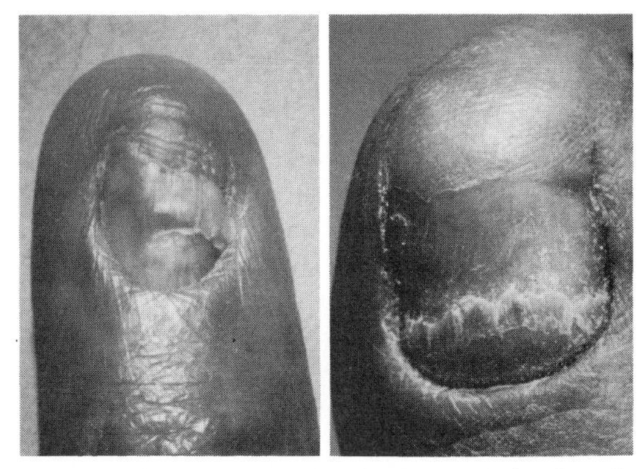

Figure 138–18. Nail changes in Cronkhite-Canada syndrome.

disease (Fig. 138–19). Fluid retention, ranging from mild peripheral edema to massive anasarca, is present in the majority of patients and correlates well with the presence of hypoalbuminemia. Chvostek's and Trousseau's signs are elicited in some patients who have hypocalcemia and hypomagnesemia. Papillary atrophy of the tongue has also been observed.

Laboratory Studies. The majority of those patients studied had anemia, protein-losing enteropathy, malabsorption, and specific serum electrolyte disturbances.[50] Mild to moderate anemia was found in 70% of patients and appeared to be secondary to enteric blood loss, malabsorption, or both. Protein loss from the gastrointestinal tract, verified in many patients by studies with one or more radiolabeled macromolecules, was also reflected by hypoproteinemia (94%) and hypoalbuminemia (87%). Impaired absorption of fat, D-xylose, vitamin B_{12}, vitamin A,

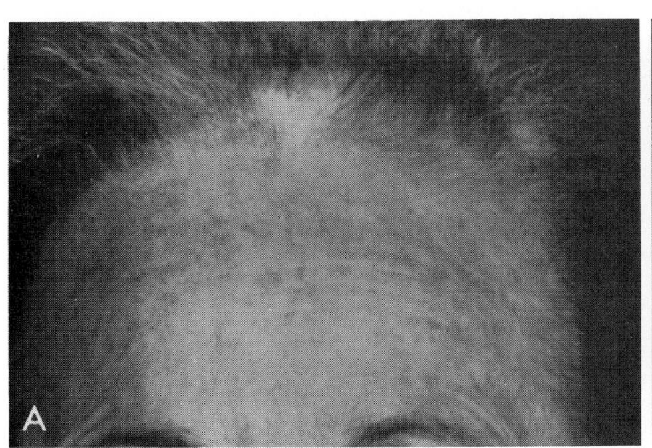

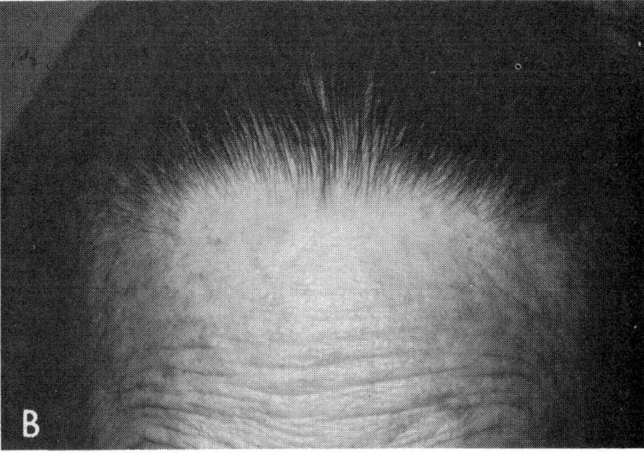

Figure 138–19. Hair loss *(A)* and regrowth *(B)* after treatment with nutritional supplements in a patient with Cronkhite-Canada syndrome. (From Daniel ES et al. Medicine 1982; 61:293–309. Reproduced with permission.)

and carotene was detected in more than two-thirds of the patients studied. The most common serum electrolyte abnormalities were hypocalcemia (93%), hypomagnesemia (54%), and hypokalemia (49%). Gastric achlorhydria or hypochlorhydria was frequently observed. A variety of tests for the evaluation of endocrine, liver, pancreatic, and renal function failed to reveal any consistent abnormalities.

Distribution of Polyps. The frequency of involvement of various segments of the gastrointestinal tract as determined from analysis of available roentgenologic, endoscopic, and necropsy data is shown in Figure 138–20. The stomach and colon were involved in all but 2 of the 55 cases cited in the literature (Fig. 138–21). Polyps in other segments of the gut were less frequently mentioned, but because appropriate examinations were not performed in every case, the frequency of small bowel and rectal involvement may have been underestimated.

Pathology. The polyps, which may be sessile or pedunculated, may appear transparent or range from red to blue on gross inspection. Superficial erosions of polyps and gross thickening of the involved mucosa are commonly observed. Histologically, the lesions have a uniform appearance, no matter where in the gastrointestinal tract they originate. The typical mucosal changes consist of proliferated, tortuous glands, often cystically dilated and filled with proteinaceous fluid and

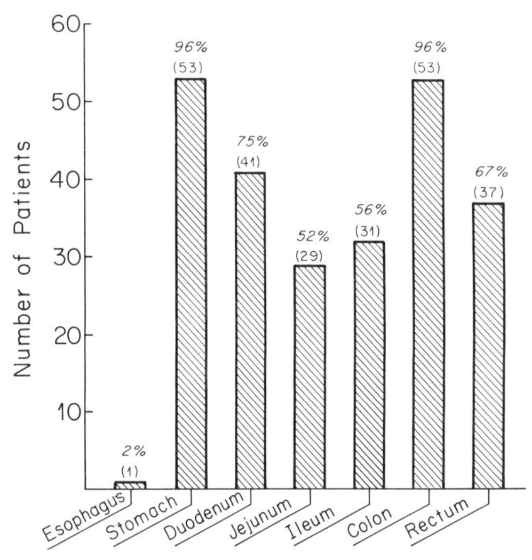

Figure 138–20. Distribution of polyps in Cronkhite-Canada syndrome. (From Daniel ES et al. Medicine 1982; 61:293–309. Reproduced with permission.)

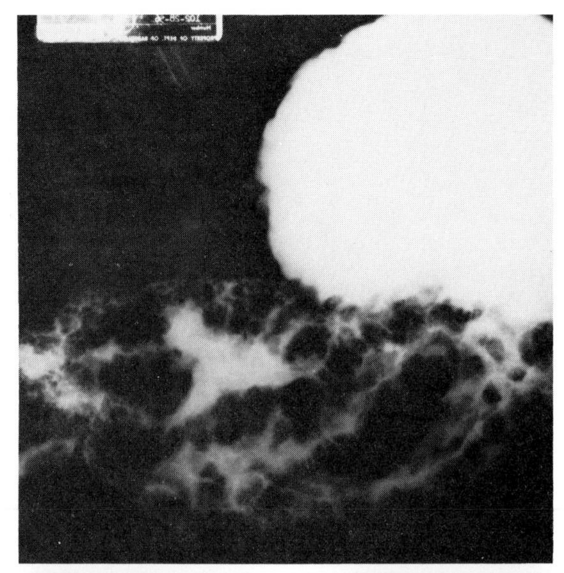

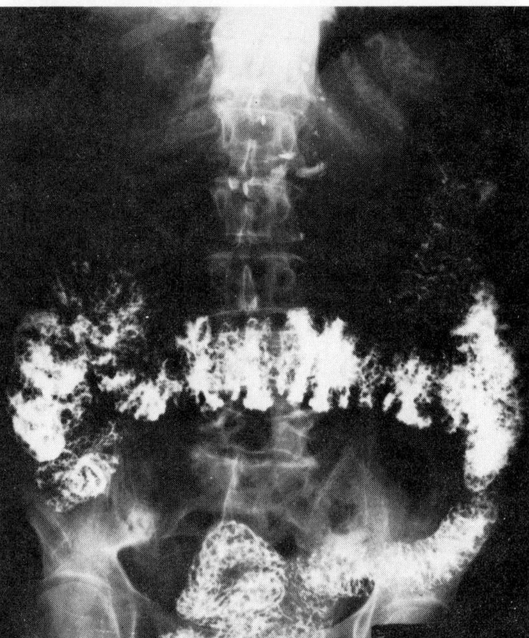

Figure 138–21. Gastric polyposis *(above)* and colonic polyposis (below) in Cronkhite-Canada syndrome. (From Daniel ES et al. Medicine 1982; 61:293–309. Reproduced with permission.)

inspissated mucus. Also seen are engorged vascular channels, eosinophilic infiltration, and surface erosions associated with an edematous, chronically inflamed lamina propria (Fig. 138–22). The mucosa between the polyps is also abnormal, revealing edema, congestion, inflammation of the lamina propria, and focal glandular ectasia. Earlier publications regarded these tumors as adenomatous,[49, 53, 54] but they are now recognized as

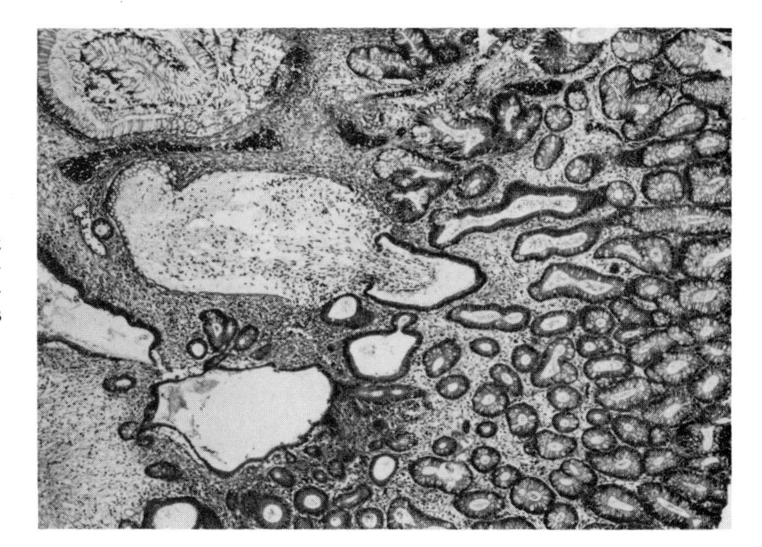

Figure 138–22. Typical colonic polyp from a patient with Cronkhite-Canada syndrome showing glandular proliferation with cystic changes and inflammation.

hamartomatous polyps of the juvenile (retention) type.[50, 51, 55] While these polyps may be indistinguishable from those found in other forms of juvenile polyposis, the abnormal intervening mucosa clearly identifies CCS histologically as a separate entity. The gastric mucosa in CCS resembles that seen in Menetrier's disease, suggesting a pathogenic relationship between these 2 entities.[54, 56]

Complications. The major complications of CCS, such as bleeding, prolapse, intussusception, and thromboembolic phenomena, are related to the size, location, and morphologic features of the polyps and to the sequelae of massive fluid, protein, and electrolyte losses. Gross gastrointestinal bleeding appears to originate from ulcerations within the diseased mucosa, particularly from erosions on the surface of the polyps. Bleeding also has been noted from discrete duodenal or jejunal ulcers in several patients. Blood loss or severe anemia was significant enough to require transfusions in 20% of the reported cases. The polyp-bearing mucosa may prolapse from the stomach into the duodenum (Fig. 138–23) or from the rectum through the anus. Jejunojejunal intussusception (Fig. 138–24) and ileocecal intussusception have been observed. Thromboembolic episodes, such as peripheral thrombophlebitis, pulmonary embolism, and cerebrovascular accidents, have occurred in approximately 15% of patients and are attributed to dehydration, heart failure, or coagulation abnormalities.

The polyps in CCS have been considered regenerative and non-neoplastic[56] and no associated malignancies were seen in the early cases. Since 1967, however, single or multiple carcinomas, often in or near the polyps, have been described in 8 patients.[50] Although the development of carcinomas in some patients with CCS may be coincidental, the possibility that a massively proliferating mucosa may have a tendency toward malignant transformation must be considered.

Treatment. Many forms of therapy, often in combination or rapid succession, have been utilized in patients with CCS. The massive fluid, electrolyte, and protein losses, as well as the high incidence of concurrent malabsorption, usually require intensive supplementation with parenteral fluids and electrolytes, albumin, amino acids, and vitamins. By means of nutritional replacement, to-

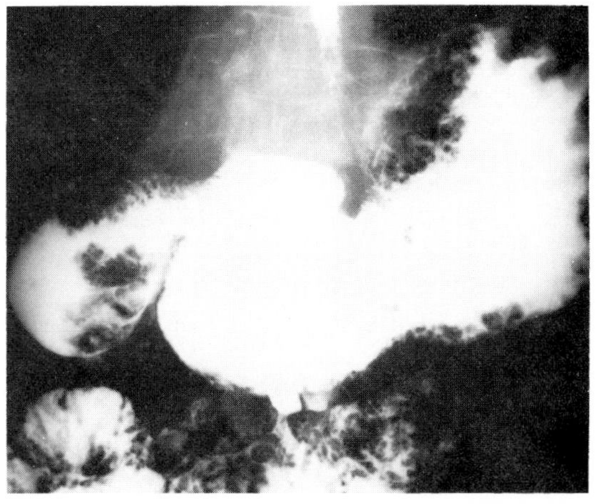

Figure 138–23. Prolapse of gastric polyps into the duodenum in a patient with Cronkhite-Canada syndrome.

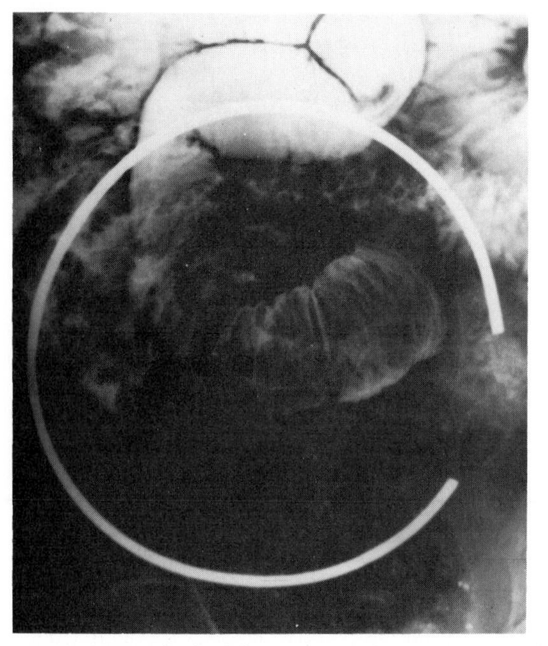

Figure 138–24. Painless jejunojejunal intussusception observed during small bowel roentgen examination in a patient with Cronkhite-Canada syndrome.

gether with symptomatic therapy for pain and diarrhea, several patients have experienced symptomatic remissions and disappearance of all ectodermal changes.[52a] Similar remissions also have been attributed in a few patients to corticosteroids, anabolic steroids, antibiotics, and surgical resections of massively involved segments of gut.[50] However, most of the patients in remission also received replacement therapy. Of 6 patients who lived 5 or more years after treatment, 1 received only nutritional and supportive therapy, 1 only tetracycline, 3 had subtotal gastrectomy, and 1 had a hemicolectomy and subtotal gastrectomy.

From these varied observations the following conclusions can be drawn: (1) All symptomatic patients should receive vigorous fluid and electrolyte replacement as well as nutritional supplementation. (2) The use of antibiotics seems reasonable when bacterial overgrowth is proved or strongly suspected and may also be tried empirically in severely ill patients who have failed to respond to supportive therapy. (3) Surgery carries a significant risk in these severely ill patients and should be reserved for those with complications such as massive bleeding, prolapse, intussusception, bowel obstruction, and obvious malignancy. In addition, surgical resection may have a place in selected patients with massive involvement of a short segment of gut.

Course and Prognosis. The causes of death, when stated, have been anemia, severe cachexia, congestive heart failure, bronchopneumonia, embolism, septicemia, shock, and complications of surgery. Although 30 of the 55 patients with CCS presently cited in the literature had died at the time of the last report, the other 25 were alive and in various stages of remission. The symptoms and ectodermal changes have been shown to be partly or completely reversible. A reduction in the size and density of polyps has also been reported, and the total disappearance of all polyps has been documented in one case.[52a] Reports of long-term survival, up to 17.5 years after therapy, challenge the initial concept that CCS is relentlessly progressive and invariably fatal.

Neurofibromatosis

Neurofibromatosis, also known as von Recklinghausen's disease, is a neuroectodermal disorder marked by pigmentary changes (café-au-lait spots), cutaneous and visceral tumors (neurofibromas), and a variety of systemic abnormalities. The disease is inherited as an autosomal dominant trait with a frequency of approximately 1 in 3000 births. It is progressive, but displays markedly variable expressivity.[57, 58]

Café-au-lait spots are usually present at birth and increase in size and number during the first decade. They occur in virtually all patients with neurofibromatosis. The presence of 6 or more café-au-lait spots larger than 1.5 cm in diameter has been suggested as a criterion for the diagnosis. Neurofibromas are nearly always present on the skin. They may also occur in deeper peripheral nerves and nerve roots and in or on viscera and blood vessels innervated by the autonomic nervous system. Associated abnormalities are pigmented hamartomas of the iris (Lisch nodules), congenital pseudarthrosis, kyphoscoliosis, benign and malignant tumors, and macrocephaly.

Gastrointestinal involvement has been estimated to occur in 25% of patients with neurofibromatosis.[57] The most common symptoms referable to lesions in the gut are hematemesis, melena, and abdominal pain. A palpable mass is occasionally present. The neurofibromas are most frequently detected in the stomach and jejunum, but all or any portion of the intestine may be involved.[57–59]

These tumors, which may be plexiform, sessile, or pedunculated, are usually found in the serosa, subserosa, and muscle layers but may protrude into the lumen. Histologically, most of them are neurofibromas consisting of an overgrowth of nerve tissue with various combinations of fibroblasts, mast cells, and vascular elements. Leiomyomas, fibromyomas, sarcomas, fibromyxosarcomas, and ganglioneuromas are occasionally seen. Malignant changes within the neurofibromas have also been reported.[57, 60]

Complications of visceral involvement are bleeding due to ulcerations of the overlying mucosa, obstruction secondary to intussusception or tumor encroachment on the lumen, small bowel perforation, and mesenteric vascular insufficiency from compression of the celiac and superior mesenteric arteries.[60] Management is directed toward the alleviation of these complications and the identification and removal of any associated malignant tumors.

Multiple Hamartoma Syndrome (MHS)

A variety of ectodermal, mesodermal, and endodermal abnormalities characterize MHS, more commonly known as Cowden's disease, after the surname of the propositi described by Lloyd and Dennis in 1963.[61] Since that time, more than 40 additional cases have appeared in the literature. These have confirmed the existence of a large number of systemic changes, particularly involving the skin, mouth, breasts, thyroid, and skeleton. The typical cutaneous lesions are multiple hyperkeratotic, verrucous papules of the face, the corners of the mouth, and the extremities.[61–63] In afflicted women massive postpubertal enlargement of the breasts with fibrocystic disease and a high rate of early malignant degeneration is notable. Oral lesions consist of gingival enlargement (fibromatosis) and a generalized hyperkeratotic papillomatosis of lips and oral and pharyngeal mucosa. Goiter, thyroid adenomas, carcinoma, or thyroiditis occurs in more than two-thirds of the patients. An extensive review of all of the systemic manifestations constituting this syndrome was presented by Nuss et al. in 1978.[63] An autosomal dominant inheritance pattern with variable expressivity has been proposed.

Gastrointestinal involvement received little attention in the initial reports, although the presence of polyps in the esophagus, stomach, duodenum, and colon was noted in a few patients studied.[63] Gentry et al.[62] performed proctosigmoidoscopy in 2 patients of a kindred and found multiple rectal and sigmoid polyps in both. Weinstock and Kawanishi[64] examined the entire gastrointestinal tract in 1 patient and found multiple sessile polyps in the esophagus, stomach, entire small bowel, sigmoid colon, and rectum. Histologically, the gastric polyps consisted of hyperplastic surface epithelium, cystically dilated glands, a thickened lamina propria infiltrated with inflammatory cells, and prominent smooth muscle bundles extending to the surface. More recently, extensive radiologic and endoscopic studies were performed in 3 patients by Hauser et al.[65] All 3 had polyps in the stomach, duodenum, and large intestine; 2 of them also had esophageal involvement, and 1 had polyps throughout the entire small intestine. The density varied from a few discrete polyps of various sizes to extensive carpet-like mamillations. In addition to the typical histologic features described, some polyps have had juvenile, lipomatous, and hyperplastic features.

While involvement of the gastrointestinal tract may be an integral component of this syndrome, the absence of thorough examinations of the gut in most of the reported cases precludes an accurate assessment of the frequency of this association.

References

1. Bussey HJR. Familial Polyposis Coli. Baltimore: Johns Hopkins University Press, 1975.
2. Welch CE, Hedberg SE. Polypoid Lesions of the Gastrointestinal Tract. 2nd Ed. Philadelphia: WB Saunders, 1975.
3. Tonnesen H. Polyposis Gastro-intestinales. Copenhagen: NYT Nordisk Forlag, 1931.
4. Shiffman MA. Familial multiple polyposis associated with soft-tissue and hard-tissue tumors. JAMA 1962; 179:514–22.
5. Pierce ER. Some genetic aspects of familial multiple polyposis of the colon in a kindred of 1,422 members. Dis Colon Rectum 1968; 11:321–9.
6. Bussey HJR, Veale AMO, Morson BC. Genetics of gastrointestinal polyposis. Gastroenterology 1978; 74:1325–30.
7. Bussey HJR. Familial polyposis coli. Pathol Annu 1979; 14:61–81.
8. Utsonomiya J, Nakamura T. The occult osteomatous changes in the mandible in patients with familial polyposis coli. Br J Surg 1975; 62:45–51.
9. Ushio K, Sasagawa M, Doi H, Yamada T, Ishikawa H, Hojo K, Koyama Y, Sano R. Lesions associated with familial polyposis coli. Studies of lesions of the stomach, duodenum, bones and teeth. Gastrointest Radiol 1976; 1:67–80.
10. Yao T, Mitsuo I, Ohsato K, Watanabe H, Omae T. Duodenal lesions in familial polyposis of the colon. Gastroenterology 1977; 73:1086–92.

10a. Sivak MV Jr, Jagelman DC. Upper gastrointestinal endoscopy in polyposis syndromes: Familial polyposis coli and Gardner's syndrome. Gastrointest Endosc 1984; 30:102–4.

11. Dorazio RA, Whelan TJ Jr. Lymphoid hyperplasia of the

terminal ileum associated with familial polyposis coli. Ann Surg 1970; 171:300–2.
12. Schwabe AD, Lewin KJ. Gastrointestinal polyposis syndromes. Viewpoints Dig Dis 1980; 12:1–4.
13. Muto T, Bussey HJR, Morson BC. The evolution of cancer of the colon and rectum. Cancer 1975; 36:2251–70.
14. Schuchardt WA Jr, Ponsky JL. Familial polyposis and Gardner's syndrome. Surg Gynecol Obstet 1979; 148:97–103.
15. Moertel CG, Hill JR, Adson MA. Surgical management of multiple polyposis. Arch Surg 1970; 100:521–6.
16. Harvey JC, Quan SH, Stearns MW. Management of familial polyposis with preservation of the rectum. Surgery 1978; 84:478–82.
17. Fonkalsrud EW. Endorectal ileal pullthrough with ileal reservoir for ulcerative colitis and polyposis. Am J Surg 1982; 144:81–7.
18. Devic A, Bussey MM. Un cas de polypose adénomateuse généralisée à tout l'intestin. Arch Mal Appar Dig 1912; 6:278–99.
19. Gardner EJ. A genetic and clinical study of intestinal polyposis—a predisposing factor for carcinoma of the colon and rectum. Am J Hum Genet 1951; 3:167–76.
20. Gardner EJ, Richards RC. Multiple cutaneous and subcutaneous lesions occurring simultaneously with hereditary polyposis and osteomatosis. Am J Hum Genet 1953; 139–47.
21. Naylor EW, Gardner EJ, Richards RC. Desmoid tumors and mesenteric fibromatosis in Gardner's syndrome. Arch Surg 1979; 114:1181–5.
22. Naylor EW, Gardner EJ. Penetrance and expressivity of the gene responsible for the Gardner syndrome. Clin Genet 1977; 11:381–93.
23. Naylor EW, Lebenthal E. Gardner's syndrome. Recent developments in research and management. Dig Dis Sci 1980; 25:945–59.
24. Gardner EJ, Burt RW, Freston JW. Gastrointestinal polyposis: Syndromes and genetic mechanisms. West J Med 1980; 132:488–99.
25. McKusick VA. Genetic factors in intestinal polyposis. JAMA 1962; 182:271–7.
26. Thomford NR, Greenberger NJ. Lymphoid polyps of the ileum associated with Gardner's syndrome. Arch Surg 1968; 96:289–91.
27. Ziter FM Jr. Roentgenographic findings in Gardner's syndrome. JAMA 1965; 192:1000–2.
28. Camiel MR, Mule JE, Alexander LL, Benninghoff DL. Association of thyroid carcinoma with Gardner's syndrome in siblings. N Engl J Med 1968; 278:1056–8.
29. Jones TR, Nance FC. Periampullary malignancy in Gardner's syndrome. Ann Surg 1977; 185:565–71.
30. Turcot J, Després JP, St. Pierre F. Malignant tumors of the central nervous system associated with familial polyposis of the colon. Dis Colon Rectum 1959; 2:465–8.
31. Baughman FA Jr, List CF, Williams JR, Muldoon JP, Segarra JM, Volkel JS. The glioma-polyposis syndrome. N Engl J Med 1969; 281:1345–6.
32. Todd DW, Christoferson LA, Leech RW, Rudolf L. A family affected with intestinal polyposis and gliomas. Ann Neurol 1981; 10:390–2.
33. Smith WG, Kern BB: The nature of the mutation in familial multiple polyposis. Papillary carcinomas of the thyroid, brain tumors, and familial multiple polyposis. Dis Colon Rectum 1973; 16:264–71.
34. Binder MC, Zablen MA, Fleischer DE, et al. Colon polyps, sebaceous cysts, gastric polyps, and malignant brain tumor in a family. Dig Dis 1978; 23:460–6.
35. Parks TG, Bussey HJR, Lockhart-Mummery HE. Familial polyposis coli associated with extracolonic abnormalities. Gut 1970; 11:323–9.
36. Jeghers H, McKusick VA, Katz KH. Generalized intestinal polyposis and melanin spots of the oral mucosa, lips and digits. N Engl J Med 1949; 241:993–1005, 1031–6.
37. Dormandy TL. Gastrointestinal polyposis with mucocutaneous pigmentation (Peutz-Jeghers syndrome). N Engl J Med 1957; 256:1093–1102, 1141–6, 1186–90.
38. McColl I, Bussey HJR, Veale AMO, Morson BC. Juvenile polyposis coli. Proc Roy Soc Med 1964; 57:896–7.
39. Veale AMO, McColl I, Bussey HJR, Morson BC. Juvenile polyposis coli. J Med Genet 1966; 3:5–16.
40. Lipper S, Kahn LB, Sandler RS, Varma V. Multiple juvenile polyposis. A study of the pathogenesis of juvenile polyps and their relationship to colonic adenomas. Hum Pathol 1981; 12:804–13.
41. Smilov PC, Pryor CA Jr, Swinton NW. Juvenile polyposis coli. Dis Colon Rectum 1966; 9:248–54.
42. Haggitt RC, Pitcock JA. Familial juvenile polyposis of the colon. Cancer 1970; 26:1232–8.
43. Grotsky HW, Rickert RR, Smith WD, Newsome JF. Familial juvenile polyposis coli. A clinical and pathologic study of a large kindred. Gastroenterology 1982; 82:494–501.
44. Goodman ZD, Yardley JH, Milligan FD. Pathogenesis of colonic polyps in multiple juvenile polyposis. Cancer 1979; 43:1906–13.
45. Sachatello CR, Pickren JW, Grace JT Jr. Generalized juvenile gastrointestinal polyposis. A hereditary syndrome. Gastroenterology 1970; 58:699–708.
46. Stemper TJ, Kent TH, Summers RW. Juvenile polyposis and gastrointestinal carcinoma. A study of a kindred. Ann Intern Med 1975; 83:639–46.
47. Cox KL, Frates RC Jr, Wong A, Gandhi G. Hereditary generalized juvenile polyposis associated with pulmonary arteriovenous malformation. Gastroenterology 1980; 78:1566–70.
48. Conte WJ, Rotter JI, Schwartz AC, Congleton JE. Hereditary generalized juvenile polyposis, arteriovenous malformations and colonic carcinoma. Clin Res 1982; 30:93A (Abstract).
49. Cronkhite LW Jr, Canada WJ. Generalized gastrointestinal polyposis: An unusual syndrome of polyposis, pigmentation, alopecia and onychotrophia. N Engl J Med 1955; 252:1011–5.
50. Daniel ES, Ludwig SL, Lewin KJ, Ruprecht RM, Rajacich GM, Schwabe AD. The Cronkhite-Canada syndrome. An analysis of clinical and pathologic features and therapy in 55 patients. Medicine 1982; 61:293–309.
51. Tokuyasu K, Takebayashi S, Takahara O, Uchiyama E. An autopsy case of Cronkhite-Canada syndrome. Gastroent Japon 1976; 11:215–23.
52. Suzuki K, Uraoka M, Funatsu T, Sakaue H, Onji M, Ohta Y, Ishikawa N. Cronkhite-Canada syndrome. A case report and analytical review of 23 other cases reported in Japan. Gastroent Japon 1979; 14:441–9.
52a. Russell DMcR, Bhathal PS, St. John DJB. Complete remission in Cronkhite-Canada syndrome. Gastroenterology 1983; 85:180–5.
53. Johnston MM, Vosburgh JW, Wiens AT, Walsh GC. Gastrointestinal polyposis associated with alopecia, pigmentation and atrophy of the fingernails and toenails. Ann Intern Med 1962; 56:935–41.
54. Gill W, Wilken BJ. Diffuse gastrointestinal polyposis associated with hypoproteinemia. J Roy Coll Surg Edinb 1967; 12:149–56.
55. Diner WC. The Cronkhite-Canada syndrome. Radiology 1971; 105:715–6.
56. Kindbloom LG, Angervall L, Santesson B, Selander S. Cronkhite-Canada syndrome. Cancer 1977; 39:2651–7.
57. Hochberg FH, Dasilva AB, Galdabini J, Richardson EP Jr. Gastrointestinal involvement in von Recklinghausen's neurofibromatosis. Neurology 1974; 24:1144–51.
58. Riccardi VM. Von Recklinghausen neurofibromatosis. N Engl J Med 1981; 305:1617–27.
59. Ghrist TD. Gastrointestinal involvement in neurofibromatosis. Arch Intern Med 1963; 112:111–6.
60. Cameron AJ, Pairolero PC, Stanson AW, Carpenter HA. Abdominal angina and neurofibromatosis. Mayo Clin Proc 1982; 57:125–8.
61. Lloyd KM, Dennis M. Cowden's disease: A possible new symptom complex with multiple system involvement. Ann Intern Med. 1963; 58:136–42.
62. Gentry WC Jr, Eskritt NR, Gorlin RJ. Multiple hamartoma syndrome (Cowden's disease). Arch Dermatol 1974; 109:521–5.
63. Nuss DD, Aeling JL, Clemons DE, Weber WN. Multiple hamartoma syndrome (Cowden's disease). Arch Dermatol 1978; 114:743–6.
64. Weinstock JV, Kawanishi H. Gastrointestinal polyposis with orocutaneous hamartomas (Cowden's disease). Gastroenterology 1978; 74:890–5.
65. Hauser H, Ody B, Plojoux O, Wettstein P. Radiological findings in multiple hamartoma syndrome (Cowden's disease). A report of 3 cases. Radiology 1980; 137:317–23.

Chapter 139

Malignant Tumors of the Colon and Rectum

Sidney J. Winawer • Warren E. Enker • Charles J. Lightdale

Malignant tumors of the colon and rectum may be classified as primary or metastatic. Primary malignant tumors are those arising within the colon and rectum. Metastatic tumors are those that (1) have spread to the colon and rectum either from distant sites or from adjacent sites by direct invasion; or (2) involve the colon and rectum as part of a disseminated process. The most common malignant tumors of the colon and rectum are primary malignancies and, within this group, adenocarcinoma is the most frequent. Epidermoid carcinomas and other primary carcinomas of the rectum arising at the squamocolumnar junction are much less frequent.

Other types of tumors that rarely originate in the large bowel include leiomyosarcomas, lymphomas, and malignant carcinoid tumors. In addition, lymphoma, leiomyosarcoma, malignant melanoma, and cancer of the breast, ovary, prostate, and lung, as well as other gastrointestinal tumors can metastasize to the large bowel. This chapter will focus on primary colorectal cancer, especially adenocarcinoma, and will touch upon the other types of primary and metastatic malignancies of the colon and rectum to a lesser extent.

Adenocarcinoma of the Colon and Rectum

Adenocarcinoma of the colon is a major health problem in the Western World. With the exception of skin cancer, carcinomas of the colon, lung, and breast are the 3 leading cancers in the United States in terms of annual new cases. The current annual incidence of more than 120,000 new cases, along with the high mortality rate of close to 60%, has stimulated interest in approaches utilizing new concepts and techniques.[1] It has become apparent that in addition to average-risk patients (identified as women and men aged 40 or older), there are subgroups in the population at increased risk for colorectal cancer.[2] These include patients who have previously had colon cancer; patients with colorectal adenomas, ulcerative colitis, or female genital cancer; and persons with a family history of polyposis, Gardner's syndrome, or the non-polyposis inherited colon cancer syndromes. Although considerable work needs to be accomplished in the identification of these high-risk groups, especially those with genetic factors, a clearer picture exists today of the spectrum of risk for colorectal cancer. There also have been technical advances in the past decade for identifying persons at risk, including new methods for fecal occult blood testing, evolution of fiberoptic flexible sigmoidoscopes and colonoscopes, and a better understanding of the application of radiologic contrast techniques.

Epidemiology

Adenocarcinoma of the colon is more prevalent in developed countries.[3] The prevalence of this carcinoma is high in North America and Europe and low in South America, Africa, and Asia. The United States has one of the highest rates for colorectal cancer in the world. Migrants to a particular geographic area have been shown to assume the colorectal cancer risk for that area and to lose the risk for some of the cancers of their country of origin. This is illustrated by the observation of a higher prevalence of colorectal cancer among blacks who have migrated to the United States as compared with those who have remained in Africa.[4] It has also been observed that Puerto Ricans who have migrated to the United States mainland acquire the risk of persons indigenous to the mainland and that first- and second-generation Japanese migrating to Hawaii and the mainland of the United States assume the risk of their new place of residence. In the United States, the frequency of colorectal cancer is higher in the North than in the South, higher in urban areas as compared with rural areas, and higher in whites than in blacks. There is a slightly higher risk among persons in certain occupations, such as automobile factory workers and woodworkers.

The geographic distribution of rectal cancer is fairly similar to that of cancer of the colon. However, rectal cancer and colon cancer may not be exactly the same epidemiologically and etiologically.[4] There is male predominance in rectal cancer, whereas the male-female ratio is approximately equal in colon cancer. In addition, there are some variations in the ratio of rectal to colon cancers from country to country.[4, 5] Moreover, the difference between rectal cancer and colon cancer is complicated by a change in the anatomic distribution of bowel cancers that has occurred in recent generations, with a proximal migration of colorectal cancer. Approximately 55% of colon cancers currently occur in the distal 25 cm of bowel, whereas 30 years ago it was approximately 75%. The incidence of colorectal cancer has been fairly stable in some countries, such as England and Wales, but has been increasing slowly in other countries, such as the United States and Denmark. The rise in incidence in the United States may reflect increases in subgroups of the population, such as residents of the southern states, blacks, and persons living in urban areas. In other countries, such as Japan, increases have been occurring substantially in the past decade, perhaps reflecting a westernization of the diet.[3]

There are variations in incidence rates for colorectal cancer within populations. In addition to variations based on race and residence, there are also variations related to different religious groups. For example, the risk among Jews is greater than in the population at large, but is decreased among Seventh Day Adventists.[5] These variations may reflect differing diet patterns.

Etiology

Migrant studies strongly suggest that environmental factors, especially diet, are important in the etiology of colon cancer.[5] In populations in which colorectal cancer is low in prevalence, there is also a low prevalence of other colonic diseases, including appendicitis, adenomas, diverticulosis, and ulcerative colitis. This has been noted in the South African Bantu and other African populations whose diets contain more fiber and less refined carbohydrates than the typical diets in populations in more developed areas such as the United States. With high-fiber diets, transit time in the intestine is reduced, so that any potential carcinogen remains in contact with the mucosa for a shorter period of time. Fiber also increases intraluminal bulk and thereby dilutes carcinogens that are normally ingested in foods and present in the intestinal tract.[4] In addition, there may be a direct association between the greater fat and animal protein intake in the Western diet and the rising incidence of colon cancer.[5] In Japan, for example, the intake of fat, mostly unsaturated, provides only 10% of dietary calories, whereas in the United States, fat represents about 40% of the total caloric intake. A diet high in fat and beef content favors the establishment of a bacterial flora with enzymatic activity such as beta-glucuronidase and azoreductase that results in increased transformation of neutral and acid sterols to carcinogenic and cocarcinogenic metabolites. Furthermore, mutagens present in feces, including nitrosamide, are increased in individuals on high-beef diets. Supplementation of the diet with ascorbic acid and alpha-tocopherol reduces mutagenicity and the levels of nitrosamide in the stool. Obviously, considerably more needs to be learned of the relationship of diet to colorectal cancer, regarding both the overall association and a specific chemical link between diet and reduction of neoplastic transformation.

Other factors have been examined regarding the etiology of colorectal cancer.[2] The role of alcoholic beverages, mainly beer, in the etiology of large bowel cancer has been an interesting issue, with detection of a possible correlation of beer drinking with colon and rectal cancer in several countries. The mechanism for a carcinogenic action of beer is speculative; beer may interact with the diet to influence either the fecal flora or the fecal steroid concentration.

Events of reproductive life may have an influence on a woman's subsequent risk of developing colon cancer. The changes accompanying pregnancy may protect against the development of colon cancer through a decrease of bile acid secretion.

Very low serum cholesterol levels may contribute to some increased risk and mortality from colorectal cancer, perhaps related to the effect of consequently increased bile acids on colon carcinogens. At the present time, the data are insufficient to draw any definite conclusions regarding a causal relationship between low cholesterol levels and cancer.

A high intake of cruciferous vegetables (i.e., plants of the mustard family) has been suggested to protect against large bowel cancer, the effect being attributed to certain indoles in the vegetables as well as their high fiber content. Controlled studies also have shown a negative association between the frequency of ingestion of vegetables and the occurrence of colorectal cancer, especially those vegetables with low concentrations of vitamin A. There is some suggestive evidence that retinol and carotene may exert a protective effect against cancer, including colorectal cancer. Several antioxidants, including ascorbic acid and selenium, are also said to protect against cancer, especially colorectal cancer.

Risk Factors

Age and Sex. In addition to the epidemiologic factors that operate on a worldwide basis to provide varying levels of risk for colorectal cancer in large populations, there are a number of risk factors that affect individuals within a given geographic area, placing them in a spectrum of greater or lesser susceptibility to the cancer (Table 139–1). One of these factors is age. The risk for colorectal

Table 139–1. COLORECTAL CANCER RISK FACTORS

Standard Risk	Age over 40, men and women
High Risk	Inflammatory bowel disease History of female genital or breast cancer History of colon cancer or adenoma Peutz-Jeghers syndrome Familial polyposis syndromes Family cancer syndromes Hereditary site-specific colon cancer History of juvenile polyps Immunodeficiency disease

cancer begins to increase slightly at age 40 and more sharply at age 50, doubling with each decade and reaching a maximum at age 75 to 80 years. There are some sex differences for colon cancer and rectal cancer that are also age-related but, in general, the risk for men and women remains much the same.[6]

Previous Colorectal Cancer. Patients who have had one colorectal cancer are at increased risk for subsequent colorectal cancer, even if they have been cured of the first cancer. A *metachronous* lesion is one that occurs at a time later than the original index lesion.[7, 8] This is distinct from recurrent carcinoma that occurs in patients who have not been cured of their original lesion and return with evidence of spread of their cancer to adjacent or distant sites. Patients with an index colorectal cancer are also at risk of harboring a *synchronous* lesion—an additional colorectal cancer occurring at the same time as their index tumor.[9] The frequency of metachronous cancers is between 5% and 10% in patients who have had an index colorectal cancer; the frequency of synchronous cancers ranges from 1.5% to 5%. A previous diagnosis of adenoma of the colon also increases the risk for subsequent colorectal cancer.[10]

Multiple Cancers. Neoplasms that occur with increased frequency in individuals with colorectal cancer include those of the breast (21%), of the gynecologic (16%) and genitourinary (11%) systems, and of other regions of the gastrointestinal tract (9%). These patients tend to develop colorectal cancer at an early age.[9,11]

Single and Multiple Sporadic Colorectal Adenomas. Colorectal adenomas, most especially those with villous features, can be associated with the development of adenocarcinoma[6, 7, 10, 12] (Chapter 138). Kindreds have been reported that show an association of single and multiple adenomas with adenocarcinomas, thus suggesting a genetic susceptibility. Observations of growth characteristics suggest that most, and possibly all, adenocarcinomas of the colon arise from preexisting adenomas.[7] The male-female distribution of adenomas and the frequency distribution of adenomas related to age correlate well with that for adenocarcinomas. In those countries where the risk of adenocarcinoma of the colon is high, the prevalence of adenomas of the colon is also high. In addition, there is increasing evidence that as adenomas grow in size, the likelihood of premalignant dysplasia and carcinoma being found in the adenoma increases. The likelihood of carcinoma being found in an adenoma is 1% for adenomas smaller than 1 cm, approximately 10% for adenomas between 1 and 2 cm, up to 50% in adenomas larger than 2 cm, and 55% in adenomas larger than 3 to 5 cm.[7] The influence of size is quite possibly a reflection of the histologic composition of the adenomas. Whereas most adenomas smaller than 1 cm are of the tubular type (Fig. 139–1), most adenomas (i.e., 75%) larger than 2 cm feature a villous component (Fig. 139–1), and it is the latter histologic feature that is most related to disposition for malignancy to develop within the adenoma.

The anatomic distribution of the adenomas bears a relationship to potential for malignancy. Adenomas in the distal descending colon and sigmoid have a greater frequency of malignancy than those elsewhere in the colon. This correlates well with the predominant distribution of colorectal cancer. As would be expected, the risk of carcinoma is greater in those patients with multiple adenomas of the colon because there are more such lesions potentially capable of undergoing malignant change. In one study,[13] the overall risk of invasive carcinoma was 8% when 1 adenoma was present, 10% when 2 adenomas were present, and 14% when 3 or more were present. The configuration of a polyp also may have some relationship to the presence of cancer. Sessile adenomas are more likely to harbor cancer (10%) than pedunculated polyps (4.5%) of the same size and histologic features. However, the absolute numbers of carcinomas are the highest in pedunculated polyps because these are the adenomas most commonly found and removed.[7] Until recently, diminutive polyps (0.5 cm or smaller) were considered to be hyperplastic. With the advent of colonoscopic polypectomy, it has come to be appreciated that a substantial proportion of these polyps are truly neoplastic adenomas.[14] However, the frequency of carcinoma in them is extremely small.

Adenomas also occur with increased frequency in the colons of patients with a discovered carcinoma (as high as 50% of cases[15]). This observation is quite important because these synchronous adenomas may harbor malignancy then or may evolve into additional adenocarcinomas years after the index carcinoma has been resected. In the preco-

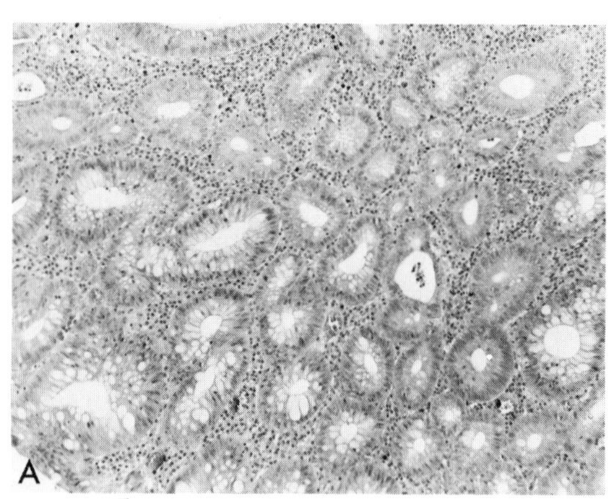

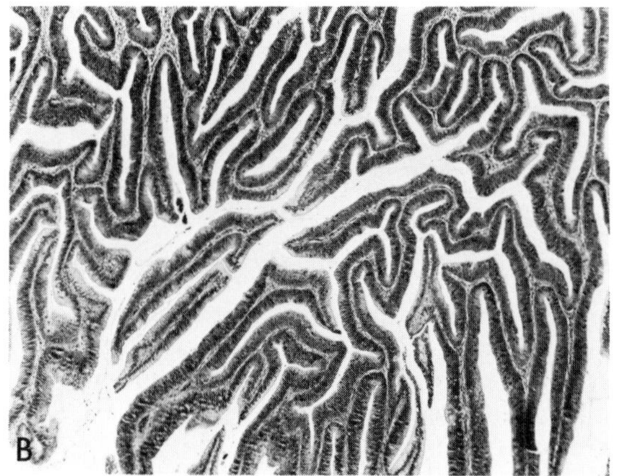

Figure 139–1. *A,* Tubular adenoma. Note orderly arrangement of glands, some with loss of mucin-producing cells. Some nuclei show hyperchromasia. *B,* Villous adenoma. Papillary projections above the surface are composed of glands with slight nuclear atypia and loss of mucin-producing cells. (Courtesy of Dr. Carlos Urmacher, Department of Pathology, Memorial Sloan-Kettering Cancer Center.)

lonoscopic era, synchronous adenomas were reported in approximately 20% or more of specimens resected for adenocarcinoma. The upward revision of frequency is based on more thorough and extensive pre- and post-operative colonoscopic examination.

Still other observations tend to relate adenomas to carcinomas. Residual adenomatous tissue has been found in a substantial number (20%) of adenocarcinomas of the colon that have been removed; it is possible that the remainder of the carcinomas also had such tissue within them that was destroyed as the cancer developed and grew.[7] If adenocarcinomas arose *de novo*, they should be detectable as pure adenocarcinomas when they are of very small size (under 1 cm and possibly under 0.5 cm). However, even with the use of meticulous screening techniques, very small carcinomas are still not found except within pre-existing adenomas. Observations in animals form the basis for the theory of *de novo* carcinomas, but as yet these have not been seen clinically.[16] Additional evidence favoring the relationship of adenomas to adenocarcinomas is (1) the reduction of risk in patients in whom search for and removal of adenomas have been performed on a regular basis,[17] and (2) the increased risk of adenocarcinoma in those patients in whom adenomas are present but are not removed.

Inflammatory Bowel Disease. Ulcerative colitis of long standing is another risk factor for colorectal cancer.[18–22] This subject is fully treated in Chapter 128. It is sufficient here to emphasize that the risk of cancer in ulcerative colitis appears to be related to 2 recognized variables: the duration of active colitis and the extent within the colon of inflammatory changes. In adults, the risk begins to rise after 7 years, and pancolitis carries a greater risk than colitis confined to the left side of the colon.[20] Colitis limited to the rectosigmoid has only minimal risk, and ulcerative proctitis appears to have no increased risk for cancer.

In recent years a small subgroup of about 10% to 15% of patients with longstanding chronic ulcerative colitis has been identified by biopsy as having colonic mucosal dysplasia as an indication of risk of cancer.[22–28] The type of dysplasia that is most related to carcinoma is severe dysplasia of the nodular or villous type.[29] Nevertheless, it must also be borne in mind that there are patients with carcinoma arising in chronic ulcerative colitis in whom pre-existing dysplasia has not been demonstrated, making early clinical diagnosis all the more difficult. There has been considerable controversy regarding the concept and terminology of dysplasia. Some pathologists are beginning to use the terms low-grade and high-grade dysplasia instead of moderate and severe, omitting the category of mild dysplasia. Patients with Crohn's disease of the colon also are at higher risk for colorectal cancer than the general population, but considerably less so than patients with chronic ulcerative colitis.[21] In these patients the risk also is related in part to the duration of disease (Chapter 128).

Hereditary Polyposis Syndromes. These syndromes are reviewed in Chapter 138. For the purposes of this discussion, therefore, comment will be confined to certain highlights of these particular syndromes.

FAMILIAL POLYPOSIS. This condition is characterized by the development of large numbers of adenomatous polyps throughout the entire colon and rectum[30,31] (Fig. 139–2). It has much bearing on carcinoma of the colon because all affected individuals will eventually develop colon carcinoma.

GARDNER'S SYNDROME. This variant of familial polyposis is an autosomal dominant disorder of variable genetic expression showing a high degree of penetrance. Adenomatous polyps are situated principally in the colon, but occasionally in the stomach and

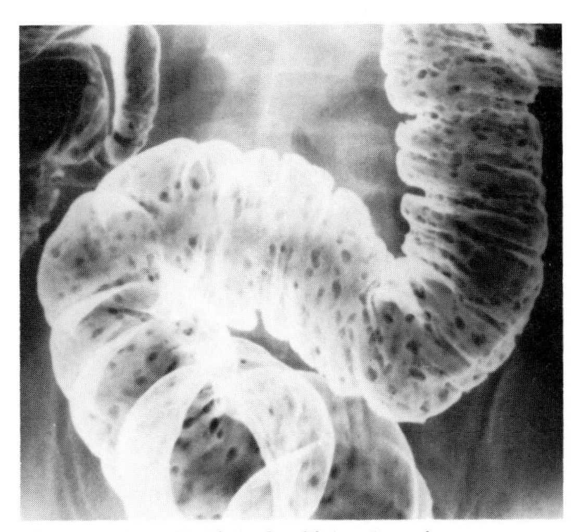

Figure 139–2. Multiple familial polyposis as seen on a double-contrast barium enema roentgenogram. This film is a coned-down view of the rectosigmoid area. (Courtesy of Dr. E. Stewart, Medical College of Wisconsin.)

small intestine as well. Classically, but not in all cases, the polyps are associated with various other lesions, including osteomas of the skull and mandible, epidermoid cysts and soft tissue tumors, and desmoid tumors of the abdominal wall and small intestinal mesentery. The polyps have a pronounced propensity to undergo carcinomatous change.

TURCOT'S SYNDROME. This syndrome consists of polyposis coli associated with malignant tumors of the central nervous system.[6, 32]

PEUTZ-JEGHERS SYNDROME. This syndrome is another autosomal dominant inherited disease with variable expression.[33] Pigmented spots appear on the lips and buccal mucosa and also on the dorsal aspect of the hands and feet. Dozens of tumors are found throughout the gastrointestinal tract, but they are usually not as numerous as in familial polyposis. Because of their composition (normal intestinal epithelium and abnormal amounts and arrangements of smooth muscle), they are considered hamartomas. The tumors originally were thought to be benign without high potential for malignancy. However, cases of cancer (of the stomach, duodenum, and colon) have been reported in association with the Peutz-Jeghers syndrome, and adenomas have been found to co-exist with the other lesions.

JUVENILE POLYPS. Distribution of the polyps in juvenile polyposis (Chapter 138) is not usually as extensive as that seen in familial polyposis.[6, 34] Although the polyps occur indiscriminately throughout the gastrointestinal tract, they are seen more often in the large intestine. The polyps are not precancerous, but adenomatous tumors have been discovered in some patients with juvenile polyposis, and a higher than normal frequency of colon carcinomas may occur in family members.

FAMILIAL COLON CANCER WITHOUT POLYPOSIS. Aside from familial polyposis, it has been difficult to identify or analyze other forms of gastrointestinal cancer that may result from hereditary predisposition. This is because members of family groups with high frequencies of colorectal and other cancers often have not allowed this information to become readily available. Despite this problem, important advances have been made in recent years toward recognition of "cancer families". Familial associations in colon cancer are higher than in control groups, suggesting that inherited factors may play a greater role in the genesis of colorectal cancer

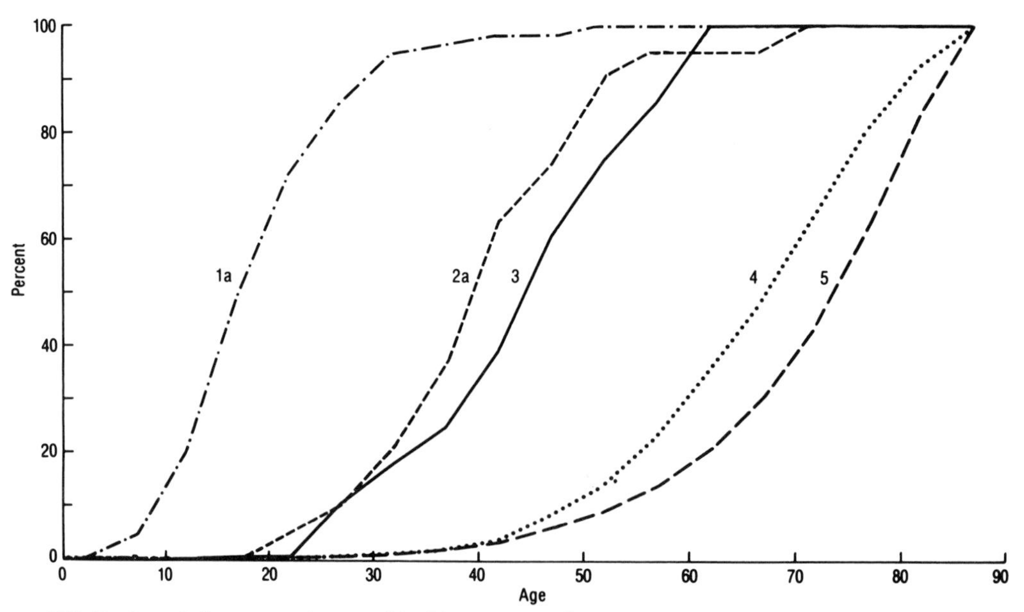

Figure 139–3. Cumulative percentages of incident cases of colon cancer at various ages. *Curve 1a,* nonmalignant polyposis; *Curve 2a,* 38 patients with familial polyposis (Memorial Hospital); *Curve 3,* 28 individuals with familial colon cancer–prone disease without polyposis (Memorial Hospital); *Curve 4,* general population of the United States (Third National Cancer Survey, NCI); *Curve 5,* general population of Japan (Dr. T. Hirayama). (From Sherlock, P et al. Am J Med 68:917, 1980. Reproduced with permission.).

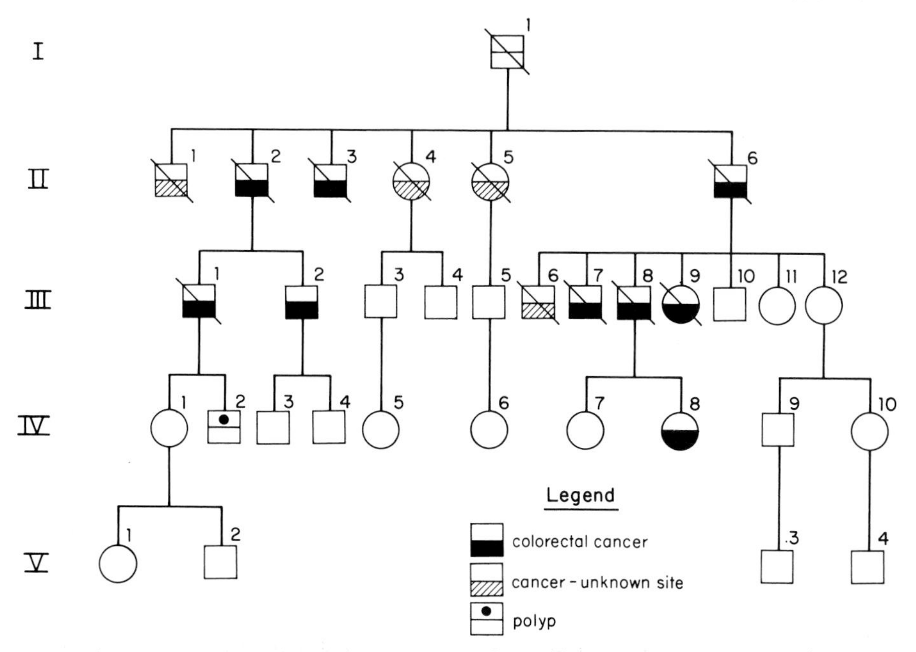

Figure 139–4. Pedigree of family with high prevalence of colorectal cancer. (From Kussin SZ et al. Am J Gastroenterol 72:448, 1979. Reproduced with permission.)

than was previously believed.[35–43] Criteria for a familial syndrome of this type include: (1) increased numbers of all types of adenocarcinomas in affected individuals, especially colon and endometrial carcinomas; (2) development of cancer at an earlier age than that noted for the same organ sites in the general population (Fig. 139–3); (3) a tendency to multiple primary malignant neoplasms in affected persons; and (4) segregation ratios consistent with an autosomal mode of inheritance (Fig. 139–4).

Many other kindreds with site-specific colon lesions have been reported. In this type of familial cancer, only colorectal cancer is present. Colon cancer risk in the "R" family described by Lynch et al.[36,37] segregated with ratios consistent with that of a single autosomal dominant gene with complete penetrance. All but 1 of 33 family members with cancer of the gastrointestinal tract had a parent with the same disease. The family as a whole showed a high risk (50%) for development of primary malignant neoplasms of the colon. Along with many "cancer family" patients, the "R" family revealed a strong tendency toward developing cancer of the proximal colon, the mean frequency in this segment being higher than in either patients with familial polyposis or the general population.

Pathology

Gross Features

Size. The size of the primary tumor appears to have little relationship to prognosis. In fact, in resected cases, a large size may be associated with a good prognosis.[44, 45] Several authors have observed that some very large, bulky colon tumors have few, if any, lymph node metastases and, hence, a correspondingly better 5-year outlook.[46]

Location. Carcinomas of the abdominal colon generally have a reasonably good prognosis. Cancers of the rectum have a significantly poorer prognosis in virtually every major surgical series. This poor outlook is almost entirely associated with cancers of the low or distal rectum (within 5 cm of the anal verge), as cancers of the mid- or upper rectum seem to have a prognosis similar, if not identical, to that of sigmoid lesions. The reasons for this difference in survival are multiple. From the standpoint of natural history, cancers of the lower rectum naturally spread both to hypogastric lymph nodes along the pelvic side walls and to mesorectal lymph nodes along the superior hemorrhoidal artery.[47] From the standpoint of therapy, the vascular pelvic dissection required to extirpate all lymph nodes associated with the potential spread of rectal cancer is a challeng-

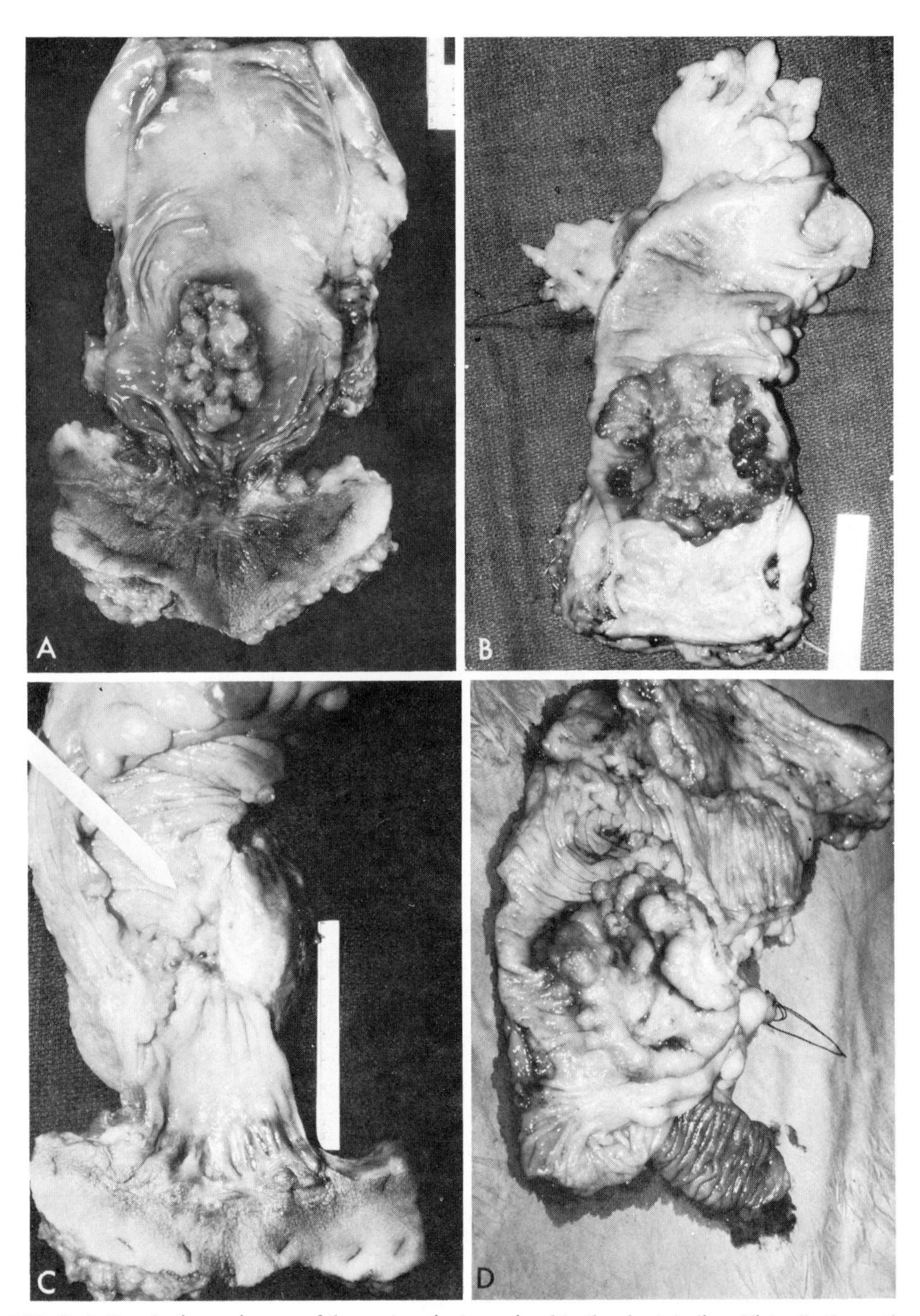

Figure 139–5. *A,* Exophytic carcinoma of the rectum just proximal to the dentate line. Virtually the entire extent of the tumor is intraluminal with little invasion of the muscularis propria. *B,* Ulcerating carcinoma of the upper rectum. The lesion is large and, in contrast to the tumor shown in *A,* has no intraluminal component and has more the appearance of a large ulcer. *C,* Ulcerating carcinoma with a significant degree of mural infiltration. *D,* Large cecal cancer.

ing operation that is rarely accomplished. Hence, the natural course of the disease, the operative limitations of pelvic dissections, treatment failures, and the recurrent pelvic disease that frequently complicates the course of rectal cancer after resection combine to produce a poorer outlook for rectal cancers. Some series have demonstrated an advantage for right-sided lesions[45, 46]; others have shown a poorer outlook, especially for ascending colon cancers, so that this issue is unresolved.[44, 48]

Gross Configuration. Carcinomas of the large bowel generally assume 1 of 4 shapes: exophytic, ulcerative, infiltrative, or annular (Fig. 139–5). It is unclear whether these are all independent shapes or whether some represent later stages of evolution, i.e., ulceration in an exophytic lesion or annular constriction by an infiltrative lesion. Rarely does site influence configuration. Exceptions include the cecum, where large polypoid carcinomas are common and may become big enough to obstruct the ileocecal junction by size alone (Fig. 139–5*D*). Exophytic or polypoid lesions project into the lumen. Although ulceration may be present, this is by no means uniformly seen. On the other hand, focal ulceration may be the gross indication of malignancy in an otherwise benign-appearing adenoma. The exophytic carcinoma may have arisen in an adenoma and in such cases a significant portion of the mass may still be a non-malignant polyp.

The shape of the cancer, whether exophytic or sessile, has been related to prognosis. Sessile or infiltrative lesions carry a poorer prognosis than do exophytic lesions.[49, 50] On cut sections, the tumor usually invades all layers of the bowel wall, exaggerating the gross features of each individual layer, whether due to infiltration or to secondary edema. The extent of circumferential involvement becomes important in relation to both symptoms and prognosis. Infiltrating or annular carcinomas cause obstruction, change in bowel habit, and bleeding. Annular carcinomas are the end product of the infiltrating type of cancer. These tumors are responsible for the clinical signs of bowel obstruction. Prognosis in such tumors is poorer, with an overall 5-year survival of less than 30%.[51] Ulcerating carcinomas may originate as polypoid tumors; however, with continued infection and necrosis the luminal component is gradually eroded. The malignant ulcer may have a clean grayish-pink nodular base that is easily biopsied for a histologic diagnosis or a necrotic, putrid lining with or without significant pericolic inflammation. Such cancers occasionally perforate, and free perforation with peritonitis generally carries an ominous prognosis.

Histology. The histologic features related to prognosis include degree of differentiation (histologic or cytologic grade); degree of mural penetration (Fig. 139–6); presence or absence of lymph node involvement; character

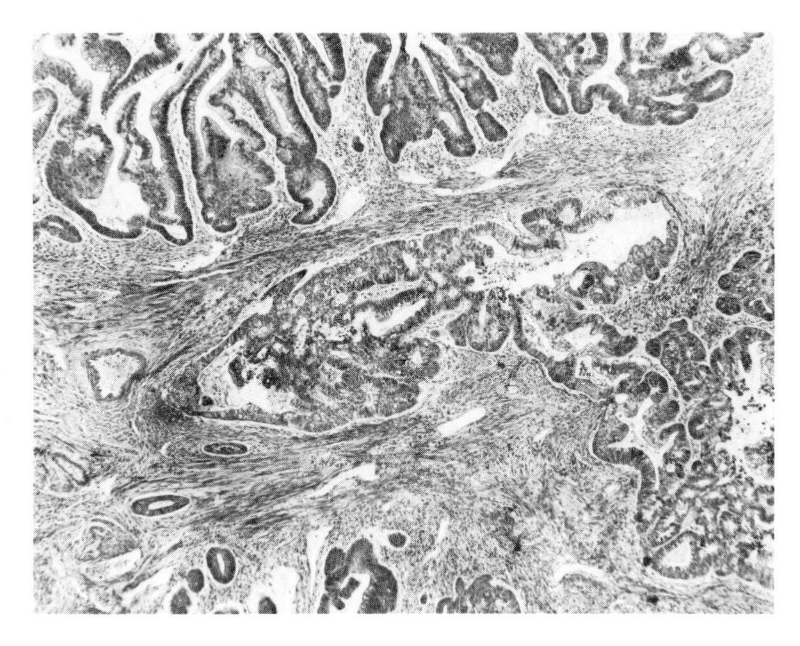

Figure 139–6. Infiltrating, well-differentiated colonic adenocarcinoma. Clusters of atypical glands extend through the muscularis propria. (Courtesy of Dr. Carlos Urmacher, Department of Pathology, Memorial Sloan-Kettering Cancer Center.)

of leading tumor margin; lymphatic, venous, or perineural infiltration; presence of an associated inflammatory response; extranodal mesenteric implants; extramesenteric nodal involvement; presence or absence of involved surgical margins; and adjacent organ involvement.

Degrees of Differentiation. Histologic grading as a tool for assessing tumor differentiation is a useful prognostic indicator.[52, 53] Most pathologists use either a numbering system (1 to 3 or 4) such as the Broders classification or a series of descriptive terms, such as "well differentiated," "moderately differentiated," "poorly differentiated," and "undifferentiated" or "anaplastic." These systems are generally interchangeable. The poorly differentiated category may include a few tumors showing minimal ability to form glandular structures, which would be included in the grade 4 category. These differences rest in part on whether the grading system is oriented more to cytology[52] or toward a description of gland-forming structures,[53] the latter being simpler to use. Well-differentiated tumors are those that are mostly or fully composed of gland-forming structures, with nuclei showing polarity and basal orientation. Moderately differentiated tumors are predominantly glandular but may demonstrate some loss of polarity and nuclear orientation. There may be some tendency for tumor cells to form solid nests. Poorly differentiated tumors are those in which the tendency to form sheets and nests predominates over the formation of glandular elements. When glandular structures are inapparent, the tumor is considered undifferentiated. The majority of colorectal tumors fit into such a grading scheme. Nevertheless, there can be sampling errors, and grading must reflect an examination of the entire tumor. Grading cannot be based on biopsy fragments alone. There may be nearly a 50% rate of error in labeling a rectal tumor as poorly differentiated by assessment of the preoperative biopsy specimen alone, since *biopsy specimens are not representative of the entire cancer.*[54]

Variants of undifferentiated carcinoma, such as signet-ring cell carcinoma or mucinous carcinoma, carry a particularly poor prognosis. Spratt and Spjut[45] reported no 5-year survivors of signet-ring cell carcinomas. The 5-year survival of patients with undifferentiated carcinomas varies from 31% to 74% when mucinous carcinoma is defined in terms of mucus occupying at least 60% of the tumor volume. The frequency of mucinous adenocarcinomas in young patients is unusually high, especially in adolescents.[55] The role of mucin in the poor prognosis of rectal lesions is unknown. Separation of tissue planes, disruption of vascular integrity, and tumor glycocalix abetting the process of metastasis, as well as impaired immunologic protection, have all been suggested. The mucin produced by tumors is histochemically different from the mucin of normal benign colonic epithelium.[56] Reports continue to characterize the changes in mucin production associated with colonic malignancy. As yet, such changes have not been proved to be of practical value as markers of specific prognosis.[57, 58] Tumor cell DNA content may be a better reflection of tumor grade and more accurately associated with prognosis. Chromatin content of an aneuploid (i.e., having other than an exact multiple of the basic haploid number of chromosomes) or heteroploid nature was associated with a poor prognosis independent of the Dukes stage.[59] These findings have been extended to observations of nuclear RNA content as well.[60]

Carcinomas, which are epithelial in origin, spread directly into and through the bowel wall. Because of this, the degree of transmural spread is recorded as one of the 2 prime features of all large bowel cancer staging methods. Severe "epithelial dysplasia," "carcinoma-in-situ," "intramucosal carcinoma," and "severe atypia," are all terms indicating restriction of the cancer to the epithelial layer of origin. The lack of systemic or nodal spread from carcinoma-in-situ is attributable to the absence of lymphatic vessels in the epithelial stroma.[61] Invasive carcinoma (requiring resection to lessen the chance of potential spread of disease) is defined as cancer that has penetrated or invaded the muscularis mucosae. Invasion of the submucosa, muscularis propria, serosa, or perirectal fat constitutes varying degrees of penetration that are recognized in the classic staging methods. Further degrees of direct extension include adherence, invasion, and fistula formation into or involving an adjacent organ. Every abdominal or retroperitoneal organ is vulnerable to direct involvement.

The presence or absence of lymph node involvement is the second prime feature of all staging methods. The prognostic significance of nodal metastases is critical.[45, 47, 48, 50, 62–64] In general, the survival of patients with nodal metastases is reduced to half that of patients without nodal disease. Correlations regarding survival have been made with the level of nodal involvement as well as with the number of involved lymph nodes. Spratt and Spjut[45] reported a 5-year survival of 49% for patients with no nodal disease, 24% for those with 1 to 5 positive nodes, 9% with 6 to 15 positive nodes, and zero with 16 or more positive nodes.

The quality of mesenteric lymph node examination varies from institution to institution and from specimen to specimen. Routine serial sectioning is probably unwarranted, but the value of serial sections of the entire lymph node has been demonstrated.[65] Although extracapsular lymph node metastases have not received the same attention in the staging of large bowel cancer as in breast cancer, such pathologic features are generally associated with poorly differentiated tumors of guarded prognosis. This feature probably has the same individual or additive prognostic significance as either an aggressive leading tumor margin or extranodal mesenteric implants. The character of the leading tumor edge or advancing margin has been correlated with survival as an independent variable.[45,49] The significance of venous invasion is another factor of clear-cut importance that has been repeatedly demonstrated.[66, 67]

The frequency of venous invasion increases with the depth of penetration by the primary tumor and the presence of lymph node metastases. The effect of venous invasion on survival is significant. In its absence, the 5-year survival may be as high as 73%; in its presence, 41%. However, in patients without nodal metastases, intramural venous invasion is not a significant prognostic factor.[51] Lymphatic invasion in the absence of nodal metastases has not been of proven prognostic significance in the management of carcinomas arising in polyps. Involvement of perineural spaces, on the other hand, does have independent prognostic significance and has been noted to relate to the frequency of local tumor recurrence. The frequency of perineural invasion may be a function of tumor grade.[68] Survival is influenced to the same degree as in venous invasion, and perineural venous lymphatic invasion seems to be an additive prognostic factor.[69]

The presence of an inflammatory response surrounding a tumor is a feature that has been associated with a good prognosis.[45] Some have considered this an immunologic response.[70] The role of lymphoid cells in an infiltrate surrounding a tumor is as yet unclear. Patt and co-workers[71] have studied the significance of regional lymph node response in sigmoid colon cancers. A well-developed paracortical immunoblast hyperplasia and an associated sinus histiocytosis segregated a group of patients so that their 5-year survival rate was 83%, regardless of the Dukes stage. Those without a significant response had a 5-year survival of 35%.

Three other histologic features merit additional mention. These include the presence of neoplastic cells at the surgical margin of resection, adjacent organ involvement, and intramural or longitudinal spread of tumor. Positive surgical margins are rarely found in adequately resected specimens. The surgeon should anticipate this possibility and should make appropriate use of frozen sections. Further resection is indicated if any conventional margin, e.g., the distal margin of resection, is positive or even questionable.

The involvement of adjacent organs is in and of itself not a limitation to curative *en bloc* resection. Given an *en bloc* resection without violation of tumor, adhesions, abscess, or fistulous involvement, cure is still possible, if not enhanced, by the appropriateness of the resection. Prognosis is generally influenced by the presence or absence of lymph node involvement and the cumulative effects of other characteristics, such as leading margins and perineural or venous invasion.[72]

Occult tumor spread within the bowel wall is not a prominent feature of large bowel carcinomas. Generally, rectal cancer will not spread microscopically more than 2 cm beyond the grossly visible tumor edge. On very rare occasions, growth may extend beyond 4 cm. Such tumor behavior is the basis for the 5-cm *in vivo* distal margin considered acceptable in the surgical treatment of rectal cancer.[73,74]

Characteristics of Cancers Arising in Adenomas. Carcinoma must penetrate the muscularis mucosae in order to metastasize.[61] There is general agreement that invasive carcinoma in a sessile adenoma should be treated by resection. Controversy exists, however, over the management of carcinoma arising in pedunculated adenomas.[75, 76] Accessible pedunculated adenomas are removable endoscopically by cautery snare. These polyps may demonstrate carcinoma-in-situ, microinvasive carcinoma (a minor penetration of the muscularis mucosae), stromal invasion (above the level of normal colonic mucosa), or invasion of the stalk. The margin of resection may be involved by tumor or may be free. Lymphatic invasion may be present in the stroma or stalk. Morson[75] has indicated that with the exception of carcinomas involving the stalk or those with an involved or unclear margin, further resection of the colon is not indicated. The overall risk of lymph node metastasis from a lesion that has not yet penetrated the bowel wall is less than 5%. As smaller and earlier lesions are removed colonoscopically, the true risk of finding lymph node metastases will probably decline proportionately.

A reasonable approach to pedunculated malignant polyps is to consider further surgical resection in those patients who have cancer that has invaded the muscularis mucosae and the stalk, especially if the lesion is poorly differentiated or associated with lymphatic or cautery line involvement. Other factors should also be taken into consideration, including the patient's age and medical status and the location of the adenoma. A prospective study of this subject is needed in order to arrive at clearer indications for resection. In the meanwhile, examination of other retrospective data would be constructive.

Age and the Pathology of Large Bowel Cancer. Cancer in patients under 30 years of age is generally considered to be aggressive.[55] An examination of certain pathologic features may help to explain this altered prognosis. Normally, histologic grade of malignancy shows the continued range of variation discussed previously. At St. Mark's Hospital, London, the grades of malignancy in any given population are distributed as approximately 20% grade 1, 60% grade 2, and 20% grade 3. Follow-up studies show that about 75% of the patients with grade 1 tumors are cured, whereas 50% of those with grade 2 tumors and only 25% with grade 3 cancers are likely to survive. Bussey[77] has demonstrated that when histologic grades are correlated with age, there is an increasing proportion of low-grade tumors in older age groups; conversely, there are proportionately more high-grade tumors in young patients. More than 50% of patients under 30 years of age have grade 3 (undifferentiated) tumors as compared with only 11% in patients over 80 years of age. The proportion of low-grade tumors in patients under 30 years of age is only 8% but increases steadily to about 30% by age 80.

Age of the patient and the Dukes classification are also seen to vary in the same way as grade. Corrected 5-year survival for rectal cancers at St. Mark's Hospital is approximately 95% for Dukes A, 72% for Dukes B, and 26% for Dukes C, with an overall survival of 50%. The proportion of A cases with favorable prognosis increases with age. In young patients, 80% of those under 30 years of age had Dukes C cancers with a cure rate of only 20%, whereas the proportion of Dukes C cases in patients 80 years old or over declined to less than 50%, with an associated increase in survival to over 70%. Thus, the poorer prognosis in the young is understandable in terms of these pathologic findings, in addition to the greater frequency of mucinous carcinomas.[77]

Staging Methods. The original Dukes classification of pathologic staging was designed to correlate survival after different types of treatment with the preoperative assessment of tumor stage. By 1932, the classification for rectal cancer took the following form: stage A, growth limited to the wall of the rectum; stage B, extension of growth into extrarectal tissue; and stage C, metastases in regional lymph nodes.[64] By 1935, the importance of proximal lymph node involvement in the resected mesentery (i.e., positive nodes in the region of the mesenteric apex or at the origin of the mesenteric vascular dissection) became apparent.[78] The stage C classification was modified to reflect this difference: C_1 represented cases in which only regional lymph glands were involved (or those in which the upward spread had not reached the point of ligation of blood vessels) and C_2 represented cases in which the glandular spread reached the point of ligature of blood vessels.[79] The validity of this staging method was borne out in the 1959 report of Dukes and Bussey[80]; each stage correlated with a significant difference in 5-year survival. In 1939, the original Dukes classification was extended for use in cases of colonic as well as rectal cancers.[81] In 1949 Kirklin et al.[82] and in 1954 Astler and Coller[62] offered modifications of the Dukes classification that combined the prognostic significance of the degree of mural penetration and/or involvement of lymph nodes. Kirklin et al.[82] proposed the Dukes A classification for lesions limited to the mucosa. In the Astler-Coller modification, B_1 and B_2 represented, respectively, incomplete and complete penetration of the muscularis propria (or the serosa where present), i.e., the entire bowel wall. Stages C_1 and C_2 represented nodal involvement in the absence (C_1) or presence (C_2) of mural penetration. Five-year survival figures for the Astler-Coller modification of the Dukes classification were: A (1 patient), 100%; B_1 (48 patients), 66.6%; B_2 (164 patients), 53.9%; C_1 (14 patients), 42.8%; and C_2 (125 patients), 22.4%. No D category for distant disease was suggested by either group. (Table 139–2).

These staging methods supported the fact that mural penetration had a prognostic significance independent of nodal metastases. Since that time, the Gastrointestinal Tumor Study Group (GITSG) of the National Cancer Institute has put into use a further modification of the Dukes classification that independently recognizes the values of both variables, i.e., the degree of mural penetration and the number of involved lymph nodes.[83] The GITSG modification of the Dukes classification combines degrees of mural penetration and the number of involved nodes; it ignores the little-used category of stage C. In addition, the GITSG classification introduces stage D (distant visceral metastases or peritoneal seeding) to the Dukes classification. This converts this staging method from a strictly postsurgical pathologic system to a combined clinicopathologic staging system.[48] In the GITSG adjuvant therapy program involving the follow-up of patients operated on for colon carcinoma, the available 4-year survival data according to this system are listed in Table 139–3.

Table 139–2. DUKES STAGING METHODS (ORIGINAL AND MODIFIED)

Dukes 1932 (Original)
- A —Cancer limited to the bowel wall
- B —Extension of growth into extrarectal tissues
- C —Metastases to regional lymph nodes

Dukes 1935 (Modified)
- C_1—Uninvolved lymph nodes at level of mesenteric vascular ligation
- C_2—Highest lymph node positive for tumor

Astler-Coller 1954
- A—Limited to mucosa (carcinoma-in-situ)
- B_1—Penetration of muscularis mucosae
- B_2—Penetration through muscularis propria
- C_1—B_1 with positive nodes
- C_2—B_2 with positive nodes

Gastrointestinal Tumor Study Group (1976)
- A—Limited to mucosa (carcinoma-in-situ)
- B_1—Penetration of muscularis mucosae
- B_2—Penetration through muscularis propria (serosa where present)
- C_1—One to four tumor-involved lymph nodes
- C_2—Five or more tumor-involved lymph nodes
- D—Distant metastases

Table 139–3. GASTROINTESTINAL TUMOR STUDY GROUP: 4-YEAR SURVIVAL ACCORDING TO THE MODIFIED DUKES STAGING FOR COLON CARCINOMAS

Dukes' Stage	No. of Patients	Recurrences	Deaths
B_2	228	40 (18%)	48 (21%)
C_1	234	76 (32%)	90 (38%)
C_2	100	57 (57%)	69 (69%)

More recent efforts to bypass the numerous modifications of the Dukes classification and provide a uniform method for staging large bowel cancer have led to the organization of the American Joint Committee (AJC) Task Force on Colon and Rectum Cancer.[84] This task force has developed a single postsurgical pathologic assessment staging system for colon and rectum cancer by an analysis of 1826 cases (924 colon and 902 rectum cancers collected from a number of institutions). Using the TNM ("*T*umor-*N*ode-*M*etastasis") classification as described by the UICC (Union International Contre le Cancer), the task force confirmed the importance of postsurgical staging (pTNM). While providing uniformity for both rectum and colon cancer, the TNM does so at the cost of being extremely complex and abandoning certain observations (i.e., degrees of mural penetration, which are of previously proven value), while emphasizing infrequent events such as adjacent organ involvement or fistula formation. Also, the number or location of positive nodes is difficult to express. Virtually all of the features incorporated into TNM derive from the Dukes classification in the first place. Therefore, while efforts may continue to simplify the TNM system, it is doubtful whether it will improve on the Astler-Coller modified Dukes classification GITSG classification. Nevertheless, the importance of attempts to achieve international uniform-

Table 139–4. TNM AND AJC PROPOSED STAGING FOR COLORECTAL CANCERS*

TNM Proposed Postsurgical Pathologic Staging

T1—Tumor confined to mucosa and submucosa
T2—Tumor invading muscularis propria but not through it
T3—Tumor through entire thickness of the bowel wall, including serosa where present
N0—No nodal metastasis identified in specimen
N1 ( )—Nodal metastasis found in specimen, ( ) the number found
M0—No known distant metastasis
M1—Distant metastasis identified

Proposed Definitions of AJC (Conform with Current UICC Except As Noted)

Tx—Depth not specified T0—No demonstrable tumor T1S—Carcinoma-in-situ (no invasion of lamina propria)	Stage 0 T1S
T1—Tumor confined to mucosa and submucosa T2—Tumor invading muscularis propria but not extending through	Stage I IA T1N0M0
T3—Tumor through entire thickness of bowel wall; through entire muscularis propria and through serosa when present; may or may not invade adjacent structures	IB T2N0M0
(UICC: 3a without fistula; 3b with fistula) (UICC adds T4 direct invasion to structures beyond those immediately adjacent)	Stage II T3N0M0
Nx—Nodes not assessed N0—No nodal metastasis identified N1—Regional node metastasis identified	Stage III T1–2N1 ( ) M0 T3N1 ( ) M0
( ) Number of nodal metastases identified (UICC: N2 Multiple nodes involved) (N3 Fixed regional nodes) (N4 Juxtaregional nodal involvement)	Stage IV Any TNM1
Mx—Distant metastases not assessed M0—Distant metastasis not identified M1—Distant metastasis reported Site ________	Subscripts Histologic grade Venous or lymphatic invasion
Stratification Age Sex Location	

TNM = "Tumor-Node-Metastasis"; AJC = American Joint Committee Task Force on Colon and Rectum Cancer; UICC = Union Internationale Contre le Cancer. (Adapted from Stearns.[51])

ity in staging cannot be overestimated (Table 139–4).

Special Considerations

Carcinoma Complicating Familial Polyposis Coli (FPC). Malignant lesions of the colon complicate virtually all cases of FPC left untreated. Malignant foci have been detected in 66.8% of patients in the St. Mark's Hospital registry[31] and in 64% of patients in the Japanese Polyposis Centre.[85] Multiplicity was observed in 47.6% and in 54% of the cases, respectively. The distribution and histology of cancers in FPC are the same as in sporadic large bowel cancer and merit no special comment.

Carcinoma Complicating Ulcerative Colitis. The mucosa of patients with ulcerative colitis seems particularly liable to produce a carcinoma in the face of relatively low grades of "premalignant" dysplasia. Blackstone et al.[29] have described the all too common appearance of an invasive carcinoma (40% of cases) beneath the epithelium manifesting only mild to moderate degrees of dysplasia, the type that might be expected to be associated with a small adenoma. It is not surprising, therefore, that carcinomas arising in ulcerative colitis are frequently found to be covered by mucosa of relatively normal appearance. Carcinomas in this setting frequently are flat, plaque-like lesions, or at most are nodular, making detection extremely difficult. Histologically, the majority of such occult lesions associated with mild dysplasia are of the Dukes B_1 stage. The prognosis of patients with carcinoma complicating ulcerative colitis is stage-dependent, as in the case of sporadic carcinomas.

Colon Carcinoma Complicating Crohn's Disease. Of the relatively small number of cases of carcinoma of the large bowel complicating Crohn's disease that have been reported to date,[21, 86] all the patients have been relatively young and all had total large bowel involvement with Crohn's disease. The frequency in reported series has been in the range of 2.2%, with an expected age-corrected incidence of carcinoma of 0.3 cases, a 20-fold increase over that expected in the general population. The 4 factors that have been associated with the advent of cancer are: (1) a long duration of Crohn's colitis (>15 years); (2) an onset before age 21; (3) total colonic involvement; and (4) surgically bypassed or excluded segments.[87] Virtually all the cancers have developed in diseased segments of bowel. Multiplicity of lesions (i.e., 2 or 3 cancers) has been more common than in sporadic cases. Right-sided lesions appear to be more common (46% of cases in the report by Keighley et al.[86]). Whereas precancer has not been pathologically identified as uniformly in Crohn's disease as in ulcerative colitis, Morson and Pang[88] have reclassified 23% of their patients as having either granulomatous or "mixed colitis," some with precancerous changes. The frequent presence of stenosis, stricture, or fistula makes a radiographic diagnosis of cancer in Crohn's colitis difficult. Similarly, colonoscopy may be limited by stricture and by previous surgical changes. Microscopically, there are no special features once invasive cancer has developed.

Clinical Features

Cancers of the rectum and colon grow and obstruct, ulcerate and bleed, invade, cause pain, and, less commonly, perforate into an adjacent organ or the peritoneal space. The clinical features in an individual patient are determined by the biologic growth characteristics of the cancer and by its location in the colon. The symptoms of colorectal cancer initially may be intermittent and subtle and all too often are overlooked or regarded as unimportant by patient and physician alike. However, when patients postpone medical attention for some time after the onset of symptoms, morbidity and the risk of mortality are greatly increased. Further delay by the physician who first sees the patient with such symptoms may be critical.

Rectal *bleeding* is a symptom most often associated with cancers of the left side of the colon and in the rectum. The passage of red blood sometimes mixed with darker blood clots is a common observation, but bleeding is usually not massive. With cancers of the right side of the colon, bleeding is more apt to be slow and blood mixed with bowel contents is more likely to be occult. Patients with cancer in this region gradually become iron-deficient and anemic because of blood loss and often present with weakness, dizziness, congestive heart failure, angina, or claudication. When right-sided colon cancers bleed more rapidly, they may produce a reddish-maroon stool. Bleeding from colon cancer tends to be intermittent, with intervals when no blood may be detected.

Cancers that occur in the more voluminous and distensible cecum and right colon, where bowel contents are liquid, usually do not cause *obstruction* until they grow to a very large size. Cancers in the ascending colon are more likely to block the lumen. In such cases, if the ileocecal valve is competent, the cecum becomes painfully dilated with gas, creating a tender right lower quadrant mass. Patients may note relief when they massage this area and force the trapped gas past the obstruction. Cecal masses that invade the ileocecal valve may produce the clinical picture of small bowel obstruction with generalized abdominal distention, nausea, and bilious vomiting.

In the left colon, where the lumen is narrower and less distensible, and the fecal stream is solid, cancers commonly obstruct the passage of feces. This is a major cause of a change in bowel habit; the gradual narrowing of the lumen slows the fecal stream to produce *constipation*. Cramping abdominal *pain* occurs when the colon is intermittently distended proximal to the lesion. Some patients may develop a paradoxical diarrhea as some colonic contents are forced past a partially obstructing cancer. Cramping may be particularly aggravated after meals as a result of increased peristaltic activity. Cramping also may be induced by laxatives used to treat the constipation caused by the malignant obstruction.

Rectal cancers characteristically produce fecal urgency, tenesmus, bright red bleeding in small amounts, change in stool caliber, and incontinence. Local invasion may be a source of perianal pain, hematuria, urinary frequency, and vaginal fistula.

Perforation of colon cancers into the peritoneal cavity usually results in localized abscess. This can be a cause of fever and intermittent sepsis. Abdominal pain and signs of localized peritoneal irritation will usually be present.

Anorexia and *weight loss* are common in advanced colon cancer. The anorexia is intensified by partially obstructing lesions that may cause cramping abdominal pain associated with meals. Weakness and malaise may be related to anemia but are often an indication of advanced and metastatic disease. Metastases from colon cancer will produce various symptoms depending on the areas affected. Local invasion of the peritoneum or retroperitoneum may produce localized abdominal or back pain. Pelvic and sciatic pain, attended by neurologic signs, may result from invasion of the lumbosacral plexus, spine, and pelvis. Ascites, bowel obstruction, and ileus may develop from intra-abdominal tumor spread. Right upper quadrant pain, a mass, or jaundice signals liver metastases. Pulmonary metastases may be a cause of cough and dyspnea.

Diagnosis

While bright red rectal bleeding can be due to a variety of benign lesions (hemorrhoids, diverticulosis, angiodysplasia, colitis, and adenomatous polyps), bleeding always should arouse suspicion of bowel cancer. The character and severity of rectal bleeding do not distinguish benign from malignant disease. However, hemorrhoids or anal fissures characteristically produce a small amount of blood streaking the toilet tissue, and profuse bleeding is more likely due to angiodysplasia, diverticulosis, or inflammatory bowel disease.

Changes in bowel habit, with constipation, crampy pain, and narrowed stool caliber, may result from diverticular disease as well as from cancer involving the left colon. It is often difficult to determine if a localized peritoneal abscess is due to a perforated diverticulum or a cancer. Inflammatory bowel disease or infectious colitis may cause bleeding, tenesmus, urgency, and diarrhea, but colorectal cancer must be considered even with these manifestations. Alternating constipation and diarrhea with left lower quadrant pain suggest an irritable bowel syndrome, but cancer of the left colon can produce the same symptoms. In most patients with an irritable bowel syndrome, on the other hand, a careful history will document longstanding symptoms. While patients with the irritable bowel syndrome do not seem to have a higher frequency of colon cancer, they are still as liable to malignancy as anyone else. Hence, a sudden worsening or change in nature of the symptoms in a patient with a known irritable bowel should suggest the possibility of a supervening colon cancer.

Digital rectal examination is a crucial part of the physical examination and should not be omitted without good reason. This examination may detect an unsuspected mass lesion. Colon cancers that become large and bulky, usually on the right side, may be palpable. Metastatic spread to the liver may cause hepatomegaly, and the liver may feel hard and nodular and be slightly tender. Peritoneal metastases may cause ascites, and peripheral lymphadenopathy may represent metastatic spread. Evidence of weight loss, cachexia, pallor, and jaundice suggests advanced disease.

Colonoscopy. Asymptomatic patients who have a positive fecal occult blood test or a positive finding on proctoscopic or barium enema examination are candidates for colonoscopy.[89–91] About 50% of patients having a positive fecal occult blood test will be found to harbor a neoplastic lesion; about 38% of these lesions will be adenomas and 12% will be cancers.[92] The predictive value of the fecal occult blood test for neoplastic lesions increases with the age of the patient.[93] Studies from around the world utilizing the fecal occult blood test for screening have demonstrated that the yield for neoplastic lesions is much higher when colonoscopy is added to barium enema examination in the diagnostic work-up. When single-column barium enema studies are used, approximately half the cancers and a majority of adenomas are missed but are detected on colonoscopy.[94] In patients having a positive proctosigmoidoscopic examination, colonoscopy is indicated as a search for additional lesions. Synchronous adenomas have been observed in about 50% of patients with cancer. When a cancer has been found, complete colonoscopy will disclose a separate synchronous cancer elsewhere in the colon in 1.5% to 5% of cases. This same high yield of synchronous adenomas has been found in patients presenting with a single adenoma at proctosigmoidoscopy.[95]

Patients who present with symptoms of neoplastic disease are usually examined first by proctosigmoidoscopy, then by barium enema, and finally by colonoscopy. If a lesion is found by proctosigmoidoscopy or barium enema, colonoscopy is needed to ascertain the nature of the lesion, to remove it if it is a benign-appearing adenoma, to obtain a tissue sample if it is a malignant lesion, and to make certain that there are no other synchronous lesions elsewhere in the colon. When a cancer has been detected by proctosigmoidoscopy or barium enema, the colonoscopic approach will vary, depending on the nature and location of the lesion. Colonoscopy can usually be safely done in patients with small to moderate-sized polypoid adenocarcinomas anywhere in the colon, the neoplasm being gently bypassed while looking for synchronous lesions. If colonoscopy requires difficult manipulation, the procedure is usually terminated. If the lesion partially obstructs the lumen, the colonoscope should not be passed beyond the lesion because of the risk of perforation. The liability to perforation may be related either to fixation of the bowel produced by the carcinoma or to segmental ischemic colitis that sometimes accompanies a neoplastic lesion and is associated with friability and loss of integrity of the bowel wall. As much of the colon as possible distal to the obstructing tumor is searched for synchronous lesions.

At times, it may be wise to omit proctosigmoidoscopy and barium enema examination and proceed directly to colonoscopy. Such an approach may be indicated in the patient with moderately severe rectal bleeding. For patients in whom rectal bleeding is not quite so severe, for whom there is no clinical urgency, a double-contrast barium enema study should precede colonoscopy. When seeing a patient with rectal bleeding for the first time, it is wise to do a proctosigmoidoscopy without a preliminary enema before attempting colonoscopy so as to exclude, insofar as possible, the presence of inflammatory bowel disease. The activity of the colitis may be such that preparation for colonoscopy should be deferred until the colitis has been treated and rendered quiescent.

It is wise to obtain a double-contrast barium enema examination before colonoscopy whenever possible (Figs. 139–7 and 139–8). Exceptions might be the patient with urgent bleeding or the patient with ulcerative colitis under surveillance. The objective is to provide the most sensitive combination of examinations for neoplasia for each patient. Although the yield of neoplastic lesions is much higher for colonoscopy than it is for barium enema examination (as the latter procedure is generally performed), false-negative results occur with colonoscopy as well. This false-negativity has not been well established for cancers. Potentially difficult for diagnosis are the areas just proximal to the hepatic and splenic flexures and the medial aspect of the ascending colon, especially the area just proximal to the ileocecal valve. The false-negativity for adenomas has been established in one study[96] in which a blinded technique for colonoscopy relative to the barium enema demonstrated that colonoscopy missed approximately 6% of adenomas 1 cm and larger.

Biopsy and *cytology* techniques have considerable value when combined with endoscopy.[97] In certain high-risk groups, lavage cytology can be done if no specific lesions are seen. Lavage cytology is routinely done during endoscopic surveillance examinations in postoperative patients with familial polyposis and in patients with longstanding ulcerative colitis. In patients with ulcerative colitis, cancers not visible by either colonos-

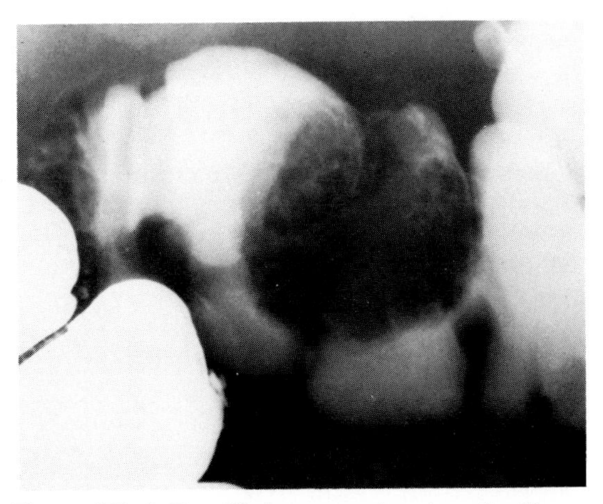

Figure 139–7. Magnified compression view of a villous adenoma in the transverse colon. The compressing gloved hand of the radiologist is seen in the film. (Courtesy of Dr. E. Stewart, Medical College of Wisconsin.)

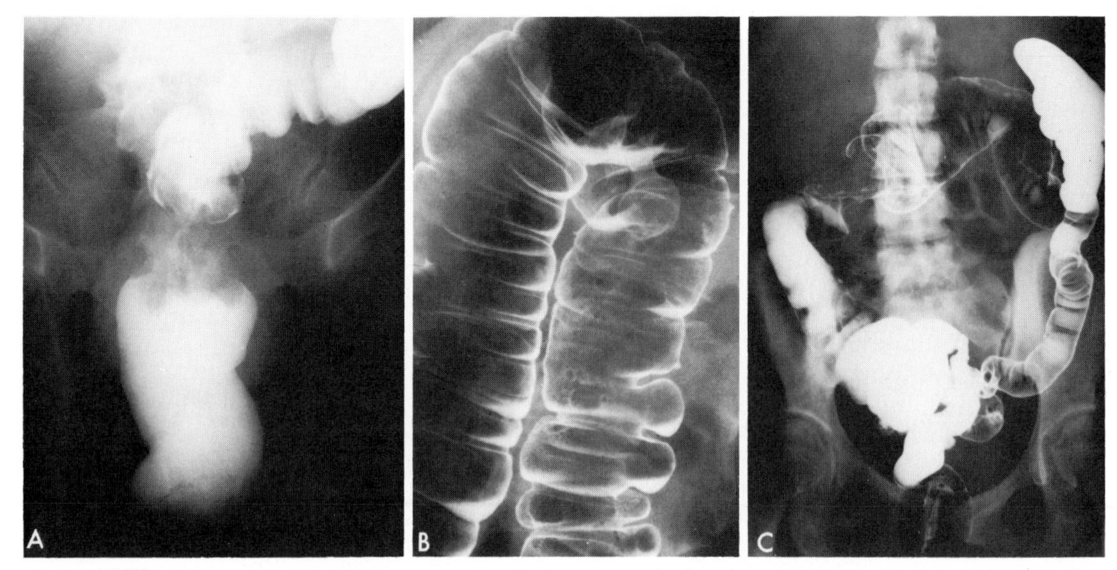

Figure 139–8. *A,* An angle view of the rectum on a single-contrast barium enema roentgenogram demonstrating an annular carcinoma at the rectosigmoid junction. *B,* A dangling pedunculated polyp is seen at the splenic flexure in this exposure taken with the patient in the erect position. *C,* In this double-contrast barium enema examination of the colon, an annular carcinoma with overhanging margins is seen in the proximal transverse colon. In addition there are diffuse blastic metastases to the skeleton. (Courtesy of Dr. E. Stewart, Medical College of Wisconsin.)

copy or barium enema examination may, on occasion, be detected by lavage cytology.

Endoscopic biopsy can be of importance in assessing the premalignant potential of the mucosa in ulcerative colitis.[22–27] In patients with distal colitis, colonoscopic biopsy of the more proximal colon may yield histologic evidence of involvement that would then place the inflammatory bowel disorder in the category of pancolitis, requiring greater surveillance for carcinoma. Also, biopsies obtained by colonoscopy may indicate the presence of dysplasia not seen on rectal biopsies (Chapter 128).

Biopsy and brush cytology are not generally used for evaluation of benign-appearing polyps. The histologic nature of benign-appearing polyps is best evaluated by total excision, either by snare and cautery or by surgical removal. We usually remove benign-appearing colonoscopic pedunculated polyps, regardless of size, by the colonscopic snare-cautery technique.[98] Also, we remove most sessile lesions that appear benign and are smaller than 2 cm. We do not attempt to remove lesions that appear malignant, whether pedunculated or sessile, and we are reluctant to remove sessile lesions that have a base larger than 2 cm, in part because of the likelihood of malignancy in such lesions. Although removal of large sessile lesions by colonoscopy has been reported, there is little follow-up information regarding recurrence, frequency of associated carcinoma, need for additional surgery, and complications. Polyps smaller than 5 mm can be removed by hot biopsy, i.e., a combination of biopsy and fulguration.

Laboratory Aids. Laboratory tests are of limited help in diagnosing and evaluating patients with colon cancer. Tests that document iron-deficiency hypochromic microcytic anemia and occult blood in the stool are basic, and both findings require consideration of colon cancer. Occult blood in the stool may be tested during the initial physical examination at the time of rectal examination by using a guaiac-impregnated slide (Hemoccult kit). A single negative test, however, should not be interpreted as ruling out cancer. Hypoalbuminemia suggests malnutrition and advanced disease. Abnormal activities of liver enzymes may indicate hepatic metastases, and elevated urea nitrogen or creatinine levels in the serum may be due to blockage of the ureters by expanding metastases.

Carcinoembryonic antigen (CEA)[99, 100] levels determined by commercially available radioimmunoassays have a sensitivity of 0.5

ng/ml (see Chapter 254 for a discussion of tumor markers and antigens). The results are also reproducible with some interlaboratory variations.[101–104] When first described, CEA appeared to be a tumor-specific test for colon cancer that would enable early diagnosis in asymptomatic patients. This has proved not to be the case.[105–108] Further, in screening large populations for colon cancer, CEA was found to have a false-positive rate of 15% and a false-negative rate of 40% to 60% in non-metastatic disease. Thus, the test lacks both the specificity and the sensitivity to allow for screening. Moreover, most asymptomatic patients with early stages of colon cancer have normal CEA values in their blood,[70, 109–111] and patients with elevated CEA tend to be those with more advanced cancer.

Prevention

Primary prevention is defined as the identification of factors, genetic or environmental, that may be responsible for colorectal cancer and eradication of these factors. *Secondary* prevention is the "early" detection of colorectal cancer previous to its more advanced, devastating, and fatal consequences, as well as detection and eradication of conditions that predispose to malignant change but do not yet show transformation into cancer.

The importance of a thorough investigation of symptomatic patients is related not only to a diagnosis of colorectal cancer but also to the discovery of a premalignant disease for which proper treatment can have an important impact on the patient's future risk for colorectal cancer. For this reason, patients with symptoms such as rectal bleeding, reduction in caliber of stools, or change in bowel habit must be studied aggressively.

For secondary prevention, the focus is on asymptomatic patients and the application of screening or case-finding techniques. *Screening* is defined as an approach to a large population and *case-finding* as an approach to individual patients and small groups within the framework of the health care system. The screening or case-finding approaches should be varied, depending on whether the patients are at average risk or in one of the high-risk groups.[32, 112]

Screening Tests

Occult Blood in Feces. The testing of stools for the presence of occult blood as an early indicator of gastrointestinal malignancy is an old concept (Chapter 24). In past years patients were asked to supply one or more stool samples without any special dietary restriction for testing. This approach was associated with a high percentage of false-positive and false-negative results.[51] *Benzidine* as a testing agent was discarded because of extremely high sensitivity, resulting in a high percentage of false-positive tests and leading to unnecessary diagnostic procedures for many patients. *Orthotoluidine* (Hematest) was shown not to yield reproducible results suited to screening. *Guaiac* has remained a reliable test agent for occult blood in the stool. In the late 1960s, Greegor[113] recommended a procedure that required the patient, while on a high-fiber, meat-free diet, to smear 2 samples of stool each day onto a paper slide impregnated with guaiac for a total of 6 smears over 3 days. The slides were then submitted for testing by a reagent consisting of hydrogen peroxide in denatured alcohol. Utilizing this approach, Greegor reported detection of colorectal cancers at an early pathologic stage in several patients. The guaiac paper slide test, as currently utilized in the Hemoccult kit, consists of filter paper impregnated with guaiac. On exposure to the reagent,[114] a positive reaction depends on the pseudo-peroxidase activity of hemoglobin; when exposed to hydrogen peroxide, there is phenolic oxidation of the guaiac reflected in a change from colorless to blue.[114] Anything having peroxidase activity, such as fresh fruits and uncooked vegetables, can produce a similar reaction. Agents that interfere with the oxidation reaction, such as ascorbic acid, may produce a false-negative reaction in the presence of hemoglobin. A positive test, therefore, can derive not only from blood but from non-hemoglobin peroxidases or from non-human hemoglobin present in foods such as meat.

A controlled clinical trial of the fecal occult blood test in screening for colorectal cancer began in 1974 at the Memorial Sloan-Kettering Cancer Center[115] (Table 139–5). In this trial, a study group of asymptomatic men and women aged 40 and older coming to the Preventive Medicine Institute received a comprehensive medical examination and a fecal occult blood kit (Hemoccult) (Smith Kline Diagnostics, Sunnyvale, California) to prepare at home and bring in at the time of re-examination. Study patients were asked to prepare 6 smears over 3 days while consuming a meat-free, high-fiber diet and avoiding

Table 139–5. FECAL OCCULT BLOOD TEST: CLINICAL DATA*

Factor	Percentage
Patient compliance	
Motivated groups	80%
Unmotivated groups	15%
Rate of positive slides (unhydrated)	1%–5%
Rate of positive slides (rehydrated)	Up to 20%
Predictive value for neoplasia	18–50%
Staging of detected cancers (Dukes A and B)	60%–80%
False positivity for cancer or adenoma	
(unhydrated slide)	2%
(rehydrated slide)	Up to 20%
False negativity for cancer	
(rehydrated slides)	7%
(unhydrated slides)	20%
False negativity for adenomas	60%–75%

*See text for significance.

vitamins and medications. If the slides were positive, double-contrast barium enema examination and colonoscopy were performed: upper gastrointestinal radiography was performed if no colonic neoplasm was found. Over 22,000 patients have been enrolled in this study to date. Compliance ranged from 70% to 80% for fecal occult blood testing and 95% for proctosigmoidoscopy. The overall rate of positive slides was 2.5%; slide positivity was 1.7% in those aged 40 to 49 and 6.6% in those over 70 years of age. The rate of positivity for the Hemoccult slide was 1%, with a predictive value for neoplasia of 50%, including 12% for cancer and 38% for adenomas. With the multiple Hemoccult II slides, the rate of positivity increased to 3.7%, with a predictive value of 44%. Analysis of daily smears indicated that only 41% of neoplastic lesions would have been detected if only 1 smear was examined rather than 2 smears. The predictive value did not correlate well with the number of positive slides. Colorectal cancer detected by slides had a more favorable pathologic staging as compared with those found in the control group.

Another controlled trial evaluating fecal occult blood testing was initiated at the University of Minnesota. In this study, 48,000 participants (age 50 or over) were assigned randomly to 1 of 3 study groups, consisting of those who received Hemoccult slide testing each year, those who received Hemoccult slide testing every other year, and a control group. The overall rate of slide positivity was 2.4%. Persons found to have positive slides were requested to have a diagnostic examination including radiography and colonoscopy. Barium enema examinations were of the solid column type. Of 873 patients who had positive tests and who underwent diagnostic evaluation, 72 (9%) had cancer of the colon or rectum, the majority (78%) of which were classified as Dukes A or B cancers. This study is now in a rescreening and follow-up stage. The highest yield of neoplastic lesions was in patients 63 years of age or older, but this may be a factor of the older age of the patients entering this study.[92, 115, 116] The essentials of these 2 studies are combined and summarized in Table 139–5.

The Hemoccult slide is sensitive to less than 1 mg/ml of hemoglobin in aqueous solution.[235] Laboratory studies also suggest that the Hemoccult II slide is more sensitive than the single Hemoccult slide previously used. Rehydration alters the apparent sensitivity of slides to hemoglobin.[91, 117] One reason for this effect is the dissolution of desiccated hemoglobin before the addition of the alcohol developing agent. However, hemoglobin is not the only component reactivated following rehydration. Other interfering compounds, such as peroxidases present in bacteria and certain foods, are also rehydrated. Our observation has been that hydration of the Hemoccult II slide does indeed increase clinical sensitivity, but this increases false-positivity to an extent unacceptable for screening. Therefore, this procedure has been eliminated within our program. Rehydration, however, is still being used in other programs. Studies reported from Australia[118] confirm an increased sensitivity of rehydrated slides and also a high rate of false-positivity. They suggest, however, that the high rate of false-positivity resulting from rehydration of slides can be reduced by the use of a low-peroxidase diet.[119]

Currently there are several products commercially available to the international medical community capable of detecting blood in the stool. In the United States, Australia, and Europe the Hemoccult slide test is the product that has received the most extensive clinical and technical evaluation. Other slides that are currently available include HemoFec (Boehringer-Mannheim, Mannheim, West Germany); Quik-Cult (Laboratory Diagnostics, Morganville, New Jersey); ColoScreen (Helena Labs., Beaumont, Texas); Colo-Rect (Roche Labs., Nutley, New Jersey); Haemoscreen (E. Merck Diagnostica, Darmstadt,

West Germany); Fe-Cult (Gamma Diagnostica, Houston, Texas); and Hema-Chek (Ames Division, Miles Laboratories, Elkhart, Indiana). Two kits now have a quality control window.

In addition to the guaiac and orthotoluidine chemical tests for peroxidase activity, an immunochemical test has been proposed that is specific for human hemoglobin, thus eliminating the false-positivity resulting from peroxidase activity derived from non-human hemoglobin and non-hemoglobin sources.[129] This test is at present more complex than the chemical fecal occult blood test but, if simplified, may become clinically applicable in the near future.

Proctosigmoidoscopy. It has been estimated that approximately 10% of colorectal cancers can be detected by rectal digital examination and that 50% of colorectal cancers and adenomas can be detected by rigid proctosigmoidoscopy. The conventional rigid proctosigmoidoscope has the potential for evaluating the distal 25 cm of colon, in which approximately 50% of colorectal neoplastic lesions occur. However, rigid proctosigmoidoscopy has never developed into a popular screening method, probably because of the discomfort it produces. Moreover, this instrument is not consistently inserted beyond 16 cm and many false-negative examinations may result from failure to visualize the region from 16 to 25 cm[121] (Chapter 42).

In recent years, flexible sigmoidoscopes 60 to 65 cm in length have been shown to give greater yield with less discomfort than the rigid proctosigmoidoscope. However, the use of the longer flexible instruments, which are sophisticated and expensive, requires considerable training and expertise. A prototype 30-cm flexible sigmoidoscope has been developed for general use as a substitute for the rigid proctosigmoidoscope (Fig. 139–9). Preliminary studies indicate that in the hands of family practice physicians and nurse practitioners, 30 cm of distal bowel can be consistently examined with this instrument with a minimum of training and minimal patient discomfort.

The value of proctosigmoidoscopy has been demonstrated in several studies. In a study of asymptomatic persons performed at the Strang Clinic–Preventive Medicine Institute, 58 cases of early rectosigmoid cancer were detected in approximately 26,000 patient examinations.[122] In this group of patients, approximately 88% of the cancers were classified as Dukes' A and B lesions; follow-up has shown 90% survival in 50 patients followed for 15 years. In another study,[123] periodic proctosigmoidoscopy resulted in mortality reduction for colorectal cancer in the screened group. At the University of Minnesota, rectosigmoid surveillance by proctosigmoidoscopy followed by identification and removal of observed polyps, practiced for over 25 years, reduced the incidence of rectosigmoid cancer expected in this group.[17] It seems, therefore, that some type of proctosigmoidoscopy has potential value in screening of patients for cancer detection as well as for detection and removal of adenomas and thus interruption of the adenoma-cancer sequence.

Tumor Markers. Additional screening tests have been evaluated as potential indicators of the presence of malignancy or the presence of phenotypic expression of a genetic trait (see Chapter 254 for a detailed outline of tumor markers and antigens). These screening tests have included (1) studies of fibroblasts in the skin of patients with familial polyposis and Gardner's syndrome; (2) tissue culture studies of chromosomal tetraploidy in epithelial cells obtained from skin biopsy specimens of patients with Gardner's syndrome; (3) studies of defects in recognitive immunity in mixed leukocyte cultures in patients with inherited colon cancer; (4) detection of proliferative abnormalities on biopsy specimens and in washings from the colon of patients with a variety of premalignant and malignant disorders, including genetic and non-genetic colon cancer; and (5) washings for carcinoembryonic antigen (CEA) from colonic lavage. To date, no such markers have been found that are clinically applicable in standard-risk patients. Markers are

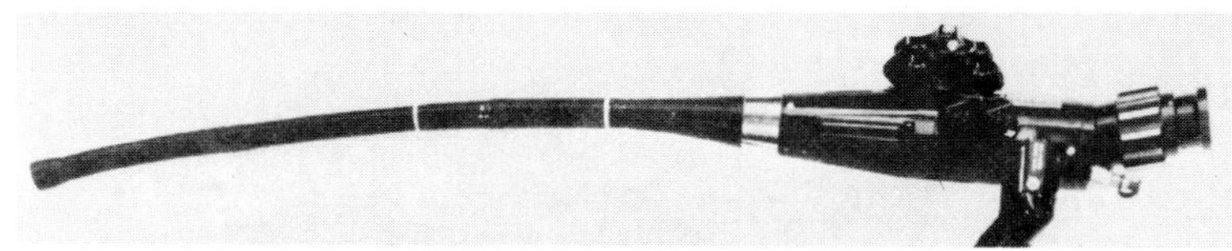

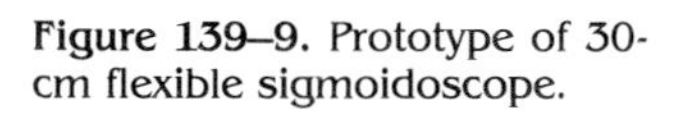

Figure 139–9. Prototype of 30-cm flexible sigmoidoscope.

needed less in the polyposis syndromes since there is good phenotypic expression of the disorder, i.e., the presence of polyps. No such phenotypic expression is present in patients with inherited colon cancer or in standard-risk patients and, thus, any marker that can be developed for application in these groups would be of utmost importance.

CEA has been studied extensively as a potential indicator of colorectal cancer.[124, 125] Unfortunately, as noted in the preceding consideration of its use as a diagnostic measure, it has not fulfilled its initial promise as a sensitive and specific biologic marker for the detection of early colorectal cancer. Most patients with elevated CEA values and colorectal cancer have advanced disease. In addition, elevated values occur in a wide variety of benign diseases. More severe disease, more extensive anatomic involvement, a younger age, and a shorter duration of disease are more likely to result in an elevation of CEA. There does not seem to be a consistent relationship between CEA elevation and known risk factors for the development of carcinoma. This applies to patients with inflammatory bowel disease who may show variations in CEA levels during the course of their disease, diminishing the value of CEA as an indicator of early carcinoma in these patients.

Guidelines for Screening and Case Finding

Average-Risk Groups. Guidelines have been developed by the American Cancer Society and also by the International Workgroup on Colorectal Cancer that address many of the issues that have been cited.[126, 127] The International Workgroup felt that analysis of available data allowed the following recommendations to be made:

1. If screening of individuals and small groups is to be promoted:
   a. Persons at risk should be encouraged to enter the health care system.
   b. Relative risk should be assessed by family and personal history questionnaires.
   c. Once patients are in the system, screening should be added to other aspects of medical evaluation.
   d. Screening should include proctosigmoidoscopy once every 3 to 5 years beginning between the ages of 40 and 50; a rigid sigmoidoscope should be used if this is the only available instrument, but flexible sigmoidoscopy (a 60-cm instrument used by a trained endoscopist or a 30-cm instrument used by a primary practicing physician or paraprofessional taught to use the instrument) is preferred.
   e. Screening should include fecal occult blood testing annually beginning between the ages of 40 and 50 (Table 139–6).
   f. Diagnostic work-up of patients with a positive screening test should include colonoscopy (Fig. 139–10).
2. Screening may be encouraged for individuals and small groups, but general or mass screening cannot be encouraged until firm mortality data pertaining to risk and cost are available from ongoing programs.
3. Screening should be accompanied by programs to educate patients and heighten physician awareness of the concepts and technology involved in screening diagnosis, treatment, and follow-up.
4. Proper record-keeping and data collection should be part of any screening program.
5. Patients with a diagnosis of colorectal neoplasia should enter a long-range follow-up surveillance program with periodic direct re-examination of the colon every 3 to 5 years.

The American Cancer Society's recommendations differ from the foregoing in that patients over the age of 40 are advised to have digital rectal examinations annually, with the stool guaiac test added at age 50 on an annual basis and with proctosigmoidoscopy every 3

Table 139–6. GUIDELINES FOR FECAL OCCULT BLOOD TEST

Not Applicable
Patients with symptoms suggesting colorectal neoplasia
Patients with familial polyposis or Gardner's syndrome
Patients with ulcerative colitis
As Primary Screen or Case Finding
Asymptomatic average-risk men and women over age 40 to 50
Suggestive family history in patients over age 20
As Adjunctive Interval Test
Patients with past history of adenoma
Patients with past history of colorectal cancer
Patients with strong history of family cancer syndrome

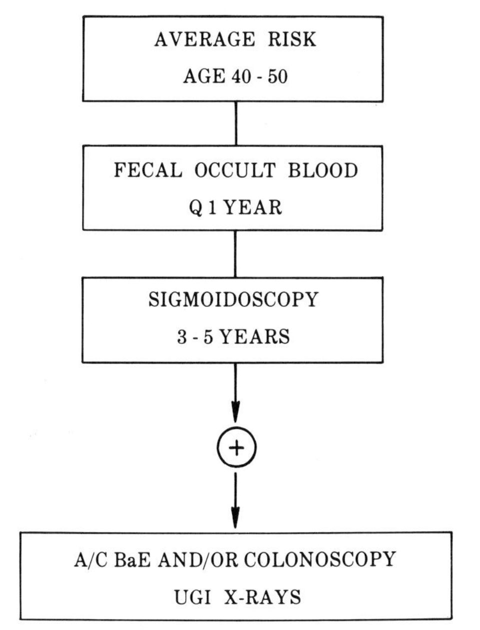

Figure 139–10. Algorithm for surveillance of average-risk patients.

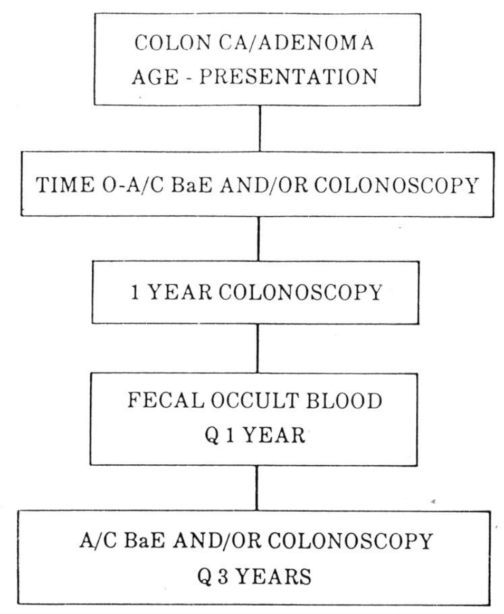

Figure 139–11. Algorithm for surveillance of patients who have had either a colon cancer or an adenoma.

to 5 years after 2 initial negative proctosigmoidoscopic examinations done 1 year apart.

The rationale for both recommendations is the suggestive evidence that the detection of colon cancer before the onset of signs and symptoms uncovers less advanced disease and should prolong survival.

High-Risk Groups. The recommendations just cited relate to average-risk patients. Patients who have already been operated on (and hopefully cured of colorectal cancer), as well as patients who have had a previous colonoscopic polypectomy, should have their colon cleared of additional synchronous lesions initially and then checked at periodic intervals thereafter (Fig. 139–11). Fecal occult blood testing may have a role as one interval examination in such high-risk groups. Fecal occult blood testing may also have some role in the non-polyposis inherited colon cancer syndromes. Patients with autosomal dominant modes of inheritance should be examined directly by radiography and/or colonoscopy at periodic intervals (Fig. 139–12). Fecal occult blood testing could serve as an interval examination in this group of patients. Patients having a suggestive family history of a non-polyposis colon cancer syndrome, but not one of an autosomal dominant form, could have fecal occult blood testing and perhaps proctosigmoidoscopy performed starting at age 20 when the risk begins. Fecal occult blood testing has no role in screening patients with familial polyposis or ulcerative colitis since the existing lesions may cause positive reactions in the absence of superimposed cancer.

Patients with ulcerative colitis of more than 7 years' duration and involving the entire colon should have annual examinations on a regularly scheduled sequential basis, as outlined later in the discussion of inflammatory bowel disease as a cancer risk factor. As also

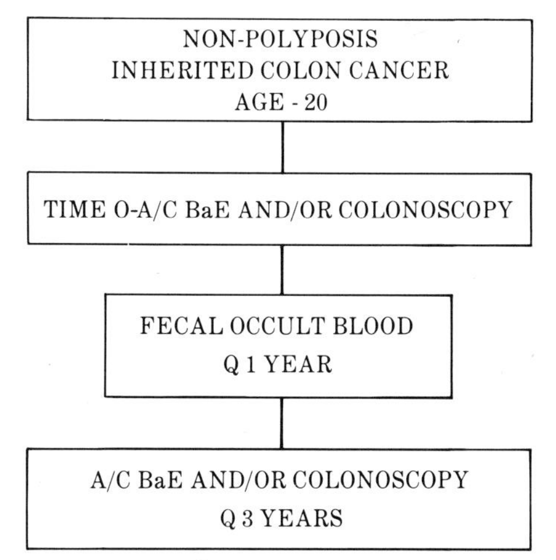

Figure 139–12. Algorithm for surveillance of patients with a family history of non-polyposis inherited colon cancer.

indicated in the discussion of inflammatory bowel disease, surveillance should be conducted as well in patients with colitis involving only the left colon, but need not be begun until later after the onset of disease.

Treatment

Surgical Treatment of the Primary Lesion

Curative Surgery. The principles guiding the curative treatment of large bowel cancer are based upon an understanding of the patterns of direct extension of tumor, the patterns of primary lymph node spread from colon or rectum cancer, and the evidence from multiple surgical series concerning the value of radical mesenteric lymphadenectomy as the guideline for adequate resection.

In 1908, Miles[128] demonstrated that the primary route of spread of rectal cancer was upward to lymph nodes along the superior hemorrhoidal artery—the "zone of upward spread"—overlying the left iliac vessels. This mesenteric route of spread was the basis upon which Miles advocated abdominoperineal resection for rectal cancer. Until that time, the common practice was excision of the primary tumor (with or without rectal amputation) and proximal colostomy, in no way treating routes of spread. Since the vast majority of lesions were classified as Dukes C cases, amputation alone offered no chance of cure, and the introduction of a mesenteric resection by Miles was a landmark in cancer therapy. In 1909, Jamieson and Dobson[129] demonstrated that lymph nodes subservient to the colon followed the named arterial blood supply. They proposed that resectable lymph node spread, at any site in the colon, could be found up to the very origins of the regional arterial blood supply. On this basis, they recommended that proper resection for rectal cancer should proceed from the origin of the inferior mesenteric artery. During the first 4 decades of the 20th century, various authors reported on the patterns of lymph node spread from primary rectal or colonic adenocarcinoma, further corroborating the value of these earlier reports.

In 1940 and 1941, Coller and co-workers[47, 50] reported on the effect of lymph node distribution from rectal and colonic carcinomas on the choice of operations. Colonic carcinomas spread to epicolic and paracolic lymph nodes before involving intermediate nodes within the regional mesentery. Rectal cancers spread in different patterns, based upon their distance from the anal verge. Cancers 5 or 6 cm above the anal verge, i.e., cancers of the middle or upper rectum, spread upward within the mesorectum to lymph nodes along the superior hemorrhoidal artery, as described by Miles. Cancers of the lower rectum have a wider spread, extending laterally as well to lymph nodes situated along the pelvic side walls (the internal iliac or hypogastric nodes) and, even more distally, to nodes along the middle hemorrhoidal arteries. In addition, Coller et al.[50] demonstrated that low-lying rectal cancers were responsible for discontinuous lymph node spread (positive proximal nodes with intervening negative nodes) to the upper sigmoid mesentery. This primary pattern of spread ensures a lower overall survival due to distant spread, a higher percentage of local recurrence, and a greater role for multidisciplinary treatment in lower rectal cancer than in cancers of the middle or upper rectum or the colon above the rectum. On the basis of these dissections, Coller and co-workers advocated that the modern abdominoperineal resection (APR) of the rectum should replace the Miles resection for cancers of the lower rectum. At the same time, the rationale for advocating sphincter-preserving operations for middle or upper rectal cancer was implicit in these data.

In 1959, Rosi[130] advocated widening the scope of resection to left hemicolectomy for left colon carcinomas, and in 1962 Rosi and Carey[131] reported an appreciable increase in 5-year survival and decline in local recurrence resulting from radical mesenteric resection. A major contribution in support of radical resection came from the Cleveland Clinic in 1967 when Turnbull et al.[132] described their experience with the "no-touch" isolation technique. Turnbull and co-workers compared the results of their radical mesenteric resection using the "no-touch" technique against the results achieved by colleagues utilizing "conventional surgery," i.e., segmental or limited resections, and found the survival rate higher following "no-touch" resections. Subsequently, Stearns[133] demonstrated that the value of Turnbull's operation probably resided in the extent of the mesenteric resection rather than just the first-step vascular interruption. Stearns and Schottenfeld,[134] as well as Enker and his associates[48] in 1979, described results supporting the value of radical mesenteric resection with high ligation or pelvic lymph node dissection.

Several misconceptions are frequently associated with the idea of radical surgery by those who advocate limited or segmental resections. The first is that the frequency of permanent colostomy is necessarily higher with radical compared with limited resection. However, the pelvic dissection can be radical yet still permit appropriately selected sphincter-preserving procedure for middle or upper rectal cancer. In our current experience at Memorial Sloan-Kettering Cancer Center, approximately 85% of the patients undergoing resections for cancer of the middle rectum have low anterior resection with radical pelvic dissection that ends in primary or colorectal or colo-anal reconstruction.

The second misconception is that the salvage of cases will be 5% to 7% overall, at most, and that this will pertain in only stage C disease. While it is hard to prove retrospectively that radical surgery is even beneficial in stage B_2 disease, recent data from one source[135] attests to a marked decrease in local recurrence. In stage C rectal cancer our data indicate that extended or sharp pelvic dissection along vascular margins is associated with a 54% 5-year survival as compared with only 29% when a limited pelvic blunt dissection had been performed. This survival advantage is manifest no matter which modification of the Dukes classification is examined (Table 139–7). Since approximately 35% to 40% of patients have positive nodes, this difference translates into the lives of 10 additional patients for each 40 patients with stage C lesions, or 10 of 100 cases of large bowel cancer overall. In a disease in which other modalities of adjuvant therapy carry serious morbidity and are still of unproven survival value, this 25% advantage in stage C lesions is an appreciable contribution to survival by a means that requires only a moderate alteration of surgical approach. This is especially true in view of the fact that colorectal cancer cannot be accurately staged intraoperatively (i.e., stage A from stage B from stage C) except in cases with obvious metastases.

The third misconception is that the operative morbidity and mortality outweigh any value ascribed to the more radical procedure. The morbidity following resection by experienced surgeons who repeatedly perform radical pelvic dissection is no higher than that occurring after limited resection. On the rectum and colon service at Memorial Sloan-Kettering Cancer Center, the operative mortality of radical resection is 2.7% for the period from 1968 to 1976. This figure is well within the lower range of operative mortality reported in all major series and is certainly no higher for radical than for less extensive procedures.

SURGICAL APPROACHES ACCORDING TO SITE OF LESION. The large bowel derives its blood supply from 3 major vessels: the superior mesenteric artery, the inferior mesenteric artery, and the hypogastric or internal iliac arteries (Chapter 131). The primary lymph nodes for any given segment of bowel are found along the named arteries and veins that are regionally related to the site of the primary tumor. The design of any given resection is based upon the anatomic site of the primary tumor and the presence or absence of adjacent organ involvement.[135]

Carcinoma of the Cecum and Ascending Colon. The appropriate operation is a right radical hemicolectomy. The right colic, ileocolic, and right branches of the middle colic arteries and veins are sacrificed at their origins. The mesentery is divided to the right of the mid-

Table 139–7. IMPROVED 5-YEAR SURVIVAL OF PATIENTS WITH DUKES C RECTAL CANCER AFTER PELVIC LYMPHADENECTOMY VS. CONVENTIONAL RESECTIONS

Staging	Extended Resection	Conventional Resection	p Value
Dukes C	54%	29%	.004
Astler-Coller			
C_1	83%	41%	.008
C_2	38%	24%	.06
GITSG*			
C_1	57%	34%	.03
C_2	41%	16%	.06

*GITSG = Gastrointestinal Tumor Study Group.

transverse colon. Posteriorly, the transverse mesocolon is dissected away from the right ureter, duodenum, and pancreas. An end-to-side or end-to-end ileocolostomy may then be performed.

Carcinoma of the Hepatic Flexure. Potentially curable spread of tumor may involve lymph nodes along the right colic vessels and the middle colic vessels. These vessels are taken at their origin. This resection sacrifices all of the right colon and most of the transverse colon. The operation is referred to as an extended right radical hemicolectomy. After its completion, the ileum may be anastomosed to the left transverse colon.

Carcinoma of the Transverse Colon. The resection is based entirely on the middle colic arteries according to their origins. The middle colic vessels may form a vascular arcade occupying the entire transverse mesocolon. The gastrocolic ligament is divided along the gastroepiploic vessels, and the transverse mesocolon is resected along its entire length at the base of the pancreas, avoiding injury to the duodenum. The right colon is generally sacrificed, and an ileocolic anastomosis is performed in the descending colon.

Carcinoma of the Splenic Flexure. This operation incorporates some features of the transverse colectomy as well as some features of the left hemicolectomy. Both the middle colic arteries and the left colic artery are at risk for nodal metastases. The left colic artery is divided, sparing the inferior mesenteric artery and its sigmoidal branches. The left branch of the middle colic artery or the origin of the entire middle colic artery is taken. While some surgeons might undertake to anastomose the right colon to the distal descending or sigmoid colon, the resulting tension would suggest that an ileo–descending colon or ileosigmoid anastomosis is safer. There is no evidence to suggest that splenectomy enhances survival in patients with cancer of the splenic flexure. In fact, splenectomy may be associated with a decreased survival. Some authors advocate left hemicolectomy, which, however, does not allow for the potential for spread along the middle colic route.

Carcinoma of the Descending Colon. Lesions situated in the descending colon below the splenic flexure are treated by left radical hemicolectomy. The resection is based on the origin of the inferior mesenteric artery at the aorta. The inferior mesenteric vein is divided above the duodenum at the inferior border of the pancreas. The line of mesenteric division follows the plane of vascular interruption up to the left branches of the middle colic artery. The inferior or distal margin of resection is in the distal sigmoid colon. Anastomosis of the transverse colon to the upper rectosigmoid or distal sigmoid is usually performed in end-to-end fashion. Care must be taken to prevent injury to the left ureter and to the spleen, as the entire left-sided mesocolon is dissected away from the retroperitoneum up to the duodenum or to the right edge of the aorta.

Cancer of the Sigmoid Colon. Resection is again based upon the origin of the inferior mesenteric artery. The procedure is tailored to the location of the lesion, i.e., lesions of the proximal sigmoid may require treatment as if they were left colon lesions, while cancers of the distal sigmoid may require dissection of the iliac and aortic bifurcation nodes along with the specimen. Ideally located lesions of the middle sigmoid are dealt with by radical sigmoid resection. The inferior mesenteric vein is again divided inferior to the pancreas. The splenic flexure is usually mobilized, allowing anastomosis of the mid-descending colon to the rectum without any tension. The remaining left colon need not be removed since the lymphatic drainage is central, i.e., along the inferior mesenteric vessels and not along the marginal vessels.

Carcinoma of the Rectum. The rectum may be defined as the distal 12 cm of the large bowel as it lies, undisturbed, in its usual place. Blood supply to the rectum is derived from the superior hemorrhoidal branches of the inferior mesenteric artery and from the middle hemorrhoidal branches of the internal iliac or hypogastric vessels. The distal rectum and the anus are supplied also by the inferior hemorrhoidal vessels. The principles guiding resection for cancer of the rectum are:

1. Cancers situated 6 to 12 cm from the anal verge usually spread to nodes along the superior hemorrhoidal artery within the mesentery overlying the left common iliac vessels.
2. Cancer within 6 cm of the anal verge may also spread laterally by way of the internal iliac nodes.
3. Only 4% of cancers of the rectum grow submucosally for a distance greater than 2 cm distally, or caudally, from the visible edge of the epithelial tumor; thus, a 5-cm distal margin is usually sufficient.[49]

Factors that influence selection of treatment include: (1) the distance of the cancer from the anal verge; (2) the size and configuration of the tumor; (3) the presence or absence of adjacent organ invasion and/or fixation; (4) an anterior or posterior location; (5) the sex of the patient, as regards to pelvic configuration; (6) the available methods of reconstruction; and (7) the degree of differentiation by preoperative biopsy.[136]

As a rule, cancers of the upper rectum are amenable to anterior resection. The scope of this operation extends from the origin of the inferior mesenteric artery. The lateral dissection involves the aortic, aortic bifurcation, and common iliac nodes, along with the entire mesentery, allowing access to the presacral space within the endopelvic fascia, i.e., peripheral to all mesorectal fat. This plane is used for the pelvic dissection. A 5-cm undistorted margin below the distal edge of the tumor is obtained *in vivo*. To achieve this length, the lateral ligaments are divided and the rectum is extensively mobilized to the posterior junction of the levator muscles. If sufficient rectum exists for reconstruction, the low anterior resection is completed by colorectal anastomosis.

In patients who are elderly, previously irradiated, or otherwise ill or if contamination, perforation, or a questionably sound anastomosis is present, a diverting colostomy should be performed.

For cancers of the distal 6 cm of rectum, *abdominoperineal resection* is the accepted and appropriate operation. The dissection of the rectum is accomplished as far as the levators from within the abdomen. The lateral ligaments are divided at the pelvic side walls; the middle hemorrhoidal arteries may be occluded without compromising the lateral dissection. The procedure is completed with the perineal phase.

Cancers in the mid-rectum may be treated by abdominoperineal resection, but a sphincter-preserving operation is preferable. Dissection of the inferior mesenteric artery begins at its origin. Sharp lateral dissection is made along pelvic vascular planes. After obtaining the necessary 5 cm of resection, reconstruction is accomplished by any of a number of satisfactory means, including use of circular anastomotic staplers. The latter device offers the possibility of reconstruction when there is little rectum remaining after resection, especially in men. Operating time, in our experience, may be slightly shorter when the EEA circular anastomotic stapler is used than when a hand-sutured anastomosis is constructed. Under certain circumstances, moreover, the EEA stapling instrument has allowed the creation of lower anastomoses than would otherwise be possible.

Other methods have been reported, including pull-through procedures of various types. These, however, may be associated with disappointingly high complication rates and with poor anorectal function. While cure rates regarding cancer may seem acceptable following pull-through procedures, unsatisfactory defecation may be more troublesome than the simple management of a well-constructed colostomy.

Colo-anal anastomoses are being employed more frequently for restoring continuity in patients when the 5-cm margin coincides with the levator-anal junction, but such procedures are still under scrutiny. The distal rectum may be sacrificed entirely to the anal verge. The proximal colon may then be mobilized into the pelvis and the primary anastomosis performed transanally.[137]

ADJACENT ORGAN INVASION. Approximately 10% of large bowel cancers, especially rectal and rectosigmoid lesions, will be found adherent to or invading an adjacent organ. Although the most common sites of invasion include the male and female genitourinary systems and the female genitalia, many other organs in the abdominal cavity may be involved by a cancer of the large bowel. Sites of adherence or invasion should be treated by resection rather than by dissection. Many of these patients will have locally extensive tumors without nodal metastases. In general, 50% or more of these patients may be cured of their disease by aggressive resection.[138]

"INOPERABLE" OR "UNRESECTABLE" CANCER OF THE LARGE BOWEL. Few cancers of the large bowel are really either inoperable or unresectable. Preoperative irradiation may convert such lesions to an operable condition. A high proportion of lesions declared inoperable after a previous laparotomy may still be resectable for cure in the hands of surgeons whose experience is concentrated in the management of this disease.[139]

Palliative Surgery. Preoperative staging, while detecting some cases of advanced disease, will fail to detect the majority with visceral metastases or peritoneal involvement. Thus, it remains for certain treatment decisions to be made at the time of operation. For those patients found with distant metastases at laparotomy, a resection of the primary tumor should be accomplished if this can be done without the obvious prospect of appreciably increased morbidity. If multi-staged operations might be needed, i.e., resection and colostomy followed by colostomy closure, it is well to consider options that avoid the second operation, if at all possible. If intra-abdominal disease involves multiple organs, e.g., a right-sided lesion that rests on or involves the duodenum, and dissection indicates that a significant risk of injury exists, bypass may prove to be the better option than resection. This is especially true when encountering widespread carcinomatosis or tumor that has infiltrated the mesentery in such a way that resection would necessitate transecting obviously neoplastic tissue. Also, a colostomy should be avoided in the presence of carcinomatosis in order to avoid exteriorizing the tumor and creating a leak of ascites.

In rectal cancer, bulky tumors should be resected despite the presence of metastatic disease in order to avoid the relentless symptoms of persistent pelvic disease, such as tenesmus, pain, mucorrhea, burning, and bleeding. These are extremely difficult to palliate otherwise. Resection and radiation therapy are of incalculable value to the patient who might otherwise suffer needlessly.

When the risk of local recurrence is deemed high, permanent colostomy is preferable to reconstruction. If resection and primary anastomosis are possible in smaller upper rectal lesions, that remains the procedure of choice. For lower rectal lesions that are small enough to be amenable to local control, repeated fulgurations with palliative intent are an acceptable means of delaying or avoiding a colostomy in selected cases.

Local Treatment of Rectal Carcinoma. The local treatment of rectal cancer has been progressively changing in emphasis from destruction *in situ* to local excision *in toto*. The majority of patients treated by local methods in the first half of this century underwent fulguration techniques. Many of these were considered palliative procedures, especially in the elderly, until Madden and Kandalaft[140] advocated the use of fulguration as the primary and preferred method of treating all rectal cancers that otherwise would require abdominoperineal resection. Objections to this broad-sweeping policy were based upon failure of this treatment to cure stage C disease, the failure of the technique to provide material suitable for pathologic evaluation, and the abuse of electrocoagulation by repeated application despite local failures.[141]

There is general agreement, however, that certain, carefully selected early rectal carcinomas do not require abdominoperineal resection. Early cancers of the rectum, distinguished by criteria such as small size and extreme mobility, are preferred lesions for local treatment. Most such cancers represent only early and localized invasion of the submucosa or local penetration of the muscularis propria and have only a 10.9% to 12.9% chance of lymph node metastases. Surgeons at Memorial Hospital in New York and at St. Mark's Hospital in London have practiced local excision *in toto* of selected rectal cancers for decades but this procedure has been used only rarely (3% of the cases treated at Memorial Hospital). The choice of local excision over fulguration is favored because excision provides the pathologist with an intact specimen for histologic examination. Criteria such as full-thickness penetration, poor differentiation, a positive margin, venous or lymphatic vessel invasion, or a significant mucinous component can be evaluated carefully. A decision can then be made whether to offer further definite resection in those cases in which local excision would be inadequate treatment.

Utilizing this approach, Stearns and colleagues[142] have reported the results of local treatment in 58 patients from 1954 to 1978. Thirty-one patients had surgical excision, while 27 patients underwent cautery snare excision. The latter was generally performed for tumors of the upper rectum in elderly patients for whom the desire to avoid general anesthesia influenced the selection of treatment. Of the 31 patients treated by local surgical excision, 25 (80%) are considered to have been cured. Cautery snare was found to be an inadequate form of treatment, with a 5-year survival of only 45%.

In Morson's review[75] in 1966 of factors influencing prognosis, the rare occurrence of lymph node metastases preceding mural penetration (10.9% to 12.9%) was mainly associated with the presence of poorly differentiated tumors. In 1977, Morson et al.[143] again reviewed the histologic findings in association with local excision at St. Mark's Hospital. Of 91 tumors that were considered completely excised, only 3 recurred; 11 of these patients had a major resection after local excision. In 18 patients in whom the completeness of the excision was in doubt, 2 patients had tumor recurrence. In 23 patients in whom the excision was clearly incomplete, 14 had no further surgery, the excision being considered palliative. Lock et al.[144] have reported on the local treatment of rectal cancer at St. Mark's Hospital between 1948 and 1972. Of 22 patients with sessile rectal cancers treated for cure, 15 patients underwent local excision; only 1 died of cancer. In selecting cases for local treatment, lesions of 3 cm or larger should be excluded; tumors of this size should be treated by definitive resection.

Morson and co-workers[143] probably have put local excision into its proper perspective. Local excision should be considered "a form of total biopsy" following which a thorough histologic examination can help determine whether the excision was complete or whether aggressive tumor characteristics indicate the advisability of a further radical operation. The combined clinical and pathologic selection of patients for local treatment offers the best chances of continued success when this treatment is considered applicable.

Treatment of Obstructing and Perforated Carcinomas. The clinical management of *obstructing* colonic carcinoma is a matter of continuing debate. Obstructing cancers have classically been handled by a staged series of 3 operations: colostomy, resection, and colostomy closure. Modern advocates propose, however, that obstructing lesions be handled by primary resection and reconstruction. They base their claim on 2 main premises: (1) the long-term survival after primary resection is better, and (2) the cumulative mortality inherent in the 3-stage procedure is prohibitive. Not clearly explained is how the surgeon selects patients for colostomy only or for resection or patients for primary anastomosis or for delay in reconstruction. There are as yet no guidelines for the correct prospective selection of which patients to manage by laparotomy and resection in preference to a diverting colostomy alone. Hopefully, such guidelines may be forthcoming from prospective studies currently in progress.

The management of colonic *perforation* generally parallels that of obstruction. The 5-year survival is very poor and is generally associated with the presence of either distant metastases or widespread lymphatic disease and/or peritoneal seeding. In the patient without obvious distant tumor spread and in whom perforation has prompted laparotomy, the best policy is immediate radical resection, if at all consistent with the patient's condition.

Treatment of Recurrent or Metastatic Disease

Surgical

LOCAL RECURRENCE. Although peri-anastomotic recurrence rarely occurs when adequate resection is practiced, such local recurrence as may develop may be amenable to further resection. In this setting, the 5-year survival of patients with resectable recurrence depends upon the extent of residual disease after operation. Patients undergoing resection for cure have been reported to have a 5-year survival of 49%; in those with microscopic residual disease, the survival rate was 12%.[145] The vast majority of patients developing recurrent disease after the adequate anatomic resections cannot undergo re-resection for cure.

In patients who have had limited or segmental resections and who present with recurrence, a careful evaluation should be conducted to exclude distant disease. Liver scan, ultrasonography, computed tomography (of the liver, abdomen, and pelvis), liver enzyme studies, CEA determination, chest radiography, and colonoscopy should be performed in the absence of obvious metastatic disease and when resection is considered a possibility. If all tests prove negative for metastases, the feasibility of exploratory surgery for resection can be discussed with the patient. Even then, the majority of patients will turn out to have distant metastases in addition to the local recurrence, preventing the possibility of cure. For this reason, cases must be carefully selected.

PELVIC RECURRENCE. Pelvic recurrence frequently complicates the course of rectal cancer. Anastomotic recurrence is rarely isolated, and more often than not it is an index of pelvic disease with broad side wall or sacral involvement. Frequently, to prevent such recurrence or to treat it, 4000 to 5000 rads of external beam radiation therapy will be administered. In the course of management, patients will frequently present with small bowel obstruction due to a combination of recurrent tumor and radiation enteritis. Dissection of the pelvis cannot achieve cure. On the contrary, it can add serious septic complications, such as abscess and fistulas to an otherwise easily handled circumstance. When recurrent rectal cancer is complicated by small bowel obstruction, especially in the presence of irradiated intestine, single or multiple enteroenterostomy bypasses achieve palliation with safety and with relative ease.

PERINEAL RECURRENCE. Perineal recurrence generally develops under 1 of 4 conditions: (1) Inadequate margins of resection following abdominoperineal resection; (2) low rectal cancer of the poorly differentiated, widely infiltrating type with separate nests of tumor in the perirectal fat; (3) delay in management of a known cancer; and (4) unjustified or repeated use of fulguration technique.

When visible tumor protrudes through the perineum, relief of pain and infection is the palliative goal, thereby allowing the patient to sit comfortably. An effective technique of palliation includes excision of obvious tumor followed by electrocoagulation to achieve tumor necrosis. This technique differs significantly from fulguration and creates a gradual slough of tumor that is not likely to bleed extensively. Topical antiseptics, such as povidone-iodine and potassium permanganate solution, are helpful adjuncts. For cases in which perineal recurrence is resectable, careful assessment will invariably demonstrate that the visible tumor is only "the tip of the iceberg." Frequently, recurrent cancer will be resectable along with virtually intact levator ani muscles as margins. Brachytherapy (short-range radiation therapy employing implanted catheters or seeds containing radioactive substances) may be of value as an adjunct to treatment when a margin of resection proves positive.

LIVER METASTASES. Approximately 20% of patients at laparotomy for resection of large bowel cancer will be found to have liver metastases. This may escape examination when the all-too-common left lower quadrant paramedian incision is employed, i.e., when the liver is not felt and seen. The extent of liver involvement should be described systematically. Metastases may be single or multiple, unilobar or multilobar, and may occupy as much as 75% of the liver substance. A histologic diagnosis of liver metastases is mandatory. Lacking such documentation in a previously operated patient may necessitate another laparotomy for biopsy only or, worse, may prevent or delay the advent of palliative therapy.

The management of liver metastases complicating large bowel cancer remains an evolving discipline. For about 3 decades, surgeons have elected to remove solitary hepatic metastases when such a procedure would render the patient clinically free of disease. This is possible because some primary tumors, i.e., the Dukes B lesion, may show no residual local disease but may have a single focus of hematogenous spread to the liver. Such an aggressive surgical approach has been rewarding in the experience at several institutions. For example, Adson,[146] at the Mayo Clinic, has reported a 5-year survival rate of 42% in 40 patients who underwent resection of apparent solitary metastases; the 10-year survival rate was 28%. At Memorial Sloan-Kettering Cancer Center, Fortner et al.[147] have indicated that of 137 liver resections, 43 have been in patients with colorectal metastases. In the stage 1 cases (no vascular or biliary invasion), the survival rates in 39 survivors are 96% at 1 year, 79% at 2 years, and 71% at 3 years. When the value of liver resection was first undergoing scrutiny at Memorial Hospital, the fate of 25 patients with resected solitary metastases was compared with the fate of 12 patients in whom solitary tumors were identified but left unresected. The 5-year survival rates were 28% and zero, respectively.[148]

Foster and Lundy,[149] in a nationwide survey, have documented 46 survivors for 5 years (22%) among 206 patients who underwent a liver resection. Today, when liver resection is being considered but laparotomy demonstrates the presence of multifocal bilobar disease, the possibilities of pump implantation to deliver therapeutic agents make the overall operative effort far more rewarding.[150] The identification of patients with early liver disease, e.g., by markers such as CEA, remains one of the critical and unsolved problems in this field.

Non-surgical

RADIATION THERAPY. Radiation therapy has been an effective means of providing palliation in localized unresectable metastatic disease[151–153] (see Chapter 256 for a more extended discussion). Radiation is used primarily for relief of pain, but has also been useful in diminishing tenesmus, bleeding, and discharge from inoperable rectal cancers. The rectum has a higher tolerance to radiotherapy than the colon, and 5000 rads over 4 to 5 weeks seems to achieve the best remission rate.[154] Implantation radiation may be applied during surgery, and areas planned for external beam radiotherapy may be marked by metallic clips. Any painful metastatic areas can be radiated, with prompt relief often after only 2000 to 3000 rads. The liver can be treated with up to 3000 rads without damage in most patients, and good palliation of painful liver metastases has been reported in a majority of those treated.[155–157] These palliative measures relieve symptoms and frequently improve performance status but do not prolong survival. Radiation is generally not effective in relieving bowel obstruction due to colorectal cancer.

In some cases, particularly of cancer of the rectum, in which surgery has been contraindicated or refused, radiation has been used as the primary treatment.[158–160] Favorable results have been obtained in early disease. To cite one example, Papillon[160] noted a 5-year survival rate of 78% after intracavitary radiation of a group of highly selected patients with small, early rectal cancers.

CHEMOTHERAPY. In unresectable colon cancer, chemotherapeutic agents are given for palliation but there is little likelihood of ameliorating symptoms and prolonging survival[161] (see Chapter 256 for more extended discussion). At the present time, there is no satisfactory, effective chemotherapy for colorectal cancer.[147a] Like most adenocarcinomas, colon cancers have slow growth rates and low rates of cell division and DNA synthesis.[162] Most chemotherapeutic drugs currently used affect dividing cells and cells undergoing DNA synthesis.[163–166]

Judging the effectiveness of chemotherapy is also difficult in patients with colorectal cancer.[167] Metastatic lesions are generally located in deep visceral areas, and response defies precise quantification. Not only is it difficult to measure response in an individual patient, but comparing responses between patients and judging reports from different investigators can be nearly impossible. Some areas of metastatic disease are easier to measure than others; e.g., metastases to skin and lymph nodes and discrete pulmonary metastases evident in chest radiographs. Liver size, on the other hand, is harder to assess because there is considerable observer variability on palpation and percussion. Computed tomography, ultrasonography, and radionuclide scans have improved the accuracy of intra-abdominal tumor measurements, but greater testing and cost containment are needed. Results of standard liver tests are non-specific. Factors such as drug toxicity or coexistent liver disease will affect these values. Assay of the activities of enzymes such as 5′-nucleotidase, gamma glutamyl transferase, and alanine aminotransferase, may be helpful in assessing the situation when there are suspected metastases to bone. CEA levels in the blood usually rise with tumor progression, fall with regression, and stay about the same when the tumor is stable. However, because of frequent exceptions to these patterns, CEA levels are best used in conjunction with other measurements of response.[168–170]

In advanced colorectal cancer, complete responses to chemotherapy are rare. Using liver size by physical examination as a major determinant of response in the presence of liver metastases, a partial response may be taken to be greater than 30% decrease in the sum of measurements of the liver edge from the costal margin, measurements being made at the xyphoid and at the midclavicular line bilaterally.[171] At the Memorial Sloan-Kettering Cancer Center, the measurements are made at the xyphoid and at 5, 10, and 15 cm to its left and right, with a partial remission defined as greater than 50% reduction in the sum of these measurements. Palliation of symptoms and determination of the quality of life in advanced colorectal cancer are even more difficult to measure, although the "performance status" developed by Karnofsky et al.[172] has been useful.

The impact of 5-fluorouracil (5-FU) on survival in colorectal cancer patients, responders and non-responders together, is marginal at best.[161] Younger patients and those with less extensive disease and higher performance status are more likely to show objective tumor response and to survive longer. There has been some indication that lung metastases are less responsive to chemotherapy than lymph node or liver lesions, but this may reflect more accurate measurement in lung disease.[167]

The response of large bowel cancer to 5-FU has been reported to range from 8% to 85%; this vast range testifies to the problems of accurate assessment of response.[161] The most widely used method is to give the drug IV. An initial loading course is given until the patient shows signs of mild toxicity consisting of stomatitis, diarrhea, or a depressed white blood count in the range of 1500 to 3500 cells/mm^3. Following recovery, a subtoxic maintenance regimen is established. Given in this way, 5-FU produces a partial response in 10% to 20% of patients for a varying period, averaging 4 to 5 months.[165] It was initially hoped that liver metastases would respond better to oral administration of 5-FU, since the absorbed drug would be carried directly to the liver by way of the portal circulation.[173, 174] Unfortunately, this did not prove to be the case. Oral administration of 5-FU is probably best reserved for the occasional instance in which IV administration is not possible.

Other single agents have been tested in colorectal cancer, but none has surpassed the minimal effectiveness of 5-FU. Notable among many are mitomycin, which produces a 10% to 15% response, but only very briefly and with limiting hematologic toxicity. Nitrosoureas, such as carmustine (BCNU) and methyl-lomustine (methyl-CCNU), yield a similar limited response. None of these agents has been effective as a salvage treatment in patients not responding to 5-FU or its analogs.[161, 167]

Combination chemotherapy, using multiple active agents at one time, has been employed, relying on adjustment of dosages and schedules to keep toxicity to a minimum.[175] A combination regimen of MOF (methyl-CCNU, vincristine [Oncovin], and 5-FU)[176] produced an overall response rate in a series of patients with colon cancer of 43% as compared with 19% among randomly chosen control subjects treated with 5-FU alone. Subsequent trials, both with and without vincristine (which by itself has no activity in colon cancer), reported responses ranging from 32% to 43%, compared with responses of 9.5% to 22% with 5-FU alone. Disappointingly, however, combination therapy has not improved survival. Indeed, one study reported that only 2 of 52 patients achieved a definite partial remission with the MOF regimen.[177] Another randomized study compared 2 different MOF schedules, one employing methyl-CCNU as a single dose and the other in divided doses over 5 days.[167] The divided dose schedule was attended by less toxicity, but both regimens produced comparable therapeutic responses and both were inferior to 5-FU alone.

Other regimens reported to show some minor advantage over 5-FU alone are combinations of BCNU and 5-FU; mitomycin and 5-FU; and 5-FU, BCNU, dacarbazine, vincristine, and methotrexate.[161] The addition of streptozotocin to the MOF regimen has been shown by Kemeny and colleagues[178] at Memorial Hospital to increase partial response rates in initial trials to the 35% range but at the price of increased gastrointestinal toxicity.

Combinations of radiation therapy and 5-FU have been used for locally metastatic disease with some limited improvement noted in symptomatic relief and survival compared with radiation alone.[179–181] Similarly, various immunostimulants have been combined with chemotherapy in patients with advanced colon cancer because chemotherapy has an immunosuppressive effect of its own. Agents such as BCG (bacille Calmette-Guérin), MER (methanol extraction residue of BCG), and levamisole have been used so far without evident benefit.[182, 183]

Despite the few small glimmerings of hope that the foregoing data might provide, it appears quite clear, as noted earlier, that adjuvant chemotherapy of colorectal cancer has little, if anything, to offer. Indeed, the most recent report to appear on this subject as of the time of this writing is quite sobering.[147a] This study, conducted by the Gastrointestinal Tumor Study Group, was prospective and randomized, was conducted at 13 institutions, involved 572 evaluable patients who entered the study between July 1975 and August 1979, and had a median follow-up time of 5½ years. The findings, compared with a control initial group of the same Dukes stage B_2, C_1 or C_2, led to the conclusion that there was no demonstrable benefit to be obtained in terms of disease-free survival or overall survival from the adjuvant use of fluorouracil/semustine chemotherapy, MER immunotherapy, or combined chemoimmunotherapy in patients with colon cancer.

Another chemotherapeutic approach to colon cancer metastatic to the liver is regional infusion of drugs directly into the hepatic circulation.[184] Theoretically, an increased antineoplastic effect may be achieved with less overall toxicity. The hepatic artery has been mainly utilized because angiographic studies indicate that most liver metastases from colon cancer get the majority of their blood supply from the hepatic artery.[185, 186] However, the vascularity of colon metastases in the liver can vary a good deal, and some investigators have also employed the portal vein for regional liver perfusion.[187, 188] The drugs used for the most part for colon cancer have been 5-FU and its analog floxuridene (FUDR).[189] Beneficial responses have been in the range of 40% to 60% but trials have been retrospective or uncontrolled against systemic therapy or have used historical controls, leaving the findings in doubt.[190–194] One prospective randomized study from the Central Oncology Group compared regional hepatic artery infusion of 5-FU with the same drug given IV in 74 patients with liver metastases from colorectal cancer.[195] No significant difference in objective response rate or survival was found and gastrointestinal toxicity was greater in the intra-arterial group.

A newer method of regional hepatic perfusion utilizes a small pump implanted subcutaneously and periodically filled by injection.[196] Catheters from the pump have been mainly placed in the hepatic artery. FUDR, which requires a smaller volume than does 5-FU, has been the drug commonly employed for hepatic metastases from colon cancer. Initial studies, while uncontrolled, have indicated that a higher response rate may be obtained with pump implantation than with systemic FUDR or 5-FU and that the former has few complications, low toxicity, and excellent patient acceptance.[196,197] One unexpected complication has been an increased incidence of gastroduodenal ulcer disease in patients receiving pump treatments.[198] Prospective randomized trials comparing hepatic artery pump perfusion with systemic FUDR are in progress.

ADJUVANT USE OF RADIATION AND CHEMOTHERAPY

Radiation. Radiation therapy as an adjuvant to surgery has been used primarily in cancers of the rectum because of the predilection for rectal cancers to extend locally into perirectal tissue and the high frequency of pelvic recurrence.[154] Treatments have been administered by external beam, intracavitary placement, or combinations of these modes. There is still no agreement, however, on the methods and benefits of radiation therapy as an adjunct to surgery in rectal cancer.

Preoperative radiation therapy was administered in the late 1930s and early 1940s at Memorial Hospital in New York. Relatively low doses of 1500 to 2000 rads were used previous to abdominoperineal resection for rectal cancer. In a retrospective review, there seemed to be definite benefit in patients with Dukes C disease.[199] However, in a prospective randomized study in 190 patients ending in 1967, no benefit from preoperative radiation could be shown.[200] This last study has been contradicted by a report from the Veterans Administration (VA) of a 5-year survival of 47% in patients treated with preoperative radiation as compared with 34% in controls.[201] In the VA study, a much lower frequency of histologically positive lymph nodes was found in the group undergoing resection after preoperative radiation, suggesting that the radiation had "sterilized" some nodes. Studies conducted at Yale University showed similar results.[202]

Other groups have subsequently reported results using higher doses of preoperative radiation in patients with rectal cancer.[203, 204] Most of these report some benefit in terms of survival and decrease in local recurrence. In general, these treatments have not been associated with significantly decreased morbidity or mortality. There is one study, still in progress by the Gastrointestinal Tumor Study Group, using either radiation alone, chemotherapy alone, or a combination of these, as adjunctive treatment in patients having surgery for rectal cancer. Preliminary data suggest that local recurrence is less and survival improved in all adjuvant treatment groups as compared with the group treated by surgery alone.

At Memorial Hospital at the present time, radiation therapy is not administered routinely before surgery for rectal cancer. Its use is reserved for selected patients with clinically inoperable or borderline lesions that are bulky and fixed. Most studies report that some patients with apparently inoperable tumors are able to undergo resection after such treatments, with a small salvage rate in terms of survival.[154]

Postoperative radiation also has been used as an adjuvant treatment for rectal cancer in an effort to improve cure rates. Results from several studies have been mixed, and complication rates have been in a tolerable range. Experience has not been as great as with preoperative radiation, doses have varied considerably, and most studies are inconclusive.[205–209] The potential advantage of reserving a decision on adjuvant therapy until after operation is to avoid unnecessary radiation in patients with very early disease or those with distant metastases. In addition, disease may be more accurately located and suspicious margins may be marked by metallic clips for guidance in determining radiation portals. Interest has developed in combining pre- and postoperative therapy to provide advantages of both—the "sandwich" technique. Experience is limited and this approach remains experimental,[208] but a therapeutic trial for rectal cancer is currently in progress at the Memorial Sloan-Kettering Cancer Center.

Chemotherapy. If there is residual disease after surgery for "cure," the number of retained tumor cells is theoretically at a low point. Most chemotherapeutic drugs act specifically in the cell cycle and are more effective against proliferating cells.[162, 175, 209] These considerations have prompted use of 5-FU postoperatively, even when all grossly visible disease has been removed. The drug has been given by various routes and in differing doses and schedules. The results have been mixed, some studies demonstrating minimal benefit in high-risk subgroups (e.g., Dukes C cancers) and others showing no benefit. Several excellent reviews on the use of 5-FU for adjuvant treatment of colorectal cancer have been published, and studies continue to be done.[210, 211] The advantages demonstrated thus far, however, appear to be so small that adjuvant chemotherapeutic treatment is not recommended for routine use. In patients with Dukes C lesions, however, many physicians do opt to treat with 5-FU postoperatively.

Several randomized control trials of adjuvant chemotherapy for colorectal cancer are currently in progress, most using combinations of agents, including 5-FU. The addition of agents such as methyl-CCNU, vincristine, mitomycin, dacarbazine, and hydroxyurea has again produced results showing only minimal benefit, if any. Toxicity has been acceptable in various combinations, but none of these agents has shown sufficient activity at this time to be recommended as a standard treatment or even as an improvement over 5-FU alone.[212]

An interesting adjuvant approach in patients undergoing resection for primary colorectal cancer is 5-FU infusion into the portal vein. The theory is to treat micrometastases that have reached the liver by way of the portal vein. In a British report,[213] 50 patients were randomized to have surgery alone or to receive 5-FU by portal vein catheter placed during operation for removal of the primary colon cancer. In the adjuvant treatment group, portal vein infusions were given for 1 week, and the catheters were then removed, with no increased morbidity. After a median follow-up of 15½ months, multiple hepatic metastases developed in 6 controls but in none of the infusion group. The study has been criticized on several technical points, and further evaluation of this method is being made.

IMMUNOTHERAPY. Lower absolute lymphocyte counts have been observed in metastatic colon cancer, and lymphocytes show decreased reactivity to non-specific mitogens, such as phytohemagglutinin (PHA). Similarly, skin reactivity to dinitrochlorobenzene (DNCB) may be impaired. Malnutrition and the postoperative state themselves depress immune function, but even when these factors are considered, patients with metastatic colorectal cancer have a decreased level of immunocompetence.

The immune response of an individual to colon cancer appears to be quite complex.[214] Specific cancer-related antigens are produced, the best known example of which is CEA.[215–217] Lymphocyte reactivity against colon cancer cells has been demonstrated *in vitro* by inhibition of the leukocyte migration test and by evidence of cytotoxicity to cultured colon cancer cells.[218–222]

The role of circulating antibodies in colon cancer is unclear. Antibodies cytotoxic to colon cancer cells have been found in some patients, but there also may be circulating factors that inhibit the action of cellular antibodies to the colon cancer.[223]

It was noted earlier that chemotherapeutic drugs tend to exert an immunosuppressive effect and that agents that stimulate the immune system, such as BCG, MER, and levamisole, have been given in conjunction with chemotherapeutic drugs for this reason.[182, 183] *Corynebacterium parvum*, thymic extract, transfer factor, and interferon have also been used, but no dramatic results have as yet been observed.

Work is under way in an attempt to stimulate an active specific immune attack against colon cancer through the use of tumor antigens or treated cancer cells to generate an immune response. In progress also is investigation of ways of eliminating suppressor cells and their inhibitory effect on immune responsiveness. This type of treatment would seem best suited to an adjuvant setting, i.e., after surgery when there are relatively fewer cancer cells to treat. Additional experimental clinical work in progress concerns the use of antibodies to CEA tagged with radioactive material to destroy cancer cells in advanced disease.[224]

SUPPORTIVE MEASURES. The optimum management of colon cancer, particularly when it has metastasized, requires multiple supportive measures in addition to therapy directed at the malignancy (see Chapter 255 for detailed consideration of these measures). The sensitive physician must be capable of communicating to the patient the nature of the disease, while at the same time offering a program of continuing treatment and supportive care. The patient's fear of being abandoned should be overcome, and he should be assured of the physician's commitment to maintaining comfort.

Anorexis is a frequent attendant of metastatic colon cancer, and good response to chemotherapy is much less often achieved in malnourished patients. Maintenance of caloric intake and avoidance of weight loss should therefore be a goal during chemotherapy. High-calorie nutritional supplements may be useful between meals. In more advanced disease with cachexia, the likelihood of a significant response to treatment theoretically may be increased if the patient's nutritional status can be improved. Supplementary enteral nutritional support (Chapter 234) or parenteral nutritional support (Chapter 235) may be required. Patients feel better when serious malnutrition is corrected and seem to better tolerate the side effects of chemotherapy.[225, 226] Stimulating tumor growth by improving nutritional status is a theoretical risk that has occurred in some laboratory models.[227] Also, the benefit of nutritional support in patients with advanced cancer who are receiving chemotherapy is controversial.

Jaundice in metastatic colon cancer usually implies large-scale replacement of liver by neoplasm. In some patients, however, the jaundice may be due to a small metastasis located in the porta hepatis that compresses the major ducts. This situation may be disclosed by ultrasonography or computed tomography and verified by retrograde endoscopic or percutaneous transhepatic cholangiography. Drains or internal stents may be placed during cholangiography to relieve the jaundice, or radiation can be directed at the lesion to shrink it sufficiently to diminish the obstruction. Radiation to the porta hepatis may also be delivered internally through a percutaneous biliary stent.[208, 228]

Ascites may develop in metastatic colon cancer from various causes. If the patient is malnourished and hypoalbuminemic, ascites may be part of generalized fluid retention; it may be associated with peritoneal or liver metastases; it may arise from portal hypertension induced by advanced metastatic liver disease; or it may be related to hepatic vein obstruction secondary to hepatic metastases. Symptomatic ascites, particularly transudates, may respond to diuretic therapy and spironolactone (Aldactone). Exudative ascites with high protein content may be removed by paracentesis without the problem of rapid reaccumulation. A surgically placed peritoneovenous (LaVeen) shunt can provide symptomatic relief in patients with ascites not associated with peritoneal carcinomatosis and not controlled by diuresis and paracentesis.[229–231]

Anemia should be corrected. Blood transfusions to maintain a hematocrit greater than 30% add considerably to patient comfort. Anemia is usually due to bone marrow suppression from chronic disease and chemotherapy. However, specific causes for anemia should be watched for, particularly occult gastrointestinal bleeding.

Patients with malignant liver disease may develop portal hypertension and esophageal varices, but hemorrhage from varices is usually massive. A large hepatic metastasis may sometimes erode into the distal stomach or duodenum and present as a malignant ulceration. Metastases to the upper gastrointestinal tract may occur. More commonly, however, upper gastrointestinal tract bleeding is from benign causes such as hemorrhagic gastritis associated with analgesics or physiologic stress, peptic ulcer, or monilial esophagitis attendant upon chemotherapy, immunosuppression, and use of antibiotics.[232] Many of these complications are treatable with appropriate addition or withdrawal of medication.

Surgical palliation is sometimes required for focal bowel obstruction due to metastatic disease other than diffuse abdominal carcinomatosis. Similarly, if bilateral ureteral obstruction develops in recurrent cancer of the pelvis, nephrostomy should not be performed, as the infiltrating cancer is often associated with severe pain that is difficult to control with narcotics. Neurosurgical procedures may be needed to relieve pain in this setting. Percutaneous spinal blocks are often the most appropriate approach to pain relief in the patient with advanced disease.

GENERAL FOLLOW-UP. After resection of a primary colorectal cancer, patients should be followed with several goals in mind: (1) detection of recurrent or metastatic cancer in a potentially curable state; (2) detection of second primary cancers at an early stage; and (3) prevention of new primary colorectal cancers by detecting and eliminating adenomas.

Once recovered from surgery, patients are usually followed at 3-month intervals for 2 years, at 6-month intervals for an additional 3 years, and then annually. At each visit, a careful history may elicit symptoms suggesting recurrence of a particular type of lesion. Questions should be directed to pain, bowel symptoms, bleeding, appetite, weight, abdominal girth, malaise, fever, chills, and cough. The patient's weight should be accurately measured and recorded at each visit. Physical examination should emphasize the condition of skin, lymph nodes, extremities, lungs, abdomen, and rectum, and a stool test for occult blood should be done. Women with colorectal cancer appear to be at increased risk for developing primary carcinomas of the breast, endometrium, and ovary. Follow-up in women should include instructions in breast self-examination, a yearly comprehensive breast examination, and an annual pelvic examination with a Papanicolaou smear. At each follow-up visit, a complete blood count and screening blood chemical examinations are obtained, including urea nitrogen, creatinine, bilirubin, and aminotransferase alkaline phosphatase activities. At the end of the first and second year, a chest radiograph, an abdominal CT scan, barium enema examination, and colonoscopy are done to search for distant metastases and local recurrence, both extracolonic and intraluminal.

The CEA test is used to follow patients after resection of colon cancer with the goal of detecting metastatic disease at an earlier resectable stage. A preoperative CEA value greater than normal seems to place the patient in a higher risk group for recurrence, even when matched stage for stage with patients having normal CEA values.[233, 234] If an elevated CEA does not fall to a normal level postoperatively, it is likely that there is residual malignant disease. If the CEA level does fall to normal 2 to 3 months after surgery, it may be followed in a serial manner at 3-month intervals. Numerous studies have shown that if the CEA level subsequently rises above normal and progresses, there is a high likelihood of tumor recurrence. This may occur months before the metastasis causes symptoms.[235–238] The non-specificity of the CEA test and its limitations, as discussed earlier, however, must be taken into account. The test additionally has definite shortcomings that sharply limit its value. For example, Beart and O'Connell[239] followed 168 patients who had undergone resection for cure of colorectal carcinoma at the Mayo Clinic. The CEA determination was of little value in the detection of locally recurrent or locally residual colorectal cancer. It was a sensitive means of identifying disseminated recurrent disease, but it did not identify the lesions at a resectable stage.

If the CEA level is found to be abnormal on a routine quarterly visit, determinations should be repeated every 2 weeks and, if a progressive rise is evident, the patient should be fully re-evaluated. If evaluation shows no evidence of disease, exploratory laparotomy has been advocated in the hope of finding resectable recurrence.[235, 236]

At the Memorial Sloan-Kettering Cancer Center, the resectability rate using the CEA test as a guide was 48%.[236] The effect on survival will require additional time to document, but some patients so treated have now been followed for 5 years and apparently are free of disease. Others[237–239] have not found CEA values to be as useful in finding resectable disease in asymptomatic patients, and further clinical data are needed to clarify this issue. In the meantime, it seems reasonable to obtain CEA tests during each follow-up visit for 5 years after surgery, with the understanding that the test, while imperfect, may be useful.

There are no good data to indicate that routine radionuclide, ultrasound, or CT scanning of the liver or abdomen is indicated in following asymptomatic patients after resection of colon cancer. These tests may be positive, but usually only in symptomatic patients. The serum alkaline phosphatase activity usually becomes elevated before an abnormality can be detected with assurance on a radionuclide scan of the liver.

Periodic endoscopic and radiologic examination of the colon is essential in postoperative follow-up. The first objective is to evaluate the colon for possible synchronous lesions. Ideally, a complete colonoscopic examination is done preoperatively to identify synchronous lesions that might be dealt with at the time of surgery. If this is not possible, e.g., when an obstructing colon cancer precludes complete examination, colonoscopy of the postoperative colon should be performed within 3 months after operation. Examination repeated 1 year after the initial colonoscopy is recommended. If polyps are encountered, they should be removed endoscopically, if possible. The surgical anastomosis should be evaluated, and biopsy and cytologic specimens should be taken from any suspicious areas. Colonoscopy should be performed yearly until the colon is free of adenomas for 2 successive years, and then the examination is recommended at 3-year intervals. This schedule is based on data indicating that the time for adenomatous tissue to grow from a microscopic lesion to a visible polyp is in the range of 3 years.[7] Two successive negative colonoscopic examinations, 1 year apart, keep the "miss rate" of significant lesions to a minimum.[240]

Air-contrast barium enema examinations are synergistic with colonoscopy in detecting polypoid lesions.[241] When used together, the procedures effectively detect nearly all polyps, including those smaller than 1 cm. This is not true with single-column barium studies, but applies only to meticulous air-contrast barium technique in a thoroughly prepared colon. Air-contrast barium enema examination is recommended before colonoscopy until the colon is cleared of polyps, and then the radiographic and endoscopic procedures should be done on alternate years.

Flexible proctosigmoidoscopy is recommended in the interval years between colonoscopic survey. In this way, the left side of the colon, the area where polyps and second cancers in non-familial colon cancer most often occur, can be followed even more closely. The 60-cm sigmoidoscope in experienced hands routinely examines the entire sigmoid segment.[242]

As noted earlier, the risk of developing metachronous cancers of the colon after resection of the index primary cancer has been estimated to be in the range of 3.5%, or 3 times higher than the risk in the general population. A single adenoma in the resected specimen has been reported to double this risk to 6 times that of the general population.[2,7] With the use of the rigid sigmoidoscope and removal of all rectal polyps found, the frequency of rectal cancer was greatly decreased and cancers were detected at an earlier stage.[17,243] Regular postoperative colonoscopy and barium enema examination appear to extend these benefits to the entire colon.[244] A comprehensive schema for follow-up of a patient after resection of a colon cancer is shown in Figure 139–11.

Management of the Patient with a Colostomy. A detailed discussion of the function and care of a colostomy is found in Chapter 130. By way of emphasis only, it may be observed here that the rehabilitation of a patient operated on for cancer of the colon or rectum and left with a colostomy must be individually fashioned. The measures taken are appreciably influenced by the location of the colostomy, whether or not the patient is free of cancer, and the physical and mental ability of the patient to cope with the mechanics of colostomy care. These factors are compounded by the attitudes of the patients and their families, and these, in turn, are conditioned by influences such as ethnic and social backgrounds. The vast majority of patients who have had a colostomy performed in the course of a curative resection for cancer of the rectum can lead normal lives. They must, however, receive competent, knowledgeable, and sympathetic instruction in the management of their colostomy and have the support of their family and physician.[245]

If the colostomy was performed in the course of a *curative* operation, the problems of adjustment are mechanical and psychological. If, however, the colostomy was established for an *inoperable* tumor, the problem of adjusting to the colostomy is of minor importance as compared with the problems of the cancer. Patients who are extremely resistant to a needed colostomy often have learned of unpleasant experiences of other patients whose colostomies, in fact, were for palliation. Their concepts of colostomy problems, therefore, are more often those associated with terminal cancer than those of a colostomy itself.

Epidermoid Carcinoma of the Anus

Squamous carcinomas and basaloid and transitional cancers are very likely all variants of the same tumor. These tumors arise in the anal canal at or above the dentate line.[246] Many of them have combined histologic features, hence names such as "basaloid." The overall prevalence of these tumors is about 3.9% of all cancers of rectum and rectosigmoid, but if only the anal canal and distal rectum (2 cm) are considered, epidermoid cancers constitute 30% of all malignant tumors. About 300 such patients were treated at Memorial Hospital (to 1975).[247]

In general, patients with this variety of cancer are slightly younger (average age 58 years) than those with adenocarcinoma of the rectum (average age 63 years). Females outnumber males 2:1, whereas in adenocarcinoma, the ratio is 1:1. Symptoms are similar to those of benign anorectal disease, i.e., bleeding, mass or lump, or "hemorrhoids." Not infrequently, squamous cancer is diagnosed after hemorrhoidectomy when histologic examination is made of excised tissue. The pattern of lymph node spread differs from rectal adenocarcinoma. Inguinal, obturator, hypogastric, and mesenteric nodes are all vulnerable to metastases.

Treatment remains controversial. Some advocate abdominoperineal and hypogastric lymph node dissection, while others advocate external beam and intracavitary radiation therapy. The trend, however, is toward use in combination of both treatment forms. The preoperative administration of radiation, in the range of 5000 rads, is followed by a decision pertaining to the needed extent of surgery.

Partly to enhance the value of radiation therapy and partly to reduce the morbidity of high-dose external beam therapy, Nigro et al.[248] have introduced combined chemotherapy and irradiation in the preoperative treatment of squamous carcinoma. They have reported on their initial experience with a small group of patients receiving systemic 5-FU (750 mg/m^2) and mitomycin C (15 mg/m^2), together with 3000 rads of external beam radiation. Favorable shrinkage of tumor was observed, suggesting the possible avoidance of radical surgery. Quan and co-workers[249] have reported on the Memorial Hospital experience with the first 21 patients treated by this preoperative protocol. In contrast to the practice of Nigro and colleagues to begin chemotherapy and radiation simultaneously, chemotherapy and radiation are given sequentially at the Memorial Hospital. In the first 21 patients, the immediate effects of treatment have been striking; 8 patients had such dramatic response that no microscopically detectable disease was found in the resected specimens. In view of these findings, 13 other patients have been initially treated by local excision rather than by abdominoperineal resection. In a follow-up study that embraced 37 patients, 31 patients with measurable lesions had major clinical responses to combined preoperative treatment. Seventeen of 32 (53%) had no evidence of residual tumor in subsequently resected specimens. Of those who had a local excision only, 4 of 17 (24%) developed local recurrence compared with 3 of 18 (17%) of those treated by abdominoperineal resection. The ultimate effects on survival remain to be seen, but this treatment program has now been employed in the management of over 100 patients, and the early dramatic results have been borne out.

So-called prophylactic groin dissection in patients with an epidermoid carcinoma of the anus failed to cure any patient with positive nodes. The current policy, therefore, is to perform only therapeutic and not prophylactic lymph node dissection. Also, the benefit accruing from local surgery after complete tumor regression has saved or delayed the need for radical surgery and colostomy in many patients.

Anorectal Melanoma

Malignant melanoma of the anal canal is an extremely aggressive tumor. Fortunately, it is also rare, with fewer than 250 cases in the English language literature. Quinn and Selah[250] in 1977, having culled the literature, reported on 9 patients who survived 5 years among the 107 patients whose case reports they had collected. At Memorial Sloan-Kettering Cancer Center, 59 patients (31 women and 28 men) were seen through 1978.[251] The average age was 55 years. Virtually all patients are white, but a few cases have been reported among blacks. Symptoms are those associated with squamous carcinoma or benign anorectal disorders. Masses are nearly always attributed to hemorrhoids, as is intermittent minor bleeding. Melanin is normally present within the anal epithelium, but there is no adequate explanation for melanoma originating in rectal mucosa.

Spread is similar to that of epidermoid carcinoma of the anal canal, with extension to inguinal, pelvic (obturator, hypogastric, iliac), and mesorectal sites.[247] Distant metastases to liver, lung, long bones, spine, and skin have also been noted.

Treatment has evolved since the 1930s from local treatment together with irradiation, through the addition of colostomy, to abdominoperineal resection, and, subsequently, to augmentation by abdominopelvic and inguinal lymph node dissection. In view of the fact that survival seems more related to stage than to treatment, it has been suggested that the primary lesion should always be excised. However, there is currently no support for one form of surgical procedure over another. A local complete excision of the primary melanoma may be as valid, in an individual case, as a radical resection.

Radiation therapy does not seem to have any effective role in the treatment of the primary tumor, but may be useful in the management of brain or bone metastases. Chemotherapy is still investigative at this time. Immunotherapy of melanoma has received much interest and attention, and local tumor immunotherapy may cause regression of local disease. There are no data, however, to support the use of non-specific immunotherapy in preventing systemic disease.

Lymphoma

Primary lymphoma of the colon is extremely rare. Of the 4234 adult patients with non-Hodgkin's lymphoma registered at Memorial Hospital before 1979, only 104 had primary lymphomas of the gastrointestinal tract,[252] and of these only 13 tumors were considered to have originated in the large bowel. Unlike small bowel lymphoma, there does not appear to be any known precursor of lymphoma in the colon. Presenting signs and symptoms are those observed in other large bowel neoplasms. Except for 7 cases of sigmoid and rectal primary lesions, most of the lymphomas were first diagnosed at laparotomy. This situation should radically change with the use of flexible fiberoptic endoscopy.

Of the 13 colorectal lymphomas seen at Memorial Hospital, the mean age of the patients was 61 (31 to 79) years and, in contrast to other gastrointestinal sites, there was a male to female ratio of 2.3:1.

Surgery and radiotherapy provided good local control in most patients. Nevertheless, 68% of patients with gastrointestinal lesions were later found with lymphomas at distant sites, thus strongly suggesting the need for systemic therapy.

Survival was significantly related to the stage and to the invasion or involvement of adjacent structures. Age, sex, site, depth of mural penetration, and number of foci involved had no bearing on survival. Stage III and IV disease was of major significance, as no patient survived past 1 year.

Because there is a distinct possibility for a second and even third or fourth malignant lesion to appear, post-treatment surveillance is of key importance.

References

1. American Cancer Society, Inc. Cancer Facts and Figures. New York: American Cancer Society, 1982.
2. Schottenfeld D, Winawer SJ. Large intestine. *In*: Schottenfeld D, and Fraumeni J Jr (eds). Cancer Epidemiology and Prevention. Philadelphia: WB Saunders, 1982: 703–27.
3. Doll R. General epidemiologic considerations in etiology of colorectal cancer. *In*: Winawer SJ, Schottenfeld D, Sherlock P (eds). Progress in Cancer Research and Therapy. Vol. 13. Colorectal Cancer: Prevention, Epidemiology, and Screening. New York: Raven Press, 1980: 3–120.
4. Burkitt DP. Fiber in the etiology of colorectal cancer. *In*: Winawer SJ, Schottenfeld D, Sherlock P (eds). Progress in Cancer Research and Therapy. Vol. 13. Colorectal Cancer: Prevention, Epidemiology and Screening. New York: Raven Press, 1980: 13–8.
5. Weisburger JH, Reddy BS, Spingarn NE, Wynder EJ. Current views on the mechanisms involved in the etiology of colorectal cancer. *In*: Winawer SJ, Schottenfeld D, Sherlock P (eds). Progress in Cancer Research and Therapy. Vol. 13 Colorectal Cancer: Prevention, Epidemiology, and Screening. New York: Raven Press, 1980: 19–41.
6. Sherlock P, Lipkin M, Winawer SJ. The prevention of colon cancer. A combined clinic and basic science seminar. Am J Med 1980; 68:917–31.
7. Morson BC. Genesis of colorectal cancer. Clin Gastroenterol 1976; 5:505–25.
8. Heald RJ, Bussey HJR. Clinical experience at St. Mark's Hospital with multiple synchronous cancers of the colon and rectum. Dis Colon Rectum 1975; 18:6.
9. Schottenfeld D, Berg JW, Vitsky B. Incidence of multiple primary cancers. II. Index cancers arising in the stomach and lower digestive system. J Natl Cancer Inst 1969; 43:77.
10. Ekelund GR. Cancer risk with single and multiple adenomas: Synchronous and metachronous tumors. *In*: Winawer SJ, Schottenfeld D, Sherlock P (eds). Progress in Cancer Research and Therapy. Vol. 13. Colorectal Cancer: Prevention, Epidemiology, and Screening. New York: Raven Press, 1980: 151–5.
11. Schoenberg BS, Greenberg RA, Eisenberg H. Occurrence of certain multiple primary cancers in females. J Natl Cancer Inst 1969; 43:15.
12. Sherlock P, Lipkin M, Winawer SJ. Predisposing factors in colon carcinoma. *In*: Stollerman GH (ed). Advances in Internal Medicine. Vol. 20. Chicago: Year Book Medical Publishers, 1975; 121–50.
13. Shinya H. Colonoscopy: Diagnosis and Treatment of Colonic Diseases. Tokyo: Igaku-Shoin, 1982.
14. Waye JD, Frankel A, Braunfeld SF. The histopathology of small colon polyps. Gastrointest Endosc 1980; 26:80.
15. Winawer SJ. Colorectal adenomas: Guidelines for detection and followup. Medical Student 1983; 9:19–20.
16. Maskens AP. Histogenesis and growth patterns of 1,2-

dimethylhydrazine-induced rat colon adenocarcinoma. Cancer Res 1976; 36:1585.
17. Gilbertsen VA, Nelms JM. The prevention of invasive cancer of the rectum. Cancer 1978; 41:1137–9.
18. Devroede G. Risk of cancer in inflammatory bowel disease. *In*: Winawer SJ, Schottenfeld D, Sherlock P (eds). Progress in Cancer Research and Therapy. Vol. 13. Colorectal Cancer: Prevention, Epidemiology, and Screening. New York: Raven Press, 1980: 325–34.
19. Gilat T, Rozen P. Risk of colon cancer in ulcerative colitis in low incidence areas—A review. *In*: Winawer SJ, Schottenfeld D, Sherlock P (eds). Progress in Cancer Research and Therapy. Vol. 13. Colorectal Cancer: Prevention, Epidemiology, and Screening. New York: Raven Press, 1980: 335–9.
20. Greenstein AJ, Sachar DD, Smith H, Pucillo A, Papatestas AE, Kreel I, Geller SA, Janowitz HD, Aufeses AH Jr. Cancer in universal and left-sided ulcerative colitis: Factors determining risk. Gastroenterology 1976; 79:290.
21. Weedon DD, Shorter RG, Ilstrup DM, Huizenga KA, Taylor WF. Crohn's disease and cancer. N Engl J Med 1973; 289:1099.
22. Lennard-Jones JW, Morson BC, Ritchie JK, Shove DC, Williams CB. Cancer in colitis: Assessment of the individual risk by clinical and histological criteria. Gastroenterology 1977; 73:1280.
23. Bayless TM, Yardley JH, Diamond MP, Paulson M. Commentary: Colon cancer and precancer in ulcerative colitis. *In*: Winawer SJ, Schottenfeld D, Sherlock P (eds). Progress in Cancer Research and Therapy. Vol. 13. Colorectal Cancer: Prevention, Epidemiology, and Screening. New York: Raven Press, 1980: 397–401.
24. Levin B, Riddell RH, Frank P, Gilpin JE. Evaluation of cancer risk in chronic ulcerative colitis: University of Chicago experience. *In*: Winawer SJ, Schottenfeld D, Sherlock P (eds). Progress in Cancer Research and Therapy. Vol. 13. Colorectal Cancer: Prevention, Epidemiology, and Screening. New York: Raven Press, 1980: 38–5.
25. Morson BC. Use of dysplasia as an indicator of risk for malignancy in patients with ulcerative colitis. *In*: Winawer SJ, Schottenfeld D, Sherlock P (eds). Progress in Cancer Research and Therapy. Vol. 13. Colorectal Cancer: Prevention, Epidemiology, and Screening. New York: Raven Press, 1980: 347–54.
26. Sheahan DG. Dysplasia: A pathologist's view of its general applicability. *In*: Winawer SJ, Schottenfeld D, Sherlock P (eds). Progress in Cancer Research and Therapy, Vol. 13. Colorectal Cancer: Prevention, Epidemiology, and Screening. New York: Raven Press, 1980: 355–73.
27. Nugent FW. Surveillance of patients with ulcerative colitis. Lahey Clinic results. *In*: Winawer SJ, Schottenfeld D, Sherlock P (eds). Progress in Cancer Research and Therapy, Vol. 13. Colorectal Cancer: Prevention, Epidemiology, and Screening. New York: Raven Press, 1980: 375–80.
28. Waye JD. The role of colonoscopy in surveillance for cancer in patients with ulcerative colitis. *In*: Winawer SJ, Schottenfeld D, Sherlock P (eds). Progress in Cancer Research and Therapy, Vol. 13. Colorectal Cancer: Prevention, Epidemiology, and Screening. New York: Raven Press, 1980: 387–92.
29. Blackstone MO, Riddell RO, Rogers BHG, Levin B. Dysplasia-associated lesion or mass (DALM) detected by colonoscopy in long-standing ulcerative colitis: An indication for colectomy. Gastroenterology 1981; 80:366–74.
30. McConnell RB. Genetics of familial polyposis. *In*: Winawer SJ, Schottenfeld D, Sherlock P (eds). Progress in Cancer Research and Therapy, vol. 13. Colorectal Cancer: Prevention, Epidemiology, and Screening. New York: Raven Press, 1980: 69–71.
31. Bussey HJR: Familial Polyposis Coli. Baltimore: Johns Hopkins University Press, 1975.
32. Winawer SJ, Sherlock P, Schottenfeld D, Miller DG. Screening for colon cancer. Gastroenterology 1976; 70:783–9.
33. Jeghers H, McKusick VW, Katz KH. Generalized intestinal polyposis and melanin spots of the oral mucosa: Lips and digits. A syndrome of diagnostic significance. N Engl J Med 1949; 241:933.
34. Stemper TJ, Kent JH, Summers RW. Juvenile polyposis and gastrointestinal carcinoma. A study of a kindred. Ann Intern Med 1975; 83:639.
35. Kussin SZ, Lipkin M, Winawer SJ. Inherited colon cancer: Clinical implications. Am J Gastroenterol 1979; 72:448–57.
36. Lynch PM, Lynch HT, Herns RE. Hereditary proximal colon cancer. Dis Colon Rectum 1977; 20:661.
37. Lynch HT, Lynch PM, Lynch JF. Analysis of genetics of inherited colon cancer. *In*: Winawer SJ, Schottenfeld D, Sherlock P (eds). Progress in Cancer Research and Therapy. Vol. 13. Colorectal Cancer: Prevention, Epidemiology, and Screening. New York: Raven Press, 1980: 117–31.
38. Anderson DE, Strong LC: Genetics of gastrointestinal tumors. *In*: Excerpts Medical International Congress. Series No. 351, Vol. 3, Amsterdam, 1974.
39. Warthin AS. Heredity with reference to carcinoma. Arch Intern Med 1913; 12:546.
40. Woolf CM, Richards RC, Gardner EJ. Occasional discrete polyps of the colon and rectum showing an inherited tendency in a kindred. Cancer 1955; 8:403.
41. Lovett E. Familial factors in the etiology of carcinoma of the large bowel. Proc Roy Soc Med 1974; 67:21.
42. Macklin M. Inheritance of cancer of the stomach and large intestine in man. J Natl Cancer Inst 1960; 24:551.
43. Woolf CM. A genetic study of carcinoma of the large intestine. Am J Hum Genet 1958; 104:42.
44. McSherry CK, Cornell GN, Glenn F. Carcinoma of the colon and rectum. Ann Surg 1969; 169:502.
45. Spratt JS Jr, Spjut HJ. Prevalence and prognosis of individual clinical and pathological variables associated with colorectal carcinoma. Cancer 1967; 20:1976.
46. Osnes S. Carcinoma of the colon and rectum. A study of 353 cases with special reference to prognosis. Acta Chir Scand 1955; 110:378.
47. Coller FA, Kay EB, MacIntyre RS. Regional lymphatic metastasis of carcinoma of the rectum. Surgery 1940; 8:294.
48. Enker WE, Laffer U Th, Block GE. Enhanced survival of patients with colon and rectal cancer is based upon wide anatomic resection. Ann Surg 1979; 190:350–60.
49. Grinnell RS. The grading and prognosis of carcinoma of the colon and rectum. Ann Surg 1939; 109:500.
50. Coller FA, Kay EB, MacIntyre RS. Regional lymphatic metastases of carcinoma of the colon. Ann Surg 1941; 114:156.
51. Stearns MW Jr. Staging colonic and rectal cancer. Int Adv Surg Oncology 1981; 4:189.
52. Broders AC. Carcinoma. Grading and practical application. Arch Pathol 1926; 2:376.
53. Dukes EC. The relation of histology to spread in intestinal cancer. Br J Cancer 1950; 4:59.
54. Nichols RJ, Ritchie JK, Wadsworth J, Parks AG. Total excision or restorative resection for carcinoma of the middle third of the rectum. Br J Surgery 1975; 66:625.
55. Enker WE, Paloyan E, Kirsner JB. Carcinoma of the colon in the adolescent. Am J Surg 1977; 133:737.
56. Felipe MI, Branfort AC. Abnormal patterns of mucus secretion in apparently normal mucosa of large intestines with carcinoma. Cancer 1974; 34:282.
57. Jirkova A. Histochemical properties of mucus in epithelial tumors of the large intestine. Cesk Patol 1981; 17:117.
58. Culling CF, Reid PE, Dunn WL, Freeman HJ. The relevance of the histochemistry of colonic mucus based upon PAS activity. Histochem J 1981; 13:889.
59. Wolley RW, Schreiber K, Karas M, Sherman MS, Koss LG. The relationship of DNA content of cells of colonic carcinomas to clinical behavior. *In*: Proceedings, Workshop of the National Large Bowel Cancer Project. Dallas, Jan 8–9, 1981: 89–90.
60. Enker WE, Melamed M. Unpublished observations.
61. Fenoglio CM, Lane N. The anatomical precursor of colorectal carcinoma. Cancer 1974; 34:819.
62. Astler VB, Coller FA. The prognostic significance of direct extension of carcinoma of the colon and rectum. Ann Surg 1954; 139:846.
63. Copeland EM, Miller LD, Jones RS. Prognostic factors in carcinoma of the colon and rectum. Am J Surg 1968; 116:875.

64. Dukes CE. The classification of cancer of the rectum. J Pathol Bacteriol 1932; 35:323.
65. Wilkinson EJ, Hause L. Probability in lymph node sectioning. Cancer 1974; 33:1269.
66. Sunderland DA. The significance of vein invasion by cancer of the rectum and sigmoid. Cancer 1949; 2:429.
67. Brown CE, Warren S. Visceral metastases from rectal carcinoma. Surg Gynecol Obstet 1938; 66:611.
68. Seefeld PH, Bargen JA. The spread of carcinoma of the rectum. Invasions of lymphatics, veins and nerves. Ann Surg 1943; 118:76.
69. Platz CE: The staging and pathology of colonic carcinoma and adenomas. *In*: Enker WE (ed). Carcinoma of the Colon and Rectum. Chicago: Year Book Medical Publishers, 1978: 21–48.
70. Zamcheck N, Doos WG, Prudente R, Lurie BB, Gottlieb LS. Prognostic factors in colon carcinoma. Correlation of serum carcinoembryonic antigen level and tumor histopathology. Hum Pathol 1975; 6:31–45.
71. Patt DJ, Byrnes RK, Vardiman JW, Coppleson LW. Mesocolic lymph node histology is an important prognostic indicator for patients with carcinoma of the sigmoid colon: An immunomorphologic study. Cancer 1975; 35:1388–97.
72. El-Domeiri A, Whiteley HW Jr. Prognostic significance of abdominal wall involvement in carcinoma of cecum. Cancer 1970; 26:552.
73. Black WA, Waugh JM. The intramural extension of carcinoma of the descending colon, sigmoid and rectosigmoid. Surg Gynecol Obstet 1948; 87:457.
74. Broders AC. The grading of carcinoma. Minn Med 1925; 8:726.
75. Morson BC. Factors influencing the prognosis in early cancer of the rectum. Proc Roy Soc Med 1966; 59:607.
76. Colacchio TA, Forde KA, Scantlebury VP. Endoscopic polypectomy: Inadequate treatment for invasive colorectal carcinoma. Ann Surg 1981; 194:704.
77. Bussey HJR. Age and cancer of the large intestine. Thule International Symposium: Cancer and Aging. Stockholm: Nordiska Bokhendelns Forlag, 1968: 203–14.
78. Donegan WL, DeCosse JJ. Pitfalls and controversies in the staging of colorectal carcinoma. *In*: Enker WE (ed). Carcinoma of the Colon and Rectum. Chicago: Year Book Medical Publishers, 1978: 49–72.
79. Gabriel WB, Dukes CE, Bussey HJR. Lymphatic spread in cancer of the rectum. Br J Surg 1935; 23:395.
80. Dukes CE, Bussey HJR. The spread of rectal cancer and its effect on prognosis. Br J Cancer 1958; 12:309.
81. Simpson WC, Mayo CW. The mural penetration of the carcinoma cell in the colon. Anatomical and clinical study. Surg Gynecol Obstet 1939; 68:872.
82. Kirklin JW, Dockerty MB, Waugh JM. The role of the peritoneal reflection in the prognosis of carcinoma of the rectum and sigmoid colon. Surg Gynecol Obstet 1949; 88:326.
83. Holyoke ED, Lokich J, Wright H. Adjuvant therapy for adenocarcinoma of the colon following clinically curative resection. *In*: Proceedings, Gastrointestinal Tumor Study Group, National Cancer Institute. Bethesda: NIH, 1975.
84. Wood DA, Robbins GF, Zippin C, Lum D, Stearns MW Jr. Staging cancer of the colon and rectum. Cancer 1979; 43:961–8.
85. Utsunomiya J, Iwama T, Hirayama R. Familial large bowel cancer. *In*: DeCosse JJ (ed). Large Bowel Cancer. Clinical Surgery International. New York: Churchill Livingstone, 1981: 16–33.
86. Keighley MR, Thompson H, Alexander-Williams J. Multifocal colonic carcinoma in Crohn's disease. Surgery 1975; 78:534.
87. Lightdale CJ, Sternberg SS, Posner G, Sherlock P. Carcinoma complicating Crohn's disease. Report of seven cases and review of the literature. Am J Med 1975; 59:262–8.
88. Morson BC, Pang LS. Rectal biopsy as an aid to cancer control in ulcerative colitis. Gut 1967; 8:423–34.
89. Hunt RH, Waye JD. Indications for colonoscopy. *In*: Hunt RH, Waye JD (eds). Colonoscopy, Techniques, Clinical Practice and Colour Atlas. London: Chapman and Hall, 1981.
90. Winawer SJ. Screening for colorectal cancer. An overview. Cancer 1980; 45:1093–8.
91. Winawer SJ. Colorectal cancer screening and early diagnosis. *In*: Brodie DR (ed). Screening and Early Diagnosis of Colorectal Cancer. Consensus Development Conference Proceedings. Washington, DC, NIH Publication No. 80–2075, 1979: 193–210.
92. Winawer SJ, Fleisher M, Baldwin M, Sherlock P. Current status of fecal occult blood testing in screening for colorectal cancer. CA 1982; 32:100–12.
93. Winawer SJ, Sherlock P. Surveillance for colorectal cancer in average-risk patients, familial high-risk groups, and patients with adenomas. Cancer 1982; 50:2609–14.
94. Tedesco FJ, Waye JD, Raskin JB, Morris SJ, Greenwald RA. Colonoscopic evaluation of rectal bleeding. Ann Intern Med 1978; 89:907–9.
95. Fox J, Andrews M, Guthrie M, Winawer SJ. Significance of the small polyp detected on proctoscopy: A preliminary report. Gastrointest Endosc 1981; 27:2:40 (Abstract).
96. Leinicke JL, Dodds WJ, Hogan WJ, Stewart ET. A comparison of colonoscopy and roentgenography for detecting polypoid lesions of the colon. Gastrointest Radiol 1977; 2:125–8.
97. Winawer SJ, Leidner SD, Hajdu SI, Sherlock P. Colonoscopic biopsy and cytology in the diagnosis of colon cancer. Cancer 1978; 42:2849–53.
98. Wolff WI, Shinya H. Polypectomy via the fiberoptic colonoscope. N Engl J Med 1973; 288:329–32.
99. Gold P, Freedman SO. Demonstration of tumor-specific antigens in human colonic carcinoma by immunological tolerance and absorption techniques. J Exp Med 1965; 121:439–62.
100. Thomson D, Krupey J, Freedman S, Gold P. The radioimmunoassay of circulating carcinoembryonic antigen of the human digestive system. Proc Natl Acad Sci USA 1969; 64:161.
101. Fleisher M, Besenfelder E, Schwartz MK, Oettgen HF. Evolution of three CEA assays. Proc Am Assoc Cancer Res 1973; 14:68.
102. LoGerfo P, Krupey J, Hansen HJ. Demonstration of a common neoplastic antigen: Assay using zirconyl gel. N Engl J Med 1971; 285:138–41.
103. Martin F, Martin MS. Demonstration of antigens related to colonic cancer in the human digestive system. Cancer 1971; 6:352–60.
104. Egan ML, Lautenschleger JT, Coligan JE, Todd CW. Radioimmunoassay of carcinoembryonic antigen. Immunochemistry 1972; 9:289–99.
105. Booth SN, King JPG, Leonard JC, Dykes PW. The significance of elevation of serum carcinoembryonic antigen (CEA) levels in inflammatory disease of the intestine. Scand J Gastroenterol 1974; 9:651–6.
106. Go VLM. Carcinoembryonic antigen. Cancer 1976; 37:562–6.
107. Moore TL, Kupchik HZ, Marcon N, Zamcheck N. Carcinoembryonic antigen assay in cancer of the colon and pancreas and other digestive disorders. Am J Dig Dis 1971; 16:1–7.
108. Reynoso G, Chu TM, Holyoke D, Cohen E, Valensuela LA, Nemoto T, Wang JJ, Chuang J, Guinan P, Murphy GP. Carcinoembryonic antigen in patients with different cancers. JAMA 1972; 220:361.
109. Cooper EH, Turner R, Steele L, Neville AM, Mackay AM. The contribution of serum enzymes and carcinoembryonic antigen to the early diagnosis of metastatic colorectal cancer. Br J Cancer 1975; 31:111–7.
110. LoGerfo P, Herter FP. Carcinoembryonic antigen and prognosis in patients with colon cancer. Ann Surg 1975; 181:81–3.
111. Kim US, Papatestas AE, Aufses AH. Prognostic significance of peripheral lymphocyte counts and carcinoembryonic antigens in colorectal carcinoma. J Surg Oncol 1976; 8:257–62.
112. Lipkin M, Winawer SJ, Sherlock P. Early identification of individuals at increased risk for cancer of the large intestine. II. Development of risk factor profiles. Memorial Sloan-Kettering Cancer Center Clin Bull 1981; 11:66–74.

113. Greegor DH. Diagnosis of large bowel cancer in the asymptomatic patient. JAMA 1967; 201:943–5.
114. Fleisher M, Schwartz MK, Winawer SJ. Laboratory studies on the Hemoccult slide for fecal occult blood testing. *In*: Winawer SJ, Schottenfeld D, Sherlock P (eds). Progress in Cancer Research and Therapy. Vol. 13. Colorectal Cancer: Prevention, Epidemiology, and Screening. New York: Raven Press, 1980: 181–7.
115. Winawer SJ, Andrews M, Flehinger B, Sherlock P, Schottenfeld D, Miller DG. Progress report on controlled trial of fecal occult blood testing for detection of colorectal neoplasia. Cancer 1980; 45:2959–64.
116. Winawer SJ. Detection and diagnosis of colorectal cancer. Cancer 1983; 51:2519–24.
117. Fleisher M, Schwartz MK, Winawer SJ. The false-negative Hemoccult test. Rapid communication. Gastroenterology 1977; 72:781–4.
118. Macrae FA, James D, St. John B. Relationship between patterns of bleeding and Hemoccult sensitivity in patients with colorectal cancers or adenoma. Gastroenterology 1982; 82:891–8.
119. Macrae FA, James D, St. John B, Caligiore P, Taylor LS, Legge JW. Optimal dietary conditions for Hemoccult testing. Gastroenterology 1982; 82:899–903.
120. Songster CL, Barrows GH, Jarrett DD. Immunochemical detection of human fecal occult blood. *In*: Winawer SJ, Schottenfeld D, Sherlock P (eds). Progress in Cancer Research and Therapy. Vol 13. Colorectal Cancer: Prevention, Epidemiology, and Screening. New York: Raven Press, 1980: 193–204.
121. Bohlman T, Katon R, Lipshutz G, McCool M, Smith F, Melnyk C. Fiberoptic pansigmoidoscopy. An evaluation and comparison with rigid sigmoidoscopy. Gastroenterology 1977; 72:644–9.
122. Hertz RE, Deddish MR, Day E. Value of periodic examination in detecting cancer of the rectum and colon. Postgrad Med 1960; 27:290–4.
123. Dales LG, Friedman GD, Ramcharan S, Siegelaub AB, Campbell BA, Feldman R, Collen MG. Multiphasic checkup evaluation study. 3. Out-patient clinic utilization, hospitalization, and mortality experience after 7 years. Prev Med 1973; 2:221–35.
124. Zamcheck N. Current status of CEA. *In*: Winawer SJ, Schottenfeld D, Sherlock P (eds). Progress in Cancer Research and Therapy. Vol. 13. Colorectal Cancer: Prevention, Epidemiology, and Screening. New York: Raven Press, 1980: 219–34.
124a. Attiyeh FF, Stearns MW Jr. Second-look laparotomy based on CEA elevations in colorectal cancer. Cancer 1981; 47:2119–35.
124b. Minton JP, Martin EW Jr. The use of serial CEA determinations to predict recurrence of colon cancer and when to do a second-look operation. Cancer 1978; 42:1422–7.
124c. Wanebo JH, Rao B, Pinsky CM, Hoffman RG, Stearns M, Schwartz MK, Oettgen HF. Preoperative carcinoembryonic antigen level as a prognostic indicator in colorectal cancer. N Engl J Med 1978; 299:448–51.
124d. Holyoke ED, Chu TM, Murphy GP. CEA as a monitor of gastrointestinal malignancy. Cancer 1975; 35:830–6.
124e. Martin EW Jr, James KK, Hurtubise PE, Catalano P, Minton JP. The use of CEA as an early indicator for gastrointestinal tumor recurrence and second-look procedures. Cancer 1977; 39:440–6.
124f. Minton JP, James K, Hurtubise PE, Rinker L, Joyce S, Martin EW Jr. The use of serial carcinoembryonic antigen determinations to predict recurrence of carcinoma of the colon and the time for a second-look operation. Surg Gynecol Obstet 1978; 147:208.
125. Sugarbaker PH, Zamcheck N, Moore FD. Assessment of serial carcinoembryonic antigen (CEA) assays in postoperative detection of recurrent colorectal cancer. Cancer 1976; 38:2310–5.
126. American Cancer Society. Guidelines for the cancer-related checkup. Recommendations and rationale. CA 1980; 30:4.
127. Winawer SJ (Chairman). Report of the International Workgroup on Colorectal Cancer. Geneva, January, 1980.
128. Miles EW. A method of performing abdomino-perineal excision for carcinoma of the rectum and of the terminal portion of the pelvic colon. Lancet 1908; 2:1812–3.
129. Jamieson JK, Dobson JF. The lymphatics of the colon: With special reference to the operative treatment of cancer of the colon. Ann Surg 1909; 50:1077–90.
130. Rosi P. Selection of operations for carcinoma of the colon. *In*: Turell R (ed). Diseases of the Colon and Rectum. Philadelphia: WB Saunders, 1959: 477.
131. Rosi P, Carey J. A ten year study of hemicolectomy in the treatment of carcinoma of the left half of the colon. Surg Gynecol Obstet 1962; 114:15–24.
132. Turnbull RP Jr, Kyle K, Watson FR, Spratt J. Cancer of the colon: The influence of the "no touch isolation" technic on survival rates. Ann Surg 1967; 166:420–5.
133. Stearns MW Jr. The choice among anterior resection, the pull-through and abdominoperineal resection of the rectum. Cancer 1974; 34:969–71.
134. Stearns MW Jr, Schottenfeld D. Techniques for the surgical management of colon cancer. Cancer 1971; 28:165–9.
135. Hojo K, Koyama Y. The effectiveness of wide anatomic resection and radical lymphadenectomy for patients with rectal cancer. Jap J Surgery 1982; 12:111–6.
136. Enker WE. Extent of operations for large bowel cancer. *In*: DeCosse JJ (ed). Large Bowel Cancer. Clinical Surgery International. New York: Churchill Livingstone, 1981: 78–93.
137. Parks AG. Per-anal anastomosis. World J Surg 1982; 6:531.
138. Polk HC. Extended resection for selected adenocarcinoma of the large bowel. Ann Surg 1972; 175:892.
139. Newman HK, Stearns MW Jr. Reexploration for "unresectable colonic cancer." Dis Colon Rectum 1975; 18:572.
140. Madden JL, Kandalaft S. Clinical evaluation of electrocoagulation in the treatment of cancer of the rectum. Am J Surg 1971; 122:347.
141. Block GE, Enker WE. Survival after operations for rectal carcinoma in patients over 70 years of age. Ann Surg 1971; 174:521.
142. Stearns MW, Jr, Sternberg SS, DeCosse JJ. Local treatment of rectal cancer. *In*: DeCosse JJ (ed). Large Bowel Cancer. Clinical Surgery International. New York; Churchill Livingstone, 1981: 144–53.
143. Morson BC, Bussey HJR, Samoorian S. Policy of local excision for early cancer of the rectum. Gut 1977; 18:1045.
144. Lock MR, Cairns DW, Ritchie JK, Lockhart-Mummey HE. The treatment of early colorectal cancer by local excision. Br J Surg 1978; 65:346.
145. Vassilopoulos PP, Yoon JM, Ledesma EJ, Mittleman A. The recurrence of adenocarcinoma of the colon and rectum at the anastomotic site. Surg Gynecol Obstet 1981; 152:777.
146. Adson MA. Diagnosis and treatment of primary and secondary solid hepatic tumors in the adult. Surg Clin North Am 1981; 61:181.
147. Fortner JG, MacLean BJ, Kim DK, Howland WS, Turnbull AD, Goldiner P, Carlon G, Beattie EJ. The seventies evolution in liver surgery for cancer. Cancer 1981; 47:2162–6.
147a. Gastrointestinal Tumor Study Group. Adjuvant therapy of colon cancer—results of a prospectively randomized trial. N Engl J Med 1984; 310:737–43.
148. Wanebo HJ, Semoglou C, Attiyeh F, Stearns MW Jr. Surgical management of patients with primary operable colorectal cancer and synchronous liver metastases. Am J Surg 1978; 135:81–5.
149. Foster JH, Lundy J. Liver metastases. Curr Probl Surg 1981; 18:160.
150. Ensminger W, Niederhuber J, Dakhil S, Thrall J, Wheeler R. Totally implanted drug delivery system for hepatic arterial chemotherapy. Cancer Treat Rep 1981; 65:393–400.
151. Smedal MT, Wright KA, Siber FJ. The palliative treatment of recurrent carcinoma of the rectum and rectosigmoid with 2 MEV radiation: Some results and description of a technique. AJR 1967; 100.904–8.
152. Whiteley HWJ, Stearns MW Jr, Leaming RH, Deddish MR. Palliative radiation therapy in patients with cancer of the colon and rectum. Cancer 1970; 25:343–6.
153. Williams IG, Schuleman IM, Todd IP. The treatment of recurrent carcinoma of the rectum by supervoltage x-ray therapy. Br J Surg 1956; 44:506–8.
154. Leaming R. Radiation therapy in the clinical management of neoplasms of the colon, rectum, and anus. *In*: Stearns MW Jr (ed). Neoplasms of the Colon, Rectum and Anus. New York: John Wiley, 1980: 143–53.

155. Phillipas R, Karnofsky DA, Hamilton LD, Nickson JJ. Roentgen therapy of hepatic metastases. AJR 1954; 71:826–34.
156. Turek-Maischeider M, Kazem I. Palliative irradiation for liver metastases. JAMA 1975; 232:625–8.
157. Lightdale CJ, Wasser J, Coleman M, Brower M, Tefft M, Pasmantier M. Anticoagulation and high dose liver radiation. Cancer 1979; 43:174–81.
158. Williams IG, Horwitz H. The primary treatment of adenocarcinoma of the rectum by high voltage roentgen rays. AJR 1956; 76:919–28.
159. Wang CC, Schultz MD. The role of radiation therapy in the management of carcinoma of the sigmoid, rectosigmoid, and rectum. Radiology 1962; 70:1.
160. Papillon J. Intracavity irradiation in early rectal cancer for cure: A series of 186 cases. Cancer 1975; 36:697–701.
161. Moertel CG, Thynne GS. Large bowel. *In*: Holland JF, Frei E III (eds). Cancer Medicine. Philadelphia: Lea & Febiger, 1981: 1830–59.
162. Lightdale CJ, Lipkin M. Cell division and tumor growth. *In*: Becker FF (ed). Cancer. A Comprehensive Treatise. Vol. 3. New York: Plenum Press, 1975: 201–15.
163. Lokich JJ. Predicting tumor response to cytotoxic therapy. Hosp Pract 1980; 7:74–80.
164. Shackney SE, McCormack GW, Cuchuaral GJ Jr. Growth rate patterns of solid tumors and their relation to responsiveness to therapy. Ann Intern Med 1978; 89:107–21.
165. Lightdale CJ, Sherlock P. Chemotherapy of gastrointestinal cancer. Drug Therapy 1979; 9:105–15.
166. Chabner BA, Myers CF, Coleman CN, Johns DG. The clinical pharmacology of antineoplastic agents. N Engl J Med 1975; 292:1107–13.
167. Yagoda A, Kemeny N. Chemotherapy of colorectal cancer: A critical analysis of response criteria and therapeutic efficacy. *In*: Lipkin M, Good R (eds). Gastrointestinal Tract Cancer. New York: Plenum Press, 1978: 554–72.
168. Bullen BR, Cooper EH, Turner R, Neville AM, Giles GR, Hall R. Cancer markers in patients receiving chemotherapy for colorectal cancer. A preliminary report. Med Pediatr Oncol 1976; 3:289–300.
169. Ravry M, Moertel CG, Schutt AJ, Go VLM. Usefulness of serum carcinoembryonic antigen (CEA) determinations during anti-cancer therapy or long term follow-up of gastrointestinal carcinoma. Cancer 1974; 34:1230–6.
170. Skarin AT, Delwiche R, Zamcheck N, Lokich JJ, Frei E III: Carcinoembryonic antigen: Clinical correlation with chemotherapy for metastatic gastrointestinal cancer. Cancer 1974; 33:1239–45.
171. Moertel CG, Reitmeier RJ. Advanced Gastrointestinal Cancer—Clinical Management and Chemotherapy. New York: Harper & Row, 1969.
172. Karnofsky DA, Ellison RR, Golbey RB. Selection of patients for evaluation of chemotherapeutic procedures in advanced cancer. Cancer Chemotherap Rep 1962; 16:73–7.
173. Bateman J, Irwin L, Pugh R, Cassidy F. Weiner J. Comparison of intravenous (IV) and oral (PO) administration of 5-fluorouracil (5-FU) for colorectal carcinoma. Proc Amer Assoc Cancer Res 1976; 16:242.
174. Hahn RG, Moertel CG, Schutt AJ, Bruckner HW. A double blind comparison of intensive course 5-fluorouracil by oral versus intravenous route in the treatment of colorectal carcinoma. Cancer 1975; 35:1031.
175. DeVita VT, Schein PS. The use of drugs in combination for the treatment of cancer: Rationale and results. N Engl J Med 1973; 288:998–1006.
176. Moertel CG, Schutt AJ, Hahn RG, Reitmeier RJ. Therapy of advanced gastrointestinal cancer with a combination of 5-FU, methyl CCNU, and vincristine. J Natl Cancer Inst 1975; 54:69.
177. Lokich J, Skarin AT, Mayer RJ, Frei E III. Lack of effectiveness of combined 5-fluorouracil and methyl-CCNU therapy in advanced colorectal cancer. Cancer 1977; 40:2792–6.
178. Kemeny N, Yagoda A, Braun D Jr, Golbey R. Therapy for metastatic colorectal carcinoma with a combination of methyl CCNU, 5-fluorouracil, vincristine, and streptozotocin (MOF-Strep). Cancer 1980; 45:876–81.
179. Moertel CG, Childs DS, Reitmeier RJ, Colby MY Jr, Holbrook MA. Combined 5-fluorouracil and supervoltage radiation therapy of locally unresectable gastrointestinal cancer. Lancet 1969; 2:865.
180. Vongtama V, Couglass HO, Moore RH, Holyoke ED, Webster JH. End results of radiation alone and combination with 5-fluorouracil in colorectal cancer. Cancer 1975; 36:2020–5.
181. Barone RM, Byfield JE, Frankel SS. Combination infusional 5-fluorouracil and radiation therapy for the treatment of metastatic carcinoma of the colon to the liver. Dis Colon Rectum 1979; 22:376–82.
182. Mavligit GM, Gutterman JU, Hersh EM. Adjuvant chemotherapy and immunotherapy in colorectal cancer. *In*: Lipkin M, Good RA (eds). Gastrointestinal Tract Cancer. New York: Plenum Press, 1978: 573–86.
183. Moertel CG, Ritts RE Jr, Schutt AJ, Hahn RG. Clinical studies of methanol extraction residue fraction of bacillus Calmette-Guerin as an immunostimulant in patients with advanced cancer. Cancer 1975; 35:3075–83.
184. Watkins E Jr, Khazei AM, Nahra KS. Surgical basis for arterial infusion chemotherapy of disseminated carcinoma of the liver. Surg Gynecol Obstet 1970; 130:581–605.
185. Suzuki T, Sarumaru S, Kawabe K, Honjo I. Study of vascularity of tumors of the liver. Surg Gynecol Obstet 1972; 134:27–34.
186. Breedis C, Young C. The blood supply of neoplasms in the liver. Am J Pathol 1954; 30:969–74.
187. Fortner JG, Kim DK, Barrett MK, Golbey RB. Intrahepatic infusional chemotherapy using multiple agents for cancer in the liver. Proc Am Soc Clin Oncol 1976; 17:293.
188. Kim DK, Watson RC, Pahnke LD, Fortner JG. Tumor vascularity as a prognostic factor for hepatic tumors. Ann Surg 1977; 185:31–4.
189. Ensminger WD, Rosowsky A, Raso V. A clinical-pharmacological evaluation of hepatic arterial infusions of 5-fluoro-2-deoxyuridine and 5-fluorouracil. Cancer Res 1978; 38:3784–92.
190. Ansfield F, Ramirez G, Skibba JL, Byran GT, Davis HL Jr, Wietmen GW. Intrahepatic arterial infusion with fluorouracil. Cancer 1971; 28:1147–58.
191. Weissman CH. Regional therapy for hepatic neoplasms. Clin Cancer Briefs 1980; 1:3–12.
192. Cady B, Oberfield RA. Regional infusion chemotherapy of hepatic metastases of carcinoma of the colon. Am J Surg 1974; 127:220–27.
193. Barone RM, Byfield JE, Goldfarb PB, Frankel S, Ginn C, Greer S. Intraarterial chemotherapy using an implantable infusion pump and liver irradiation for the treatment of hepatic metastases. Cancer 1982; 50:850–62.
194. Herter RP, Markowitz AM, Flind CR. Cancer chemotherapy by continuous intraarterial infusion of antimetabolites. Am J Surg 1963; 105:628–39.
195. Grage TB, Vasilopoulos PP, Shingleton WW, Jubert AV, Elias ZG, Aust JB, Moss SE. Results of a prospective randomized study of hepatic artery infusion with 5-fluorouracil versus intravenous 5-fluorouracil in patients with hepatic metastases from colorectal cancer. A central oncology group study. Surgery 1979; 86:550–5.
196. Ensminger WD, Niederhuber J, Dakhil S, Thrall J, Wheeler R. A totally implanted drug delivery system for hepatic arterial chemotherapy. Cancer Treat Rep 1981; 65:393–400.
197. Barone RM, Byfield JE, Goldfarb PB, Frankel S, Ginn C, Greer S. Intra-arterial chemotherapy using an implantable infusion pump and liver irradiation for the treatment of hepatic metastases. Cancer 1982; 50:850–62.
198. Narsete T, Ansfield FJ, Wirtanen G, Ramirez G, Wolberg W, Jarrett F. Gastric ulceration in patients receiving intrahepatic infusion of 5-fluorouracil. Ann Surg 1977; 186:739.
199. Leaming RH, Stearns MW Jr, Deddish MR. Preoperative irradiation in rectal carcinoma. Radiology 1961; 77:257–63.
200. Stearns MW, Deddish MR, Quan SHQ, Leamong RH. Preoperative roentgen therapy for cancer of the rectum and rectosigmoid. Surg Gynecol Obstet 1974; 138:584–6.
201. Roswit B, Higgins GA Jr, Keehn RJ. Preoperative irradiation for carcinoma of the rectum and rectosigmoid colon: Report of a national Veterans Administration randomized study. Cancer 1975; 35:1597–1602.
202. Kligerman MM. Preoperative radiation therapy in rectal cancer. Cancer 1975; 36:691–5.

203. Tepper M, Vidone RA, Hayes MA. Preopertive irradiation in rectal cancer: Initial comparison of clinical tolerance, surgical and pathologic findings. AJR 1968, 102:587–95.
204. Stevens KR, Allen CV, Fletcher WS. Preoperative radiotherapy for adenocarcinoma of the rectosigmoid. Cancer 1976; 37:2866–74.
205. Gunderson L, Votava C, Brown RC, Plenk HP. Colorectal carcinoma: Combined treatment with surgery and postoperative radiation—LDS Hospital experience. Int J Radiat Oncol Biol Phys 1976; 2(Suppl 1):64.
206. Withers HR, Romsdahl M. Adjuvant postoperative radiotherapy for carcinoma of the rectum. Int J Radiat Oncol Biol Phys 1976; 2(Suppl 1):62.
207. Turner SS, Vieira EF, Ager PJ, Ghossein NA. Elective postoperative radiotherapy for locally advanced colorectal cancer. Cancer 1977; 40:105–8.
208. Sischy B. The place of radiotherapy in the management of rectal adenocarcinoma. Cancer 1982; 50:2631–7.
209. Frei E, Canellos G. Dose: A critical factor in cancer chemotherapy. Am J Med 1980; 69:585–94.
210. Carter SK. The adjuvant chemotherapy of large bowel cancer. *In*: Carter SK, Glatstein E, Livingston RB (eds). Principles of Cancer Treatment. New York: McGraw-Hill, 1982: 397–401.
211. Moertel CG. Adjuvant therapy of gastrointestinal carcinoma: An overview. *In*: Salmon SE, Jones SE (eds). Adjuvant Therapy of Cancer. III. New York: Grune & Stratton 1981; 559–67.
212. Davis HL. Chemotherapy of large bowel cancer. Cancer 1982; 50:2638–46.
213. Taylor I, Brooman P, Rowling JT. Adjuvant liver perfusion in colorectal cancer: Initial results of a clinical trial. Br Med J 1977; 2:1320–2.
214. Baldwin RW, Embleton MJ, Jones JSP, Langman MJS. Cell-mediated and humoral immune reactions to human tumours. Int J Cancer 1973; 12:73–83.
215. Lejtenyi MC, Freedman SO, Gold P. Response of lymphocytes from patients with gastrointestinal cancer to the carcinoembryonic antigen of the human digestive system. Cancer 1971; 28:115–20.
216. LoGerto P, Herter FP, Bennett SJ. Absence of circulating antibodies to carcinoembryonic antigen in patients with gastrointestinal malignancies. Int J Cancer 1972; 9:344–8.
217. MacSween JM. The antigenicity of carcinoembryonic antigen in man. Int J Cancer 1975; 25:246–52.
218. Bull DM, Leibach JR, Williams MA, Helms RA. Immunity to colon cancer assessed by antigen-induced inhibition of mixed mononuclear cell migration. Science 1973; 181:957–9.
219. Hellstrom I, Hellstrom KE. Newer concepts of cancer of the colon and rectum: Cellular immunity to human colonic carcinomas. Dis Colon Rectum 1972; 15:100–5.
220. Lauder I, Bone G. Lymphocyte transformation in large bowel cancer. Br J Cancer 1973; 27:409–13.
221. McIllmurray MB, Price MR, Langman MJS. Inhibition of leucocyte migration in patients with large intestinal cancer by extracts prepared from large intestinal tumors and from normal colonic mucosa. Br J Cancer 1974; 29:305–11.
222. Nind APP, Matthews N, Pihi EAV, Rolland JM, Nairn RC. Analysis of inhibition of lymphocyte cytotoxicity in human colon carcinoma. Br J Cancer 1975; 31:620–9.
223. Schultz RM, Woods WA, Chirigos MA. Detection in colorectal carcinoma patients of antibody cytotoxic to establish cell strains derived from carcinoma of the human colon and rectum. Int J Cancer 1975; 16:16–23.
224. Order SE, Klein JE, Ettinger D, Alderson P, Siegelman S, Leichner P. The use of isotopic immunoglobulin in therapy. Cancer Res 1980; 40:3001–7.
225. Shils ME. Principles of nutritional therapy. Cancer 1979; 2093–2102.
226. Copeland EM III, Daly JM, Dudrick SJ. Nutrition and cancer. Int Adv Surg Oncol 1981; 4:1–13.
227. Daly JM, Copeland EM III, Dudrick SJ, Delaney JM. Nutritional repletion of malnourished tumor-bearing and non-tumor-bearing rats. Surg Res 1980; 28:507–18.
228. Laurence BH, Cotton PB. Endoscopic placement of palliative drainage tubes in malignant biliary obstruction. Br Med J 1980; 280:522–6.
229. Raaf JH, Stroehlein JR. Palliation of malignant ascites by the LeVeen peritoneo-venous shunt. Cancer 1980; 45:1019–24.
230. Straus AK, Roseman DL, Shapiro TM. Peritoneo-venous shunting in the management of malignant ascites. Arch Surg 1978; 114:489–91.
231. Pollock AV. The treatment of resistant malignant ascites by insertion of a peritoneo-atrial Holter valve. Br J Surg 1975; 62:104–7.
232. Lightdale CJ, Kurtz RC, Boyle CC, Sherlock P, Winawer SJ. Cancer and upper gastrointestinal tract hemorrhage. Benign causes of bleeding demonstrated by endoscopy. JAMA 1973; 226:139–41.
233. Wanebo HJ, Rao B, Pinsky CH, Hoffman RG, Stearns M Jr, Schwartz MK, Oettgen HF. Preoperative carcinoembryonic antigen level as a prognostic indicator in colorectal cancer. N Engl J Med 1978; 299:448.
234. Goslin R, Steele G, MacIntyre J, Mayer R, Sugarbaker P, Cleghorn K, Wilson R, Zamcheck N. Preoperative CEA stratification of Dukes' C tumors. Ann Surg 1980; 192:747.
235. Mach JP, Jaeger P, Bertholet MM, Ruegsegger CH, Loo Loosli RM, Pettavel J. Detection of recurrence of large bowel carcinoma by radioimmunoassay of circulating carcinoembryonic antigen (CEA). Lancet 1974; 2:535–40.
236. Attiyeh FF, Stearns MW Jr. Second-look laparotomy based on CEA elevations in colorectal cancer. Cancer 1981; 47:2119.
237. Wedell J, Meier zu Eissen P, Luu TH, Fiedler R, van Calker H, Koldowski P, Schlipkoter H. A retrospective study of serial CEA determinations in the early detection of recurrent colorectal cancer. Dis Colon Rectum 1981; 24:618.
238. Beart RW Jr, Metzger PP, O'Connell MJ, Schutt AJ. Postoperative screening of patients with carcinoma of the colon. Dis Colon Rectum 1981; 24:585.
239. Beart RW Jr, O'Connell MJ. Postoperative follow-up of patients with carcinoma of the colon. Mayo Clin Proc 1983; 58:361–3.
240. Shani A, O'Connell MJ, Moertel CG, Schutt AJ, Silvers A, Go VLW. Serial plasma carcinoembryonic antigen measurements in the management of metastatic colorectal carcinoma. Ann Intern Med 1978; 88:627.
241. Fork FT. Double contrast enema and colonoscopy in polyp detection. Gut 1981; 22:971–7.
242. Winawer SJ, Leidner SD, Boyle C, Kurtz RC. Comparison of flexible sigmoidoscopy with other diagnostic techniques in the diagnosis of rectocolon neoplasia. Am J Dig Dis 1979; 24:277.
243. Hertz RE, Deddish MR, Day E. Value of periodic examination in detecting cancer of the rectum and colon. Postgrad Med 1960; 27:290.
244. Enker WE, Kramer RG. The follow-up of patients after definitive resections for large bowel cancer. World J Surg 1982; 6:578–84.
245. Stearns MW Jr. The care of the patient with a colostomy. *In*: Stearns MW Jr (ed). Neoplasms of the Colon, Rectum, and Anus. New York: John Wiley, 1981: 185–92.
246. Sternberg SS. Pathological aspects of colon and anorectal cancer. *In*: Stearns MW Jr (ed). Neoplasms of the Colon, Rectum, and Anus. New York: John Wiley, 1980: 37–62.
247. Stearns MW Jr, Urmacher C, Sternberg SS, Woodruff J, Attiyeh F. Cancer of the anal canal. Curr Probl Surg 1980; 4:1–44.
248. Nigro N, Vaitkevicius VK, Considine BJ. Combined therapy for cancer of the anal canal. A preliminary report. Dis Colon Rectum 1974; 17:354.
249. Quan SH, Magill GB, Leaming RH, Hajdu SI. Multidisciplinary preoperative approach to the management of epidermoid carcinoma of the anus and anorectum. Dis Colon Rectum 1978; 21:89.
250. Quinn D, Selah C. Malignant melanoma of the anus in a Negro: Report of a case and review of the literature. Dis Colon Rectum 1977; 20:627.
251. Wanebo HJ, Woodruff JM, Farr GH, Quan SHQ. Anorectal melanoma. Cancer 1981; 47:1891–1900.
252. Weingrad D, DeCosse JJ, Sherlock P, Straus D, Lieberman PH, Filippa DA. Primary gastrointestinal lymphoma. Cancer 1982; 49:1258–65.

Chapter 140

Injuries of the Colon and Rectum

Alexander J. Walt

Penetrating wounds of the colon and rectum due to gunshots or stabs are now common entities in the emergency rooms of urban hospitals and account for over 90% of all injuries of the large bowel. Whereas the mortality rate of these injuries used to range between 12% and 15%, the rate has tended to fall over the past decade to as low as 6.5% (Table 140–1). Only a third of the deaths are due to the colonic injury; the others are ascribable to initial blood loss or to the complications of extracolonic damage. Other factors affecting the outcome include: (1) the time elapsing between injury and treatment (more than 6 hours is highly undesirable); (2) the age of the patient (the 5% who are over 60 years of age do less well); (3) the cardiopulmonary status prior to injury; and (4) the presence of diabetes, alcoholism, malnutrition, or immunologic depression.

In addition to the more common stabs and gunshots, iatrogenic perforations resulting from proctosigmoidoscopy, colonoscopy, barium enema, biopsy, or fulguration of mucosal lesions are occasionally encountered. More rarely, patients incur injury from jets of compressed air, foreign bodies, or accidental impalement on protruding objects. Blunt injuries, occuring in falls from heights or in association with automobile accidents, con-

Table 140–1. COLLECTED SERIES: COLORECTAL INJURIES

Institution	Date	Patients (N)	Mortality (%)	Gunshot Wounds::Stabs
Wayne State	1959–70	340	15.0	3::1
	1971–73	113	12.0	5::1
Vietnam[1]	1968–69	220	11.8	All gunshot wounds
Baylor[3]	1949–64	328	12.8	2::1
	1965–70	424	14.2	6::1
University of California–San Francisco[14]	1960–70	147	15.0	2::1
University of California–San Francisco[6]	1970–75	124	6.5	2::1
Grady[11]	1975–79	268	8.0	—
Louisville[4]	1976–80	137	16.0	9::1
Henry Ford Hospital[35]	1975–80	114	5.3	4::1
University of Natal[2]	1977–82	394	6.6	1::9

stitute about 5% of colonic injuries and are becoming more common as seat belts are increasingly worn.

Whatever the primary etiologic factor, certain fundamental principles apply to the management of all patients with colonic or rectal injuries. The mortality rates for these lesions during the First and Second World Wars and the Korean conflict were approximately 70%, 25%, and 15%, respectively. From these experiences the view developed that all penetrating wounds of the large bowel should be either exteriorized, locally repaired with the addition of a defunctioning proximal colostomy, or resected, although never with primary anastomosis of the colon. In the Vietnam action (where about 7% of all war wounds were abdominal and approximately one-third of these involved the large intestine) a more flexible approach to the problem evolved in conjunction with improved transport and hospital facilities. However, the surgical approach was inevitably influenced by the extensive tissue damage caused by high-velocity missiles.[1] The validity of extrapolating the results from a military series to injuries sustained in civilian life has been challenged and has become largely discredited. Even now, however, in the treatment of civilian injuries insufficient attention is given to the differences in the nature and velocity of the wounding object, the availability of rapid transport to the emergency room, and the prognostic impact of early administration of appropriate antibiotics, fluids, and other resuscitative measures.

Types and Sites of Injury

Some representative modern approaches to the treatment of colorectal injuries in civilians have been reported from many institutions.[2–7] The data must be interpreted with caution, however, as the morbidity, mortality, and selection of patients for simple closure of the colonic wound or for resection and primary anastomosis of the bowel depend in large measure on the nature of the wounding agent in each series (Table 140–2). It is noteworthy that because of the increased use of firearms by the civilian population, the frequency of primary resection and anastomosis has actually decreased in many institutions committed by tradition and experience to a more aggressive surgical approach.[8] Jordan,[9] for example, reports that at the Ben Taub Hospital in 1980 only 46% of the patients with colonic injury had primary repair, which represented a decline. Weiner et al.,[10] on the other hand, performed primary repair in 105 of 181 patients (59%), with a 7% mortality. Whereas the mortality rate for stab wounds of the colon approximates 2% to 3% and for handgun wounds is about 12%, the figure rises to 50% in the case of shotgun wounds and blunt injuries.

Table 140–2. PROCEDURES FOR COLORECTAL INJURIES AT WAYNE STATE UNIVERSITY, FEBRUARY 1972 TO FEBRUARY 1974 (Prospective Study)*

	Patients	Mortality (%)	Average No. Organs Injured†
Primary closure (with or without resection)	49	4	1.8
Primary closure with proximal colostomy	51	16	2.1
Exteriorization or resection with end colostomy	34	9	2.5
Exteriorized anastomosis	31	3	2.5
	145‡	10	

*Adapted from Kirkpatrick JR, Rajpal SC. Am J Surg *129*:187, 1975.

†Average number of organs injured in those who died was 5.2 in contrast to 2.1 in the survivors.

‡80% missile injuries.

Only about 20% of colonic injuries are isolated, and the great majority of patients with single lesions survive. Gunshot wounds are equally distributed throughout the colon. Stab wounds involve the transverse colon disproportionately because of its length and anatomic position. In a review of injuries of the large bowel in our institution, extracolonic organs were involved in 100% of shotgun wounds, 80% of handgun injuries, 46% of stab wounds, and 80% of blunt injuries. In descending order of frequency, the organs most likely to be injured are the small intestine, liver, stomach, major vessels, kidney, chest, spleen, extremities, duodenum, pancreas, and central nervous system. Mortality is much more likely to be related to the injured extracolonic organs, rising in proportion to the number of structures injured. It cannot be stressed too strongly that while morbidity and length of hospitalization vary considerably with the extent and site of the colorectal injury, the colonic lesion is seldom the main determinant of death. About 40% of surviving patients develop postoperative complications, the most common of which are wound infections, intra-abdominal abscesses (in the pelvis or subphrenic area or between loops of intestines), intestinal obstruction, wound disruptions, and pulmonary insufficiency (especially in patients who have required large quantities of blood).

Initial Examination

It is vital that all hospital emergency personnel have a distinct but flexible plan of management for the severely injured patient suspected of having a traumatic perforation of the intestine. Details of history obtained from the patient or a bystander may be of value in determining the type or direction of injury. As soon as feasible, the patient is completely stripped and carefully examined back and front for concomitant injuries, both abdominal and extra-abdominal. Particular search is made for thoracic complications, since these are often the most immediately life-threatening. The anal and gluteal regions should be examined with special care, because small puncture wounds may create lethal internal injuries and are easily missed if the examination is cursory. Digital examination of the anorectum is performed and, if blood is present on the examining finger, proctoscopy and sigmoidoscopy should follow. Plain radiographs of the abdomen, posteroanterior and lateral, are important in outlining free air, a retroperitoneal hematoma, fractures of the pelvis and spine, or the position and track of any residual missile. Where only an entrance wound is seen and no intra-abdominal bullet is visible on the radiograph, it is essential to obtain films of the chest, the neck, and the limbs, because missiles occasionally pursue bizarre and unpredictable courses. A reasonably thorough neurologic examination should be conducted and the state of the anal sphincters noted, especially in cases of damage to the sacral area in which concomitant neurologic damage is more likely to occur. Accurate recording is essential both for initial assessment and for possible later medicolegal evidence. In automobile accidents, the presence of ecchymoses and abrasions of the abdominal skin or transverse rupture of the rectus muscles often serves as a clue to associated intestinal rupture by a seat belt.

General Principles of Management

Many patients will have multiple injuries, and immediate attention must be given to resuscitation. A penetrating wound anywhere from the neck to the buttocks, anterior or posterior, must be regarded as having possibly entered the large intestine. The provision of adequate ventilation and blood volume takes precedence. One or 2 large IV cannulas are inserted into arm veins, so that fluids may be given rapidly if necessary. The central venous pressure is monitored. Blood is drawn for typing and cross matching, and balanced salt solution is administered.

A nasogastric tube is inserted to empty the stomach and reduce the hazard of subsequent aspiration and ileus. A Foley catheter is placed in the bladder to detect any hematuria and to assess continuing adequate urinary output. Whenever hematuria is present, investigation of the urinary tract is essential. An IV pyelogram should be obtained as soon as possible and followed, if necessary, by cystography. In selected patients in whom a bladder injury is suspected, cystography may precede or supersede pyelography.

Whenever a perforation of the intestine is suspected, gross contamination of the peritoneal cavity should be assumed, and IV administration of antibiotics is begun in the emergency department immediately. The pathogenic organisms most often cultured are *Escherichia coli*, enterococci, and *Bacteroides*. There is no unanimity about the initial selection of antibiotics, whether these turn out to be prophylactic or therapeutic, but if a colonic injury is suspected, a combination of an aminoglycoside and clindamycin or cefoxitin alone is most often used. Some surgeons, however, favor the initial administration IV of cefazolin and a change to broader coverage if fecal contamination is found at operation. Any antibiotics ordered should be precisely detailed on the order sheet, given intraoperatively and in the immediate postoperative period, and modified to reflect renal function. All patients should receive a booster dose of tetanus toxoid or, if never immunized, 250 units of tetanus immune globulin (Hyper-Tet).

Treatment of Specific Injuries

Stab Wounds. These wounds in most instances have clean edges requiring little or no debridement and may be oversewn with 1 or 2 layers of sutures. Where there has been modest contamination, soft rubber drains may be placed close to but not against the area of injury if the repaired bowel is returned to the peritoneal cavity. Any deaths in this group of patients are usually due to associated transection of a large vessel, such as the inferior vena cava or aorta. As in any colonic injury, the apparent presence of a single intestinal wound must be viewed with great suspicion. In all intestinal wounds, it is vital that an exit wound be assiduously searched for, special attention being directed to the mesenteric area of the adjacent bowel wall where lacerations may easily be hidden. Failure to take this precaution may result in subsequent leakage of fecal contents and generalized peritonitis.

Gunshot Wounds. These wounds pose many problems, since it is usual to have one or more organs, sometimes at a distance, injured simultaneously. The extent of the visceral damage is determined by the nature and velocity of the missile. Damage to the adjacent organs, such as the liver and pancreas or large vessels, is more likely to determine the final outcome than is the colonic lesion. Hence, priority is given to the most life-threatening lesions after first rapidly applying tissue forceps to the colonic laceration to prevent continuing fecal spillage. When attention is finally directed to the colon, decisions may need to be tempered by the degree and duration of shock, the extent of peritoneal contamination, the character of any severe concomitant injuries, and the age of the patient (if more than 60 years old). These are all factors that may adversely affect both the prognosis and the healing of intraperitoneal anastomoses.

Absolute contraindications to primary repair of the colon and return of the anastomosis to the peritoneal cavity are:[11]

1. Persistent hypovolemic shock, pre- or intraoperatively.
2. A lapse of more than 6 hours before the colonic repair is completed.
3. Gross feces in the peritoneal cavity.
4. The presence of more than 1000 ml of blood in the peritoneal cavity.
5. Two or more concomitant visceral injuries, allowing for the fact that a massive single visceral injury may also preclude primary closure.
6. Extensive damage to the muscles of the posterior abdominal wall, such as the psoas, or destruction of the anterior abdominal wall of a degree to make reliable repair uncertain.
7. A younger patient whose physiologic age seems to be greater than that associated with the average 60-year-old patient.
8. The presence of substantial cirrhosis or evidence of marked immunodepression.

In most small wounds of the bowel wall caused by low-velocity bullets, the edges may be trimmed, the adequacy of the blood supply confirmed, and primary repair performed without a defunctioning colostomy, provided contamination is minimal and concomitant hazards (see previous list) are absent. This approach is regarded as unwarrantably aggressive by some, but is accepted on the basis of the number of excellent results in the hands of experienced surgeons.[4,7,11] When primary repair is contemplated, sound clinical judgment is vital. Increasingly, most surgeons eschew the use of drains alone for the colonic repair. In the patient severely injured by a gunshot wound, however, the simplest, quickest, and safest procedure is the time-honored exteriorization of the lesion when feasible or resection and the establishment of a proximal colostomy. Wide local drainage of the contaminated area is advisable after reduction of the bacterial load by local irrigation and the removal of any foreign materials.

With injuries of the right side of the colon, the technical decision is less difficult, since right hemicolectomy followed by primary anastomosis is relatively easy to accomplish and ordinarily carries low morbidity and mortality rates.[12] The alternative to anastomosis is an ileostomy and colonic mucous fistula, dislike for which tempts some surgeons to attempt primary anastomosis at almost any cost. This latter approach can be disastrous, however, when selection of patients is faulty. Patients who have been in shock and have required massive blood transfusions or who have serious intra-abdominal injuries associated with gross contamination or severe retroperitoneal muscle damage are best treated by removal of the injured area of colon, wide drainage of the retroperitoneal region, and the establishment of an ileostomy and colonic mucous fistula. With the patient fully resuscitated, free of sepsis, and in a favorable metabolic state, definitive re-establishment of intestinal continuity can be much more safely performed 2 to 12 weeks later, depending on the patient's progress. The difficulties of management of a temporary ileostomy in such cases have been grossly exaggerated.

Some surgeons have tried to avoid the morbidity and the subsequent operation for closure necessitated by a proximal colostomy.[2, 13, 14] Seeking to steer a middle course in questionable cases, these surgeons have advocated primary repair of the damaged bowel with exteriorization of the anastomosis. This is based on animal experiments that have shown that exteriorized anastomoses heal as satisfactorily as those placed intraperitoneally.[15] The exteriorized anastomosis can then be observed on the abdominal wall and, if intact, simply returned to the abdominal cavity on about the sixth postoperative day if the patient's general condition is satisfactory. Alternatively, if it seems desirable at any time, the colostomy can be opened at the bedside without difficulty.[13] When successful, this approach obviates the need for subsequent closure of a colostomy initially established to protect the intraperitoneal suture line, a procedure that carries a morbidity rate of about 29%.[16]

If the technique of extraperitonealization of the anastomosis is attempted, it is important that an adequate passage through the abdominal wall of about 8 cm be established so that there is no kinking of the exteriorized segment with consequent iatrogenic obstruction of the already unavoidably edematous segment.[14] Using this technique, Okies et al.[17] have avoided formal colostomy in 49% of 37 patients. Schrock et al.,[18] however, reported a success rate of only 21%. In contrast, Kirkpatrick[13] successfully avoided colostomy in 62% of a series of 61 patients, but surprisingly found that hospitalization was not significantly reduced, largely because of the delay in healing of associated injuries.

Injuries to the descending colon seldom are suitable for resection and primary anastomosis, since the bowel is unprepared in terms of fecal content and the blood supply is more precarious than on the right side. The conservative surgical approach, which avoids the temptation to attempt definitive repair in any other than minor fresh wounds, continues to prevail for lesions distal to the splenic flexure.[19]

Special precautions are necessary in dealing with injuries of the extraperitoneal rectum.[20, 21] Not infrequently, the extent of the damage is virtually impossible to assess adequately at the initial operation because of an obscuring pelvic hematoma and the relative anatomic inaccessibility of the area. In many cases, the situation is further complicated by vesical, sacral, neurologic, and major vascular injuries. Attempts to achieve initial definitive repair are hazardous and lead to a high mortality rate. An attempt should be made to visualize and repair all lacerations of the rectum, but the assumption should also be made that lesions may be missed and that repairs may fail to remain sealed. Consequently, the best results are obtained by the addition of:

1. A proximal diverting sigmoid colostomy.
2. Thorough cleansing of the bowel between the colostomy and the anus by saline irrigations at the time of operation to reduce the bacterial load and to obviate subsequent leakage of stool into the damaged extraperitoneal planes.
3. Adequate debridement of the pelvic tissues.
4. Extensive drainage of the extraperitoneal area with drains emerging through an adequate precoccygeal incision.
5. Administration of systemic antibiotics, most often penicillin, gentamicin, and clindamycin.
6. Instillation of antibiotics, such as neomycin or kanamycin, into the defunctioned bowel.
7. Four-finger anal dilation at the end of the operation.
8. General supportive measures.

Whenever there has been gross contamination of the peritoneal cavity by intestinal contents, the abdomen should be thoroughly washed with saline at the end of the operation and widely drained. The insertion of irrigating catheters for the purpose of instilling antibiotics, such as kanamycin, remains controversial. Neomycin and kanamycin should at least not be used until the effects of muscle relaxants given at the time of anesthesia have been completely eliminated, because of the risk of respiratory paralysis. The subcutaneous tissues are best left open initially and closed by secondary suture after approximately 5 days. Primary wound closure results in an inordinate number of wound abscesses, with increased morbidity and hospitalization.

Perforation Incident to Endoscopy or Barium Enema

Instrument Perforation. The frequency of perforation during the passage of a sigmoidoscope or following biopsy, with or without fulguration, is not fully reflected in the literature. The majority of these perforations occur because of technical ineptitude, and the injury is usually above the peritoneal reflection. Although in many instances the patient immediately experiences acute abdominal or shoulder tip pain, accentuated when air is insufflated, discomfort and subsequent peritonitis may not develop in some patients for a number of hours. Free air in the peritoneal cavity on plain radiographs of the abdomen or visualization of the rent by the leakage of contrast material is pathognomonic.

In the past, mortality rates of approximately 50% were described following instrument perforation. The outcome is largely related to the time permitted to elapse between the injury and formal operation. When this is less than 6 hours, there should be virtually no deaths, as the bowel is usually clean from the preparation preliminary to the endoscopy. Most of these injuries can be repaired primarily.

The burgeoning use of the colonoscope (Chapter 43) has resulted in an increased number of perforations. The true frequency of these perforations is difficult to assess and is obviously influenced by the skill of the endoscopist, the state of the colon (the attenuated bowel of chronic ulcerative colitis, especially during an acute episode, is unnaturally friable), and whether or not a biopsy or polypectomy is performed. It seems likely that the occurrence rate of perforation is less than 2% while experience is being obtained by the endoscopist, about 0.4% once expertise has been attained, and a little less than 1% when biopsy is performed by an experienced colonoscopist.[22, 23] Perforation is most likely to occur (1) when the tip of the instrument is pushed too firmly against the bowel wall, usually the sigmoid, and especially if there is some underlying disease of the bowel, such as diverticulitis or ulcerative colitis; (2) when the base of a polyp is excessively fulgurated; (3) at the rectosigmoid junction when the instrument is fed into the bowel but does not advance, resulting in acute bow-stringing with laceration of the antimesenteric border of the rectosigmoid just above the peritoneal reflection; and (4) when inappropriate quantities of air are insufflated. Another rare but dire complication of colonoscopy that may occur with or without perforation is disruption of the phrenicosplenic ligament as the transverse colon is straightened.

Symptoms following perforation may be minimal or severe. Although the need for immediate surgical intervention is generally agreed upon for those with severe symptoms, some physicians advocate meticulous observation of patients with minimal symptoms. The latter group is simultaneously protected by an umbrella of heavy antibiotic coverage that includes gentamicin and clindamycin. However, the proponents of watchful waiting accept a grave responsibility. Justification advanced for this approach is the occasional observation that the perforation may be too small to be found even at operation and that it is, in effect, sometimes self-sealing. Surgeons, on the other hand, sensitized to the high and sometimes unpredictable morbidity of colonic injuries, prefer routine abdominal exploration and appropriate repair of the colonic laceration as soon after diagnosis as possible.

Perforation by Enema. Perforations associated with barium enemas (Chapter 33) are far more serious than purely instrument perforations. The combination of barium and feces is a potentially virulent mixture causing severe infection. Subsequent granulomas and widespread dense adhesions with resulting intestinal obstruction may follow. Most of these lesions are the result of carelessness with the large intrarectal balloon or enema tip and may take the form of extensive lacerations, often extraperitoneal. It is highly questionable whether a barium enema performed gently can be held responsible for the perforation of a diverticulum, as is sometimes claimed. Immediate operation is essential to cleanse the peritoneal cavity of barium and feces to prevent further leakage. The mortality rate of barium peritonitis approaches 50%, in part due to failure in the early stages to recognize the accident and later to administer large quantities of electrolyte solutions to combat the third-space loss of fluid caused by the irritating barium.

In patients who have had colonoscopic biopsy, barium enema should probably be avoided for 7 to 10 days if perforations are to be reduced in frequency. The radiologist should always be informed that biopsy has been done so that appropriate technical adjustments may be made.

Perforation of the colon through a colostomy by a carelessly employed catheter or enema tip is extremely dangerous. Few such victims survive, presumably because of delay in seeking surgical attention.

Jet Air Perforation. Extensive lesions may result from the passage of a jet of compressed air up the anal canal. This injury usually follows a prank when the nozzle is held a few inches from the victim's buttocks and the pressure suddenly turned on. It has been estimated that about 4 lb/square inch of pressure is needed to rupture the bowel; compressed air jets may generate up to 125 lb/ square inch.[24] The laceration of the bowel usually occurs in the rectosigmoid area and may extend for 10 cm or more. Early operative treatment is essential.

Perforations from Within the Bowel

Rectal impalement by a wide variety of objects, such as pickets, broomsticks, or hydraulic jacks, has been described.[25, 26] These wounds may extend into any abdominal organ and even into the chest. The principles of treatment are the same as for all penetrating injuries, with the additional caveat that the impaling object be left in situ while the patient is transported to the hospital and removed only at operation under direct vision with the abdomen open. This assists in the identification of the injured organs, reduces fecal spillage, and facilitates immediate control of hemorrhage, which may otherwise be catastrophic on withdrawal of the impaling object.

Current mores are reflected in an increasing number of incidents in which patients are seen with ruptured bowels following insertion into the rectum of bottles, fists, or other firm objects. After removal of the offending object, careful sigmoidoscopic inspection should always be made to exclude the presence of an occult laceration. If a perforation has occurred, the principles delineated earlier should be followed.

Non-penetrating Injuries

Blunt trauma is responsible for about 8% of all colonic injuries and poses special problems inasmuch as its occurrence is rarely recognized in the early stages.[27] An isolated colonic injury occurs in only about 10% of these patients; concomitant head, chest, or limb injuries usually dominate the clinical picture. Of our 35 patients, 22 were involved in automobile accidents, either as pedestrians or as passengers; the remainder suffered falls or direct assaults. The responsible mechanism is most often a shearing injury or an increased intraluminal bursting pressure. In a few cases, the injury seems to be due to a direct crush, especially when the patient is wearing a seat belt. The severity of the blow is not necessarily reflected in the degree of intestinal damage, and the ultimate colonic injury is greatly influenced by the degree of tension of the abdominal muscles at the moment of impact. Damage to the spinal column, such as fractured lumbar pedicles, or rupture of the rectus muscles may occur concomitantly and should serve as a clinical warning.

Although the use of seat belts has significantly reduced the frequency of injury in automobile accidents, it has produced intestinal injury in some patients, especially when the belt is incorrectly worn above the iliac crests.[28, 29] Although the ileum is the organ most often affected, tears of the colonic mesentery or of the colon itself may occur. The symptoms and signs of serious intra-abdominal injury may be delayed for up to a week, as the ischemic bowel becomes more necrotic before finally perforating into the free peritoneal cavity or, rarely, into the retroperitoneal tissues with formation of a colocutaneous fistula.[30]

Intramural hematomas of the colon probably occur more often than has been recognized.[31] Most of these will regress spontaneously, but in a few cases sudden rupture with intraperitoneal hemorrhage or chronic inflammatory changes leading to later colonic stenosis may occur.[32]

An uncommon form of crush injury has been described in pedestrians run over by a vehicle. These unfortunates sustain a sudden rise in intra-abdominal pressure followed by an abrupt release that results in rupture of the pelvic muscular diaphragm.[33, 34] In some, the anorectal apparatus may be left intact but torn from the levator ani sling, as has also been described in some blast injuries from below. This complex injury is recognized by the proximal retraction of the anal canal and rectum above the levators or by the gross eccentric displacement of the anus in the perineum. The patient will often be in shock and may have associated genitourinary injuries. These patients require early operation, with debridement and drainage of the perineum, repair of the bowel where a laceration has occurred, establishment of a proximal colostomy in many cases, and, finally, anchoring of the anal canal both to the levators and to the perineal skin.

References

1. Ganchrow MI, Lavenson GS, McNamara JJ. Surgical management of traumatic injuries of the colon and rectum. Arch Surg 1970; 100:515.
2. Baker LW, and Robbs JV. Selective management of penetrating injuries of the colon. S Afr J Surg 1982; 20:275.
3. Beall AC, Bricker DL, Alessi FJ, et al. Surgical considerations in the management of civilian colon injuries. Ann Surg 1971; 173:971.
4. Flint LM, Vitale GC, Richardson JD, et al. The injured colon: Relationships of management to complications. Ann Surg 1981; 193:619.
5. Garfinkle SE, Cohen SE, Matolo NM, et al. Civilian colonic injuries: Changing concepts of management. Arch Surg 1974; 109:402.
6. Steele M, Blaisdell FW. Treatment of colon injuries. J Trauma 1977; 17:557.
7. Walt AJ. Management of injuries of the colon and rectum. *In*: MacLean LD, ed. Advances in Surgery, Vol 16. Chicago: Year Book Medical Publishers, 1983: 277–97.
8. Jordan GL, Jr. Abdominal trauma Texas style. Am J Surg 1971; 121:503.
9. Jordan G. Colonic injuries. Presentation at the Spring Meeting, American College of Surgeons, 1982.
10. Wiener I, Rojas P, Wolfman FJ. Traumatic colonic perforation: Review of 16 years' experience. Am J Surg 1975; 131:705.
11. Stone HH, Fabian TC. Management of perforating colon trauma: Randomization between primary closure and exteriorization. Ann Surg 1979; 190:430.
12. Chilimindris C, Boyd DR, Carlson LE, et al. A critical review of management of right colon injuries. J Trauma 1971; 11:651.
13. Kirkpatrick JR, Rajpal SG. The injured colon: Therapeutic considerations. Am J Surg 1975; 129:187.
14. Lou MA, Johnson AP, Atik M, et al. Exteriorized repair in the management of colon injuries. Arch Surg 1981; 116:926.
15. Kirkpatrick JR, Rajpal SG. Management of a high-risk intestinal anastomosis. Am J Surg 1973; 125:362.
16. Smit R, Walt AJ. The morbidity and cost of the temporary colostomy. Dis Colon Rectum 1978; 21:558.
17. Okies JE, Bricker DL, Jordan GL, et al. Exteriorized primary repair of colon injuries. Am J Surg 1972; 124:807.
18. Schrock TR, Christensen N. Management of perforating injuries of the colon. Surg Gynecol Obstet 1972; 135:65.
19. Bartizal JF, Boyd DF, Folk FA, et al. A critical review of management of 392 colonic and rectal injuries. Dis Colon Rectum 1974; 17:313.
20. Lavenson GS, Cohen A. Management of rectal injuries. Am J Surg 1971; 122:226.
21. Trunkey D, Hayes RJ, Shires GT. Management of rectal trauma. J Trauma 1973; 13:411.
22. Smith LE, Nivatvongs S. Complications in colonoscopy. Dis Colon Rectum 1975; 18:214.
23. Spencer RJ, Coates HL, Anderson MJ. Colonoscopic polypectomies. Mayo Clin Proc 1974; 49:40.
24. Weigel CJ. Traumatic injuries to the large bowel and rectum in industry. Am J Proctol 1962; 13:155.
25. Kaufer N, Shein S, Levowitz BS. Impalement injury of the rectum: An unusual case. Dis Colon Rectum 1967; 10:394.
26. Weckesser EC, Putnam TC. Perforating injuries of the rectum and sigmoid colon. J Trauma 1962; 2:474.
27. Howell HS, Bartizal JF, Freeark RJ. Blunt trauma involving the colon and rectum. J Trauma 1976; 16:624.
28. Editorial. Seat belt injuries to the colon. Br Med J 1974; 1:85.
29. Towne JB, Coe JD. Seat belt trauma of the colon. Am J Surg 1971; 122:683.
30. Wightman JAK. Delayed traumatic rupture of colon with colocutaneous fistula. Br Med J 1967; 2:93.
31. Nance FC, Crowder VH. Intramural hematoma of the colon following blunt trauma to the abdomen. Am Surg 1968; 34:85.
32. Altner PC. Constrictive lesions of the colon due to blunt trauma to the abdomen. Surg Gynecol Obstet 1964; 118:1257.
33. Morton JH. Perineal and rectal damage following nonpenetrating abdominal trauma. J Trauma 1972; 12:347.
34. Stein A. Ano-rectal avulsion associated with crush injuries. S Afr J Surg 1964; 2:43.
35. Obeid FN, Sorensen V, Vincent G, et al. Management of colonic trauma; 6-year experience at Henry Ford Hospital. Henry Ford Hosp Med J 1983; 31:17.

Chapter 141

Antibiotic-Associated Injury to the Gut

Te-Wen Chang

Antimicrobial agents may produce injury to the gastrointestinal tract either by direct toxicity or indirectly by a change of intestinal microbial flora. Most antimicrobials may give rise to some irritation of the gastrointestinal tract. While most side effects are minor and do not interfere with continued administration of the drug, certain reactions are serious. A list of adverse reactions involving the gastrointestinal tract is shown in Table 141–1. The list includes antibacterial, antifungal, antiparasitic, and antiviral agents.

Teeth

Yellow discoloration and hypoplasia of the enamel of the teeth occur frequently in children who received tetracycline during the period of mineralization of the teeth. The drug is deposited as a calcium complex in the mineralizing zones of the teeth. The discolored teeth fluoresce with a yellow color under ultraviolet light; this is of diagnostic value in differentiation from other causes of tooth discoloration.[1]

Mineralization of the deciduous teeth occurs from the fourth month of intrauterine life until 7 months after birth. Calcification of the permanent teeth, with the exception of the third molars, begins at birth and continues through the eighth year of life.[2]

Concentrations of oxytetracycline and chlortetracycline in cord blood are about one-half of those in maternal blood.[3] Not surprisingly, therefore, about half of all children exposed to tetracyclines during the third trimester will develop tooth discoloration. Tetracycline may also be ingested through the mother's milk and produce similar damage. A total dose of 3 g or therapy over 10 days produces visible dental changes in about one-third of children given tetracycline.[4]

Because of these observations, pregnant women should not be given tetracycline after the fourth month of pregnancy. Nursing mothers should not be treated with tetracycline. No tetracycline should be given to children from the time of birth through 8 years of age. As a matter of fact, the discoloration of the permanent teeth and enamel hypoplasia in children taking tetracycline have led the Food and Drug Administration to propose to withdraw marketing licenses for concentrated forms of tetracyclines for pediatric use.[5]

Oral Mucosa

Glossitis and/or stomatitis has been seen occasionally following the administration of metronidazole, sulfonamides, trimethoprim-sulfamethoxazole, chloramphenicol, gentamicin, cephradine, and sulfasalazine. Black hairy tongue, glossitis, stomatitis, and other reactions of the oropharynx have been described following the use of tetracyclines and penicillins, but their pathogenesis remains unclear. These same manifestations have also been seen without exposure to antibiotics. In occasional cases, *Candida albicans* is found.[6]

Esophagus

Esophageal ulcerations due to ingestion of capsules of various tetracyclines are appar-

Table 141–1. ADVERSE REACTIONS TO ANTIMICROBIAL AGENTS INVOLVING THE GASTROINTESTINAL TRACT

Drug	Anorexia	Nausea	Vomiting	Diarrhea	Glossitis	Stomatitis	Dysphagia	Entero-colitis	Others*
Tetracyclines	+	+	+	+	+	+	+	+	1, 5, 11, 16, 17
Minocycline	+	+	+	+	+		+	+	16
Erythromycin		+	+	+				+	6, 13
Cefazolin	+	+	+	+				+	5, 13
Cephalexin	+	+	+	+ +				+	6, 13
Cephradine		+	+	+ +	+			+	6, 7, 13
Cefoxitin		+	+	+				+	13
Cefaclor		+ +	+ +	+ +				+	13
Cephadroxil		+ +		+ +				+	
Gentamicin		+	+			+			13, 15
Neomycin		+ +	+ +	+ +					14
Kanamycin		+	+	+					14
Amikacin, tobramycin		+	+						
Chloramphenicol		+	+	+	+	+		+	
Clindamycin, lincomycin		+	+	+ +			+	+	6, 13
Ampicillin		+	+	+ +	+	+		+	1, 2, 13
Amoxicillin		+	+	+	+	+		+	2, 13
Penicillin G and V		+	+	+				+	1, 2
Oxacillin					+	+		+	13
Cloxacillin		+		+				+	13
Nafcillin		+	+	+				+	13
Carbenicillin		+	+	+				+	6, 9, 13
Metronidazole	+ +	+ +	+ +	+ +	+	+		+	2, 6, 8, 9, 10
Sulfonamides	+	+	+	+	+	+		+	4, 6, 12
Trimethoprim-sulfamethoxazole		+	+	+	+	+		+	4, 6, 12
Sulfasalazine	+ +	+ +	+ +	+		+		+	4, 6, 12
Amphotericin B	+ +	+ +	+ +	+ +					2, 3, 4
Flucytosine, griseofulvin		+	+	+					
Miconazole	+	+ +	+ +	+					
Ketoconazole		+ +	+ +	+					
Nystatin		+	+	+					
Nitrofurantoin, nalidixic acid	+ +	+ +	+ +	+					6
Isoniazid		+	+						2, 4
Rifampin	+	+	+	+				+	2, 4, 6
Para-aminosalicylic acid	+ +	+ +	+	+					2
Pyrantel pamoate	+ +	+ +	+ +	+					2, 6, 7
Thiabendazole	+ +	+ +	+ +	+					2
Piperazine, pyrvinium pamoate		+	+	+					6
Vidarabine	+	+	+	+					
Amantadine	+	+	+						9, 10

Frequency of adverse reactions: + + commonly observed, + less common.

*1. Black hairy tongue. 2. Epigastric pain or distress. 3. Melena or acute hemorrhagic gastroenteritis. 4. Hepatitis. 5. Oral candidiasis. 6. Abdominal pain. 7. Tenesmus. 8. Metallic taste. 9. Dry mouth. 10. Constipation. 11. Hepatic cholestasis. 12. Pancreatitis. 13. Abnormal liver function tests. 14. Malabsorption. 15. Transient hepatomegaly. 16. Candidiasis in anogenital region. 17. Discoloration of teeth.

ently not uncommon, especially if esophageal motility is disturbed. It is recommended that patients should not lie down immediately after taking a tetracycline capsule, that the capsules be swallowed with an ample amount of water, and that these capsules should probably be avoided in patients with dysphagia.[7]

Delayed passage of oral tablets of clindamycin or lincomycin has been incriminated in causing esophageal ulceration.[8] These tablets should be taken with a meal or with a glass of water.

Upper Gastrointestinal Tract

Nausea, vomiting, and *epigastric discomfort* are the most common side effects seen with antibiotic therapy. Such side effects have been observed following oral administration of practically all antimicrobial agents, including antibacterial, antifungal, antiparasitic, and antiviral drugs, but the most frequent offenders are metronidazole, neomycin, cefaclor, amphotericin B, sulfasalazine, miconazole, ketoconazole, nitrofurantoin, nalidixic acid, para-aminosalicylic acid (PAS), pyrantel pamoate, and thiabendazole. Nausea is frequently seen with tetracycline therapy. *Anorexia* has been observed frequently following the administration of metronidazole, sulfasalazine, amphotericin B, nitrofurantoin, nalidixic acid, PAS, pyrantel pamoate, and thiabendazole. Occasionally, anorexia is seen with the tetracyclines, cefazolin, cephalexin, sulfonamides, miconazole, rifampin, vidarabine, and amantadine.

To alleviate these complications, the antimicrobial agents may be taken after meals, with an antacid, or with a glass of milk. However, tetracyclines should not be taken with milk, antacids containing calcium or magnesium, and/or iron because they are chelated by these divalent or trivalent cations to form complexes that are either poorly absorbed or not absorbed at all.[9, 10] The combination of oral administration of tetracycline and iron leads to poor absorption of both as a result of chelation and blockage of mucosal reabsorption from tetracycline. To avoid this undesirable interaction, a time interval of 2 to 3 hours should separate the administration of tetracycline and iron preparations.

Malabsorption

Neomycin, when taken orally in doses of 3 to 12 g daily, produces malabsorption of fat, protein, and carbohydrates. Within 1 week of therapy, the following events have been observed: striking shortening of villi, round cell infiltration in the mucosa of the upper small intestine, and crypt cell damage resembling mitochondrial degeneration and vesiculation of the outer cell membrane of the organ of Corti.[11] The crypt cell damage may lead to a decrease of serum cholesterol, which is synthesized to some degree by these cells.[12] The major cause of malabsorption is probably a direct toxic effect of neomycin on the mucosa. A minor contributory factor is an interaction between neomycin and bile salts, leading to interference with fat digestion.[13]

Kanamycin also occasionally produces malabsorption, but to a lesser extent.

Diarrhea and Enterocolitis

Diarrhea is a frequent complication of antimicrobial therapy. While the cause of diarrhea is not completely known, many of the cases appear to be related to overgrowth of *Clostridium difficile,* which produces 2 distinct toxins that cause diarrhea and enterocolitis.

Before the discovery of *C. difficile* as a cause of intestinal disease, only *pseudomembranous colitis* (PMC) was known to be associated with use of antibiotics, especially clindamycin. Since the etiologic role of *C. difficile* has been revealed and its presence is capable of being made precisely by laboratory testing, the spectrum of antimicrobial-associated diarrhea has greatly expanded. It is now clear that PMC is only one form, albeit the most severe, of the diarrheal complications of antimicrobial usage. Since many drugs with antibacterial activity have been implicated, the broader term *antimicrobial-associated diarrhea and enterocolitis* more accurately describes this condition.[13a]

PMC was first described in 1893 by Finney[14] as a surgical complication. During the pre-antibiotic era, the disease was associated with a number of conditions, chiefly intestinal surgery, but also spinal fracture, intestinal obstruction, colon carcinoma, heavy metal poisoning, and others. The frequency rate was low, but the death rate was high. PMC is characterized by plaque-like lesions on the intestinal mucosa and was usually diagnosed at surgery or necropsy. During the early 1950s, it was first related to use of antibiotics, chiefly tetracycline and chloramphenicol. These agents were thought to suppress sensitive intestinal organisms, allowing resistant *Staphylococcus aureus* to overpopulate and become the predominant stool organism.[15] The terms *antimicrobial-induced pseudomembranous enterocolitis, postoperative colitis, diphtheritic enteritis,* and *staphylococcal enterocolitis* were often used interchangeably. Vancomycin was used successfully for therapy during the 1970s. However, while "staphylococcal enterocolitis" practically vanished, PMC remained.

Etiology and Pathogenesis. While animal studies had established an etiologic role for *C. difficile,* a clear-cut demonstration of toxins in the stools of humans with PMC required tissue-culture studies. As it happened, the toxin was discovered almost a year before the bacterial source was identified.[16–19]

Evidence for the role of *C. difficile* in PMC in man is now convincing. The organism is seldom isolated from the stools of normal healthy adults, but is nearly always found in patients with PMC. Also present in the stools of patients with this disease are toxins with the same characteristics as those produced by the organism and which cause colitis when introduced into laboratory animals. When the toxins are eliminated from the stools of patients with PMC, the symptoms subside and the lesions resolve.

C. difficile is not considered a usual part of the normal gut flora in healthy adults, and therefore the organism must be acquired exogenously. While the process is not completely understood, a change of intestinal flora due to antimicrobial administration is probably the most important factor in permitting *C. difficile* to overpopulate. It has been shown that certain stool organisms can inhibit the growth of *C. difficile,* whereas others enhance its multiplication.[20] When the effect of various antibiotics on the intestinal flora is examined, it appears that suppression of "inhibitors" is the important effect that allows overgrowth of *C. difficile* in the gut. When diarrhea stops, either spontaneously or after treatment, most patients are able to eliminate the organism from the gut. Occasionally, *C. difficile* may persist and multiply, causing clinical relapse.

The mechanism of the diarrhea that is induced is still being investigated. *C. difficile* does not appear to be invasive; blood cultures are negative, and no organisms have been detected in the mucosa. All available evidence points to the importance of toxins in the disease process. At least 2 distinct toxins, A and B, have been isolated and purified from cultures of *C. difficile.*[21–23] Animal studies have shown that toxin A is 2 to 3 times more potent than toxin B in inducing fluid accumulation, an inflammatory exudate, and erythema. On the other hand, toxin B is much more potent than toxin A in causing cytopathic effects in cell cultures, as well as lethality in mice. However, either toxin A or toxin B alone may cause fatal colitis in the hamster. Immunization with a single toxoid produces protection against challenge by homologous but not by heterologous toxin. Only a combined toxoid A and B gives protection against challenge with a culture of *C. difficile* (which contains both toxin A and toxin B).[24] These studies indicate that in spite of some differences in biologic activities, both toxins are probably important in the disease process. There is some evidence that the toxin(s) may stimulate guanine cyclase to produce increased intracellular levels of cyclic guanine monophosphate with concomitant decrease of cyclic adenosine monophosphate.[25] There is also evidence showing that both toxins cause microscopic as well as ultrastructural changes of the cell membrane.[26,27] All these changes probably contribute to the pathogenesis of the disease.

Nearly all antimicrobial agents have been implicated in *C. difficile*–associated diarrhea or enterocolitis. Interestingly, the organism remains generally sensitive to the implicated antimicrobial agents.[28–30] The most common antimicrobials are ampicillin or amoxicillin, clindamycin, and the cephalosporins (Table 141–2). These agents account for 80% of all prescribed antimicrobials. Occasionally, other penicillins, erythromycin, or trimethoprim-sulfamethoxazole (Bactrim) is to blame;

Table 141–2. ANTIMICROBIAL AGENTS IMPLICATED IN *C. difficile*–INDUCED DIARRHEA AND ENTEROCOLITIS

Common	Occasional	Rare
Ampicillin or amoxicillin	Erythromycin	Metronidazole
Clindamycin	Penicillins	Sulfasalazine
Cephalosporins	Carbenicillin	Tetracyclines
Cefamandole	Dicloxacillin	Rifampin
Cefoperazone	Nafcillin	Chloramphenicol
Cefazolin	Oxacillin	Anticancer agents
Cefoxitin	Penicillin G	
Cephalexin	Penicillin V	
Cephradine	Ticarcillin	
Moxalactam	Trimethoprim-sulfamethoxazole	

rarely, tetracycline, chloramphenicol, rifampin, sulfasalazine, metronidazole, and anticancer agents have been found to be the inciting agents. With the exception of clindamycin, oral administration is associated with the highest risk. Whereas topical application is apparently safe, a case of PMC following topical clindamycin therapy for acne has been reported.[31]

Pathology. The demonstration of *C. difficile* and its toxins as a cause of PMC led to the discovery of a number of other drug-related intestinal complications of varying severity. The mildest form of toxin-positive diarrhea is simple diarrhea with negligible mucosal changes. Non-specific ulcers may be seen by endoscopic examination, or the mucosa may show only redness and/or edema without ulcers.[32] In contrast, in patients with PMC, elevated, cream-colored plaques measuring 2 to 8 mm in diameter are seen superimposed on a red, friable, edematous mucosa. These plaques are composed of fibrinoid material, polymorphonuclear leukocytes, and epithelial debris, but contain no bacteria or fungi. They are usually confined to the rectum and sigmoid, but may involve the entire colon or a part of the ascending colon. Histologic changes include polymorphonuclear cell infiltration in the lamina propria and overlying mucosa. Similar mucosal changes have been observed in biopsy specimens of the small intestine.[33]

Epidemiology. The prevalence of toxin-positive diarrhea and enterocolitis varies from time to time and from place to place. The same applies to the positive isolation rate of *C. difficile*. We have examined over 25,000 stools of patients with antibiotic-associated diarrhea submitted to us from some 150 hospitals scattered throughout the eastern half of the United States. The toxin-positive rate was about 13%. With both culture and toxin assay, the positive yield was higher by about an additional 10%.[34]

From 0% to 3% of healthy adults carry *C. difficile* in their stools. Toxin, on the other hand, has not been detected.[35,36] In infants, the carriage rate is much higher, varying in different locations from <10% to 90%. Nevertheless, these infants remain healthy, an enigma that is still unclear. The bacterial counts in infants may reach high levels with detectable toxin in stools. The frequency rate of asymptomatic toxin excretions varies from 0% to 14%.[37, 38–41] The carriage rate of *C. difficile* in older children also varies from place to place, but in general is much lower than that observed during infancy and is only slightly higher than that observed in healthy adults.[39, 40]

Patients receiving anticancer chemotherapy or bone marrow transplantation not uncommonly acquire *C. difficile*. Although the majority of the patients either are symptomatic or will develop diarrhea later on, some remain free of intestinal complaints.[42, 43]

Besides human sources, *C. difficile* has been recovered from contaminated soil.[44] In hospitals, outbreaks of PMC or toxin-positive diarrhea have been observed repeatedly. An exogenous source has been identified by culturing environmental samplings from case-associated hospital wards. Positive cultures were obtained from toilet seats, bedpans, floors, and hands and stools of asymptomatic personnel working in areas in which these disorders appeared.[45, 46] In another study, the use of unsterilized sigmoidoscopes may have contributed to the appearance of multiple cases in a single ward. While environmental dissemination of *C. difficile* may be important in some hospitals, it is not a universal phenomenon.[47] In 3 clusters of cases of *C. difficile* infection in different hospitals known to us, no evidence for a nosocomial origin could be detected.

Clinical Aspects. The clinical manifestations of *C. difficile* infection of the gastrointestinal tract vary widely.[30, 32, 48–51] *Diarrhea* is present in almost all patients. About one-third to one-half of patients develop diarrhea during the course of antibiotic therapy, while the rest begin to have diarrhea 4 to 6 weeks after cessation of antimicrobial administration. In most instances, diarrhea is not associated with colitis and will stop within a few days after the antimicrobial agent is discontinued. In some patients, diarrhea may persist for weeks or even months without appropriate therapy. In severe cases, as many as 30 bouts of watery diarrhea may occur in a single day.

Most patients with antimicrobial-associated colitis suffer from *diarrhea, fever, leukocytosis,* and *abdominal cramps.* Some patients may have only diarrhea without systemic symptoms or signs. Temperature as high as 41°C has been reported, but the usual range is between 38 and 39°C. *White blood cell counts* usually range from 10,000 to 20,000/mm^3; occasionally, counts as high as 40,000/mm^3

or greater may occur. *Abdominal tenderness* is a frequent finding. The *stools* are usually watery, offensive, large in volume, and without gross evidence of mucus or blood. However, leukocytes are usually present in the stools. A recent study from our laboratory on the characteristics of 71 consecutive toxin-positive stools is shown in Table 141–3. Our data indicate a correlation between toxin titer and the severity of diarrhea.

In milder conditions, *proctosigmoidoscopic examination* may show the mucosa to be normal or erythematous and edematous, with or without non-specific ulcers at various levels of the accessible rectosigmoid or sigmoid colon or limited to the rectum. On *colonoscopic examination* or *surgical exploration*, lesions may be found to be limited to the cecum or ascending colon or may be widespread. Typical cream-colored, plaque-like lesions (pseudomembranes) of 2 to 8 mm in diameter are seen on a red, friable, edematous mucosa. They are usually confined to the rectum or sigmoid, but may be present in other parts of the colon. Histologic changes include polymorphonuclear cell infiltration in the lamina propria and the overlying mucosa.

Barium enema study with air contrast may reveal plaque-like mucosal lesions, which are the characteristic feature of PMC. More often than not, however, radiographic findings are non-specific.

Diagnosis and Differential Diagnosis. Diarrhea developing during or within 2 to 6 weeks of antimicrobial chemotherapy should lead to suspicion of the diagnosis of *C. difficile*–induced disease. Frank blood may be present in the stools on rare occasions. As a rule, less than 10 white cells are seen per high power field. Shreds of mucus are present in about one-fourth of stools (Table 141–3).

Endoscopy is indicated in more serious or refractory cases. While proctosigmoidoscopy is sufficient to visualize colonic changes in the majority of cases, colonoscopy may sometimes be necessary in those patients with segmental involvement of the proximal colon.

Sudden onset of abdominal pain, with or without fever and chills and often without diarrhea at the onset, may bring the patient to the emergency room. The findings here of abdominal tenderness and leukocytosis may suggest an "acute abdomen" and lead to emergency surgery. At laparotomy, the entire colon, or just a portion of it, is found to be inflamed, and a small amount of fluid is accumulated in the abdominal cavity. Lacking any other obvious explanation for the findings, it is important to consider the diagnosis of antimicrobial-associated colitis and not to perform unnecessary resections. Colotomy with visualization of the characteristic mucosal plaques on the inflamed mucosa may help identify the true nature of the condition.

Chronic diarrhea of more than 2 months' duration is a puzzling problem in children. Some of these children are found to excrete *C. difficile* toxin and to show a good response to vancomycin therapy. Unfortunately, multiple relapses have been observed in some children despite repeated vancomycin therapy.[52]

Because of occasional bloody diarrhea with the presence of ulcers, antimicrobial colitis may be confused with idiopathic ulcerative colitis. Treatment with steroids not only fails to improve the symptoms, but may actually make the condition worse. Rarely, rectal bleeding without diarrhea is the first symptom, and the disease is limited to the involvement of the rectum. In these circumstances,

Table 141–3. CHARACTERISTICS OF TOXIN-POSITIVE STOOLS

Consistency	Watery	Soft	Formed*	Total
No. examined	37	32	2	71
GMT† of toxin	1062	248	142	
Leukocytes	13(35%)	0	0	13
Epithelial cells	5(14%)	6(18%)	0	11
Mucus shreds	9(24%)	6(18%)	0	15
Occult blood	10(27%)	3(9%)	0	13
pH (average)	6.6	6.8	7.2	

*Post-treatment stool samples from patients with pseudomembranous colitis who completed 10-day course of vancomycin therapy.

†Geometric mean titer of *C. difficile* toxin; the number represents reciprocal of stool dilution.

the condition has to be differentiated from other causes of proctitis.

Conflicting reports have appeared in the literature on the role of *C. difficile* in relapsing chronic inflammatory bowel diseases[53, 54] (Chapter 126). Based on the examination of over 100 stools from patients with chronic inflammatory bowel disease, we have been unable to find any significant contribution of *C. difficile* toxin to the activation of these diseases. An association between *C. difficile* and enterocolitis in Hirschsprung's disease, and between the organism and necrotizing enterocolitis in neonates, has been reported.[41,55,56] However, more data are needed for confirmation.

The presence of *C. difficile* can be established by tissue culture assay for *C. difficile* toxin. This is the preferred test at present, since culture for *C. difficile* is time-consuming and impractical as a routine diagnostic test. Using tissue culture assay, virtually 100% of patients with PMC are toxin-positive, while only 13% of patients with antimicrobial-associated diarrhea other than PMC are toxin-positive. About 2% of antibiotic recipients who do not have diarrhea and another 2% of patients with miscellaneous diarrheal conditions who are not taking antibiotics have been found to excrete *C. difficile* toxin in their stools.[30, 57, 58]

While toxin assay can be completed in a day, isolation of *C. difficile* requires at least a week. A selective medium has been developed to allow recognizable colonies to form in 2 to 3 days,[59] but the identification process takes longer. A recent report on a rapid identification procedure has made it possible to complete the isolation of *C. difficile* in 3 to 4 days.[34] When both toxin assay and bacterial isolation are performed, the disorder in an additional 10% of patients with antimicrobial-associated diarrhea can be diagnosed as related to *C. difficile* overgrowth. As a rule, toxin-negative, culture-positive patients either are asymptomatic or have mild diarrhea.

Several simplified diagnostic tests have been studied, including counterimmunoelectrophoresis, enzyme-linked immunosorbent assay, and radioimmunoassay. So far, only the enzyme-linked immunosorbent assay has been shown to be dependable and reproducible.[60] Although this method is somewhat more sensitive than tissue culture assay, it does not save time when used as a routine diagnostic test.

Complications. PMC, if untreated, carries a death rate of 15% to 30%. In patients with protracted diarrhea, electrolyte imbalance and hypoalbuminemia may develop. Toxic megacolon has also been reported.[61] In mild cases, with or without colitis, complications are uncommon. Occasionally, however, diarrhea may persist for weeks or months in the absence of specific therapy.

Treatment. Once the diagnosis is made, the most important step is to discontinue the implicated antibiotic. Many patients will improve spontaneously with just this measure. As a general rule, antiperistaltic drugs, such as diphenoxylate hydrochloride with atropine sulfate (Lomotil), should be avoided, as toxic dilatation of the colon may result. Patients with *C. difficile* infection, PMC, or diarrhea should be isolated and placed on enteric precautions to prevent the organism from spreading and causing focal outbreaks within institutions.

If diarrhea continues or if it begins after the antimicrobials have been discontinued, additional treatment is needed. Specific treatment has been aimed at either removal of the toxin by an anionic exchange resin or elimination of the toxin-producing organism by *vancomycin*. The latter approach has proved to be more successful. Controlled studies clearly show that oral vancomycin produces clinical improvement and eradicates the toxin.[62–66] Because of its poor absorption, vancomycin by mouth does not cause systemic toxicity. However, it is expensive and has a bitter taste.

Indications for vancomycin treatment include persistent symptoms after the implicated antimicrobial agent is discontinued; severe diarrhea, especially with systemic symptoms; and the need to continue the implicated antimicrobial or a substitute that is likely to cause the disease. The recommended dosage of vancomycin is 150 to 500 mg 4 times daily orally for at least 5 days. Generally, however, the duration of treatment extends from 7 to 14 days. One practical guide is the rapidity of response to vancomycin treatment. If diarrhea stops in 2 to 3 days, treatment for 5 days is probably sufficient. If it is not, treatment should be continued for at least 1 week.

Relapses of diarrheal disease have been observed in 15% to 20% of patients treated with vancomycin; about one-third of patients who suffer a relapse will have a second relapse. Occasionally, a third or fourth relapse has been observed. The relapse rate does not correlate with the total duration of treatment, the total amount of vancomycin administered, or the rapidity of initial clinical response. However, the persistence of toxin in the stool at the completion of treatment is significantly associated with future relapse. For this reason, a second stool toxin determination is recommended after the completion of therapy. Inasmuch as the organism remains sensitive to vancomycin, re-treatment with the drug will again bring about a prompt response.

Other antimicrobial agents that have been reported to be effective for PMC include *metronidazole*,[67] *tetracycline*,[68] and *bacitracin*.[69] Metronidazole, which is much less expensive than vancomycin, has been used as an alternative to vancomycin. Inasmuch as it is almost completely absorbed, the drug levels in the colon are unpredictable. In severe cases, therefore, vancomycin is still the drug of choice. It should also be kept in mind that both metronidazole and tetracycline have been implicated in causing *C. difficile* disease. In contrast to these 2 absorbable drugs, bacitracin, like vancomycin, is poorly absorbed when given by mouth and thus does not cause systemic symptoms. The suggested dosage is 25,000 units 4 times daily for 1 week. Our experience in patients with PMC and other forms of antimicrobial-associated diarrhea has indicated that bacitracin is effective in producing a clinical response as well as eliminating toxin from the stools. For severe cases of PMC, however, bacitracin seems to be less efficacious clinically than vancomycin.

Cholestyramine, which binds toxin, has been used as a single agent to treat PMC, but its efficacy is less convincing. The suggested dosage is 4 g/day orally for 5 days.[63, 70] *Colestipol*, another anionic exchange resin with more toxin-binding capacity than cholestyramine, is not effective in treating PMC.[64, 71]

Surgery has no place in the treatment of *C. difficile* colitis except in rare instances, such as intestinal perforation or megacolon. We have successfully treated one patient with megacolon complicating PMC with vancomycin alone. Occasionally, patients with segmental colitis may present with acute abdominal symptoms, and laparotomy is often unavoidable. However, when unexplained inflammation of the colon is detected, a diagnosis of *C. difficile* colitis should be suspected and resection avoided if at all possible.

Prognosis. Antimicrobial-associated diarrhea without colitis is for the most part a self-limited condition. With treatment, even severe and protracted cases have a good prognosis. When there is associated colitis, the situation is much more serious. If not appropriately treated, the disorder may even be fatal, although improvement after the institution of specific therapy is the rule. Relapses are not uncommon, with or without colitis. Relapses occur especially in children who have a prolonged period of diarrhea before diagnosis. Except for repeated treatment with vancomycin, there is at present no effective method to terminate these relapses. An attempt may be made to restore normal fecal flora by introducing fecal organisms through the rectum.[72] This approach, however, is not without risk of introducing pathogens. Another treatment program, also aimed at restoring normal intestinal flora, is to administer cholestyramine immediately following vancomycin or concomitantly with vancomycin and progressively reducing the latter.

References

1. Witkop CJ, Wolf RO. Hypoplasia and intrinsic staining of enamel following tetracycline therapy. JAMA 1963; 185:1008–11.
2. Rebdle-Short TJ. Tetracycline in teeth and bone. Lancet 1962; 1:1188–9.
3. Charles D, Bost D. Placental transmission of antibiotics. J Obstet Gynecol 1954; 61:750–7.
4. Cochie JM, Munroe JD, Anderson DO. Incidence of staining of permanent teeth by the tetracyclines. Can Med Assoc J 1970; 103:451–6.
5. Tetracycline pediatric drops to be withdrawn from the market. FDA Drug Bull 1978; May-June: 23.
6. Shwachman G, Schuster A. The tetracyclines. Applied pharmacology. Pediatr Clin North Am 1956; 3:295–303.
7. Stillman E, Martin J. Tetracycline-induced esophageal ulcerations. Arch Dermatol 1979; 115:1005.
8. Sutton DR, Gosnold JK. Oesophageal ulceration due to clindamycin. Br Med J 1977; 1:1598.
9. Neuvonen PJ, Gothoni G, Hackman R, Bjorksten K. Interference of iron with the absorption of tetracyclines in man. Br Med J 1970; 4:532–4.
10. Weisbren BA, Hueckel JS. Reduced absorption of aureomycin caused by aluminum hydroxide gel. Proc Soc Exp Biol Med 1950; 73:73–4.
11. Dobbins WO III, Herrepo BA, Mansbach CM. Morphologic alterations associated with neomycin induced malabsorption. Am J Med Sci 1968; 255:63–7.
12. Dietschy JM, Siperstein M. Cholesterol synthesis by the gastrointestinal tract: Localization and mechanisms of control. J Clin Invest 1965; 44:1311–27.
13. Hardison WG, Rosenberg IH. The effect of neomycin on bile salt metabolism and fat digestion in man. J Lab Clin Med 1969; 74:564–73.

13a. Bartlett JG. Antibiotic-associated colitis. Viewpoints Dig Dis 1984; 16:9–12.

14. Finney JMT. Gastroenterostomy for cicatrizing ulcer of the pylorus. Bull Johns Hopkins Hosp 1893; 4:53–5.
15. Editorial: Antibiotics, staphylococcal enteritis, and pseudomembranous enterocolitis. N Engl J Med 1953; 249:37–40.
16. Larson HE, Parry JV, Price AB, Davies DR, Dolby J, Tyrrell DAJ. Undescribed toxin in pseudomembranous colitis. Br Med J 1977; 1:1246–8.
17. Chang TW. *Clostridium difficile* toxin and antimicrobial agent-induced diarrhea. J Infect Dis 1978; 137:854.
18. Larson HE, Price AB, Honour P, Borriello SP. *Clostridium difficile* and the aetiology of pseudomembranous colitis. Lancet 1978; 1:1063–6.
19. George RH, Symonds JM, Dimock F, Brown JD, Arabi Y, Shinagava N, Alexander-Williams J, Burdon DW. Identification of *Clostridium difficile* as a cause of pseudomembranous colitis. Br Med J 1978; 1:695.
20. Rolfe RD, Helebian S, Finegold SM. Bacterial interference between *Clostridium difficile* and normal fecal flora. J Infect Dis 1981; 143:470–5.
21. Taylor NS, Thorne GM, Bartlett JD. Comparison of two toxins by *Clostridium difficile*. Infect Immun 1981; 34:1036–43.
22. Libby JM, Wilkins TD. Production of two toxins of *Clostridium difficile* and immunological comparison of the toxins by cross-neutralization studies. Infect Immun 1982; 35:374–6.
23. Lyerly DM, Lockwood DE, Richardson SH, Wilkins TD. Biological activities of toxin A and B of *Clostridium difficile*. Infect Immun 1982; 35:1147–50.
24. Libby JM, Wilkins TD. Effects of two toxins of *Clostridium difficile* in antibiotic-associated cecitis in hamsters determined by active immunization and intracecal injection. Abstract No 716. Presented at the 21st Interscience Conference on Antimicrobial Agents and Chemotherapy. Chicago, November, 1981.
25. Vesely DL, Straub KD, Nolan CM, Rolfe RD, Finegold SM, Monson TP. Purified *Clostridium difficile* cytotoxin stimulates guanylate cyclase activity and inhibits adenylate cyclase activity. Infect Immun 1981; 33:285–91.
26. Chang TW, Lin PS, Gorbach SL, Bartlett GS. Ultrastructural changes of cultured human amnion cells by *Clostridium difficile* toxin. Infect Immun 1979; 23:795–8.
27. Donta ST, Shaffer SJ. Effects of *Clostridium difficile* toxin on tissue cultured cells. J Infect Dis 1980; 141:218–20.
28. Bartlett JG. Antimicrobial agents implicated in *Clostridium difficile* toxin-associated diarrhea or colitis. Johns Hopkins Med J 1981; 149:6–9.
29. Chang TW. Antimicrobial-associated diarrhea and enterocolitis. Drug Ther 1981; 6:71–8.
30. Bartlett JG, Taylor NS, Chang TW. Clinical and laboratory observations in *Clostridium difficile* colitis. Am J Clin Nutr 1980; 33:2521–6.
31. Milstone EB, McDonald AJ, Scholhamer CF Jr. Pseudomembranous colitis after topical application of clindamycin. Arch Dermatol 1981; 117:154–5.
32. Cohen LE, McNeil CJ, Wells RF. Clindamycin-associated colitis. JAMA 1973; 223:1379–80.
33. Hyams JS, Berman MM, Helgason H. Nonantibiotic-associated enterocolitis caused by *Clostridium difficile* in an infant. J Pediatr 1981; 99:750–2.
34. Chang TW, Gorbach SL. Rapid identification of *Clostridium difficile* by toxin detection. J Clin Microbiol 1982; 15:465–7.
35. Viscidi R, Willey S, Bartlett JG. Isolation rates and toxigenic potential of *Clostridium difficile* isolates from various patient populations. Gastroenterology 1981; 81:5–9.
36. George WL, Sutter VL, Citron D, Finegold SM. Toxicity and antimicrobial susceptibility of *Clostridium difficile*, a cause of antimicrobial agent-associated colitis. Curr Microbiol 1978; 1:55–8.
37. Sheretz RJ, Marshall RL, Sarubbi FA. *Clostridium difficile*: A pathogen in neonates? Abstract No 707. Presented at 21st Interscience Conference on Antimicrobial Agents and Chemotherapy. Chicago, November, 1981.
38. Thompson CM, Gilligan PH, Fisher MC, Long SS. *Clostridium difficile* in the pediatric population. Abstract No 724. Presented at 21st Interscience Conference on Antimicrobial Agents and Chemotherapy. Chicago, November 1981.
39. Holst E, Helin I, Mardh P-A. Recovery of *Clostridium difficile* from children. Scand J Infect Dis 1981; 13:41–5.
40. Stark PL, Lee A, Parsonage BD. Colonization of the large bowel by *Clostridium difficile* in healthy infants: Quantitative study. Infect Immun 1982; 35:895–9.
41. Chang TW, Areson P. Neonatal necrotizing enterocolitis: Absence of enteric bacterial toxins. N Engl J Med 1978; 299:424.
42. Fainstein V, Bodey GP, Fekety R. *Clostridium difficile* colonization in cancer patients admitted to laminar air flow units. Clin Res 1982; 30:365A.
43. Yolken TR, Bishop CA, Townsend TR, Bolyard EA, Bartlett JG, Sabtos GW, Saral R. Infectious gastroenteritis in bone-marrow-transplant recipients. N Engl Med 1982; 306: 1009–12.
44. Smith LDS. The Pathogenic Anaerobic Bacteria. 2nd Ed. Springfield, Ill: Charles C Thomas, 1975.
45. Mulligan ME, Rolfe RD, Finegold SM, George WL. Contamination of a hospital environment with *Clostridium difficile*. Curr Microbiol 1979; 3:173–5.
46. Kim R-H, Fekety R, Batts DH, Brown D, Cudmore M, Silva J Jr, Waters D. Isolation of *Clostridium difficile* from the environment and contacts of patients with antibiotic-associated colitis. J Infect Dis 1981; 143:42–50.
47. Pierce PF Jr, Wilson R, Silva J Jr, Garagusi VF, Rifkin GD, Fekety R, Nunez-Montiel O, Dowell VR Jr, Hughes JM. Antibiotic-associated pseudomembranous colitis: An epidemiologic investigation of a cluster of cases. J Infect Dis 1982; 145:269–74.
48. Mogg GAG, Keighley MRB, Burdon DW, Alexander-Williams J, Youngs D, Johnson M, Bentley S, George RH. Antibiotic-associated colitis: A review of 66 cases. Br J Surg 1979; 70:738–42.
49. Totten MA, Gregg JA, Fremont-Smith P, Legg M. Clinical and pathological spectrum of antibiotic-associated colitis. Am J Gastroenterol 1978; 69:311–19.
50. Tedesco FJ, Stanley RJ, Alpers DH. Diagnostic features of clindamycin-associated pseudomembranous colitis. N Engl J Med 1974; 290:841–3.
51. Gorbach SL, Bartlett JG. Pseudomembranous colitis: A review of its diverse forms. J Infect Dis 1977; 135(Suppl):89–94.
52. Stephen JL, Grand RJ, Flores A, Chang TW, Bartlett JG. Chronic diarrhea associated with *Clostridium difficile* in children. Am J Dis Child 1983; 137:275–8.
53. Meyers S, Mayer L, Bottone E, Desmond E, Janowitz HD. Occurrence of *Clostridium difficile* toxin during the course of inflammatory bowel disease. Gastroenterology 1981; 80:697–700.
54. Trnka YM, Lamont JT. Association of *Clostridium difficile* toxin with symptomatic relapse of chronic inflammatory bowel disease. Gastroenterology 1981; 80:693–6.
55. Thomas DFM, Fernie DS, Malone M, Bauston R, Spitz L. Association between *Clostridium difficile* and enterocolitis in Hirschsprung's disease. Lancet 1982; 1:78–9.
56. Sayed H, Han V, Chance G. *C. difficile* and toxin(s) in neonatal necrotizing enterocolotis. Abstract No C316. Presented at the Annual Meeting of the American Society of Microbiology. Atlanta, May, 1982.
57. Chang TW, Lauermann M, Bartlett JG. Cytotoxicity assay in antibiotic-associated colitis. J Infect Dis 1979; 140:765–70.
58. Bartlett JG, Chang TW, Gurwith M, Gorbach SL, Onderdonk AB. Antibiotic-associated colitis. J Infect Dis 1979; 140:765–70.
59. George WL, Sutter VL, Citron D, Finegold SM. Selective and differential medium for isolation of *Clostridium difficile*. J Clin Microbiol 1979; 9:214–9.
60. Yolken RH, Whitcomb LS, Marien G, Bartlett JG, Libby J, Ehrich M, Wilkins T. Enzyme immunoassay for the detection of *Clostridium difficile* antigen. J Infect Dis 1981; 144:378.
61. Axelrod M, Allon O, Felton M, Goldfinger M. Clindamycin-associated colitis with toxic megacolon. JAMA 1975; 233:419–20.
62. Keighley MRB, Burdon DW, Arabi Y, Alex Y, Alexander-Williams J, Thompson H, Youngs D, Johnson M, Bentley S, George RH, Mogg GAG. Randomized controlled trial of vancomycin for pseudomembranous colitis and postoperative diarrhea. Br Med J 1978; 2:1667–9.
63. Tedesco FJ, Napier J, Gamble W, Chang TW, Bartlett JG.

Therapy of antibiotic-associated pseudomembrancous colitis. J Clin Gastroenterol 1979; 1:51–4.
64. Mogg GAG, Arabi Y, Youngs D, Johnson M, Bentley S, Burdon DW, Keighley MR. Therapeutic trials in antibiotic associated colitis. Scand J Infect Dis 1980; 22(Suppl):41–5.
65. Tedesco FJ, Markham R, Gurwith M, Christie D, Bartlett JG. Oral vancomycin therapy for antibiotic-associated pseudomembranous colitis. Lancet 1978; 2:226–8.
66. Bartlett GJ, Tedesco FJ, Shull S, Lowe B, Chang TW. Relapse following oral vancomycin therapy of antibiotic-associated pseudomembranous colitis. Gastroenterology 1979; 78:431–43.
67. Pashby NL, Bolton RP, Sherriff RJ. Oral metronidazole in *Clostridium difficile*. Br Med J 1979; 1:1605–6.
68. Dejesus R, Peternel WW. Antibiotic-associated diarrhea treated with oral tetracycline. Gastroenterology 1978; 74:818–20.
69. Chang TW, Gorbach SL, Bartlett JG, Saginur R. Bacitracin treatment of antibiotic-associated colitis and diarrhea caused by *Clostridium difficile* toxin. Gastroenterology 1980; 78:1584–6.
70. Kreutzer EW, Milligan FD. Treatment of antibiotic-associated pseudomembranous colitis with cholestyramine resin. Johns Hopkins Med J 1978; 143:67–72.
71. Chang TW, Onderdonk AB, Bartlett JG. Anion-exchange resins in antibiotic-associated colitis. Lancet 1978; 2:257–8.
72. Bowden TA Jr, Mansberger AR, Lykins LE. Pseudomembranous enterocolitis: Mechanism for restoring floral homeostasis. Am Surg 1981; 47:178–83.

Chapter 142

Radiation Injury to the Gut

S. Philip Bralow • Gerald Marks

Susceptibility
Pathology
Clinical Aspects
Diagnostic Studies
Treatment
Risk of Cancer

Radiation enterocolitis is an insidious, progressive disease that is seen with increasing frequency with the utilization of supervoltage. The dose of radiation now can be increased to levels that are truly curative without injuring the skin.[1] Radiation treatment is rarely used as a single mode of therapy; more often it is given preoperatively or postoperatively as adjunctive therapy. It may be combined with chemotherapy[2] and possibly with immunotherapy. It is estimated that radiation is used in 50% of cancer patients at some time during their course of treatment.[3] Tissue damage and functional integrity follow a bimodal curve and usually return to normal within 2 weeks after cessation of therapy. The clinical spectrum of radiation-induced injury to the intestine ranges from mild gastrointestinal symptoms to malabsorption, obstruction, perforation, fistulization, hemorrhage, and the development of neoplasms. In about 10% of patients, the damage may become devastating and life threatening.[4]

Susceptibility

Radiosensitivity varies along the gastrointestinal tract.[5] The small bowel and descending colon can tolerate doses from 4500 to 6500 rads,* and the rectum can withstand 5500 to 8000 rads (Table 142–1). The oral cavity and pharynx appear to be the most sensitive, owing to the rapid epithelial cell renewal rate and the abundant lymphatic tissue of Waldeyer's ring in the submucosa. Minor salivary glands are largely of the mucous type and are more radioresistant. The squamous epithelium of the esophagus may be damaged when neoplasms in the lung, mediastinum, or vertebrae are irradiated. The submucosa of the esophagus will respond to radiation by edema and vascular dilatation, leading to progressive fibrosis and telangiectasia. Esophageal strictures may occur when doses reach 6000 rads over a 6-week period. Esophageal, aortic, and tracheoesophageal fistulas have been reported.[6]

Radiation effects vary from one area of the stomach to the other, depending upon cell kinetics. The isthmus of the gastric glands and the surface epithelium show acute effects of radiation injury, while the convoluted glands with their parietal and chief cells are much more resistant.[6] Therapeutic doses exceeding 4800 rads have been reported to produce radiation ulceration with low gastric acidity. Doses between 1500 and 2000 rads were once used to treat intractable peptic ulcers without significant mucosal damage other than atrophy.[7]

Permanent injury to the small intestine may occur during therapeutic radiation for malignant tumors of the upper abdomen or retroperitoneum or for periaortic metastatic carcinoma. The small intestine is the most radiosensitive of all the intra-abdominal organs. Significant damage usually is avoided by the mobility of the small intestine. The duodenum and upper jejunum are fixed by

Table 142–1. TOLERANCE TO X-IRRADIATION OF DIGESTIVE ORGANS ACCORDING TO SITE*

Organ	Tolerance Doses (in rads)	
	Minimal Dose	*Maximal Dose*
Liver	3500	4500
Esophagus	6000	7500
Stomach	4500	5000
Small bowel	4500	6500
Colon	4500	6500
Rectum	5500	8000

*Minimal dose produces injury in 1% to 5% of patients in 5 years; maximal dose produces injury in 50% of patients within 5 years.

Rad is an acronym for "*r*adiation *a*bsorbed *d*ose."

the ligament of Treitz, and the terminal ileum is held fast by its attachment to the immobile cecum. Damage to the terminal ileum should be considered in any patient developing gastrointestinal symptoms following radiation to the pelvis. It is estimated that 2.4% to 25% of patients treated for pelvic and intra-abdominal malignancy have damage to the ileum as well as to the distal colon.[8]

Patients who face a high risk of serious radiation damage are those presenting with diabetes, a thin physique, previous surgical procedures with adhesions fixing the bowel to the pelvic area, or pelvic sepsis. Patients with generalized diseases, aortic aneurysms, or hypertension are also at increased risk for intestinal damage by radiation. Patients receiving chemotherapy also may be at increased risk for intestinal damage by radiotherapy.[2]

Pathology

Radiation suppresses cell proliferation in the crypts of the intestinal epithelium. The cells in the G_1 postmitotic phase of the cell cycle are the most radiosensitive, and the cells in the late S-synthetic phase are the most resistant.[9] Mitotic activity returns to normal levels a few days after radiation exposure, restoring cellular homeostasis. The existing cells usually maintain the integrity of the mucosal surface unless radiation exposure is prolonged or when repeated doses destroy the proliferating zone population. The endothelial cells of the small submucosal arterioles are exceedingly radiosensitive and respond to injury with swelling and proliferation. The vessel wall may continue to undergo degeneration for several weeks after the acute damage. Vascular thrombosis leads to an obliterative endarteritis and endophlebitis, producing graded ischemic changes (Fig. 142–1). These findings contribute to mucosal ulceration and necrosis (Fig. 142–2). Intestinal bacteria can invade the necrotic tissue and cause further damage. Microabscesses within the crypts can be seen during the third and fourth weeks of radiation treatment. Electron microscopic changes occur: microvilli become shortened, nucleoli enlarged, mitochondria and endoplasmic reticulum dilated, and cytoplasmic secretory granules markedly decreased.[3] These ultrastructural changes disappear within 3 days following cessation of radiation, and the shortened villi return to normal within 2 weeks.

A subacute period occurs between 2 and 12 months after radiotherapy. The intestinal mucosa regenerates and heals to a variable extent, but the endothelial cells of the small arteries are still swollen and detached from the basement membrane. Fibrin plugs cause thrombosis with attempts at recannulization. Large foam cells are seen beneath the intima, and these cells are thought to be diagnostic of radiation-induced vascular injury.[10] Ischemia becomes progressive, leading to severe chronic changes with collagen degeneration and atrophy of the glandular mucosa. The submucosa becomes thickened and fi-

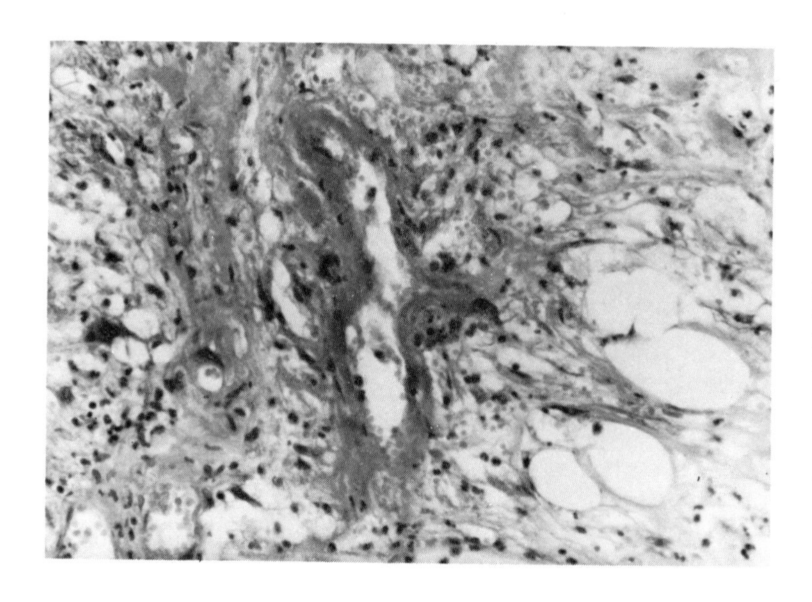

Figure 142–1. Histologic section of rectal wall showing fibrinoid necrosis and atypical fibroblastic proliferation. (× 100.)

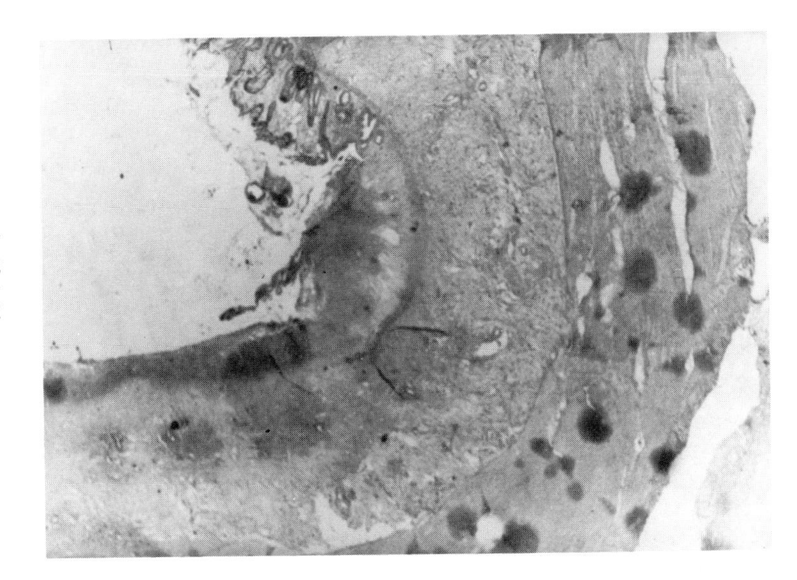

Figure 142–2. Low power view of rectal wall demonstrating marked ulceration and extensive submucosal fibrosis and thickening.

brotic with large and bizarre fibroblasts.[11] Edema of the submucosa and serosa leads to atypical hyperplastic glands and cyst formation. Focal venous and lymphatic dilation is prominent. Normal lymphatic tissue seldom regenerates completely after irradiation, causing lymphatic ectasia.

The marked morphologic changes in the irradiated small bowel result in disturbed absorption of fat, carbohydrate, and protein and lead to malnutrition.[3] Diarrhea may be secondary to decreased bile salt reabsorption in the damaged terminal ileum. Reduction in the bile salt pool causes an increased liver synthesis of unconjugated bile salts, producing cholanorrheic enteropathy and increased diarrhea or steatorrhea.[12] Alterations in intraluminal fat and bile salt metabolism can be measured by fecal fat analysis and by breath tests (Chapter 27). During the first week of pelvic irradiation, 9% of the patients have abnormal breath tests; by the fifth week, 45% of tests are abnormal. Gradually, resolution occurs and by 1 year, bile salt absorption is normal unless extended damage has occurred.

Carbohydrate malabsorption also contributes to radiation-induced diarrhea. Disaccharidases of the brush border of the jejunal and ileal mucosa are decreased by radiation injury. The unabsorbed carbohydrates produce a marked osmotic effect in the small bowel lumen, and bacterial fermentation releases organic acids, carbon dioxide, hydrogen, and methane. The lowered colonic pH impairs water and electrolyte transport. Small bowel biopsy and histochemical assays can identify deficiencies in lactase, sucrase, and maltase. Carbohydrate malabsorption can also be quantitated by labeled CO_2 and hydrogen breath tests. During the first and fifth weeks of treatment, the frequency of abnormal breath test results using carbon-labeled lactose was 13%, and by the fifth week 50% of tests were abnormal.[13] The D-xylose test can detect carbohydrate malabsorption in patients with normal liver and renal function, but abnormalities do not correlate well with the morphologic changes in the intestinal mucosa.[14] Tamura et al.[15] irradiated various exteriorized segments of rat small bowel using a sublethal dose of 700 rads by direct exposure (Fig. 142–3). When

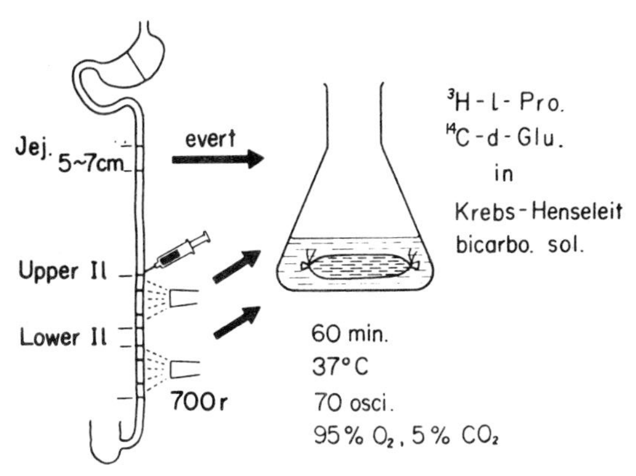

Figure 142–3. Irradiated (700 rads) segments of upper and lower ileum tested for absorption of 3H-L-proline and 14C-D-glucose using everted sac technique. (From Tamura et al.[15])

both the upper and lower ileum were irradiated, impaired absorption of labeled D-glucose and L-proline lasted approximately 90 days. Non-irradiated segments from the jejunum and the upper and lower ileum showed decreased absorption for only 3 to 7 days after irradiation of other segments. Absorption from the irradiated segments seems to be bimodally affected with impairment during the acute and late periods; the periods of impaired absorption correlate with the inflammatory changes in the histopathologic specimen (Fig. 142–4).

Many attempts have been made to develop agents that can protect normal tissue from adverse effects of x-irradiation. Stryker and Albert[16] demonstrated that pretreatment with metronidazole may reduce the severity of radiation injury to the normal canine rectal mucosa. With this pretreatment, the number of hypoxic tumor cells, which are radioresistant, would be decreased and, thus, smaller doses of radiation could be employed. Pretreatment with cytosine arabinoside protects intestinal epithelial stem cells against radiation[17] and enhances cell survival in experimental animal studies.

A liquid elemental diet taken for 3 days preceding and then throughout the period of intensive abdominal and pelvic radiotherapy can maintain body weight and serum protein levels of seriously ill cancer patients, especially children.[18] Elemental nutrients may be absorbed more efficiently than ordinary foodstuffs by the irradiated mucosa. Gluten-free, milk-free, low-fat, and low-residue diets have been given to children at high risk for bowel damage by radiation.

Clinical Aspects

Early symptoms usually occur during the first or second week of x-radiation therapy.

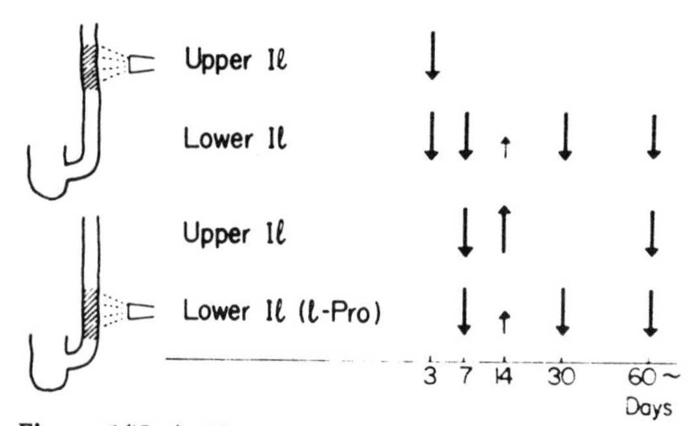

Figure 142–4. Bimodal pattern of impaired absorption of L-proline by everted intestinal sacs following irradiation. (From Tamura et al.[15])

Nausea, vomiting, and diarrhea are the most common presenting complaints. *Nausea* is usually related to the central nervous system effects of the radiation. The Court-Brown syndrome occurs 40 to 90 minutes following massive x-ray exposure.[19] The initial post-radiation feeling of well-being disappears with onset of *vomiting*, recurring hourly over an 8-hour period. As yet, no known therapeutic agent is able to control these symptoms, but large doses of metaclopromide or cannabis may be helpful. Rectal mucosal injury produces *mucoid rectal discharge*, a sensation of *incomplete rectal evacuation*, and *rectal bleeding*. A dusky, edematous pattern is seen on proctosigmoidoscopy. With continued irradiation, mucosal ulceration and friability may occur, accompanied by marked tenesmus and rectal bleeding. *Lower abdominal cramps* suggest involvement of the small bowel.

Following cessation of the acute injury pattern, a latent period of 2 months to many years may pass before symptoms again appear. The overall frequency of late radiation effects has been estimated to range from 0.5% to 15%, but less than 2% of patients require surgical intervention.[13] The spectrum of late effects includes (in order of decreasing frequency): proctitis, colitis, enteritis, and pancolitis. *Decreasing stool caliber*, *tenesmus*, and *progressive constipation* may herald a rectal stricture. *Fistula formation* between pelvic and abdominal organs may present as a feculent vaginal discharge, pneumaturia, or rapid passage of undigested food in the stool. Intra-abdominal abscesses usually occur in the pelvis. Frank peritonitis can develop, but free perforation of the involved bowel is uncommon. Recurrent massive *hemorrhage* from the ileum may be the only presenting problem following pelvic radiotherapy, the bleeding coming from multiple telangiectatic vessels in the crests of the mucosal villi.[20]

Diagnostic Studies

Radiation necrosis can be present with only minimal symptoms and findings since the bowel is frequently encased in a fibrinous envelope preventing the physical signs of peritonitis. *Malabsorption* and significant *weight loss* may be the only presenting complaints of patients suffering from the late effects of irradiation. If small bowel strictures or colonic fistulas are present, intraluminal bacterial overgrowth may occur, producing severe *steatorrhea* and malabsorption of vitamin B_{12}. Irradiation can also release plasmogen activators from the intestine and increase mucosal fibrinolysins, which promotes *rectal bleeding*.[21]

Proctosigmoidoscopic findings of late radiation injury are variable and range from a granular, friable mucosa with multiple telangiectasia to ulcerations and necrosis. The ulcerations vary in size and are transverse in orientation. They usually occur on the anterior rectal wall, about 4 to 6 cm above the pectinate line. Rectal strictures tend to be located higher than the ulcerations, at about 8 to 10 cm above the anal verge. *Barium contrast examinations* are helpful in assessing the extent of radiation damage. Irregularity, spasm, and possibly fine serrations of the anterior wall of the rectosigmoid may suggest acute ulcerative colitis. Localized areas of radiation injury in the colon may present as strictures resembling carcinoma (Fig. 142–5). *Colonoscopy* is helpful in the differentiation of strictured areas as well as for long-term follow-up of patients with radiation colitis.[22] Widening of the presacral space, increase in perirectal fat, thickening of the perirectal fibrous tissue, and visualization of the fibrotic connection between the sacrum and rectum may occur following irradiation of the bladder, but less often in irradiation of the cervix.[23] These findings are similar to those encountered in patients with perirectal abscess, ulcerative colitis, pelvic lipomatoses, syphilis, tuberculosis, and lymphopathia venereum. In the absence of radiodermatitis, the observed changes lacking specificity may cause diagnostic delay and contribute to increased mortality and morbidity rates. Later, the small bowel may develop a stricture and show a distorted mucosal pattern and a thickened wall with a narrowed lumen (Fig. 142–6). The presence of fistulas can simulate Crohn's ileocolitis.

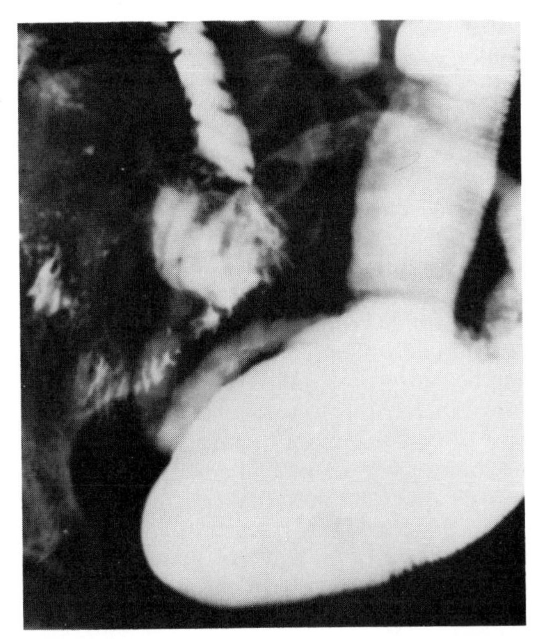

Figure 142–6. Involvement of a long segment of terminal ileum with fixation in the pelvic area of irradiation.

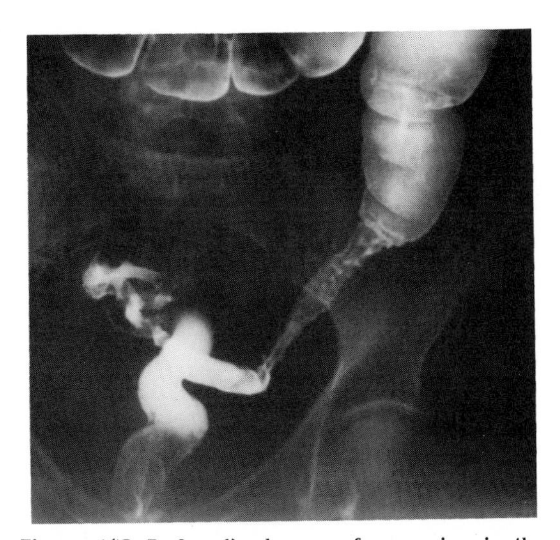

Figure 142–5. Localized area of narrowing in the sigmoid colon secondary to pelvic irradiation for cancer of cervix 15 years previously in a 72-year-old woman.

Treatment

Radiotherapy demands careful planning to minimize possible complications. The dose and delivery of small increments of radiation at spaced intervals tend to reduce colonic complications.

In acute injury, symptomatic benefit can frequently be accomplished with antispasmodics, anticholinergic drugs, or opiates. Diarrhea and rectal pain usually respond to hydrophilic colloids, local analgesics, and warm sitz baths. Cholestyramine, a bile acid–sequestering resin, may be helpful in controlling refractory diarrhea. Buffered acetylsalicylic acid frequently is effective in relieving abdominal distention and diarrhea, presumably by inhibiting prostaglandin E synthesis. In severe diarrhea, an elemental diet free of gluten and lactose may have dramatic beneficial effects. Children may require hospitalization for IV fluids and hyperalimentation.[24] Corticosteroids and sulfasalazine may be helpful.[25] Occasionally, rectal bleeding may become massive and unrelenting, requiring multiple blood transfusions. Symptoms of acute enteritis abate shortly after the completion of irradiation, when repopulation of the intestinal crypt cells has occurred. The absence of acute effects, however, offers no assurance that late changes will not develop. In one study, 53% of those patients who were asymptomatic during the irradiation period suffered late small bowel and rectal complications.[26]

Severe late radiation injury is infrequent, but radiation injuries are usually greater than anticipated and progression of the disease postoperatively must be kept in mind. An estimated 2% of patients receiving abdominal or pelvic irradiation will require surgery for complications. Small bowel injuries account for 30% to 50% of all severe late radiation problems.[27]

There is no single surgical approach to these problems.[28] A patient who has lost more than 10 pounds (4.5 kg) should have either an elemental diet or parenteral alimentation before operation to improve nitrogen balance and decrease morbidity. Partial obstruction of the small bowel secondary to stricture formation should initially be treated conservatively if possible; complete obstruction will necessitate prompt surgery. Intestinal intubation is necessary prior to surgical intervention. Antibiotic treatment should be administered several days before operation together with mechanical cleansing of the colon (especially of defunctionalized segments), using topical antibiotic solutions. Although rectovaginal *fistulas* may close spontaneously or after diversion of the fecal stream with a transverse colostomy, enterocolic and enterorectal vesicle fistulas frequently need to be treated surgically. The genitourinary tract must be thoroughly investigated by cystoscopy and pyelography. If the ureters are involved, diversion of urine may become necessary. The condition of the vaginal wall should be inspected and coincidental cancer or recurrence must be ruled out.

Complete exploration of the abdominal cavity should be made at the time of surgery with lysis of adhesions. The risk of intestinal fistulization is exaggerated under these conditions.[28, 29] The length of resected bowel is determined by the condition of the bowel wall being used for anastomosis. Anastomotic leak may be a potentially lethal complication. When the bowel is unsuited for anastomosis, a colostomy is indicated. Since the terminal ileum and cecum are frequently injured by radiation, ileo-ileal anastomosis or ileocecal anastomosis is best avoided. When radiation injury necessitates resection of the terminal ileum, the cecum and the major portion of the right colon should be included as well, and anastomosis should be made to the hepatic flexure, which is undamaged.

Previous anorectal disease or impaired sphincter activity should be considered before initiating an anorectal continuity procedure. A permanent diverting colostomy may be successful in relieving pain, but this does not control radiation-induced bleeding. Furthermore, retained injured bowel leads to progression of the disease and its malignant potential. Reconstitution with an abdominal trans-sacral method has been reported to be reasonably safe, surgically sound, and physiologically effective.[29] The use of stapling devices to allow for low anorectal anastomosis is controversial. The upper rectum and rectosigmoid are fibrotic, elastic, and thickened as a result of the previous irradiation, and the anastomosis may not be as secure as desired.[30]

If the possibility of a short bowel syndrome exists after operation, home parenteral nutrition should be discussed with the patient preoperatively.[31]

Risk of Cancer

The overall risk of colorectal cancer from radiation is small, accounting for only 1% of all cancers in that area.[32] Cancer arising in irradiated small bowel has not been reported. A true assessment of the risk is difficult.[33] The risk of a second cancer in patients with gynecologic carcinoma is high even without irradiation. Women who have received pelvic irradiation have 1.2 to 8 times greater risk for colorectal cancer than the rest of the age-adjusted population. This risk estimate is based on a 10-year latency period. Individuals subjected to irradiation that involves the colorectal area should be screened actively after the 10-year period by flexible proctosigmoidoscopy yearly or biennially.

References

1. Localio SA, Pachter HL, Gouge TH. The radiation injured bowel. *In*: Nyhus L (ed). Surgery Annual, Vol. II. Chicago: Year Book Medical Publisher, 1979: 181–205.
2. Danjoux GE, Catton GE. Delayed complications in colorectal carcinoma treated by combination radiotherapy and 5-fluorouracil. E.C.O.G. Pilot Study. Int J Radiol Oncol Bio Phys 1979; 5:311–5.
3. Kinsella TJ, Bloomer WD. Tolerance of the intestine to radiation therapy. Surg Gynecol Obstet 1980; 151:273–84.
4. DeCosse JJ, Rhodes RS, Wentz WB, et al. The natural history and management of radiation induced injury of the gastrointestinal tract. Ann Surg 1969; 170:369–84.
5. Berthrong M, Fajardo LF. Radiation injury in surgical pathology. Part II. Alimentary tract. Am J Surg Pathol 1981; 5:153–78.
6. Fajardo LF, Lee A. Rupture of major vessels after radiation. Cancer 1975; 36:904–13.
7. Clayman CB, Palmer WL, Kirsner JB. Gastric irradiation in the treatment of peptic ulcer. Gastroenterology 1968; 55: 403–7.
8. Mason GR, Guernsey JM, Hanks GE, Nelson TS. Surgical therapy for radiation enteritis. Oncology 1968; 22:241–59.
9. Earnest DL, Trier JS. Radiation enteritis and colitis. *In*: Sleisenger M, Fordtran J (eds). Gastrointestinal Disease. 2nd Ed. Philadelphia: WB Saunders, 1978: 1736–45.
10. Sheehan JF. Foam cell plaques in intima of irradiated small arteries. Arch Pathol 1944; 37:297–308.
11. Trier JS, Browning TH. Morphologic response of human small intestine to x-ray exposure. J Clin Invest 1966; 45:194–204.
12. Hofmann AF. The syndrome of ileal disease and the broken enterohepatic circulation; cholerheic enteropathy. Gastroenterology 1967; 52:752–7.
13. Stryker JA, Hepner GW, Mortel R. The effect of pelvic irradiation on ileal function. Radiology 1977; 124:213–6.
14. Tarpila S. Morphological and functional responses to the human small intestinal mucosa to ionizing radiation. Scand J Gastroenterol 1971; 6(Suppl 12):1–52.
15. Tamura K, Bralow SP, Kramer S. Unpublished data, 1975.
16. Stryker JA, Albert AB. The radio-protective effect of misonidazole on normal canine rectum. Strahlen Therapie 1980; 156:719–24.
17. Phelps TA, Blackett NM. Protection of intestinal damage by pretreatment with Cytarabine (cytosine arabinoside). Int J Radiation Oncol Biol Phys 1979; 5:1617–20.
18. Bounous G. Protection of gastrointestinal mucosa by elemental diets. Clin Invest Med 1980; 3:237–44.
19. Danjouz CE, Rider WD, Fitzpatrick PJ. The acute radiation syndrome. A memorial to William Michael Court-Brown. Clin Radiol 1979; 30:581–4.
20. Taverner D, Talbott IC, Carr-Locke MB, Wicks ACB. Massive bleeding from the ileum: A late complication of pelvic radiotherapy. Am J Gastroenterol 1982; 77:29–31.
21. Steinberg B, Risberg B, Petersen HI. Irradiation and gastrointestinal fibrinolysis, an experimental study in the rat. Europ J Clin Invest 1980; 10:139–41.
22. Reicheldelderfer M, Morrissey JF. Colonoscopy in radiation colitis. Gastrointest Endosc 1980; 26:41–3.
23. Doubleday LC, Bernardino ME. CT findings in the perirectal area following radiation therapy. J Comput Assist Tomogr 1980; 4:634–8.
24. Donaldson SS. Nutritional consequences of radiotherapy. Cancer Res 1977; 37:2407–13.
25. Goldstein F, Khoury J, Thornton JJ. Treatment of chronic radiation enteritis and colitis with salicylazosulfapyridine and systemic corticosteroids. Am J Gastroenterol 1976; 65:201–8.
26. Kline JC, Buchler DA, Boone ML, et al. The relationship of reactions to complications in the radiation therapy of cancer of the cervix. Radiology 1972; 105:413–6.
27. Cram AE, Pearlman NW, Jochimsen PR. Surgical management of complications of radiation-injured gut. Am J Surg 1977; 133:551–3.
28. Marks G, Mohiudden M. The surgical management of the radiation-injured intestine. Surg Clin North Am 1983; 63:81–96.
29. Marks G. Combined abdominotranssacral reconstruction of the radiation-injured rectum. Am J Surg 1976; 131:54–9.
30. Bricker EM, Johnston WD, Patwardhan RV. Repair of post-irradiation damage to colorectum, a progress report. Am Surg 1981; 193:555–64.
31. Lavery IC, Steiger E, Fazio VW. Home parenteral nutrition in management of patients with severe radiation enteritis. Dis Colon Rectum 1980; 23:91–3.
32. Schottenfeld D. Radiation as a risk factor in the natural history of colorectal cancer. Editorial. Gastroenterology 1983; 84:186–90.
33. Sandler RS, Sandler DP. Radiation-induced cancers of the colon and rectum: assessing the risk. Gastroenterology 1983; 84:51–7.

Chapter 143

Anorectal Diseases

Stanley M. Goldberg • Santhat Nivatvongs

Hemorrhoids

In the upper anal canal are cushions of submucosal tissues composed of connective tissue containing venules and smooth muscle fibers. Usually there are 3 cushions: left lateral, right anterior, and right posterior. This anatomic arrangement is remarkably constant and bears no relationship, as previously thought, to the terminal branches of the superior rectal vessels, which are quite inconstant.[1] The function of these cushions is speculative. By their bulk, they aid in anal continence, and during the act of defecation, when they become engorged with blood, they cushion the anal canal and support the lining. "Hemorrhoid" is the term used for the situation in which there is a downward displacement of the anal cushions causing dilatation of the venules.[1]

External Skin Tag. This refers to redundant fibrotic skin at the anal verge. It is usually the result of a previous thrombosed external hemorrhoid or previous anal surgery. Excision is indicated only if the skin tag causes pain or irritation or interferes with anal hygiene.

External Hemorrhoids. External hemorrhoids are dilated venules of the inferior hemorrhoidal plexus located below the pectinate or dentate line. Intravascular clotting of blood results in thrombosis of these vessels,[2] an occurrence that causes extreme pain during the first 48 hours. Excision is the treatment of choice and is usually done under local anesthesia as an office or outpatient procedure (Fig. 143–1). Incision alone should be discouraged because the clots are multiloculated. If the pain starts to subside, excision is unnecessary, and warm sitz baths will speed up the resolution.

Internal Hemorrhoids. Internal hemorrhoids are dilated venules of the superior hemorrhoidal plexus situated above the pectinate line. They most commonly are manifested by painless, bright red rectal bleeding associated with a bowel movement. The patient commonly describes the bleeding episode as "blood drips into the toilet bowl." When these dilated venules are chronically prolapsed, mucorrhea may develop, which frequently causes perianal irritation. A feel-

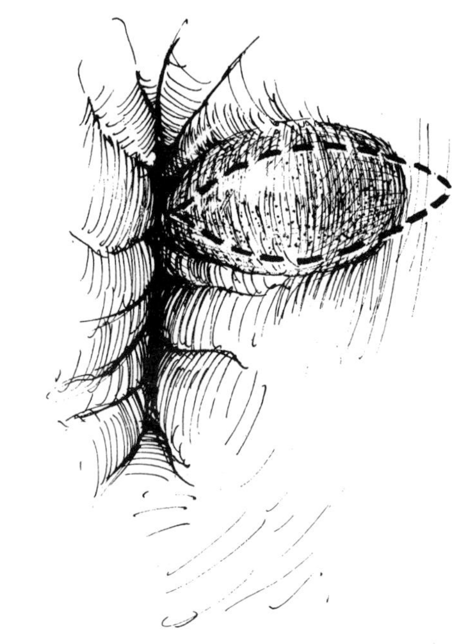

Figure 143–1. Excision of thrombosed external hemorrhoid.

ing of incomplete evacuation also is common in severe hemorrhoids.

Pain is not a common symptom of internal hemorrhoids unless they are complicated by an anal fissure, stenosis, or thrombosis. For the patient complaining of anal pain, there is a temptation to prescribe local anesthetic agents. We do not recommend these because of the high frequency of anal irritation thereby induced. The only medication that we think is of symptomatic benefit is pramoxine. This is a surface anesthetic agent that is chemically unrelated to the benzoate esters of the "-caine" type. It is contained in the preparation Tronolane, which is available as a cream or suppository.

The severity of internal hemorrhoids is graded according to the degree of prolapse:[3]

First degree. The anal cushions slide down beyond the dentate line on straining. The most common symptom is painless rectal bleeding. Treatment consists of bulk-forming agents, such as bran or psyllium seed. If bleeding persists, rubber band ligation should be done (Fig. 143–2).

Second degree. The anal cushions prolapse through the anus on straining but can be spontaneously reduced. Rubber band ligation is the treatment of choice,[4,5] along with bran or psyllium seed.

Third degree. The anal cushions prolapse through the anus upon straining or walking and require manual replacement into the anal canal. Hemorrhoidectomy gives the best results.[6]

Fourth degree. The prolapse has become strangulated and irreducible. Severe anal pain is the rule. Urgent or emergency hemorrhoidectomy is indicated.

Postpartum Hemorrhoids. Patients have usually had some difficulty with hemorrhoids before or during pregnancy. Prolonged straining during labor leads to thrombosis and often to strangulation. Hemorrhoidectomy is the treatment of choice for most cases.[7] If only a thrombosed external hemorrhoid occurs, excision is all that is necessary.

Hemorrhoids in Portal Hypertension. Although the portal system communicates with the systemic system by way of the superior rectal, middle rectal, and inferior rectal veins, the frequency of hemorrhoids in patients with portal hypertension is not higher than in the normal population.[8] Active bleeding usually occurs from ulceration of a hemorrhoid. A "stick-tie" at the bleeding site will solve the problem. In some cases, hemorrhoidectomy at the site of bleeding is necessary.[8] Any bleeding diathesis related to the associated liver disease must be corrected.

Anal Fissure

An anal fissure is a tear of the skin-lined part of the anal canal, i.e., the area from the pectinate or dentate line to the anal verge. Its length is usually a few mm and rarely exceeds 1 cm. Most anal fissures are initiated by the passage of a large hard stool. Because

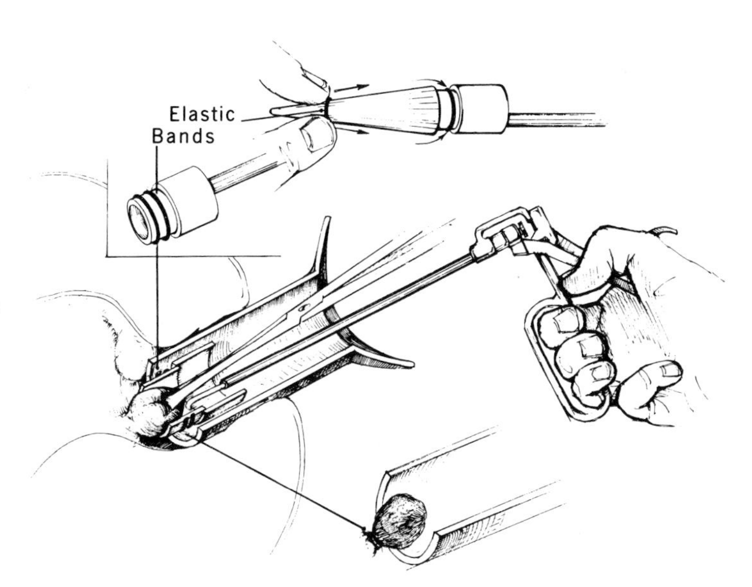

Figure 143–2. Rubber band ligation of an internal hemorrhoid.

of poor muscular support of the anal canal posteriorly, the majority of the fissures occur in the posterior midline and less frequently in the anterior midline. An anal fissure off the midline, either posterior or anterior, arouses the suspicion of another underlying disease (Fig. 143–3).

Anal fissures occur mostly in young and middle-aged adults. The characteristic symptom is a sharp burning pain during and after a bowel movement. Another common complaint is bright red blood on the toilet paper upon wiping. Identification often may be made simply by separating the buttocks gently. This usually reveals the fissure, but digital and anoscopic examination may be necessary to establish the diagnosis. Proctosigmoidoscopic examination will also exclude any associated abnormalities of the anal canal and rectum, especially inflammatory bowel disease.

Conservative treatment will improve or heal many acute anal fissures. Such treatment consists of anal hygiene; use of bulk-producing agents, such as bran and psyllium seed; warm sitz baths; and application of a local anesthetic jelly. Once the fissure becomes chronic, surgical treatment is ordinarily required. The treatment of choice is usually a lateral internal sphincterotomy.[9] Fissurectomy may occasionally be indicated.

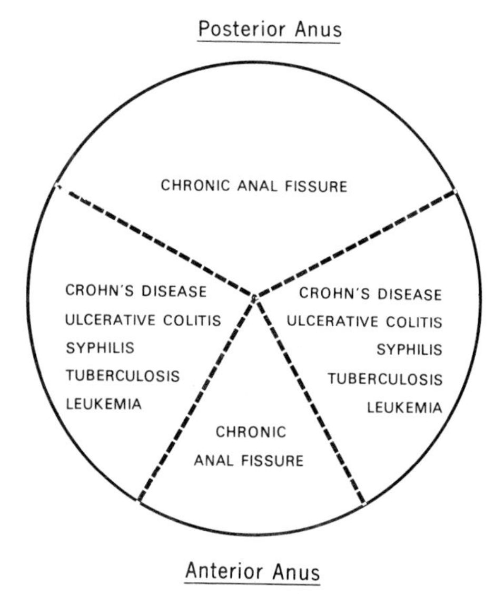

Figure 143–3. Common locations of chronic anal fissures and other anorectal conditions.

Anorectal Abscesses

Anorectal abscesses are infections of the potential spaces around the anorectum. The infection starts in the anal glands that lie between the internal and external sphincter muscles. The initial formation, therefore, is an *intersphincteric abscess.* This abscess may rupture into the anal lumen and the infection may then subside. However, the infection may extend instead into the perianal space to form a *perianal abscess,* or through the external sphincter to form an *ischioanal* or *ischiorectal abscess,* or above the levator ani muscle to form a *pelvirectal* or *supralevator abscess* (Fig. 143–4).

Diagnosis. Anorectal abscesses characteristically present with severe anal pain and tenderness and commonly with high fever. The throbbing anal pain is acute and is aggravated by sitting, coughing, sneezing, and straining. The less common intersphincteric abscess causes dull aching or throbbing pain in the anorectum, rather than the perianal area. Extreme tenderness usually precludes an adequate examination without anesthesia. Rectal examination reveals a soft or indurated mass in the wall of the upper anal canal, usually in the posterior quadrant. The existence of the more common perianal and ischioanal abscesses is made apparent by tender swelling in the perianal area. The rare supralevator abscess is difficult to diagnose. The patient may present with fever of unknown origin or signs of peritonitis simulating an intra-abdominal process. Induration of the supralevator spaces suggests the diagnosis.

Treatment. The standard treatment of anorectal abscesses is incision and drainage,[10–13] even in the absence of fluctuation. Antibiotics should never constitute the principal therapy, but may be used adjunctively. Most perianal abscesses can be drained under local anesthesia as an outpatient procedure (Fig. 143–5). Intersphincteric, ischioanal, and supralevator abscesses, however, should be drained in the operating room with the aid of adequate anesthesia.

Fistula-in-ano

Fistula-in-ano is a track lined by granulation tissue resulting from incomplete healing of a drained anorectal abscess. The primary

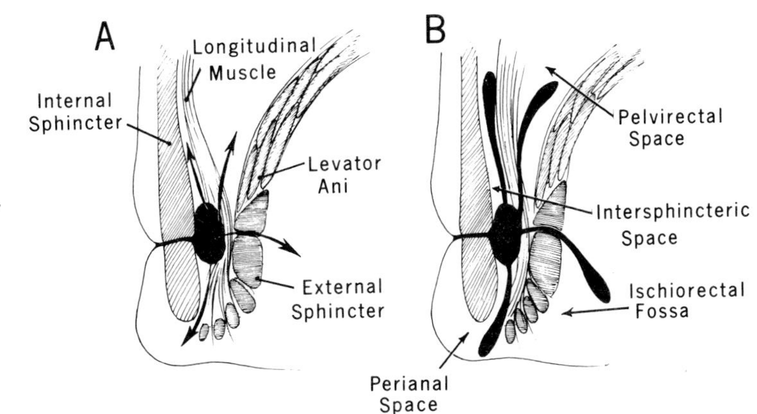

Figure 143–4. Avenues of extension in perianal abscess.

opening is in the cryptoglandular area of the anal canal at the dentate line, and the secondary opening is in the perianal skin where the abscess ruptured or drained.[14]

Diagnosis. Most, but not all, patients with fistula-in-ano give a history of previous anorectal abscesses. Intermittent purulent or serosanguineous discharge is the main complaint. Pain is unusual, but itching and irritation of the perianal area from the fistulous discharge are common.[15] The external opening is usually apparent in the perianal area as a red elevation of granulation tissue with discharge on compression. The internal opening can be identified in the anal canal in most cases when the examination is conducted in the operating room.[15] With a simple fistula, the track can be palpated as an indurated cord.

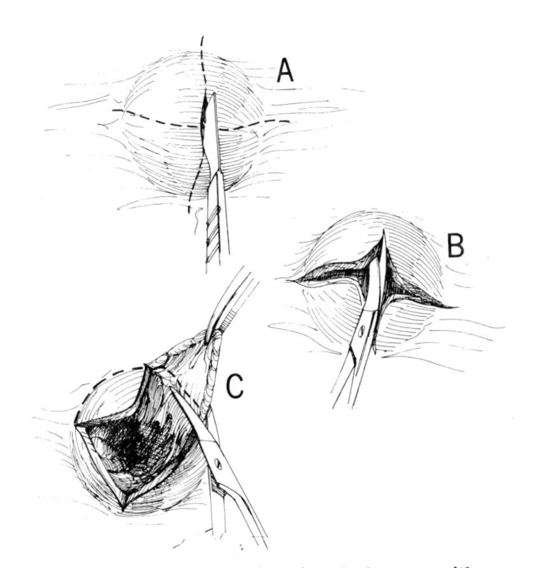

Figure 143–5. Drainage of perianal abscess with cruciate incision.

Several disorders must be considered in the differential diagnosis of fistula-in-ano. It is important to rule out fistulas associated with *Crohn's disease* and *ulcerative colitis,* in which case extensive operative procedures on the fistulas are contraindicated because of poor wound healing. The differential diagnosis may necessitate complete study of the gastrointestinal tract. *Sigmoid diverticulitis* with perforation and fistulization to the perineum occurs rarely. *Hidradenitis suppurativa* (infection of sweat glands) is apparent by the presence of multiple openings in the perianal skin. *Pilonidal sinus with perianal extension* and *infected perianal sebaceous cysts* must be considered. Rarely, a *carcinoma* may develop in longstanding fistulas, but rectal and anal carcinomas rarely present as a fistula in the perineum.

Treatment. Once established, fistula-in-ano rarely heals spontaneously. The basic principle of treatment is to lay open the fistulous track. Deep or high fistulas may require a 2-stage operation. In order to prevent anal incontinence, a seton or a silk suture is placed around the sphincter muscle overlying the fistula to create fibrosis and fixation.[16] The muscle is then cut 6 to 8 weeks later to lay open the fistulous track.

Prolapse of the Rectum

Prolapse of the rectum (procidentia) is an uncommon condition in which the full thickness of the rectal wall turns inside out into or through the anal canal. Typically, the extruded rectum is seen as concentric rings of mucosa (Fig. 143–6). This should not be confused with rectal mucosal prolapse or prolapsed hemorrhoids in which the radial folds of mucosa extrude through the anus. Although prolapse of the rectum can occur at any age, the peak occurrence in women is in the seventh decade; in men the age distribution is more constant.[17] The female to male ratio is 5:1.[17] For years, the theory of sliding hernia had been put forth as the causative mechanism. More recently, however, with the use of cineradiography, intussusception has been demonstrated.[18–21] The intussusception begins circumferentially about 6 to 7 cm from the anal verge.

The early symptoms are minor and include anorectal pain or discomfort during defecation. Difficulty in initiating a bowel movement and a feeling of incomplete evacuation also are common. Diagnosis is easy if the prolapse comes through the anus. When the prolapse remains in the upper anal canal ("hidden prolapse"), the diagnosis can be difficult. Redness of the rectal mucosa, especially anteriorly at about the 6- to 7-cm level gives a clue. Straining of the anorectum with an anoscope in place is also helpful. In the advanced stage, fecal and urinary incontinence are common. Parks et al.[22] have shown that the incontinence is the consequence of entrapment or stretching of the pudendal or perineal nerve, resulting in neuromuscular dysfunction. Therefore, it is essential to repair the prolapse before this mishap occurs.

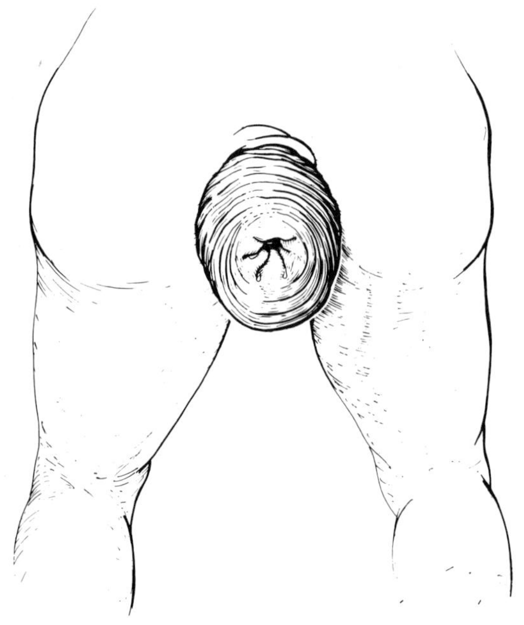

Figure 143–6. Concentric circular rings of mucosa in prolapse of rectum.

Treatment. Over the years there have been more than 50 methods for the repair of rectal prolapse, all with varying rates of success. The modern concept of the repair is to remove the intussusception or to prevent the intussusception from occurring. Most methods of repair are by the transabdominal or transperineal approach.

The rectal sling operation, introduced by Ripstein,[23] consists of a sling of Teflon or Marlex that fixes the fully mobilized rectum to the sacrum. *The Ivalon sponge wrap operation*, devised by Wells,[24] has been popular in the United Kingdom. The fully mobilized rectum is fixed to the sacrum with a rectangular sheet of Ivalon sponge (polyvinyl alcohol). *Anterior resection of the rectum*, first described by Muir[25] in 1955, consists of full mobilization of the rectum, as for abdominoperineal resection or for low anterior resection of carcinoma of the rectum. The midrectum along with the redundant sigmoid colon is resected and an anastomosis is made. *Transabdominal proctopexy* is another method of fixing the mobilized rectum to the sacrum, but without the necessity of using a foreign material.[26] *Perineal rectosigmoidectomy* is a perineal approach in which the rectum and rectosigmoid colon are resected through the prolapse itself.[27] It is very well tolerated by the patients, and general or regional anesthesia can be used.

Our choice of procedure has been the *transabdominal proctopexy* for good-risk patients. For patients who are not suitable for an intraabdominal procedure but who can withstand general or regional anesthesia, *perineal rectosigmoidectomy* is the method of choice. In elderly patients and those whose general condition precludes a definitive repair, the *Thiersch wire procedure* may be used, in which the anus is encircled with wire or other suture materials under local anesthesia. The procedure is simple and is well tolerated, but the success rate is poor and is associated with a high rate of recurrence, fecal impaction, and suture breakage. A modification of the Thiersch procedure using Marlex or Silastic strips has been found to be superior.[28]

Pruritus Ani

Pruritus ani is a common problem and difficult to treat. The perianal skin is sensitive; any condition causing soiling or moisture to the area can produce itching. Pruritus ani may be a manifestation of local or systemic disease. The surgically correctable conditions contributing to this disorder include prolapsing hemorrhoids, ectropion, anal fissure, fistula-in-ano, condyloma acuminatum, and neoplasm of the anal canal or perineum. Other predisposing conditions include diarrhea, dermatitis, severe diabetes mellitus, severe jaundice, lymphomas, and leukemia. In children, *Enterobius vermicularis* (pinworm) infection is a common cause. In most cases, no specific cause is found, and the pruritus is called "idiopathic." This common form can be particularly vexing to the patient and therapist alike.

The diagnosis of pruritus ani is simple. In the acute and subacute stages, the anal and perianal skin is red, excoriated, and moist, frequently owing to a fungus infection, especially Candida and Epidermophyton. Mycostatin powder or gentian violet will rapidly improve the condition. When pruritus ani has become chronic, the affected surfaces are thickened and white with multiple radial and irregular folds. There has been no specific treatment for chronic idiopathic pruritus ani. Anal hygiene, consisting of gentle cleansing of the anal area with moist tissue and then thorough drying, is the cornerstone of successful control. Bowel habit regulation, to prevent incomplete evacuation and soiling, must be emphasized.[29] All other possible causes, such as sensitivity to certain kinds of toilet paper, various dyes in underclothing, and allergy to soap, cream, or ointment, should be excluded. Certain foods and beverages have been postulated to cause pruritus ani, although this is unproved. Among these are coffee, tea, cola, beer, chocolate, and tomatoes.[30]

Hydrocortisone in a 0.5% preparation applied locally gives temporary symptomatic relief. An undercutting operation, subcutaneous injection of alcohol, tattooing with mercury sulfate, and topical irradiation for chronic idiopathic pruritus ani have been abandoned as methods of treatment. They are ineffective and achieve only transient relief.

Proctalgia Fugax and the Levator Syndrome

Proctalgia fugax is a severe spasmodic rectal pain lasting a few minutes or longer. The exact cause is unknown, but the condition may be due to levator ani muscle spasm.[31] The characteristic history is that of severe pain awakening the patient at night.[32] The pain usually is located in the midrectum and disappears spontaneously without residual symptoms. Proctoscopic examination is indicated to rule out anorectal diseases. Treatment to relieve the pain during an acute attack consists of firm pressure on the anus, a warm sitz bath, or a heating pad applied to the perineum. Many of these patients are anxious and fear cancer; hence, reassurance is an important aspect of therapy. Further information pertaining to proctalgia fugax is to be found in Chapter 134.

Another group of patients have chronic vague pain in the anorectum. Examination reveals tenderness of the levator ani muscle, more often on the left side. This is termed the *levator syndrome*. Digital masssage of the tender muscle at weekly intervals may provide effective relief.[33]

Condylomata Acuminata

Anal condylomata acuminata, or warts, are caused by a papilloma virus. The condition is most commonly found in male homosexuals.[34,35] In the majority of patients, the warts involve the perianal skin and anal verge. Occasionally, the lesions also involve the mucosa of the upper anal canal and the lower rectum. The extent of the disease varies from a few small excrescences to an extensive mass occluding the anus. The diagnosis is usually obvious by the characteristic papillary appearance. Anoscopic examination is essential to detect intra-anal involvement. As most cases are transmitted by sexual contact, other co-existing venereal diseases, especially gonorrhea and syphilis, should be excluded.

Small perianal warts can be destroyed by applying podophyllin solution or bichloracetic acid.[35] Extensive warts in the perianal area or in the anal canal require electrocoagulation or excision under anesthesia.[36] Frequent postoperative follow-up is necessary because these lesions recur in as many as 65% of patients.[37] Immunotherapy, using autogenous wart-tissue vaccine, in conjunction with excision of the lesions has been found to be effective and has reduced the recurrence rate to within 10%.[34, 37] The role of immune mechanisms in recurrent wart formation is yet to be determined. Immunotherapy should be used with caution because the vaccine contains oncogenic virus.

Gonococcal Proctitis

Gonococcal proctitis is found most commonly among homosexuals. In women, the anorectum may be infected by the spread of discharge from a gonococcal cervicitis or urethritis. Patients are generally asymptomatic but may have mild anal burning, pain, discharge, or bleeding in the acute phase. Proctoscopic examination reveals hyperemic and edematous anorectal mucosa with purulent discharge in the anal crypts. In the chronic phase, the anorectum may appear normal. Diagnosis is confirmed by observing the infecting organisms on stained smears of the discharge and plating the exudate immediately onto the Thayer-Martin culture medium.

Penicillin remains the antibiotic of choice.[38] When penicillin is contraindicated, oral tetracycline or IM injection of spectinomycin hydrochloride may be used. In patients who fail to respond to penicillin, spectinomycin should be given.[38,39] Smears and cultures from the anorectum should be taken after 1 week of treatment to confirm the response.

Herpes Simplex

Anorectal herpes is caused by *herpes virus hominis type II*, the same organism implicated in genital herpes.[40] It is less common than gonorrhea but more common than syphilis. The clinical presentation usually begins with itching and soreness in or around the anus, followed by severe anorectal pain.[39, 41] The pain may be so intense that the patient is reluctant to have a bowel movement, leading to constipation and impaction. Examination reveals erythematous areas with small groups of vesicles that rupture and become ulcerated. The diagnosis is confirmed by viral culture of the vesicular fluid.[39, 41] The lesions should be kept clean by frequent sitz baths. Symptomatic relief is obtained by the use of analgesic drugs and the local application of soothing agents. Topical 5% acyclovir ointment is effective in shortening the duration of viral shedding and the clinical course of primary genital herpes.[9a] At the present time, the Federal Food and Drug Administration has approved its use for primary but not for recurrent herpes simplex infection.

Imperforate Anus

Imperforate anus is a rare congenital anomaly in which there is no opening of the anus at the normal position in the perineum (Chapter 87). The anomaly results from failure of migration of the rectal opening during the developmental period of the embryo.[42] Although there are several classifications, the simplest one is to classify the problem in relation to the levator ani muscle. When the blind pouch is above the levator ani muscle, the anomaly is called supralevator or high imperforate anus, and if the blind pouch is below the levator muscle, the term used is infralevator or low imperforate anus.[43,44] Before planning for surgery, it is imperative to know whether the imperforate anus is the high or low type, since treatment is different for each type. Associated anomalies are common, and it is important to search for them.

Diagnosis. The diagnosis of imperforate anus is made by examination of the perineum. If a dimple or fistula is seen in the perineum, or a vaginal fourchette in females, the imperforate anus is the low type. If no fistula or dimple is seen, it is important to determine the position of the blind pouch. The upside-down (Wangensteen-Rice technique) radiographic view, which is taken after the swallowed air has had time to reach the rectum (12 to 24 hours), provides a useful diagnostic technique.[45] If the blind rectal pouch is above the "pubococcygeal line" (a line drawn on the lateral film, between the pubis and lowermost segment of the sacrum), the anomaly is the supralevator type. Similarly, if the blind rectal pouch is below this line, it is the infralevator type.[46] Unfortunately, the Wangensteen-Rice technique may be misleading if there is meconium in the large bowel. Respiration and crying may also cause the blind rectal pouch to be at variable levels. Instillation of 5 ml of Gastrografin into the stomach by way of a nasogastric tube can determine the level of the blind pouch in about half the cases.[43] Radiopaque material can also be injected into the blind pouch through the perineum.[43]

Urologic anomalies are common in these patients; IV pyelogram and urinalysis to detect meconium in the urine are therefore essential. Esophageal atresia, malrotation of midgut, and intestinal atresia are the most common gastrointestinal complications. An anteroposterior roentgenograph of the vertebral column will easily reveal abnormality of the sacrum. Absence or abnormality of the sacrum may imply failure of innervation of the pelvic musculature. Studies should also be made that are directed at detecting cardiac anomalies.[43]

Treatment. For the infralevator type, opening of the perineum and anoplasty should be done without delay. For the supralevator type, staged operation is necessary. A diverting transverse colostomy is first established. The second stage should be deferred until the infant is about a year old to allow the pelvis to enlarge and the pelvic musculature to develop better. A pull-through procedure is then performed to bring the rectum through the opening in the perineum. It is important that the rectum be brought through the puborectalis muscle sling to achieve good anal continence.[46] The procedure is performed through a sacroabdominoperineal approach.[47]

Solitary Ulcer of the Rectum

Solitary ulcer of the rectum is an uncommon chronic ulceration of the rectum. The term is misleading because there may be more than one ulcer, and there is a stage of the disease when no ulceration is present.[48–51] Moreover, the lesion can occur in the bowel elsewhere than the rectum (Chapter 126). The gross appearance of the lesion may be misinterpreted by clinicians as proctitis, Crohn's ulceration, villous adenoma, or even carcinoma.[50–52]

Etiology. The etiology of solitary rectal ulcer is unknown. Electromyography of puborectalis and superficial anal sphincter muscles in patients with solitary ulcer of the rectum suggests that during bearing-down efforts the puborectalis muscle behaves paradoxically, i.e., it goes into a state of tight contraction instead of relaxation.[51] In some cases, self-induced trauma has been suspected.[53]

Clinical Aspects. Solitary ulcer of the rectum occurs most commonly in young adults, with an equal distribution between men and women. The common symptoms include slight to moderate bleeding on defecation, passage of mucus on defecation, anal or rectal pain and discomfort, irregular bowel habit, and lower abdominal pain.[48–51] Massive bleeding from the ulcer is rare but has been reported.[54, 55]

Diagnosis. Most ulcers are about 2 cm in diameter, but they may be no larger than a match head or as large as 5 cm. The distance of the ulcer from the anal verge varies from 3 to 12 cm, with an average of 8 cm.[49] Proctoscopy is essential for diagnosis. Most (about 85%) of the ulcers are located in the anterior part of the rectum.[48] The base of the ulcer is characteristically covered with a white, gray, or yellowish slough. The ulcer is shallow, with a sharply demarcated hyperemic edge.[50] It is believed that in some cases there is a non-ulcer stage[50] in which the rectal mucosa appears red and granular and resembles a localized proctitis, but gross ulceration is not present. Histologically, the appearance is not different from the ulcerative type whose most characteristic histologic features are: (1) obliteration of the lamina propria of the mucosal layer in the region of the ulcer by fibroblasts and muscle fibers derived from the muscularis mucosae; (2) thickening of the muscularis mucosae and extension of its fibers into the lamina propria; (3) absence of a large number of inflammatory cells in the lamina propria; and (4) occasionally, cystic dilatation of the tubules and sometimes displacement of the tubules into the submucosa.[50] Most of the time, the diagnosis can be made from the gross appearance of the lesion.[49,50] Nevertheless, a diagnosis of solitary ulcer of the rectum should not be made without considering and excluding disorders such as carcinoma, Crohn's disease, proctitis, and lymphogranuloma venereum.

Treatment. Treatment of this condition consists essentially of correcting the associated problems, particularly full-thickness rectal prolapse (procidentia) and rectal mucosal prolapse.[56] Neither medical treatment nor local excision of the lesion consistently achieves relief of symptoms or healing of the ulcer.[48] Adjustment of diet to avoid straining at stool may be helpful.

Tuberculosis

Tuberculosis affecting the anus and rectum is covered in Chapter 120, to which the reader is referred.

References

1. Thomson WHF. The nature of hemorrhoids. Br J Surg 1975; 62:542–52.
2. Ganchrow MI, Bowman HB, Clark JF. Thrombosed hemorrhoids: A clinicopathologic study. Dis Colon Rectum 1971; 5:331–40.
3. Marino MAW Jr, Mazier WP, Morgan B, Salvati EP, Smith LE. Anorectal surgery—hemorrhoids. Dis Colon Rectum 1980; 23:211–22.
4. Alexander-Williams J, Crapp AR. Conservative management of hemorrhoids. Part I: Injection, freezing and ligation. Clin Gastroenterol 1975; 4:595–618.
5. Wrobleski DE, Corman ML, Veidenheimer MC, Coller JA. Long-term evaluation of rubber ring ligation in hemorrhoidal disease. Dis Colon Rectum 1980; 23:478–82.
6. Buls JG, Goldberg SM. Modern management of hemorrhoids. Surg Clin North Am 1978; 58:469–78.
7. Schottler JL, Balcos EG, Goldberg SM. Post partum hemorrhoidectomy. Dis Colon Rectum 1973; 16:395–6.
8. Jacobs DM, Bubrick MP, Onstad GR, Hitchcock CR. The relationship of hemorrhoids to portal hypertension. Dis Colon Rectum 1980; 23:567–9.
9. Abcarian H. Surgical correction of chronic anal fissure: Results of lateral internal sphincterotomy vs fissurectomy–mid-line sphincterotomy. Dis Colon Rectum 1980; 23:31–6.

9a. Corey L. The diagnosis and treatment of genital herpes. JAMA 1982; 248:1041–9.

10. Goldberg HS. Supralevator abscess: Diagnosis and treatment. Surgery 1982; 91:164–7.
11. Prasad ML, Read DR, Abcarian H. Supralevator abscess: Diagnosis and treatment. Dis Colon Rectum 1981; 24:456–61.
12. Read DR, Abcarian H. A prospective survey of 474 patients with anorectal abscess. Dis Colon Rectum 1979; 22:566–8.
13. Scoma JA, Salvati EP, Rubin RJ. Incidence of fistulas subsequent to anal abscesses. Dis Colon Rectum 1974; 17:357–9.
14. Parks AG. Etiology and surgical treatment of fistula-in-ano. Dis Colon Rectum 1963; 6:17–22.
15. Lilius HG. Fistula-in-ano. An investigation of human faecal anal ducts and intramuscular glands and a clinical study of 150 patients. Acta Chir Scand 1968; Suppl 383, 18–82.
16. Goldberg SM, Gordon PH, Nivatvongs S. Essentials of Anorectal Surgery. Philadelphia: JB Lippincott, 1980: 123.
17. Kupfer CA, Goligher JC. One hundred consecutive cases of complete prolapse of the rectum treated by operation. Br J Surg 1970; 57:481–7.
18. Broden B, Snellman B. Procidentia of the rectum studied with cineradiography: A contribution to the discussion of causative mechanisms. Dis Colon Rectum 1968; 11:330–47.
19. Devadhar DSC. A new concept of mechanism and treatment of rectal procidentia. Dis Colon Rectum 1965; 8:75–7.
20. Theuerkauf FJ Jr, Beahrs OH, Hill JR. Rectal prolapse: Causation and surgical treatment. Ann Surg 1970; 171:819–35.
21. Ihre T, Seligson U. Intussusception of the rectum—internal procidentia: Treatment and results in 90 patients. Dis Colon Rectum 1975; 18:391–6.
22. Parks AG, Swash M, Urich H. Sphincter denervation in anorectal incontinence and rectal prolapse. Gut 1977; 18:656–65.
23. Ripstein CB, Lanter B. Etiology and surgical therapy of massive prolapse of the rectum. Ann Surg 1963; 157:259–64.
24. Wells C. New operation for rectal prolapse. Proc R Soc Med 1959; 52:602–3.
25. Muir EG. Rectal prolapse. Proc R Soc Med 1955; 48:33–44.
26. Goldberg SM, Gordon PH. Treatment of rectal prolapse. Clin Gastroenterol 1975; 4:489–504.
27. Altemeier WA, Culbertson WR, Schowengerdt C, Hunt J. Nineteen years' experience with one-stage perineal repair of rectal prolapse. Ann Surg 1971; 173:993–1006.
28. Labow S, Rubin RJ, Hoexter B, Salvati EP. Perineal repair of rectal procidentia with an elastic fabric sling. Dis Colon Rectum 1980; 23:467–9.
29. Smith LE, Henrichs D, McCullah RD. Prospective studies on the etiology and treatment of pruritus ani. Dis Colon Rectum 1982; 25:358–63.
30. Friend WG. The cause and treatment of idiopathic pruritus ani. Dis Colon Rectum 1977; 20:40–2.
31. Douthwaite AH. Proctalgia fugax. Br Med J 1962; 2:164–5.
32. Neill ME, Swash M. Chronic perianal pain: An unsolved problem. J R Soc Med 1982; 75:96–101.
33. Grant SR, Salvati EP, Rubin RJ. Levator syndrome: An analysis of 316 cases. Dis Colon Rectum 1975; 18:161–3.
34. Abcarian H, Sharon N. The effectiveness of immunotherapy in the treatment of anal condyloma acuminatum. J Surg Res 1977; 22:231–6.
35. Swerdlow DB, Salvati EP. Condylomata acuminatum. Dis Colon Rectum 1971; 14:226–31.
36. Thomson JPS, Grace RH. The treatment of perianal and anal condylomata acuminata: A new operative technique. J R Soc Med 1978; 71:180–5.
37. Eftaiha MS, Amshel AL, Shonberg IL, Batshon B. Giant and recurrent condylomata acuminatum: Appraisal of immunotherapy. Dis Colon Rectum 1982; 25:136–8.
38. Sands M. Treatment of anorectal gonorrhea infections in men. JAMA 1980; 243:1143–4.
39. Fiumara NJ. The treatment of gonococcal proctitis. An evaluation of 173 patients treated with 4 g of spectinomycin. JAMA 1978; 239:735–7.
40. Catterall RD. Sexually transmitted diseases of the anus and rectum. Clin Gastroenterol 1975; 4:659–69.
41. Jacobs E. Anal infections caused by herpes simplex virus. Dis Colon Rectum 1976; 19:151–7.
42. Bill AH Jr, Johnson RJ. Failure of migration of the rectal opening as the cause for most cases of imperforate anus. Surg Gynecol Obstet 1958; 106:643–51.
43. Kiesewetter WB. Rectum and anus—malformations. *In*: Ravich MM, Welch KJ, Benson CD, Aberdeen E, Randolph JG, eds. Pediatric Surgery, 3rd Ed. Chicago: Year Book Medical Publishers, 1979: 1059–72.
44. McGill CW, Polk HC Jr. The clinical basis for a simplified classification of anorectal agenesis. Surg Gynecol Obstet 1978, 146:177–81.
45. Wangensteen OH, Rice CO. Imperforate anus. Ann Surg 1930; 92:77–81.
46. Stephens FD. Congenital imperforate rectum, rectourethral and rectovaginal fistulae. Aust NZ J Surg 1953; 22:161–72.
47. Adkins JC, Kiesewetter WB. Imperforate anus. Surg Clin North Am 1976; 56:379–94.
48. Ford MJ Jr, Anderson JR, Gilmour HM, Holt S, Sircus W, Heading RC. Clinical spectrum of "solitary ulcer" of the rectum. Gastroenterology 1983; 84:1533–40.
49. Kennedy DK, Hughes ESR, Masterton JP. The natural history of benign ulcer of the rectum. Surg Gynecol Obstet 1979; 144:718–20.
50. Madigan MR, Morson BC. Solitary ulcer of the rectum. Gut 1969; 10:871–81.
51. Rutter KRP, Riddell RH. The solitary ulcer syndrome of the rectum. Clinic Gastroenterol 1975; 4:505–30.
52. Thomson G, Clark A, Handyside J, Gillespie G. Solitary ulcer of the rectum—or is it? A report of 6 cases. Br J Surg 1981; 68:21–4.
53. Thomson H, Hill D. Solitary rectal ulcer: Always a self-induced condition? Br J Surg 1980; 67:784–5.
54. Goldberg M, Hoffman GC, Wombo HDG. Massive hemorrhage from rectal ulcers in chronic renal failure. Ann Intern Med 1984; 100:397.
55. Delaney H, Hitch WS. Solitary rectal ulcer: A cause of life-threatening hemorrhage. Surgery 1974; 76:830–2.
56. Schweiger M, Alexander-Williams J. Solitary-ulcer syndrome of the rectum. Its association with occult rectal prolapse. Lancet 1977; 1:170–1.

Chapter 144

The Appendix

Gordon McHardy

Anatomy and Development

The gross anatomy of the appendix is described in Chapter 131, and the various positions that it may occupy in the abdomen are illustrated in Figure 131–6.

On section, the lumen usually is Y-shaped. The wall consists of a mucosa of variable thickness in relation to the degree of lymphoid tissue mass; a thin muscularis; a somewhat open, delicate, vascular submucosa; circular and longitudinal muscle layers; and extremely thin subserosal and peritoneal coats. Two sympathetic nerve plexuses are identified—Meissner's plexus in the submucosa and Auerbach's plexus in the muscularis. Lymphatics are prominent in the mucosa and submucosa; in the submucosa, they tend to longitudinal distribution, explaining the frequency of submucosal spread of infection.

The microscopic anatomy of the organ has little clinical significance other than the predominance of lymphoid tissue in the first 3 decades of life. This has been proposed as a potential source for subsequent adenocarcinoma. Electron microscopic studies have developed 3 morphologic zones in the appendiceal structure[1]: (1) subepithelial, i.e., the lymphoid lamina propria; (2) parafollicular; and (3) follicular. Two types of lymphocytes are encountered, "light" and "dark." The former are abundant in clusters in the epithelium and parafollicular postcapillary venules, clustering around epithelial cells. They may mature into plasma cells in the subepithelial areas and are possibly T or B lymphocytes or both.

Anomalies. Anomalies that may be found include agenesis (related in one case to thalidomide therapy,[2] malrotation of the large bowel resulting in a left-sided position of the appendix[3,4] (Chapter 88), duplication,[5] and diverticular formation[6] (Fig. 144–1). Vascular malformations may occur in the appendix and may predispose to bleeding.[7]

Physiology

The appendix is not generally credited with substantial function. However, current evidence tends to involve it in the immunologic mechanism.[8,9–13] The studies of Gorgollon[1] suggest that the appendix is a well-developed lymphoid organ with immunologic functions. Fichtelius[14] conceived of the appendix as a central lymphoid organ concerned with the maturation process of B lymphocytes. Calkins and his associates[15] concluded that the appendix complements receptor B lymphocytes, and Craig and Cebra[16] indicated the existence in the appendix of an IgA precursor B lymphocyte.

Lymphoid tissue accumulation appears shortly after birth and increases to a peak between the second and third decades, decreasing rapidly thereafter and practically disappearing in individuals beyond age 60. Fibrosis occurs with the decrease in lymphoid tissue, creating luminal constriction and, in many instances, obliteration. It may be significant that the period of highest prevalence

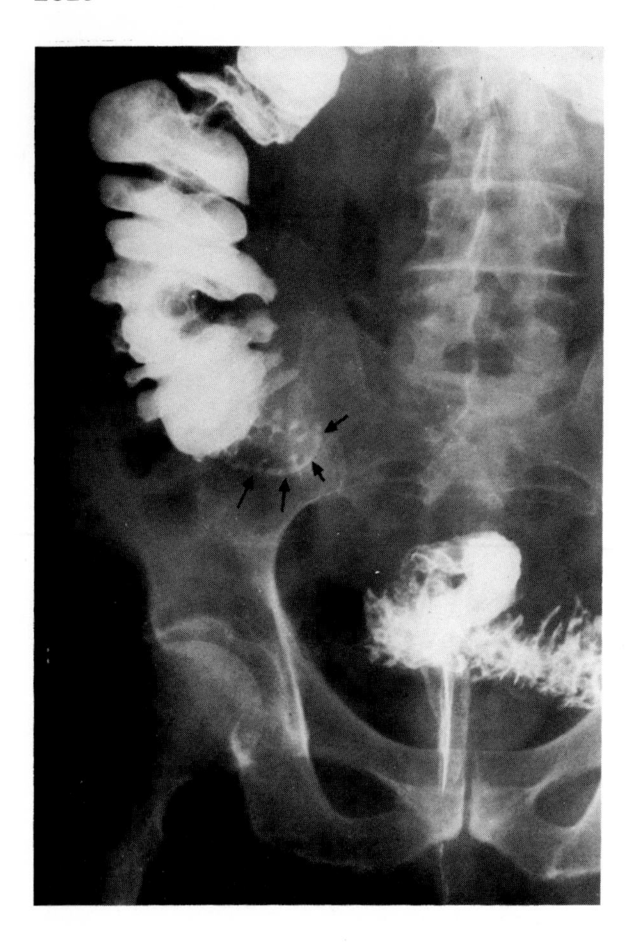

Figure 144–1. Diverticulosis of the appendix *(arrows).*

of acute appendicitis parallels the peak period of lymphoid aggregates. A relationship between the appendix and the development of colonic neoplasm has also been hypothesized on the basis of the lymphoid aggregates.[17,18] The concept that appendectomy predisposes to Hodgkin's disease, however, has been discounted.[19]

Physiologically, the appendix secretes an alkaline fluid containing amylase, erepsin, and mucin; in the presence of an obstruction, this may create a mucocele (Fig. 144–2). A minimal degree of motor activity occurs in the appendix.

Acute Appendicitis

Historical Background. Fitz,[20] in 1886, is properly accredited with establishing appendicitis as a clinical and pathologic entity, correctable by surgery. McBurney's[21] description of operative correction of appendiceal disease, published in 1889, led to the use of his name for a localization point. Murphy,[22] in 1904, published the first extensive surgical survey of 2000 operations for appendicitis. In the interval from this notable contribution until the present, surgical proficiency, anesthetic advancement, effective chemotherapy, and proven supportive measures have favorably altered the outlook in acute and complicated disease states.[23] The present challenge primarily relates to diagnostic accuracy and investigation of complications, but as the disease is still associated with appreciable morbidity and mortality, it continues to demand the interest and attention of clinicians and investigators alike.[24,25]

Etiology and Pathogenesis. Acute appendicitis has been noted to result from appendiceal obstruction by fecaliths,[26] hypertrophy of lymphoid tissue,[27] neoplasm,[28, 29] foreign bodies,[30–32] and parasites.[33] It has also been recorded in association with a large variety of other disorders and changes that presumably bear some etiologic relationship to the appendicitis. Included among these are Crohn's disease,[34] cecal diaphragms,[35] and

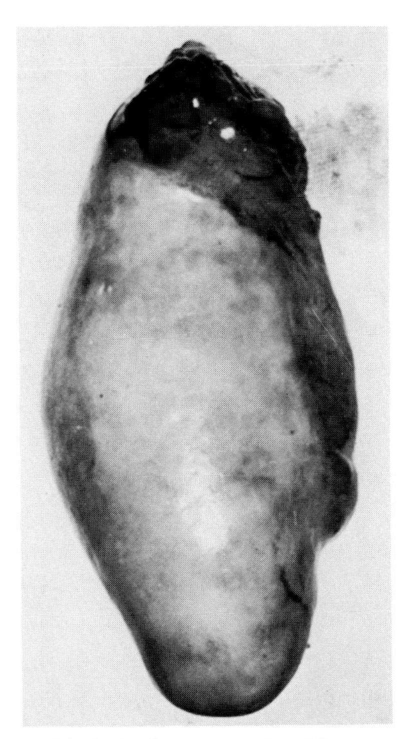

Figure 144–2. Benign mucocele of the appendix.

parasites such as *Schistosoma japonicum*,[36] *Strongyloides stercoralis*,[37] and *Trichuris trichiura*.[38] Acute appendicitis has similarly occurred with measles,[39] other viruses,[40,41] *Shigella sonnei*,[42,1] and Legionnaire's disease.[43] Barium retention after upper gastrointestinal study or enema has also been incriminated as a cause for inflammatory change in the appendix.[44] Foreign bodies of all sorts[45] (pins, lead shots, seeds, bones, eggshells, glass, teeth, nails, and even a thermometer) have been recovered from the appendix, and these must be viewed as potential inciters of an acute inflammatory response.

Burkitt and his associates[28] and Westlake et al.[46] include appendicitis among the disorders that may be induced by exaggerated muscle contractions associated with low-fiber diets and a resultant small volume of colon content. In a similar vein, Anderssen and his associates,[47] pointing to a disproportionate share of appendicitis among persons in the higher social classes, hypothesize that patients in this category eat more refined foods.

The inflammatory process is considered to arise when the appendix, with a luminal capacity of 0.1 to 0.2 ml, continues its mucosal secretion in the face of an obstruction at its outlet. This results in distention. When the increased intraluminal pressure so produced exceeds the venous pressure, occlusion of the capillaries and venules occurs. This, coupled with continued arterial blood flow, results in engorgement of the organ and vascular congestion. Bacterial invasion occurs secondarily in the congested tissue, followed by infiltration by polymorphonuclear cells with microabscess formations throughout the wall. If the process continues, the arterial circulation becomes compromised, infarction develops, and perforation may occur.

Spontaneous subsidence of the acute process is a possibility and probably occurs in some cases. When this does happen, the acute inflammatory reaction and the granular degeneration of the smooth muscle that may occur[48] are apt to be succeeded by fibrous tissue. Indeed, a history of prior episodes typical of appendicitis may occasionally be elicited from patients found to have extensive fibrosis of the appendix.

Frequency. Despite a seeming decrease in frequency of occurrence, acute appendicitis remains one of the most common causes of the acute surgical abdomen. The apparent decline in prevalence of the disorder may be related to improved nutrition, changing intestinal flora, decreased parasitic and dysenteric disease, commonly employed antimicrobial therapy, and the inclination to remove the appendix during the course of other abdominal surgery or concomitant with gynecologic operative procedures.[49, 50]

Clinical Manifestations. Acute appendicitis occurs equally in both sexes and at all ages, with a peak rate in the second and third decades.[51–57]

Symptoms. The acute disease is heralded primarily by pain (Chapter 3). This manifestation may be descriptively sequenced into the acute obstructive phase, the inflammatory phase, and the final period of complications.

During the initial obstructive phase, pain results from distention and/or exaggerated contraction of the appendix and has the characteristics of visceral pain. It lasts perhaps 4 to 6 hours; may be persistent or intermittent, resembling intestinal colic; is ordinarily not of great severity; and is poorly localized over the midabdominal and epigastric areas. With the development of inflammation, pain grows more intense. As the serosa becomes involved and parietal nerves are affected, the pain also focalizes at the location of the appendix, typically the right lower quadrant of the abdomen. If the appendix is situated retrocecally, the pain tends to concentrate in the right flank. Likewise, an appendix that lies in the pelvis may create suprapubic pain, a left-sided appendix gives rise to pain focalized in the left abdomen, a retroileal appendix induces testicular pain, and a subhepatic positioned appendix causes pain predominantly located in the right upper quadrant of the abdomen.

There is often an urge to defecate.[58] Nausea and vomiting commonly occur early. Constipation is frequent, but diarrhea may occur.

With progression of the process to the stage of impending or actual complication, pain is severe and is aggravated by movement of the body, particularly extension of the extremities. At this phase, chills may appear.

Physical Signs. During the early obstructive phase, physical findings in the abdomen are most often minimal. With the development of inflammation, however, distinct signs become evident. The patient may prefer to lie supine with the thighs, especially the right thigh, drawn up to the abdomen in flexion. Muscle guarding and tenderness to palpation at the appendiceal site are the classic findings. Right abdominal cutaneous hyperesthesia, corresponding to T10, T11, and T12, is an inconstant but significant finding. When the appendix is located in the pelvis, rectal examination may reveal tenderness in the cul-de-sac and excite suprapubic pain. When the appendix is retrocecal, maximum tenderness and muscle contraction are present posteriorly, extending toward, but rarely as high as, the costovertebral angle.

The temperature is usually elevated, but the degree of elevation is variable. Urinary symptoms in the form of frequency, with or without urgency, and alteration in bowel function correspond to the degree of extension of the inflammatory process to the genitourinary tract and upper sigmoid segment. When the inflammation advances to incite peritonitis or becomes complicated, as by abscess formation or perforation, rotation and extension of the right leg may accentuate the abdominal pain, both direct and indirect rebound tenderness are present, and fever becomes more pronounced.

Laboratory Findings. Leukocytosis (10,000 to 15,000 cells/mm^3)[52] accompanied by polymorphonuclear predominance (above 70%) is commonplace. A white blood cell count of approximately 18,000 cells/mm^3 with a marked shift of neutrophils to the left, accompanying appendiceal symptoms lasting 4 hours or longer, favors peritoneal extension of the inflammatory process. Leukocytosis greater than 29,000 cells/mm^3 is more likely to be the result of a suppurative process of other than appendiceal origin.[52]

Urinalysis is ordinarily negative in acute appendicitis. However, leukocytes and blood may appear in the urine when the appendiceal inflammatory process extends to the ureteral or vesical areas.

The presence of a parasite on stool study, especially if the eosinophil count is increased, would raise the possibility of a parasitic basis for the appendicitis. Stool examination is imperative in areas where parasitic infection is endemic, and specific therapy is an essential adjunct to appendectomy.

Roentgenologic Features. Roentgen studies usually include supine and upright films of the abdomen, but these are not diagnostic *per se*.[59,60] Multiple radiologic findings are diagnostically more helpful than a single finding. Distention of small bowel loops with fluid levels confined to the right lower quadrant ("appendiceal ileus") may be noted on a *plain film of the abdomen*. Also seen on plain abdominal films in some cases are radiopaque foreign bodies occupying the appendiceal area, appendiceal calculi, or a gas-filled appendix. When the entire appendiceal lumen is distended by gas and accompanied by a surrounding soft tissue mass, the roentgen diagnosis of acute appendicitis may be ventured with reservation, since an air-filled appendix is not a specific finding[61] and may be found as well in individuals with abdominal complaints of other than appendiceal origin.[62] Frank adynamic ileus may occur when there is impending or actual perforation. Pneumoperitoneum in association with an acute abdomen is rarely caused by appendiceal rupture. Interstitial emphysema dissecting the psoas muscle structure as high as the renal area may occasionally be seen on plain films in patients with advanced and usually complicated disease.

A *chest film* may disclose a right basal pneumonitis, some degree of atelectasis, or even fluid in the right pleural space, depending on the acuteness and severity of the inflammation and the presence or absence of a subdiaphragmatic infiltration or a subhepatically located appendix.

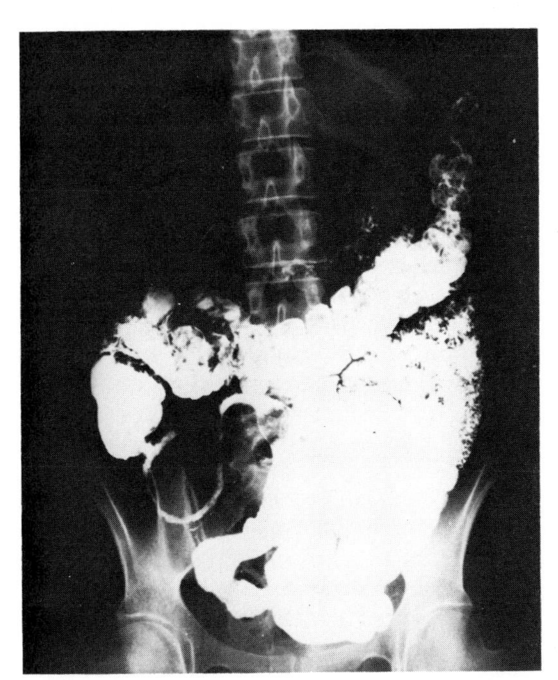

Figure 144–3. Appendiceal abscess with ileocecal displacement.

Most physicians are hesitant to have a *barium enema examination* performed. When this study is made, or a *barium meal study* of the gut is carried out, Shimkin[63] has described the changes that may be seen: (1) cecal flattening, destroying the convexity between the origin of the appendix and the ileocecal valve; (2) a smooth or irregular filling defect in the region of the appendix; (3) a bilobed cecal filling defect representing indentation between 2 cecal lobes caused by filling of the most proximal portion of an obstructed appendix; and (4) large cecal filling defects and terminal ileal displacement indicating abscess formation (Fig. 144–3). Displacement of other structures has also been reported. A retrocecal appendix characteristically affects the ascending colon; a pelvic abscess may impinge on the rectosigmoid; or the bladder and right ureter may be displaced. The acutely inflamed and obstructed appendix will not fill with barium. As the disease process progresses, the wall of the cecum becomes thick and edematous, producing an irregular or fluffy pattern.

Ultrasonography (Fig. 144–4) and *computed tomography* used selectively may be of help in the diagnosis of acute appendicitis, especially when complicated by abscess formation. Although *arteriography* has been employed to depict appendiceal abscess, the use of this examination in cases of acute appendicitis is rarely warranted.

Diagnosis and Differential Diagnosis. When the appendix occupies its usual anatomic position and responds to obstruction and inflammation in characteristic evolutionary fashion, a conclusive and prompt diagnosis is usually achieved. Diagnostic difficulties are created primarily by anatomic variations in appendiceal position; the presence of other intra-abdominal disorders, the effects of self-medication, especially analgesics and purgatives; and delay before consulting a physician. As will be discussed later, the pattern of pain and the clinical

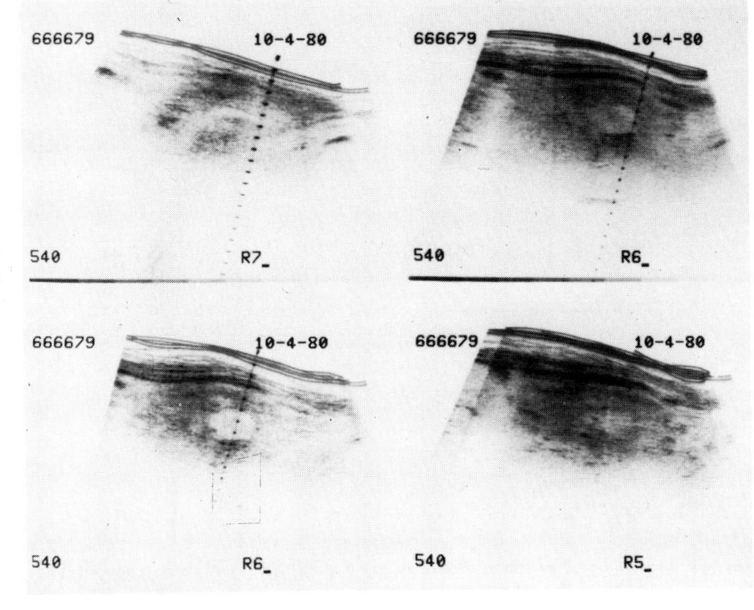

Figure 144–4. Ultrasonic demonstration and localization of appendiceal abscess.

picture are less orthodox in the very young[64,65] and the very old.[66] Because of diagnostic uncertainty and surgical delay, complications develop and contribute to higher mortality in infants, children of preschool age, and those beyond age 50.[67]

Pelvic adnexal disease often enters into differential consideration in women, especially when the appendix is situated in the pelvis. The problem of distinguishing pelvic inflammatory disease from acute appendicitis is heightened in the patient with vulvovaginal gonorrhea because of the occurrence in such patients of gonococcal appendicitis and periappendicitis.[68] *Laparoscopy* may be of value in these instances. This examination is favored by some[69] in all cases of acute abdomen to identify the underlying cause.

Complications. In most instances, complications are an expression of disease progression. The frequency of complications is proportionate to the duration of delay in performing a definitive operation,[70] but there is some evidence that early use of antimicrobial drugs may forestall the development of some of the more serious complications that may ensue.[71]

Extra-appendiceal Inflammation. Transmural inflammation and infection may extend along the subserosa and serosa to the periappendiceal area and adjacent peritoneum. Progressive severity of appendiceal symptoms, with more diffuse pain, accentuated systemic manifestations, and paralytic ileus, may be evidenced. At times, diarrhea may occur despite abdominal distention and ileus, making differential diagnosis from Crohn's disease quite difficult.

Perforation. Reports in the literature suggest an occurrence rate of appendiceal perforation as high as 32%[72] and a startling frequency in children (conservative estimates of 30% to 42%,[73] with extremes as high as 50% to 83% being reported[74]). Obstruction close to the tip of the appendix seems to predispose to early perforation and obstruction at the base of the appendix to delayed occurrence.[67]

Abscess. Abscess formation is most often periappendiceal in location but may develop elsewhere, especially in the pelvis or beneath the liver or diaphragm. Paralytic ileus with abdominal distention and signs of peritonitis are common features, and a tender mass may be palpable. Systemic manifestations become progressively worse. When there is subdiaphragmatic localization, right subcostal pain radiating to the subscapular and interscapular areas and shoulder tip may be described, often with accentuation of pain on respiration. The diaphragm may become elevated along with impaired aeration of the right lung base. On examination of the chest, there may be signs of pulmonary congestion and a pleural effusion. Abscesses may present as a bladder tumor or pelvic mass, cause hematuria or ureteral obstruction, or precipitate massive gastrointestinal bleeding. Abscess formation in the right thigh, perinephric area, and right groin has been encountered.[75]

Plain roentgenograms of the chest and abdomen may demonstrate pneumonitis or pleural effusion, hepatic displacement, and, at times, a partially air-filled abscess. Ultrasonography or computed tomography may aid further in delineating and focalizing the location of an abscess.

Fistulization. This is primarily the end result of unresolved appendiceal perforation with abscess formation.[76-79] The abscess extends to contiguous structures to create a communication with the bowel (small or large), bladder, vagina, or abdominal wall. The fistulous communication may actually result in evacuation of the abscess into the bladder or vagina or externally through the abdominal wall. Radiologic opacification of the fistulous tract is helpful in determining its extent and communication.[80] To be noted is the possibility that the abscess may persist despite drainage of the fistula and that multiple loculations may occur.

Pyelophlebitis (Chapter 169). This complication is the result of septic thrombosis of the appendiceal venous drainage.[81,82] Spread occurs by way of the ileocolic vasculature to the superior mesenteric circulation and ultimately to the portal vein. Hepatomegaly with tenderness, jaundice, and an altered liver profile suggests this development. Chills, marked hyperpyrexia, leukocytosis, and, at times, a shock-like state, frequently ensue.[83] Multiple hepatic abscesses may follow and are often revealed by hepatic scintigraphy, ultrasonography, or computed tomography.

Mucocele. This is the end result of continued appendiceal mucosal secretion of mucus in the face of appendiceal obstruction (see Fig. 144–2).[66,84] A tender mass may be felt, which may be depicted radiologically by a compression defect in the ileocecal area if barium is used. On scintigraphy and ultrasonography the contour may permit differentiation from an abscess. The precise diagnosis may require exploratory laparotomy. Not all mucoceles are benign, so that malignancy should be suspected in all instances.

Systemic Sepsis. Septicemia has been reported to occur in approximately 10% of patients with acute appendicitis and perforation in whom there is diffuse peritonitis and in 1% of such patients in whom peritonitis is localized. This complication is not seen in acute appendicitis without perforation.

Wound Infection. Wound infection is the most common complication and the most frequent contributor to morbidity following appendectomy for acute appendicitis. Its frequency rate varies from 1.8% to 9% in appendicitis without perforation, rising to 8% to 25% in patients with a perforated appendix, and approaching the extreme of 35% in the presence of appendiceal abscess.[51] The type of incision and suture material used, the use of drains,[85] the technical aspects of management of the appendiceal stump,[86] the choice of primary vs. delayed closure, and the prophylactic use of topical, systemic, and intraperitoneal antibiotics are all determining factors in the occurrence of postoperative wound infection.

Adhesions. Appendiceal serosal inflammation, operation, and tissue trauma are prone to create adhesions of structures adjacent to the appendix. After a clean appendectomy, the occurrence rate of small bowel obstruction due to adhesions is minimal (0.2%), but increases to 1.7% after contaminated appendectomies and to 4.6% if the appendix has perforated. Most adhesions are asymptomatic, but Simonowitz and White[87] have estimated that symptoms accredited to adhesions account for 4% of the morbidity following appendectomy. Numerous measures have been tried to prevent adhesions, but each has proved futile. From the surgical standpoint, it seems universally agreed that adhesion formation may be minimized by limited and gentle tissue handling, avoidance of surface drying, and use of omental coverage as needed.

Appendiceal Granuloma of the Cecum. This may develop as an aftermath of rupture of an appendiceal abscess into the cecum and may simulate a cecal neoplasm. A rarity, it is more frequent in the elderly and has been associated with intussusception. Decreased lymphoid tissue and vascular sclerosis are thought to contribute to its occurrence. Differentiation from a neoplasm or an ameboma is facilitated by colonoscopy as an adjunct to barium study.

Ileocecal Intussusception. Intussusception in the adult, caused by granuloma of the appendiceal stump and a variety of benign and malignant neoplasms, has been reported.[88] The intussusception may be asymptomatic.

Treatment

Medical Management. The treatment of acute appendicitis and its complications involves timed appendectomy, management of concomitant disease, and whatever additional procedures may be required to correct the complications that may have developed.

Delay in surgery may be necessitated because of the need to manage co-existent disease (e.g., diabetes mellitus), to restore fluid, chemical, and electrolyte balance, or for other reasons. During this period the patient should be prepared for eventual surgery as follows: immobilization in Fowler's position, avoidance of all oral intake, nasogastric suction if nausea and vomiting are present, parenteral fluids and electrolytes as required to correct deficiencies and ensure adequate renal output, and administration of broad spectrum antibiotics as well as appropriate analgesics. Antibiotics, in the absence of determinable bacterial sensitivity, would be in order of preference: penicillin in combination with streptomycin, cephalothin sodium, ampicillin, or cephaloridine. Massive dosage and continuous IV coverage are imperative in the presence of perforation.[89] Relief of pain, once the diagnosis is established, may be achieved through the use of meperidine hydrochloride (Demerol), 75 to 100 mg every 4 hours. Concomitant use of an agent such as hydroxyzine pamoate (Vistaril) may be helpful by relieving anxiety, nausea, and vomiting and reinforcing the action of the analgesics. In exceptional circumstances, as when the disease develops in a remote area or on shipboard where a surgeon or surgical facilities are not available, or when the patient refuses to consent to surgery, or when operation imposes an inordinate risk, the conservative measures just outlined may be used alone in the hope of controlling or resolving the acute process.

Surgical Management. The type of surgical management of acute appendicitis is determined by the phase of the disease process at the time of laparotomy. The type of incision is influenced by the surgeon's preference and experience and his evaluation of the desired exposure. Appendectomy in the early phases of acute, uncomplicated appendicitis, or when there is only localized peritonitis, most often is attended by negligible morbidity and mortality and a rapid, uncomplicated convalescence. The appendiceal stump, unligated or ligated, is commonly inverted and, depending on the philosophy of the surgeon, a drain is or is not inserted.

When the process has advanced to the point where an appendiceal abscess has formed that is localized by the omentum and neighboring bowel, surgical management requires individualization. Surgical intervention may disrupt protective natural barriers, resulting in generalized peritonitis. Conservatism may lead to a satisfactory resolution but, on the other hand, may permit progression to even more severe complications. The decision generally is for operative intervention in the high-risk instances of children, elderly patients, pregnant women, and those in whom the diagnosis of abscess is questionable. In all patients, adequate antibiotic coverage is imperative in the pre-, inter-, and postoperative periods. When indecision or circumstances demand a period of observation, antibiotic coverage and bowel immobilization are imperative and the patient must be closely observed. Should there be accentuation of pain and worsening of systemic manifestations beyond 24 hours, appendectomy with drainage, or perhaps drainage alone, must be done. If, however, the clinical manifestations appear to be subsiding, further delay may be justified before appendectomy is ultimately carried out.

Whether percutaneous catheter drainage of an appendiceal abscess under guidance by computed tomography and/or ultrasonography should be attempted is unsettled. Welsh[90] expressed the view that surgical responsibility probably precludes such an endeavor.

When the disease is even further advanced with generalized peritonitis, paralytic ileus, and severe systemic manifestations, a complexity of complications is usually present. In such instances, adequate parenteral administration of antibiotics, replacement of electrolytes and fluids, nasogastric tube decompression, and complete bowel immobilization are all important measures. Drainage, with or without appendectomy, awaits the restoration of the patient to an adequate operative status. Decision on procedure depends upon the operative findings. A perforated, gangrenous appendix, open to the peritoneal cavity, demands removal supplemented by drainage. Abscesses (subphrenic, pelvic, or elsewhere) add to the complexity of management.

Interval appendectomy should be done when the acute phase of the disease has subsided with conservative measures or when simple drainage has been judiciously elected in the presence of appendiceal abscess. Appendectomy is imperative in these situations because recurrence has been experienced as early as 60 days in 10% to 20% of individuals and in up to 50% in 5 years.

If a portion of the appendix is left at the time of primary surgery, recurrent disease may eventuate, with attendant problems in diagnosis and therapy. Recurrent appendicitis, rupture of the appendiceal stump, and appendiceal abscesses have all been reported.[91–95] Despite Rose's[94] statement, "When removing a friable appendix, care must be taken that no remnants are left behind," such occurrences persist, as is exemplified in the finding at endoscopy of an ulcerated appendiceal stump.[95] Because there is a history of appendectomy, the possibility of recurrent appendicitis may not be considered. Furthermore, a defect in the cecum caused by the presence of a viable, sizable appendiceal stump within the cecum may closely simulate a polyp or growth, and an inverted appendiceal stump, visualized on colonoscopy, may be inadvertently excised during this examination.[96]

Prognosis. Simple appendectomy in uncomplicated acute appendicitis still carries a mortality approaching 0.2%.[42] Pearson's survey[97] in the New Haven metropolitan area revealed only 2 deaths in 1000 appendectomies for acute appendicitis. Regardless of the phase of disease, the overall mortality of primary appendectomy is appreciably under 1%,[98] although it was 1.4% in the series of Mittlepunkt and Nora.[99] The average hospital stay following an uncomplicated appendectomy for acute appendicitis approximates 6.4 days, but the complications of gangrene and perforation extend the average stay to 14.5 days.

Anesthesia, age, infirmity, and associated disease influence the outcome with respect to both morbidity and mortality. In one study, 85% of the deaths were in the patient population beyond 50 years of age. A mortality rate of 15% that has been noted in patients beyond 70 years of age is disturbing, considering that the prevalence of appendicitis is on the rise in the aged.[100]

Improved surgical techniques, antimicrobials, gastroenteric immobilization with adequate nasogastric intubation and decompression, pre- and postoperative fluid and electrolyte replacement to normal levels, and the application of supportive aids in recovery and intensive care units have contributed appreciably to the reduction in morbidity and mortality from the complications inherent in delayed diagnosis, i.e., perforation, abscess, fistula, and pyelophlebitis.

Special Situations

Neonatal Appendicitis. Acute appendicitis in the neonate is extremely rare and unexpected because the appendix is characteristically funnel-shaped for the first 9 to 12 months of life. Hence, luminal obstruction by fecaliths, edema, or lymphoid hyperplasia is unlikely. Manifestations are non-specific, consisting of anorexia, vomiting, and diarrhea with related dehydration.

Fever is often absent and the leukocytic response may not be significant. As a consequence, diagnosis is often delayed and the reported mortality rates range between 70% and 83%. Perforation increases the mortality rate to 85%.[101] Expertise in the fluid and electrolyte management of the neonate, careful neonatal anesthesia technique, early investigation of abdominal distention, and meticulous surgery may reduce mortality.

Acute Appendicitis in Children. Acute appendicitis is relatively uncommon in infants and children under the age of 4 years. In infants and young children, the disease is a most serious process, is more difficult to diagnose, and is accompanied by a high frequency of perforation[73] and increased morbidity and mortality.[64,102] The inability of an undeveloped omentum to assume its protective role contributes to the high rate of perforation. In infants, fever, refusal to eat, and vomiting occur during the early disease state. With retention of the cecum in a high position, there is poor localization of tenderness. When well localized tenderness and actual muscle guarding are demonstrable, the disease state is advanced and complicated by peritoneal involvement. In preschool-aged children, the frequency of abdominal complaints encourages decreased parental awareness and the frequent tendency for the parents to give the child a cathartic. This not only occasions delay, but additionally predisposes the acutely inflamed appendix to perforation.[65,103]

There is no definitive correlation between leukocytosis and the disease state. Normal urinary findings tend to exclude pyelitis, and a chest film aids in eliminating pleuropulmonary disease.

Because of the diagnostic complexity and the ominous prognosis, it is considered advisable to hospitalize all "suspect" patients for closer observation over a 24-hour period. This will hopefully preclude unnecessary surgery and at the same time avoid the morbidity and mortality of complications resulting from unduly delayed surgery. Statistics on perforation, varying from 15% to 85%, and a mortality rate of 40% to 60% stress the difficulty of evaluating and managing this disease state in this age group.[104,105]

Controversial management areas in children continue to be antibiotic usage, primary closure, and drainage.[106] Antibiotics effective against both aerobic and anaerobic organisms are indicated in patients with proven or suspected perforation. Delayed wound closure is favored in appendicitis with perforation because of the lower incidence of wound infection. The routine use of drains in children with perforation is plagued by wound infection and by intra-abdominal abscess. Graham and his associates[107] stress preoperative correction of dehydration, systemic use of broad-spectrum antibiotics when perforation is suspected, antibiotic peritoneal irrigation when there is frank perforation, and carefully managed delayed wound closure. These measures helped them avoid any deaths in 155 patients.

Acute Appendicitis in the Aging. Acute appendicitis is less frequent in individuals beyond 60 years of age. The earlier frequency estimate of less than 2% has more recently been altered to 4.2% and as high as 6.8%, possibly reflecting the increase in older persons in the general population. Diagnosis in the elderly is a challenge because of atypical manifestations, increased occurrence of complications (35%), greater morbidity, and accentuated mortality (8%), all attributed to therapeutic delay.

Anticipated concomitant disease in late life (cardiovascular disease, pulmonary insufficiency, diabetes), coupled with renal insufficiency and proneness to pneumonia, contributes to lowered physiologic reserve. Clinically, the illness tends to be insidious and deceptive. Mild symptoms, readily interpreted as previously experienced digestive distress and bowel dysfunction, render the initial complaints less significant. Neoplastic and diverticular disease often will be uppermost in the mind of the physician.

Self-medication is frequent, especially in the form of cathartics with their unfavorable sequelae. Positive findings on abdominal examination, with the exception of tenderness, are frequently absent until late in the course of the disease. Fever and leukocytosis are also less commonly encountered.[108,109] Additionally, diminished lymphoid tissue, fibrous appendiceal alteration, and impaired visceral vascularity potentiate development of complications.

Appendiceal perforation is frequently encountered at exploration (67% to 90%).[110] Postoperative complications, inherent in surgery in the elderly, further alter the prognosis; ileus, wound infection, dehiscence with subsequent herniation, and urinary difficulty (in men) are prone to prolong hospitalization and morbidity. Owens and Hamit[111] accept this as a challenge, contending that while the elderly tend to have less fever, less reliable symptoms, and possibly a diminished leukocyte response, acute appendicitis should nevertheless be diagnosed with sufficient dispatch to minimize morbidity and mortality.

Presenting findings are essentially the same as those encountered in more youthful patients: localized pain (92% to 100%), right lower quadrant tenderness (88% to 99%), fever (74%), and leukocytosis (78% to 94%). Progressive, uncontrolled infection and a high frequency rate of concurrent disease, rather than delay in operative intervention, were found by Owens and Hamit[111] to be the principal factors affecting outcome. In their group, 73% of the patients were operated upon within 6 hours of admission. While the occurrence of non-lethal complications does not appreciably increase in patients beyond 65 years of age, perforation is encountered more frequently (as high as 87.5%), contributing to a mortality figure approximating 23%.

Appendicitis During Pregnancy. Although acute appendicitis during pregnancy is infrequent (estimated to be 1 in 1500 deliveries),[112] it is the most common non-gynecologic parturition emergency encountered.[113] The disease is no different in pregnant women than it is in non-pregnant women, but diagnostic difficulty and delay and the severity of complications add to its significance.[114] Appendicitis is more prone to occur in the first 6 months (74%).[115] During this period, symptoms such as anorexia, nausea, vomiting, and abdominal pain may be attributed to the pregnancy. Physical findings of localized tenderness, rebound tenderness, and muscle guarding are not altered by cephalad displacement of the cecum by the enlarging uterus; cecal displacement, progressively cephalad after the initial 6 months, tends to localize pain and tenderness to the right upper quadrant and flank when inflammation extends to the parietal peritoneum.[116] Stretched abdominal musculature alters the reflex responses, and there is inability to examine the abdomen satisfactorily. All of these contribute to the diagnostic dilemma[117] and to delay in surgery. Additionally, uterine displacement of structures essential to the walling-off process within the abdomen predisposes to spread of the inflammatory process, thereby increasing morbidity, mortality, and the potential for fetal loss.

Leukocytosis as high as 15,000 cells/mm^3 is often a normal accompaniment of pregnancy. This lessens its value as a diagnostic aid.[114]

Laparoscopy has been added to the diagnostic armamentarium in the patient with acute abdominal pain of unknown cause. Its use may resolve the question of acute appendicitis and avoid unnecessary laparotomy.[118]

Early diagnosis obviously is important because of the frequency of abortion and fetal mortality with appendiceal complications. Progesterone administration to prevent premature labor has been proposed with reservation.[114] Appendectomy in the absence of peritonitis should not enhance the occurrence rates of abortion, morbidity, or mortality.[115] A progressive decline in maternal mortality to a projected 0.01% is credited to early diagnosis,[112] improved anesthesia, and enhanced surgical care and pre- and postoperative support, including the use of antibiotics.[114] Antibiotic coverage, however, should not be considered routine, other than in the pre- and postoperative care of an individual with appendiceal gangrene or perforation.[115] Fetal loss has been reduced to an approximate figure of 8.5% in the absence of peritonitis; however, abortion has been estimated to occur in as high as 35.7% of individuals with peritonitis.[119]

Stress and Appendicitis. Acute appendicitis has been reported to occur within hours of emotional stress.[120] Theoretically, stress and altered psychologic factors, because of their effect on the immune system, may create a situation conducive to infection and hypertrophy of lymphoid tissues; luminal obstruction of the appendix and secondary bacterial invasion may result in appendicitis. On the other hand, it should be borne in mind that emotional and psychologic disturbances are commonplace in patients with abdominal pain, perhaps especially in children. Thus, psychologic elements have been recorded in some two-thirds of a group of young people who were operated on for appendicitis but found to have a normal appendix at surgery.[121] Also, a carefully conducted study of psychologic variables in relation to appendectomy led Creed[122] to conclude: "In some cases removal of a mildly inflamed appendix will not cure the abdominal pain."

Recurrent and Chronic Appendicitis

The pathophysiology of recurrent and/or chronic appendicitis is not well understood, and the very existence of such an entity continues to be a matter of debate and controversy.[123] The term "chronic appendicitis" is unsavory today. Yet, recurrent attacks of appendicitis do appear to occur,[124] and pathologic evidence considered supportive of such a process has been advanced by Befeler[125] and Ferrier.[126]

Clinical experience would suggest that mild attacks of acute appendiceal inflammatory disease that resolves spontaneously do occur. The likelihood that they do is fortified by the frequency with which a history of previous episodes of abdominal pain that seem compatible with appendiceal inflammation is obtained from a patient with bona fide acute appendicitis.[127] On the other hand, when appendectomy is carried out some weeks after subsidence of a typical acute inflammatory episode, chronic inflammatory cells, chiefly lymphocytes and large numbers of eosinophils, are found to have replaced the polymorphonuclear cells in the submucosal and serosal coats. The lymphocytes in the subserosa are primarily perivascular in distribution. Foreign body giant cells may also be seen in the wall of the appendix. These alterations may be readily interpreted as evidence of chronic inflammation, but perhaps the designation "healing appendicitis" would be more applicable.

Appendiceal fibrosis is characterized by thickening and firmness of the appendix. The cut surface shows a rigid, circular, patulous lumen. There may be luminal stenosis proximally with distal dilatation. Microscopically, there is general fibrotic thickening along with a variety of non-specific alterations, i.e., increased submucosal fat, evidence of former mucosal hemorrhage represented by brown pigmentation, and serosal accumulation of lymphocytes with dilated lymphatics. These changes, however, are not proof-positive of previous inflammation because the same findings may be encountered in appendices removed incidental to other operative procedures in individuals who never had a suspicious episode of appendicitis. Probably the term "fibrosis of the appendix" should be used without reference to chronic appendicitis or inference that the fibrosis represents chronic appendicitis.

Obliteration of the appendiceal lumen with all coats fused into a fibrous mass is seen usually in older persons, although it may occur in a younger age group. While fibrosis, luminal constriction, and prominence of neural elements suggest the possibility of chronic inflammation, they more likely represent a normal process of involution. This is supported by a 65% occurrence of "fibrotic appendix" in necropsy studies by Collins,[128] and the presence of neuromas in 86% of obliterative fibrotic appendices studied by Masson.[129]

Thus, the matter remains unsettled with the likelihood that the entity probably exists. However, a diagnosis of chronic appendicitis as the basis for primary appendectomy is defensible only if the clinical and histologic features appear to be incontrovertible.

Incidental Appendectomy

Removal of the appendix during intra-abdominal or gynecologic surgery for other conditions is common.[49,50] This practice is readily rationalized when the appendix appears to be diseased, as in carcinoid involvement. It also seems reasonable at exploratory laparotomy for Crohn's disease, when the appendix and cecum are not involved in the inflammatory process, because of the recurrence rate and chronicity of the primary process and its tendency to simulate appendicitis.

Incidental appendectomy should not be done in the face of other inflammatory intraperitoneal disease, and its performance concomitantly with cesarean section is definitely questionable. Whether incidental removal of the appendix is justified in other situations rests on an assumed favorable benefit-risk ratio, but this assumption requires proof. The question of increased cancer risk as a consequence of incidental appendectomy appears to have been resolved by the studies of Berndt.[17]

Neoplasms of the Appendix

Tumors of the appendix of all categories are rarities and are for the most part devoid of manifestations. They may cause appendiceal intussusception[130] and by causing luminal obstruction are a potential source of acute appendicitis and mucocele formation.[131]

Benign Tumors. Among the benign tumors that may be found in the appendix in order of frequency are leiomyomas, fibromas, neuromas, lipomas, neurofibromas, and ganglioneuromas. *Carcinoids* occur more frequently in the appendix than elsewhere. When they are confined to the appendix and appear histologically benign, their inclusion among the benign neoplasms of the appendix is justified. Carcinoids usually are very small and are situated most often in the distal third of the appendix. Hence, they rarely initiate appendicitis. An instance of Cushing's syndrome presumably cured by removal of a benign appendiceal carcinoid has been reported.[132] Adenocarcinoid, a mucin-producing lesion, has also been described.[133]

Epithelial neoplasms (cystadenomas, papillary adenomas, and adenomatous polyps) are other rare growths that may develop in the appendix.[134,134a] When such lesions are encountered, the colon should be thoroughly explored for additional neoplasms because of the frequent concurrence of such growths.

Endometriosis involving the appendix and benign epidermoid cysts and mucoceles may be interpreted as tumors, but this classification is probably not correct.[135,136]

Malignant Tumors. Included among the malignant neoplasms affecting the appendix are adenocarcinoma (crypt cell carcinoma),[137] reticuloendothelial sarcoma, follicular lymphoblastoma, lymphosarcoma, malignant mucosal polyps, fibrosarcoma, malignant carcinoids, malignant mucocele, and invasive carcinoma arising from a villous adenoma.[138]

Burkitt's lymphoma of the appendix, a true rarity, has been thought to have an infectious etiology. Cases of this type of lymphoma have been reported mainly from equatorial Africa but also from elsewhere in the world. Extensive removal of the bulk tumor and initiation of chemotherapy have been shown to improve survival significantly.[139]

Carcinoids that are clinically and histologically malignant present the problem of whether simple appendectomy is an adequately effective measure or whether there is justification for right hemicolectomy and excision of the node-bearing mesentery. More detailed consideration of carcinoid tumors is found in Chapter 113.

Adenocarcinoma, classified as colonic in type because of its behavior and gross microscopic appearance, is found more frequently in the form of mucous papillary cystadenocarcinoma.[140] When carcinoma of the appendix is encountered, a search for a second colonic lesion is requisite.

Malignant mucoceles, by virtue of mucosal and neoplastic secretion and cellular proliferation, distend the appendiceal lumen. Since appendiceal lymphatic drainage is rather diffuse, right hemicolectomy is frequently required. Malignant mucoceles are prone to perforate (25%), with peritoneal seeding and the production of pseudomyxoma peritonei. Careful surgical handling is therefore essential. Postoperative radiation and chemotherapy are frequently utilized. Prognosis depends upon the extent of the disease process and its responsiveness to therapy.

A preoperative diagnosis of a tumor of the appendix, possibly malignant, may be suspected if, on barium enema examination, an extracecal mass deforms the cecal contour (Fig. 144–5). However, diagnosis is uncommon before operation, and 18% of the cancers have already metastasized at the time of surgery. A right hemicolectomy is the procedure of choice, with a 5-year survival rate of 61% when this is done compared with a survival rate of 21/% after simple appendectomy.[141] The prognosis of adenocarcinoma of the appendix is about the same as that for cecal carcinoma (Chapter 139). Supplementing surgery with nitrogen mustard or mechlorethamine hydrochloride irrigation has been suggested; 5-fluorouracil systemically is also advocated.

Pseudomyxoma peritonei occurs when cystic neoplasms containing mucus-producing cells rupture, whether the neoplastic lesion is benign or malignant. The result is seeding of

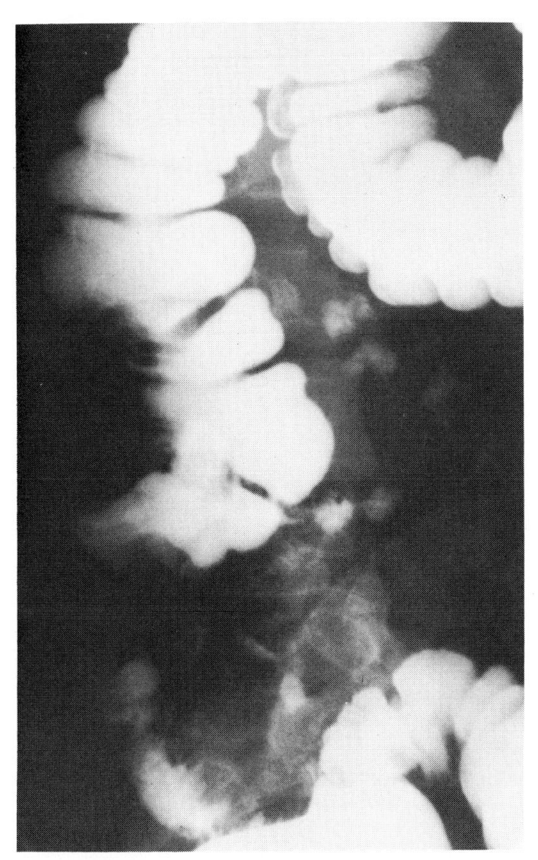

Figure 144–5. A 37-year-old physician was seen because of pain in the right abdomen for 10 days. There was no fever and no symptoms of gastrointestinal or urinary disturbance. Physical examination disclosed a tender mass in the right flank and rectal induration suggesting a Blumer's shelf. Barium enema examination showed an extrinsic impingement of the lateral wall of the cecum and ascending colon. Intravenous pyelogram showed caliceal dilatation on the right. Operation revealed an adenocarcinoma of the vermiform appendix with confined perforation and extensive inflammatory reaction. A right hemicolectomy was performed. (Courtesy of Dr. Parviz Foroozan. The Scripps Clinic and Research Foundation, La Jolla, California.)

the peritoneal surfaces with cells that continue to secrete mucus into the peritoneal cavity. The degree of effectiveness of removal of the appendix and tumor together with chemotherapy is variable.

Miscellaneous Appendiceal Entities

Appendiceal torsion, presenting as appendicitis, is the subject of isolated case reports.[142] *Crohn's disease of the appendix* as a primary entity is gaining increased reference in the literature.[143] Appendectomy as a possible curative procedure is questionable; involvement elsewhere is difficult to rule out. *Whipple's disease* involving the appendix has also been reported.[144] *Acute tuberculous appendicitis* is a true rarity and is likely a component of enterocolonic tuberculosis (Chapter 120). Conservative resection and antituberculous therapy over 9 to 12 months is advocated.[145] Fistulization after simple appendectomy is a feared complication. *Barium appendicitis* probably has the same significance as appendicolithiasis, occurring many months after barium study of the gastrointestinal tract. Sakover and Del Fava[146] have reported on 7 cases, 5 with gangrene and perforation.

Another peculiar tumor that has been found in the appendix is *myxoglobulosis*.[147] This is a cystic condition in which the cysts characteristically contain globoid bodies of mucinous character.

Appendiceal perforation resulting from ingested foreign bodies is a rarity. *Externally produced perforation of the appendix by injury* is also extremely unusual because the appendix is protected by its small size and position in the abdomen. The appendix also tends to escape injury in cases of *penetrating wounds* of the abdomen unless the abdominal wounds are multiple.[148]

Diverticula of the appendix (see Fig. 144–1) are classified as congenital (true or acquired) faults, as are diverticula elsewhere in the alimentary tract. Minute in size and often distally located, they are usually single. It has been speculated that they may occur as a component of luminal obstruction by neoplasm and that, as with appendicitis, they are a consequence of low-fiber intake.[149] Appendiceal diverticula are conceded to have little, if any, clinical manifestations and in general are simply an incidental finding without clinical significance. Conceivably, they can contribute to obstruction when accompanied by hypertrophy of the muscle wall or by fibrosis, but no such occurrence has been authenticated. Also, appendiceal diverticulitis has been described, with clinical manifestations resembling diverticulitis of the colon but with milder pain that is intermittent for days.

Periappendicitis has been defined as a clinical entity in which a fibropurulent involvement is confined to the appendiceal serosa without histologic evidence of transmural disease. In the absence of a generalized inflammatory peritoneal reaction, this lesion, on surgical inspection, is thought probably to represent a healing stage of acute appendicitis rather than an appendiceal serosal entity. In a study by O'Neil and Moore,[150] the finding proved to be more common in women with a history of possible appendiceal symptoms of fairly long duration. Postoperative follow-up indicated that it could be satisfactorily managed by appendectomy.

References

1. Gorgollon P. The normal human appendix: a light and electron microscopic study. J Anat 1978; 126:87–101.
2. Shand JEG, Bremner DN. Agenesis of the vermiform appendix in a thalidomide child. Br J Surg 1977; 64:203–4.
3. Holgersen LO, Kulkner CR, Stanley-Browne EG. Acute appendicitis in a child with complete situs inversus. J Pediatr Surg 1970; 5:379–80.
4. Owen-Smith MD. Acute left-sided appendicitis. Br J Surg 1969; 56:233–4.
5. Bonk U. Double appendix. Pathol Res Pract 1980; 167:400–1.
6. Payan HM. Diverticular disease of the appendix. Dis Colon Rectum 1977; 20:473–6.
7. Foster JH, Morgan CV, Therlkell JB, Yune HY. Vascular malformation of the appendiceal stump. JAMA 1971; 215:636–8.
8. Dawson M. The role of the human appendix in immunity to infections. J Pharm Pharmacol 1978; 30(Suppl):90P.
9. Toma VA, Reteif FP. Human vermiform appendix. Immunocompetent topography and cell-to-cell interactions in situ. J Immunol Methods 1978; 20:333–47.
10. Draper LR, Sussdorf DH. Roles of the liver and appendix in the serum hemolysin response in rabbits. J Immunol 1965; 95:306–13.
11. Hanoaka M, Nomato K, Waksman BH. Appendix and gamma M antibody formation. I. Immune response to tolerance to bovine gamma globulin in irradiated appendix-shielded rabbits. J Immunol 1970; 104:616–25.
12. Konda S, Harris TN. Effect of appendectomy and of the thymectomy, with x-irradiation, on the production of antibodies to two protein antigens in young rabbits. J Immunol 1966; 97:805–14.
13. Ozer H, Waksman BH. Appendix and gamma-M antibody formation: IV. Synergism of appendix and bone marrow cells in early antibody response to sheep erythrocytes. J Immunol 1970; 105:791–2.
14. Fichtelius KE. The gut epithelium—a first level lymphoid organ. Exp Cell Res 1968; 46:231–4.
15. Calkins CE, Ozer H, Waksman BH. B cells in the appendix and other lymphoid organs of the rabbit: stimulation of DNA synthesis by antiimmunoglobulin. Cell Immunol 1975; 18:187–98.
16. Craig SW, Cebra JJ. Rabbit Peyer's patches. Appendix and popliteal lymph node B lymphocytes: A comparative analysis of their membrane immunoglobulin components and plasma cell precursor potential. J Immunol 1975; 144:492–502.
17. Berndt H. Is appendectomy followed by increased cancer risk? Digestion 1970; 3:187–91.
18. Bierman HR. Human appendix and neoplasia. Cancer 1968; 21:109–18.
19. Ruuskanen O, Vanha-Perttula T, Kouvalainen K. Tonsillectomy, appendicectomy and Hodgkin's disease. Lancet 1971; 1:1127–8.
20. Fitz RN. Perforating inflammation of the vermiform appendix, with special reference to its early diagnosis and treatment. Am J Med 1886; 92:321–46.
21. McBurney C. Experience with early operative interference in cases of disease of the vermiform appendix. NY State J Med 1889; 50:676–84.
22. Murphy JB. Two thousand operations for appendicitis, with deductions from his personal experiences. Am J Med Sci 1904; 128:187–94.
23. Kazarain KK, Roeder WJ, Mersheimer WL. Decreasing mortality and increasing morbidity from acute appendicitis. Am J Surg 1970; 119:681–5.
24. Jess P, Bjerregaard MD, Brynitz S, Holst-Christensen J, Kalaja E, Lund-Kristensen J. Acute appendicitis: Prospective trial concerning diagnostic accuracy and complications. Am J Surg 1981; 141:232–4.
25. Murray HW. Is the appendix boring? Arch Intern Med 1981; 141:571–2.
26. Faegenburg D. Fecaliths of the appendix: incidence and significance. AJR 1963; 89:752–9.
27. Bohrod MG. The pathogenesis of acute appendicitis. Am J Clin Pathol 1946; 16:752–70.
28. Burkitt DP, Moolgaokar AS, Tovey FI. Aetiology of appendicitis (letter). Br Med J 1979; 1:620.
29. Latchis KS, Canter JW. Acute appendicitis secondary to metastatic carcinoma. Am J Surg 1966; 111:220–3.
30. Carey LS. Lead shot appendicitis in northern native people. J Can Assoc Radiol 1977; 28:171–4.
31. Maganini RJ. Two foreign bodies of the appendix. A case report. Ill Med J 1966; 129:137–8.
32. Rydell WB Jr. Bullet appendicitis. A new form of lead poisoning. Rocky Mt Med J 1970; 67:48–50.
33. Smedresman P. *Ascaris lumbricoides* as an unusual cause of appendicitis in an 8-year-old girl. Clin Pediatr 1977; 16:197.
34. Hall JH. Crohn's disease of the appendix presenting as acute appendicitis. Br J Surg 1969; 56:390–2.
35. Jenkins JD, Rack JH. Caecal diaphragms causing mucocele of the appendix and acute appendicitis. Br J Surg 1967; 54:155–6.
36. Palmieri JR, Lestadi J, Purnomo, Lim HS, Tedjasukmana T. *Schistosoma japonicum*-like eggs in the appendix of an inhabitant of Java, Indonesia. Am J Trop Med Hyg 1981; 30:92–5.
37. Noodleman JS. Eosinophilic appendicitis. Demonstration of *Strongyloides stercoralis* as a causative agent. Arch Pathol Lab Med 1981; 105:148–9.
38. Haines DO. A cryptic infection of an appendix with the whipworm *Trichuris trichiura* in Britain. J Helminthol 1968; 42:289–94.
39. White AS, MacBain GC. Acute appendicitis and measles. J R Coll Edinb 1977; 22:428–9.
40. Forbes GB, Lloyd-Davies RW. Calculous disease of the vermiform appendix. Gut 1966; 7:583–92.
41. Reif RM. Viral appendicitis. Human Pathol 1981; 12:193–6.
42. Piltokallio P, Tykke H. Evolution of the age distribution and mortality of acute appendicitis. Arch Surg 1981; 116:153–6.
43. Holt P. Legionnaire's disease and abscess of appendix. Br Med J 1981; 2:1035–6.
44. Vukmer GJ, Trummer MJ. Barium appendicitis. Report of a case. Arch Surg 1965; 91:630–2.
45. Balch CM, Silver D. Foreign bodies in the appendix. Report of eight cases and review of the literature. Arch Surg 1971; 102:14–20.
46. Westlake CA, St. Leger AS, Burr ML. Appendicectomy and dietary fibre. J Hum Nutr 1980; 34:267–72.
47. Anderssen N, Cockroft A, Murphy JF. Acute appendicitis and social class. Br J Clin Pract 1981; 35:272–3.
48. Sobel HJ, Marquet E, Schwarz R: Granular degeneration of appendiceal smooth muscle. Arch Pathol 1971; 92:427–32.
49. Miranda R, Johnson AD, O'Leary JP. Incidental appendectomy: Frequency of pathologic abnormalities. Am Surg 1980; 46:355–7.
50. Cromartic AD, Kavalacek PJ. Incidental appendectomy at the time of surgery for ectopic pregnancy. Am J Surg 1980; 139:244–6.
51. Lewis FR, Holcroft JW, Boey J, Dunphy JE. Appendicitis: A critical review of diagnosis and treatment in 1,000 cases. Arch Surg 1975; 110:677–82.
52. Appendicitis in recent years. Statist Bull Metrop Life Insur Co 1969; 50:4–5.
53. Dieter RA Jr. Appendicitis in the male veteran: A 5-year review. Milit Med 1968; 133:804–10.
54. Howorth MB Jr. Acute appendicitis in a small community hospital. South Med J 1969; 62:548–50.
55. Leffall LD Jr. Appendicitis. A continuing surgical challenge. Am J Surg 1967; 113:654–9.

56. Wiles CE. Current attitude toward appendicitis. NY J Med 1967; 67:787–9.
57. Willoughby DV, Davis MJ. A five-year review of appendectomy at Canadian Forces Hospital, Halifax. Med Serv J Can 1967; 23:27–31.
58. Keyes EL. Symposium on clinical surgery: New method for early diagnosis of acute appendicitis in absence of localization. Surg Clin North Am 1950; 30:1447–56.
59. Thorpe JA. The plain abdominal radiograph in acute appendicitis. Ann R Coll Surg Engl 1979; 61:45.
60. Leonidas JC, Harris DJ, Amoury RA. How accurate is the roentgen diagnosis of acute appendicitis in children? Ann Radiol (Paris) 1975; 18:479–87.
61. Shaffer HA, Harrison RB. Gas in the appendix: A sometimes significant but not diagnostic sign. Arch Surg 1979; 114:586–9.
62. Lim MS. Gas-filled appendix: Lack of diagnostic specificity. AJR 1977; 128:209–10.
63. Shimkin PM. Radiology of acute appendicitis. Am J Radiol 1978; 130:1001–4.
64. Holder TM, Leape LL. The acute surgical abdomen in children. N Engl J Med 1967; 277:921–3.
65. Jackson RH. Parents, family doctors and acute appendicitis in childhood. Br Med J 1963; 1:277–81.
66. Kuehn PG, Speer CS. Mucocele of the appendix associated with profound anemia. Report of a case. Dis Colon Rectum 1966; 9:283–5.
67. Deck KB, Pettit BJ, Harrison MR. The length-time correlate in appendicitis. JAMA 1980; 244:806–7.
68. Allman GL, Waldenburg LM. Gonococcal periappendicitis in a prepubertal girl. Pediatrics 1977; 58:287–8.
69. Llanio R. Laparoscopia en Urgencias. Havana: Editorial. Cientifico-Technica, 1977.
70. Campbell WB. Prophylaxis of infection after appendectomy. Survey of current surgical practice. Br Med J 1980; 2:1597–1600.
71. Burke JF. The effective period of preventive antibiotic action in experimental incisions and dermal lesions. Surgery 1981; 50:161–8.
72. Scher KS, Coil JA. Appendicitis: Factors that influence the frequency of perforation. South Med J 1980; 73:1561–3.
73. Savrin RA, Chatworthy HW. Appendiceal rupture. Pediatrics 1979; 63:37–43.
74. Stone HH, Sanders SL, Martin JD Jr. Perforated appendicitis in children. Surgery 1971; 69:673–9.
75. Cauble WG. Unusual complications. Report of a case of appendicitis. J Kansas Med Soc 1978; 79:247–8.
76. Arlen M. Appendicojejunal fistula secondary to appendiceal calculus. Arch Surg 1970; 101:94.
77. Cook GT. Appendiceal abscess causing urinary obstruction. J Urol 1969; 101:212–5.
78. Pairolero PC, Judd ES, Hodgson JR. Appendicoenterosigmoid fistula. Surgery 1969; 66:695–7.
79. Walker LG Jr, Rhame DW, Smith RB III. Enteric and cutaneous appendiceal fistulae. Arch Surg 1969; 99:585–8.
80. Way S. The use of the "sac" technique in pelvic exenteration. Gynecol Oncol 1974; 2:476–81.
81. Rex JC, Harrison EG Jr, Priestley JT. Appendicitis and ligneous perisyphilitis. Arch Surg 1961; 82:735–45.
82. Witte CL. Mesenteric venous thrombosis from nonperforated acute appendicitis. Report of a case resembling acute hemorrhagic pancreatitis with more diffuse pain. Am J Surg 1969; 117:739–41.
83. Grayer SP. Nonperforated appendicitis presenting as shock and liver abscess. Am J Surg 1969; 35:461–2.
84. Watne AL, Trevino E. Diagnostic features of mucocele of the appendix. Arch Surg 1962; 84:516–24.
85. Everson NW, Fossard DP, Nash JR, MacDonald RC. Wound infection following appendectomy: The effect of extraperitoneal wound drainage and systemic antibiotic prophylaxis. Br J Surg 1977; 64:236–8.
86. Sculco TP, Priebe CJ. Management of the appendiceal stump in children. Surg Gynecol Obstet 1973; 136:182–4.
87. Simonowitz DA, White TT. The colon. Part III: Postoperative complications of appendectomy (including adhesions). Clin Gastroenterol 1979; 8:429–41.
88. Hanson EL, Goodkin L, Pfeffer RB. Ileocolic intussusception in an adult caused by a granuloma of the appendiceal stump: Report of a case. Ann Surg 1967; 166:150–2.
89. Raffensperger JG, Metzger W. Antibiotic therapy for perforated appendicitis in children. Chicago Med Sch Q 1969; 28:179–83.
90. Welsh CE. Catheter drainage of abdominal abscesses. N Engl J Med 1981; 305:694–5.
91. Baumgardner LO. Rupture of appendiceal stump three months after uneventful appendectomy with repair and recovery. Ohio State Med J 1949; 45:476–7.
92. Greene JM, Peckler D, Schumer M, Greene EI. Incomplete removal of the appendix: Its complications. J Int Coll Surg 1958; 29:141–6.
93. Siegel SA. Appendiceal stump abscess: Report of stump abscess 23 years postappendectomy. Am J Surg 1954; 88:630–2.
94. Rose TF. Recurrent appendiceal abscess. Thirteen cases of recurrent appendiceal abscess; two due to incomplete removal of appendix. Med J Austral 1945; 32:659–62.
95. Maas LC, Gelzayd EA, Uppaputhangkule V, Silberberg B. Endoscopic removal of an ulcerated appendiceal stump. JAMA 1978; 240:248–9.
96. Gaylord SF. Colonoscopic appendectomy. Gastrointest Endosc 1981; 27:203.
97. Pearson RJC. Acute appendicitis in the New Haven standard metropolitan area in 1958 and 1959. Conn Med 28:807–10, 1964.
98. Zollinger RM, Howe CT. Small and large intestines. *In*: Davis L, ed. Christopher's Textbook of Surgery. 9th Ed. Philadelphia: WB Saunders, 1968.
99. Mittlepunkt A, Nora PF. Current features in the treatment of acute appendicitis. An analysis of 1,000 consecutive cases. Surgery 1966; 60:971–5.
100. Thorbjarnarson B, Loehr WJ. Acute appendicitis in patients over the age of 60. Surg Gynecol Obstet 1967; 124:1277–80.
101. Fowkes GL. Neonatal appendicitis. Br Med J 1976; 1: 997–8.
102. Fields IA, Cole NM. Acute appendicitis in infants thirty-six months of age or younger. Ten year survey at the Los Angeles County Hospital. Am J Surg 1967; 113:269–75.
103. Smith EI, Shopfner CE. The acute abdomen in the preschool child. South Med J 1966; 59:1260–7.
104. Abel WG, Allen PD. Acute appendicitis in children. A review of 1165 cases. Ann Surg 1950; 132:1093–1102.
105. Benson CD, Coury JJ Jr, Hagge DR. Acute appendicitis in infants: 15 year study. AMA Arch Surg 1952; 64:561–70.
106. Bower RJ, Morton JB, Ternberg JC. Controversial aspects of appendicitis management in children. Arch Surg 1981; 116:885–7.
107. Graham JM, Pokorny WJ, Harberg FJ. Acute appendicitis in preschool age children. Am J Surg 1980; 139:247–50.
108. Boyce FF. Nonsurgical mortality of acute appendicitis. J La State Med Soc 1964; 106:430–7.
109. Hubbell DS, Barton WK, Solomon DD. Leukocytosis in appendicitis in older persons. JAMA 1961; 175:139–41.
110. Swartz SI. Principles of Surgery. New York: McGraw-Hill, 1969.
111. Owens BJ, Hamit HF. Appendicitis in the elderly. Ann Surg 1978; 187:392–6.
112. Babaknia A, Parsa H, Woodruff JD. Appendicitis during pregnancy. Obstet Gynecol 1977; 50:40–4.
113. O'Neill JP. Surgical conditions complicating pregnancy. I. Acute appendicitis—real and simulated. Aust NZ J Obstet Gynaecol 1969; 9:94–9.
114. Sarason EL, Bauman S. Acute appendicitis in pregnancy: Difficulties in diagnosis. Obstet Gynecol 1963; 22:382–6.
115. Gomez A, Wood M. Acute appendicitis during pregnancy. Am J Surg 1979; 137:180–3.
116. Black WP. Acute appendicitis during pregnancy. Br Med J 1960; 1:1938–41.
117. Cunningham FG, McCubbin JH. Appendicitis complicating pregnancy. Obstet Gynecol 1975; 45:415–20.
118. Robinson HB, Smith GW. Applications for laparoscopy in general surgery. Surg Gynecol Obstet 1976; 143:829–34.
119. Townsend JM, Greiss FC. Appendicitis in pregnancy. South Med J 1976; 69:1161–3.
120. Paulley JW. Psychosomatic factors in aetiology of acute appendicitis. Arch Middlesex Hosp 1955; 5:35–41.

121. Harding HE. A notable source of error in the diagnosis of appendicitis. Br Med J 1962; 2:1028–9.
122. Creed F. Life events and appendicectomy. Lancet 1981; 1:1381–5.
123. Savrin RA, Clausen K, Marten EW, Cooperman M. Chronic and recurrent appendicitis. Am J Surg 1979; 137:355–7.
124. Talbert JL, Zuidema GD. Appendicitis—a reappraisal of an old problem. Surg Clin North Am 1966; 46:1101–12.
125. Befeler D. Recurrent appendicitis: Incidence and prophylaxis. Arch Surg 1964; 89:666–8.
126. Ferrier PK. Acute appendicitis in university students: A 20-year study of 1,028 cases. Am Coll Health Assoc J 1972; 20:287–90.
127. Boyce FF. Role of atypical disease in continuing mortality of acute appendicitis. Ann Intern Med 1954; 40:669–93.
128. Collins DC. Seventy-one thousand human appendix specimens: A final report summarizing 40 years study. Am J Proctol 1963; 14:356–81.
129. Masson P. Carcinoids (argentaffin-cell tumors) and nerve hyperplasia of the appendicular mucosa. Am J Pathol 1928; 4:181–211.
130. Barry R, Visser JD, Nel CJ. Intussusception as a result of adenoma of the appendix. S Afr J Surg 1980; 19:133–7.
131. Darby AJ, Doctor A. Villous papilloma of the appendix associated with mucocele and intussusception. Postgrad Med J 1974; 50:650–4.
132. Miller T, Bernstein J, Van Herle A. Cushing's syndrome cured by resection of appendiceal carcinoid. Arch Surg 1971; 103:770–3.
133. Warkel RL, Cooper PH, Helwig EB. Adenocarcinoid, a mucin producing tumor of the appendix. A study of 39 cases. Cancer 1978; 42:2781–93.
134. Wolff M, Ahmed N. Epithelial neoplasms of the appendix (exclusive of carcinoid). I. Adenocarcinoma of the appendix. Cancer 1976; 37:2493–2510.
134a. Wolff M, Ahmed N. Epithelial neoplasms of the appendix (exclusive of carcinoid). II. Cystadenomas, papillary adenomas and adenomatous polyps of the appendix. Cancer 1976; 37:2511–22.
135. Langman J, Rowland R, Vernon-Roberts B. Endometriosis of the appendix and epidermoid cysts which may be interpreted as tumors. Br J Surg 1981; 68:121–4.
136. Piserchia NE, Davey RB. Epidermoid cyst of the appendix. J Pediatr Surg 1980; 15:674–5.
137. Isaacson P. Crypt cell carcinoma of the appendix. Am J Surg Pathol 1981; 5:213–24.
138. Pettigrew RA. Invasive carcinoma arising in villous adenomata of the appendix. Aust NZ J Surg 1980; 50:627–9.
139. Sin IC, Laing ET, Prentice RSA. Burkitt's lymphoma of the appendix. Report of 2 cases. Pathology 1980; 11:465–70.
140. Menon NK. Primary carcinoma of the appendix. Postgrad Med J 1980; 56:448–50.
141. Hopkins GB, Tullis RH, Kristensen KA. Primary adenocarcinoma of the vermiform appendix: Report of seven cases and review of the literature. Dis Colon Rectum 1973; 16:140–4.
142. Killam AR. An unusual case of appendicitis: Torsion produced by a mesoappendiceal lipoma. Am Surg 1969; 35:648–9.
143. Nugent FW: Editorial: Crohn's disease of the appendix. Am J Gastroenterol 1976; 65:83.
144. Misra PS, Lebwohl P, Laufer H. Hepatic and appendiceal Whipple's disease with negative jejunal biopsies. Am J Gastroenterol 1981; 75:302–6.
145. Bhasin V, Chopra P, Kapur BM. Acute tubercular appendicitis. Int Surg 1977; 62:563–4.
146. Sakover RP, Del Fava RL. Frequency of visualization of the normal appendix with the barium enema examination. AJR 1974; 121:312–7.
147. Rolon PA. Myxoglobulosis of the appendix. Int Surg 1977; 62:355–6.
148. Simstein NL, Mattix KL. Penetrating injuries of the appendix. Am J Surg 1977; 134:415.
149. Painter NS, Burkitt DP. Diverticular disease of the colon: A deficiency disease of Western civilization. Br Med 1971; 2:450–4.
150. O'Neil B, Moore DB. Periappendicitis: Clinical reality or pathologic curiosity. Am J Surg 1977; 134:356–7.

Bockus

GASTROENTEROLOGY

INDEX

Index

Note: Page numbers in *italics* refer to illustrations; those followed by (t) refer to tables.